Sixth Edition

Tuberculosis
and **Nontuberculous Mycobacterial Infections**

NOTICE

Sixth Edition

Tuberculosis
and **Nontuberculous Mycobacterial Infections**

Edited by

David Schlossberg, MD, FACP

Professor of Medicine
Temple University School of Medicine

and

Medical Director
Tuberculosis Control Program
Philadelphia Department of Public Health
Philadelphia, Pennsylvania

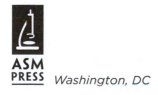
ASM PRESS *Washington, DC*

Copyright © 2011   ASM Press
American Society for Microbiology
1752 N St., N.W.
Washington, DC 20036-2904

Library of Congress Cataloging-in-Publication Data

Tuberculosis and nontuberculous mycobacterial infections / edited by David Schlossberg. — 6th ed.
   p. ; cm.
  Rev. ed. of: Tuberculosis & nontuberculous mycobacterial infections / edited by
David Schlossberg. 5th ed. c2006.
  Includes bibliographical references and index.
  ISBN-13: 978-1-55581-513-4 (hardcover : alk. paper)
  ISBN-10: 1-55581-513-8 (hardcover : alk. paper) 1. Tuberculosis. 2. Mycobacterial
diseases. I. Schlossberg, David. II. Tuberculosis & nontuberculous mycobacterial infections.
  [DNLM: 1. Tuberculosis. 2. Mycobacterium Infections. WF 200]
  RC311.T824 2011
  616.9′95—dc22

                                        2010053868

10   9   8   7   6   5   4   3   2   1

Address editorial correspondence to ASM Press, 1752 N St., N.W., Washington, DC 20036-2904, USA

Send orders to ASM Press, P.O. Box 605, Herndon, VA 20172, USA
Phone: 800-546-2416; 703-661-1593
Fax: 703-661-1501
E-mail: books@asmusa.org
Online : http://estore.asm.org

Cover image: The light micrograph in the petri plate design reveals some of the histopathologic cytoarchitectural characteristics in a mycobacterial skin infection. An unidentified gram-positive *Mycobacterium* sp. (rod-shaped bacilli) is visible throughout the cutaneous tissue sample. Courtesy of the Centers for Disease Control and Prevention, Atlanta, GA, and Dr. Roger Feldman.

This book is dedicated to the memory of John Weil Uhlmann, who fought valiantly against an implacable foe. His wife, children, grandchildren, and loyal friends miss him profoundly. We hope he is finally at peace.

"The Captain of all these men of death that came against him to take him away, was the consumption; for it was that that brought him down to the grave."

John Bunyan
The Life and Death of Mr. Badman

The weariness, the fever, and the fret
   Here, where men sit and hear each other groan;
Where palsy shakes a few, sad, last gray hairs,
   Where youth grows pale, and spectre-thin, and dies;
Where but to think is to be full of sorrow
   And leaden-eyed despairs,
Where beauty cannot keep her lustrous eyes,
   Or new love pine at them beyond tomorrow.

John Keats
Ode to a Nightingale

There is a dread disease which so prepares its victim, as it were, for death . . . a dread disease, in which the struggle between soul and body is so gradual, quiet, and solemn, and the results so sure, that day by day, and grain by grain, the mortal part wastes and withers away, so that the spirit grows light . . . a disease in which death and life are so strangely blended that death takes the glow and hue of life, and life the gaunt and grisly form of death—a disease which medicine never cured, wealth warded off, or poverty could boast exemption from—which sometimes moves in giant strides, or sometimes at a tardy sluggish pace, but, slow or quick, is ever sure and certain.

Charles Dickens
Nicholas Nickleby

CONTENTS

III.   Nontuberculous Mycobacteria

CONTRIBUTORS

Ritesh Agarwal
Department of Pulmonary Medicine
Postgraduate Institute of Medical Education &
Research
Sector-12, Chandigarh 160012, India

José M. Aguado
Unit of Infectious Diseases
University Hospital 12 de Octubre
Madrid, Spain

Daniel M. Albert
Department of Ophthalmology and Visual Sciences
University of Wisconsin School of Medicine and
Public Health
Madison, WI 53792-3284

Noelia Alonso-Rodríguez
Department of Clinical Microbiology,
IIS-Fundación Jiménez Díaz
28040 Madrid, Spain

Stephen C. Aronoff
Department of Pediatrics
Temple University School of Medicine
Philadelphia, PA 19140

Alexandra Aubry
Centre National de Référence pour la résistance
des Mycobactéries aux antituberculeux
Université Pierre et Marie Curie
AP-HP Hôpital Pitié-Salpêtrière, Paris, France

Marvin J. Bittner
Department of Medicine
Creighton University School of Medicine
Omaha, NE 68131

Emily A. Blumberg
Division of Infectious Diseases
University of Pennsylvania School of Medicine
Philadelphia, PA 19104

Henry M. Blumberg
Division of Infectious Diseases
Emory University School of Medicine
Atlanta, GA 30303

Barbara A. Brown-Elliott
Department of Microbiology
University of Texas Health Science Center
Tyler, TX 75708

Emmanuelle Cambau
Centre National de Référence pour la résistance
des Mycobactéries aux antituberculeux (laboratoire
associé)
Laboratoire de Bactériologie, Université Paris
Diderot,
AP-HP Hôpital Saint Louis, Paris, France

Eric H. Choi
Division of Gastroenterology and Hepatology
Scripps Clinic Torrey Pines
10666 N. Torrey Pines Road, N203
La Jolla, CA 92037

Preston Church
Ralph H. Johnson VAMC
Charleston, SC 29425

Paul J. Converse
Department of Medicine, School of Medicine
The Johns Hopkins University
Baltimore, MD 21205

Walter J. Coyle
Division of Gastroenterology and Hepatology
Scripps Clinic Torrey Pines
10666 N. Torrey Pines Road, N203
La Jolla, CA 92037

John A. Crocco
Department of Medicine
UMDNJ—Robert Wood Johnson Medical School
New Brunswick, NJ 08854

Thomas M. Daniel
Department of Medicine
Case Western Reserve University
Cleveland, OH 44106

Arthur M. Dannenberg, Jr.
Bloomberg School of Public Health
The Johns Hopkins University
Baltimore, MD 21205

Thomas E. Dobbs
Mississippi State Department of Health
University of Mississippi Medical Center
Jackson, MI 39215

Asim K. Dutt
Chief, Medical Service (retired)
Alvin C. York Veterans Administration Medical
Center, Murfreesboro, Tennessee
Professor and Vice Chairman (retired)
Department of Medicine
Meharry Medical College, Nashville, Tennessee
4117 SW 30th Court
Ocala, FL 34474

Kevin Elwood
Division of Tuberculosis Control
British Columbia Centre for Disease Control
655 West 12th Avenue
Vancouver, BC V5Z 4R4, Canada

Marcos A. Espinal
Health Surveillance, Disease Control & Prevention
Pan American Health Organization
525 23rd St., NW
Washington, DC 20037

Jaime Esteban
Department of Clinical Microbiology
Fundación Jiménez Díaz
Av. Reyes Católicos 2
28040 Madrid, Spain

André A. Figueiredo
Núcleo Interdisciplinar de Pesquisa em Urologia
and Department of Morphology, Federal University
of Juiz de Fora, Minas Gerais—Brazil
Rua Irineu Marinho 365, apto 801—bloco 3
Bom Pastor—Juiz de Fora, MG 36021-580, Brazil

David M. Fleece
Department of Pediatrics
Temple University School of Medicine
Philadelphia, PA 19140

Connie A. Haley
Division of Infectious Diseases
Vanderbilt University Medical Center
Nashville, TN 37203

Carol D. Hamilton
Family Health International
Duke University Medical Center
Durham, NC 27710

Michael K. Hill
56 Starbrush Circle
Covington, LA 70433

Edward A. Horowitz
Department of Medicine
Creighton University School of Medicine
Omaha, NE 68131

W. Garrett Hunt
Section of Infectious Diseases
Nationwide Children's Hospital
Columbus, OH 43205

Dalia Ibrahim
Department of Internal Medicine
Georgetown University Hospital
Washington, DC 20007

Kashef Ijaz
Division of Tuberculosis Elimination
Centers for Disease Control and Prevention
Mail Stop E-10, 1600 Clifton Road
Atlanta, GA 30333

Surinder K. Jindal
Department of Pulmonary Medicine
Postgraduate Institute of Medical Education
& Research, Sector-12
Chandigarh 160012, India

James C. Johnston
Division of Tuberculosis Control
British Columbia Centre for Disease Control
655 West 12th Avenue
Vancouver, BC V5Z 4R4, Canada

Marc A. Judson
Division of Pulmonary and Critical Care Medicine
Medical University of South Carolina
Charleston, SC 29425

Gregory C. Kane
Department of Pulmonary and Critical Care
Medicine
Thomas Jefferson University
Philadelphia, PA 19107

Midori Kato-Maeda
Division of Pulmonary and Critical Care Medicine
San Francisco General Hospital
University of California, San Francisco
1001 Potrero Avenue
San Francisco, CA 94110

Mary E. Kreider
Pulmonary and Critical Care Section
Hospital of the University of Pennsylvania
Philadelphia, PA 19104-4283

Timothy Lahey
Section of Infectious Diseases and International
Health
Department of Medicine
Dartmouth Medical School
Lebanon, NH 03756

Alfred A. Lardizabal
New Jersey Medical School Global Tuberculosis
Institute
University of Medicine and Dentistry of New Jersey
Newark, NJ 07103

John M. Leonard
Department of Medicine—Infectious Disease
Vanderbilt University Medical Center
1161 21st Avenue South—A 2200 MCN
Nashville, TN 37232-2582

Michael K. Leonard, Jr.
Division of Infectious Diseases
Emory University School of Medicine
Atlanta, GA 30303

James H. Lewis
Division of Hepatology
Department of Medicine
Georgetown University Hospital
Washington, DC 20007

Philip LoBue
Division of Tuberculosis Elimination
Centers for Disease Control and Prevention
Mail Stop E-10, 1600 Clifton Road
Atlanta, GA 30333

Robert N. Longfield
Heartland National TB Center
University of Texas Health Science Center
2303 Southeast Military Drive
San Antonio, TX 78223

Antônio M. Lucon
Division of Urology
University of São Paulo Medical School
Av Dr. Enéas de Carvalho Aguiar, 255
7 Andar, sala 710 F.
São Paulo, SP 05403-000, Brazil

Annie Luetkemeyer
HIV/AIDS Division
San Francisco General Hospital
University of California, San Francisco
995 Potrero Avenue
San Francisco, CA 94110

Beverly Metchock
Division of Tuberculosis Elimination
Centers for Disease Control and Prevention
Mail Stop F-08, 1600 Clifton Road
Atlanta, GA 30333

Alladi Mohan
Department of Medicine
Sri Venkateswara Institute of Medical Sciences
Tirupati 517 507, India

Randall A. Oyer
Oncology Program
Lancaster General Hospital
Lancaster, PA 17604-3555

George A. Pankey
Infectious Diseases Research
Ochsner Clinic Foundation
1514 Jefferson Highway
New Orleans, LA 70121

Robert J. Peralta
Department of Ophthalmology and Visual Sciences
University of Wisconsin School of Medicine and
Public Health
Madison, WI 53792-3284

Laurel C. Preheim
Department of Medicine
Creighton University School of Medicine
Omaha, NE 68131

Gary W. Procop
Clinical Pathology/L40
Cleveland Clinic
9500 Euclid Avenue
Cleveland, OH 44195

Mario C. Raviglione
Stop TB Department
World Health Organization
Geneva 1211, Switzerland

Lee B. Reichman
New Jersey Medical School Global Tuberculosis
Institute
University of Medicine and Dentistry of New Jersey
Newark, NJ 07103

Glenn D. Roberts
Laboratory Medicine and Pathology
Mayo Clinic College of Medicine
200 First Street Southwest
Rochester, MN 55905

Milton D. Rossman
Pulmonary and Critical Care Section
Hospital of the University of Pennsylvania
Philadelphia, PA 19104-4283

Charles V. Sanders
Department of Medicine
Louisiana State University School of Medicine
1542 Tulane Avenue, Suite 421, Box T4M-2
New Orleans, LA 70112

David Schlossberg
Department of Medicine
Temple University School of Medicine
Philadelphia Department of Public Health
Philadelphia, PA 19140

Barbara J. Seaworth
Heartland National TB Center
University of Texas Health Science Center
2303 Southeast Military Drive
San Antonio, TX 78223

Sorana Segal-Maurer
Division of Infectious Diseases
New York Hospital Queens
Flushing, NY 11355

Surendra K. Sharma
Department of Medicine
All India Institute of Medical Sciences
New Delhi 110 029, India

Alan D. L. Sihoe
Department of Cardiothoracic Surgery
Queen Mary Hospital
University of Hong Kong
Hong Kong, China

Nina Singh
University of Pittsburgh Medical Center
2A 137 Infectious Diseases Section
VA Pittsburgh Healthcare System and University of
Pittsburgh
University Drive C
Pittsburgh, PA 15240

Peter M. Small
Institute for Systems Biology
1441 N. 34th Street
Seattle, WA 98103-8904

Miguel Srougi
Division of Urology
University of São Paulo Medical School
Av Dr. Enéas de Carvalho Aguiar, 255
7 Andar, sala 710 F.
São Paulo, SP 05403-000, Brazil

Jeffrey R. Starke
Department of Pediatrics
Baylor College of Medicine
Houston, TX 77030

Jason E. Stout
Division of Infectious Diseases and International
Health
Duke University Medical Center
Durham, NC 27710

Thomas H. Taylor
Division of Gastroenterology
Georgetown University Hospital
Washington, DC 20007

Melisa Thombley
Division of Tuberculosis Elimination
Centers for Disease Control and Prevention
Mail Stop E-10, 1600 Clifton Road
Atlanta, GA 30333

Matthew J. Thompson
Tower Clock Eye Center
1087 West Mason Street
Green Bay, WI 54303

Urvashi Vaid
Department of Pulmonary and Critical Care
Medicine
Thomas Jefferson University
Philadelphia, PA 19107

Christopher Vinnard
Division of Infectious Diseases
University of Pennsylvania School of Medicine
Philadelphia, PA 19104

C. Fordham von Reyn
Section of Infectious Diseases and International
Health
Department of Medicine
Dartmouth Medical School
Lebanon, NH 03756

Richard J. Wallace, Jr.
Department of Microbiology
University of Texas Health Science Center
Tyler, TX 75708

Risa M. Webb
Department of Infectious Diseases
G. V. "Sonny" Montgomery VA Medical Center
University of Mississippi Medical Center
Mississippi State Department of Health
Jackson, MS 39216

Henry Yeager
Department of Medicine
Georgetown University Medical Center
Washington, DC 20007

Wing Wai Yew
Tuberculosis and Chest Unit
Grantham Hospital
Hong Kong, China

PREFACE

I am pleased to present the sixth edition of *Tuberculosis and Nontuberculous Mycobacterial Infections*.

Tuberculosis remains epidemic in much of the world, causing several million deaths each year. Although most of these deaths occur in developing nations, the developed world continues to struggle with tuberculosis, with evolving challenges from drug resistance, immigration, immunosuppression, and the expanding awareness of nontuberculous mycobacterial infection.

The previous structure of this book has been maintained. Section I presents basic concepts of epidemiology, pathophysiology, diagnosis, medical and surgical therapy, resistant tuberculosis, vaccines, tuberculosis in enclosed populations, and the role of the Health Department. Section II describes both classic and more recently described clinical manifestations of tuberculous infection. Virtually every organ system is included, as are the endocrinologic and hematologic complications of tuberculosis. Separate chapters address issues unique to pregnancy, infants and children, human immunodeficiency virus infection, and the immune reconstitution syndrome. Section III comprises nontuberculous mycobacterial infections, with an overview of clinical syndromes produced by these organisms as well as individual chapters on *Mycobacterium avium-intracellulare*, *Mycobacterium fortuitum*, and other rapidly growing mycobacteria; *Mycobacterium kansasii*; *Mycobacterium marinum*; *Mycobacterium scrofulaceum*; and additional, less common, pathogenic mycobacteria.

Three new chapters have been added. "Tuberculosis in History: Did It Change the Way We Live?"

explores the influence of tuberculosis on our civilization's history and culture, "Tuberculosis and Organ Transplantation" defines the challenges of tuberculous infection in the expanding world of transplantation, and "*Mycobacterium bovis* and Other Uncommon Members of the *Mycobacterium tuberculosis* Complex" updates the clinical significance of these mycobacteria.

In addition to the new chapters, every chapter has been thoroughly updated. New clinical data affect our understanding of gamma interferon release assays, the human immunodeficiency virus-tuberculosis interaction, immune reconstitution inflammatory syndrome, and extensively drug-resistant tuberculosis. The protean facets of pulmonary and extrapulmonary tuberculosis continue to challenge the clinician, as does the growing list of nontuberculous mycobacterial pathogens. Epidemiological issues include airline-associated infection, the explosion of tuberculosis in areas of the developing world, and the critical roles of the World Health Organization and departments of public health in tuberculosis control.

I hope that this text continues to provide a complete and user-friendly resource for everyone—clinician, scientist, and epidemiologist—involved in the diagnosis and treatment of tuberculosis.

I am grateful for the guidance and support of the editorial staff at ASM Press, particularly Jeff Holtmeier, Ken April, Greg Payne, and John Bell.

David Schlossberg, MD, FACP

I. GENERAL CONSIDERATIONS

Tuberculosis and Nontuberculous Mycobacterial Infections, 6th ed.
Edited by David Schlossberg
© 2011 ASM Press, Washington, DC

Chapter 1

Tuberculosis in History: Did It Change the Way We Live?

THOMAS M. DANIEL

INTRODUCTION

Tuberculosis is one of the oldest of humankind's plagues (10). The genus of the causative organism, *Mycobacterium*, may be millions of years old. *Mycobacterium tuberculosis* probably emerged as a pathogen of our early ancestors 20,000 to 15,000 years ago in east Africa. As humans peopled the globe, they took their diseases with them, including tuberculosis. DNA of *M. tuberculosis* and typical tuberculous lesions containing acid-fast bacilli have been identified in both Egyptian and Peruvian mummies. Further documentation of the ancient spread of tuberculosis is contained in ancient texts and is documented at archeological sites.

As Europe emerged from the Middle Ages and the Industrial Revolution swept into Europe and North America, the lives of inhabitants of those regions changed dramatically. As computer chips, automobiles, and cell phones dominate our age, machines and urban living dominated in the 18th and 19th centuries. The writings of classical Greek and Roman physicians make it clear that they recognized tuberculosis. Regarding the Middle Ages, little is known of most diseases, including tuberculosis, although royal touching for scrofula began with Clovis in 496 and archeological sites have revealed bony evidence of the disease. During the 17th and 18th centuries, tuberculosis exploded with soaring prevalence. In 1680 John Bunyan described it as "the Captain among these men of death" (6). During the next 200 years this sobriquet would hold, as tuberculosis became a leading cause of death in Europe and North America. Then tuberculosis waned, as have all disease epidemics, for reasons that remain unclear.

A unified concept of tuberculosis first emerged with the work of Laënnec in the early 19th century, and from that time forward one can recognize the impact that this disease has had on the way we live. This impact can be illustrated by the life stories of many individuals, some often told, others less commonly recounted. A few have been selected for this account.

IMPACT ON THE PRACTICE OF MEDICINE

For scores of years the treatment of tuberculosis pervaded the practice of nearly every physician. Early therapeutic regimens were intended to remove malevolent humors and included bleeding, leeches, cupping, and vesicants. Sir James Clark, physician to Queen Victoria and to the dying John Keats, estimated that pulmonary tuberculosis caused about one-fifth of all deaths in Europe and North America in his era, the early 19th century. Clark was a moderate, and his therapy was largely palliative. He urged restraint in bloodletting and advocated travel to salubrious climates. "The change of scene and the constant succession of new objects exert a direct and most beneficial influence," he wrote (8). Later in that century Sir William Osler recommended optimum nutrition and palliation of symptoms (26). He also argued for removing patients to favorable environments, citing the Adirondack experience of Edward Livingston Trudeau, who retreated to the wilderness, recovered his health, and opened his famous Adirondack Cottage Sanitarium at Saranac Lake, New York. Trudeau ultimately succumbed to tuberculosis.

In the first half of the 20th century, tuberculosis sanatoria assumed a major position in medical care. In fact, by the mid-1950s, when the advent of chemotherapy would lead to the rapid closing of these nearly ubiquitous institutions, there were 839 sanatoria in the United States, comprising more than 130,000 beds for tuberculosis patients (11). The world's first voluntary health agency, the National Association for the Study and Prevention of Tuberculosis, now the American Lung Association, was founded as an advocacy agency for sanatorium patients in 1904.

The modern science of epidemiology owes much of its gestation to the work of Wade Hampton Frost. Frost developed tuberculosis in 1918 and recovered in Asheville, North Carolina, a much-favored location at that time. In elegant studies of tuberculosis

Thomas M. Daniel • Department of Medicine, Case Western Reserve University, University Hospitals Case Medical Center, Cleveland, OH 44106.

in Williamson County, Tennessee, Frost first developed the concept of the index case, now known to every epidemiologist and public health investigator (29). Mass radiographic surveys were a prominent part of American and Canadian public health efforts for two decades, from the mid-1940s until they were abandoned in the face of rapidly declining disease incidence.

Modern clinical practice relies upon data collected in randomized, controlled clinical trials to establish its standards of care. The studies of tuberculosis treatment protocols conducted by the British Medical Research Council are often cited as pioneering in this arena (17, 22). In fact, the first randomized, placebo-controlled, double-blind clinical trial in the history of medicine was conducted in 1926 and 1927 at the William H. Maybury Sanatorium in Detroit, Michigan, by J. Burns Amberson, B. T. McMahon, and Max Pinner to evaluate the efficacy of sanocrysin, a gold salt, in treatment of tuberculosis (1). Twenty-four patients with tuberculosis were randomly assigned by the flip of a coin to receive injections of either sanocrysin or a saline placebo. Only the one nurse giving the injections knew which patients were in which group. When the results were analyzed, sanocrysin was found to have no therapeutic benefit but significant toxicity.

The life stories of many pioneering tuberculosis physicians enrich our understanding of the era of great tuberculosis prevalence. Some of them had enormous influence on the practice of medicine in their times and later. Early in the van of these exceptional men of medicine was René Théophile Hyacinthe Laënnec (9, 12). Laënnec was born on 17 February 1781 in Quimper on the Brittany coast of France. Because his mother was too ill with tuberculosis to care for him, he was placed with an uncle. When the latter died of tuberculosis, Laënnec was sent to the home of a physician uncle in Nantes. There he began his studies of medicine in 1795, moving to Paris in 1801 to study at the École de Médicine at the Hôpital Charité under the tutelage of pioneering anatomist Jean Nicolas Corvisart. In 1804, while near the end of his medical studies but still a student, he presented a paper in which he challenged existing concepts and argued that disease manifested by tubercles in whatever part of the body they were found was one disease that should be called tuberculosis.

In 1816 Laënnec invented the stethoscope, for which he was widely acclaimed. Using his instrument he described most of the physical signs of pulmonary disease, coining such terms as "ronchus" and "egophany," which are still taught to medical students. Laënnec published his work in 1819 under the title *De l'Auscultation Médiate*; it was translated into English and extensively reworked by John Forbes in 1821 (16). The publication of this work and especially its translation into English mark the beginning of pulmonary medicine as a clinical specialty.

Laënnec suffered from tuberculosis. He was undoubtedly infected as a child. While in Nantes he incurred a prosector's wart when he inadvertently inoculated his hand while performing an autopsy on an individual who had died of tuberculosis. In Paris he increasingly suffered from respiratory disease. He returned to his native Brittany in 1918 and recovered somewhat. Later he imported bottles of air from Brittany to his Paris apartment. Famous in his time and much sought for his clinical expertise, he was elected to the French Academy of Medicine and, in 1824, made a Chevalier of the Legion of Honor. His tuberculous disease progressed, however, and in April 1826 he returned to his beloved Brittany for the last time. Tuberculosis claimed his life at age 45 on 13 August 1826. It took from the world one of the greatest physicians of the time, a man of then-unequaled clinical skills. One can only speculate on what more he might have contributed to medicine.

IMPACT ON WORLD POLITICS

Tuberculosis is not prominent in the personal histories of many of the world's historically notable politicians and leaders. It took the life of France's Louis XIII. So, also, did tuberculosis bring premature death to Charles IX of England. More notably, in modern times, South Africa's Nelson Mandela developed tuberculosis while a prisoner but recovered with drug therapy. In none of these instances can one assert that the course of world history was altered.

The British Empire would seem to owe much to its explorers who went to Africa seeking relief from tuberculosis. James Bruce, a Scotsman, discovered the Ethiopian source of the Blue Nile in 1770. Mungo Park explored West Africa in 1795. Both of these men set off on their adventurous journeys seeking relief from tuberculosis; travel was a common prescription for consumptives at that time.

Cecil Rhodes brought South Africa under British hegemony; he had a lasting impact on the future course of sub-Saharan Africa. When the 17-year-old Rhodes arrived in South Africa in 1870, the region included two Boer republics, two British colonies, two independent states, and a number of indigenous territories that England controlled as protectorates. Three years earlier diamonds had been discovered, and the region was booming with prospectors. Rhodes's oldest brother, Herbert, had preceded him to South Africa by a year and become a planter. In the diamond frenzy, Herbert had staked a claim that was to yield enormous numbers of the precious gems.

Cecil Rhodes was born in Hertfordshire, England, on 5 July 1853 (21). He developed tuberculosis at age 16 and went to South Africa to join his brother because a sea voyage and change in climate were considered likely to benefit his health. Indeed, he did regain vigorous health and within 2 years was managing his brother's diamond mine. Herbert Rhodes sold his claim in 1873. Cecil Rhodes, now a wealthy young man, returned to England to study at Oxford. His tuberculosis recurred about 6 months later, and within the year he was back in South Africa and once more recovering his well-being.

Rhodes's business acumen was extraordinary. By his 35th birthday, he controlled more than 90% of South Africa's diamond production and held a dominant position in its gold mining industry. With some of his business colleagues, he founded the British South Africa Company. By force or negotiation, he obtained concessions from local tribal chiefs. In October 1889, Queen Victoria granted the company a royal charter. Investors eagerly subscribed to its stock offerings. Rhodes envisioned expansion of his and England's realms northwards, but the Boer settlers fought this expansion vigorously. Some native tribes revolted. Much of Rhodes's time and efforts went into consolidating and securing the company's holdings. He traveled between England and South Africa to negotiate and lead the empire-building effort.

In 1902 the 49-year-old Rhodes became ill. The nature of this illness is not clear, although it was thought that his heart was failing. Indeed, some biographers dispute the generally held belief that Rhodes had tuberculosis, arguing that he suffered from congenital heart disease (31); that assertion seems difficult to reconcile with what is known of the course of his disease during an often very active life. Rhodes died in South Africa, a land he loved, on 26 March 1902.

Taking place in more recent times, the story of Manuel Quezon and his leadership of the people of the Philippines reflects his battle with tuberculosis. Afflicted with the disease since his youth, he defied it and ignored it through an active life of leadership that resulted in his election as the first president of the Philippine Commonwealth in 1935. In fact, in his autobiography, completed during his terminal illness and published posthumously in 1946, Quezon makes but scant reference to his illness (30). In 1927, while in the United States lobbying for the appointment of a Philippine governor, he was found to have tuberculosis. Quezon was hospitalized at the Pottenger Sanatorium in Monrovia, California, but was unhappy with his treatment there and left after a short stay. After the Japanese invasions of the Philippines in World War II, he left his country to lead a government in exile, initially in Australia and then in the United States. With his tuberculosis again active, he conducted his government's affairs from a cottage at Saranac Lake, where he died following a massive hemoptysis in July 1944 (34).

Josephine Baker, an African-American dancer, chanteuse, and comic who exiled herself to France because of racial segregation in American entertainment venues, was a remarkable woman, sometimes remembered for dancing at the Folies-Bergère wearing only a bunch of bananas (2). During the World War II Nazi occupation of France, she was entertaining in Marseilles. The French underground approached her with a request that she serve as a courier of secret messages, exploiting her freedom to travel and carry music on which information was transcribed in invisible ink. Having a cough, she sought a physician's order to be released from the obligations of a contract and go to Morocco. The physician obtained a chest radiograph that showed bilateral tuberculosis. He told her to go to Morocco and to rest. She left Marseilles but did not rest: she embarked on an espionage career that supported the French resistance effort throughout the German occupation of France. Her selfless effort was recognized by the French government after the war with the award of Chevalier of the Legion of Honor. Her tuberculosis remained quiescent throughout the rest of her life.

Rhodes was an exceptional empire builder. Had he lived longer, the British hegemony over much of Africa might have been extended further. Quezon and Baker played roles in sustaining the resistance of those living under Japanese and German wartime occupation.

IMPACT ON CIVIL SOCIETY

Not all history is political. The lives of ordinary citizens are often affected by the actions of not-so-ordinary individuals. There are numerous instances in which tuberculosis played a role in these actions and their impact. Francis of Assisi emerged from prison wasted and an apparent victim of tuberculosis (23). During the next decade he led a life of poverty and ministry to the poor that led to his sainthood and the founding of the Franciscan order. He succumbed in 1226. Saint Thérèse of Lisieux died of tuberculosis in 1897 at age 24. John Harvard, whose 1638 bequest of 400 books and half of his estate put his name on one of America's most prestigious universities, died of tuberculosis. Tuberculosis claimed the life of 43-year-old Louis Braille, who made writing available to blind persons, in 1852. Alexander Graham Bell, the telephone's inventor, moved with his parents from Edinburgh, Scotland, to the putatively more salubrious Nova Scotia, Canada, in 1870 following the death of his two older brothers from tuberculosis. Six years later he made the world's first telephone call. Desmond Tutu developed tuberculosis as a teenager and spent 2 years at the Rietfontein Chest Hospital in South Africa, where he underwent collapse therapy with pneumothorax. George Balanchine was ill with tuberculosis in 1935. Eleanor Roosevelt was hospitalized with tuberculosis in France as a young woman. Ignoring the advice to seek further treatment upon her return to the United States, she embarked on a disease-free, remarkable humanitarian life, only to succumb to disseminated tuberculosis at age 75 in 1962.

John Batterson Stetson was born in Orange, New Jersey, in 1830, the seventh of 12 children of Stephen Stetson, a hatter (14, 18, 27). Apprenticed to the family hat business as a youth, he developed tuberculosis at about age 21. A standard prescription of the day was travel to the American West. Thus, Stetson headed west, settling first in St. Joseph, Missouri, were he worked in and later became owner of a brickyard. The business flourished, but his health did not, so after about 2 years he headed further west to Colorado. There he began making hats. He knew the art of felting, and he applied his skill to fur from pelts his hunting friends discarded. Soon he had made a broad-brimmed felt hat, which he sold for a five-dollar gold piece. The Stetson hat was born. Today, no Western movie is complete without Stetson-wearing cowboys and cattle rustlers, white hats for heroes and black ones for villains.

Stetson relocated to Philadelphia, Pennsylvania, where he founded the John B. Stetson Company and built a factory. By 1906 he was producing two million hats a year. He wintered in DeLand, Florida, and in 1887 he became a trustee of DeLand College. Two years later he became president of the board of trustees. He donated generously to the college, and in 1889 DeLand College was renamed Stetson University (18).

Athletes who made lasting marks on their sports also suffered from tuberculosis. It took the life of Christopher "Christy" (also called "Matty") Mathewson, perhaps the greatest baseball pitcher in the history of the sport (32). Pitching for the New York Giants in 1905, Mathewson won 31 games out of 39 starts. His earned run average that year was 1.27. He worked 339 innings, striking out 206 batters and walking only 64. In the World Series against Philadelphia that year, he pitched 27 innings, won three shutouts, and had an earned run average of 0.00. Mathewson slumped the following year; he was

not well and was plagued by a cough. By 1909 he was back in form, winning 37 games, 12 of them shutouts, and losing only 11. His earned run average for the year was 1.43.

Mathewson was born in Factoryville, Pennsylvania, in 1880. In high school and on sandlots, he played baseball whenever the opportunity arose. At Bucknell University he starred on both football and baseball teams and also distinguished himself academically. In 1900 he joined the New York Giants to begin his record-setting career in major league baseball. Mathewson was an instant star on the baseball diamond, success following success.

In 1915, however, Mathewson began a slump that seemed irreversible. One bad year followed another; he was often tired, coughing, and unwell. He dropped from the lineup to become a coach. In 1920 his doctors gave him the diagnosis of tuberculosis, and in July he went to Saranac Lake, hoping to recover his health. In 1923 he was well enough to assume the position of president of the Boston Braves, but the following year found him back at Saranac Lake. He passed the remainder of his life there, succumbing to tuberculosis on 7 October 1925. Tuberculosis had claimed one of baseball's greatest legends, a 30-game winner in four seasons and a Hall-of-Famer from the first year that institution opened.

Alice Marble was one of the most outstanding female competitors in the history of tennis. Her life was also touched by tuberculosis (20). Growing up in San Francisco, California, she was a tomboy who loved sports—baseball initially but then tennis. Given a racquet while in high school, she soon became the top female player on the West Coast. At age 18 she made her debut at Forest Hills in New York City, losing miserably in singles but winning the women's doubles championship with fellow Californian Bonnie Miller. The following year she began working with Eleanor "Teach" Tennant, the coach and lifelong friend who would shape her raw talent into the form and skills that made her the greatest female tennis player of her time.

In May 1934 Marble collapsed during a tournament in France. She was carried from the court to the American Hospital at Neuilly, where she learned she had tuberculosis. She would never play tennis again, was her doctor's prognosis. She returned to her native California and entered Pottenger's Sanatorium in Monrovia. An initial 6 weeks stretched to 8 months. Marble, gaining weight and losing the physical fitness that had graced her athletic form, was despondent. Then one day she received a letter from Carol Lombard, whom "Teach" Tennant also coached and who had learned of Marble's illness from Tennant. Glamorous movie star Lombard had suffered disfiguring wounds to her face in an automobile accident but regained her movie stardom after multiple surgical procedures. "I made my career come true, just as you can—if you'll fight. If I can do it, so can you," Lombard wrote (20). Soon thereafter, Marble walked out of the sanatorium. In 1936 she won the U.S. women's championship at Forest Hills. Her disease never recurred.

IMPACT ON CREATIVITY IN LITERATURE AND THE ARTS

Creative works of art, music, dance, and literature all express the lives of their creators, and thus tuberculosis in these lives affected their works. Some were greatly afflicted by the disease, others less so or were treated and fared well. And so it is that while the works of some reflect their struggles with tuberculosis, the creativity of others was little affected. George Balanchine developed tuberculosis shortly after his 1933 arrival in New York City, but it had little influence on his life and creativity. Igor Stravinsky suffered recurrent bouts of tuberculosis before being treated and cured with newly developed drugs; he lived to be 88 years old. Sarah Bernhardt was given a diagnosis of tuberculosis as a 15-year-old but recovered to star on the stage and live to be 78. Andrew Wyeth was ill as a child. Tuberculosis, the doctor said. Yet he lived to be 91 without further evidence of the disease.

Stephen Crane died at age 28 of tuberculosis, but he had produced his masterpiece, *The Red Badge of Courage*, 4 years earlier. Amadeo Modigliani died of tuberculous meningitis in 1920 at age 35. Finnish composer Ernst Mielck was said to have been Max Bruch's favorite student. He succumbed to tuberculosis when he was 21 years old. Band leader Chick Webb, "First King of Swing," died of tuberculosis at age 34. What works might the genius of these talented persons have yielded had their lives not been taken by tuberculosis?

Frédéric Chopin developed tuberculosis while a young émigré in Paris. He struggled with his illness, constantly sick, slowly losing ground to the "Captain of Death" but always productive. While seeking relief in Mallorca, Spain, with Georges Sand, his paramour, he wrote despairingly to his publisher:

> I can't send you the manuscript, for it's not finished. I have been sick as a dog these last two weeks; I caught cold in spite of 18 degrees of heat, roses, oranges, palms, figs and three most famous doctors of the island. One sniffed at what I spat up, the second tapped where I spat it from, the third poked about and listened how I spat it. One said I had died, the second that I am dying, the 3rd that I shall die (25).

Yet Chopin did compose while in Mallorca. He struggled on, increasingly disabled, writing music and performing on the piano until he died at age 39 of pulmonary insufficiency resulting from the destruction of his lungs by tuberculosis.

Norwegian painter Edvard Munch was born in 1863 (28). Two weeks after his 13th birthday, tuberculosis entered his life with a frightening episode of hemoptysis. He later wrote:

> The illness followed me all through my childhood and youth—the germ of consumption placed its blood-red banner victoriously on the white handkerchief (28).

In fact, he recovered and was then relatively well for the next several years, until tuberculosis recurred when he was 36. One lung was badly damaged, his doctor told him, the other less so. He was repeatedly confined to tuberculosis sanatoria during his middle thirties. Often ill, he lived on to reach the age of 80.

The effect of tuberculosis on Munch's art is complicated by his recurrent depression—probably manic-depressive bipolar disease—which also almost certainly affected his work. There is no doubt that these two illnesses, tuberculosis prominently of the two, had a great impact on his work. In his words:

> I must retain my physical weaknesses; they are an integral part of me. I don't *want* to get rid of illness, however unsympathetically I may depict it in my art. . . . My sufferings are a part of my self and my art (28).

Munch often portrayed death. *The Sick Child*, dating to 1885–1886, when Munch had recovered from his adolescent bout with tuberculosis and not yet been again stricken, evokes sympathy and serenity. The pale-faced, red-headed child smiles at her grieving mother, a look of serenity on the girl's face. *Death in the Sickroom* (1893), *The Deathbed* (1895), and *Dead Mother and Child* (1899) portray quite different images of death. They are somber, with gray and black tones, and evoke grief and despair. Their mood is one of unremitting sorrow. Munch was ill, in and out of tuberculosis sanatoria, during the years these paintings came from his palette.

Literature is replete with descriptions of tuberculosis, often reflecting the authors' lives. John Keats, Anton Chekhov, and W. Somerset Maugham all suffered from the disease, and it is reflected in their writings. Katherine Mansfield, on the other hand, was recurrently ill before dying following a massive hemoptysis, but she did not mention tuberculosis in any of her many short stories.

Striking examples of tuberculosis in literature are provided by the novels of the Brontë sisters. The

Reverend Patrick Brontë was plagued with cough throughout the 84 years of his life. He almost certainly had chronic tuberculosis (13, 19). He probably infected his wife and six children, all of whom succumbed to the disease. The three of his five daughters who survived to adulthood wrote both prose and poetry. Their novels are icons of Victorian Age literature.

Emily Brontë died in December 1848. Her death certificate stated that her illness was of 2 months' duration, but the letters of her sister, Charlotte, make it clear that her illness was well established at an earlier date (33). Emily Brontë's novel, *Wuthering Heights*, was published in 1847. She may have been ill as she was writing; certainly she knew tuberculosis well, for she had watched her mother and two sisters, Maria and Elizabeth, succumb while she was a child. *Wuthering Heights* is an extraordinary literary work. A complex tale of the struggle of good to overcome evil, the work is pervaded by tuberculosis. Malevolent Heathcliff mourns the loss of Catherine Earnshaw, who dies of tuberculosis early in the book.

> The doctor says she must go: he says she's been in a consumption these many months. . . . One night . . . a fit of coughing took her—a very slight one . . . her face changed, and she was dead (5).

Death from tuberculosis is also described in *Jane Eyre* by Charlotte Brontë in a passage set in a Cowan Bridge School.

> I am very happy, Jane; and when you hear that I am dead, you must be sure and not grieve; there is nothing to grieve about. We must all die one day, and the illness which is removing me is not painful; it is gentle and gradual: my mind is at rest (4).

This part of *Jane Eyre* is considered by most scholars to be autobiographical, the dying Helen representing Charlotte Brontë's sister Maria.

Eugene O'Neill was America's greatest dramatist. His plays won four Pulitzer Prizes and the Nobel Prize. Critics uniformly acclaimed him. He had tuberculosis, and the disease figures prominently in two of his plays. *The Straw* was written while he was a sanatorium patient, and it is loosely based on his experiences there. It has not been considered one of his better works. *Long Day's Journey into Night* is frankly autobiographical and deals with the time when O'Neill was told he must go to a tuberculosis sanatorium. It is a universally acclaimed masterpiece.

O'Neill was born on 16 October 1888, the youngest of two surviving sons of successful actor James O'Neill and Ellen O'Neill. The O'Neills were an Irish immigrant family with strong roots in Catholicism, but their family life was disrupted by James O'Neill's tours with theatrical companies. As in many Irish families in America at that time, alcohol consumption was frequent and copious. Ellen O'Neill was addicted to opiates (3).

Eugene O'Neill's life was marked by a variety of excesses and tragedies. Educated initially in boarding schools, he entered Princeton University in 1906. He married a casual girlfriend, whom he had impregnated—this would be the first of three marriages—but then deserted her, left Princeton, and spent more than a year as a seaman and wanderer in South America. He returned to divorce his wife and soon thereafter was stricken with tuberculosis. In a sanatorium he began writing plays (7).

O'Neill's powerful, autobiographical drama, *Long Day's Journey into Night*, is set in 1912, the year in which O'Neill was found to have tuberculosis, in an oceanfront house presumably in New London, Connecticut, the O'Neill family residence (24). The play was written in 1940. Initially he asked that it not be published until 25 years after his death, but he later relaxed this injunction, and it was produced in 1956, 3 years after his death. The action of the drama takes place in one day, beginning with a sunny noon and progressing through a foggy afternoon to a dark midnight. True to the actual O'Neill family history, the Tyrone family of the play consists of father James, an actor who cannot quite deal with the multiple problems in his family; mother Mary, fading from reality during the day and night as she takes additional amounts of opiates; their oldest son, James, Jr., a drunkard; and their youngest son, Edmund, who has just been given a diagnosis of tuberculosis and told he must go to a sanatorium. Putting aside much of the powerfully presented multiple dynamics of this dysfunctional family, Edmund's tuberculosis is central to the tense interactions of the Tyrone family throughout the long day and night chronicled in the play (24). His plight is that his penurious father wants to send him to the "state farm" to avoid paying the $7.00 per day cost of a private sanatorium, where Edmund feels he would be better treated. "So why waste money? That's why you're sending me to a state farm—," Edmund challenges his father. His mother refuses to accept the diagnosis. "A summer cold makes anyone irritable. . . . It *is* just a cold! Anyone can tell that!"

In actuality, Eugene O'Neill was initially hospitalized at Laurel Heights, a Connecticut state farm for consumptives, for 2 days before being transferred to highly regarded Gaylord Farm Sanatorium on

Christmas Eve of 1912. O'Neill's disease had begun about 2 months earlier. It presented as pleurisy with effusion, a form of tuberculosis with a relatively favorable prognosis. And O'Neill did well, being discharged after 6 months as "arrested" (at that time, no patient was ever considered cured, as relapses were common). O'Neill's tuberculosis did not recur. However, he never forgot it during his often tumultuous life, and it was three decades later that he wrote his dramatic account of the diagnosis. After an enormously productive if often anguished life, O'Neill died in November 1953 of what was then called Parkinsonism but from a modern perspective sounds more like Alzheimer's disease.

CONCLUSIONS

Reflecting on the history of tuberculosis, let us now ask again, did it affect the way we lived? One must conclude that it did, variously at various times, and sometimes only subtly. During the 19th century, the "Captain of Death" was present in the lives of many. Scarcely did a family not count a member or relative who was afflicted. The tuberculous deaths of all six Brontë children and their mother may have been remarkable—perhaps the family carried one of the genetic polymorphisms that decrease native resistance—but it was not out of keeping with the epidemiology of tuberculosis at that time. Chopin struggled with his disease but continued to compose and perform. As the course of history moved into the 20th and 21st centuries, tuberculosis incidence declined. Fewer dramatic instances of disease occurred. Yet it robbed baseball of the life of one of its greatest athletes in 1925.

The practice of medicine has reflected the prevalence of tuberculosis over the course of time. During the sanatorium era, an entire parallel health system devoted itself to the care of consumptives. Tuberculosis has intruded upon the political arena, but its impact has been minor. That Quezon conducted the Philippine government in exile from his bed in Saranac Lake cannot be said to have changed the course of war in the Pacific. Josephine Baker's espionage efforts were commendable, but the Allies would have won the war without them. Civilian life produced more notable examples. Can one imagine John Wayne without a Stetson hat?

In the world of creative arts, the impact of tuberculosis is most readily seen and was often dramatic. The Brontë novels presented it prominently, but also as something not exceptional—as an ordinary, 19th-century, life-ending event. Edvard Munch's depictions

of death certainly reflected his continuing struggle with the disease. No short life taken by tuberculosis is better known than that of John Keats. Three months after the hemoptysis that led him to make his own diagnosis of tuberculosis, he wrote:

> Darkling I listen, and, for many a time
> I have been half in love with easeful death,
> Call'd him soft names in many a mused rhyme,
> To take into the air my quiet breath (15).

REFERENCES

1. **Amberson, J. B., B. T. McMahon, and M. Pinner.** 1931. A clinical trial of sanocrysin in pulmonary tuberculosis. *Am. Rev. Tuberc.* **24:**401–434.
2. **Baker, J.-C., and C. Chase.** 1993. *Josephine. The Hungry Heart.* Random House, New York, NY.
3. **Bowen, C.** 1959. *The Curse of the Misbegotten. A Tale of the House of O'Neill.* McGraw-Hill Book Company, Inc., New York, NY.
4. **Brontë, C.** 2003. *Jane Eyre.* Barnes & Noble Classics, New York, NY.
5. **Brontë, E.** 1946. *Wuthering Heights.* Random House, New York, NY.
6. **Bunyan, J.** 1900. *The Life and Death of Mr. Badman.* R. H. Russell, New York, NY.
7. **Carpenter, F. I.** 1979. *Eugene O'Neill.* Twayne Publishers, Boston, MA.
8. **Clark, J.** 1835. *A Treatise on Pulmonary Consumption; Comprehending an Inquiry into the Causes, Nature, Prevention, and Treatment of Tuberculous and Scrofulous Diseases in General.* Carey, Lea, and Blanchard, Philadelphia, PA.
9. **Daniel, T. M.** 2004. René Theophile Hyacinthe Laennec and the founding of pulmonary medicine. *Int. J. Tuberc. Lung Dis.* **8:**517–518.
10. **Daniel, T. M.** 2006. The history of tuberculosis. *Respir. Med.* **100:**1862–1870.
11. **Davis, A. L.** 1996. History of the sanatorium movement, p. 40–54. *In* W. N. Rom and S. M. Garay (ed.), *Tuberculosis.* Little, Brown and Company, New York, NY.
12. **Duffin, J.** 1998. *To See with a Better Eye. A Life of R. T. H. Laennec.* Princeton University Press, Princeton, NJ.
13. **Gaskin, E. C.** 1857. *The Life of Charlotte Brontë.* D. Appleton and Company, New York, NY.
14. **Hubbard, E.** 1911. *A Little Journey to the Home of John B. Stetson.* The Roycrofters, East Aurora, NY.
15. **Keats, J.** 1935. *Ode to a Nightingale* (orig. pub. 1812), p. 841–842. *In* H. F. Lowry and W. Thorp (ed.), *An Oxford Anthology of English Poetry.* Oxford University Press, New York, NY.
16. **Laennec, R. T. H.** 1962. *A Treatise on the Disease of the Chest with Plates Translated from the French of R. T. H. Laennec with a Preface and Notes by John Forbes.* Hafner Publishing Company, New York, NY.
17. **Lilienfeld, A. M.** 1982. *Ceteris paribus:* the evolution of the clinical trial. *Bull. Hist. Med.* **56:**1–18.
18. **Lycan, G. L.** 1983. *Stetson University: the First 100 Years.* Stetson University Press, DeLand, FL.
19. **Macnalty, A. S.** 1934. The Brontës: a study in the epidemiology of tuberculosis. *Br. J. Tuberc.* **28:**4–7.

20. **Marble, A., with D. Leatherman.** 1991. *Courting Danger: My Adventures in World-Class Tennis, Golden Age Hollywood, and High Stakes Spying.* St. Martin's Press, New York, NY.

21. **Maurois, A.** 1953. *Cecil Rhodes. Translated from the French by Rohan Wadham.* Collins, London, United Kingdom.

22. **Medical Research Council.** 1948. Streptomycin treatment of pulmonary tuberculosis. *Br. Med. J.* 2:769–782.

23. **Moorman, L. J.** 1940. *Tuberculosis and Genius.* The University of Chicago Press, Chicago, IL.

24. **O'Neill, E.** 1956. *Long Day's Journey into Night.* Yale University Press, New Haven, CT.

25. **Opienski, H.** 1931. *Chopin's Letters. Translated from the Original Polish and French.* Alfred A. Knopf, New York, NY.

26. **Osler, W.** 1892. *The Principles and Practice of Medicine.* D. Appleton and Company, New York, NY.

27. **Parker, V.** August 1976. John B. Stetson. *SANTA News,* p. 6.

28. **Prideaux, S.** 2005. *Edvard Munch. Behind the Scream.* Yale University Press, New Haven, CT.

29. **Puffer, R. R., J. A. Doull, R. S. Glass, W. J. Murphy, and W. C. Williams.** 1942. Use of the index case in the study of tuberculosis in Williamson County. *Am. J. Public Health* 32:601–605.

30. **Quezon, M. L.** 1946. *The Good Fight.* D. Appleton-Century Company, New York, NY.

31. **Roberts, B.** 1987. *Cecil Rhodes. Flawed Colossus.* W. W. Norton & Company, New York, NY.

32. **Robinson, R.** 1993. *Matty. An American Hero. Christy Mathewson of the New York Giants.* Oxford University Press, New York, NY.

33. **Spake, M. (ed.).** 1954. *The Letters of the Brontës. A Selection.* University of Oklahoma Press, Norman, OK.

34. **Taylor, R.** 1986. *Saranac. America's Magic Mountain.* Houghton Mifflin Company, Boston, MA.

Tuberculosis and Nontuberculous Mycobacterial Infections, 6th ed.
Edited by David Schlossberg
© 2011 ASM Press, Washington, DC

Chapter 2

Epidemiology and Host Factors

ASIM K. DUTT

Tuberculosis is an ancient infection that has plagued humans throughout recorded and archeological history. It is always a surprise to those of us who live in Western countries that even today the infection remains the cause of higher rates of morbidity and mortality than any other infection in the world. This is because of its great prevalence in the densely populated developing countries; however, the incidence of tuberculosis is grossly underreported in these countries. According to estimates of the World Health Organization (WHO), in 2008 there were approximately 9.3 million active cases, of which 3 to 4 million cases were infectious, with positive sputum smears (115). Deaths due to tuberculosis occur in 1.8 million people worldwide each year (115). The estimates are that a death from tuberculosis occurs every minute. Thus, tuberculosis is still a major cause of disease and death, and its elimination will be extremely difficult as long as poverty, overpopulation, and multidrug-resistant (MDR) disease characterize large portions of the earth. Human immunodeficiency virus (HIV) is already deemed the number one preventable cause of death in developing countries (83).

The tubercle bacillus was discovered in 1882 and has been the subject of extensive research ever since. There is still much to be learned about the nature of the organism, its virulence, its genetic characteristics, and the response of the host to the infection.

HISTORY

Tuberculosis appears to be as old as humanity itself. Skeletal remains of prehistoric humans dating back to 8000 BC, found in Germany, show clear evidence of the disease. Egyptian skeletons dating back from 2500 to 1000 BC have revealed evidence of Pott's disease of the spine. Ancient Hindu and Chinese writings have documented the presence of the disease. From these descriptions, however, it is impossible to differentiate tuberculosis from diseases that produce similar pathology. Perhaps the best proof of tuberculosis has come from an Inca mummy of an 8-year-old boy who lived about 700 AD. The radiographic picture of the lumbar spine showed evidence of Pott's disease, and the smears of the lesion revealed acid-fast bacilli (AFB), most likely *Mycobacterium bovis*.

Tubercle bacilli can remain in viable form for many years in the tissues of healthy persons. When they produce disease, it runs a chronic and protracted course that gives ample time for transmission to susceptible hosts. The infection can produce disease in a human being after decades of dormancy. Thus, the infection becomes endemic when a large proportion of the population is infected. It can produce an epidemic, however, when introduced into a population of which only a small portion is immunologically protected by already having been infected. The history of tuberculosis in Europe and North America is better known for the past 150 years; however, there is a paucity of historic information on the epidemiology of tuberculosis in other parts of the world (14).

"EPIDEMIC WAVES" OF TUBERCULOSIS

When a new infection is introduced into a susceptible population, the morbidity and mortality rates take the predictable form of an epidemic wave (57). There is a sharp rise to a peak, followed by a more gradual descent. For many infectious diseases this curve is measured in weeks or months, but for tuberculosis it is measured in decades and centuries. Epidemiological information, though incomplete, reflects the incidence and prevalence of disease over a period of two or three centuries.

The waveform of the tuberculosis epidemic occurs by natural selection of susceptible persons and runs its course in about 300 years. Grigg (57) has described, on hypothetical grounds, three separate curves of mortality (elimination of susceptible

Asim K. Dutt • 4117 SW 30th Court, Ocala, FL 34474.

persons), morbidity (disease in the more resistant), and inapparent infections (infection without disease in the highly resistant) (Fig. 1). The three curves peak successively at 50- to 100-year intervals. With the decline of the epidemic, the death rate declines first, followed by morbidity and, finally, by inapparent infections.

In England the present epidemic wave began in the 16th century and probably reached its peak in about 1780 as a result of the Industrial Revolution and the growth of cities, which allowed the spread of disease from person to person. The epidemic then rapidly spread from England to other large cities in Western Europe, reaching a peak in the early 1800s. In Eastern Europe the peaks came in about 1870 and 1888, and by 1900 North American and South American epidemic waves had peaked. In the developing countries of Asia and Africa the wave has not peaked yet. Thus, as a global phenomenon, the epidemic is declining in one geographic area while still rising or just reaching its peak in another.

Industrialization and overcrowding of the cities can produce an epidemic of tuberculosis by bringing together large numbers of susceptible people and promoting transmission of *Mycobacterium tuberculosis* to new hosts. In addition, psychological stresses of urban life may lower individual resistance to infection. Grigg (57) has published curves to show the major tuberculosis waves in two contrasting imaginary settings, rural and urban (Fig. 2). These communities are assumed to remain isolated and to have a constant degree of urbanization. From the graph, one can conclude that after elimination of the susceptible persons, the survivors become relatively resistant and the epidemic starts to decline. The rate of decline is exponential, though factors such as war, famine, or flood may temporarily interrupt it. The overall decline in morbidity and mortality is persistent and is still continuing, though it may have leveled off some in the Western countries, owing to immigration; however, it is difficult to separate the considerable influence of socioeconomics and cultural improvement from racial and genetic factors in the dramatic improvement in tuberculosis in the developed world (78).

In the United States tuberculosis was increasing in the 17th century. The first available mortality figures from Massachusetts in 1876 indicated 300 deaths per 100,000 population. The peak mortality figure reached in New England was 1,600/100,000 per year in 1800. With industrial development, the epidemic traveled to the Midwest years later. The peak was reached in New Orleans, Louisiana, in 1840 and in the West in 1880. Though the disease occurred in blacks at a lower rate than in whites before the Civil War, thereafter, the increase was massive among blacks, with a peak of 650/100,000 per year in 1890, when emancipation and urbanization created an ideal atmosphere for transmission of tuberculosis. There is controversial evidence of the

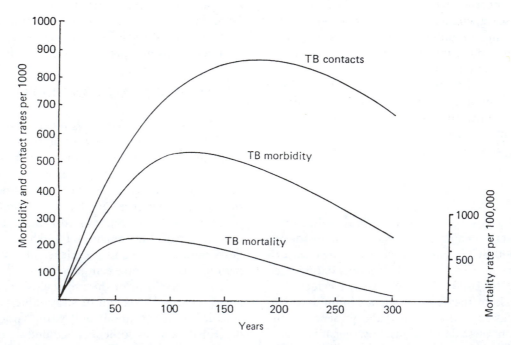

Figure 1. Theoretical concept of the development of tuberculosis (TB) in a community. Tuberculosis is assumed to appear for the first time at zero. The death rate, rate of morbidity, and rate of contacts are shown in reference to a living population. All these curves show a steep ascending limb and a prolonged exponentially decelerated descending limb. (Adapted from reference 57 with permission of the American Thoracic Society.)

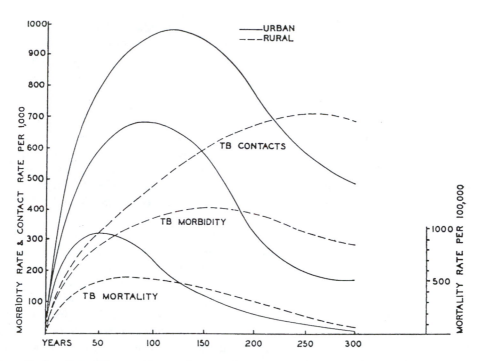

Figure 2. Rate of tuberculosis (TB) mortality, morbidity, and contacts at two extreme theoretical urban and rural settings. These two imaginary communities are assumed to remain isolated from the rest of the world. The variation in death rates between countries or communities can be explained by the difference in urbanization, both in time and in space. (From reference 57 with permission of the American Thoracic Society.)

presence of tuberculosis among the Native Americans until they were concentrated on reservations. This group reached the peak in about 1910 as a consequence of urbanization and crowding, which favored easy spread of the infection.

Thus, the epidemic of the disease in North America started with the earliest peak in the Northeast and then traveled to the Midwest, Southwest, and West. The Native Americans and Alaskans were the last American populations to become involved. From the data from the original epidemic it is obvious that the disease has been in steady decline for more than 100 years, even though the mortality rate was 113/100,000 per year in 1920. At that time tuberculosis was the second most common cause of death in the United States. The impact of isolation of tubercle bacilli, tuberculin testing, vaccination with bacilli Calmette-Guérin (BCG), and chemotherapy on the decline of the incidence of tuberculosis has often been exaggerated; the rate of decline was well established before the advent of any of these factors (Fig. 3). It does appear that discovery of isoniazid (INH) has considerably sharpened the natural decline in both the morbidity and mortality rates of tuberculosis and has led to a decline in the prevalence of the infection in the population (83).

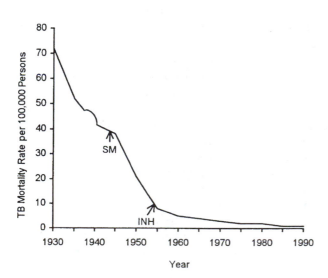

Figure 3. Tuberculosis (TB) mortality rates per 100,000 persons in the United States. SM, streptomycin. (Adapted from reference 93 with permission.)

TRANSMISSION OF TUBERCULOSIS

Although tuberculosis can affect any organ of the body, the lungs are virtually always the portal of entry. The bacilli are most commonly discharged into the atmosphere by aerosolization of pulmonary secretions by a diseased pulmonary patient in coughing, sneezing, speaking, and singing. Aerosol droplets dry rapidly, leaving tiny droplet nuclei, some of which contain a few bacilli (111). Large droplets fall to the floor, but droplet nuclei in the range of 1 to 10 μm can be inhaled, with the larger ones trapped in the upper nasal passages or expelled into the pharynx by the mucociliary mechanism of the lower respiratory tract and harmlessly swallowed and digested; smaller droplet nuclei may reach the alveoli and establish infection. Droplet nuclei carrying tubercle bacilli are produced by patients with active pulmonary tuberculosis in proportion to the liquidity of the secretions and the number of bacilli excreted; i.e., they are most numerous in persons with a productive cough and positive sputum smears (77). In several classic studies, Riley and others (87) show that droplet nuclei from smear-positive tuberculosis patients could infect guinea pigs in the environment. The number of organisms in the airborne aerosol also depends on the expulsive force of the cough and the presence of cavitation in the lungs (77, 87, 111) (Fig. 4).

Other methods of transmission are rare. In the past, transmission of infection with *Mycobacterium bovis* through consumption of milk from infected cows was common, but this means has been brought under control in all developed countries by elimination of diseased cattle and pasteurization of milk

and milk products. Transmission is still prevalent in developing countries due to consumption of unpasteurized milk, poorly heat-treated meat, and closer contact with infected animals (8). A recent genetic fingerprinting technique has revealed human-to-human transmission of *M. bovis* among HIV-infected persons in hospitals. Although less frequent, *M. bovis* as a causative organism for tuberculosis is identified also in developed countries. Approximately 7% of tuberculosis cases in San Diego, California, are caused by *M. bovis* (73). The national TB Genotyping Service isolated *M. bovis* in 1.4% of 11,860 linked cases during the period from 1995 to 2003. Mostly involved was extrapulmonary disease in young, U.S.-born Hispanics, indicating that infection was possibly related to food-borne exposure (61). Tuberculin skin test (TST) conversions among contacts revealed the same airborne transmission as in *M. tuberculosis*, regardless of the route of infection (74).

Although aerosolization of organisms during manipulation of tuberculosis lesions has been implicated in new infections among health care workers (52, 108), such infection from handling contaminated fomites is not a problem; however, infection can occur by way of inoculation when bacilli are introduced into or through the skin. Infection from this source is an occupational hazard among pathologists and laboratory workers who must handle infected issues and tuberculosis cultures. Fomites such as books, clothes, bedding, and eating utensils are not involved in the spread of infection and need no special attention.

Tuberculosis is clearly an airborne disease due to infection via droplet nuclei in the majority of patients (88). The close contacts of a smear-positive patient are at maximum risk of being infected; however, the disease is not as highly infectious as some of the viral infections. The ability of the bacilli to cause infection in newly exposed contacts depends on the adequacy of the innate antibacterial defenses of the person. Studies have shown that the infection rate among close contacts ranges from 25 to 50% even in the worst overcrowded and substandard conditions (104, 105). In one study the infection rate of 8.9% in close contacts of smear-negative, culture-positive patients was comparable to that in the community (58); however, prolonged close contact with such a person can be dangerous. On the basis of epidemiological data, it appears that exposure generally must be close and sustained, the environment heavily laden with droplet nuclei, and the prospective host unprotected by inborn defenses, previously activated immune mechanisms, or both if an infection sufficient to produce disease is to be established (see Fig. 4).

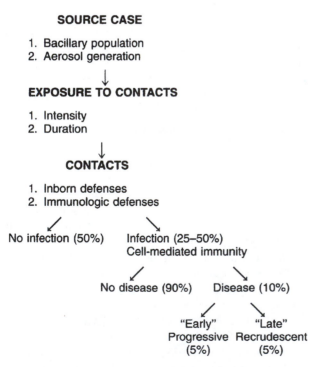

Figure 4. Major factors that determine transmission of infection from a source case to contacts and natural history of tuberculosis in infected contacts.

IMMUNOLOGIC CONSIDERATIONS

Infection with tubercle bacilli evokes cell-mediated immunity (CMI) 2 to 8 weeks after infection. Activated T lymphocytes and macrophages form granulomas. Granulomas inhibit replication and spread of organisms (89). The organisms become sequestered in the granulomas as dormant foci, which remain contained, and active disease may not occur in the majority of infected persons. CMI against *M. tuberculosis* evokes development of a positive TST. Alveolar macrophages infected with *M. tuberculosis* interact with T lymphocytes through several important cytokines. The macrophages release interleukins, which stimulate T lymphocytes (most CD4-positive lymphocytes) to release gamma interferon (16, 89, 94). Gamma interferon stimulates phagocytosis of *M. tuberculosis* in the macrophage (50, 51). It may not directly kill *M. tuberculosis* in the macrophages, partly because the organisms inhibit the cytokines' transcriptional responses (109, 113). Gamma interferon is essential for the control of *M. tuberculosis* infection (49). The major histocompatibility complex influences T-cell response, which is antigenic specific (49, 89). The initial host immune response contains *M. tuberculosis* infection. Depending on the adequacy of CMI, the organisms become sequestered in dormant foci and cause no clinical disease in approximately 90% of infected persons. Such a person is infected with these bacilli but not diseased. If the immune response fails, active disease may occur in some of the remaining 10% of infected persons; 5% may experience early progressive disease within 5 years of exposure. In heavy exposures in hospital personnel, the risk of tuberculosis has been shown to be 15% within the first year if not treated prophylactically with isoniazid (95). The remaining 5% may experience late recrudescent disease after several decades of infection (Fig. 4) (48). Subsequent development of active disease from reactivation of remote infection depends upon several factors affecting the host immune response. Immunosuppression with HIV is the greatest single risk factor. Other medical conditions affecting the immune system, such as uncontrolled diabetes mellitus, chronic renal failure, and vitamin D deficiency, may lead to progression of the disease (5, 68, 112). Studies on the immune system are unraveling defects which may influence susceptibility and development of disease. Researchers have detected defects in the production of gamma interferon (60, 94), tumor necrosis factor (TNF) (2, 103) deficiency in the gamma interferon receptor (66), and interleukin-12 receptor B1 (4). Clinical implications of these findings should be excitingly informative.

RISK FACTORS FOR TUBERCULOSIS

Various factors may influence the risk of developing tuberculosis in an individual or a population. The age and sex variables are also influenced by the timing of the epidemic in the population (Fig. 5). In the developing world tuberculosis rates are highest among young adults, indicating primary transmission in this age group.

As tuberculosis was declining until 1984 in the United States, the increased morbidity in elderly patients was remarkable (the end of epidemic wave). The age distribution of tuberculosis cases in Arkansas over the previous 20 years had undergone a dramatic shift from more cases in the first decade of life to almost no first-decade cases and more than 50% of cases over the age of 65 (96). The great majority of these cases result from recrudescence of infection acquired many years earlier (97). Between 1985 and 1992, persons 25 to 44 years of age accounted for more than 80% of the total increase in the number of cases (23). Considerable evidence has documented the linkage of tuberculosis with HIV/AIDS (54, 107). Dormant tuberculosis infection progresses to active disease in persons infected with HIV at a rate of 10% per year. Furthermore, HIV-infected persons are highly susceptible to exposure to tuberculosis (29).

With further decline in tuberculosis rates in the United States between 1993 and 2008, there is a declining trend in tuberculosis rates in all age groups. In 2008, the rates tended to increase with age from a low of less than 2 per 100,000 in children to a high of 9 per 100,000 in men 65 years and older. The rates in men 45 years and older were approximately twice those in same-age women (35) (Fig. 6).

Industrialization and urbanization provide optimal conditions for transmission owing to crowded living conditions with deplorable sanitation and housing. In all phases of an epidemic the urban areas show higher rates, and the peak is earlier there than in rural areas. Overcrowding of poor and ill-nourished people in the ghetto areas of large cities continues to produce a relatively high incidence of disease owing to a greater ease of transmission of the infection. In the United States there was a 20% increase in reported cases from 1985 to 1992. Most of the increase of tuberculosis occurred in cities with populations greater than 500,000 (21). Among the urban poor, the homeless have been identified as another risk group (21, 40).

Socioeconomic status and tuberculosis morbidity have an inverse relationship, although there are many factors involved, such as racial differences, crowding, and availability of health care. The case

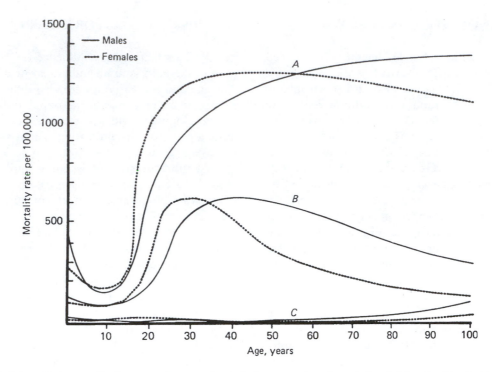

Figure 5. Tuberculosis mortality by age and sex—a theoretical presentation. *A*, period at height of epidemic; *B*, period at intermediate state; *C*, period at end of wave. (Adapted from reference 57 with permission of the American Thoracic Society.)

rate of those in the lowest median income group is approximately eight times that of persons in the highest median income group (20). The increased incidence in prisons reflects several of these factors: the prevalence of infection is higher among new prisoners than in the general population of similar age because there is a weighting of prisoners toward the lower end of the socioeconomic scale. The close living arrangements also make transmission to new hosts more likely than in normal living. Prisoners are at a greater risk for both tuberculosis and HIV infection because of socioeconomic status and overcrowding. This

combination of circumstances increases tuberculosis reactivation and person-to-person transmission (20). Indeed, for several years, 12% of new prisoners were infected each year in one prison before the epidemic was discovered and terminated by wide application of prophylactic treatment with INH (98). Patients in chronic mental hospitals and nursing homes experience a 10 times greater incidence of tuberculosis than does the general population (99). Danish workers found that among natural tuberculin reactors, the case rate was 29/100,000 per year, but the risk was 30 times greater in persons with abnormal results on

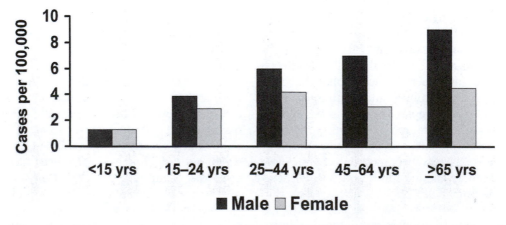

Figure 6. Tuberculosis (TB) case rates by age group and sex, United States, 2008. Rates tended to increase with age. The rates in men 45 years or older were approximately twice those in women of the same age. (Reprinted from reference 35 with permission of the CDC.)

chest radiographs (62). The risk was only two times greater in persons with nothing more than calcified residuals of a primary infection.

Substance abuse is a common behavioral risk factor among patients with tuberculosis in the United States (84). Injection drug abuse contributes to the high prevalence of tuberculosis among drug users (43, 90).

Alcoholics have been found to have a 10 times higher risk of developing tuberculosis than the general population in urban areas (46). This risk of active tuberculosis is substantially elevated in persons who consume more than 40 g of alcohol per day (75).

Cigarette smoking increases a relative risk of 1.5 to 2.0 for the development of tuberculosis (15). Smoking has been found to be associated with both risk of relapse of tuberculosis and tuberculosis morbidity (63).

Other factors associated with an increased risk of developing tuberculosis are HIV infection, diabetes mellitus, lymphoma, any chronic debilitating disease, gastrectomy, cancer, silicosis, and immunosuppressive therapy. Presently, however, HIV infection is the strongest risk factor (28, 42, 45).

GENETIC FACTORS

Patients may have a genetic predisposition toward tuberculosis. Studies among monozygotic and dizygotic twins (38) and observations in tuberculosis risk according to ancestral history (100) have raised consideration of genetic susceptibility. It also appears that race may play a role in individual risk of infection. In studies of both nursing homes and prison populations, blacks were twice as likely to become infected as whites under similar conditions of exposure (101). In vitro studies support these observations: monocytes from black donors are relatively permissive of mycobacterial growth (41, 44). Some correlation of histocompatibility types with development of tuberculosis has been observed (1). Associations between tuberculosis and some HLA alleles have been found, and also polymorphisms in the genes for natural resistance-associated macrophage protein (NRAMPI), the vitamin D receptor, and interleukin 1 (17, 55, 112). Although the role is not clear, NRAMPI polymorphism could influence tuberculosis susceptibility by regulation of interleukin 10 (7). This may differ with ethnic origin. To what extent these observations have influenced the global tuberculosis burden remains unclear. It is difficult to separate lifelong environmental influences from genetic predisposition, and this should be a fruitful area for future research.

MORTALITY AND MORBIDITY DATA

Global Epidemiology

The global epidemiology of tuberculosis is discussed in detail in chapter 10.

Epidemiology in the United States

In the United States, tuberculosis mortality and morbidity rates have been falling steadily, as shown in Fig. 3 and 7. The mortality rate has shown a steeper decline since the introduction of chemotherapy in 1945. The number of tuberculosis cases declined

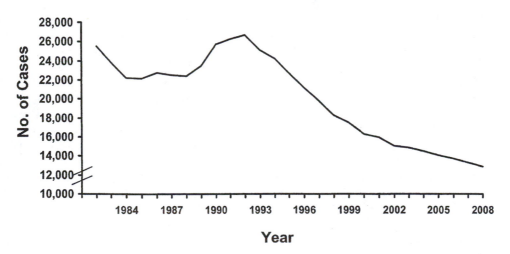

Figure 7. Tuberculosis cases, United States, 1982 to 2008, reported by the National Tuberculosis Surveillance System (35) (prepared by the Division of Tuberculosis Elimination, CDC). The resurgence of tuberculosis in the mid-1980s peaked in 1992. Cases started declining from 1993 to 2008 (12,904 cases), approximately 50% from 1992.

from 84,304 in 1953 to 22,255 in 1984 at a rate of 5% per year, for a rate of 9.3/100,000 population. The trend reversed dramatically in 1985. The number rose by 3% in 1986, by 5% in 1989, and by 6% in 1990. In 1992, there were 26,673 reported cases, for a rate of 10.5/100,000 population, a 9.4% increase from the previous year. As a result, it was estimated that over 52,100 excess cases occurred between 1985 and 1992 (23).

The resurgence of tuberculosis between 1985 and 1992 depended on several factors, including knowledge of the physician, social forces (poverty, homelessness, drug abuse, and incarceration), evidence of drug-resistant cases, increase in immigration from countries that had a high prevalence of disease, and the political and economic priorities of the nation, i.e., availability of the resources of tuberculosis control (19). As tuberculosis declined in the country, several factors were responsible for the resurgence in 1992 at its peak. Limited public health programs due to federal funding for tuberculosis control decreased. New public health programs resulted in diversion of funds, and many state and city governments downgraded their tuberculosis control program and supervision of chemotherapy. The excess cases of tuberculosis shook the authorities, public, and physicians; however, this unprecedented resurgence of tuberculosis was also due to tuberculosis occurring in persons with HIV infection. HIV infection had become the most important risk factor for tuberculosis (6, 23). In tuberculin-positive persons, tuberculosis is the first infection to develop, long before the common opportunistic infections occur. It is important to note that tuberculosis is one of the very few diseases of HIV-infected persons that can be transmitted to healthy persons. Utilizing a new molecular epidemiology technique of restriction fragment length polymorphism (RFLP) showed that 40% of cases were due to recent transmission rather than reactivation of previously acquired infection (64). A subsequent RFLP study indicated a decrease in recent transmission to 19 to 32% in many parts of the country (53).

Other important factors were the size of the population and the social organization of the community. Case rates were twice as high in large cities as in smaller ones and rural areas. Tuberculosis rates in urban areas increased 28.6% during this 8-year period (22 cases/100,000), while the rate of tuberculosis in nonurban areas fell by 3% (6.5 cases/100,000) (30).

Tuberculosis in the United States progressively had become a disease of the elderly, the foreign born, and minorities (25). The proportion of cases among minorities rose from 24% in 1953 to 49% in 1987. The ratio of incidence rate in nonwhites to that in whites had risen steadily from 2.9 in 1953 to 5.3 in

1987 (25). The age distribution of tuberculosis cases indicated profound changes in the racial and ethnic composition. For all age groups under 65, tuberculosis was predominately a disease of the minorities, while cases involving non-Hispanic whites predominated in persons above age 65 (31). Between 1985 and 1992, 62% of the cases occurred in black and Hispanic populations. The rate of tuberculosis among blacks rose to 37.8% (31.7/100,000 population) (30). According to the Centers for Disease Control and Prevention (CDC), 47% of U.S.-born persons with tuberculosis in the 25- to 44-year-old age group were HIV seropositive (29).

Although the largest increase in tuberculosis cases occurred in blacks and Hispanics aged 25 to 44 years, the age group in which excess AIDS cases also occur, an increase among foreign-born persons was also reported. Thus, factors other than HIV infection had also contributed to the increase in morbidity. Between 1986 and 1993, the tuberculosis case rate among the foreign-born increased to 30.1/100,000, compared with 8.1/100,000 for native residents (22, 30).

Fortunately, the case rate of tuberculosis in the United States resumed declining steadily in 1992, from 10.5/100,000, which represents a peak after 7 years of resurgence, to 4.2/100,000 population in 2008 (Fig. 7) (35). This decline most likely resulted from reinfusion of federal funds for tuberculosis control programs, improved public health efforts, physician and patient education, and implementation of directly observed therapy; however, in 2008, 59% of the reported patients were born in another country or in United States territory. Half of them had developed disease within 5 years of their arrival to the United States, and most of them were under the age of 35 years (35). The tendency of tuberculosis to be concentrated in younger age groups among minorities consisting of blacks, Hispanics, and the foreign-born is an ominous epidemiological sign. From 1992 through 2008, tuberculosis case rates declined every year. This was achieved by starting four appropriate drug regimens (72 to 87%, 1993 to 2008) and given as directly observed therapy, which rose from 36% in 1993 to 88% in 2008. Completion of treatment was in less than a year (from 64 to 84%, 1993 to 2008) (35). Reporting of new cases improved during this period (35). There was also considerable improvement in HIV testing (from 46 to 72% in persons between 25 and 44 years old and 30 to 62% in persons of all ages). Coinfection of tuberculosis and HIV was reduced from 29 to 10% in persons aged between 25 and 44 years and from 15 to 6% at all ages (Fig. 8). Also, drug-resistant cases declined between 1993 and 2008. MDR (resistance to INH

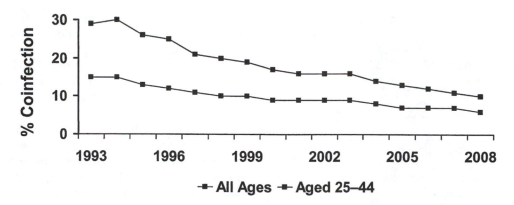

Figure 8. Estimated HIV coinfections in person reported with tuberculosis, 1993 to 2008. For all ages the estimated rate of coinfection of HIV and TB decreased from 15 to 6% overall; the rate decreased from 29 to 10% in persons aged 25 to 44 years during this period. (Reprinted from reference 35 with permission of the CDC.)

and rifampin) declined from 402 cases in 1993 to 86 in 2008. Primary MDR tuberculosis decreased from 2.3% in 1993 to approximately 1.1% in 2007 to 2008. There is no apparent trend in the number of extremely drug-resistant tuberculosis cases between 2003 and 2008. Ten cases were reported in 1993, and four cases were reported in 2008. In 2008, the number of reported cases of tuberculosis decreased in every age group, race, and ethnicity and for both sexes; however, despite improvement in rates of directly observed therapy, timely completion of treatment, and equalization of MDR tuberculosis rates, there are still disparities in the group (Fig. 9).

In 2008, the number of tuberculosis cases dropped to 12,904, a case rate of 4.2/100,000 population, which was a 3.8% decrease from 2007. The rate decreased in 35 states (3.5/100,000). Among 11 states that supplied information on cases during the period from 2003 to 2009, California, New York, and Texas accounted for 49% of cases. The data indicate a decreased number of tuberculosis cases among U.S.-born persons and an increased number among foreign-born persons (35). In 2008, the proportion of tuberculosis cases in persons born outside of the United States further increased to 59% (Fig. 10); this figure accounted for 47% of the total reported cases nationally.

The tuberculosis mortality rate has been decreasing in the United States since the middle of the 20th century. During the prechemotherapy period, the

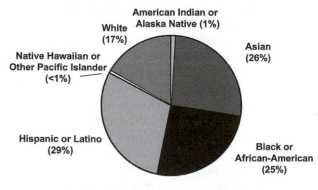

Figure 9. Tuberculosis cases by race/ethnicity in the United States, 2008. A total of 83% of reported cases occurred in racial ethnic minorities, whereas 17% of cases occurred in non-Hispanic whites. Hispanics are the largest group. (Reprinted from reference 35 with permission of the CDC.)

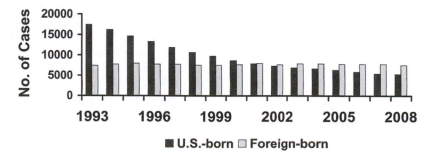

Figure 10. Number of tuberculosis cases in U.S.-born versus foreign-born people, United States, 1993 to 2008. The percentage of cases increased from 29% in 1993 to 59% in 2008. Overall, the number of cases in foreign-born persons remained virtually level (7,000 to 8,000) each year, whereas the number in U.S.-born persons decreased from 17,000 in 1993 to less than 5,300 in 2008. (Reprinted from reference 35 with permission of the CDC.)

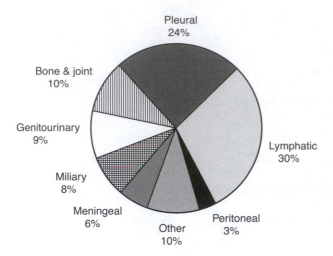

Figure 11. Reported cases of tuberculosis by anatomic site. (Reprinted from reference 92a with permission of McGraw-Hill.)

rate declined from 194.4/100,000 persons in 1900 to 70/100,000 in 1930 and then to 40/100,000 persons in 1943. The natural decline may be due to the epidemic wave and natural history of the disease, in addition to improved socioeconomic conditions and public health intervention. As noted above, the mortality rate has shown a steeper decline since the introduction of chemotherapy in 1945 (27). After 1954, it reached a low single-digit figure by 1965 (see Fig. 7), and the rate continues to be low.

The case rate for extrapulmonary tuberculosis in the United States did not decline in past years; it remained constant at about 2/100,000 per year from 1969 to 1979 (47). The proportion of extrapulmonary tuberculosis increased from 7% in 1963 to 18% in 1987 and slowly increased in recent years to 20% of reported cases (23, 86, 91). More than half of the extrapulmonary cases are due to involvement of the pleura and lymphatic system, followed by bone and joint diseases, genitourinary involvement, miliary disease, meningitis, and peritonitis (Fig. 11). This increase is due to HIV infection. Extrapulmonary tuberculosis can be seen in more than 50% of patients with concurrent AIDS and tuberculosis (81, 92). Also, minorities and the foreign-born are disproportionately more likely to have extrapulmonary disease (22, 91).

Detection of Tuberculosis Infection and Disease

In the past, mass radiographic surveys were productive in identifying diseased persons in populations with a high prevalence of infection, but they have little place in the United States today. In prisons and nursing homes it is more practical first to identify those who are infected by the use of the TST and to perform X-ray examinations on all reactors to search

for active disease. Thereafter, new infections can be determined by purified protein derivative (PPD) conversion in the event of an exposure. Skin testing (TST) with PPD (the Mantoux test) thus remains the most cost-effective method for recognizing and detecting new infection (10, 39). Later follow-up testing in the population gives evidence of new infection and the disease following the infection. Details of skin testing are presented in chapter 5.

TST for detection of latent tuberculosis infection, however, has major limitations in that it requires two visits and skilled staff for the test placement and interpretation. In addition, TST does not reliably separate reactions from previous immunization with *Mycobacterium bovis* BCG and infection with other environmental mycobacteria (4, 79). With advancement in immunology and genomics, T-cell-based in vitro assays of interferon released by T cells after stimulation with *Mycobacterium tuberculosis* antigens have been developed to identify tuberculosis infection. Two gamma interferon release assays are available in commercial kits: the QuantiFERON-TB Gold assay (Cellestis Ltd.) and the TB-SPOT-TB (Oxford Immunotec).

Gamma interferon detection has higher specificity for *M. tuberculosis* and less cross-reactivity with BCG vaccination than TST. The test is unreliable in the subgroup of patients with immunosuppression, including HIV/AIDS patients, those with extrapulmonary tuberculosis, children, and populations in high-incidence countries. The CDC recommends detection of latent infection via either the PPD or a gamma interferon release assay, the latter having the advantage of a single test for patients (5). Cost-effectiveness needs further evaluation.

The prevalence of infection varies according to the geographic areas and ranges from 2 to 8% according to the socioeconomic factors. The infection rate is higher in urban areas (4.1%) and is highest in the poor and disadvantaged residents of large cities; however, with the present reduction in incidence of tuberculosis, the infection rate is much lower now. Tuberculin testing is most effective in detecting infection among the close contacts of newly diagnosed patients. Only about 15 to 20% of the contacts are found to be infected in such situations, indicating that tuberculosis is less infectious than many other communicable diseases. In rare instances the attack rate of new infection may be as high as 80 to 90% if a heavy exposure is also a prolonged one. Infectiousness of the index case is rapidly decreased by the institution of proper chemotherapy. This fact has been amply demonstrated in controlled trials of chemotherapy in the hospital versus the home in Chennai (formerly Madras), India (67). There was no greater infection rate in the close contacts of patients treated at home. Most of the spread of infection to contacts occurs before the discovery of disease and institution of chemotherapy.

In 1999 to 2000, 4.2% of the United States population aged 1 year or older showed tuberculosis infection. Among subjects aged 25 to 74 years, the prevalence of tuberculosis infection decreased from 14.4% in 1971 to 1972 to 5.6% in 1999 to 2000. The decline was greater in the U.S.-born population (12.6 to 2.5%) than in foreign-born populations (35.6 to 21.3%). The prevalence of infection among foreign-born persons was more than eight times that of U.S.-born persons (70). Higher prevalences of tuberculosis infection were found in foreign-born persons (18.7%), non-Hispanic blacks/African Americans (70%), Mexican Americans (9.4%), and individuals living in poverty (6.1%) (18). A total of 63% of cases of latent tuberculosis infection (LTBI) were found among foreign-born persons. A targeted evaluation and treatment of individuals in high-prevalence groups shall be needed for prevention and control of tuberculosis (5).

The risk of developing disease after acquiring infection has been observed among Navy recruits, in nursing homes, and in a prison. It was found to be in the range of 5% in the first year, and although it declines rapidly thereafter, an additional 5% develop disease at some future time (48). The rate of developing disease after recent infection varies considerably in different geographic areas. Although tuberculosis rates have dropped for all racial and ethnic groups, disparities still remain. Poverty and malnutrition are important risk factors for tuberculosis (37). Malnutrition deeply affects CMI, which is the key host

Table 1. Incidence of active tuberculosis in persons with a positive tuberculin test by selected risk factors[a]

Risk factor	No. of TB cases/1,000 person-years
Recent TB infection	
Infection <1-yr past	12.9
Infection 1–7-yr past	1.6
HIV infection	35.0–162
Injection drug use	
HIV positive	76.0
HIV negative or unknown	10.0
Silicosis	68
Radiographic findings consistent with prior TB	2.0–13.6
Weight deviation from standard	
Underweight by ≥15%	2.6
Underweight by 10%–14%	2.0
Underweight by 5%–9%	2.2
Weight within 5% of standard	1.1
Overweight by ≥5%	0.7

[a]Adapted from the *American Journal of Respiratory and Critical Care Medicine*, Official Journal of the American Thoracic Society; American Thoracic Society.

Table 2. Relative risk for developing active tuberculosis by selected clinical conditions[a]

Clinical condition	Relative risk
Silicosis	30
Diabetes mellitus	2.0–4.1
Chronic renal failure/hemodialysis	10.0–25.3
Gastrectomy	2–5
Jejunoileal bypass	27–63
Solid-organ transplantation	
Renal	37
Cardiac	20–74
Carcinoma of head or neck	16

[a]Relative to control population, independent of tuberculin test status. Table 2 was adapted from reference 37a.

defense against tuberculosis. Primary or latent infection may progress to active disease in malnourished persons (71). In latent infection, the presence of malnutrition may be an important reactivating factor for the incidence of tuberculosis (13, 24, 71). This may be one of the reasons that tuberculosis incidence is high among immigrants from developing countries.

HIV-infected persons are highly susceptible to acquiring infection and progressing from infection to clinical tuberculosis to a degree that is unprecedented in recent history (59). Also, there is often considerable concern regarding the diagnosis of tuberculosis infection in HIV-infected individuals because of the high prevalence of anergy, which is dependent on the presence of CD4 T lymphocytes (27). Since 1993 there has been progressive improvement in the rates of HIV testing and a decrease in coinfection with tuberculosis and HIV (see Fig. 8). The risk of developing tuberculosis after acquiring infection in various groups is shown in Tables 1 and 2.

SPECIAL HIGH-RISK GROUPS

Tuberculosis in the Foreign-Born

Since 1986, tuberculosis disease has been reported increasingly in foreign-born persons every year. The number and proportion of cases among the foreign-born increased from 29% in 1993 to 58% in 2008. Five countries that commonly accounted for the cases were Mexico (23%), the Philippines (11%), Vietnam (8.0%), India (8%), and China (5.0%); however, the countries varied according to local epidemiological profile (Fig. 12). The tuberculosis rate among foreign-born persons was 25.3/100,000 population, which was 5.3 times greater than among U.S.-born persons (4.8 cases/100,000 population) (80). Tuberculosis case rates in foreign-born persons remain higher than those of the U.S.-born population. From 1993 through 2008, the ratio in U.S.-born persons decreased from 7.4/100,000 to 2.0, whereas the ratio in foreign-born persons increased from 5.4/100,000 to

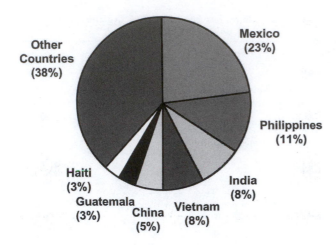

Figure 12. Countries of birth for foreign-born persons reported with tuberculosis in the United States, 2008. (Reprinted from reference 35 with permission of the CDC.)

20.3 (Fig. 13). From 1998 to 2008, among the three top reporting states, California, New York, and Texas, there were decreases in cases among U.S.-born persons (57%) which were far greater than the decreases among foreign-born persons (25.3%) (22, 31).

The majority of immigrants were from countries with a very high presence of tuberculosis, with a case rate of 100 to 250/100,000 population. Most of them were infected in their country of origin. During 2008, tuberculosis in immigrants was diagnosed in 27.7% of those who had resided in the United States for 1 to 4 years, 16% of those who had resided there for <1 year, and 52% of those who had resided there for ≥5 years (35).

Because the disease develops mostly within 5 years of arrival and the rate is high among children, most of the tuberculosis cases in foreign-born persons represent reactivation or progression of previous disease acquired in the country of origin. RFLP analysis often reveals that most of these cases are due to

reactivation of latent infection rather than transmission within communities. Generally, HIV infection is not a factor contributing to the development of disease among foreign-born immigrants. Another major issue is that these developing countries have higher rates of drug resistance than the United States. Several reports have documented higher rates of resistance in immigrants from Haiti, Latin America, and Southeast Asia (12, 39).

The most common resistance found is to INH and streptomycin. Primary drug resistance was approximately two times higher among foreign-born than among U.S.-born persons. In foreign-born persons resistance declined from 12.9% in 1993 to 10.3% in 2008; the rate declined from 6.8 to 4.9% in U.S.-born persons. Resistance to rifampin is generally low. During 2003, drug resistance among initial isolates of *M. tuberculosis* in persons with no previous tuberculosis episodes was more common for foreign-born patients than for U.S.-born patients. The rate of MDR (resistance to INH and rifampin) among foreign-born persons was 1.4% (for U.S.-born persons, 0.6%). This has an implication for treatment of the disease, which should be initiated with at least four bactericidal drugs. The cost of caring for patients with MDR tuberculosis is high. Inadequate screening of immigrants for tuberculosis infection and disease before they enter the United States or inadequate follow-up of those persons who had abnormal chest radiographic results with negative sputum smears are reasons for increases in cases among the foreign born which should be strengthened through improved screening by immigration services, both overseas and in the United States (117), by prompt reporting of suspected cases to public health programs, and by early identification and treatment of tuberculosis in foreign-born persons. Preventive therapy for infected persons, even when vaccinated with BCG, is highly indicated to reduce their incidence of disease.

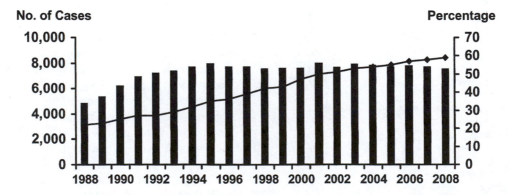

Figure 13. Trends in tuberculosis cases in foreign-born persons, 1988 to 2008. The number of cases among foreign-born persons increased from nearly 5,000 in 1998 to 7,000 to 8,000 each year since 1991. The percentage of tuberculosis cases accounted for by foreign-born persons increased from 22% in 1988 to 59% in 2008. (Reprinted from reference 35 with permission of the CDC.)

Tuberculosis in Health Care Workers

With the rapid decline of tuberculosis cases, the risk of disease among health care workers had decreased accordingly; however, several outbreaks of MDR tuberculosis and nosocomial transmission of drug-sensitive disease in hospital patients and health care workers have occurred (42, 45, 82). In outbreaks of tuberculosis among hospital personnel, many become infected (PPD changed from 0 to ≥15 mm). In such situations, 20% of persons may develop culture-positive tuberculosis within 2 to 4 months, suggesting a large inoculation (95). It is alarming that health care workers are at increased risk of contracting tuberculosis in the profession (Table 3). Several factors were identified that increase exposure and risk of tuberculosis in hospitals. Tuberculosis control measures in hospitals have not been appropriately followed (failure of respiratory isolations and ineffective or absent ventilation and positive-pressure isolation rooms).

With the decline in tuberculosis (4.2/100,000 population in 2008), delay in diagnosis and in initiation of early therapy will enhance transmission of infection. In the United States, between 1993 and 2006, an increasing proportion of cases of advanced pulmonary tuberculosis with cavitary lung disease and sputum positive for AFB was reported, indicating delays in the diagnosis (110) (Fig. 14). These patients are more likely to transmit disease. Physicians often lack a high index of suspicion for the presence of tuberculosis in their patients or hesitate to start therapy without microbiological confirmation of the disease, thus prolonging exposure of the staff (110). Patients with active tuberculosis may have smears negative for AFB in 25 to 50% of cases, resulting in diagnostic delays. In 1992, a survey found that 27% of the hospitals did not have isolation rooms and did not meet recommended standards of U.S. hospitals (34). Facilities to perform tests for AFB examination were not available in 16% of U.S. hospitals caring for patients with tuberculosis. The CDC reported that only 14% of 2,862 mycobacteriology laboratories in the United

States performed culture identification and drug susceptibility testing (33). For these reasons, diagnosis of tuberculosis was delayed considerably, resulting in prolonged exposure to infection for patients and hospital workers. Moreover, comorbidity with HIV infection in some of the population increased further risk of infection and rapid progression of disease with a high mortality rate.

Appropriate implementation of guidelines recommended by the CDC for isolation and treatment of suspected cases of tuberculosis consisting of early diagnostic laboratory procedures, provision of negative-pressure or UV-equipped isolation rooms (102), and the use of particulate respirators by health care workers (27) have fortunately minimized outbreaks of tuberculosis among health care workers since 1993. Heightened awareness and vigilance of hospital staff are required to identify and treat suspected patients with tuberculosis promptly. Hospital infection control programs should develop protocols and implement them administratively. Initial PPD skin tests of the employees should be performed and recorded in their files, and these tests should be repeated on the negative reactors at intervals. The rate of conversions should reflect appropriate tuberculosis control in the facility. Local tuberculosis control programs of health departments can assist in contact investigations of persons in the community.

Tuberculosis and Air Travel

Transmission of tuberculosis infection during air travel has been observed. Between 1993 and 1995, the CDC investigated seven instances when passengers or flight crew with infectious tuberculosis traveled on commercial flights. Six passengers and a crew member were symptomatic, with sputum smears positive for AFB and cavitary pulmonary tuberculosis. One had laryngeal tuberculosis. In two instances strains of *M. tuberculosis* were resistant to INH and rifampin (MDR tuberculosis) (36).

The studies indicated transmission of *M. tuberculosis* infection during the flight in three instances.

Table 3. Risk factors for TST conversion in Canadian hospitals[a]

Risk factor	Adjusted-odds ratio	95% Confidence interval
Respiratory therapist	6.1	3.1–12.0
Nursing	4.3	2.7–6.9
Housekeeping	4.2	2.3–7.6
<2 air changes per h (nonisolation patient rooms)	3.4	2.1–5.8
Physiotherapy	3.3	1.5–7.2
Inadequate ventilation (isolation rooms)	1.0	0.8–1.3

[a]Data from references 82a and 83a.

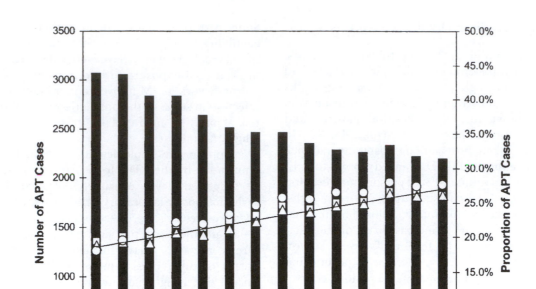

Figure 14. Trends in advanced pulmonary tuberculosis (APT) adjusted for selected risk factors, 1993 to 2006. Bars, APT; squares, age adjusted; triangles, foreign-born adjusted; circles, HIV adjusted; line, unadjusted. (Reprinted from reference 110 with permission.)

Most of the infected individuals were among passengers in seating proximity. Clinical evidence indicates a low risk of transmission of tuberculosis in aircraft and that the exposure needs to be prolonged, with the duration of flight exceeding 8 h. The risk may be similar to that for other confined places. On shorter flights there is minimal risk of transmission of infection, with no cases of clinical or bacteriologically confirmed tuberculosis. For prevention and control of transmission of tuberculosis, the WHO has provided guidelines which need be followed by patients, airlines, and various governmental bodies (116).

Tuberculosis and Iatrogenic Immunosuppression

Glucocorticosteroid

Increased risk of tuberculosis may occur with the use of prolonged steroid therapy. Receiving a dosage of ≥15 mg of prednisone (or equivalent) per day administered for ≥1 month is a risk factor for tuberculosis (5). The dosage primarily may suppress tuberculin reaction (5). Glucocorticosteroids have depressive effects on the cellular immune response, which tuberculosis requires for its control. A case-controlled study demonstrated that patients with tuberculosis were 4.9 times more likely to have been treated with glucocorticosteroids than those without tuberculosis (65).

TNF inhibitors

TNF alpha inhibitors are an effective treatment in immune-mediated inflammatory diseases such as rheumatoid arthritis, ankylosing spondylitis, Crohn's disease, and psoriatic arthritis. However, TNF is a protective cytokine for host defense against *Mycobacterium tuberculosis*. It has an important role in association with other cytokines for the development and maintenance of granulomas to localize bacilli during infection. Although baseline elevation of the tuberculosis incidence ratio is documented for rheumatoid arthritis, inhibition of TNF with anti-TNF therapy with infliximab may cause a four- to fivefold-higher incidence of tuberculosis in patients with latent infection (56, 59, 114). Development of tuberculosis is rapid with initiation of infliximab, with a median onset of 12 weeks and 98% of cases occurring within 6 months. There is a higher incidence of life-threatening extrapulmonary and disseminated diseases (69). Incidence of TB has been reported also with use of TNF receptor antagonist etanercept and monoclonal antibody adalimumab. Prior to initiation of infliximab therapy, it is imperative to exclude latent or active tuberculosis infection. Appropriate prophylactic therapy reduces the incidence of active disease. The TST is often falsely negative, and testing with QuantiFERON-TB Gold in association with TST may be beneficial in detecting latent infection in some of these patients.

Antineoplastic agents

Antineoplastic agents have immunosuppressive effects but also decrease the number of lymphocytes, monocytes, and granulocytes. The changes in the ratio of CD4$^+$ to CD8$^+$ lymphocytes predispose patients to intracellular pathogens like *Mycobacterium tuberculosis*. However, the most common infectious complication due to granulocytopenia is bacterial infection (106).

Tuberculosis in other special high-risk groups is discussed in chapters 12 and 32.

REFERENCES

1. **Al-Arif, L. I., R. A. Goldstein, L. F. Attronti, et al.** 1979. HLA-BW and tuberculosis in North America black population. *Am. Rev. Respir. Dis.* **120:**1275–1278.
2. **Algood, H. M., P. L. Lin, and J. L. Flynn.** 2005. Tumour necrosis factor and chemokine interaction in the formation and maintenance of granuloma in tuberculosis. *Clin. Infect. Dis.* **41**(Suppl. 3):S189–S193.
3. **Alland, D., G. E. Kalkut, A. R. Moss, R. A. McAdam, J. A. Hahn, W. Bosworth, E. Drucker, and B. R. Bloom.** 1994. Transmission of tuberculosis in New York City—an analysis by DNA fingerprinting and conventional epidemiologic methods. *N. Engl. J. Med.* **330:**1710–1716.
4. **Altare, F., A. Ensser, and A. Brieman.** 2001. Interleukin-12 receptor beta l deficiency in a patient with abdominal tuberculosis. *J. Infect. Dis.* **184:**231–236.
5. **American Thoracic Society and Centers for Disease Control and Prevention.** 2000. Targeted tuberculin testing and treatment of latent tuberculosis infection. *Am. J. Respir. Crit. Care Med.* **161:**221–247.
6. **Antonucci, G., E. Girardi, M. C. Raviglione, and G. Ippolito for the Gruppo Italiano di Studio Tubercolosi e AIDS (GISTA).** 1995. Risk factors for tuberculosis in HIV-infected persons. A prospective cohort study. *JAMA* **274:**143–148.
7. **Awomoyi, A., A. Merchant, and J. M. M. Howson.** 2002. Interleukin-10 polymorphism in SLC11A1 (formerly NRAMPI), and susceptibility to tuberculosis. *J. Infect. Dis.* **186:**1808–1814.
8. **Ayele, W. Y., S. D. Neill, and J. Zingstag.** 2004. Bovine tuberculosis: an old disease but a new threat to Africa. *Int. J. Tuberc. Lung Dis.* **8:**924–937.
9. **Baker, S. H., and K. Sorensen.** 1968. The epidemiology of tuberculosis infection in a closed environment. *Arch. Environ. Health* **16:**26–32.
10. **Barnes, P. F.** 2004. Diagnosing latent tuberculosis infection: turning glitter to gold. *Am. J. Respir. Crit. Care Med.* **170:** 5–6.
11. **Barnes, P. F., Z. Yang, and P. M. Pogoda.** 1999. Foci of tuberculosis transmission in central Los Angeles. *Am. J. Respir. Crit. Care Med.* **159:**1081.
12. **Barnes, P. F.** 1987. The influence of epidemiologic factors on drug resistance rates in tuberculosis. *Am. Rev. Respir. Dis.* **136:**325–328.
13. **Barr, R. G., A. V. Diez-Roux, and C. A. Knirsch.** 2001. Neighborhood poverty and resurgence of tuberculosis in New York City, 1989–1992. *Am. J. Public Health* **91:**1487–1493.
14. **Bates, J. H., and W. W. Stead.** 1993. The history of tuberculosis as a global epidemic. *Med. Clin. N. Am.* **77:**1205–1217.
15. **Bates, M. N., A. Khakdina, M. Pai, L. Chang, F. Lessa, and K. R. Smith.** 2007. Risk of tuberculosis from exposure to tobacco smoke: a systemic review and meta analysis. *Arch. Intern. Med.* **107:**335–342.
16. **Bean, A. G., D. R. Roach, and H. Briscoe.** 1991. Structural deficiencies in granuloma formation in TNF gene targeted mice underlie the heightened susceptibility to aerosol *Mycobacterium tuberculosis* infection, which is not compensated for by lymphotoxin. *J. Immunol.* **162:**3504–3561.
17. **Bellamy, R., C. Ruwende, and T. Corrah.** 1998. Variations in the NRAMPI gene and susceptibility to tuberculosis in West Africans. *N. Engl. J. Med.* **338:**640–644.
18. **Bennett, D. E., J. M. Courval, I. Onorato, T. Agerton, J. P. Gibson, L. Lambert, G. M. McQuillan, B. Lewis, T. R. Navin, and K. G. Castro.** 2008. Prevalence of tuberculosis infection in the United States population; the national health and nutrition examination survey, 1999–2000. *Am. J. Respir. Crit. Care Med.* **177:**348–355.
19. **Bloom, B. R., and C. J. Murray.** 1992. Tuberculosis: commentary on a re-emergent killer. *Science* **257:**1055–1064.
20. **Braun, M. M., B. I. Truman, and B. Maguire.** 1980. Increasing incidence of tuberculosis in a prison inmate population associated with HIV infection. *JAMA* **261:**393–397.
21. **Brudney, R., and J. Dobkin.** 1991. Resurgent tuberculosis in New York City. *Am. Rev. Respir. Dis.* **144:**745–749.
22. **Cain, K. P., C. A. Haley, L. R. Armstrong, et al.** 2007. Tuberculosis among foreign-born persons in the United States: achieving tuberculosis elimination. *Am. J. Respir. Crit. Care Med.* **175:**75–79.
23. **Cantwell, M. F., D. E. Snider, and G. M. Cauthen.** 1994. Epidemiology of tuberculosis in the United States, 1985 through 1992. *JAMA* **272:**535–539.
24. **Cegielski, J. P., and D. N. McMurray.** 2004. The relationship between malnutrition and tuberculosis: evidence from studies in humans and experimental animals. *Int. J. Tuberc. Lung Dis.* **8:**286–298.
25. **Centers for Disease Control.** 1987. Tuberculosis in minorities—United States. *MMWR Morb. Mortal. Wkly. Rep.* **36:** 77–80.
26. **Centers for Disease Control.** 1981. Drug resistance among Indochinese refugees with tuberculosis. *MMWR Morb. Mortal. Wkly. Rep.* **30**(22):273–275.
27. **Centers for Disease Control.** 1991. Purified protein derivative (PPD)-tuberculin anergy testing and management of anergic persons at risk for tuberculosis. *MMWR Morb. Mortal. Wkly. Rep.* **40**(RR-5):27–32.
28. **Centers for Disease Control.** 1989. Tuberculosis and human immunodeficiency virus infection: recommendations of the Advisory Committee for the Elimination of Tuberculosis (ACET). *MMWR Morb. Mortal. Wkly. Rep.* **38:**236–238, 243–250.

29. Centers for Disease Control and Prevention. 1993. Tuberculosis mortality—United States. *MMWR Morb. Mortal. Wkly. Rep.* **42**:696–704.

30. Centers for Disease Control and Prevention. 1995. Tuberculosis morbidity—United States, 1995. *MMWR Morb. Mortal. Wkly. Rep.* **45**:365–369.

31. Centers for Disease Control and Prevention. 2009. Trends in tuberculosis—United States, 2008. *MMWR Morb. Mortal. Wkly. Rep.* **58**:249.

32. Centers for Disease Control and Prevention. 2003. Trends in tuberculosis—United States, 1998–2003. *MMWR Morb. Mortal. Wkly. Rep.* **53**:209–214.

33. Centers for Disease Control and Prevention. 1995. Laboratory practices for diagnosis of tuberculosis—United States, 1994. *MMWR Morb. Mortal. Wkly. Rep.* **44**:587–590.

34. Centers for Disease Control and Prevention. 1994. Guidelines of preventing transmission of *Mycobacterium tuberculosis* in health care facilities. *MMWR Morb. Mortal. Wkly. Rep.* **43**(RR-13):1–132.

35. Centers for Disease Control and Prevention. 2009. Tuberculosis in the United States: Natural Tuberculosis Surveillance System highlights from 2008. http://www.cdc.gov/tb/statistics/surv/surv2008/default.htm.

36. Centers for Disease Control and Prevention. 1995. Exposure of passengers and flight crew to *Mycobacterium tuberculosis* in commercial aircraft, 1992–1995. *MMWR Morb. Mortal. Wkly. Rep.* **44**:137–140.

37. Chandran, R. K. 1991. Nutrition and immunity. Lesson for the past and new insights into the future. *Am. J. Clin. Nutr.* **53**:1087–1107.

37a. Cohn, D. L. 2003. Treatment of latent tuberculosis infection. *Semin. Respir. Infect.* **189**:249–259.

38. Comstock, G. W. 1978. Tuberculosis in twins: a reanalysis of Prophit survey. *Am. Rev. Respir. Dis.* **117**:621–629.

39. Comstock, G. W., and S. F. Woolport. 1978. Tuberculin conversions: true or false? *Am. Rev. Respir. Dis.* **118**:215–217.

40. Concato, J., and W. N. Rom. 1994. Endemic tuberculosis among homeless men in New York City. *Arch. Intern. Med.* **154**:2069–2107.

41. Crowle, A. J., and N. Elkins. 1990. Relative permissiveness of macrophages from black and white people for virulent tubercle bacilli. *Infect. Immun.* **58**:632–638.

42. Daley, C. L., P. M. Small, and G. F. Schecter. 1992. An outbreak of tuberculosis with accelerated progression among persons infected with HIV. *N. Engl. J. Med.* **326**:231–235.

43. Deiss, R. G., T. C. Rodwell, and R. S. Garfein. 2009. Tuberculosis and illicit drug use: review and update. *Clin. Infect. Dis.* **48**:72–82.

44. Delgado, J. C., A. Beena, and S. Thim. 2002. Ethnic-specific genetic associations with pulmonary tuberculosis. *J. Infect. Dis.* **186**:1463–1468.

45. Dooley, S. W., M. E. Villarino, and M. Lawrence. 1992. Nosocomial transmission of tuberculosis in a hospital unit for HIV infected patients. *JAMA* **267**:2632–2635.

46. Ellner, J. J. 1997. Review: the human response in human tuberculosis—implications for tuberculosis control. *J. Infect. Dis.* **176**:1351–1359.

47. Farer, L. S., A. M. Lowell, and M. P. Meador. 1979. Extrapulmonary tuberculosis in the United States. *Am. J. Epidemiol.* **109**:205–209.

48. Ferebee, S. H. 1970. Controlled chemoprophylaxis trials in tuberculosis: a general review. *Adv. Tuberc. Res.* **17**:28–106.

49. Flynn, J. L., J. Chan, K. J. Triebold, D. K. Dalton, T. A. Stewart, and B. R. Bloom. 1993. An essential role for interferon γ in resistance to *Mycobacterium tuberculosis* infection. *J. Exp. Med.* **178**:2249–2254.

50. Flynn, J. L., and J. D. Ernst. 2000. Immune response in tuberculosis. *Curr. Opin. Immunol.* **12**:432–436.

51. Flynn, J. L., M. M. Goldstein, and J. Chan. 1995. Tumor necrosis factor-α is required on the protective immune response against *Mycobacterium tuberculosis* in mice. *Immunity* **2**:561–572.

52. Frampton, M. W. 1992. An outbreak of tuberculosis among hospital personnel caring for a patient with skin ulcer. *Ann. Intern. Med.* **117**:312–313.

53. Geng, E., B. Kreisworth, C. Driver, J. Li, J. Burzynski, P. Della-Latta, A. LaPaz, and N. W. Schluger. 2002. Changes in the transmission of tuberculosis in New York City from 1990 to 1999. *N. Engl. J. Med.* **340**:1453–1458.

54. Glynn, J. R. 1998. Resurgence of tuberculosis and the impact of HIV infection. *Br. Med. Bull.* **54**:579–593.

55. Goldfeld, A. E., J. C. Delgado, and S. Thim. 1998. Association of an HLA-DQ allele with clinical tuberculosis *JAMA* **279**:226–228.

56. Gomez-Reino, J. J., L. Carmona, V. R. Valverde, E. M. Mola, and M. D. Montero. 2003. Treatment of rheumatoid arthritis with tumor necrosis factor inhibitors may predispose to significant increase in tuberculosis risk: a multicenter active surveillance report. *Arthritis Rheum.* **48**:2122–2127.

57. Grigg, E. R. N. 1958. Arcana of tuberculosis. *Am. Rev. Respir. Dis.* **78**:151–172.

58. Gryzbowski, L., G. D. Barnett, and K. Styblo. 1975. Contacts of cases of active tuberculosis. *Bull. Int. Union Tuberc. Lung Dis.* **50**:80–106.

59. Guelar, A., J. M. Gatell, J. Verdejo, D. Podzamczer, L. Lozano, E. Aznar, J. M. Miró, J. Mallolas, L. Zamora, J. González, et al. 1993. A prospective study of the risk of tuberculosis among HIV-infected patients. *AIDS* **7**:1345–1349.

60. Hirsch, C. S., Z. Toosi, and C. Othieno. 1999. Depressed T-cell interferon-gamma response in pulmonary tuberculosis: analysis of underlying mechanism and modulation with therapy. *J. Infect. Dis.* **180**:2069–2073.

61. Hlvasa, M. C., P. K. Moonan, L. S. Cowan, T. R. Navin, J. S. Kammerer, G. P. Merlock, J. T. Crawford, and P. A. Lobue. 2008. Human tuberculosis due to *Mycobacterium bovis* in the United States, 1995–2005. *Clin. Infect. Dis.* **47**:1608–1609.

62. Horwitz, O. 1970. The risk of tuberculosis in different groups of the general population. *Scand. J. Respir. Dis.* **72**(Suppl.):55–60.

63. Hsien-Ho, L., M. Ezzati, H. Y. Chang, and M. Murray. 2009. Association between tobacco smoking and active tuberculosis in Taiwan: prospective cohort study. *Am. J. Respir. Crit. Care Med.* **180**:475–480.

64. Jasmer, R. M., J. A. Hahn, P. M. Small, C. L. Daley, M. A. Behr, A. R. Moss, J. M. Creasman, G. F. Schechter, E. A. Paz, and P. C. Hopewell. 1999. A molecular epidemiologic analysis of tuberculosis trends in San Francisco, 1991–1997. *Ann. Intern. Med.* **130**:971–978.

65. Jick, S. S., E. S. Liberman, E. I. J. Rahman, and H. Choi. 2006. Glucocorticoid use, other associated factors and the risk of tuberculosis. *Arthritis Rheum.* **55**:19.

66. Jouanguy, E., S. Lamhamedi-Cherradi, F. Altare, M. C. Fondanèche, D. Tuerlinckx, S. Blanche, J. F. Emile, J. L. Gaillard, R. Schreiber, M. Levin, A. Fischer, C. Hivroz, and J. L. Casanova. 1997. Partial interferon-gamma receptor 1 deficiency in a child with tuberculoid bacillus Calmette-Guérin infection and a sibling with clinical tuberculosis. *J. Clin. Investig.* **100**:2658–2664.

67. Kamat, S. R., S. J. Y. Dawson, and S. Devadatta. 1966. A controlled study of the influence of segregation of tuberculosis patients for one year on the attack rate of tuberculosis in close family contacts in south India. *Bull. W. H. O.* **34**:577–632.

68. Karyadi, E., C. E. West, and W. Schultink. 2002. A double blind, placebo controlled study of vitamin A and zinc supplementation in persons with tuberculosis in Indonesia: effects on clinical response and nutritional status. *Am. J. Clin. Nutr.* **75:** 720–727.

69. Keane, J., S. Gershon, R. P. Wise, E. Mirabile-Levens, J. Kasznica, and W. D. Schwietermann. 2001. Tuberculosis associated with infliximab, a tumor necrosis factor alpha-neutralizing agent. *N. Engl. J. Med.* **345:**1098–1104.

70. Khan, K., J. Wang, W. Hu, A. Bierman, Y. Li, and M. Gardam. 2008. Tuberculosis infection in the United States: national trend over three decades. *Am. J. Respir. Crit. Care Med.* **177:** 455–460.

71. Kvale, G. 2001. Tackling the disease of poverty. *Lancet* **358:** 845–846.

72. Lademarco, M. F., and K. G. Castro. 2003. Epidemiology of tuberculosis. *Semin. Respir. Infect.* **18:**225–240.

73. LoBue, P. A., W. Betancourt, and C. Peter. 2003. Epidemiology of *Mycobacterium bovis* disease in San Diego County, 1994–2000. *Int. J. Tuberc. Lung Dis.* **7:**180–185.

74. LoBue, P. A., J. J. LeClair, and K. S. Moser. 2004. Contact investigation for cases of pulmonary *Mycobacterium bovis*. *Int. J. Tuberc. Lung Dis.* **8:**868–872.

75. Lonnroth, K., B. G. William, S. Stadlin, E. Jaramillo, and C. Dye. 2008. Alcohol use as a risk factor to tuberculosis—a systematic review. *BMC Public Health* **8:**289.

76. Lopez De Fede, A., J. E. Stewart, M. J. Harris, and K. Mayfield-Smith. 2008. Tuberculosis in socio-economically deprived neighborhoods. *Int. J. Tuberc. Lung Dis.* **12:**1425–1436.

77. Louden, R. G., and R. M. Roberts. 1966. Droplet expulsion from the respiratory tract. *Am. Rev. Respir. Dis.* **95:**435–442.

78. Marais, B. J., R. P. Gie, and H. S. Schaaf. 2004. The clinical epidemiology of childhood pulmonary tuberculosis: a critical review of literature from the pre-chemotherapy era. *Int. J. Tuberc. Lung Dis.* **8:**278–285.

79. Mazurek, G. H., P. A. LoBue, and C. L. Daley. 2001. Comparison of whole blood interferon γ assay with tuberculin skin testing for detecting latent mycobacterial tuberculosis infection. *JAMA* **286:**1740–1747.

80. McKenna, M. J., E. McCray, and I. Onorato. 1995. The epidemiology of tuberculosis among foreign-born persons in the United States, 1986–1993. *N. Engl. J. Med.* **232:**1071–1076.

81. Mehta, J. B., A. K. Dutt, and L. Harvill. 1991. Epidemiology of extrapulmonary tuberculosis: a comparative analysis with pre-AIDS era. *Chest* **99:**1134–1138.

82. Menzies, D., A. Fanning, and G. Juan. 1995. Tuberculosis among health care workers. *N. Engl. J. Med.* **332:**92–98.

82a. Menzies, D., A. Fanning, L. Yuan, and J. M. FitzGerald for the Canadian Collaborative Group in Nosocomial Transmission of TB. 2000. Hospital ventilation and risk for tuberculous infection in Canadian health care workers. *Ann. Intern. Med.* **133:**779–789.

83. Murray, C. J. L., K. Styblo, and A. Rouillion. 1990. Tuberculosis in developing countries: burden, intervention and cost. *Bull. Int. Union Tuberc. Lung Dis.* **65:**6–24.

83a. Nardell, E. A. 2003. Environmental infection control of tuberculosis. *Semin. Respir. Infect.* **18:**307–319.

84. Oeltmann, J. E., J. S. Kammerez, and E. S. Pavzner. 2009. Tuberculosis and substance abuse in the United States, 1997–2006. *Arch. Intern. Med.* **169:**189.

85. Pitchenik, A. E., B. W. Russell, and T. Cleary. 1982. The prevalence of tuberculosis and drug resistance among Haitians. *N. Engl. J. Med.* **307:**162–165.

86. Reider, H. L., D. E. Snider, and G. M. Cauthen. 1990. Extrapulmonary tuberculosis in the United States. *Am. Rev. Respir. Dis.* **141:**347–351.

87. Riley, R. L. 1957. The J. Burns Amberson Lecture: aerial dissemination of pulmonary tuberculosis. *Am. Rev. Tuberc.* **76:** 931–941.

88. Rouillion, A., S. Predrizet, and R. Parrot. 1976. Transmission of tubercle bacilli: the effects of chemotherapy. *Tubercle* **57:** 275–299.

89. Schluger, N. W., and W. N. Rom. 1998. The host immune response to tuberculosis. *Am. J. Respir. Crit. Care Med.* **157:** 679–691.

90. Selwyn, P. A., D. Hartel, V. A. Lewis, E. A. Schoenbaum, S. H. Vermund, R. S. Klein, A. T. Walker, and J. H. Friedland. 1989. A prospective study of the risk of tuberculosis among intravenous drug users with human immunodeficiency virus infection. *N. Engl. J. Med.* **320:**545–550.

91. Shafer, R. W., D. S. Kim, J. P. Weiss, and J. M. Quale. 1991. Extrapulmonary tuberculosis in patients with human immunodeficiency virus infection. *Medicine* (Baltimore) **70:** 384–397.

92. Small, P. M., P. C. Hopewell, S. P. Singh, A. Paz, J. Parsonnet, D. C. Ruston, G. F. Schecter, C. L. Daley, and G. K. Schoolnik. 1994. The epidemiology of tuberculosis in San Francisco: a population-based study using conventional and molecular methods. *N. Engl. J. Med.* **330:**1703–1709.

92a. Snider, D. E., and M. Onorato. 1995. Epidemiology, p. 3–17. *In* M. D. Rossman and R. R. MacGregor (ed.), *Tuberculosis: Clinical Management and New Challenges.* McGraw Hill, New York, NY.

93. Snider, G. L. 1997. Tuberculosis then and now: a personal perspective on the last 50 years. *Ann. Intern. Med.* **126:**237–243.

94. Sodhi, A., J. Gong, and C. Silva. 1997. Clinical correlates of interferon-gamma production in patients with tuberculosis. *Clin. Infect. Dis.* **25:**617–620.

95. Stead, W. W. 1995. Management of health care workers after inadvertent exposure to tuberculosis: a guide for the use of preventive therapy. *Ann. Intern. Med.* **122:**906–912.

96. Stead, W. W., and J. P. Lofgren. 1983. Does the risk of tuberculosis increase in old age? *J. Infect. Dis.* **147:**951–955.

97. Stead, W. W., J. P. Lofgren, and E. Warren. 1985. Tuberculosis as an epidemic and nosocomial infection among the elderly in nursing homes. *N. Engl. J. Med.* **312:**1483–1487.

98. Stead, W. W. 1978. Undetected tuberculosis in prison: source of infection of community at large. *JAMA* **240:**2544–2547.

99. Stead, W. W. 1981. Tuberculosis among elderly persons: an outbreak in a nursing home. *Ann. Intern. Med.* **94:**606–610.

100. Stead, W. W. 1992. Genetics and resistance to tuberculosis. *Ann. Intern. Med.* **116:**937–941.

101. Stead, W. W., J. W. Senner, and W. J. Reddick. 1990. Racial differences in susceptibility to infection by *Mycobacterium tuberculosis*. *N. Engl. J. Med.* **322:**422–427.

102. Stead, W. W., C. Young, and C. Hartnett. 1996. Probable role of ultraviolet irradiation in preventing transmission of tuberculosis: a case study. *Infect. Control Hosp. Epidemiol.* **17:** 11–13.

103. Sterling, T. R., S. E. Dorman, and R. E. Chaisson. 2001. HIV-seronegative adults with extrapulmonary tuberculosis have abnormal innate immune responses. *Clin. Infect. Dis.* **25:** 976–982.

104. Styblo, K. 1984. *Epidemiology of Tuberculosis*, p. 82–100. VEB Gustav Fischer Verlag Jena, Hague, Germany.

105. Sutherland, I. 1976. Recent studies in the epidemiology of tuberculosis based on the risk of being infected with tubercle bacilli. *Adv. Tuberc. Res.* **19:**1–63.

106. Taiwo, B. O., and R. L. Murphy. 2008. Corticosteroids, cytotoxic agent and infection: 2008. *In* D. Schlossberg (ed.), *Clinical Infectious Disease.* Cambridge, United Kingdom.

107. Telzak, E. E. 1997. Tuberculosis and HIV infection. *Med. Clin. N. Am.* **81:**345–360.

108. Templeton, G. L., L. N. Illing, and L. Young. 1995. The risk of transmission of *Mycobacterium tuberculosis* at the bedside and during autopsy. *Ann. Intern. Med.* **122:**922–925.

109. Ting, L. M., A. C. Kim, and A. Cattamanchi. 1999. *Mycobacterium tuberculosis* inhibits IFN-gamma transcriptional responses without inhibiting activation of STAT1. *J. Immunol.* **163:**3898–3906.

110. Wallace, R. M., J. S. Kammerer, M. F. Lademarco, S. P. Athomsons, C. A. Winston, and T. R. Navin. 2009. Increasing proportions of advanced pulmonary tuberculosis reported in the United States. Are delays in diagnosis on the rise? *Am. J. Respir. Crit. Care Med.* **180:**1016–1022.

111. Wells, W. F. 1934. On airborne infection: study 11, droplets & droplet nuclei. *Am. J. Hyg.* **20:**611–618.

112. Wilkinson, R. J., M. Llewelyn, and Z. Toossi. 2000. Influence of vitamin D deficiency and vitamin D receptor polymorphisms on tuberculosis among Gujarati Asians in West London: a case control study. *Lancet* **355:**618–621.

113. Wilkinson, R. J., P. Petal, and M. Llewelyn. 1999. Influence of polymorphism in the genes for the interleukin (IL)-1 receptor antagonist and IL-1 beta on tuberculosis. *J. Exp. Med.* **189:**1863–1874.

114. Wolfe, F., K. Michaud, J. Anderson, and K. Urbansky. 2004. Tuberculosis infection in patients with rheumatoid arthritis and the effect of infliximab therapy. *Arthritis Rheum.* **50:**372–379.

115. World Health Organization. 2009. *Global Tuberculosis Control: Epidemiology, Strategy, Financing.* WHO publication WHO/HTM/TB/2009.411. World Health Organization, Geneva, Switzerland.

116. World Health Organization. 2006. *Tuberculosis and Air Travel: Guidelines for Prevention and Control*, 2nd ed. WHO publication WHO/HTM/TB/2006.363. World Health Organization, Geneva, Switzerland.

117. Yecai Liu, M. S., M. S. Weinberg, L. S. Ortega, J. A. Painter, and M. D. Maloney. 2009. Overseas screening for tuberculosis in U.S. bound immigrants and refugees. *N. Engl. J. Med.* **360:**2406–2415.

Tuberculosis and Nontuberculous Mycobacterial Infections, 6th ed.
Edited by David Schlossberg
© 2011 ASM Press, Washington, DC

Chapter 3

Pathophysiology and Immunology

Arthur M. Dannenberg, Jr., and Paul J. Converse

PART I: PATHOGENESIS OF TUBERCULOSIS

Host-Parasite Interactions

The pathogenesis of human pulmonary tuberculosis can be considered as a series of battles between the host and the tubercle bacillus. Each of these participants has its own weapons which can be used against the other. In addition, both the host and the bacillus have sites of vulnerability where the adversary can get the upper hand.

The weapons of the host are (i) the activated macrophage—a phagocyte powerful enough to kill (or inhibit) the tubercle bacilli that it ingests—and (ii) the ability to stop intracellular bacillary growth in nonactivated macrophages by killing those macrophages, thereby transforming a favorable intracellular environment into the inhibitory environment of solid caseous tissue. (Bacillary growth means bacillary replication, i.e., an increase in their number; their size remains constant.)

The weapons of the bacillus are (i) the ability to multiply logarithmically within nonactivated macrophages, i.e., within the monocytes that emigrate from the bloodstream into the tissues at the sites of infection, and (ii) the ability to multiply extracellularly (often reaching tremendous numbers) in liquefied caseous material, especially the liquefied caseum on the inner surface of pulmonary cavities.

The vulnerabilities of the host are (i) nonactivated macrophages, which provide a favorable environment for the intracellular growth of the bacillus, and (ii) liquefied caseous material, the only menstruum in the host that supports the extracellular growth of the bacillus.

The vulnerabilities of the bacillus are (i) the inability to survive within fully activated macrophages and (ii) the inability to multiply in solid caseous tissue.

Methods To Prevent Contagion

The following measures would reduce the incidence of new cases of clinical tuberculosis (42a, 60, 82, 87): (i) instructing all patients—during a cough or sneeze—to turn their heads away from others and to cover their mouth and nose with their hands or, preferably, a cloth or tissue; (ii) wearing of tight-fitting effective masks by attending personnel; (iii) vaccination of tuberculin-negative persons with an effective bacillus Calmette Guérin (BCG) strain, if such persons are likely to be exposed to tubercle bacilli; and (iv) increasing the air exchange in rooms containing tuberculous individuals by means of an exhaust fan, by purifying the air through a HEPA filter, by means of a UV light (aimed at the ceiling and shielded to protect the eyes of personnel), or, preferably, by combinations of any or all of these methods. Prophylaxis is especially important for persons who may be exposed to antimicrobial-resistant tubercle bacilli.

Contracting Tuberculosis by the Respiratory Route (62, 78, 146)

Size of infectious particle

When inhaled, only fine particles or "droplet nuclei" containing one to three tubercle bacilli are capable of starting the infection, because they remain suspended in the airstream that enters the alveolar spaces (146, 200). The heavier droplet nuclei containing more bacilli (and/or bits of caseous material) impinge upon the mucosal surfaces of both the nasopharynx and the bronchial tree. The impinged bacillary particles are moved up the bronchial tree by cilia and are eventually swallowed. The mucosal surfaces of the respiratory and gastrointestinal systems are not easily infected by tubercle bacilli: very large numbers of bacilli are required to achieve such infection.

Arthur M. Dannenberg, Jr. • Departments of Environmental Health Sciences, Molecular Microbiology and Immunology, and Epidemiology, Bloomberg School of Public Health, and Department of Pathology, School of Medicine, The Johns Hopkins University, Baltimore, MD 21205. **Paul J. Converse** • Department of Medicine, School of Medicine, The Johns Hopkins University, Baltimore, MD 21205.

Virulence of bacillary strain

Tubercle bacilli may vary in virulence, both genetically and phenotypically. Genetically, BCG, human-type tubercle bacilli (e.g., H37Rv), and bovine-type tubercle bacilli (e.g., Ravenel S), in that order, are of increasing virulence for rabbits (146, 148). The entry of tubercle bacilli into monocytes/macrophages and their survival within such host cells are reviewed in references 188, 210, and 213.

The pathogenicity of a specific strain of tubercle bacillus is due to its genotype, the response of the host, and the way in which the bacillus was cultivated in the laboratory. Common measures of virulence are the number of bacilli in a particular organ, the pathology produced, and the time of death of the host.

The entire genome of *Mycobacterium tuberculosis* (which has now been sequenced) has changed relatively little over the years, i.e., it has had a low rate of synonymous and nonsynonymous base substitutions (95, 223). However, some deletions and insertions have caused evolutionary changes in the virulence of various members of the *M. tuberculosis* complex (35). For example, despite 99% genomic identity, *M. microti* is naturally attenuated for humans, due to several gene deletions (33, 158). BCG (which was derived from virulent *M. bovis*) was attenuated by serial passage in media containing ox bile (22–24). Similarly, the virulence of H37Rv can sometimes be reduced by repeated subculturing (54a, 84a, 146), by desiccation, or by exposure to sunlight.

The virulence of clinical isolates of *M. tuberculosis* has also been found to be variable: several strains, isolated from humans with active tuberculosis in India, Southeast Asia, and Hong Kong, were reduced in virulence for guinea pigs (50, 83, 167).

The degrees of virulence of various mycobacterial strains for rabbits and mice may differ, probably because these strains contain (or produce) slightly different antigens (157, 159, 160). For example, the HN878 strain of tubercle bacilli, which caused an epidemic in humans in Houston, Texas, was hypervirulent in rabbits (160). In mice, it caused a delay in the host's Th1 lymphocyte response—a property that may have contributed to its hypervirulence (160).

Number of tubercle bacilli inhaled and microbicidal power of AM

When many infectious units of one to three bacilli are inhaled, a phenotypically hardy bacillus is likely to be among them. In addition, the alveolar macrophages (AM) apparently vary in their capacity to destroy bacilli (146, 148). Evidently, some AM are rich in enzymes (72) and microbicidins; others are poor in both. The ratio of "rich" to "poor" AM seems to be determined by the native genetic resistance of each individual, as well as phenotypic factors. In humans, pulmonary infection begins only after a strongly endowed bacillus is ingested by a weakly endowed AM. The average number of inhaled bacillary particles required to establish a primary pulmonary tubercle is not known for humans. The range is probably between 5 and 200 for virulent human-type tubercle bacilli (see reference 223a). Among the common laboratory animals, the range is 600 to 1,200 for New Zealand White rabbits and 3 to 15 for mice, guinea pigs, and nonhuman primates (71).

Overview of the Five Stages of Pulmonary Tuberculosis (64, 65, 76, 146)

In stage 1, the stage of no bacillary growth, the bacillus is usually destroyed or inhibited by the mature resident AM that ingests it (Fig. 1A). If, however, the bacillus is not destroyed or inhibited, it multiplies and the AM allowing this multiplication eventually dies.

In stage 2, the symbiotic stage, the bacilli multiply logarithmically (Fig. 2) within the immature (nonactivated) macrophages of the developing lesion (now called a tubercle) (Fig. 1B). These nonactivated macrophages have entered the tubercle from the bloodstream (where they were called monocytes). This stage is called symbiotic (146), because (i) in this early lesion the bacilli multiply without apparent damage to the host, and (ii) increasing numbers of nonactivated macrophages accumulate there.

In stage 3, the stage in which caseous necrosis first occurs, the number of viable bacilli becomes stationary (Fig. 2), because bacillary growth is inhibited by the immune response to tuberculin-like antigens released from the bacilli (64). At this stage, the immune response is mainly tissue-damaging delayed-type hypersensitivity (DTH), which kills the bacillus-laden macrophages of the symbiotic stage (see "Part II: Immunology of Tuberculosis," below). The lesion then contains a solid caseous center within which the (now extracellular) bacilli do not multiply. Surrounding this center are both nonactivated macrophages, which permit intracellular bacillary multiplication, and partly activated macrophages (immature epithelioid cells) produced by cell-mediated immunity (CMI) (Fig. 1C).

In stage 4, the stage which usually determines whether the disease becomes clinically apparent, CMI plays a major role (see "Part II: Immunology of Tuberculosis," below). If only weak CMI develops, bacilli escaping from the edge of the caseous

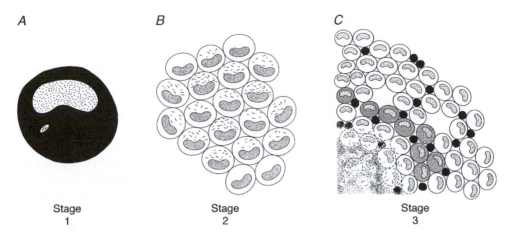

Figure 1. Stages in pulmonary tuberculosis. (A) Stage 1: an AM that has ingested and is destroying the two tubercle bacilli in the phagocytic vacuole. The cytoplasm of this macrophage is darkly shaded to depict the high degree of AM activation, i.e., high levels of lysosomal and oxidative enzymes (72). (B) Stage 2: an early primary tubercle, in which tubercle bacilli have multiplied logarithmically within macrophages that have emigrated from the bloodstream into the developing lesion. These newly arriving phagocytes are nonactivated, so the cytoplasm of these macrophages is unshaded to depict the lack of activation. In fact, virulent tubercle bacilli grow well within the phagocytic vacuoles of these nonactivated macrophages. Stage 2 is called the stage of symbiosis (64, 65, 146) since the bacilli are multiplying, the macrophages are accumulating, and neither is destroyed. (C) Stage 3: a tubercle 3 weeks of age with a caseous necrotic center and a peripheral accumulation of partly activated macrophages (lightly shaded) and lymphocytes (small dark cells). The first stages of caseation occur when the tissue-damaging DTH response (to the tuberculin-like products of the bacilli) kills the nonactivated macrophages that have allowed the bacilli to grow logarithmically within them. The dead and dying macrophages are depicted as fragmented cell membranes. Intact and fragmented bacilli are present, both within macrophages and within the caseum. Reprinted with permission from *Tuberculosis: Pathogenesis, Protection, and Control* (76) (see also pages 23 to 29 in reference 69).

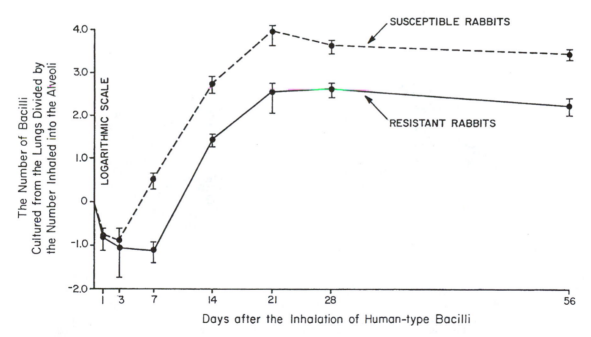

Figure 2. Changes in the number of virulent human-type tubercle bacilli in the lungs of natively resistant rabbits and natively susceptible rabbits at different intervals after the quantitative airborne inhalation of these bacilli (150). By 7 days after infection, the resistant animals had inhibited the growth of the bacilli 20 to 30 times more effectively than did the susceptible animals, but from then on, the two curves were parallel. At 4 to 5 weeks, susceptible animals had about 13 times the number of primary pulmonary tubercles present in the resistant animals. Means and standard errors are shown. The number of bacilli in the lungs of the resistant group failed to decrease during the period illustrated, because liquefaction with extracellular multiplication of the bacilli readily occurred in the resistant rabbits but only rarely occurred in the susceptible rabbits (146, 150). The macrophages of the resistant rabbits apparently developed higher levels of hydrolytic enzymes (70). Reprinted with permission from *American Review of Tuberculosis and Pulmonary Diseases* (150) (see also page 23 in reference 69).

necrosis multiply again in the surrounding nonactivated (and partly activated) macrophages present. The cytotoxic DTH immune response again kills these macrophages, causing enlargement of the caseous center and progression of the disease (Fig. 3A). If strong CMI develops, a mantle containing highly activated macrophages surrounds the caseous necrosis (Fig. 3B). These macrophages ingest and destroy (or inhibit) the escaping bacilli, often arresting the development of the lesion at a subclinical stage.

In stage 5, the stage of liquefaction, the bacilli evade the host defenses. When liquefaction of the caseous center occurs, the bacilli can multiply extracellularly for the first time, frequently reaching tremendous numbers (Fig. 4). Even a well-developed CMI is often ineffective in controlling such large numbers of bacilli. The high local concentration of tuberculin-like products released by these bacilli causes a tissue-damaging DTH response, which erodes the bronchial wall and thereby forms a cavity. Then, the bacilli enter the bronchial tree and spread to other parts of the lung, and also to the outside environment—most commonly during spells of coughing. Arrest of the disease at this stage depends on whether the antigenic load (of both the bacilli and their products) remains small enough for the host to control.

The First Stage of Pulmonary Tuberculosis: Its Establishment

After a unit of one to three bacilli is inhaled into an alveolus, the first stage of tuberculosis begins (64, 65, 76, 78, 146). An AM ingests the inhaled bacillary unit and often destroys it. This destruction depends on the inherent microbicidal power of the AM and the genetic and phenotypic virulence of the ingested bacilli (discussed above). Most AM are activated cells (Fig. 1A). They have been activated nonspecifically by many stimulating factors, including the ingestion and digestion of a variety of inhaled particles and occasional extravasated erythrocytes.

Seven days after inhalation of human tubercle bacilli, the lungs of Lurie's inbred susceptible rabbits contained 20- to 30-fold more viable bacilli than did the lungs of his resistant rabbits (146, 150) (Fig. 2). Therefore, the AM of the resistant host must have destroyed more inhaled bacilli and inhibited the growth of others more effectively than did the AM of the susceptible host. In other words, the ability to activate macrophages—in a nonspecific as well as in an immunologically specific manner—is one of the genetic factors that affect host resistance to tuberculosis.

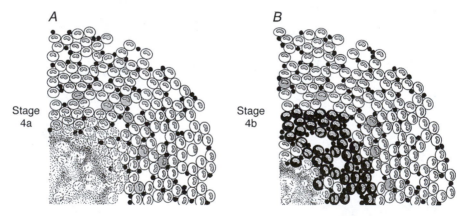

Figure 3. (A) Stage 4a: an established tubercle 4 to 5 weeks of age representing that found in Lurie's susceptible rabbits. It has an enlarging caseous center. The bacilli escaping from the edge of this center are ingested by nonactivated (incompetent) macrophages. In such macrophages, the bacilli again find a favorable intracellular environment in which to multiply. They do so until again the tissue-damaging immune response kills these new bacillus-laden macrophages and the area of caseous necrosis enlarges. This sequence may be repeated many times. The living tissue is destroyed, and the bacilli spread by the lymphatic and hematogenous routes to other sites, where the tissue destruction continues. Several partly activated macrophages (lightly shaded) are included to show that these susceptible rabbits develop only weak CMI. This pattern of tuberculosis is seen in immunosuppressed individuals, including nonterminal HIV/AIDS patients. (B) Stage 4b: an established tubercle 4 or 5 weeks of age representing those found in Lurie's resistant rabbits. The caseous center remains small because the bacilli escaping from its edge are ingested by highly activated (competent) macrophages (darkly shaded) that surround the caseum. In such activated macrophages, the bacilli cannot multiply and are eventually destroyed. Such effective macrophages are the result of activation by T cells and their cytokines. If the caseous center remains solid and does not liquefy, the disease will be arrested by this CMI process, because further tissue destruction does not occur. This scenario occurs in healthy immunocompetent human beings who show positive tuberculin reactions and yet no clinical and often no X-ray evidence of the disease. Reprinted with permission from *Tuberculosis: Pathogenesis, Protection, and Control* (76) (see also page 27 in reference 69).

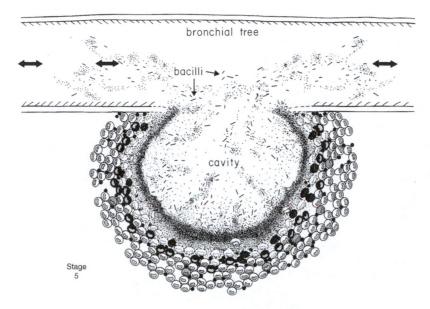

Figure 4. Stage 5: a recently formed small cavity discharging liquefied caseous material into a bronchus. In this liquefied material, the bacilli have multiplied profusely and extracellularly. With such large numbers of bacilli, there is an increased likelihood of a mutation resulting in antimicrobial resistance. Also, the large quantities of bacilli and their antigens in the liquefied caseum are too much for even a formerly effective CMI to control, and the DTH reaction to them destroys nearby tissues, including the wall of an adjacent bronchus (illustrated here). The bacilli are then discharged into the airways, where they disseminate to other parts of the lung and to the environment. Reprinted with permission from *Tuberculosis: Pathogenesis, Protection, and Control* (76) (see also page 29 in reference 69).

The Second Stage of Tuberculosis: Symbiosis

If the original AM fails to destroy or inhibit the inhaled particle of one to three bacilli, the bacilli multiply until that macrophage (or its progeny) bursts. Its bacillary load is then ingested by other AM and by nonactivated blood-borne monocytes/macrophages. Both types of macrophages are attracted to the site by chemotactic factors from the bacilli, e.g., fMet-Leu-Phe (formylmethionyl-leucyl-phenylalanine), and by chemotactic factors from the host, e.g., the complement component C5a and the cytokine monocyte chemoattractant protein (MCP-1) (138). In time, nonactivated macrophages from the bloodstream become completely responsible for the fate of the early lesion. In such a lesion, the AM rarely participate, because they remain peripherally (Fig. 5) rather far from the bacilli, which are almost always located more centrally.

The entering immature macrophages from the bloodstream readily ingest the bacilli released from AM. Then, a symbiotic relationship develops (4, 64–67, 76, 146, 150) in which neither the macrophages of the host nor the bacilli injure each other: the new macrophages have not yet been activated, so they cannot inhibit or destroy the bacilli, and the bacilli cannot injure the macrophages (Fig. 6), since the host has not yet developed tissue-damaging DTH. With time, more and more macrophages and more and more bacilli accumulate in the lesion.

In this symbiotic stage, between 7 and 21 days after infection, the bacilli grow logarithmically, at the same rate in Lurie's resistant and susceptible rabbits (Fig. 2). Evidently, intracellular tubercle bacilli inhibit the microbicidal mechanisms of immature macrophages equally well in both the resistant and the susceptible hosts (see "Phagocytosis and Killing of Tubercle Bacilli by Macrophages," below). Smith and Harding (220) observed the same parallelism in BCG-vaccinated and control guinea pigs. The bacilli contain sulfatides which (in vitro) inhibit the activation of macrophages (37, 187). Other mechanisms by which tubercle bacilli inhibit the microbicidal ability of macrophages are listed in references 38 and 120.

Only the activated macrophages of resistant and susceptible rabbits show differences in their ability to inhibit the growth of tubercle bacilli. AM are activated nonspecifically before inhalation of tubercle bacilli. Blood-borne monocytes/macrophages are mainly activated by specific CMI involving lymphocyte (T-cell) cytokines.

Histologically, macrophages in the lesions of the susceptible host tend to be located intra-alveolarly and contain more visible bacilli (Fig. 6) (146). Macrophages in the lesions of the resistant host are usually located interstitially (i.e., within the alveolar walls)

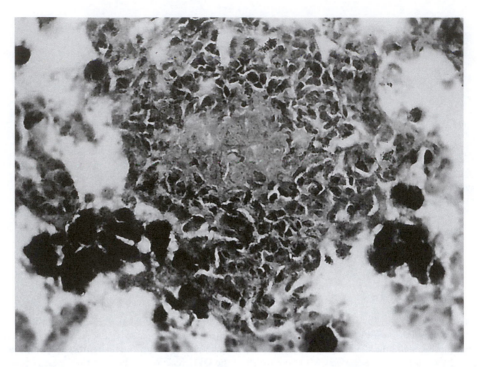

Figure 5. A tissue section of a 10-day (rabbit) pulmonary BCG lesion. In the caseous center are disintegrated β-galactosidase-negative epithelioid cells and more than 10 faintly stained tubercle bacilli. (β-Galactosidase activity is our histochemical marker for activated macrophages that are capable of destroying tubercle bacilli [9, 59, 74].) Around the caseous center are viable, poorly activated β-galactosidase-negative mononuclear cells (DCs, macrophages, and lymphocytes) from the bloodstream, which control the fate of the lesion. The highly activated pulmonary AM, staining 3+ and 4+ for β-galactosidase, have accumulated in the surrounding alveolar spaces, rather far from the bacilli in the center. Although this lesion was produced by the intravenous injection of tubercle bacilli, tubercles produced by the inhalation of bacilli should show the same pattern. Specifically, bacilli are released from weakly activated pulmonary AM that failed to control the initial bacillary multiplication. These bacilli and host cytokines chemotactically attract new nonactivated macrophages (from the bloodstream), which cannot control the multiplication of tubercle bacilli in their cytoplasm (until they become activated by antigen-specific T lymphocytes). This photograph clearly demonstrates that pulmonary AM play a minor role in controlling the fate of established pulmonary tubercles, but these AM play a major role in destroying endogenous and exogenous tubercle bacilli that enter the alveolar spaces. Magnification, ×400. Reprinted with permission from *American Journal of Pathology* (219a) (see also page 25 in reference 69).

and contain fewer visible bacilli (150). However, during this symbiotic stage, these differences have no apparent effect on the rate of bacillary growth (Fig. 2). In both resistant and susceptible rabbits, the newly arrived macrophages from the bloodstream support bacillary multiplication equally well in their cytoplasm. The interstitial inflammatory areas in the resistant rabbits contain greater numbers of lymphocytes, attracted there by chemoattractants, especially the chemokines (see "Cytokines," below). Such lymphocytes play a major role in the CMI and tissue-damaging DTH that terminate the second (i.e., the symbiotic) stage of this disease.

The Third Stage of Tuberculosis: the Early Stages of Caseous Necrosis

In rabbits, the third stage of the disease takes place 2 to 3 weeks after infection, when the early specific immune response occurs (65, 76). Tissue-damaging DTH (the major response at this stage) kills the macrophages that have allowed the tubercle bacillus to grow logarithmically in their cytoplasm, thereby producing caseous necrosis in humans, rabbits, and guinea pigs. The favorable intracellular environment for bacillary multiplication is eliminated and replaced by the extracellular environment of solid caseum, in which the bacillary multiplication is inhibited. The logarithmic bacillary growth in the pulmonary tubercle is stopped (Fig. 2) and is replaced by bacillary dormancy in its caseous center and a balance between bacillary growth and bacillary destruction in the surrounding viable tissues.

During the second (symbiotic) stage, and at its end, the lungs of Lurie's susceptible rabbits contained 20 to 30 times more bacilli than did the lungs of his resistant rabbits (Fig. 2). Most of these bacilli were probably located in developing tubercles.

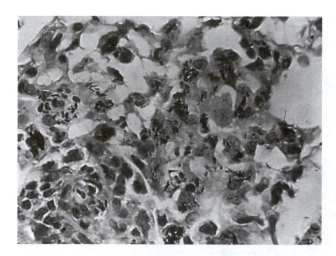

Figure 6. Tissue section of a tuberculous lesion from one of Lurie's genetically susceptible rabbits 2 weeks after the inhalation of virulent human-type tubercle bacilli. The nonactivated macrophages from the bloodstream contain numerous (rod-shaped) acid-fast bacilli. Two weeks is near the end of stage 2, the stage of symbiosis: the bacilli have grown logarithmically within these nonactivated macrophages with no apparent damage to the cells. Magnification, ×855. Reprinted with permission from *American Review of Tuberculosis and Pulmonary Diseases* (150) (see also page 25 in reference 69).

Unexpectedly, the susceptible hosts inhibited further bacillary growth just as effectively as did the resistant hosts (Fig. 2). CMI could not be responsible, because the susceptible hosts developed only weak CMI, and at this stage of the disease, the strong CMI of the resistant hosts was not yet fully developed. The marked inhibition of bacillary growth in both strains of rabbits must therefore be due to another mechanism, i.e., the tissue-damaging DTH that occurs in the third stage of pulmonary tuberculosis.

As stated above, such DTH kills the nonactivated macrophages in which the bacilli are growing, thereby eliminating the intracellular environment that is so favorable to such growth. This concept was advocated by several research groups (30, 38, 117, 119, 120, 144, 186) and had been predicted many years ago (39, 191). In fact, Robert Koch (the discoverer of the tubercle bacillus) described it before the terms DTH and CMI were in our vocabulary (127).

But why did the susceptible rabbits, which are known to develop weak CMI responses, i.e., to develop only weakly activated macrophages (146), stop the logarithmic growth of the bacillus just as effectively as did the resistant rabbits? The answer is that two immune mechanisms (CMI and tissue-damaging DTH) control the growth of tubercle bacilli. Lurie's susceptible rabbits developed weak CMI, but they developed strong tuberculin reactions, especially when

numerous tubercle bacilli were present in their bodies: a large number of bacilli provided a greater antigenic stimulus than did a smaller number. When the bacillary growth curves became level (Fig. 2), the susceptible rabbits often had tuberculin reactions equal to those of the resistant rabbits (146). The caseous centers of the lesions were larger in the susceptible rabbits than in resistant rabbits, apparently because more bacillus-laden macrophages had been present and were killed (150).

The tubercle bacillus can survive in this solid caseous material, but it cannot multiply, probably due to the anoxic conditions, reduced pH, and the presence of inhibitory fatty acids (107, 191). In fact, some bacilli may survive for years in solid caseous tissue. In this dormant state, the bacilli are not metabolizing and therefore are rather resistant to antimicrobial therapy (206).

In brief, the host locally destroys its own tissues to control the uninhibited growth of bacilli within nonactivated macrophages, which otherwise would be lethal to the host (39, 191). Only after such control is established can CMI (producing highly activated macrophages around the caseous focus) prevent the progression of the disease (Fig. 7).

Caseous necrosis in tuberculosis is a DTH reaction produced by T cells, including cytotoxic T cells (30, 38, 117, 119, 120, 130, 144, 185, 186, 202) (Table 1). Contributing to this necrosis are clotting factors (anoxia), cytokines (e.g., tumor necrosis factor [TNF]) (92, 114, 205–207), reactive oxygen and nitrogen intermediates (103, 126, 136, 169, 226) (from macrophages and other cells), and possibly antigen-antibody complexes, complement, and toxic products released from dead bacilli.

Tuberculin-like products seem to play a major role in the caseous process. These products (143), and other antigens (3, 8, 121), seem to be secreted or released from the live (and perhaps dead) intracellular tubercle bacilli. T-cell sensitivity (DTH) to tuberculin-like products probably occurs before T-cell sensitivity to the other antigens of the bacillus, because the release of other antigens may require killing and lysis of this microorganism. Thus, tuberculin-like proteins (and other early-released bacillary products) probably play major roles in stopping the logarithmic microbial growth of the symbiotic stage, whereas in later stages of the disease, the necrosis that these proteins produce may be more harmful than beneficial. (See "Development of Better Vaccines for Tuberculosis" below.)

If cytotoxic DTH is directed against tuberculin-like products of the bacillus on the surface of bacillus-laden macrophages, why is there so much damage

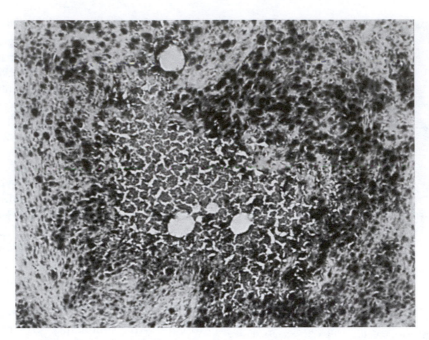

Figure 7. Tissue section of a 12-day (rabbit) dermal BCG lesion. Highly activated macrophages (stained dark blue for β-galactosidase) surround the caseous center. Therefore, bacilli released from dead and dying macrophages will now be ingested by macrophages able to inhibit intracellular bacillary growth. Magnification, ×120. Reprinted with permission from *American Journal of Pathology* (219a) (see also page 101 in reference 69).

to adjacent tissues? An answer to this question was suggested in an article from our laboratory (1b). In all inflammatory reactions, the postcapillary venule endothelium is activated by cytokines that upregulate ICAM-1, ELAM-1, VCAM-1, and other adhesion molecules (1b, 118, 131, 218, 227, 236), as well as major histocompatibility complex (MHC) class I and class II molecules (1b, 190). Such activated endothelial cells, therefore, would then be capable of presenting tuberculin-like antigens to cytotoxic T cells, which, in

turn, could injure the endothelium and thereby initiate the clotting cascade. Increased sensitivity to the toxic effects of TNF seems to be involved (91), as well as other factors (142). Local thrombosis would follow endothelial cell injury (155), and the thrombosis would cause ischemia and necrosis to nearby tissues. The use of anticoagulants to reduce the amount of caseous necrosis has not been investigated.

The Fourth Stage of Tuberculosis: Interplay of CMI and Tissue-Damaging DTH

During the fourth stage, the caseous tuberculous lesion may become clinically apparent (at least by radiograph), or it may be arrested with little visible evidence remaining, except for a positive tuberculin skin test. The fate of the lesion is mainly controlled by CMI. If CMI is weak, as in Lurie's susceptible rabbits, the bacilli escaping from the edge of the caseous centers again multiply intracellularly in poorly activated macrophages. Again, such infected macrophages are killed by tissue-damaging DTH, and the caseous center enlarges (Fig. 3A).

If the lesion is regressing, as in Lurie's resistant rabbits, the bacilli escaping from the caseous center are ingested and destroyed (or inhibited) by the highly activated macrophages that have accumulated perifocally (Fig. 3B and 7). These macrophages were previously activated (173) by the strong CMI that develops in these resistant hosts.

Table 1. Causes of tissue damage and caseous necrosis[a]

Cytotoxic T cells and NK cells
  Involving apoptosis and other mechanisms

Anoxia
  Produced by thrombosis—macrophages produce clotting factors

Toxic cell products
  Reactive oxygen and nitrogen intermediates; certain cytokines, such as TNF; hydrolytic enzymes; complement

Toxic bacillary products
  Intact tubercle bacilli are nontoxic, but when they are broken down, toxic products, such as "cord factor" (trehalose dimycolate), may be released

Overview
  Caseous necrosis is initiated by a tissue-damaging DTH reaction to high local concentrations of tuberculin-like bacillary products. Th1-type lymphocytes are responsible for the specificity of this reaction.

[a]Reprinted with permission from reference 78.

In each case, the number of viable bacilli is stationary (Fig. 2) (i) because of bacillary dormancy and slow death in the caseous material of the tubercle and (ii) because of a balance between growth of bacilli in some macrophages and their destruction by other macrophages. Also, the tubercle bacillus might become dormant in some macrophages, with no growth or destruction.

Histologically, the tuberculous lesions are quite different in the resistant and susceptible rabbits. The lesions in the resistant ones have less necrosis and many strongly activated macrophages (mature epithelioid cells). Those in the susceptible ones have more necrosis and many weakly activated macrophages (immature epithelioid cells). Large numbers of perifocal mature epithelioid cells, i.e., strongly activated macrophages (Fig. 7), enable the resistant host to control the disease (146, 148). (Fifty years ago, Lurie had no histochemical test for activated macrophages capable of destroying tubercle bacilli, but he identified them histologically as mature epithelioid cells.) We found that such cells contained high levels of β-galactosidase (9, 59, 74) and other histochemically demonstrable marker enzymes (74).

Resistant rabbits and the majority of immunocompetent adult humans develop the so-called adult-type tuberculosis. The caseous center of the lesion becomes surrounded by many such microbicidal macrophages (activated by T-cell cytokines) (Fig. 7). The bacilli that escape the caseous center are, therefore, ingested and destroyed. Eventually, the tubercle is walled off, the caseous center inspissates, and the disease is arrested, usually for a lifetime. The few bacilli that enter the lymphatics or the bloodstream are rapidly destroyed at their site of lodgment by accelerated tubercle formation, i.e., a rapid CMI response producing many locally activated macrophages (Fig. 7) (47, 59, 62, 152, 178) with relatively little caseous necrosis.

Susceptible rabbits, human infants, and immunosuppressed persons develop the so-called childhood-type tuberculosis. The caseous center is surrounded by many poorly activated macrophages, which permit the bacillus to grow intracellularly (78, 146, 148). These macrophages are usually killed (because of tissue-damaging DTH), and the caseous center enlarges. Thus, throughout the fourth stage of this disease in susceptible rabbits, DTH stops the intracellular growth of tubercle bacilli in the poorly activated macrophages, and this process results in further caseous necrosis.

In susceptible rabbits infected with virulent bovine-type tubercle bacilli, the bacilli lodging in the draining tracheobronchial lymph nodes (and often elsewhere) are not destroyed. The same is true for humans who develop only weak CMI when they are infected with virulent human-type bacilli. In both cases, multiple progressing caseous tubercles (of hematogenous origin) develop throughout the body, especially in the lungs, and the host eventually succumbs (78, 146, 148).

In hosts with such weak CMI, most of the secondary lesions in the lungs originate from bacilli in the caseous tracheobronchial lymph nodes. The lymph from these nodes drains the bacilli into the great veins leading to the right side of the heart, from which the bacilli are distributed directly into the lungs. Bacilli entering the bloodstream from primary pulmonary lesions are carried via the pulmonary veins to the left side of the heart, from which these bacilli are distributed throughout the body, but not directly into the lungs.

In general, the hilar lymph nodes in adult-type tuberculosis remain small and arrest the progress of the disease within them, whereas the hilar lymph nodes in childhood-type tuberculosis become large and caseous, in some cases giving rise to miliary tuberculosis in which tubercle bacilli are spread throughout the host via the bloodstream.

The Fifth Stage of Tuberculosis: Liquefaction and Cavity Formation

Overview

Unfortunately, even if CMI is well developed, progression of the disease may still occur in resistant hosts (including immunocompetent adult humans). Such progression is caused by liquefaction and cavity formation, which perpetuate the disease in humankind (39, 78, 146, 148, 199).

The liquefied material is frequently, but not always (53), an excellent growth medium for the tubercle bacillus (39, 70, 77, 118a, 146). In liquefied caseum, the bacillus often multiplies extracellularly (for the first time during the course of the disease), sometimes reaching tremendous numbers (Fig. 8). Because of the presence of DTH, the tuberculin-like antigens (produced by this large bacillary load) are toxic to tissues and may cause the wall of a nearby bronchus to become necrotic. If the necrotic bronchial wall ruptures, a cavity is formed. Then, the bacilli and the liquefied caseous material are discharged into the airways and are distributed to other parts of the lung and also to the outside environment. This adult-type tuberculosis occurs when a large number of tubercle bacilli from a cavity overwhelms the strong immunity that is usually present in the host.

Because the liquefied caseous material is so rich in tuberculin-like antigens, an exudate forms when

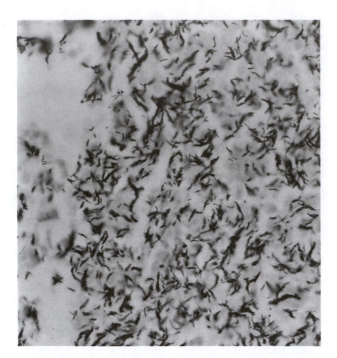

Figure 8. Tubercle bacilli growing profusely in the liquefied caseum in the wall of an early rabbit pulmonary cavity. Such bacillary growth occurs when the metabolism of the bacilli changes from dormancy in solid caseum to extracellular growth in liquefied caseum. For bacillary growth to occur, the composition of the liquefied caseum must be favorable. Also, oxygen (from the airways) enhances such growth (54). Similar bacillary growth has been found in many human tuberculosis cavities. Magnification, ×600. Reprinted with permission from *Clinical and Diagnostic Laboratory Immunology* (54) (see also page 45 in reference 69).

this material is aspirated into the alveolar spaces. Therefore, caseous bronchopneumonia will occur whenever this aspiration is extensive (Fig. 9). The bacilli need not multiply in the exudate, because the high concentration of tuberculin-like antigens in liquefied caseum is usually sufficient to cause this form of the disease.

Mutant bacilli resistant to antimicrobial agents may be present among the large number of bacilli in the liquefied caseum of the inner cavity wall. For this reason, tuberculosis is usually treated with several antimicrobials simultaneously. Liquefied caseous foci and cavities do not occur in Lurie's susceptible rabbits (146, 148) and are not common in infants or in fully immunosuppressed individuals infected with *M. tuberculosis* (15, 78).

Macrophages do not survive in solid caseous material, and even when it liquefies, the entering macrophages do not function effectively (146). Possibly, they have been passively sensitized to tuberculin and other antigens, which are present there in high (lethal) concentrations. Possibly, the entering macrophages are killed by toxic fatty acids originating from host cells, the bacilli, or both (107, 191).

Thus, even activated macrophages (produced by well-developed CMI) are completely ineffective in controlling the extracellular multiplication of bacilli within a cavity.

The cause of liquefaction is largely unknown. See references 70, 77, 245, and 247 for reviews of the subject and references 53, 54, 176, and 247 for recent experiments on cavity formation in rabbits. Hydrolytic enzymes (77) and DTH to the tuberculin-like products of the bacillus (245, 246) are involved (Table 2). At present, no therapeutic agent exists to prevent liquefaction, but if developed, such agents would greatly aid antimicrobial therapy in reducing the number of viable bacilli and controlling the disease (70).

Preventing liquefaction and cavity formation

The development of drugs to inhibit liquefaction and cavity formation has been hampered by the lack of a convenient animal model in which to produce these conditions. Mice and guinea pigs are the most common animals in which to study tuberculosis, but neither readily form pulmonary cavities. Only rabbits readily do so, but they are more expensive to purchase and care for and do not fit into the aerosol chambers used to infect the other two species.

A very simple method to speed up research in liquefaction and cavity formation was recently proposed (70), namely, the use of liquefaction and ulceration in the skin of rabbits as a surrogate model for the liquefaction and cavity formation in the lungs (Fig. 10). The lesions produced in the skin caseate, liquefy, ulcerate, and discharge liquefied caseum. The host cells in these skin lesions are the same types as cells in cavitary pulmonary lesions, i.e., macrophages, lymphocytes, dendritic cells (DCs), and others.

Once found, of course, effective liquefaction inhibitors in the skin should be evaluated for their effects on liquefaction and cavity formation in the lungs, in order to determine whether the inherent difference between the two organs affects the process.

Table 2. Causes and results of liquefaction[a]

Causes
  DTH to tuberculin-like bacillary products
  Hydrolytic enzymes: proteases, DNases and RNases, and
    probably lipases
Results
  Extracellular multiplication (sometimes tremendous) of the
    bacilli, resulting in antimicrobial drug-resistant mutants
  Erosion of bronchial walls, resulting in spread of bacilli
    through the air passages to other parts of the lung and to
    other persons

[a]Reprinted with permission from reference 78.

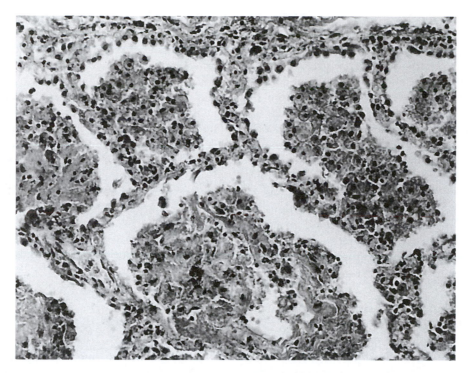

Figure 9. Tissue section of an area of tuberculous pneumonia in a lung of a 47-year-old man. A large proportion of the cellular exudate in the alveolar spaces has undergone caseous necrosis, and infiltrating cells thicken the alveolar septa. Magnification, ×266. From the collection of the late A. R. Rich and W. G. MacCallum, Department of Pathology, School of Medicine, The Johns Hopkins University (see also page 41 in reference 69).

In the surrogate model, an intradermal dose of live or dead BCG, dead (or live) virulent *M. tuberculosis*, or dead (or live) virulent *M. bovis* is titrated in the skin of rabbits to find the threshold dose required for liquefaction and ulceration: 10^3 to 10^8 bacilli is probably the best initial dose range, but the range will be decreased after the threshold number of tubercle bacilli is determined. The threshold bacillary dose is the lowest dose that would produce liquefaction and ulceration in the skin. Effective liquefaction inhibitors would raise the threshold dose, so liquefaction and ulceration would occur only at relatively high bacillary doses.

This method could be used to find drugs (probably inhibitors of proteinases, DNases, RNases, and/ or lipases) that would increase the threshold dose required for live or dead virulent tubercle bacilli (or BCG) to cause liquefaction and ulceration in the skin. If dead or attenuated tubercle bacilli were used, a biosafety level 3 facility would not even be required. In rabbits already sensitive to tuberculin, the lesions will ulcerate more quickly. See references 70, 176, and 246.

Once found, effective antiliquefaction drugs could then be tested in the rabbit model for their ability to prevent liquefaction and cavity formation in the lungs (53, 70, 146, 176, 246).

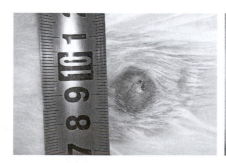
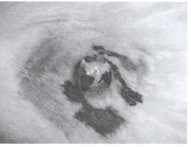

Figure 10. An example of liquefaction and ulceration in the skin of a rabbit produced by the intradermal injection of BCG. In the photograph on the right, the lesion contents were exposed by cutting it with a scalpel. Reprinted with permission from *Tuberculosis* (Edinburgh) (70).

Causes of the Subapical Localization of Adult Tuberculosis

Adult-type tuberculosis usually occurs in the subapical regions of the lungs, whereas childhood-type tuberculosis usually occurs in the middle or lower lung lobes. Adults spend most of the day in an upright position. Infants spend most of the day sleeping in a horizontal position. Common laboratory animals are also horizontal, and following the inhalation of a few tubercle bacilli, the tuberculous lesions develop preferentially in the dorsal regions.

How position affects the place of tuberculous lesions has been the subject of much debate for many years. Reference 172 gives the clearest insight, and reference 69 gives a few more.

The following is a brief overview.

1. In upright humans, less air is breathed into the apical part of the lungs than in the lower parts. (The bronchi reaching the lower lungs tend to be straighter and larger than those that branch to the upper lungs.) Therefore, with normal breathing, fewer dust and microbial particles reach the apical regions than reach the rest of the lungs, so the apical AM population may be less activated and less able to destroy the few inhaled *M. tuberculosis* organisms that land there. (AM are nonspecifically activated by most particles that they ingest.)

2. In the apices, the blood pressure is lower (because of gravity), and therefore the blood flow is less. Consequently, fewer macrophages and antigen-specific lymphocytes enter the apices to keep a beginning tuberculous lesion there from progressing.

3. Also, because of less blood flow, inhaled oxygen in the alveoli remains at higher concentrations at the apex, and carbon dioxide in the blood is removed less efficiently there. Both oxygen and carbon dioxide enhance the growth of tubercle bacilli.

4. Tubercle bacilli and the bits of caseous tissues (which surround many of the bacilli) contain lipids and tend to float. Therefore, in upright adult humans, the blood-borne tubercle bacilli would preferentially be distributed by the pulmonary arteries to the upper parts of the lungs. Endogenous blood-borne tubercle bacilli could reach a lung apex from a caseous hilar lymph node during a primary *M. tuberculosis* infection in childhood and remain dormant in the apex for years. Alternatively, endogenous blood-borne tubercle bacilli could reach a lung apex after a recent reactivation of a tuberculous hilar lymph node, followed by lymphatic drainage of *M. tuberculosis* into the great veins to the right side of the heart and then into the lungs. (See the section above on the fourth stage of tuberculosis.)

Clinical Tuberculosis

Pulmonary tuberculosis, once developed in humans, often shows a composite picture (39, 78, 191, 199). Tuberculosis is a local disease influenced by the local concentration of antigen, the amount of local macrophage activation, and the number of local lymphocytes with receptors for the antigens of the bacillus. Each lesion is handled by the host almost as if other lesions did not exist. Thus, lesions in one area of the lung may liquefy and progress, while lesions in another area of the same lung may stabilize or may regress. Even parts of a single lesion may progress, while other parts of the same lesion remain stable or regress. Finally, the disease as a whole may fluctuate between periods of exacerbation and remission (Table 3).

The childhood and adult types of tuberculosis are described above (see the sections above on the fourth and fifth stages of tuberculosis).

Tuberculosis in Common Laboratory Animals

The rabbit is the only common laboratory animal in which tuberculosis closely resembles the typical chronic cavity form found in the majority of adult humans (61, 70, 71, 73, 100, 146). Mice develop only weak tuberculin sensitivity and have much less necrosis in their tuberculous lesions than do humans and rabbits. Tuberculosis in mice is essentially a progressive granulomatous disease. Liquefaction and cavity formation never occur in mice (Table 4) (61, 71, 100).

Guinea pigs develop relatively strong tuberculin sensitivity and are the most susceptible of the group (61, 73, 100, 146). They usually develop a progressive hematogenously disseminated disease similar to that developed by infants and immunosuppressed persons. Cavity formation is not common in guinea pigs but can occur (220).

Lurie infected his inbred resistant and also susceptible strains of rabbits by the inhalation of virulent

---

Table 3. Basic types of pulmonary tuberculosis[a]

Types of lesions
  Encapsulated caseous, liquefied, or calcified nodules
  Proliferative type of pulmonary lesions
  Exudative type of pulmonary lesions
  Cavities

Types of disease
  Small discrete tubercles of hematogenous origin; focally localized or scattered diffusely throughout both lungs (miliary tuberculosis)
  Liquefied caseous lesions with cavity formation and bronchogenic spread
  Progressive, locally destructive lesions

[a]Modified from reference 199.

Table 4. Tuberculosis in various animal species[a]

Species	Response			
	Susceptibility	Tuberculin sensitivity	Caseous necrosis	Cavity formation
Mice[b]	++	+	+	0
Guinea pigs	+++++	+++	+++++	+
Rabbits[c]	++	++	+++++	++++
Humans	++	+++++	+++++	++++

[a]Adapted from *Tuberculosis in Animals and Man* (100) and reproduced in references 60 and 61.
[b]However, C3HeB/FeJ mice seem to make caseous tuberculous lesions (79a, 187a).
[c]Rabbits are fairly resistant to virulent human-type tubercle bacilli but rather susceptible to virulent bovine-type tubercle bacilli. The other species are more equally susceptible to both types.

tubercle bacilli (146). These studies are the main ones on record in which the onset, development, and progression (or healing) of primary pulmonary tubercles have been studied histopathologically. They provide insight (not obtainable by any other means) into host-parasite interactions that also occur in the human disease.

When evaluated at 5 and 12 months, pulmonary lesions caused by the inhalation of virulent human-type bacilli were regressing in both the resistant and the susceptible rabbits. At those times, the susceptible rabbits showed distinct primary lesions and often metastatic lesions of hematogenous origin, and the resistant rabbits showed either small almost-healed primary lesions or larger (primary) cavitary lesions. In these resistant animals, no grossly visible metastatic lesions were found, even though some bacilli must have spread from the cavitary lesions into the airways (146).

In both strains of rabbits, the pulmonary lesions produced by the inhalation of virulent bovine-type bacilli did not heal but caused progressive disease (67, 146). The susceptible rabbits died of a disease spread by the hematogenous route, and the resistant rabbits died of a disease spread through the airways by bacilli from pulmonary cavities (4, 146, 148). Lurie's susceptible rabbits did not form cavities (146).

Animal studies have also confirmed the genetic basis of susceptibility to tuberculosis. The resistant C57BL/6 and BALB/c mouse strains survived much longer than did the susceptible C3H, CBA, and DBA/2 mouse strains (165). Studies of genetic linkages in mice have found a possible susceptibility locus on chromosome 1 (128, 129).

Multiple genetic differences existed among Lurie's resistant and susceptible rabbits (146, 151). Unfortunately, these strains are now extinct. However, a strain of inbred rabbits (recently developed by the late Jeanette Thorbecke) was found to be more susceptible to tuberculosis than commercial outbred New Zealand White rabbits (85). (The outbred rabbits are almost as resistant as Lurie's inbred resistant strains [53].) The Thorbecke rabbits had larger tuberculous lesions that showed more bacilli, fewer mature epithelioid cells, and more extensive caseous necrosis than did those of the commercial rabbits, but the tuberculin skin tests of the Thorbecke rabbits were smaller. Unfortunately, because of a fire, the Thorbecke rabbits are no longer available.

New tuberculosis vaccines should always be evaluated in rabbits, mice, and guinea pigs before they are used in clinical trials, because each species develops different amounts of DTH and CMI when infected by *M. tuberculosis* (71) (see "Development of Better Vaccines for Tuberculosis" below). Mice develop weak DTH, guinea pigs develop weak CMI, and rabbits (and humans) usually develop the right amounts of DTH and CMI.

DTH kills poorly activated macrophages containing more viable tubercle bacilli than CMI can control, and tubercle bacilli do not grow in the solid caseous necrosis that results. Therefore, DTH and CMI are both necessary for the host to survive infection with *M. tuberculosis*. Some bacillus-laden poorly activated macrophages exist in every tuberculous lesion (68), and without adequate DTH, the host will eventually die of the disease (71).

In brief, mice eventually die of infection with *M. tuberculosis* because of weak DTH. Guinea pigs eventually die of this infection because of weak CMI. And, rabbits and most humans usually arrest infection with *M. tuberculosis* because they develop adequate DTH and CMI.

Both rhesus monkeys (*Macaca mulatta*) and cynomolgus monkeys (*Macaca fascicularis*) are very susceptible to *M. tuberculosis*—similar to isolated human populations that have never been exposed before to *M. tuberculosis* (71). Cynomolgus monkeys (140a) are somewhat more resistant than rhesus monkeys but not nearly as resistant as modern-day humans (and rabbits) (71).

Human Susceptibility to Tuberculosis

The average number of infectious particles of one to three bacilli that humans must inhale before converting their tuberculin skin test is unknown. Estimates vary from 5 to 200. However, only 1 in about 10 individuals who convert their tuberculin skin test will develop active tuberculosis during their lifetime. In other words, the majority of these individuals completely arrest the infection.

Arrest of the infection depends on a fully functional cell-mediated immune response. Persons coinfected with human immunodeficiency virus (HIV) or immunosuppressed from other causes are more likely to develop clinical disease from exogenously inhaled tubercle bacilli and also from endogenous (latent) tubercle bacilli that were inhaled years previously. A total of 5 to 10% of tuberculin-positive HIV-infected individuals reactivate this disease in a given year. In contrast, 5 to 10% of tuberculin-positive non-HIV-infected individuals reactivate this disease in their entire lifetime.

Even in the absence of immunosuppression, a spectrum of human susceptibility to tuberculosis clearly exists. Monozygotic twins show higher rates of concordance of the disease than do dizygotic twins (146). Population-based studies of susceptibility to tuberculosis have identified several genetic polymorphisms that may be associated with an increased risk of tuberculosis, including genes for NRAMP-1 (natural-resistance-associated macrophage protein 1), the vitamin D receptor, and the MHC (26, 27, 42, 156, 214, 215, 244).

An overview of genetic variations in different human populations is presented in references 42, 99a, and 223a.

PART II: IMMUNOLOGY OF TUBERCULOSIS

Comments

In this part, we briefly review the innate and acquired (adaptive) immune factors that play a role in tuberculosis. The reader is referred to textbooks of immunology for more details than those given here. Additional references were published in our chapter in the fourth and fifth editions of this book. The immunology of tuberculosis is reviewed in references 46, 71, 96, 123, 179, and 210c.

Most of the recent literature on the immunology of tuberculosis has discussed analysis of the mechanisms that start the immunological process and keep it from being excessive and even detrimental in the host. Cell surface receptors and mechanisms of transduction from the cell surface to its cytoplasm and nucleus are involved. There are so many checks and balances, as well as enhancing and diminishing mechanisms, that the system was likened to a spiderweb (155) with wires (spokes) from the outside to the center and wires circling these spokes at all levels. If one wire is broken, the whole web readjusts to a different configuration. This analogy explains why genetically knocking out one receptor, one cytokine, or one transduction factor can globally affect the function of the entire host. In other words, *each* receptor, cytokine, or transduction factor is important and must function properly to control an infection.

Overview of the Immunology of Tuberculosis

CMI and DTH play key roles in the pathogenesis of tuberculosis (64, 65, 71, 76). The tubercle bacillus apparently is not injurious to the host until these immune responses develop.

DTH and CMI are both mediated by Th1 lymphocytes. DTH to tuberculin-like antigens kills non-activated macrophages within which tubercle bacilli have multiplied extensively, because the local concentration of the tuberculin-like products soon reaches toxic levels (65, 69). CMI prevents such bacillary multiplication by activating macrophages (65, 69). Macrophages that are activated by CMI before they ingest tubercle bacilli are probably more effective than macrophages that are activated by CMI after they have ingested tubercle bacilli.

The antigens of *M. tuberculosis* that produce DTH are active at very low concentrations, whereas those that produce CMI are active at higher concentrations. For skin testing of people, 1 tuberculin unit (1 TU) of purified protein derivative (PPD) (first strength) or 5 TU (intermediate strength) is frequently used. One TU contains 0.00002 mg of PPD in the 0.1 ml used for intradermal injection. If second-strength PPD (250 TU, i.e., 0.005 mg) is injected intradermally in a person who is known to be strongly tuberculin positive, caseous necrosis will develop at the site of the tuberculin injection. In other words, the concentration of tuberculin is still very low when it is able to stop the intracellular multiplication of the bacillus by killing bacillus-laden macrophages.

The antigens producing CMI have not been fully identified or quantified (71). In general, the tuberculoproteins, peptides and carbohydrates in tuberculin, favor DTH, whereas other proteins complexed with carbohydrates and lipids favor CMI (reviewed in reference 69 on page 345).

To date, no laboratory has analyzed the known tuberculosis antigens for the amount of DTH and the amount of CMI that each antigen produces. For DTH, such an investigation would involve determining the minimal concentration of each antigen that elicits a positive (antigen-specific) skin test in tuberculous rabbits or guinea pigs and, possibly, the minimal concentration of each antigen required in vitro to kill macrophages containing live tubercle bacilli. For CMI, such an investigation would involve determining the concentration of each antigen that activates macrophages sufficiently to inhibit the intracellular growth of virulent tubercle bacilli. Unfortunately, the concentrations found in vitro may or may not match those found locally in vivo.

Note that the amount of caseous necrosis in the pulmonary lesions themselves reflects the ability of DTH to kill macrophages containing too many tubercle bacilli for CMI to inhibit. Therefore, we consider the amount of caseous necrosis produced in mice, guinea pigs, and rabbits to be a measure of the ability of these hosts to produce DTH. The tuberculin skin test does not reflect DTH function as well as does the amount of necrosis in pulmonary lesions, because laboratory animal species vary in skin composition and in skin thickness.

Cell-Mediated Immunity

CMI is characterized by an expanded population of antigen-specific T lymphocytes (Th1 cells) which, in the presence of these antigens, produce cytokines locally. These cytokines attract lymphocytes, monocytes/macrophages, and DCs from the bloodstream into the lesion and activate them. Gamma interferon (IFN-γ) and TNF-α are major macrophage-activating cytokines. IFN-γ also induces interleukin 2 (IL-2) receptors in monocytes/macrophages (111, 231, 241), following which IL-2 (from T lymphocytes exposed to specific antigens) becomes an additional activating cytokine for these phagocytes. Activated macrophages produce reactive-oxygen and reactive-nitrogen intermediates (103, 126, 169, 226), lysosomal enzymes, and other factors that kill and digest tubercle bacilli.

Acquired cellular resistance is characterized by the presence of a local population of activated (microbicidal) macrophages, produced by CMI, i.e., by the cytokines of antigen-stimulated lymphocytes (16). Monocytes/macrophages enter the tuberculous lesion in a nonimmune, nonactivated state. They readily ingest the tubercle bacillus and provide a favorable intracellular environment for its multiplication. These macrophages become activated and develop their microbicidal ability only where the bacillary antigens are located (Fig. 11 and 12). The greater the local accumulation of highly activated macrophages, the greater will be the host's ability to destroy tubercle bacilli (Fig. 7).

In this chapter, we include "acquired cellular resistance" in our definition of CMI, even though in the absence of antigen, CMI (i.e., an expanded specific T-cell population) can exist systemically before acquired cellular resistance (i.e., activated macrophages) develops locally within tuberculous lesions.

Delayed-Type Hypersensitivity

DTH is immunologically the same process as CMI, involving Th1-type T cells and their cytokines. As stated above, the main difference between DTH and CMI is the concentration of the antigens required to produce their effects: DTH antigens kill bacillus-laden macrophages at very low local concentrations, whereas CMI antigens evidently require larger concentrations to activate macrophages and thereby prevent intracellular bacillary growth. CMI antigens in very large concentrations would produce necrosis, and tuberculin-like DTH antigens in very small concentrations do, in fact, activate macrophages without necrosis (10). Tuberculin-like antigens are the major type producing DTH.

In this chapter, we use the term tissue-damaging DTH for the immunological reaction that causes necrosis. In a tuberculin-positive host, such necrosis develops wherever the tuberculin-like antigens from the bacilli reach a concentration that elicits a very strong DTH reaction. Such concentrations occur in tuberculous lesions whenever large concentrations of tubercle bacilli (or their products) are present.

Synergism between CMI and DTH

The role of CMI and DTH in the control of facultative intracellular microorganisms was debated for most of the 20th century. From the bacillary growth curves (Fig. 2) and the histology of tuberculous lesions (4, 64, 65, 146, 150), it is quite apparent that both CMI and DTH inhibit the multiplication of tubercle bacilli rather well. However, CMI does so by activating macrophages to kill the bacilli they ingest, and tissue-damaging DTH does so by destroying bacillus-laden (nonactivated) macrophages and nearby tissues, thereby eliminating the intracellular environment that is so favorable to bacillary growth.

Thus, both tuberculin-positive hosts with strong CMI and tuberculin-positive hosts with weak CMI can arrest bacillary growth, but the host with weak CMI does so with much damage to its own tissues. Humans (and rabbits) with adequate CMI usually recover, but humans (and rabbits) with weak CMI will usually die from excessive tissue destruction. Interestingly, mice have weak DTH but strong CMI, and

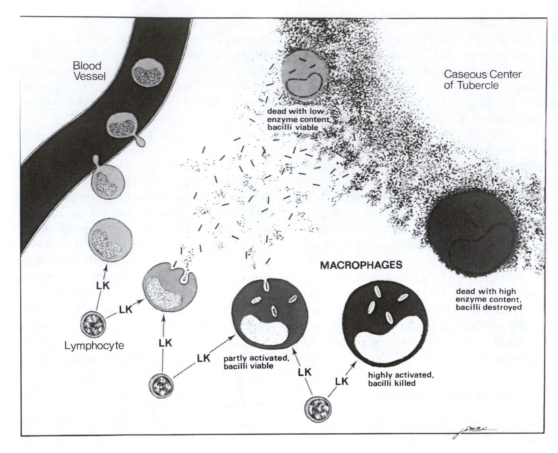

Figure 11. CMI activating macrophages in a tuberculous lesion. Mononuclear phagocytes that entered the lesion from the bloodstream are activated by the cytokines of antigen-specific T lymphocytes that had also entered the lesion. ("LK" stands for lymphokines, the former name for lymphocyte cytokines.) Antigen-specific lymphocytes produce these cytokines when stimulated by the bacillus and its products. Only activated macrophages seem capable of destroying the tubercle bacillus. Reprinted with permission from *Mycobacterial Infections of Zoo Animals* (60) (see also page 100 in reference 69).

guinea pigs have strong DTH but weak CMI, and both mice and guinea pigs usually die when infected with virulent *M. tuberculosis* (71).

Tissue-damaging DTH causing local necrosis stops the initial bacillary growth within nonactivated macrophages (Fig. 1C and Fig. 2), but such cytotoxic DTH is not sufficient to stop the progression of the disease. This is because viable tubercle bacilli escape from the edge of the necrotic areas and are ingested by perifocal macrophages. Only if the perifocal macrophages have been sufficiently activated by CMI will the ingested tubercle bacilli be destroyed and disease be arrested.

However, as stated above, nonactivated macrophages from the bloodstream are continually entering tuberculous lesions (68), and some ingest local tubercle bacilli. Since these macrophages have not yet been activated by CMI, the bacilli will again grow intracellularly, and tissue-damaging DTH is required to stop such growth. Therefore, DTH works synergistically

with CMI throughout the whole course of tuberculosis—not only in its initial stages.

It is not known whether nonactivated macrophages containing only a few tubercle bacilli can be activated by CMI to prevent further intracellular multiplication. The main function of CMI seems to be the activation of uninvolved nearby macrophages (Fig. 7) (59, 64, 65, 76). These activated perifocal macrophages ingest and destroy the bacilli escaping from the caseous center, as well as the bacilli released from macrophages that are killed by DTH (Fig. 13).

Phagocytosis of Tubercle Bacilli by Macrophages

In order to recognize a microorganism, phagocytes must first recognize patterns on the bacillary surface (171a). The pattern recognition receptors of macrophages and DCs include mannose receptors, complement receptors, fibronectin receptors, and

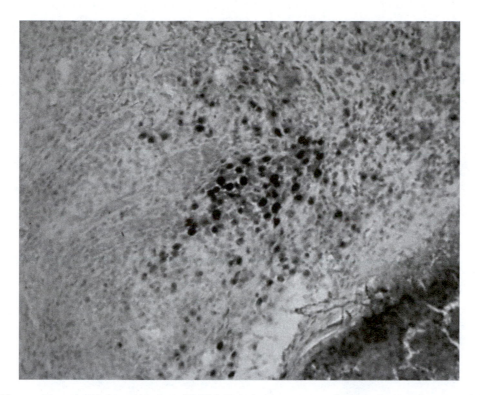

Figure 12. Tissue section of a 21-day rabbit dermal BCG lesion, showing a group of activated macrophages (epithelioid cells) stained darkly for the lysosomal enzyme β-galactosidase. (As stated in the legend to Fig. 5, β-galactosidase activity is our histochemical marker for activated macrophages that are capable of destroying tubercle bacilli [9, 59, 74].) Although perifocal tuberculous granulation tissue contains hundreds of macrophages, only those macrophages in locations where tubercle bacilli (and their products) are present become activated and develop the power to destroy the bacillus. In other words, the acquired cellular resistance (produced by CMI) is a local phenomenon. The darker the macrophage is stained for β-galactosidase, the more it resembles the mature epithelioid cell that Lurie identified with the destruction of the tubercle bacillus (9, 146). Magnification, ×160. Reprinted with permission from *Bacteriological Reviews* (59) (see also page 103 in reference 69).

Toll-like receptors (TLRs), all of which are involved in the host's innate immune response (90a).

Extensive studies have been made on TLRs (90a, 96, 164, 179). This receptor family is comprised of 10 members, some of which recognize various mycobacterial cell wall components, including lipoproteins and glycolipids (e.g., lipoarabinomannan). Engagement of human macrophage TLRs by 19-kDa mycobacterial lipoproteins activates NF-κB, induces IL-12 secretion, and increases the transcription of inducible nitric oxide synthase (NOS) (31), all of which participate in killing or inhibiting tubercle bacilli. TLR knockout mice produced conflicting results (2, 198, 219), possibly due to differences in the infecting dose or species differences between mice and humans.

After acquired (adaptive) immunity develops, macrophages also recognize antibody-opsonized microorganisms by Fc receptors and by complement receptors (90a, 155).

Killing of Tubercle Bacilli by Macrophages

Because of the receptors just mentioned, *M. tuberculosis* is easily bound to macrophages and internalized into phagosomes. Ordinarily, such phagosomes fuse with lysosomes, undergo acidification, and receive an abundance of lysosomal enzymes that can degrade the ingested microorganisms. However, *M. tuberculosis* subverts phagosome-lysosome fusion and subsequent maturation of the phagosome into an acidic, microbicidal, and hydrolytic compartment (210a). *M. tuberculosis* also resists degradation by lysosomal enzymes. Although the bacillus inhibits the entry of many microbicidal factors into the phagosome (11), it allows nutrients (such as iron carried by transferrin) to enter. See reviews in references 188, 210, and 210a.

The intracellular growth of virulent tubercle bacilli is currently an active field of investigation. One interesting recent development is the

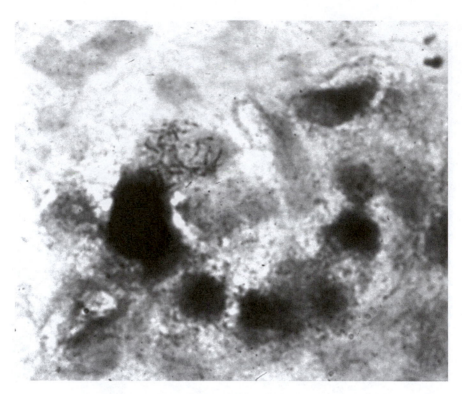

Figure 13. Macrophages stained both for β-galactosidase activity and for acid-fast bacilli in a BCG lesion of a rabbit injected intradermally 21 days previously. The macrophage near the center shows negligible β-galactosidase activity. It contains numerous bacilli and has ruptured. Another macrophage (just adjacent) shows high β-galactosidase activity. It contains no bacilli but apparently is ingesting the bacilli released from the ruptured cell. These two cells illustrate how CMI works; i.e., CMI produces locally many highly activated macrophages that can ingest (and destroy) bacilli released from ineffectual macrophages (9). Several other activated macrophages are also shown in this photograph. Magnification, ×1,600. Reprinted from reference 59 (see also page 102 in reference 69).

finding of a mycobacterial eukaryotic-like serine/threonine protein kinase G (PknG) that modulated the signal transduction pathways involved in the trafficking of host cell organelles (242) and thereby inhibited lysosome-phagosome fusion. Tetrahydrobenzothiophene specifically inhibited PknG and is a promising candidate for developing another class of antimicrobials to combat tuberculosis (242).

In mice, isocitrate lyase (ICL) is produced by inhibited mycobacteria within activated macrophages, but ICL is not produced in multiplying mycobacteria within nonactivated macrophages (163, 210). This lyase enables the bacillus to persist on the fatty acids released from lipids and thereby avoid being destroyed by the microbicidins of activated macrophages (reviewed in references 163 and 210). ICL is present in mycobacteria but not in mammalian hosts, and it is therefore a potential target for new antimicrobials.

Macrophage defenses include the formation of reactive nitrogen intermediates (RNIs) and reactive oxygen intermediates to which *M. tuberculosis* is exquisitely susceptible (43a, 143a). In mice, chemical inhibition of NOS or deletion of the NOS gene exacerbates tuberculosis (153, 153a, 211, 212). The proteasomes of the tubercle bacillus are also involved in its resistance against host RNIs, possibly by activating transcription factors for bacillary genes that produce RNI resistance products (79, 189).

Innate Immunity and Its Relation to Acquired (Adaptive) Immunity

In innate immunity, the host recognizes substances that are present in the pathogen but not in the host itself (171a). Such foreign-substance recognition (also existing in invertebrates) is used in higher animals to upregulate the costimulatory molecules of antigen-presenting cells (APCs). These costimulatory molecules must be upregulated for the antigen-specific immune response of T lymphocytes to occur in vertebrates.

Most self-antigens do not upregulate costimulatory molecules on APCs. Therefore, autoimmune reactions are rare. Not only are there costimulatory surface molecules but also there are coinhibitory surface molecules that control and limit the specific immune response. Coinhibition to self-antigens seems to be defective in some autoimmune diseases. The intricacies of APC, T-cell, and B-cell interactions have been clearly presented by Matzinger (161).

In acquired immunity, APCs first recognize lipopolysaccharides and other specific microbial products by means of innate receptors (171a). Then, the APCs upregulate their B7 costimulatory factors and their MHC class I and class II surface molecules. Both B7s and MHCs are needed for the APCs to present antigens to T cells. The T-cell ligand CD28 binds to B7, and the antigen-specific α/β T-cell receptor binds to the antigen-MHC complex. These T cells then become activated and clonally expand, producing the antigen-specific immunity found in vertebrates. The activated T cells also secrete various cytokines (see below) and express other surface molecules, e.g., ligands for CD40, a major costimulatory molecule, and ligands for Fas, a major cell surface death receptor.

A major cytokine activating the innate immune pathway of host resistance is the IL-12 produced by macrophages and DCs stimulated by microbial products. IL-12 activates both natural killer (NK) cells and Th1 lymphocytes. Subsequently, IL-12 induces IL-10 production in lymphocytes and phagocytes, and the IL-10, in turn, inhibits or regulates IL-12 production (232). IL-10 also activates Th2 lymphocytes. Patients infected with HIV are often deficient in their ability to produce IL-12, and this deficiency seems to play a role in the susceptibility of these patients to tuberculosis (232).

APCs and the MHC

The main APCs for T cells are the DCs (Table 5) (12, 14, 165a, 171a, 224) located in the marginal zones of lymph nodes. They are produced in the bone marrow, reside in various tissues, and mature by a two-step process: initially for antigen processing and subsequently for T-cell stimulation. The main APCs for B cells are the DCs in the lymphoid follicles. Macrophages, B cells, and other cells (222) can also present antigens, but they do so less effectively than DCs.

DC subsets determine the type and the extent of the acquired (adaptive) immune response. The differentiation of immature DCs into a particular subset is influenced by the organ in which the infectious agent resides (161).

DCs circulate in the blood and are recruited to sites of inflammation (36), such as tuberculous lesions. Not only do DCs initiate and enhance the immune response but also "tolerogenic" DCs exist that turn off or suppress the immune response (225).

APCs present antigens to most T cells as specific peptides in the context of the MHC, which means that a given T cell will recognize the antigen only when its peptide fragments are bound to a self-MHC molecule. In general, MHC class I molecules present peptides (generated in the APC cytosol) to (cytotoxic) CD8 T cells, and MHC class II molecules present peptides (from proteins degraded in APC endosomes) to (helper) CD4 T cells. (CD stands for clusters of differentiation, specifically cell surface molecules recognized by monoclonal antibodies with the designated number.) The MHC class I molecules can react with stimulatory as well as inhibitory receptors on T cells. Thus, the immune response is carefully controlled.

MHCs differ from person to person. Therefore, the responses to various antigens also differ from person to person, in part depending on the affinity of a person's own MHC molecules for each antigenic peptide. Thus, some people will produce a strong immune response to the antigens of the tubercle bacillus, and other people will produce a weaker response.

Mycolic acid and lipoarabinomannan are cell wall components of the tubercle bacillus. Such lipid and glycolipid antigens have also been found to be presented to T cells in association with CD1 surface molecules (19, 116, 192, 194) rather than in association with MHC class I and II molecules. CD1-restricted T cells appear to play an important role in the control of many microbial infections, especially those caused by the tubercle bacillus (20, 116, 165a, 170, 193, 194). Such CD1-restricted T cells can lyse macrophages infected with virulent *M. tuberculosis* (116). These CD1 T cells also produce high levels of IFN-γ (116), a major Th1 cytokine that activates macrophages, so that they can destroy or inhibit the growth of tubercle bacilli (81, 173).

In humans infected with *M. tuberculosis*, circulating CD8 T cells have been identified that are classically restricted (MHC class Ia) (139, 238) and also nonclassically restricted (group 1 CD1) (209) and HLA-E (HLA Ib) (106).

Lymphocytes: T Cells, B Cells, CD4 Cells, CD8 Cells, and γ/δ T Cells

Overview

Lymphocytes provide the immunological specificity for the host's CMI and DTH responses to tubercle bacilli. Lymphocyte "memory" is synonymous with an expanded specific lymphocyte population that enables (because of their increased number) a rapid recall of local CMI and DTH at sites where

Table 5. Major cell types involved in specific and nonspecific host defense reactions against the tubercle bacillus[a]

Macrophages

Macrophages are the effector cells of the mononuclear phagocyte system. They are produced in the bone marrow, circulate as monocytes in the bloodstream, and are called macrophages when they emigrate from the blood into the tissues. Nonactivated monocytes/macrophages allow tubercle bacilli to multiply within them. Highly activated macrophages destroy or inhibit tubercle bacilli.

Lymphocytes (T cells and B cells)

T cells (from the thymus) and B cells (from the bone marrow in mammals or bursa in birds) provide immunological specificity to the host's defense against tubercle bacilli. In tuberculous lesions, antigen-activated T cells activate macrophages by producing cytokines.
T cells have been subdivided in a variety of ways based on (i) their surface markers (CD4 and CD8 T cells), (ii) their receptors (α/β, γ/δ, and CD1), (iii) the cytokines they produce (Th1, Th2, and Th17 cells), and (iv) their functions (helper, regulatory, inflammatory, and cytotoxic T cells).
Antigen-activated B cells produce antibodies, especially when they differentiate into plasma cells. In tuberculous lesions, antigen-antibody reactions hasten the local accumulation of DCs, macrophages, and antigen-specific T cells, i.e., antibodies enhance the local cell-mediated immune response.

APCs

DCs are the main APCs. DCs migrate from the site of infection to the draining lymph nodes, where they initiate the immune response by presenting antigens to the recirculating lymphocytes that had entered these nodes. DCs, macrophages, and B cells can also present antigens to lymphocytes within tuberculous lesions.

NK cells

NK cells, both local and circulating, are an important early defense against intracellular microorganisms (viruses, bacteria, fungi, and protozoa). In tuberculosis, NK cells can kill bacillus-laden macrophages and can produce IFN-γ, which activates macrophages and stimulates a Th1 cytokine immune response.

[a]Adapted from reference 78.

endogenous or exogenous tubercle bacilli infect the host. The major types of lymphocytes (listed in Table 5) are described in more detail in this section.

Lymphocytes originate in the bone marrow and follow two paths of differentiation (171a). T lymphocytes (usually called T cells) enter the thymus, where they develop their antigen-specific receptors (by DNA rearrangements and/or deletions). In contrast, B lymphocytes (usually called B cells) develop their antigen-specific receptors in the bone marrow. When exposed to the antigen for which they have a receptor, these T and B cells respond by clonal proliferation, greatly increasing their number.

T cells

In tuberculosis, T cells appear to have two main functions: (i) killing poorly activated macrophages in which the bacilli are multiplying and (ii) producing cytokines that activate macrophages so that these macrophages can now kill or inhibit ingested bacilli.

T cells can be divided into two subsets, Th1 and Th2, on the basis of the cytokines they produce, although some T cells show a mixed (i.e., heterogeneous) cytokine pattern (1). (Th1 and Th2 have also been called type 1 and type 2, respectively.) Th1 cells suppress Th2 cells, and Th2 cells suppress Th1 cells.

The Th1 subset produces IL-2 (which causes T-cell proliferation), as well as IFN-γ and TNF-β (both of which activate macrophages). IFN-γ downregulates

the Th2 response. The Th2 subset produces IL-4, IL-5, IL-6, IL-9, IL-10, and IL-13, which promote antibody production by B cells. IL-4, IL-10, and IL-13 downregulate the Th1 response.

Macrophages produce IL-12, a major Th1 cell activator, and later they produce IL-10, a major Th1 cell inhibitor. Th2 cells also seem to have a role in keeping the Th1 response from becoming excessive.

B cells

B cells produce antibodies, especially when they differentiate into plasma cells. Plasma cells are frequently found in tuberculous lesions. B cells (when activated) also increase the production of IFN-γ by NK cells (see next section). NK cells can kill antibody-coated, bacillus-laden macrophages by antibody-dependent cell-mediated cytotoxicity.

CD4 cells

MHC class II-restricted CD4 lymphocytes are key players in the immune response against tuberculosis, because they produce IFN-γ and other activating cytokines. HIV-infected persons with reduced CD4 cells have increased susceptibility to tuberculosis and a more severe form of the disease (43). In mice, the importance of CD4 cells was confirmed by depletion (with CD4-specific antibodies) (171), adoptive transfer (181, 182), and knockout procedures (40).

CD8 cells

The primary role of CD8 lymphocytes is cell-mediated cytotoxicity, but they also produce IFN-γ (which activates macrophages) (96, 123, 179). Mice deficient either in CD8 cells (221) or in MHC class I-restricted cells (204) are less able to control infection with *M. tuberculosis*. CD8 cells can kill infected cells by producing perforin, granzymes, and Fas ligand. Perforin punches holes in the cell membranes, and granzymes and Fas ligands cause apoptosis (55, 109). Cytotoxic CD8 lymphocytes can also be divided into Th1 and Th2 subsets on the basis of the cytokines they produce.

Additional information on the role of CD8 T cells in tuberculosis can be found in references 21, 45, 96, 98, and 216. See the section on APCs above for information on CD1-restricted CD8 cells.

$\gamma\delta$ T cells

$\gamma\delta$ T cells have receptors that are composed of $\gamma\delta$ chains rather than the usual $\alpha\beta$ chains (reviewed in reference 105). $\gamma\delta$ T cells seem to have a much wider influence on the host's response to microorganisms than was previously expected, because they affect functions of NK cells, B cells, and other T cells, in part by producing IFN-γ and other cytokines (29, 105).

$\gamma\delta$ T cells are activated before $\alpha\beta$ T cells and have been postulated to play an early role in host defense against tuberculosis (88, 133). At least some of the $\gamma\delta$ T cells have receptors that combine directly with intact antigens without the usual processing and presentation by DCs. $\gamma\delta$ T cells are present in high percentages in mucosal epithelium and play a role in bronchial sensitivity to antigens (1, 134). They recognize lipid antigens bound to CD1 (described above).

$\gamma\delta$ T cells expressing the Vγ2Vδ2 T-cell receptor are the majority of circulating $\gamma\delta$ T cells in humans and nonhuman primates (217) but are absent in mice (96, 123). Humans with active *M. tuberculosis* infection, or health care professionals recently exposed to patients with tuberculosis, have increased numbers of $\gamma\delta$ T cells in their blood (13, 41, 44, 101, 113, 140, 239).

NK Cells

NK cells (see Table 5) comprise 5 to 10% of the peripheral blood lymphocyte population. They proliferate in response to both macrophage- and T-cell-derived cytokines. NK cells have the morphology of large granular lymphocytes and are defined as cytotoxic cells that do not express surface CD3 or many other T-cell receptors but do express CD56.

NK cells have both MHC class I and non-MHC-requiring receptors, whereas the cytotoxic T (CD8) cells recognize only specific antigenic peptides in association with MHC class I molecules. In fact, engagement of NK-cell surface receptors with the MHC class I molecules of host cells usually turns off the lytic machinery of the NK cell. Cells infected by viruses and other intracellular microorganisms have reduced (or absent) MHC class I expression and will be lysed by NK cells, whereas healthy cells (expressing normal levels of MHC-I) will not be lysed. Since NK cells can kill infected host cells without prior sensitization, they are considered part of the innate immune system (195). In tuberculosis, NK cells are an early source of IFN-γ, which activates macrophages and enhances Th1 immunity.

NK T cells (really NK1.1 T cells) are CD4-negative and CD8-negative cells that have both $\alpha\beta$ T-cell receptors and CD1 T-cell receptors (171a). Since they mostly respond to lipid and glycolipid antigens, they probably play a role in the early host response to tubercle bacilli.

Only a few studies have been made on NK cells and mycobacteria. Human peripheral blood mononuclear cells (PBMC) kill more intracellular *M. tuberculosis* organisms when cocultured with NK cells (248). Also, human NK cells (stimulated in vitro with IL-12) activate macrophages to inhibit the intracellular growth of *M. avium* (28). In mice, NK cell depletion enhances the growth of *M. avium* (104).

Role of Antibodies in Tuberculosis

Antibodies have never been thought to play a significant role in the pathogenesis of tuberculosis, because the passive transfer of antibodies to uninfected animals had no observable effect on the course of a subsequent infection with tubercle bacilli (146, 197).

However, studies in our laboratory (218) suggest a role for antibodies that had not previously been considered. Namely, in hosts with strong CMI, an antigen-antibody reaction causes a more rapid infiltration of DTH- and CMI-producing cells into sites where tubercle bacilli are located. In other words, antibodies enhance the local cell-mediated host response (218).

Circulating antibodies to the various antigens of the tubercle bacillus exist in all tuberculin-positive individuals (57, 58, 132, 141), including BCG-vaccinated hosts and healthy persons with inapparent tuberculous lesions. Such antibodies rapidly combine with tubercle bacilli of exogenous (or endogenous) reinfection. The resulting antigen-antibody reaction produces chemotaxins (e.g., the C5a component of complement and probably chemokines). These chemotaxins rapidly bring circulating DCs, macrophages, and the expanded antigen-specific memory T-cell population to sites of bacillary lodgment.

The rapidity with which DTH and CMI are locally produced can prevent many developing microscopic tubercles from reaching clinically apparent size. In brief, antibodies are beneficial in tuberculosis whenever an expanded antigen-specific T-cell population exists.

Cytokines

Cytokines (94, 175, 210c, 240) are proteins made by cells that affect the behavior of other cells that are usually nearby in the tissues (171a). They can be considered local hormones and include chemokines, ILs, IFNs, and TNFs. IL-1 and TNF-α are often considered primary cytokines (130a, 131), because they tend to upregulate the production of other cytokines. Cytokines interact with each other: one concentration of a cytokine may stimulate, and a higher concentration of the same cytokine may suppress (69, 175).

Once secreted from cells, cytokines bind to the glycosaminoglycans in the extracellular matrix (155), which usually keeps the cytokines nearby. However, TNF-α is even carried to the draining lymph nodes bound to heparin-based particles produced by local mast cells. Cytokines have been mostly evaluated in the mouse model of tuberculosis, but a few cytokines have been evaluated in guinea pigs (151a) and rabbits (218, 227).

Kaplan and colleagues (25, 234, 235) have published a series of papers that underscore the critical importance of the balance of various cytokines in the control of tuberculosis in both rabbits and mice. They have developed a rabbit model of mycobacterial meningitis that resembles tuberculous meningitis in humans. The level of TNF in the cerebrospinal fluid was correlated with the severity of the disease and was probably due to the greater numbers of granulocytes and macrophages present.

Details on several of these cytokines follow. For a more thorough discussion of these and numerous other cytokines, see references 1, 171a, and 210c.

(i) Chemokines are chemotactic cytokines. MCP-1 is a chemokine that plays a major role in the formation of tuberculous lesions (210c, 218, 227). MCP-1 attracts macrophages and lymphocytes into sites where the tubercle bacilli are located (69).

(ii) IL-12 is a cytokine that is produced primarily by phagocytes, including DCs (165a, 210c), in response to ingested microorganisms (43a, 165a, 233). IL-12 activates both NK cells and Th1 lymphocytes, causing them to produce IFN-γ and TNF-β.

Therefore, IL-12 is a key cytokine in the cell-mediated immune response to tubercle bacilli. IL-12 is a covalent dimer of 35- and 40-kDa peptides (p35 and p40). Mice deficient in p40 are more susceptible to *M. tuberculosis* than those deficient in p35 (56). The administration of IL-12 to mice increases their survival time with this disease (99, 177). Supplemental IL-12 was also beneficial to one patient with *M. abscessus* and one patient with drug-resistant *M. tuberculosis* (103a, 110a).

(iii) Recently, IL-17 (produced by Th17 cells) has been shown to play an important early role during infections (171a). It stimulates local fibroblasts and epithelial cells to produce cytokines that recruit granulocytes and possibly macrophages into the site. Additional roles of IL-17 are briefly summarized in reference 250.

(iv) TNF-α is predominantly secreted by monocytes and tissue macrophages. It is a powerful inducer of the inflammatory response and plays a critical role in host resistance to tuberculosis (168, 201, 210c). TNF-α knockout mice, TNF-receptor knockout mice, and mice receiving anti-TNF antibody all had more severe disease (18, 97, 125), and TNF therapy was beneficial to mice infected with BCG (201a). Also, patients with rheumatoid arthritis or Crohn's disease who were treated with anti-TNF-α monoclonal antibodies showed a high incidence of reactivation tuberculosis and greater dissemination of the disease (124, 154). The cachexia found in advanced cases of human tuberculosis is at least partly due to systemic TNF-α (18).

(v) IFN-γ is secreted by CD4 and CD8 T cells as well as NK cells (135, 184, 210c, 243). IFN-γ knockout mice have impaired activation of macrophages with low levels of NOS. In these mice, bacillary growth is not contained, and rapid death occurred. Although IFN-γ reduced the infection in mice, it did not clear the infection. Humans with IFN-γ receptor defects have higher rates of atypical mycobacterial disease (42, 86). Because of the critical role of IFN-γ in host resistance, patients with multidrug-resistant tuberculosis have been treated with adjunctive IFN-γ by aerosol, with some benefit (52, 86).

Systemic Immunity

Greater numbers of T lymphocytes with specific receptors for the antigens of the tubercle bacillus are present in the blood and lymphoid tissues of individuals infected with virulent or avirulent tubercle bacilli than are present in the blood and tissues of individuals who have never been exposed to such bacilli. The clonal expansion of these antigen-specific T cells is the basis of the immunizing process. When these "immune" individuals are exposed to exogenous or endogenous tubercle bacilli, greater numbers of specific (and also nonspecific) T cells accumulate at sites where the bacilli are deposited. The large number of local T cells produces high concentrations of cytokines that accelerate the local accumulation and activation of macrophages, so that the bacillus is destroyed before it multiplies appreciably. The developing lesion usually remains small and heals rapidly. Such accelerated tubercle formation is the reason why small endogenous tubercles of hematogenous, lymphogenous, and bronchogenic origins do not usually progress in immunocompetent adult humans.

In brief, tuberculin-positive and disease-free individuals have an expanded antigen-specific T-cell population, as well as antigen-specific circulating antibodies (132). In these individuals, macrophages are activated locally at an accelerated rate at sites wherever exogenous or endogenous tubercle bacilli are deposited. These systemic manifestations of cellular immunity exist to enable local acquired (adaptive) resistance to occur at a higher rate (227). Systemic immunity has little or no effect on the disease until it does so.

M. tuberculosis Virulence Factors

This is the age of molecular microbiology in which the genomes of microorganisms are providing clues to their virulence, as well as guides for the development of new antimicrobial agents. The genomic sequence of M. tuberculosis is now known (32a), and this sequence enables the identification of every product that M. tuberculosis manufactures. The genome of M. tuberculosis transcribes two product categories: (i) those that maintain the life of the bacillus and allow it to reproduce wherever it thrives and (ii) those that enable it to withstand the innate and acquired (adaptive) defenses of the host. Here are a few examples of the latter category: (i) phthiocerol dimycocerosate, which makes the mycobacterial cell wall resistant to destruction by macrophages (172a); (ii) the early-secreted antigenic target 6-kDa protein (ESAT-6), produced by the RD1 gene region (35, 100a, 103b), which (among other functions) induces the recruitment of nonactivated macrophages in which intracellular bacillary growth readily occurs (240a) (the absence of ESAT-6 production contributes to the avirulence of both BCG [the widely used TB vaccine] and H37Ra [a common avirulent laboratory strain]); (iii) cell surface lipids that enable M. tuberculosis to survive within the phagosome and prevent its acidification and maturation (210a); and (iv) factors that enable the bacillus to survive in solid caseous necrosis in the guinea pig model of tuberculosis (1a, 54a, 115).

Antimicrobials that inhibit products that enable the survival and growth of M. tuberculosis anywhere may be effective against many other virulent microorganisms. However, antimicrobials that enable M. tuberculosis to withstand the innate and acquired (adaptive) defenses of the host are usually more specific for M. tuberculosis.

The genomic field is still in its infancy, and many more factors involved in host-parasite interactions will be discovered in the next few years.

Turnover of Macrophages in Tuberculous Lesions

Macrophages and lymphocytes have a continual turnover in the caseous tuberculous lesions. Numerous lymphocytes enter these lesions, and numerous lymphocytes die there (or leave via the lymphatics) (68).

After an intravenous injection of BCG, acquired (adaptive) cellular resistance decreases with time. Such resistance, however, can be rapidly recalled to full strength by reinjection of BCG. From the first exposure, the host retains increased numbers of (clonally expanded) T cells with specific receptors for these antigens. Upon reexposure to BCG antigens, these T cells rapidly produce cytokines, which cause local macrophage (and lymphocyte) accumulation and activation.

The injection of other types of facultative intracellular bacilli (e.g., listeriae or salmonellae) does not rapidly recall immunity to BCG (152). However, once macrophages have been activated in local sites by BCG (the specific antigen), these macrophages can nonspecifically destroy a variety of facultative intracellular microorganisms (in the same local sites). *The specificity of CMI resides entirely in the T lymphocyte, not in the macrophage. Macrophages kill facultative intracellular microorganisms only nonspecifically.*

The Mackaness group (152) administered the immunizing (and recalling) BCG intravenously. In this case, most of the bacilli were deposited in the liver and spleen, where many local sites containing activated macrophages developed. Such macrophages could readily destroy other types of facultative intracellular bacilli that were deposited in the liver and spleen by a subsequent intravenous injection.

The number of specific T cells in the blood and tissues decreases with time, and a positive tuberculin reaction may even disappear. These events may occur if the tubercle bacilli and their antigens have been eliminated from the host. Nonetheless, increased numbers of antigen-specific T cells still remain in the host, so upon reinfection, antigen-specific CMI and DTH (i.e., tuberculin sensitivity) are rapidly recalled.

Prognostic Significance of the Tuberculin Skin Test

The size of the dermal tuberculin reaction has little or no prognostic significance, either during the disease or after it is arrested. During the disease, a large reaction may signify a host of high native and acquired resistance to tuberculosis, because such resistant hosts are able to accumulate large numbers of lymphocytes and macrophages, both in tuberculous lesions and at the site of tuberculin injection. A large tuberculin reaction may also signify a host of low native and acquired resistance, because the lesions of such susceptible hosts contain numerous bacilli that provide a high dose of antigen for sensitization.

A large tuberculin reaction, remaining years after the primary disease has healed, probably signifies that a few dormant bacilli are still present in inapparent caseous foci. Such bacilli seem to be released from time to time and then are rapidly destroyed, which gives a booster effect to the whole immune system, including the level of tuberculin sensitivity.

Booster Effect of a Repeat Tuberculin Skin Test

Individuals who have recently been infected with the tubercle bacillus can, in time, become tuberculin negative with or without antimicrobial treatment. In many of these individuals, a recall of tuberculin sensitivity is produced by antigens in the tuberculin (PPD) that was just injected for skin testing. Therefore, when such an individual is retested again with intermediate-strength PPD, he or she who was negative 3 weeks earlier may now be tuberculin positive as a result of the booster effect of the tuberculin itself (51, 229). The previous injection of PPD expands the tuberculin-sensitive T-cell population (i.e., memory T cells) to a level where the number of these cells is now sufficient to produce a positive tuberculin test when a repeat skin test is performed. Details on this booster effect of tuberculin are reviewed in reference 166.

Clinicians should be aware of the booster effect, so that they do not assume that the conversion of the tuberculin skin test means a recently acquired active infection with *M. tuberculosis*.

Negative Tuberculin Test for Patients with Active Tuberculosis

Individuals who are clinically ill with this disease may have a negative tuberculin skin test. When they are recovering, however, they again develop a positive skin test. Compartmentalization could be the cause of this skin test anergy. The pulmonary tuberculous lesions may collect most of the antigen-specific circulating T cells, so that few are available to participate in the dermal tuberculin reaction. This concept receives support from the fact that lymphocytes from diseased tissues obtained by bronchoalveolar lavage, or from pleural exudates, contain a greater proportion of antigen-specific T cells, secrete greater quantities of cytokines, and show a greater tendency to proliferate (in the presence of specific antigens) than do the T lymphocytes in peripheral blood (16, 17, 203, 237).

Tuberculin-negative patients with active tuberculosis also have a greater number of suppressor monocytes and lymphocytes in their peripheral blood (89, 102, 108, 110, 162, 203, 230, 237). This fact, however, does not prove that T cells within tuberculous lesions are suppressed. In such lesions, the composition of the cell population is different from that present in peripheral blood, as indicated by the studies (just mentioned) of the cells in both blood and pleural fluids from patients with tuberculous pleurisy.

In peripheral blood of such patients, mononuclear cells produce transforming growth factor beta (TGF-β) and IL-10, which are (at least in part) responsible for the immunosuppressive effects on tuberculin sensitivity.

In summary, many patients with active tuberculosis have a negative PPD skin test. This immunosuppression was correlated with a decrease in the ability of their peripheral blood lymphocytes to undergo clonal expansion and to produce IFN-γ and IL-2 when these cells were cultured in vitro with PPD (90, 237). The suppressive effect is in part due to the production of TGF-β and IL-10 by circulating mononuclear cells.

Whether such studies on PBMC can predict the future course of the disease remains to be determined. At least during effective antimicrobial therapy, the return of a positive PPD skin test and the return of increased PPD-induced peripheral blood lymphocyte blastogenesis and IFN-γ production are good prognostic signs (90).

Improved Diagnostic Tests for Active Tuberculosis

The tuberculin skin test cannot reliably differentiate between (i) DTH from a progressive tuberculous lesion and (ii) DTH from environmental mycobacteria or BCG vaccination or a nonprogressive arrested lesion. Since ESAT-6 is produced by virulent human-type tubercle bacilli and not by BCG or by many environmental mycobacteria, an in vitro diagnostic test on human PBMC was developed and evaluated in Ethiopia (80, 196). This test measures the amount of IFN-γ produced by PBMC after 5 days in culture and stimulation with ESAT-6.

At the beginning of this study, the amount of IFN-γ produced by PBMC from tuberculin-positive

household contacts of active (sputum-positive) tuberculous persons was determined (84). Two years
later these contacts were evaluated for clinically active tuberculosis. The household contacts who developed clinically active tuberculosis in 2 years were
those whose PBMC originally produced high levels
of IFN-γ, whereas those contacts whose PBMC originally produced low levels of IFN-γ remained healthy.
Parallel studies with tuberculin (PPD) as the in vitro antigen showed no difference between these two
groups. Evidently, the contacts with early progressive tuberculosis could be identified by an increase
in the number of circulating lymphocytes capable of
responding to ESAT-6.

This was the first study in which a laboratory test
could distinguish tuberculin-positive persons with
progressive early tuberculous lesions (who should be
treated with antimicrobials) from persons with nonprogressive lesions (who would not need antimicrobial therapy). If further studies confirm these results,
the ESAT-6 in vitro test would be a major addition to
the control of this disease.

Details on the QuantiFERON and similar TB
tests are presented in chapter 5.

Effect of Vaccines on Establishment of Pulmonary Tuberculous Lesions

Vaccination cannot prevent the establishment of
an infection with the tubercle bacillus (228). It can
only prevent progression of the disease after a microscopic tubercle is established. In vaccinated (usually
tuberculin-positive) individuals, the inhaled virulent
tubercle bacillus is ingested by an AM. These highly
activated cells usually destroy the inhaled tubercle
bacillus before it has a chance to multiply in both
vaccinated and nonvaccinated individuals. One or
two years after vaccination with BCG, all but a small
residual of the BCG has been eliminated. At that time,
one would expect both the vaccinated and nonvaccinated individuals to show no difference in the number
of AM or in their microbicidal abilities. Therefore,
both the vaccinated and nonvaccinated hosts would
initially destroy the same number of inhaled virulent
bacilli, or initially allow the same number to multiply.

When first inhaled, a bacillary unit of one to
three bacilli (which is the only quantity that can stay
suspended in the airstream long enough to reach the
alveolar spaces) contains insufficient antigen to stimulate the immune system. However, once this bacillary
unit begins to multiply, sufficient antigen is present
to be recognized by lymphocytes. From this point
on, the vaccinated and the nonvaccinated individuals
show different responses. In the vaccinated hosts an
accelerated tubercle formation occurs; i.e., there is a

rapid local accumulation of lymphocytes and macrophages and a rapid activation of these cells. This
accelerated immune response often arrests the early
focus of infection, thereby preventing its development
into clinical disease (66, 71). In the nonvaccinated
hosts, lymphocyte and macrophage activation develops at a much slower pace, so clinical disease occurs
more frequently.

Small arrested tuberculous lesions of humans
and rabbits have different characteristics. Humans
are so sensitive to the tuberculin products of the bacillus that even microscopic tuberculous lesions soon
caseate. In practically all tuberculin-positive humans
(without clinically apparent disease), a calcified arrested caseous lesion (usually 0.5 to 1.0 mm) can be
found at necropsy many years later (228).

The tuberculin sensitivity of rabbits is much
lower than the tuberculin sensitivity of humans.
Therefore, in rabbits, following the inhalation of virulent human-type tubercle bacilli, many microscopic
tuberculous lesions resolve without caseation (or calcification) and become undetectable at a later time.
However, in both humans (228) and rabbits (63, 66,
71, 146, 149), BCG vaccination reduces the progress
of tuberculous lesions once they are established.

Development of Better Vaccines for Tuberculosis (see chapter 10)

The challenge to researchers engaged in vaccine
development for tuberculosis is to find (i) antigens
that are *more potent* than BCG in producing T-cell
populations that activate macrophages to destroy
the bacillus (CMI) and (ii) antigens that are *less potent* than BCG in producing T-cell populations that
cause caseous necrosis and liquefaction (70), which
we define "pathologically" as tissue-damaging DTH.
In other words, a vaccine is needed that produces a
higher "CMI/tissue-damaging DTH ratio" than do
currently available BCG vaccines.

Both CMI and DTH are immunological processes produced by T lymphocytes with specific receptors for the various antigens of the tubercle bacillus.
These specific T cells attract macrophages and other
lymphocytes to sites of antigen deposition. There, the
macrophages and T lymphocytes activate each other,
as well as other members of their own cell type.

In rabbits, guinea pigs, and humans, some tissue
necrosis (DTH) is apparently necessary to stop the
logarithmic growth of tubercle bacilli within nonactivated macrophages. Would, therefore, vaccines that
produce reduced tuberculin sensitivity be just as effective as other vaccines? The answer seems to be yes.

In the British Medical Research Council trials, one lot of vole bacillus vaccine produced a high

incidence of tuberculin positivity and another lot did not. Yet, the two lots showed equally high protective potencies against tuberculosis (49). This and other studies with different strains of BCG (93) clearly demonstrate that the antigens causing strong tuberculin positivity were not required to protect humans.

When applied to the pathogenesis of tuberculosis, these findings indicate that the killing of non-activated macrophages (in which the bacilli grow intracellularly in a logarithmic fashion) is due not only to tuberculin-like antigens. It can apparently be produced by a DTH response to other antigens of the bacillus when these antigens reach the appropriate concentration. In fact, in the mouse model, lymphocytes transferring protective immunity can be dissociated from those that transfer tuberculin sensitivity (182).

A vaccine superior to present strains of BCG would be one that produces strong CMI with little or no sensitivity to tuberculin. Favorable antigenic fractions of the tubercle bacillus (probably certain proteins complexed with certain carbohydrates and lipids) would stimulate CMI with minimal tissue-damaging DTH, whereas detrimental antigens (probably the tuberculoproteins that produce the tuberculin reaction) would produce more tissue-damaging DTH (caseation and liquefaction) with less CMI.

Tuberculoproteins that cause the tuberculin reaction have never been shown to be protective (56a, 146, 197a). In fact, they can produce severe necrosis in the tuberculin-positive host if their concentration exceeds that which is safe for a given host (199). Other fractions may be effective immunogens without producing tuberculin sensitivity. These principles, however, still remain to be established. The roles of the carbohydrate fractions of these bacilli and of the proteins secreted by living tubercle bacilli need further investigation (213a).

Additional insight has recently been gained into the adjuvanticity of tuberculosis vaccines (227). In dermal BCG lesions, the percentage of mononuclear cells containing cytokine (especially chemokine) mRNA and protein was highest during the first 3 days. This finding suggests that the most effective tuberculosis vaccines would contain not only the most appropriate mycobacterial antigens but also mycobacterial adjuvants that recruit the largest number of macrophages, lymphocytes, and DCs into local sites of antigen deposition.

It is possible that recombinant BCG vaccines will be better than existing BCG vaccines (5, 32, 48, 71, 112, 112a, 180). To produce such vaccines, the DNAs for additional antigens are added to the BCG genome. These antigens may increase the virulence of the BCG, so careful evaluation in animal models should be performed before human trials are begun.

DNA vaccines are those in which the DNAs of one or more mycobacterial antigens are incorporated into a plasmid and usually injected intramuscularly. Such DNA vaccines increased the immunity of mice and guinea pigs to virulent tubercle bacilli, but not more than did BCG, and the immunity produced was shorter lived (reviewed in references 5 and 32). DNA vaccines or vaccines incorporating mycobacterial protein, lipid, and/or glycolipid antigens (in adjuvants) may be useful in HIV patients, because these nonviable vaccines cannot cause tuberculosis in immunosuppressed individuals.

A substantial percentage of the world's human population is already tuberculin positive from inhaling virulent tubercle bacilli. Therefore, postinfection immunization to prevent endogenous (and exogenous) reinfection would be especially useful. Subunit vaccines are probably the safest type to use for this purpose (reviewed in references 32 and 48).

Finally, combination vaccines which consist of BCG and one or more booster immunizations with important mycobacterial antigens (including those produced by DNA vaccines [145]) will probably provide the most effective protection against active disease (5, 6, 32, 34, 48, 71, 112a). The antigens in such boosters would expand the appropriate T-lymphocyte population almost as well as if these antigens had been incorporated into the live vaccine itself. They would, however, probably require one or more repeat injections.

Because BCG tends to persist in the host for many years, recombinant BCG vaccines containing specific antigens from various viral, bacterial, and parasitic microorganisms are being evaluated (179a).

References 5, 6, 32, 48, 122, 183, 208, and 249 and chapter 10 review some of the newly developed vaccines for tuberculosis.

All new tuberculosis vaccines should first be evaluated in all common laboratory animals, because each species responds to each antigen in its own specific manner (71). Mice respond poorly to the *M. tuberculosis* antigens in vaccines that elicit DTH but respond well to the *M. tuberculosis* antigens that elicit CMI, and they eventually die of the disease. Guinea pigs respond well to the *M. tuberculosis* antigens in vaccines that elicit DTH but respond poorly to the *M. tuberculosis* antigens that elicit CMI, and they eventually die of the disease. However, rabbits and humans respond well to both DTH and CMI antigens and usually control infection with *M. tuberculosis*. Because of these animal differences in the response to various *M. tuberculosis* antigens, new vaccines in only one laboratory animal species might miss some antigens that are important in immunizing human populations. Therefore, all three animal models (and perhaps monkeys) should always be used in the preclinical testing of candidate tuberculosis vaccines (71).

Advantages of Vaccines Containing Little or No Tuberculin-Like Antigens

There are many benefits in eliminating tuberculin-like antigens from BCG (Table 6) (63). (i) Vaccinated individuals would not be appreciably tuberculin positive, so tuberculin testing of such persons would still be a useful procedure for diagnosing infection with virulent tubercle bacilli.

ESAT-6 and culture filtrate protein 10 (CFP-10) antigens are not present in BCG (6, 7). In vitro IFN-γ production by peripheral blood leukocytes stimulated with ESAT-6 and CFP-10 identifies individuals who are tuberculin positive due to BCG and individuals who are tuberculin positive from virulent tubercle bacilli. The use of these antigens to enhance immunity to tuberculosis is currently being investigated (6, 7).

(ii) Such a vaccine could even be given to tuberculin-positive individuals with less harm, and probably with true benefit. It would expand the T-cell population responding to protective antigens of the tubercle bacillus and not expand the T-cell population responding to antigens in tuberculin that are often detrimental. Thus, existing latent (or even active) foci of tuberculosis would be less apt to progress, because these foci would become surrounded by a population rich in beneficial T cells and macrophages.

(iii) Because it produces little or no DTH, a vaccine without tuberculin-like antigens could be given more than once to create high levels of immunity (especially in high-risk groups).

(iv) When available, such a vaccine might replace isoniazid (INH) in preventive therapy of persons who recently became tuberculin positive. Substituting such a vaccine for INH would eliminate the danger of INH hepatotoxicity and INH bacillary resistance.

Table 6. Advantages of tuberculosis vaccines producing strong CMI and weak tissue-damaging DTH (especially those producing little or no tuberculin sensitivity)

To prevent clinical tuberculosis (prophylaxis)
To treat clinical tuberculosis (immunotherapy)
To vaccinate PPD-positive persons without possible harm
To further enhance immunity by repeated vaccinations (not advised with current BCG vaccines)

*Adapted from reference 63. Reprinted with permission from Elsevier.

Tuberculosis Vaccines and Immunity to Critical Antigens

Critical antigens are the antigens of the major factors that enable *M. tuberculosis* to survive in the host (71). Unfortunately, the use of critical antigens for both prophylactic immunization and immunotherapy is still in developmental stages (reviewed in references 6, 7, 83a, 112a, 208, and 208a).

Prophylactically, vaccines containing critical antigens would expand the corresponding Th1 lymphocyte population, so during a subsequent exposure to virulent *M. tuberculosis*, this Th1 population would be increased even further, even though the infecting virulent strain contained only small amounts of such critical antigens. Therefore, prophylactic vaccination with critical antigens would increase host resistance above that produced during an active TB infection in unvaccinated individuals. Immunotherapy with critical antigens in patients who already have active tuberculosis would have similar beneficial effects, because these antigens are so necessary for *M. tuberculosis* survival in the host.

The effects of primary vaccination with live attenuated tubercle bacilli (often BCG) followed by a booster vaccination with critical antigens months or years later are currently being evaluated (see chapter 10). This two-step vaccination regimen is most promising, because it combines the multiple antigens of intact viable tubercle bacilli with the critical antigens that are found to have the greatest effect on host resistance.

Modified vaccinia virus Ankara expressing the immunodominant secreted antigen 85A (MVA85A) is already in clinical trials as a booster for persons who had a positive tuberculin skin test from BCG or a naturally acquired (arrested or latent) tuberculosis infection (83a, 163a, 163b, 210b). It is too soon to know whether individuals receiving an MVA85A booster vaccination will develop less clinical tuberculosis than BCG-vaccinated individuals who did not receive the booster.

ESAT-6, CFP-10, recombinant fusion protein Mtb72F, and others listed in references 6, 7, and 103c might be promising critical antigens to boost the host's immune response (208a). To date, however, ESAT-6 and CFP-10 have mainly been used with human PBMC (i) to diagnose latent and active tuberculosis and (ii) to assess the immune response to new tuberculosis vaccines (83a, 163a, 163b, 210b).

With the genome of *M. tuberculosis* now known, many possible critical antigens should soon become available for testing (discussed in reference 180a). Some of these *M. tuberculosis* antigens may be more effective (or critical) than others in controlling the growth of the tubercle bacillus. The best tuberculosis vaccine would enhance those critical antigens the most. The addition of pulmonary tubercle counting in rabbits to the current methods of antigen selection for tuberculosis vaccines should make such selections more precise (71).

PART III: CONCLUSIONS

1. In humans beings, most pulmonary AM are nonspecifically activated to a high degree. Such activated macrophages soon ingest and kill inhaled tubercle bacilli and prevent them from infecting the host. This is the most common situation, and the tuberculin skin test remains negative.

2. However, if the inhaled bacillus is ingested by a poorly activated AM, it multiplies and eventually kills that macrophage. Then, most of the released bacilli are ingested by nonactivated macrophages (from the bloodstream) within which the bacillus multiplies logarithmically. In this case, a small tubercle is formed, and the tuberculin skin test becomes positive.

3. Tissue-damaging DTH (to the antigens of the bacilli) is the main mechanism by which the host stops the bacillary growth in these nonactivated macrophages. DTH does so by killing these macrophages and nearby tissues. Tubercle bacilli do not multiply appreciably in the resulting (solid) caseous necrotic tissue.

4. If tubercle bacilli frequently escape from the edge of the caseous focus, nonactivated macrophages may ingest them and allow the bacilli to multiply intracellularly. Then, DTH will kill these macrophages and nearby tissues. The released bacilli can enter the bloodstream and may form progressing lesions throughout the body. This is the childhood-type miliary tuberculosis that often kills the host.

5. However, simultaneously with DTH, CMI develops. CMI activates the macrophages that surround the caseous center. These activated macrophages can ingest and destroy tubercle bacilli, thereby stopping the progression of the disease. (CMI is caused by an expanded antigen-specific T-lymphocyte population that produces macrophage-activating cytokines.) Therefore, continued destruction of host tissue will no longer occur, because the bacilli now reside in highly activated macrophages that prevent bacillary growth and arrest the disease.

6. Finally, if the solid caseous tissue liquefies, the tubercle bacilli can multiply extracellularly (for the first time during the course of the disease), sometimes reaching tremendous numbers. Such large numbers cannot be killed or inhibited, even in a highly immune host. Due to the presence of tissue-damaging DTH, the bacilli and/or their tuberculin-like products erode a bronchial wall and form a cavity. The bacilli can then spread throughout the airways to other parts of the lung and to the outside environment. Also, antimicrobial-resistant mutants may arise among the numerous actively growing bacilli.

7. If developed, recombinant BCG strains that produce high CMI with little or no sensitivity to tuberculin could be more effective than currently available BCG strains. Such a BCG vaccine would expand the T-cell population capable of producing CMI with less expansion of the T-cell population capable of producing DTH (caseous necrosis). Lesions caused by virulent bacilli in such vaccinated hosts would therefore contain more T cells (from the memory population) that cause activated macrophages (CMI) and relatively few tuberculin-reactive T cells that cause tissue necrosis (and liquefaction) with little CMI. The same result could be accomplished by giving (some time after an initial BCG immunization) booster immunizations with antigens, such as ESAT-6 and/or CFP-10, which cause CMI but do not cause tuberculin sensitivity.

8. Therapeutic drugs that reduce the amount of liquefaction would be of considerable help in the treatment of tuberculosis and in limiting the spread of this disease to other persons. Yet, to our knowledge, little or no research to develop such drugs is currently underway. We recently proposed a simple method to recognize potential antiliquefaction drugs, namely, to measure the reduction in the liquefaction and ulceration produced by live or dead tubercle bacilli in the skin of rabbits (70).

9. The pathogenesis of tuberculosis (Part I) with respect to the bacillary multiplication is summarized in Table 7.

10. The major research advances in immunology that have direct bearing on the pathogenesis of tuberculosis are described in Part II. They include interactions between innate immunity and acquired immunity, interactions among the cytokines, and up-regulating and downregulating mechanisms of both inflammatory and immune responses.

Table 7. Multiplication of tubercle bacilli and the host immune response

No multiplication of bacilli: no disease, no CMI, no DTH

Bacilli dormant in caseous focus: arrested disease; strong CMI; strong, weak, or nearly absent DTH

Intracellular multiplication of bacilli: caseous foci, hematogenous spread, weak CMI, often strong DTH

Extracellular multiplication of bacilli: cavity formation, bronchial spread, caseous bronchopneumonia, strong CMI (sometimes overwhelmed by the large number of bacilli), usually strong DTH

Acknowledgments. Many of these principles of the pathogenesis of tuberculosis were established by Max B. Lurie, with whom A.M.D. spent 12 years at the University of Pennsylvania. Dr. Lurie's insight into the mechanisms of this disease was both penetrating and comprehensive.

The help of Lori Rosman and Ivy L. Garner at our Welch Library in formatting the manuscript is greatly appreciated. Figures 1, 3, and 4 were drawn by Roberta R. Proctor and Lester J. Dyer, and Fig. 11 was drawn by Joseph M. Dieter, Jr. Figure 10 was provided by Bingdong Zhu of Lanzhou University, Lanzhou, China, and Ying Zhang of The Johns Hopkins University, Baltimore, MD.

REFERENCES

1. **Abbas, A. K., and A. H. Lichtman.** 2008. *Basic Immunology: Functions and Disorders of the Immune System*, 3rd ed. Saunders/Elsevier, Philadelphia, PA.

1a. **Abdul-Majid, K.-B., L. H. Ly, P. J. Converse, D. E. Geiman, D. N. McMurray, and W. R. Bishai.** 2008. Altered cellular infiltration and cytokine levels during early *Mycobacterium tuberculosis sigC* mutant infection are associated with late-stage disease attenuation and milder immunopathology in mice. *BMC Microbiology* **8:**151.

1b. **Abe, Y., K. Sugisaki, and A. M. Dannenberg, Jr.** 1996. Rabbit vascular endothelial adhesion molecules: ELAM-1 is most elevated in acute inflammation, whereas VCAM-1 and ICAM-1 predominate in chronic inflammation. *J. Leukoc. Biol.* **60:**692–703.

2. **Abel, B., N. Thieblemont, V. J. Quesniaux, N. Brown, J. Mpagi, K. Miyake, F. Bihl, and B. Ryffel.** 2002. Toll-like receptor 4 expression is required to control chronic *Mycobacterium tuberculosis* infection in mice. *J. Immunol.* **169:**3155–3162.

3. **Abou-Zeid, C., I. Smith, J. M. Grange, T. L. Ratliff, J. Steele, and G. A. Rook.** 1988. The secreted antigens of *Mycobacterium tuberculosis* and their relationship to those recognized by the available antibodies. *J. Gen. Microbiol.* **134:**531–538.

4. **Allison, M. J., P. Zappasodi, and M. P. Lurie.** 1962. Host-parasite relationships in natively resistant and susceptible rabbits on quantitative inhalation of tubercle bacilli. Their significance for the nature of genetic resistance. *Am. Rev. Respir. Dis.* **85:**553–569.

5. **Andersen, P.** 2001. TB vaccines: progress and problems. *Trends Immunol.* **22:**160–168.

6. **Andersen, P.** 2007. Tuberculosis vaccines—an update. *Nat. Rev. Microbiol.* **5:**484–487.

7. **Andersen, P.** 2007. Vaccine strategies against latent tuberculosis infection. *Trends Microbiol.* **15:**7–13.

8. **Andersen, P., D. Askgaard, L. Ljungqvist, J. Bennedsen, and I. Heron.** 1991. Proteins released from *Mycobacterium tuberculosis* during growth. *Infect. Immun.* **59:**1905–1910.

9. **Ando, M., A. M. Dannenberg, Jr., M. Sugimoto, and B. S. Tepper.** 1977. Histochemical studies relating the activation of macrophages to the intracellular destruction of tubercle bacilli. *Am. J. Pathol.* **86:**623–634.

10. **Ando, M.** 1973. Macrophage activation in tuberculin reactions of rabbits with primary BCG infection and reinfection. *J. Reticuloendothel. Soc.* **14:**132–145.

11. **Armstrong, J. A., and P. D. Hart.** 1971. Response of cultured macrophages to *Mycobacterium tuberculosis*, with observations on fusion of lysosomes with phagosomes. *J. Exp. Med.* **134:**713–740.

12. **Austyn, J. M.** 1996. New insights into the mobilization and phagocytic activity of dendritic cells. *J. Exp. Med.* **183:**1287–1292.

13. **Balbi, B., M. T. Valle, S. Oddera, D. Giunti, F. Manca, G. A. Rossi, and L. Allegra.** 1993. T-lymphocytes with gamma delta+ V delta 2+ antigen receptors are present in increased proportions in a fraction of patients with tuberculosis or with sarcoidosis. *Am. Rev. Respir. Dis.* **148:**1685–1690.

14. **Banchereau, J., and R. M. Steinman.** 1998. Dendritic cells and the control of immunity. *Nature* **392:**245–252.

15. **Barnes, P. F., A. B. Bloch, P. T. Davidson, and D. E. Snider, Jr.** 1991. Tuberculosis in patients with human immunodeficiency virus infection. *N. Engl. J. Med.* **324:**1644–1650.

16. **Barnes, P. F., S. J. Fong, P. J. Brennan, P. E. Twomey, A. Mazumder, and R. L. Modlin.** 1990. Local production of tumor necrosis factor and IFN-gamma in tuberculous pleuritis. *J. Immunol.* **145:**149–154.

17. **Barnes, P. F., S. D. Mistry, C. L. Cooper, C. Pirmez, T. H. Rea, and R. L. Modlin.** 1989. Compartmentalization of a CD4+ T lymphocyte subpopulation in tuberculous pleuritis. *J. Immunol.* **142:**1114–1119.

18. **Bean, A. G., D. R. Roach, H. Briscoe, M. P. France, H. Korner, J. D. Sedgwick, and W. J. Britton.** 1999. Structural deficiencies in granuloma formation in TNF gene-targeted mice underlie the heightened susceptibility to aerosol *Mycobacterium tuberculosis* infection, which is not compensated for by lymphotoxin. *J. Immunol.* **162:**3504–3511.

19. **Beckman, E. M., and M. B. Brenner.** 1995. MHC class I-like, class II-like and CD1 molecules: distinct roles in immunity. *Immunol. Today* **16:**349–352.

20. **Beckman, E. M., A. Melian, S. M. Behar, P. A. Sieling, D. Chatterjee, S. T. Furlong, R. Matsumoto, J. P. Rosat, R. L. Modlin, and S. A. Porcelli.** 1996. CD1c restricts responses of mycobacteria-specific T cells. Evidence for antigen presentation by a second member of the human CD1 family. *J. Immunol.* **157:**2795–2803.

21. **Behar, S. M., C. C. Dascher, M. J. Grusby, C. R. Wang, and M. B. Brenner.** 1999. Susceptibility of mice deficient in CD1D or TAP1 to infection with *Mycobacterium tuberculosis. J. Exp. Med.* **189:**1973–1980.

22. **Behr, M. A., and P. M. Small.** 1997. Has BCG attenuated to impotence? *Nature* **389:**133–134.

23. **Behr, M. A., and P. M. Small.** 1999. A historical and molecular phylogeny of BCG strains. *Vaccine* **17:**915–922.

24. **Behr, M. A., M. A. Wilson, W. P. Gill, H. Salamon, G. K. Schoolnik, S. Rane, and P. M. Small.** 1999. Comparative genomics of BCG vaccines by whole-genome DNA microarray. *Science* **284:**1520–1523.

25. **Bekker, L. G., A. L. Moreira, A. Bergtold, S. Freeman, B. Ryffel, and G. Kaplan.** 2000. Immunopathologic effects of tumor necrosis factor alpha in murine mycobacterial infection are dose dependent. *Infect. Immun.* **68:**6954–6961.

26. **Bellamy, R., C. Ruwende, T. Corrah, K. P. McAdam, M. Thursz, H. C. Whittle, and A. V. Hill.** 1999. Tuberculosis and chronic hepatitis B virus infection in Africans and variation in the vitamin D receptor gene. *J. Infect. Dis.* **179:**721–724.

27. **Bellamy, R., C. Ruwende, T. Corrah, K. P. McAdam, H. C. Whittle, and A. V. Hill.** 1998. Variations in the NRAMP1 gene and susceptibility to tuberculosis in West Africans. *N. Engl. J. Med.* **338:**640–644.

28. **Bermudez, L. E., M. Wu, and L. S. Young.** 1995. Interleukin-12-stimulated natural killer cells can activate human macrophages to inhibit growth of *Mycobacterium avium. Infect. Immun.* **63:**4099–4104.

29. **Boismenu, R., and W. L. Havran.** 1997. An innate view of gamma delta T cells. *Curr. Opin. Immunol.* **9:**57–63.

30. **Boom, W. H., R. S. Wallis, and K. A. Chervenak.** 1991. Human *Mycobacterium tuberculosis*-reactive CD4+ T-cell clones: heterogeneity in antigen recognition, cytokine production, and

cytotoxicity for mononuclear phagocytes. *Infect. Immun.* **59:** 2737–2743.

31. **Brightbill, H. D., D. H. Libraty, S. R. Krutzik, R. B. Yang, J. T. Belisle, J. R. Bleharski, M. Maitland, M. V. Norgard, S. E. Plevy, S. T. Smale, P. J. Brennan, B. R. Bloom, P. J. Godowski, and R. L. Modlin.** 1999. Host defense mechanisms triggered by microbial lipoproteins through Toll-like receptors. *Science* **285:**732–736.

32. **Britton, W. J., and U. Palendira.** 2003. Improving vaccines against tuberculosis. *Immunol. Cell Biol.* **81:**34–45.

32a.**Brodin, P., C. Demangel, and S. T. Cole.** 2005. Introduction to functional genomics of the *Mycobacterium tuberculosis* complex, p. 143–153. *In* S. T. Cole, K. D. Eisenach, D. N. McMurray, and W. R. Jacobs, Jr. (ed.), *Tuberculosis and the Tubercle Bacillus.* ASM Press, Washington, DC.

33. **Brodin, P., K. Eiglmeier, M. Marmiesse, A. Billault, T. Garnier, S. Niemann, S. T. Cole, and R. Brosch.** 2002. Bacterial artificial chromosome-based comparative genomic analysis identifies *Mycobacterium microti* as a natural ESAT-6 deletion mutant. *Infect. Immun.* **70:**5568–5578.

34. **Brooks, J. V., A. A. Frank, M. A. Keen, J. T. Bellisle, and I. M. Orme.** 2001. Boosting vaccine for tuberculosis. *Infect. Immun.* **69:**2714–2717.

35. **Brosch, R., S. V. Gordon, M. Marmiesse, P. Brodin, C. Buchrieser, K. Eiglmeier, T. Garnier, C. Gutierrez, G. Hewinson, K. Kremer, L. M. Parsons, A. S. Pym, S. Samper, D. van Soolingen, and S. T. Cole.** 2002. A new evolutionary scenario for the *Mycobacterium tuberculosis* complex. *Proc. Natl. Acad. Sci. USA* **99:**3684–3689.

36. **Brown, K. A., P. Bedford, M. Macey, D. A. McCarthy, F. Leroy, A. J. Vora, A. J. Stagg, D. C. Dumonde, and S. C. Knight.** 1997. Human blood dendritic cells: binding to vascular endothelium and expression of adhesion molecules. *Clin. Exp. Immunol.* **107:**601–607.

37. **Brozna, J. P., M. Horan, J. M. Rademacher, K. M. Pabst, and M. J. Pabst.** 1991. Monocyte responses to sulfatide from *Mycobacterium tuberculosis*: inhibition of priming for enhanced release of superoxide, associated with increased secretion of interleukin-1 and tumor necrosis factor alpha, and altered protein phosphorylation. *Infect. Immun.* **59:**2542–2548.

38. **Bryk, R., C. D. Lima, H. Erdjument-Bromage, P. Tempst, and C. Nathan.** 2002. Metabolic enzymes of mycobacteria linked to antioxidant defense by a thioredoxin-like protein. *Science* **295:**1073–1077.

39. **Canetti, G.** 1955. *The Tubercle Bacillus in the Pulmonary Lesion of Man: Histobacteriology and Its Bearing on the Therapy of Pulmonary Tuberculosis.* Springer Publishing Co., New York, NY.

40. **Caruso, A. M., N. Serbina, E. Klein, K. Triebold, B. R. Bloom, and J. L. Flynn.** 1999. Mice deficient in CD4 T cells have only transiently diminished levels of IFN-gamma, yet succumb to tuberculosis. *J. Immunol.* **162:**5407–5416.

41. **Carvalho, A. C., A. Matteelli, P. Airo, S. Tedoldi, C. Casalini, L. Imberti, G. P. Cadeo, A. Beltrame, and G. Carosi.** 2002. γδ T lymphocytes in the peripheral blood of patients with tuberculosis with and without HIV co-infection. *Thorax* **57:**357–360.

42. **Casanova, J. L., and L. Abel.** 2002. Genetic dissection of immunity to mycobacteria: the human model. *Annu. Rev. Immunol.* **20:**581–620.

42a.**Centers for Disease Control and Prevention.** 2005. Guidelines for preventing the transmission of *Mycobacterium tuberculosis* in health-care settings. *MMWR Morb. Mortal. Wkly. Rep.* **54**(RR-17):1–147.

43. **Chaisson, R. E., and G. Slutkin.** 1989. Tuberculosis and human immunodeficiency virus infection. *J. Infect. Dis.* **159:**96–100.

43a.**Chan, J., R. F. Silver, B. Kampmann, and R. S. Wallis.** 2005. Guidelines for preventing the transmission of *Mycobacterium tuberculosis* infection, p. 437–449. *In* S. T. Cole, K. D. Eisenach, D. N. McMurray, and W. R. Jacobs, Jr. (ed.), *Tuberculosis and the Tubercle Bacillus.* ASM Press, Washington, DC.

44. **Chen, Z. W., and N. L. Letvin.** 2003. Vγ2-Vδ2+ T cells and anti-microbial immune responses. *Microbes Infect.* **5:**491–498.

45. **Cho, S., V. Mehra, S. Thoma-Uszynski, S. Stenger, N. Serbina, R. J. Mazzaccaro, J. L. Flynn, P. F. Barnes, S. Southwood, E. Celis, B. R. Bloom, R. L. Modlin, and A. Sette.** 2000. Antimicrobial activity of MHC class I-restricted CD8+ T cells in human tuberculosis. *Proc. Natl. Acad. Sci. USA* **97:**12210–12215.

46. **Cole, S. T., K. D. Eisenach, D. N. McMurray, and W. R. Jacobs, Jr. (ed.).** 2005. *Tuberculosis and the Tubercle Bacillus.* ASM Press, Washington, DC.

47. **Collins, F. M., and S. G. Campbell.** 1982. Immunity to intracellular bacteria. *Vet. Immunol. Immunopathol.* **3:**5–66.

48. **Collins, H. L., and S. H. Kaufmann.** 2001. Prospects for better tuberculosis vaccines. *Lancet Infect. Dis.* **1:**21–28.

49. **Comstock, G. W.** 1988. Identification of an effective vaccine against tuberculosis. *Am. Rev. Respir. Dis.* **138:**479–480.

50. **Comstock, G. W., and R. J. O'Brien.** 1991. Tuberculosis, p. 745–771. *In* A. S. Evans and P. S. Brachman (ed.), *Bacterial Infections of Humans: Epidemiology and Control*, 2nd ed. Plenum Medical Book Co., New York, NY.

51. **Comstock, G. W., and S. F. Woolpert.** 1978. Tuberculin conversions: true or false? *Am. Rev. Respir. Dis.* **118:**215–217.

52. **Condos, R., W. N. Rom, and N. W. Schluger.** 1997. Treatment of multidrug-resistant pulmonary tuberculosis with interferon-gamma via aerosol. *Lancet* **349:**1513–1515.

53. **Converse, P. J., A. M. Dannenberg, Jr., J. E. Estep, K. Sugisaki, Y. Abe, B. H. Schofield, and M. L. Pitt.** 1996. Cavitary tuberculosis produced in rabbits by aerosolized virulent tubercle bacilli. *Infect. Immun.* **64:**4776–4787.

54. **Converse, P. J., A. M. Dannenberg, Jr., T. Shigenaga, D. N. McMurray, S. W. Phalen, J. L. Stanford, G. A. Rook, T. Koru-Sengul, H. Abbey, J. E. Estep, and M. L. Pitt.** 1998. Pulmonary bovine-type tuberculosis in rabbits: bacillary virulence, inhaled dose effects, tuberculin sensitivity, and *Mycobacterium vaccae* immunotherapy. *Clin. Diagn. Lab. Immunol.* **5:**871–881.

54a.**Converse, P. J., K. D. Eisenach, S. A. Theus, E. L. Nuermberger, S. Tyagi, L. H. Ly, D. E. Geiman, H. Guo, S. T. Nolan, N. C. Akar, L. G. Klinkenberg, R. Gupta, S. Lun, P. C. Karakousis, G. Lamichhane, D. N. McMurray, J. H. Grosset, and W. R. Bishai.** 21 April 2010. The impact of mouse passaging of *Mycobacterium tuberculosis* strains prior to virulence testing in the mouse and guinea pig models. *PLoS One* 5(4):e10289. doi:10.1371/journal.pone.0010289.

54b.**Converse, P. J., P. C. Karakousis, L. G. Klinkenberg, A. K. Kesavan, L. H. Ly, S. S. Allen, J. H. Grosset, S. K. Jain, G. Lamichhane, Y. C. Manabe, D. N. McMurray, E. L. Nuermberger, and W. R. Bishai.** 2009. Role of the *dosR-dosS* two-component regulatory system in *Mycobacterium tuberculosis* virulence in three animal models. *Infect. Immun.* **77:**1230–1237.

55. **Cooper, A. M., C. D'Souza, A. A. Frank, and I. M. Orme.** 1997. The course of *Mycobacterium tuberculosis* infection in the lungs of mice lacking expression of either perforin- or granzyme-mediated cytolytic mechanisms. *Infect. Immun.* **65:** 1317–1320.

56. **Cooper, A. M., A. Kipnis, J. Turner, J. Magram, J. Ferrante, and I. M. Orme.** 2002. Mice lacking bioactive IL-12 can generate protective, antigen-specific cellular responses to mycobacterial infection only if the IL-12 p40 subunit is present. *J. Immunol.* **168:**1322–1327.

56a.**Crowle, A. J.** 1988. Imunization against tuberculosis: what kind of vaccine? *Infect. Immun.* **56:**2769–2773.

57. **Daniel, T. M.** 1988. Antibody and antigen detection for the immunodiagnosis of tuberculosis: why not? What more is needed? Where do we stand today? *J. Infect. Dis.* **158:**678–680.

58. **Daniel, T. M.** 1989. Rapid diagnosis of tuberculosis: laboratory techniques applicable in developing countries. *Rev. Infect. Dis.* **11**(Suppl. 2)**:**S471–S478.

59. **Dannenberg, A. M., Jr.** 1968. Cellular hypersensitivity and cellular immunity in the pathogenesis of tuberculosis: specificity, systemic and local nature, and associated macrophage enzymes. *Bacteriol. Rev.* **32:**85–102.

60. **Dannenberg, A. M., Jr.** 1978. Pathogenesis of pulmonary tuberculosis in man and animals: protection of personnel against tuberculosis, p. 65–75. *In* R. Montali (ed.), *Mycobacterial Infections of Zoo Animals*. Smithsonian Institution Press, Washington, DC.

61. **Dannenberg, A. M., Jr.** 1984. Pathogenesis of tuberculosis: native and acquired resistance in animals and humans, p. 344–354. *In Microbiology—1984*. American Society for Microbiology, Washington, DC.

62. **Dannenberg, A. M., Jr.** 1989. Immune mechanisms in the pathogenesis of pulmonary tuberculosis. *Rev. Infect. Dis.* **11**(Suppl. 2)**:**S369–S378.

63. **Dannenberg, A. M., Jr.** 1990. Controlling tuberculosis: the pathologist's point of view. *Res. Microbiol.* **141:**192–196; discussion, 262–263.

64. **Dannenberg, A. M., Jr.** 1991. Delayed-type hypersensitivity and cell-mediated immunity in the pathogenesis of tuberculosis. *Immunol. Today* **12:**228–233.

65. **Dannenberg, A. M., Jr.** 1993. Immunopathogenesis of pulmonary tuberculosis. *Hosp. Pract.* (Off. Ed.) **28:**51–58.

66. **Dannenberg, A. M., Jr.** 1998. Lurie's tubercle-count method to test TB vaccine efficacy in rabbits. *Front. Biosci.* **3:**27–33.

67. **Dannenberg, A. M., Jr.** 2001. Pathogenesis of pulmonary *Mycobacterium bovis* infection: basic principles established by the rabbit model. *Tuberculosis* (Edinburgh) **81:**87–96.

68. **Dannenberg, A. M., Jr.** 2003. Macrophage turnover, division and activation within developing, peak and "healed" tuberculous lesions produced in rabbits by BCG. *Tuberculosis* (Edinburgh) **83:**251–260.

69. **Dannenberg, A. M., Jr.** 2006. *Pathogenesis of Human Tuberculosis: Insights from the Rabbit Model*. ASM Press, Washington, DC.

70. **Dannenberg, A. M., Jr.** 2009. Liquefaction and cavity formation in pulmonary TB: a simple method in rabbit skin to test inhibitors. *Tuberculosis* (Edinburgh) **89:**243–247.

71. **Dannenberg, A. M., Jr.** 2010. Perspectives on clinical and preclinical testing of new tuberculosis vaccines. *Clin. Microbiol. Rev.* **23:**781–794.

72. **Dannenberg, A. M., Jr., M. S. Burstone, P. C. Walter, and J. W. Kinsley.** 1963. A histochemical study of phagocytic and enzymatic functions of rabbit mononuclear and polymorphonuclear exudate cells and alveolar macrophages. I. Survey and quantitation of enzymes, and states of cellular activation. *J. Cell Biol.* **17:**465–486.

73. **Dannenberg, A. M., Jr., and F. M. Collins.** 2001. Progressive pulmonary tuberculosis is not due to increasing numbers of viable bacilli in rabbits, mice and guinea pigs, but is due to a continuous host response to mycobacterial products. *Tuberculosis* (Edinburgh) **81:**229–242.

74. **Dannenberg, A. M., Jr., O. T. Meyer, J. R. Esterly, and T. Kambara.** 1968. The local nature of immunity in tuberculosis, illustrated histochemically in dermal BCG lesions. *J. Immunol.* **100:**931–941.

75. Reference deleted.

76. **Dannenberg, A. M., Jr., and G. A. Rook.** 1994. Pathogenesis of pulmonary tuberculosis: an interplay of tissue-damaging and macrophage-activating immune responses—dual mechanisms that control bacillary multiplication, p. 459–483. *In* B. R. Bloom (ed.), *Tuberculosis: Pathogenesis, Protection, and Control*. ASM Press, Washington, DC.

77. **Dannenberg, A. M., Jr., and M. Sugimoto.** 1976. Liquefaction of caseous foci in tuberculosis. *Am. Rev. Respir. Dis.* **113:**257–259.

78. **Dannenberg, A. M., Jr., and J. Tomashefski.** 1998. Pathogenesis of pulmonary tuberculosis, p. 2447–2471. *In* A. P. Fishman and J. A. Elias (ed.), *Fishman's Pulmonary Diseases and Disorders*, 3rd ed. McGraw-Hill, Health Professions Division, New York, NY.

79. **Darwin, K. H., S. Ehrt, J. C. Gutierrez-Ramos, N. Weich, and C. F. Nathan.** 2003. The proteasome of *Mycobacterium tuberculosis* is required for resistance to nitric oxide. *Science* **302:**1963–1966.

79a. **Davis, S. L., E. L. Nuermberger, P. K. Um, C. Vidal, B. Jedynak, M. G. Pomper, W. R. Bishai, and S. K. Jaim.** 2009. Noninvasive pulmonary [18F]-2-fluoro-deoxy-D-glucose positron emission tomography correlates with bactericidal activity of tuberculosis drug treatment. *Antimicrob. Agents Chemother.* **53:**4879–4884.

80. **Demissie, A., P. Ravn, J. Olobo, T. M. Doherty, T. Eguale, M. Geletu, W. Hailu, P. Andersen, and S. Britton.** 1999. T-cell recognition of *Mycobacterium tuberculosis* culture filtrate fractions in tuberculosis patients and their household contacts. *Infect. Immun.* **67:**5967–5971.

81. **Denis, M.** 1991. Interferon-gamma-treated murine macrophages inhibit growth of tubercle bacilli via the generation of reactive nitrogen intermediates. *Cell. Immunol.* **132:**150–157.

82. **Department of Health and Mental Hygiene.** 1991. *Guidelines for Preventing the Transmission of Tuberculosis in Health-Care Settings*. State of Maryland Communicable Diseases Bulletin.

83. **Dickinson, J. M., M. J. Lefford, J. Lloyd, and D. A. Mitchison.** 1963. The virulence in the guinea-pig of tubercle bacilli from patients with pulmonary tuberculosis in Hong Kong. *Tubercle* **44:**446–451.

83a. **Dockrell, H. M., and Y. Zhang.** 2009. A courageous step down the road toward a new tuberculosis vaccine. *Am. J. Respir. Clin. Care Med.* **179:**628–629.

84. **Doherty, T. M., A. Demissie, J. Olobo, D. Wolday, S. Britton, T. Eguale, P. Ravn, and P. Andersen.** 2002. Immune responses to the *Mycobacterium tuberculosis*-specific antigen ESAT-6 signal subclinical infection among contacts of tuberculosis patients. *J. Clin. Microbiol.* **40:**704–706.

84a. **Domenech, P., and M. B. Reed.** 2009. Rapid and spontaneous loss of phthiocerol dimycocerosate (PDIM) from *Mycobacterium tuberculosis* grown in vitro: implications for virulence studies. *Microbiology* **155:**3532–3543.

85. **Dorman, S. E., C. L. Hatem, S. Tyagi, K. Aird, J. Lopez-Molina, M. L. Pitt, B. C. Zook, A. M. Dannenberg, Jr., W. R. Bishai, and Y. C. Manabe.** 2004. Susceptibility to tuberculosis: clues from studies with inbred and outbred New Zealand White rabbits. *Infect. Immun.* **72:**1700–1705.

86. **Dorman, S. E., and S. M. Holland.** 1998. Mutation in the signal-transducing chain of the interferon-gamma receptor and susceptibility to mycobacterial infection. *J. Clin. Investig.* **101:**2364–2369.

87. **Dowdle, W. R., for the Centers for Disease Control.** 1989. A strategic plan for the elimination of tuberculosis in the United States. *MMWR Morb. Mortal. Wkly. Rep.* **38**(Suppl. 3)**:**1–25.

88. **D'Souza, C. D., A. M. Cooper, A. A. Frank, R. J. Mazzaccaro, B. R. Bloom, and I. M. Orme.** 1997. An anti-inflammatory

role for gamma delta T lymphocytes in acquired immunity to *Mycobacterium tuberculosis. J. Immunol.* **158**:1217–1221.

89. Ellner, J. J. 1996. Immunosuppression in tuberculosis. *Infect. Agents Dis.* **5**:62–72.

90. Ellner, J. J. 1997. Regulation of the human immune response during tuberculosis. *J. Lab. Clin. Med.* **130**:469–475.

90a. Fenton, M. J., L.W. Riley, and L. S. Schlesinger. 2005. Receptor-mediated recognition of *Mycobacterium tuberculosis* by host cells, p. 405–426. *In* S. T. Cole, K. D. Eisenach, D. N. McMurray, and W. R. Jacobs, Jr. (ed.), *Tuberculosis and the Tubercle Bacillus.* ASM Press, Washington, DC.

91. Filley, E. A., H. A. Bull, P. M. Dowd, and G. A. Rook. 1992. The effect of *Mycobacterium tuberculosis* on the susceptibility of human cells to the stimulatory and toxic effects of tumour necrosis factor. *Immunology* **77**:505–509.

92. Filley, E. A., and G. A. Rook. 1991. Effect of mycobacteria on sensitivity to the cytotoxic effects of tumor necrosis factor. *Infect. Immun.* **59**:2567–2572.

93. Fine, P. E. 1989. The BCG story: lessons from the past and implications for the future. *Rev. Infect. Dis.* **11**(Suppl. 2): S353–S359.

94. Fitzgerald, K. A., L. O'Neill, and A. Gearing. 2001. *The Cytokine Factsbook.* Elsevier Academic Press, San Diego, CA.

95. Fleischmann, R. D., D. Alland, J. A. Eisen, L. Carpenter, O. White, J. Peterson, R. DeBoy, R. Dodson, M. Gwinn, D. Haft, E. Hickey, J. F. Kolonay, W. C. Nelson, L. A. Umayam, M. Ermolaeva, S. L. Salzberg, A. Delcher, T. Utterback, J. Weidman, H. Khouri, J. Gill, A. Mikula, W. Bishai, W. R. Jacobs, Jr., J. C. Venter, and C. M. Fraser. 2002. Whole-genome comparison of *Mycobacterium tuberculosis* clinical and laboratory strains. *J. Bacteriol.* **184**:5479–5490.

96. Flynn, J. L., and J. Chan. 2001. Immunology of tuberculosis. *Annu. Rev. Immunol.* **19**:93–129.

97. Flynn, J. L., M. M. Goldstein, J. Chan, K. J. Triebold, K. Pfeffer, C. J. Lowenstein, R. Schreiber, T. W. Mak, and B. R. Bloom. 1995. Tumor necrosis factor-alpha is required in the protective immune response against *Mycobacterium tuberculosis* in mice. *Immunity* **2**:561–572.

98. Flynn, J. L., M. M. Goldstein, K. J. Triebold, B. Koller, and B. R. Bloom. 1992. Major histocompatibility complex class I-restricted T cells are required for resistance to *Mycobacterium tuberculosis* infection. *Proc. Natl. Acad. Sci. USA* **89**: 12013–12017.

99. Flynn, J. L., M. M. Goldstein, K. J. Triebold, J. Sypek, S. Wolf, and B. R. Bloom. 1995. IL-12 increases resistance of BALB/c mice to *Mycobacterium tuberculosis* infection. *J. Immunol.* **155**:2515–2524.

99a. Fortin, A., L. Abel, J. L. Casanova, and P. Gros. 2007. Host genetics of mycobacterial diseases in mice and men: forward genetic studies of BCG-osis and tuberculosis. *Annu. Rev. Genomics Hum. Genet.* **8**:163–192.

100. Francis, J. 1958. *Tuberculosis in Animals and Man: a Study in Comparative Pathology*, p. 293–318. Cassell, London, United Kingdom.

100a. Frigui, W., D. Bottai, L. Majlessi, M. Monot, E. Josselin, P. Brodin, T. Garnier, B. Gicquel, C. Martin, C. Leclerc, S. T. Cole, and R. Brosch. 2008. Control of *M. tuberculosis* ESAT-6 secretion and specific T cell recognition by PhoP. *PLoS Pathog.* **4**:e33.

101. Gioia, C., C. Agrati, R. Casetti, C. Cairo, G. Borsellino, L. Battistini, G. Mancino, D. Goletti, V. Colizzi, L. P. Pucillo, and F. Poccia. 2002. Lack of CD27-CD45RA-Vγ 9V-δ2+ T cell effectors in immunocompromised hosts and during active pulmonary tuberculosis. *J. Immunol.* **168**:1484–1489.

102. Gong, J. H., M. Zhang, R. L. Modlin, P. S. Linsley, D. Iyer, Y. Lin, and P. F. Barnes. 1996. Interleukin-10 downregulates *Mycobacterium tuberculosis*-induced Th1 responses and CTLA-4 expression. *Infect. Immun.* **64**:913–918.

103. Green, S. J., C. A. Nacy, and M. S. Meltzer. 1991. Cytokine-induced synthesis of nitrogen oxides in macrophages: a protective host response to *Leishmania* and other intracellular pathogens. *J. Leukoc. Biol.* **50**:93–103.

103a. Greinert, U., M. Ernst, M. Schlaak, and P. Entzian. 2001. Interleukin-12 as successful adjuvant in tuberculosis treatment. *Eur. Respir. J.* **17**:1049–1051.

103b. Guinn, K. M., M. J. Hickey, S. K. Mathur, K. L. Zakel, J. E. Grotzke, D. M. Lewinsohn, S. Smith, and D. R. Sherman. 2004. Individual RD1-region genes are required for export of ESAT-6/CFP-10 and for virulence of *Mycobacterium tuberculosis. Mol. Microbiol.* **51**:359–370.

103c. Gupta, U. D., V. M. Katoch, and D. N. McMurray. 2007. Current status of TB vaccines. *Vaccine* **25**:3742–3751.

104. Harshan, K. V., and P. R. Gangadharam. 1991. In vivo depletion of natural killer cell activity leads to enhanced multiplication of *Mycobacterium avium* complex in mice. *Infect. Immun.* **59**:2818–2821.

105. Hayday, A. C. 2000. Gamma-delta cells: a right time and a right place for a conserved third way of protection. *Annu. Rev. Immunol.* **18**:975–1026.

106. Heinzel, A. S., J. E. Grotzke, R. A. Lines, D. A. Lewinsohn, A. L. McNabb, D. N. Streblow, V. M. Braud, H. J. Grieser, J. T. Belisle, and D. M. Lewinsohn. 2002. HLA-E-dependent presentation of Mtb-derived antigen to human CD8+ T cells. *J. Exp. Med.* **196**:1473–1481.

107. Hemsworth, G. R., and I. Kochan. 1978. Secretion of antimycobacterial fatty acids by normal and activated macrophages. *Infect. Immun.* **19**:170–177.

108. Hirsch, C. S., R. Hussain, Z. Toossi, G. Dawood, F. Shahid, and J. J. Ellner. 1996. Cross-modulation by transforming growth factor beta in human tuberculosis: suppression of antigen-driven blastogenesis and interferon gamma production. *Proc. Natl. Acad. Sci. USA* **93**:3193–3198.

109. Hirsch, C. S., Z. Toossi, J. L. Johnson, H. Luzze, L. Ntambi, P. Peters, M. McHugh, A. Okwera, M. Joloba, P. Mugyenyi, R. D. Mugerwa, P. Terebuh, and J. J. Ellner. 2001. Augmentation of apoptosis and interferon-gamma production at sites of active *Mycobacterium tuberculosis* infection in human tuberculosis. *J. Infect. Dis.* **183**:779–788.

110. Hirsch, C. S., Z. Toossi, C. Othieno, J. L. Johnson, S. K. Schwander, S. Robertson, R. S. Wallis, K. Edmonds, A. Okwera, R. Mugerwa, P. Peters, and J. J. Ellner. 1999. Depressed T-cell interferon-gamma responses in pulmonary tuberculosis: analysis of underlying mechanisms and modulation with therapy. *J. Infect. Dis.* **180**:2069–2073.

110a. Holland, S. M. 2000. Cytokine therapy of mycobacterial infections. *Adv. Intern. Med.* **45**:431–452.

111. Holter, W., C. K. Goldman, L. Casabo, D. L. Nelson, W. C. Greene, and T. A. Waldmann. 1987. Expression of functional IL 2 receptors by lipopolysaccharide and interferon-gamma stimulated human monocytes. *J. Immunol.* **138**:2917–2922.

112. Horwitz, M. A., G. Harth, B. J. Dillon, and S. Maslesa-Galic. 2000. Recombinant bacillus Calmette-Guerin (BCG) vaccines expressing the *Mycobacterium tuberculosis* 30-kDa major secretory protein induce greater protective immunity against tuberculosis than conventional BCG vaccines in a highly susceptible animal model. *Proc. Natl. Acad. Sci. USA* **97**:13853–13858.

112a. Horwitz, M. A., G. Harth, B. J. Dillon, and S. Maslesa-Galic. 2005. Enhancing the protective efficacy of *Mycobacterium bovis* BCG vaccination against tuberculosis by boosting with *Mycobacterium tuberculosis* major secretory protein. *Infect. Immun.* **73**:4676–4683.

113. Ito, M., N. Kojiro, T. Ikeda, T. Ito, J. Funada, and T. Kokubu. 1992. Increased proportions of peripheral blood gamma delta T cells in patients with pulmonary tuberculosis. *Chest* **102:**195–197.

114. Jaattela, M. 1991. Biologic activities and mechanisms of action of tumor necrosis factor-alpha/cachectin. *Lab. Investig.* **64:**724–742.

115. Jain, S. K., S. M. Hernandez-Abanto, Q.-J. Cheng, P. Singh, L. H. Ly, L. G. Klinkenberg, N. E. Morrison, P. J. Converse, E. Nuermberger, J. Grosset, D. N. McMurray, P. C. Karakousis, G. Lamichhane, and W. R. Bishai. 2007. Accelerated detection of *Mycobacterium tuberculosis* genes essential for bacterial survival in guinea pigs, compared with mice. *J. Infect. Dis.* **195:**1634–1642.

116. Jullien, D., S. Stenger, W. A. Ernst, and R. L. Modlin. 1997. CD1 presentation of microbial nonpeptide antigens to T cells. *J. Clin. Investig.* **99:**2071–2074.

117. Kaleab, B., T. Ottenoff, P. Converse, E. Halapi, G. Tadesse, M. Rottenberg, and R. Kiessling. 1990. Mycobacterial-induced cytotoxic T cells as well as nonspecific killer cells derived from healthy individuals and leprosy patients. *Eur. J. Immunol.* **20:**2651–2659.

118. Kansas, G. S. 1996. Selectins and their ligands: current concepts and controversies. *Blood* **88:**3259–3287.

118a. Kaplan, G., F. A. Post, A. L. Moreira, H. Wainwright, B. N. Kreiswirth, M. Tanverdi, B. Mathema, S. V. Ramaswamy, G. Walther, L. M. Steyn, C. E. Barry III, and L. G. Bakker. 2003. *Mycobacterium tuberculosis* growth at the cavity surface: a microenvironment with failed immunity. *Infect. Immun.* **71:**7099–7108.

119. Kaufmann, S. H. 1988. CD8+ T lymphocytes in intracellular microbial infections. *Immunol. Today* **9:**168–174.

120. Kaufmann, S. H. 1989. In vitro analysis of the cellular mechanisms involved in immunity to tuberculosis. *Rev. Infect. Dis.* **11**(Suppl.)2:S448–S454.

121. Kaufmann, S. H. 1989. Leprosy and tuberculosis vaccine design. *Trop. Med. Parasitol.* **40:**251–257.

122. Kaufmann, S. H. 2001. How can immunology contribute to the control of tuberculosis? *Nat. Rev. Immunol.* **1:**20–30.

123. Kaufmann, S. H. 2003. Immunity to intracellular bacteria, p. 1229–1261. *In* W. E. Paul (ed.), *Fundamental Immunology*, 5th ed. Lippincott Williams & Wilkins, Philadelphia, PA.

124. Keane, J., S. Gershon, R. P. Wise, E. Mirabile-Levens, J. Kasznica, W. D. Schwieterman, J. N. Siegel, and M. M. Braun. 2001. Tuberculosis associated with infliximab, a tumor necrosis factor alpha-neutralizing agent. *N. Engl. J. Med.* **345:**1098–1104.

125. Kindler, V., A. P. Sappino, G. E. Grau, P. F. Piguet, and P. Vassalli. 1989. The inducing role of tumor necrosis factor in the development of bactericidal granulomas during BCG infection. *Cell* **56:**731–740.

126. Klebanoff, S. 1988. Phagocytic cells: products of oxygen metabolism, p. 391–444. *In* R. Snyderman, J. I. Gallin, and I. M. Goldstein (ed.), *Inflammation: Basic Principles and Clinical Correlates.* Raven Press, New York, NY.

127. Koch, R. 1891. Fortsetzung der Mitteilungen über ein Heilmittel gegen Tuberkulose. *Dtsch. Med. Wochenschr.* **Jan. 15:**101–102.

128. Kramnik, I., P. Demant, and B. R. Bloom. 1998. Susceptibility to tuberculosis as a complex genetic trait: analysis using recombinant congenic strains of mice. *Novartis Found. Symp.* **217:**120–131; discussion, 132–137.

129. Kramnik, I., W. F. Dietrich, P. Demant, and B. R. Bloom. 2000. Genetic control of resistance to experimental infection with virulent *Mycobacterium tuberculosis. Proc. Natl. Acad. Sci. USA* **97:**8560–8565.

130. Kumararatne, D. S., A. S. Pithie, P. Drysdale, J. S. Gaston, R. Kiessling, P. B. Iles, C. J. Ellis, J. Innes, and R. Wise. 1990. Specific lysis of mycobacterial antigen-bearing macrophages by class II MHC-restricted polyclonal T cell lines in healthy donors or patients with tuberculosis. *Clin. Exp. Immunol.* **80:**314–323.

130a. Kupper, T. S. 1990. Immune and inflammatory processes in cutaneous tissues: mechanisms and speculations. *J. Clin. Investig.* **86:**1783–1789.

131. Kupper, T. S., and R. W. Groves. 1995. The interleukin-1 axis and cutaneous inflammation. *J. Investig. Dermatol.* **105:**62S–66S.

132. Laal, S., and Y. Skeiky. 2005. Immune-based methods, p. 71–83. *In* S. T. Cole, K. Eisenach, D. N. McMurray, and W. R. Jacobs, Jr. (ed.), *Tuberculosis and the Tubercle Bacillus.* ASM Press, Washington, DC.

133. Ladel, C. H., C. Blum, A. Dreher, K. Reifenberg, and S. H. Kaufmann. 1995. Protective role of gamma/delta T cells and alpha/beta T cells in tuberculosis. *Eur. J. Immunol.* **25:**2877–2881.

134. Lahn, M., A. Kanehiro, K. Takeda, J. Terry, Y. S. Hahn, M. K. Aydintug, A. Konowal, K. Ikuta, R. L. O'Brien, E. W. Gelfand, and W. K. Born. 2002. MHC class I-dependent Vγ4+ pulmonary T cells regulate αβ T cell-independent airway responsiveness. *Proc. Natl. Acad. Sci. USA* **99:**8850–8855.

135. Lalvani, A., R. Brookes, R. J. Wilkinson, A. S. Malin, A. A. Pathan, P. Andersen, H. Dockrell, G. Pasvol, and A. V. Hill. 1998. Human cytolytic and interferon gamma-secreting CD8+ T lymphocytes specific for *Mycobacterium tuberculosis. Proc. Natl. Acad. Sci. USA* **95:**270–275.

136. Laskin, D. L., and K. J. Pendino. 1995. Macrophages and inflammatory mediators in tissue injury. *Annu. Rev. Pharmacol. Toxicol.* **35:**655–677.

137. Reference deleted.

138. Leonard, E. J., and T. Yoshimura. 1990. Human monocyte chemoattractant protein-1 (MCP-1). *Immunol. Today* **11:**97–101.

139. Lewinsohn, D. M., L. Zhu, V. J. Madison, D. C. Dillon, S. P. Fling, S. G. Reed, K. H. Grabstein, and M. R. Alderson. 2001. Classically restricted human CD8+ T lymphocytes derived from *Mycobacterium tuberculosis*-infected cells: definition of antigenic specificity. *J. Immunol.* **166:**439–446.

140. Li, B., M. D. Rossman, T. Imir, A. F. Oner-Eyuboglu, C. W. Lee, R. Biancaniello, and S. R. Carding. 1996. Disease-specific changes in gamma-delta T cell repertoire and function in patients with pulmonary tuberculosis. *J. Immunol.* **157:**4222–4229.

140a. Lin, P. L., A. Myers, L. Smith, C. Bigbee, M. Bigbee, C. Fuhrman, H. Grieser, I. Chiosea, N. N. Voitenek, S. V. Capuano, E. Klein, and J. L. Flynn. 2010. Tumor necrosis factor neutralization results in disseminated disease in acute and latent *Mycobacterium tuberculosis* infection with normal granuloma structure in a cynomolgus macaque model. *Arthritis Rheum.* **62:**340–350.

141. Lind, A., and M. Ridell. 1984. Immunologically based diagnostic tests: humoral antibody methods, p. 221–248. *In* G. P. Kubica and L. G. Wayne (ed.), *The Mycobacteria: a Sourcebook.* Dekker, New York, NY.

142. Lindner, H., E. Holler, B. Ertl, G. Multhoff, M. Schreglmann, I. Klauke, S. Schultz-Hector, and G. Eissner. 1997. Peripheral blood mononuclear cells induce programmed cell death in human endothelial cells and may prevent repair: role of cytokines. *Blood* **89:**1931–1938.

143. Long, E. R. 1958. *The Chemistry and Chemotherapy of Tuberculosis*, 3rd ed., p. 106–108 and 122–124. Lippincott Williams & Wilkins, Baltimore, MD.

143a.Long, R., B. Light, and J. A. Talbot. 1999. Mycobacteriocidal action of exogenous nitric oxide. *Antimicrob. Agents Chemother.* **43**:403–405.

144. Lowrie, D. B. 1990. Is macrophage death on the field of battle essential to victory, or a tactical weakness in immunity against tuberculosis? *Clin. Exp. Immunol.* **80**:301–303.

145. Lowrie, D. B. 2003. DNA vaccination: an update. *Methods Mol. Med.* **87**:377–390.

146. Lurie, M. B. 1964. *Resistance to Tuberculosis: Experimental Studies in Native and Acquired Defensive Mechanisms.* Published for the Commonwealth Fund by Harvard University Press, Cambridge, MA.

147. Reference deleted.

148. Lurie, M. B., and A. M. Dannenberg, Jr. 1965. Macrophage function in infectious disease with inbred rabbits. *Bacteriol. Rev.* **29**:466–476.

149. Lurie, M. B., P. Zappasodi, E. Cardona-Lynch, and A. M. Dannenberg, Jr. 1952. The response to the intracutaneous inoculation of BCG as an index of native resistance to tuberculosis. *J. Immunol.* **68**:369–387.

150. Lurie, M. B., P. Zappasodi, and C. Tickner. 1955. On the nature of genetic resistance to tuberculosis in the light of the host-parasite relationships in natively resistant and susceptible rabbits. *Am. Rev. Tuberc. Pulmon. Dis.* **72**:297–329.

151. Lurie, M. B., P. Zappasodi, A. M. Dannenberg, Jr., and G. H. Weiss. 1952. On the mechanism of genetic resistance to tuberculosis and its mode of inheritance. *Am. J. Hum. Genet.* **4**:302–314.

151a.Ly, H. L., M. I. Russell, and D. N. McMurray. 2008. Cytokine profiles in primary and secondary pulmonary granulomas of guinea pigs with tuberculosis. *Am. J. Respir. Cell. Mol. Biol.* **38**:455–462.

152. Mackaness, G. B. 1968. The immunology of antituberculous immunity. *Am. Rev. Respir. Dis.* **97**:337–344.

153. MacMicking, J., Q. W. Xie, and C. Nathan. 1997. Nitric oxide and macrophage function. *Annu. Rev. Immunol.* **15**:323–350.

153a.MacMicking, J. D., R. J. North, R. LaCourse, J. S. Mudgett, S. K. Shah, and C. F. Nathan. 1997. Identification of nitric oxide synthase as a protective locus against tuberculosis. *Proc. Natl. Acad. Sci. USA* **94**:5243–5248.

154. Maini, R., E. W. St. Clair, F. Breedveld, D. Furst, J. Kalden, M. Weisman, J. Smolen, P. Emery, G. Harriman, M. Feldmann, and P. Lipsky for the ATTRACT Study Group. 1999. Infliximab (chimeric anti-tumour necrosis factor alpha monoclonal antibody) versus placebo in rheumatoid arthritis patients receiving concomitant methotrexate: a randomised phase III trial. *Lancet* **354**:1932–1939.

155. Majno, G., and I. Joris. 2004. *Cells, Tissues, and Disease: Principles of General Pathology*, 2nd ed. Oxford University Press, New York, NY.

156. Malik, S., and E. Schurr. 2002. Genetic susceptibility to tuberculosis. *Clin. Chem. Lab. Med.* **40**:863–868.

157. Manabe, Y. C., A. M. Dannenberg, Jr., S. K. Tyagi, C. L. Hatem, M. Yoder, S. C. Woolwine, B. C. Zook, M. L. Pitt, and W. R. Bishai. 2003. Different strains of *Mycobacterium tuberculosis* cause various spectrums of disease in the rabbit model of tuberculosis. *Infect. Immun.* **71**:6004–6011.

158. Manabe, Y. C., C. P. Scott, and W. R. Bishai. 2002. Naturally attenuated, orally administered *Mycobacterium microti* as a tuberculosis vaccine is better than subcutaneous *Mycobacterium bovis* BCG. *Infect. Immun.* **70**:1566–1570.

159. Manca, C., L. Tsenova, C. E. Barry III, A. Bergtold, S. Freeman, P. A. Haslett, J. M. Musser, V. H. Freedman, and G.

Kaplan. 1999. *Mycobacterium tuberculosis* CDC1551 induces a more vigorous host response in vivo and in vitro, but is not more virulent than other clinical isolates. *J. Immunol.* **162**:6740–6746.

160. Manca, C., L. Tsenova, A. Bergtold, S. Freeman, M. Tovey, J. M. Musser, C. E. Barry III, V. H. Freedman, and G. Kaplan. 2001. Virulence of a *Mycobacterium tuberculosis* clinical isolate in mice is determined by failure to induce Th1 type immunity and is associated with induction of IFN-alpha/beta. *Proc. Natl. Acad. Sci. USA* **98**:5752–5757.

161. Matzinger, P. 2002. The danger model: a renewed sense of self. *Science* **296**:301–305.

162. Maw, W. W., T. Shimizu, K. Sato, and H. Tomioka. 1997. Further study on the roles of the effector molecules of immunosuppressive macrophages induced by mycobacterial infection in expression of their suppressor function against mitogen-stimulated T cell proliferation. *Clin. Exp. Immunol.* **108**:26–33.

163. McKinney, J. D., K. Honer zu Bentrup, E. J. Munoz-Elias, A. Miczak, B. Chen, W. T. Chan, D. Swenson, J. C. Sacchettini, W. R. Jacobs, Jr., and D. G. Russell. 2000. Persistence of *Mycobacterium tuberculosis* in macrophages and mice requires the glyoxylate shunt enzyme isocitrate lyase. *Nature* **406**:735–738.

163a.McShane, H., A. A. Pathan, C. R. Sander, N. P. Goonetilleke, H. A. Fletcher, and A. V. S. Hill. 2005. Boosting BCG with MVA85A: the first candidate subunit vaccine for tuberculosis in clinical trials. *Tuberculosis* **85**:47–52.

163b.McShane, H., A. A. Pathan, C. R. Sander, S. M. Keating, S. C. Gilbert, K. Huygen, H. A. Fletcher, and A. V. Hill. 2004. Recombinant modified vaccinia virus Ankara expressing antigen 85A boosts BCG-primed *and* naturally acquired antimycobacterial immunity in humans. *Nat. Med.* **10**:1240–1244.

164. Means, T. K., S. Wang, E. Lien, A. Yoshimura, D. T. Golenbock, and M. J. Fenton. 1999. Human Toll-like receptors mediate cellular activation by *Mycobacterium tuberculosis*. *J. Immunol.* **163**:3920–3927.

165. Medina, E., and R. J. North. 1998. Resistance ranking of some common inbred mouse strains to *Mycobacterium tuberculosis* and relationship to major histocompatibility complex haplotype and Nramp1 genotype. *Immunology* **93**:270–274.

165a.Mendelson, M., W. Hanekom, and G. Kaplan. 2005. Dendritic cells in host immunity to *Mycobacterium tuberculosis*, p. 451–461. *In* S. T. Cole, K. D. Eisenach, D. N. McMurray, and W. R. Jacobs, Jr. (ed.), *Tuberculosis and the Tubercle Bacillus*. ASM Press, Washington, DC.

166. Menzies, D. 1999. Interpretation of repeated tuberculin tests. Boosting, conversion, and reversion. *Am. J. Respir. Crit. Care Med.* **159**:15–21.

167. Mitchison, D. A., A. L. Bhatia, S. Radakrishna, J. B. Selkon, T. V. Subbaiah, and J. Wallace. 1961. The virulence in the guinea-pig of tubercle bacilli isolated before treatment from South Indian patients with pulmonary tuberculosis. I. Homogeneity of the investigation and a critique of the virulence test. *Bull. W. H. O.* **25**:285–312.

168. Mohan, V. P., C. A. Scanga, K. Yu, H. M. Scott, K. E. Tanaka, E. Tsang, M. M. Tsai, J. L. Flynn, and J. Chan. 2001. Effects of tumor necrosis factor alpha on host immune response in chronic persistent tuberculosis: possible role for limiting pathology. *Infect. Immun.* **69**:1847–1855.

169. Moncada, S., R. M. Palmer, and E. A. Higgs. 1991. Nitric oxide: physiology, pathophysiology, and pharmacology. *Pharmacol. Rev.* **43**:109–142.

170. Moody, D. B., T. Ulrichs, W. Muhlecker, D. C. Young, S. S. Gurcha, E. Grant, J. P. Rosat, M. B. Brenner, C. E. Costello,

G. S. Besra, and S. A. Porcelli. 2000. CD1c-mediated T-cell recognition of isoprenoid glycolipids in *Mycobacterium tuberculosis* infection. *Nature* **404**:884–888.

171. Müller, I., S. P. Cobbold, H. Waldmann, and S. H. Kaufmann. 1987. Impaired resistance to *Mycobacterium tuberculosis* infection after selective in vivo depletion of L3T4+ and Lyt-2+ T cells. *Infect. Immun.* **55**:2037–2041.

171a.Murphy, K., P. Travers, and M. Walport. 2008. *Janeway's Immunobiology*, 7th ed. Garland Science, Taylor & Francis Group, New York, NY.

172. Murray, J. F. 2003. Bill Dock and the location of pulmonary tuberculosis: how bed rest might have helped consumption. *Am. J. Respir. Crit. Care Med.* **168**:1029–1033.

172a.Murry, J. P., A. K. Pandey, C. M. Sassetti, and E. J. Rubin. 2009. Phthiocerol dimycocerosate transport is required for resisting interferon-γ-independent immunity. *J. Infect. Dis.* **200**:774–782.

173. Nathan, C. 1991. Mechanisms and modulation of macrophage activation. *Behring Inst. Mitt.* **88**:200–207.

174. Reference deleted.

175. Nathan, C. 2002. Points of control in inflammation. *Nature* **420**:846–852.

176. Nedeltchev, G., T. R. Raghunand, M. S. Jassal, S. Lun, Q. J. Cheng, and W. R. Bishai. 2009. Extrapulmonary dissemination of *Mycobacterium bovis*, but not *Mycobacterium tuberculosis*, in a bronchoscopic rabbit model of cavitary tuberculosis. *Infect. Immun.* **77**:598–603.

177. Nolt, D., and J. L. Flynn. 2004. Interleukin-12 therapy reduces the number of immune cells and pathology in lungs of mice infected with *Mycobacterium tuberculosis*. *Infect. Immun.* **72**:2976–2988.

178. North, R. J. 1974. Cell-mediated immunity of antituberculous immunity in the pathogenesis of tuberculosis: specificity and local nature, and associated macrophage enzymes, p. 418. *In* R. T. McCluskey and S. Cohen (ed.), *Mechanisms of Cell-Mediated Immunity*. Wiley, New York, NY.

179. North, R. J., and Y. J. Jung. 2004. Immunity to tuberculosis. *Annu. Rev. Immunol.* **22**:599–623.

179a.O'Donnell, M. A. 1997. The genetic reconstitution of BCG as a new immunotherapeutic tool. *Trends Biotechnol.* **15**:512–517.

180. Ohara, N., and T. Yamada. 2001. Recombinant BCG vaccines. *Vaccine* **19**:4089–4098.

180a.Olsen, A. W., and P. Andersen. 2003. A novel TB vaccine; strategies to combat a complex pathogen. *Immunol. Lett.* **85**:207–211.

181. Orme, I. M., and F. M. Collins. 1983. Protection against *Mycobacterium tuberculosis* infection by adoptive immunotherapy. Requirement for T cell-deficient recipients. *J. Exp. Med.* **158**:74–83.

182. Orme, I. M., and F. M. Collins. 1984. Adoptive protection of the *Mycobacterium tuberculosis*-infected lung. Dissociation between cells that passively transfer protective immunity and those that transfer delayed-type hypersensitivity to tuberculin. *Cell. Immunol.* **84**:113–120.

183. Orme, I. M., D. N. McMurray, and J. T. Belisle. 2001. Tuberculosis vaccine development: recent progress. *Trends Microbiol.* **9**:115–118.

184. Orme, I. M., A. D. Roberts, J. P. Griffin, and J. S. Abrams. 1993. Cytokine secretion by CD4 T lymphocytes acquired in response to *Mycobacterium tuberculosis* infection. *J. Immunol.* **151**:518–525.

185. Ottenhoff, T. H., B. K. Ab, J. D. Van Embden, J. E. Thole, and R. Kiessling. 1988. The recombinant 65-kD heat shock protein of *Mycobacterium bovis* bacillus Calmette-Guerin/M.

tuberculosis is a target molecule for CD4+ cytotoxic T lymphocytes that lyse human monocytes. *J. Exp. Med.* **168**:1947–1952.

186. Ottenhoff, T. H., and R. R. de Vries. 1990. Antigen reactivity and autoreactivity: two sides of the cellular immune response induced by mycobacteria. *Curr. Top. Microbiol. Immunol.* **155**:111–121.

187. Pabst, M. J., J. M. Gross, J. P. Brozna, and M. B. Goren. 1988. Inhibition of macrophage priming by sulfatide from *Mycobacterium tuberculosis*. *J. Immunol.* **140**:634–640.

187a.Pan, Y., B. S. Yan, M. Rojas, Y. V. Shebzukhov, H. Zhou, L. Kobzik, D. E. Higgins, M. J. Daly, B. R. Bloom, and I. Kramnik. 2005. Ipr1 gene mediates innate immunity to tuberculosis. *Nature* **434**:767–772.

188. Pieters, J. 2001. Entry and survival of pathogenic mycobacteria in macrophages. *Microbes Infect.* **3**:249–255.

189. Pieters, J., and H. Ploegh. 2003. Microbiology. Chemical warfare and mycobacterial defense. *Science* **302**:1900–1902.

190. Pober, J. S., and R. S. Cotran. 1990. The role of endothelial cells in inflammation. *Transplantation* **50**:537–544.

191. Poole, J., and H. Florey. 1970. Chronic inflammation and tuberculosis, p. 1183–1224. *In* H. Florey (ed.), *General Pathology*, 4th ed. Saunders, Philadelphia, PA.

192. Porcelli, S. A. 1995. The CD1 family: a third lineage of antigen-presenting molecules. *Adv. Immunol.* **59**:1–98.

193. Porcelli, S. A., and R. L. Modlin. 1999. The CD1 system: antigen-presenting molecules for T cell recognition of lipids and glycolipids. *Annu. Rev. Immunol.* **17**:297–329.

194. Porcelli, S. A., C. T. Morita, and R. L. Modlin. 1996. T-cell recognition of non-peptide antigens. *Curr. Opin. Immunol.* **8**:510–516.

195. Raulet, D. H. 2003. Natural killer cells, p. 365–391. *In* W. E. Paul (ed.), *Fundamental Immunology*, 5th ed. Lippincott Williams & Wilkins, Philadelphia, PA.

196. Ravn, P., A. Demissie, T. Eguale, H. Wondwosson, D. Lein, H. A. Amoudy, A. S. Mustafa, A. K. Jensen, A. Holm, I. Rosenkrands, F. Oftung, J. Olobo, F. von Reyn, and P. Andersen. 1999. Human T cell responses to the ESAT-6 antigen from *Mycobacterium tuberculosis*. *J. Infect. Dis.* **179**:637–645.

197. Reggiardo, Z., and G. Middlebrook. 1974. Failure of passive serum transfer of immunity against aerogenic tuberculosis in rabbits. *Proc. Soc. Exp. Biol. Med.* **145**:173–175.

197a.Reggiardo, Z., and G. Middlebrook. 1974. Delayed-type hypersensitivity and immunity against aerogenic tuberculosis in guinea pigs. *Infect. Immun.* **9**:815–820.

198. Reiling, N., C. Holscher, A. Fehrenbach, S. Kroger, C. J. Kirschning, S. Goyert, and S. Ehlers. 2002. Cutting edge: Toll-like receptor (TLR)2- and TLR4-mediated pathogen recognition in resistance to airborne infection with *Mycobacterium tuberculosis*. *J. Immunol.* **169**:3480–3484.

199. Rich, A. R. 1951. *The Pathogenesis of Tuberculosis*, 2nd ed. Charles C Thomas, Springfield, IL.

200. Riley, R. L., C. C. Mills, F. O'Grady, L. U. Sultan, F. Wittstadt, and D. N. Shivpuri. 1962. Infectiousness of air from a tuberculosis ward. Ultraviolet irradiation of infected air: comparative infectiousness of different patients. *Am. Rev. Respir. Dis.* **85**:511–525.

201. Roach, D. R., A. G. Bean, C. Demangel, M. P. France, H. Briscoe, and W. J. Britton. 2002. TNF regulates chemokine induction essential for cell recruitment, granuloma formation, and clearance of mycobacterial infection. *J. Immunol.* **168**:4620–4627.

201a.Roach, D. R., H. Briscoe, K. Baumgart, D. A. Rathjen, and W. J. Britton. 1999. Tumor necrosis factor (TNF) and a TNF-mimetic peptide modulate the granulomatous response to

Mycobacterium bovis BCG infection in vivo. *Infect. Immun.* 67:5473–5476.

202. **Rock, K. L.** 1996. A new foreign policy: MHC class I molecules monitor the outside world. *Immunol. Today* 17:131–137.

203. **Rohrbach, M. S., and D. E. Williams.** 1986. T-lymphocytes and pleural tuberculosis. *Chest* 89:473–474.

204. **Rolph, M. S., B. Raupach, H. H. Kobernick, H. L. Collins, B. Perarnau, F. A. Lemonnier, and S. H. Kaufmann.** 2001. MHC class Ia-restricted T cells partially account for β2-microglobulin-dependent resistance to *Mycobacterium tuberculosis. Eur. J. Immunol.* 31:1944–1949.

205. **Rook, G. A.** 1988. Role of activated macrophages in the immunopathology of tuberculosis. *Br. Med. Bull.* 44:611–623.

206. **Rook, G. A.** 1990. Mycobacteria, cytokines and antibiotics. *Pathol. Biol.* (Paris) 38:276–280.

207. **Rook, G. A., and R. al Attiyah.** 1991. Cytokines and the Koch phenomenon. *Tubercle* 72:13–20.

208. **Rook, G. A., G. Seah, and A. Ustianowski.** 2001. *M. tuberculosis*: immunology and vaccination. *Eur. Respir. J.* 17:537–557.

208a. **Rook, G. A.W., K. Dheda, and A. Zumla.** 2005. Immune response to tuberculosis in developing countries: implications for new vaccines. *Nat. Rev. Immunol.* 5:661–667.

209. **Rosat, J. P., E. P. Grant, E. M. Beckman, C. C. Dascher, P. A. Sieling, D. Frederique, R. L. Modlin, S. A. Porcelli, S. T. Furlong, and M. B. Brenner.** 1999. CD1-restricted microbial lipid antigen-specific recognition found in the CD8+ alpha beta T cell pool. *J. Immunol.* 162:366–371.

210. **Russell, D. G.** 2001. *Mycobacterium tuberculosis*: here today, and here tomorrow. *Nat. Rev. Mol. Cell Biol.* 2:569–577.

210a. **Russell, D. G.** 2005. *Mycobacterium tuberculosis*: the indigestible microbe, p. 427–435. *In* S. T. Cole, K. D. Eisenach, D. N. McMurray, and W. R. Jacobs, Jr. (ed.), *Tuberculosis and the Tubercle Bacillus.* ASM Press, Washington, DC.

210b. **Sander, C. R., A. A. Pathan, N. E. R. Beveridge, I. Poulton, A. Minassian, N. Alder, J. Van Wijgerden, A. V. S. Hill, F. V. Gleeson, R. J. O. Davies, G. Pasvol, and H. McShane.** 2009. Safety and immunogenicity of a new tuberculosis vaccine, MVA85A, in *Mycobacterium tuberculosis*-infected individuals. *Am. J. Respir. Crit. Care Med.* 179:724–733.

210c. **Sasindran, S. J., and J. B. Torrelles.** 2011. *Mycobacterium tuberculosis* infection and inflammation: what is beneficial for the host and for the bacterium? *Front. Microbiol.* 2:2. doi:10.3389/fmicb.2011.00002.

211. **Scanga, C. A., V. P. Mohan, H. Joseph, K. Yu, J. Chan, and J. L. Flynn.** 1999. Reactivation of latent tuberculosis: variations on the Cornell murine model. *Infect. Immun.* 67:4531–4538.

212. **Scanga, C. A., V. P. Mohan, K. Tanaka, D. Alland, J. L. Flynn, and J. Chan.** 2001. The inducible nitric oxide synthase locus confers protection against aerogenic challenge of both clinical and laboratory strains of *Mycobacterium tuberculosis* in mice. *Infect. Immun.* 69:7711–7717.

213. **Schlesinger, L. S.** 1996. Role of mononuclear phagocytes in *M. tuberculosis* pathogenesis. *J. Investig. Med.* 44:312–323.

213a. **Seibert, F. B.** 1960. A theory of immunity in tuberculosis. *Perspect. Biol. Med.* 3:264–281.

214. **Selvaraj, P., P. R. Narayanan, and A. M. Reetha.** 1999. Association of functional mutant homozygotes of the mannose binding protein gene with susceptibility to pulmonary tuberculosis in India. *Tuberc. Lung Dis.* 79:221–227.

215. **Selvaraj, P., P. R. Narayanan, and A. M. Reetha.** 2000. Association of vitamin D receptor genotypes with the susceptibility to pulmonary tuberculosis in female patients & resistance in female contacts. *Indian J. Med. Res.* 111:172–179.

216. **Serbina, N. V., C. C. Liu, C. A. Scanga, and J. L. Flynn.** 2000. CD8+ CTL from lungs of *Mycobacterium tuberculosis*-infected mice express perforin in vivo and lyse infected macrophages. *J. Immunol.* 165:353–363.

217. **Shen, Y., D. Zhou, L. Qiu, X. Lai, M. Simon, L. Shen, Z. Kou, Q. Wang, L. Jiang, J. Estep, R. Hunt, M. Clagett, P. K. Sehgal, Y. Li, X. Zeng, C. T. Morita, M. B. Brenner, N. L. Letvin, and Z. W. Chen.** 2002. Adaptive immune response of Vγ2-Vδ2+ T cells during mycobacterial infections. *Science* 295:2255–2258.

218. **Shigenaga, T., A. M. Dannenberg, Jr., D. B. Lowrie, W. Said, M. J. Urist, H. Abbey, B. H. Schofield, P. Mounts, and K. Sugisaki.** 2001. Immune responses in tuberculosis: antibodies and CD4-CD8 lymphocytes with vascular adhesion molecules and cytokines (chemokines) cause a rapid antigen-specific cell infiltration at sites of bacillus Calmette-Guerin reinfection. *Immunology* 102:466–479.

219. **Shim, T. S., O. C. Turner, and I. M. Orme.** 2003. Toll-like receptor 4 plays no role in susceptibility of mice to *Mycobacterium tuberculosis* infection. *Tuberculosis* (Edinburgh) 83:367–371.

219a. **Shima, K., A. M. Dannenberg, Jr., M. Ando, S. Chandrasekhar, J. A. Seluzicki, and J. I. Fabrikant.** 1972. Macrophage accumulation, division, maturation, and digestive and microbicidal capacities in tuberculous lesions. I. Studies involving their incorporation of tritiated thymidine and their content of lysosomal enzymes and bacilli. *Am. J. Pathol.* 67:159–180.

220. **Smith, D. W., and G. E. Harding.** 1977. Animal model of human disease. Pulmonary tuberculosis. Animal model: experimental airborne tuberculosis in the guinea pig. *Am. J. Pathol.* 89:273–276.

221. **Sousa, A. O., R. J. Mazzaccaro, R. G. Russell, F. K. Lee, O. C. Turner, S. Hong, L. Van Kaer, and B. R. Bloom.** 2000. Relative contributions of distinct MHC class I-dependent cell populations in protection to tuberculosis infection in mice. *Proc. Natl. Acad. Sci. USA* 97:4204–4208.

222. **Sprent, J.** 1995. Antigen-presenting cells. Professionals and amateurs. *Curr. Biol.* 5:1095–1097.

223. **Sreevatsan, S., X. Pan, K. E. Stockbauer, N. D. Connell, B. N. Kreiswirth, T. S. Whittam, and J. M. Musser.** 1997. Restricted structural gene polymorphism in the *Mycobacterium tuberculosis* complex indicates evolutionarily recent global dissemination. *Proc. Natl. Acad. Sci. USA* 94:9869–9874.

223a. **Stead, W. W.** 2001. Variation in vulnerability to tuberculosis in America today: random or legacies of different ancestral epidemics? *Int. J. Tuberc. Lung Dis.* 5:807–814.

224. **Steinman, R. M.** 1991. The dendritic cell system and its role in immunogenicity. *Annu. Rev. Immunol.* 9:271–296.

225. **Steinman, R. M., D. Hawiger, and M. C. Nussenzweig.** 2003. Tolerogenic dendritic cells. *Annu. Rev. Immunol.* 21:685–711.

226. **Stuehr, D. J., and M. A. Marletta.** 1987. Induction of nitrite/nitrate synthesis in murine macrophages by BCG infection, lymphokines, or interferon-gamma. *J. Immunol.* 139:518–525.

227. **Sugisaki, K., A. M. Dannenberg, Jr., Y. Abe, J. Tsuruta, W. J. Su, W. Said, L. Feng, T. Yoshimura, P. J. Converse, and P. Mounts.** 1998. Nonspecific and immune-specific upregulation of cytokines in rabbit dermal tuberculous (BCG) lesions. *J. Leukoc. Biol.* 63:440–450.

228. **Sutherland, I., and I. Lindgren.** 1979. The protective effect of BCG vaccination as indicated by autopsy studies. *Tubercle* 60:225–231.

229. **Thompson, N. J., J. L. Glassroth, D. E. Snider, Jr., and L. S. Farer.** 1979. The booster phenomenon in serial tuberculin testing. *Am. Rev. Respir. Dis.* 119:587–597.

230. **Toossi, Z., P. Gogate, H. Shiratsuchi, T. Young, and J. J. Ellner.** 1995. Enhanced production of TGF-beta by blood monocytes from patients with active tuberculosis and presence of TGF-beta in tuberculous granulomatous lung lesions. *J. Immunol.* **154:**465–473.

231. **Toossi, Z., J. R. Sedor, J. P. Lapurga, R. J. Ondash, and J. J. Ellner.** 1990. Expression of functional interleukin 2 receptors by peripheral blood monocytes from patients with active pulmonary tuberculosis. *J. Clin. Investig.* **85:**1777–1784.

232. **Trinchieri, G.** 1997. Cytokines acting on or secreted by macrophages during intracellular infection (IL-10, IL-12, IFN-gamma). *Curr. Opin. Immunol.* **9:**17–23.

233. **Trinchieri, G.** 2003. Interleukin-12 and the regulation of innate resistance and adaptive immunity. *Nat. Rev. Immunol.* **3:**133–146.

234. **Tsenova, L., A. Bergtold, V. H. Freedman, R. A. Young, and G. Kaplan.** 1999. Tumor necrosis factor alpha is a determinant of pathogenesis and disease progression in mycobacterial infection in the central nervous system. *Proc. Natl. Acad. Sci. USA* **96:**5657–5662.

235. **Tsenova, L., K. Sokol, V. H. Freedman, and G. Kaplan.** 1998. A combination of thalidomide plus antibiotics protects rabbits from mycobacterial meningitis-associated death. *J. Infect. Dis.* **177:**1563–1572.

236. **Tsuruta, J., K. Sugisaki, A. M. Dannenberg, Jr., T. Yoshimura, Y. Abe, and P. Mounts.** 1996. The cytokines NAP-1 (IL-8), MCP-1, IL-1 beta, and GRO in rabbit inflammatory skin lesions produced by the chemical irritant sulfur mustard. *Inflammation* **20:**293–318.

237. **Tsuyuguchi, I.** 1996. Regulation of the human immune response in tuberculosis. *Infect. Agents Dis.* **5:**82–97.

238. **Turner, J., and H. M. Dockrell.** 1996. Stimulation of human peripheral blood mononuclear cells with live *Mycobacterium bovis* BCG activates cytolytic CD8+ T cells in vitro. *Immunology* **87:**339–342.

239. **Ueta, C., I. Tsuyuguchi, H. Kawasumi, T. Takashima, H. Toba, and S. Kishimoto.** 1994. Increase of gamma/delta T cells in hospital workers who are in close contact with tuberculosis patients. *Infect. Immun.* **62:**5434–5441.

240. **Vaddi, K., R. C. Newton, and M. Keller.** 1997. *The Chemokine Factsbook.* Academic Press, San Diego, CA.

240a. **Volkman, H. E., T. C. Pozos, J. Zheng, J. M. Davis, J. F. Rawls, and L. Ramakrishnan.** 2010. Tuberculosis granuloma induction via interaction of a bacterial secreted protein with host epithelium. *Science* **327:**466–469.

241. **Wahl, S. M., N. McCartney-Francis, D. A. Hunt, P. D. Smith, L. M. Wahl, and I. M. Katona.** 1987. Monocyte interleukin 2 receptor gene expression and interleukin 2 augmentation of microbicidal activity. *J. Immunol.* **139:**1342–1347.

242. **Walburger, A., A. Koul, G. Ferrari, L. Nguyen, C. Prescianotto-Baschong, K. Huygen, B. Klebl, C. Thompson, G. Bacher, and J. Pieters.** 2004. Protein kinase G from pathogenic mycobacteria promotes survival within macrophages. *Science* **304:**1800–1804.

243. **Wang, J., J. Wakeham, R. Harkness, and Z. Xing.** 1999. Macrophages are a significant source of type 1 cytokines during mycobacterial infection. *J. Clin. Investig.* **103:**1023–1029.

244. **Wilkinson, R. J., P. Patel, M. Llewelyn, C. S. Hirsch, G. Pasvol, G. Snounou, R. N. Davidson, and Z. Toossi.** 1999. Influence of polymorphism in the genes for the interleukin (IL)-1 receptor antagonist and IL-1β on tuberculosis. *J. Exp. Med.* **189:**1863–1874.

245. **Yamamura, Y.** 1958. The pathogenesis of tuberculous cavities. *Bibl. Tuberc.* **9:**13–37.

246. **Yamamura, Y., Y. Ogawa, H. Maeda, and Y. Yamamura.** 1974. Prevention of tuberculous cavity formation by desensitization with tuberculin-active peptide. *Am. Rev. Respir. Dis.* **109:**594–601.

247. **Yoder, M., G. Lamichhane, and W. Bishai.** 2004. Cavitary tuberculosis: the "Holey Grail" of disease transmission. *Curr. Sci.* **86:**74–81.

248. **Yoneda, T., and J. J. Ellner.** 1998. CD4+ T cell and natural killer cell-dependent killing of *Mycobacterium tuberculosis* by human monocytes. *Am. J. Respir. Crit. Care Med.* **158:**395–403.

249. **Young, D. B., and G. R. Stewart.** 2002. Tuberculosis vaccines. *Br. Med. Bull.* **62:**73–86.

250. **Zenaro, E., M. Donini, and S. Dusi.** 2009. Induction of Th1/Th17 immune response by *Mycobacterium tuberculosis*: role of dectin-1, mannose receptor, and DC-SIGN. *J. Leukoc. Biol.* **86:**1393–1401.

Tuberculosis and Nontuberculous Mycobacterial Infections, 6th ed.
Edited by David Schlossberg
© 2011 ASM Press, Washington, DC

Chapter 4

Laboratory Diagnosis and Susceptibility Testing

GARY W. PROCOP AND GLENN D. ROBERTS

INTRODUCTION

Clinical microbiology laboratories currently have a number of methods available that will provide for an accurate and rapid laboratory diagnosis of tuberculosis. Molecular methods are now part of the diagnostic algorithm in many laboratories and have dramatically shortened the time to diagnosis. However, the sensitivity of all methods is dependent on the selection and collection of an appropriate clinical specimen source. It is important for the clinician to request the specimen(s) that will most likely contain *Mycobacterium tuberculosis only when the patient is actually suspected to have active tuberculosis*; this ensures that the laboratory has the best opportunity to detect and identify this important microorganism and increases the sensitivity and positive predictive value of testing methods, especially molecular assays. The control of tuberculosis is dependent on a number of factors; the laboratory plays an important role in making a definitive diagnosis in as short a time as possible, thereby often setting into motion a series of infection control activities that will help diminish the spread of disease.

SPECIMEN COLLECTION

The specimens submitted for mycobacterial culture include a wide variety of body fluids, as well as tissues from sundry locations. When pulmonary tuberculosis is suspected, the most common specimen submitted for culture is sputum. Collection in the early morning is preferable, and patients should be instructed to expectorate a deep respiratory specimen with no nasal secretions or saliva. Ideally, the sputum should be obtained on three consecutive days. Sample volumes of 5 to 10 ml are appropriate. Specimens with less volume should be processed and a notation made on the report that a "less than optimal amount of specimen was submitted." Sample collection with swabs should be discouraged because the amount of material collected is limited and negative culture results may be misleading (i.e., the negative predictive value is low in such instances). For patients who are unable to produce sputum, hypertonic saline (5 to 15%) can be nebulized for induction. When nebulization is ineffective or an immediate diagnosis is needed, bronchoscopy with a bronchoalveolar lavage is the next best choice, because these procedures provide additional material for study (washings and brushing and biopsy specimens), which can help obtain a rapid diagnosis of tuberculosis. Pooled respiratory tract specimens are unacceptable due to bacterial overgrowth and contamination.

For children and some adult patients who are unable to expectorate sputum, gastric lavage provides a specimen of alternative choice, although it may not be as good as induced sputum for culturing (43). These specimens should be processed within 4 h, because the gastric acidity is potentially harmful to the mycobacteria. If rapid processing is not possible, gastric aspirates must be neutralized with sodium carbonate or another buffer salt to a pH of 7.0.

The diagnosis of renal tuberculosis is made by culturing three to five first morning midstream urine specimens. A pooled urine specimen is inappropriate because pooling increases bacterial contamination and decreases the recovery rate for mycobacteria.

Mycobacterial culture of stool specimens may be of value in intestinal tuberculosis cases, but these are rare. This type of culture has been requested to detect *Mycobacterium avium-M. intracellulare* infections in patients with AIDS; however, given that intestinal involvement with *M. avium-M. intracellulare* is thought to be a component of disseminated disease, a blood culture for mycobacteria is the specimen of choice in this setting.

Gary W. Procop • Cleveland Clinic, 9500 Euclid Avenue, Clinical Pathology/L40, Cleveland, OH 44195.
Glenn D. Roberts • Mayo Clinic and Mayo Clinic College of Medicine, 200 First Street Southwest, Rochester, MN 55905.

If extrapulmonary tuberculosis is suspected, several specimen sources may be cultured, including blood, cerebrospinal fluid, pleural fluid, pericardial fluid, peritoneal fluid, aspirates, joint fluids, and/or biopsy tissues such as synovial or pleural specimens, lymph nodes, liver, and bone marrow.

Generally, all the specimens should be collected in clean, sterile containers and transported to the laboratory in a rapid manner. Specimens must be refrigerated if they cannot be processed immediately; this prevents overgrowth by other bacteria. Specimens should be collected before antimycobacterial chemotherapy is initiated; even a few days of therapy may obscure the diagnosis because of the failure to recover mycobacteria.

DECONTAMINATION AND PROCESSING OF SPECIMENS

Some species of mycobacteria are slow growing and have an extended generation time (20 to 22 h) compared with that of common members of the bacterial microbiota (40 to 60 min); overgrowth of cultures by other bacteria and fungi can occur in specimens obtained from nonsterile sources. The high lipid content of the cell wall makes mycobacteria more resistant to strong acids and alkalis than other bacteria. This property has been used to develop decontamination procedures to eliminate common members of the bacterial microbiota while ensuring the mycobacterial viability. Specimens that require decontamination include sputum, urine, and bronchial and gastric aspirates, among others.

A number of alkaline digestion-decontamination solutions are commonly used for eliminating bacteria from contaminated specimens. Benzalkonium (Zephiran) chloride with trisodium phosphate or 4% NaOH is usually effective in reducing contamination. If specimens are transported promptly, N-acetyl-L-cysteine—2% NaOH is a suitable alternative. Excessive amounts of mucus may interfere with centrifugation-concentration procedures. Dithiothreitol (Sputolysin; Calbiochem, La Jolla, CA) or N-acetyl-L-cysteine should be added to the alkali solution as a mucolytic agent. A refrigerated centrifuge and a speed of at least 3000 × g are necessary to counteract the buoyant quality of the cell wall lipids and to permit optimal sedimentation and concentration of mycobacteria (45). All liquid specimens should be centrifuged prior to culturing. If the sterility of the specimen is in question, aliquots of the specimen should be cultured onto bacteriological media and incubated prior to culturing for mycobacteria.

CULTURE OF MYCOBACTERIA

Solid Media

The growth requirements of mycobacteria on artificial media include simple compounds such as potassium, magnesium, phosphorus, and sulfur. Ammonium salts or egg ingredients provide a nitrogen source, and glucose or glycerol supplies a carbon source. The optional pH range for growth is 6.5 to 7.0. Although mycobacteria are strict aerobes, a CO_2 concentration between 5 and 10% is necessary for their primary recovery on solid media. The incubation conditions should include high humidity and a temperature of 35 to 37°C for noncutaneous sources.

Traditional mycobacterial culture media include egg-based, agar-based, liquid, and selective media. Examples of egg-based media are Löwenstein-Jensen (L-J), Petragnani, and American Thoracic Society media. Of these, Petragnani medium is the most inhibitory to contaminating bacteria because of the high content of malachite green (an antibacterial agent). All are complex media and include whole eggs, potato flour, salts, glycerol, and malachite green. L-J is the most common egg-based medium used for primary culture. It has been noted that it has a lower recovery rate (40%) than 7H11 agar-based medium (81%), and therefore it is not recommended as a primary recovery medium for mycobacteria by some authors (57). Middlebrook 7H10 and 7H11 are well-defined agar-based media containing agar, organic compounds, salts, glycerol, and albumin. 7H11 also contains 0.1% casein hydrolysate, which is incorporated to improve the recovery rate and enhance the growth of mycobacteria that exhibit resistance to isoniazid. Selective media are made with the base media plus the addition of antimicrobials to inhibit contaminating bacteria that survived the decontamination procedure. Among them, L-J Gruft medium contains penicillin, nalidixic acid, and malachite green. Middlebrook selective 7H11 (S7H11) contains carbenicillin, polymyxin B, trimethoprim lactate, amphotericin B, and malachite green.

After processing, 0.25 ml of the sediment from the decontaminated specimen is inoculated onto the surface of solid media contained in tubes, 0.5 ml is inoculated onto the media contained in culture plates, or both. The caps on media in tubes should be left slightly loose to provide adequate aeration of the culture. Culture plates should be placed in CO_2-permeable polyethylene plastic bags and sealed by heat pressure. All media should be incubated for up to 8 weeks at 35°C; the first 3 to 4 weeks of incubation should be in an atmosphere of 5 to 10% CO_2.

Specimens yielding positive acid-fast smears and negative cultures for mycobacteria after 8 weeks of incubation on solid media should be incubated for an additional 8 weeks. Young cultures (0 to 4 weeks old) should be examined twice weekly for visible evidence of growth. Older cultures (4 to 8 weeks old) should be examined at least once weekly. When colonies resembling mycobacteria are observed, an acid-fast smear and subculture for identification and susceptibility testing should be made. Nucleic acid probe testing or another comparable molecular method of identification can be performed on colonies as soon as they appear, and the definitive identification can be made if results are consistent with *Mycobacterium tuberculosis* complex (*M. tuberculosis*, *M. bovis*, *M. bovis* BCG, *M. africanum*, *M. microti*, and "*M. canetti*").

Broth Media

The MGIT tube system (Becton Dickinson, Sparks, MD) contains a 7H9-based medium with enrichment, antibiotics, and an oxygen-labile fluorescent indicator at the bottom of each tube. As mycobacteria grow and use oxygen, the indicator compound is excited, and the resulting fluorescence can be visually examined with a UV source. It was designed to replace the BACTEC 460 TB system to eliminate the use of ^{14}C. The MGIT system is automated and continuously monitors tubes inoculated with clinical specimens for evidence of growth. It is now a suitable alternative to the BACTEC 460. However, published results vary in their conclusions as to recovery rates and times for *M. tuberculosis*. Recovery rates of 91.5% (48), 88% (15), and 88% (54) for the MGIT system are reported, compared to 95.7% (48), 90% (15), and 90.5% (54) for the BACTEC 460 TB system. The reading times are different for the two systems, and the MGIT 960 is read more often. Recovery times for the MGIT 960 ranged from 12.5 to 13.4 days for acid-fast smear-positive and -negative specimens, respectively (48), while others reported recovery times of 12.5 and 19.6 days for smear-positive and -negative specimens (54). The MGIT 960 has a higher contamination rate ($\geq 10\%$) than does the BACTEC 460 TB system, which could result in a decrease in the rate of recovery by this system. One advantage for the MGIT 960 is that DNA probe identification and antibiotic susceptibility testing can be performed from broth tubes.

Currently, in addition to the BACTEC MGIT 960 TB system, other commercial systems are available. They have been evaluated for their ability to recover mycobacteria from clinical specimens and determine the antimicrobial susceptibility or resistance profile of an organism. All appear to be suitable alternatives

to the BACTEC 460 TB system, which was the prior "gold standard" but is no longer available.

The VersaTREK Myco system for mycobacterial recovery and susceptibility testing is the newer name for the ESP Myco system (Trek Diagnostic Systems, Cleveland, OH) and consists of a bottle containing a modification of Middlebrook 7H9 broth and oleic acid-albumin-dextrose-catalase enrichment in addition to the automated hardware. Bottles contain the medium and a cellulose sponge, which is thought to increase the surface area for growth, reminiscent of the airspaces of the human lung. Each bottle is supplemented with an antibiotic mixture used to prevent bacterial contamination. The VersaTREK Myco system is automated and measures a change in oxygen consumption as growth occurs.

Only limited retrospective data are available for the VersaTREK Myco system compared to the MGIT 960 system. Basically, the two systems, when used with a solid medium, were equivalent for the recovery of *M. tuberculosis*; any difference was slight. The time to detection for *M. tuberculosis* using the VersaTREK was 17.5 days, compared to 13.3 days for the MGIT 960 system (K. Chapin and L. Binns, presented at the 108th General Meeting of the American Society for Microbiology, Boston, MA, 1 to 5 June 2008). However, the number of isolates of *M. tuberculosis* compared was relatively small, and other studies will provide more definitive data in the future.

The BacT/Alert MP (bioMérieux, Durham, NC) uses bottles containing modified Middlebrook 7H9 medium and growth factors. Numerous studies have shown that the BacT/Alert MP system for the recovery of mycobacteria is satisfactory but should be used in combination with a solid medium, which is true for all of the automated systems. Recovery rates for *M. tuberculosis* were 98.7% (34), 96.7% (33), and 91.3% (42) for the BacT/Alert MP in three studies. Recovery rates for the BACTEC 460 were 89.8, 96.7, and 90.0%, respectively, by comparison. The mean recovery times for the BacT/Alert MP were 11.6 and 17.8 days for acid-fast smear-positive and -negative specimens, respectively.

STAINING PROCEDURES AND BIOCHEMICAL IDENTIFICATION

Staining followed by microscopic observation is applied to both direct smear examinations of patient specimens and organisms growing from the culture. If an organism is present in sufficient numbers, this is the most rapid procedure for the detection of mycobacteria in clinical samples. It has been estimated that at least 10^5 organisms/ml of sputum must be present to be detected by staining of a smear, and the sensitivity of the smear is related to the type of infection (i.e., advanced cavitary disease), relative centrifugal force used to concentrate the specimen, and other factors. Overall, the acid-fast smear used with clinical specimens is not an adequate diagnostic tool to exclude an infection caused by mycobacteria (i.e., there are smear-negative but culture-positive specimens). Furthermore, it does not provide information concerning the identification or viability of the organism, since all species of mycobacteria are acid fast.

Two procedures are commonly used for acid-fast staining: carbol fuchsin methods, including the Ziehl-Neelsen and Kinyoun procedures, and a fluorochrome method using auramine O or auramine-rhodamine dye.

The Ziehl-Neelsen and Kinyoun staining procedures differ in their staining principles. The former procedure requires heating the carbol fuchsin to penetrate the mycobacterial cell wall. The latter is a "cold" staining method using an increased amount of phenol in the solution to enhance penetration of the cell wall. Both methods stain the mycobacterial cells red against a methylene blue counterstain. The stained smears must be viewed using a 100× oil immersion objective.

Auramine O-stained mycobacteria are bright yellow against a dark background and are easily visualized using a 25× objective. Modification of the auramine O technique includes the use of rhodamine, which gives a golden appearance to the cells. Auramine-rhodamine is the method of choice for clinical specimens, including tissue sections, when trying to detect mycobacteria.

Fluorochrome staining has the advantage of being more sensitive than carbol fuchsin techniques. Fluorochrome-stained smears can be scanned using a 25× objective, whereas an oil immersion objective is required for viewing smears stained with carbol fuchsin. A disadvantage of all these different staining methods is the indiscriminate staining of nonviable organisms. Therefore, mycobacteria rendered nonviable by chemotherapy may be stained. It has been noticed that blood present in the sputum can sometimes cause false-positive auramine stains. In addition, variable staining of Mycobacterium fortuitum and possibly other rapidly growing mycobacteria occurs. Because of the ease of reading, it is recommended that a fluorochrome staining method of detecting acid-fast bacilli (AFB) in clinical specimens be used. If desired, a carbol fuchsin procedure may then be employed to confirm questionable fluorochrome results. It is also necessary to perform a culture. Clinicians should be aware that a negative smear does not exclude the possibility of an infection caused by a Mycobacterium sp.

In addition, the presence of mycobacteria as seen on direct examination does not establish the specific diagnosis of tuberculosis, since nontuberculous mycobacteria stain virtually indistinguishably. Also, weakly decolorized acid-fast stains sometimes yield positive results (i.e., the organism appears "acid-fast") with nonmycobacteria such as Rhodococcus, Nocardia, Legionella micdadei, and the cysts of Cryptosporidium, Cystoisospora (Isospora), and Cyclospora.

Traditionally, the identification of M. tuberculosis complex has relied on acid fastness, niacin production, nitrate reduction, and inactivation of catalase at 68°C. Generally, the recovery time for M. tuberculosis complex varies; on solid media, colonies can be observed in as short a time as 12 days or as long as 4 to 6 weeks, with an average of about 3 to 4 weeks. The colonies are rough, "cauliflower-like," and colorless. Unlike most mycobacterial species, M. tuberculosis complex lacks the enzyme to convert free niacin to niacin ribonucleotide, and niacin accumulates in the medium, resulting in a positive niacin test result. Mycobacterium tuberculosis complex possesses nitroreductase and yields a positive result using nitrate reduction testing. Among mycobacteria, the quantity of catalase produced and its stability at 68°C are species dependent. Mycobacterium tuberculosis complex produces a column measuring less than 50 mm in the quantitative catalase production test performed with L-J medium. This organism also produces a heat-labile catalase that is inactivated after 20 min of exposure to 68°C (32).

MOLECULAR METHODS FOR DETECTION OF M. TUBERCULOSIS COMPLEX

Identification by Nucleic Acid Probe

Since the beginning of the 1990s, nucleic acid probes have been used for the identification of mycobacteria. At present, these commercially available probes (AccuProbe; Gen-Probe, Inc., San Diego, CA) can identify M. tuberculosis complex, Mycobacterium kansasii, Mycobacterium avium-M. intracellulare, and Mycobacterium gordonae. After lysis of mycobacterial cells, an acridinium ester-labeled, single-stranded DNA probe hybridizes with the rRNA of the target organism and forms a stable DNA-rRNA hybrid. After chemically degrading the unhybridized DNA-acridinium ester probes, the acridinium present on the DNA-rRNA hybrid is detected when chemiluminescence of the acridinium ester is measured in a luminometer.

The M. tuberculosis complex nonisotopic probe has demonstrated sensitivity and specificity of 100% compared with its isotopic predecessor (24).

The procedure is quick and can be finished in 1 h. Originally, this probe test was designed to be used for culture confirmation of organisms growing on solid media. However, this test has successfully used broth culture, such as the BACTEC 12B medium and MGIT system (2, 18, 35). Mycobacteria growing in the culture broth vials are concentrated by centrifugation, lysed, and subjected to nucleic acid probe hybridization, as previously described. The combination of nucleic acid probe identification and BACTEC 12B culture system makes the *M. tuberculosis* complex culture times and reporting times as short as 15.5 days (50) or 16.4 to 10 days (17), depending on the study. The only drawback reported is the possibility of false-positive reactions caused by members of the *M. terrae* complex and *M. celatum* (9, 19). However, this problem can be eliminated by extending the selection time to 8 to 10 min. Clinical laboratories may use the nucleic acid probes alone or in combination with other identification methods (7, 27), including nucleic acid sequencing (25, 56).

Nucleic Acid Amplification, Postamplification Analysis, and Typing

Because of the slow-growing nature of *M. tuberculosis* complex, prompt detection and identification have been a challenge for clinical microbiology laboratories. Extensive studies have shown that molecular diagnostics are a good solution to the problem (12, 29).

These methods include *M. tuberculosis* complex-specific nucleic acid amplification systems, as well as broad-range mycobacterial amplification assays that are followed by some type of postamplification analysis, such as DNA sequencing or microarray hybridization. Genes that encode rRNA or RNA polymerase are commonly used genetic targets. Although many laboratory-developed tests reported in the literature hold promise, commercial tests have also demonstrated good performance. The newer, rapid-cycle PCR systems have less chance of carryover contamination, are more amenable to quantification, and provide very high specificity, and some are capable of being automated (47, 49).

The FDA-approved assays include the Amplified *Mycobacterium tuberculosis* Direct (AMTD) test by Gen-Probe and the Amplicor *M. tuberculosis* test by Roche Diagnostic Systems (Branchburg, NJ). The AMTD test is approved for use with both acid-fast smear-positive and -negative respiratory tract specimens, whereas the Amplicor assay is approved only for smear-positive respiratory specimens.

The AMTD test uses a transcription-mediated amplification system. It is an isothermal test and uses a single temperature during the amplification step. The target is the 16S RNA. After the nucleic acids are released from mycobacterial cells by sonication, specimens are heated to disrupt the secondary structure of the rRNA. At a constant 42°C temperature, the reaction generates multiple copies of the mycobacterial RNA. The *M. tuberculosis* complex-specific sequences are then detected by the Gen-Probe chemiluminescence-labeled DNA probes, and results are measured in a luminometer. The test has several advantages: it detects rRNA, which theoretically exists in concentrations several thousandfold more than that found in genomic DNA of the organism, so the sensitivity is high, and it uses a single temperature and a single-tube format, which makes the test easier to perform and contamination less likely to occur. Specimens for testing should be obtained from untreated patients. It has been shown that the test result can remain positive after cultures become negative during therapy (36). The usefulness of the system on nonrespiratory specimens has been studied by different investigators. Specimens included urine, feces, tissue, pleural exudates, cerebrospinal fluids, ascitic fluid, and bone marrow. Generally, the specificity was high (97.7 to 100%), whereas the sensitivity was greater than or equal to 83.9% (17, 20, 39). Users of the AMTD test should be aware that a false-positive test, although rare, may occur for patients infected with *Mycobacterium celatum* (13, 51). A useful and informative review of the AMTD test is presented by Piersimoni and Scarparo (41).

The Roche Amplicor *M. tuberculosis* test is a PCR-based assay. Instead of detecting rRNA, it detects the rRNA gene in the genome (DNA). After amplification using biotinylated oligonucleotide primers, the products are hybridized with a specific probe that is bound to a microwell plate. The avidin-horseradish peroxidase conjugate and the substrates are then added for color development. The kit is approved for use with acid-fast, smear-positive respiratory specimens. Bergmann and Woods evaluated the method using 956 respiratory tract specimens from 502 patients and compared results with those of the culture and the medical history (6). They found that although the specificity was very high (99.5 to 100%), the sensitivities were 97.6 and 40% for AFB smear-positive and -negative specimens, respectively. The results reported by Bennedsen et al. in 1996 were similar, with sensitivities of 91.4 and 60.9% for AFB smear-positive and -negative specimens, respectively (5). Even for those culture-positive, smear-negative samples, the sensitivity of this test is reported as 46% (10). So far, smear-positive samples are optimal and the method is not recommended for use with nonrespiratory specimens (28). Therefore, although the AMTD test and

Amplicor *M. tuberculosis* tests use different amplification techniques and are manufactured by different companies, both methods are rapid and specific. The sensitivity of the AMTD test is similar to or slightly greater than that of the Amplicor test (40). There have been numerous reports on the use of the Amplicor *M. tuberculosis* test for detection and identification of *M. tuberculosis* in BACTEC 12B and ESP II broth cultures. A comprehensive review of the performance of this test is presented by Piersimoni and Scarparo (41).

It should be mentioned that although these nucleic acid amplification methods provide rapid results, mycobacterial cultures are still required. Cultures are essential to exclude the possibility of mixed infections, which exist although are rare; in some instances, for further characterization or identification (most amplification tests give results only at the *M. tuberculosis* complex level); and, most importantly, for complete antimicrobial susceptibility testing. Furthermore, an international survey that evaluated the reliability and performance of nucleic acid amplification for the detection of *M. tuberculosis* complex showed that among the 30 laboratories in 18 countries using different tests (including both in-house and commercial kits), only 5 laboratories were able to identify correctly the presence or absence of mycobacterial nucleic acid in all 20 samples distributed (38). These results emphasize the variation of tests and results from laboratory to laboratory and the need for good laboratory practice. Hundreds of "laboratory-developed" assays including real-time PCR (16, 31) are mentioned in the literature, most of which have not been compared.

In general, amplified tests currently are not "stand-alone" tests. They must still be used in conjunction with conventional cultures. When the specimen volume is an issue, conventional cultures are preferred over amplified tests. To date, these methods are not commonly used to detect *M. tuberculosis* in paraffin block sections, but this is possible when there is an appropriate quantity of organism in the specimen. These tests are expensive, which must be considered when they are ordered, given the current state of limited health care resources. The American Thoracic Society provided a statement in 1997 on the specific uses for these tests, and the information is still relevant today (11). When used on properly selected patients and on appropriate specimens, the FDA-approved nucleic acid amplified tests for the detection of *M. tuberculosis* can be powerful diagnostic tools that can have a great impact on patient care and the control of tuberculosis.

Guidance is provided in the updated guidelines for the use of nucleic acid amplification tests in the diagnosis of tuberculosis from the Centers for Disease Control and Prevention (12). These guidelines state that nucleic acid amplification tests should be performed on at least one respiratory specimen from each patient with signs and symptoms of pulmonary tuberculosis *for whom the diagnosis of tuberculosis is being considered but is not yet established*. They also state that testing should be performed for those for *whom the test result would alter case management or tuberculosis control activities, such as contact investigations*. These recommendations are excellent guidelines which should work to both optimize the clinical impact of these tests and reduce unnecessary testing and costs; a complete review of this document is recommended to those interested in this matter (12).

Broad-range PCR assays are different from species-specific PCR assays in that they amplify nucleic acid from an entire group of organisms. A broad-range PCR assay for mycobacteria will amplify DNA from all members of the genus. The amplified product can then be differentiated by various methods of postamplification analysis, which include probe hybridization, reverse hybridization, traditional sequencing, pyrosequencing, and microarray analysis, among others (44, 49, 55). In addition to using these technologies to determine the identity of the microorganism present, these may also be used in associated with PCR to determine the presence of genetic variations that encode drug resistance (1).

Postamplification analysis may also be used for a variety of microbial typing methods. In general, typing methods evaluate the presence, absence, or differences between genetic elements of microorganisms of the same species that are being compared. The comparison may denote that the strains are distinguishable (i.e., different from one another) or indistinguishable (i.e., cannot be proven to be different based on the genetic elements studied). Demonstrating that strains are indistinguishable does not necessarily prove that the strains are definitively derived from the same parent strain but is supportive evidence of that possibility. A variety of methods have been used to type strains of the *M. tuberculosis* complex, but the method most commonly used is spoligotyping. This method uses PCR to amplify a polymorphic direct repeat locus in the genome of *M. tuberculosis* (22, 23). The amplified products differ in size and sequence content, so they may be separated by gel electrophoresis or probe/microarray analysis. Although the former is the standard of practice, the liquid microarray application appears to be an easy-to-perform alternative which may provide quicker times to results (14). Prior to the development of spoligotyping, restriction fragment length polymorphism, with the IS*6110* insertion element used as a probe, was the most commonly used method to type *M. tuberculosis* (22, 23).

ANTIMICROBIAL SUSCEPTIBILITY TESTING OF *M. TUBERCULOSIS* COMPLEX (see also chapter 8)

The reemergence of *M. tuberculosis* complex as a cause of disease and the increasing percentage of cases with drug resistance have made antimicrobial susceptibility testing more important (26). Susceptibility tests should be performed on all isolates of *M. tuberculosis* complex recovered from previously untreated patients and also on isolates from patients on therapy who have positive acid-fast smears or cultures after 2 months of treatment. Patients at increased risk for drug resistance also include those with a history of treatment failure for tuberculosis, contacts of patients with resistant tuberculosis, and residents of high-prevalence areas, including countries outside of the United States.

The traditional susceptibility test method is a 1% agar proportion method. Resistance is defined as mycobacteria with greater than 1% of the population exhibiting growth in the presence of the critical concentration of drug tested. Based on clinical experience, a correlate has been found between the 1% resistance in vitro to in vivo chemotherapeutic failure. Organisms are inoculated onto 7H10 or 7H11 agar plates containing the various antibiotic concentrations and incubated; results may be obtained after 14 to 21 days.

Subsequently, the BACTEC 460 TB system was used to obtain results much earlier. In this assay, an organism was inoculated into BACTEC 12B bottles that contained antimicrobials, and the susceptibility was detected by failure of the test organism to produce $^{14}CO_2$ in the presence of an antibiotic. This method not only correlates well with the 1% proportion method (90 to 100% agreement) but also significantly shortened the turnaround time of antibiotic susceptibility testing (4 to 7 days, compared with 14 to 21 days) (46). Antimicrobials available for testing include the primary drugs, which are streptomycin, isoniazid, rifampin, ethambutol, and pyrazinamide, and the secondary drugs, which include capreomycin, ethionamide, amikacin, levofloxacin, ofloxacin, *p*-aminosalicylic acid, and streptomycin.

Three commercially available, broth-based automated systems can also perform antimycobacterial susceptibility testing (3, 4, 30, 53). The Clinical and Laboratory Standards Institute document *Susceptibility Testing of Mycobacteria, Nocardiae, and Other Aerobic Actinomycetes* (approved standard M-24A, 2nd ed.) indicates that the MGIT 960, BacT/AlertMP, and VersaTREK systems have been approved by the FDA for use in susceptibility testing (58). It appears that all automated systems are suitable alternatives to the now infrequently used BACTEC 460 TB system for susceptibility testing of *M. tuberculosis* complex.

The molecular mechanisms of drug resistance for many of the more important antimycobacterial agents have been elucidated (8, 21, 37). The molecular detection of some of these key determinants of resistance offers promise because this can potentially shorten the time to detection of resistance from weeks to days and may be subject to automation. One of the more thoroughly studied targets for drug resistance to rifampin is *rpoB*, which encodes the β-subunit of RNA polymerase; *katG*, *inhA*, *imabA*, and *ahpC* are genes associated with isoniazid resistance. A real-time PCR assay has been developed to detect important mutations in the *inhA* and *rpoB* genes associated with resistance (52). The characterization of genes important in resistance to antimycobacterial agents is currently most thoroughly accomplished by traditional Sanger sequencing. These genetic indicators of resistance may, however, be detected through pyrosequencing or microarray analysis, among other techniques. The markers of resistance to other drugs, including streptomycin (*rpsL* and *rrs*), ethambutol (*embCAB*), and fluoroquinolones (*gyrA*), have also been studied. Although the advantages of genetic testing of antibiotic susceptibility are obvious, it is unlikely that the conventional methods will soon be fully replaced. The clinical correlation of genetic testing to clinical treatment outcomes must still be determined before this testing is routinely used. To date, there are no FDA-approved molecular assays for the detection of resistance to antimycobacterial agents.

REFERENCES

1. Abdelaal, A., H. A. El-Ghaffar, M. H. Zaghloul, N. El Mashad, E. Badran, and A. Fathy. 2009. Genotypic detection of rifampicin and isoniazid resistant *Mycobacterium tuberculosis* strains by DNA sequencing: a randomized trial. *Ann. Clin. Microbiol. Antimicrob.* 8:4.
2. Alcaide, F., M. A. Benitez, J. M. Escriba, and R. Martin. 2000. Evaluation of the BACTEC MGIT 960 and the MB/BacT systems for recovery of mycobacteria from clinical specimens and for species identification by DNA AccuProbe. *J. Clin. Microbiol.* 38:398–401.
3. Angeby, K. A., J. Werngren, J. C. Toro, G. Hedstrom, B. Petrini, and S. E. Hoffner. 2003. Evaluation of the BacT/ALERT 3D system for recovery and drug susceptibility testing of *Mycobacterium tuberculosis*. *Clin. Microbiol. Infect.* 9:1148–1152.
4. Bemer, P., T. Bodmer, J. Munzinger, M. Perrin, V. Vincent, and H. Drugeon. 2004. Multicenter evaluation of the MB/BACT system for susceptibility testing of *Mycobacterium tuberculosis*. *J. Clin. Microbiol.* 42:1030–1034.
5. Bennedsen, J., V. O. Thomsen, G. E. Pfyffer, G. Funke, K. Feldmann, A. Beneke, P. A. Jenkins, M. Hegginbothom, A. Fahr, M. Hengstler, G. Cleator, P. Klapper, and E. G. Wilkins. 1996. Utility of PCR in diagnosing pulmonary tuberculosis. *J. Clin. Microbiol.* 34:1407–1411.

6. **Bergmann, J. S., and G. L. Woods.** 1996. Clinical evaluation of the Roche AMPLICOR PCR *Mycobacterium tuberculosis* test for detection of *M. tuberculosis* in respiratory specimens. *J. Clin. Microbiol.* **34:**1083–1085.

7. **Bird, B. R., M. M. Denniston, R. E. Huebner, and R. C. Good.** 1996. Changing practices in mycobacteriology: a follow-up survey of state and territorial public health laboratories. *J. Clin. Microbiol.* **34:**554–559.

8. **Blanchard, J. S.** 1996. Molecular mechanisms of drug resistance in *Mycobacterium tuberculosis. Annu. Rev. Biochem.* **65:**215–239.

9. **Butler, W. R., S. P. O'Connor, M. A. Yakrus, and W. M. Gross.** 1994. Cross-reactivity of genetic probe for detection of *Mycobacterium tuberculosis* with newly described species *Mycobacterium celatum. J. Clin. Microbiol.* **32:**536–538.

10. **Cartuyvels, R., C. De Ridder, S. Jonckheere, L. Verbist, and J. Van Eldere.** 1996. Prospective clinical evaluation of Amplicor *Mycobacterium tuberculosis* PCR test as a screening method in a low-prevalence population. *J. Clin. Microbiol.* **34:**2001–2003.

11. **Catanzaro, A., B. Davidson, P. Fujiwara, M. Goldberger, F. Gordin, M. Salfinger, J. Sbarbaro, N. Schluger, M. Sierra, and G. Woods.** 1997. Rapid diagnostic tests for tuberculosis. *Am. J. Respir. Crit. Care Med.* **155:**1804–1814.

12. **Centers for Disease Control and Prevention.** 2009. Updated guidelines for the use of nucleic acid amplification tests in the diagnosis of tuberculosis. *MMWR Morb. Mortal. Wkly. Rep.* **58:**7–10.

13. **Christiansen, D. C., G. D. Roberts, and R. Patel.** 2004. *Mycobacterium celatum*, an emerging pathogen and cause of false positive amplified *Mycobacterium tuberculosis* direct test. *Diagn. Microbiol. Infect. Dis.* **49:**19–24.

14. **Cowan, L. S., L. Diem, M. C. Brake, and J. T. Crawford.** 2004. Transfer of a *Mycobacterium tuberculosis* genotyping method, Spoligotyping, from a reverse line-blot hybridization, membrane-based assay to the Luminex multianalyte profiling system. *J. Clin. Microbiol.* **42:**474–477.

15. **Cruciani, M., C. Scarparo, M. Malena, O. Bosco, G. Serpelloni, and C. Mengoli.** 2004. Meta-analysis of BACTEC MGIT 960 and BACTEC 460 TB, with or without solid media, for detection of mycobacteria. *J. Clin. Microbiol.* **42:**2321–2325.

16. **Drosten, C., M. Panning, and S. Kramme.** 2003. Detection of *Mycobacterium tuberculosis* by real-time PCR using pan-mycobacterial primers and a pair of fluorescence resonance energy transfer probes specific for the *M. tuberculosis* complex. *Clin. Chem.* **49:**1659–1661.

17. **Ellner, P. D., T. E. Kiehn, R. Cammarata, and M. Hosmer.** 1988. Rapid detection and identification of pathogenic mycobacteria by combining radiometric and nucleic acid probe methods. *J. Clin. Microbiol.* **26:**1349–1352.

18. **Evans, K. D., A. S. Nakasone, P. A. Sutherland, L. M. de la Maza, and E. M. Peterson.** 1992. Identification of *Mycobacterium tuberculosis* and *Mycobacterium avium-M. intracellulare* directly from primary BACTEC cultures by using acridinium-ester-labeled DNA probes. *J. Clin. Microbiol.* **30:**2427–2431.

19. **Ford, E. G., S. J. Snead, J. Todd, and N. G. Warren.** 1993. Strains of *Mycobacterium terrae* complex which react with DNA probes for *M. tuberculosis* complex. *J. Clin. Microbiol.* **31:**2805–2806.

20. **Gamboa, F., J. M. Manterola, B. Vinado, L. Matas, M. Gimenez, J. Lonca, J. R. Manzano, C. Rodrigo, P. J. Cardona, E. Padilla, J. Dominguez, and V. Ausina.** 1997. Direct detection of *Mycobacterium tuberculosis* complex in nonrespiratory specimens by Gen-Probe Amplified Mycobacterium Tuberculosis Direct Test. *J. Clin. Microbiol.* **35:**307–310.

21. **Garcia de Viedma, D.** 2003. Rapid detection of resistance in *Mycobacterium tuberculosis*: a review discussing molecular approaches. *Clin. Microbiol. Infect.* **9:**349–359.

22. **Gori, A., A. Bandera, G. Marchetti, A. Degli Esposti, L. Catozzi, G. P. Nardi, L. Gazzola, G. Ferrario, J. D. van Embden, D. van Soolingen, M. Moroni, and F. Franzetti.** 2005. Spoligotyping and *Mycobacterium tuberculosis. Emerg. Infect. Dis.* **11:**1242–1248.

23. **Gori, A., A. D. Esposti, A. Bandera, M. Mezzetti, C. Sola, G. Marchetti, G. Ferrario, F. Salerno, M. Goyal, R. Diaz, L. Gazzola, L. Codecasa, V. Penati, N. Rastogi, M. Moroni, and F. Franzetti.** 2005. Comparison between spoligotyping and IS*6110* restriction fragment length polymorphisms in molecular genotyping analysis of *Mycobacterium tuberculosis* strains. *Mol. Cell. Probes* **19:**236–244.

24. **Goto, M., S. Oka, K. Okuzumi, S. Kimura, and K. Shimada.** 1991. Evaluation of acridinium-ester-labeled DNA probes for identification of *Mycobacterium tuberculosis* and *Mycobacterium avium-Mycobacterium intracellulare* complex in culture. *J. Clin. Microbiol.* **29:**2473–2476.

25. **Hall, L., K. A. Doerr, S. L. Wohlfiel, and G. D. Roberts.** 2003. Evaluation of the MicroSeq system for identification of mycobacteria by 16S ribosomal DNA sequencing and its integration into a routine clinical mycobacteriology laboratory. *J. Clin. Microbiol.* **41:**1447–1453.

26. **Heifets, L. B.** 1996. Clinical mycobacteriology. Drug susceptibility testing. *Clin. Lab. Med.* **16:**641–656.

27. **Herold, C. D., R. L. Fitzgerald, and D. A. Herold.** 1996. Current techniques in mycobacterial detection and speciation. *Crit. Rev. Clin. Lab. Sci.* **33:**83–138.

28. **Huang, T. S., Y. C. Liu, H. H. Lin, W. K. Huang, and D. L. Cheng.** 1996. Comparison of the Roche AMPLICOR MYCOBACTERIUM assay and Digene SHARP Signal System with in-house PCR and culture for detection of *Mycobacterium tuberculosis* in respiratory specimens. *J. Clin. Microbiol.* **34:**3092–3096.

29. **Jonas, V., and M. Longiaru.** 1997. Detection of *Mycobacterium tuberculosis* by molecular methods. *Clin. Lab. Med.* **17:**119–128.

30. **Kontos, F., M. Maniati, C. Costopoulos, Z. Gitti, S. Nicolaou, E. Petinaki, S. Anagnostou, I. Tselentis, and A. N. Maniatis.** 2004. Evaluation of the fully automated Bactec MGIT 960 system for the susceptibility testing of *Mycobacterium tuberculosis* to first-line drugs: a multicenter study. *J. Microbiol. Methods* **56:**291–294.

31. **Kraus, G., T. Cleary, N. Miller, R. Seivright, A. K. Young, G. Spruill, and H. J. Hnatyszyn.** 2001. Rapid and specific detection of the *Mycobacterium tuberculosis* complex using fluorogenic probes and real-time PCR. *Mol. Cell. Probes* **15:**375–383.

32. **Kubica, G. P., and G. L. Pool.** 1960. Studies on the catalase activity of acid-fast bacilli. I. An attempt to subgroup these organisms on the basis of their catalase activities at different temperatures and pH. *Am. Rev. Respir. Dis.* **81:**387–391.

33. **Laverdiere, M., L. Poirier, K. Weiss, C. Beliveau, L. Bedard, and D. Desnoyers.** 2000. Comparative evaluation of the MB/BacT and BACTEC 460 TB systems for the detection of mycobacteria from clinical specimens: clinical relevance of higher recovery rates from broth-based detection systems. *Diagn. Microbiol. Infect. Dis.* **36:**1–5.

34. **Manterola, J. M., F. Gamboa, E. Padilla, J. Lonca, L. Matas, A. Hernandez, M. Gimenez, P. J. Cardona, B. Vinado, and V. Ausina.** 1998. Comparison of a nonradiometric system with Bactec 12B and culture on egg-based media for recovery of mycobacteria from clinical specimens. *Eur. J. Clin. Microbiol. Infect. Dis.* **17:**773–777.

35. Metchock, B., and L. Diem. 1995. Algorithm for use of nucleic acid probes for identifying *Mycobacterium tuberculosis* from BACTEC 12B bottles. *J. Clin. Microbiol.* **33**:1934–1937.

36. Moore, D. F., J. I. Curry, C. A. Knott, and V. Jonas. 1996. Amplification of rRNA for assessment of treatment response of pulmonary tuberculosis patients during antimicrobial therapy. *J. Clin. Microbiol.* **34**:1745–1749.

37. Musser, J. M. 1995. Antimicrobial agent resistance in mycobacteria: molecular genetic insights. *Clin. Microbiol. Rev.* **8**:496–514.

38. Noordhoek, G. T., J. D. van Embden, and A. H. Kolk. 1996. Reliability of nucleic acid amplification for detection of *Mycobacterium tuberculosis*: an international collaborative quality control study among 30 laboratories. *J. Clin. Microbiol.* **34**:2522–2525.

39. Pfyffer, G. E., P. Kissling, E. M. Jahn, H. M. Welscher, M. Salfinger, and R. Weber. 1996. Diagnostic performance of amplified *Mycobacterium tuberculosis* direct test with cerebrospinal fluid, other nonrespiratory, and respiratory specimens. *J. Clin. Microbiol.* **34**:834–841.

40. Piersimoni, C., A. Callegaro, D. Nista, S. Bornigia, F. De Conti, G. Santini, and G. De Sio. 1997. Comparative evaluation of two commercial amplification assays for direct detection of *Mycobacterium tuberculosis* complex in respiratory specimens. *J. Clin. Microbiol.* **35**:193–196.

41. Piersimoni, C., and C. Scarparo. 2003. Relevance of commercial amplification methods for direct detection of *Mycobacterium tuberculosis* complex in clinical samples. *J. Clin. Microbiol.* **41**:5355–5365.

42. Piersimoni, C., C. Scarparo, A. Callegaro, C. P. Tosi, D. Nista, S. Bornigia, M. Scagnelli, A. Rigon, G. Ruggiero, and A. Goglio. 2001. Comparison of MB/BacT ALERT 3D system with radiometric BACTEC system and Löwenstein-Jensen medium for recovery and identification of mycobacteria from clinical specimens: a multicenter study. *J. Clin. Microbiol.* **39**:651–657.

43. Pomputius, W. F., III, J. Rost, P. H. Dennehy, and E. J. Carter. 1997. Standardization of gastric aspirate technique improves yield in the diagnosis of tuberculosis in children. *Pediatr. Infect. Dis. J.* **16**:222–226.

44. Procop, G. W. 2007. Molecular diagnostics for the detection and characterization of microbial pathogens. *Clin. Infect. Dis.* **45**(Suppl. 2):S99–S111.

45. Rickman, T. W., and N. P. Moyer. 1980. Increased sensitivity of acid-fast smears. *J. Clin. Microbiol.* **11**:618–620.

46. Roberts, G. D., N. L. Goodman, L. Heifets, H. W. Larsh, T. H. Lindner, J. K. McClatchy, M. R. McGinnis, S. H. Siddiqi, and P. Wright. 1983. Evaluation of the BACTEC radiometric method for recovery of mycobacteria and drug susceptibility testing of *Mycobacterium tuberculosis* from acid-fast smear-positive specimens. *J. Clin. Microbiol.* **18**:689–696.

47. Sandin, R. L. 1996. Polymerase chain reaction and other amplification techniques in mycobacteriology. *Clin. Lab. Med.* **16**:617–639.

48. Scarparo, C., P. Piccoli, A. Rigon, G. Ruggiero, P. Ricordi, and C. Piersimoni. 2002. Evaluation of the BACTEC MGIT 960 in comparison with BACTEC 460 TB for detection and recovery of mycobacteria from clinical specimens. *Diagn. Microbiol. Infect. Dis.* **44**:157–161.

49. Shrestha, N. K., M. J. Tuohy, G. S. Hall, U. Reischl, S. M. Gordon, and G. W. Procop. 2003. Detection and differentiation of *Mycobacterium tuberculosis* and nontuberculous mycobacterial isolates by real-time PCR. *J. Clin. Microbiol.* **41**:5121–5126.

50. Telenti, M., J. F. de Quiros, M. Alvarez, M. J. Santos Rionda, and M. C. Mendoza. 1994. The diagnostic usefulness of a DNA probe for *Mycobacterium tuberculosis* complex (Gen-Probe) in Bactec cultures versus other diagnostic methods. *Infection* **22**:18–23.

51. Tjhie, J. H., A. F. van Belle, M. Dessens-Kroon, and D. van Soolingen. 2001. Misidentification and diagnostic delay caused by a false-positive amplified *Mycobacterium tuberculosis* direct test in an immunocompetent patient with a *Mycobacterium celatum* infection. *J. Clin. Microbiol.* **39**:2311–2312.

52. Torres, M. J., A. Criado, M. Ruiz, A. C. Llanos, J. C. Palomares, and J. Aznar. 2003. Improved real-time PCR for rapid detection of rifampin and isoniazid resistance in *Mycobacterium tuberculosis* clinical isolates. *Diagn. Microbiol. Infect. Dis.* **45**:207–212.

53. Tortoli, E., M. Benedetti, A. Fontanelli, and M. T. Simonetti. 2002. Evaluation of automated BACTEC MGIT 960 system for testing susceptibility of *Mycobacterium tuberculosis* to four major antituberculous drugs: comparison with the radiometric BACTEC 460TB method and the agar plate method of proportion. *J. Clin. Microbiol.* **40**:607–610.

54. Tortoli, E., P. Cichero, C. Piersimoni, M. T. Simonetti, G. Gesu, and D. Nista. 1999. Use of BACTEC MGIT 960 for recovery of mycobacteria from clinical specimens: multicenter study. *J. Clin. Microbiol.* **37**:3578–3582.

55. Tuohy, M. J., G. S. Hall, M. Sholtis, and G. W. Procop. 2005. Pyrosequencing as a tool for the identification of common isolates of *Mycobacterium* sp. *Diagn. Microbiol. Infect. Dis.* **51**:245–250.

56. Turenne, C. Y., L. Tschetter, J. Wolfe, and A. Kabani. 2001. Necessity of quality-controlled 16S rRNA gene sequence databases: identifying nontuberculous *Mycobacterium* species. *J. Clin. Microbiol.* **39**:3637–3648.

57. Wilson, M. L., B. L. Stone, M. V. Hildred, and R. R. Reves. 1995. Comparison of recovery rates for mycobacteria from BACTEC 12B vials, Middlebrook 7H11-selective 7H11 biplates, and Lowenstein-Jensen slants in a public health mycobacteriology laboratory. *J. Clin. Microbiol.* **33**:2516–2518.

58. Woods, G., B. Brown-Elliot, E. Desmond, G. Hall, L. Heifets, G. Pfyffer, J. Ridderhof, R. J. Wallace, N. Warren, and F. Witebsky. 2010. *Susceptibility Testing of Mycobacteria, Nocardiae, and Other Aerobic Actinomycetes*. Approved standard M-24A, 2nd ed. Clinical and Laboratory Standards Institute, Wayne, PA.

Chapter 5

Diagnosis of Latent Tuberculosis Infection

ALFRED A. LARDIZABAL AND LEE B. REICHMAN

OVERVIEW

During 2009, there were a total of 11,540 tuberculosis (TB) cases (3.8 cases per 100,000 population) in the United States. The 2009 rate showed the greatest single-year decrease ever recorded. Despite a decline in TB nationwide, foreign-born and racial/ethnic minorities continued to have TB disease disproportionate to their respective populations (9). This is a trend observed in the United States and many other industrialized nations with a low incidence of TB. In these countries, most new, active cases have occurred among persons who were once infected, contained the infection, and then later developed active disease (27). Where TB case rates have declined significantly over the past decade, the elimination of TB will increasingly depend on diagnosing and treating latent TB infection (LTBI) to prevent development of disease. This chapter reviews the tuberculin skin test (TST) and the newer blood tests to detect LTBI.

TUBERCULIN SKIN TESTING

TST is currently still the most widely used and available test for the diagnosis of tuberculous infection. Following infection with *Mycobacterium tuberculosis*, a cascade of immune responses ensues triggered by activated macrophages and carried out by T cells. Two different cell-mediated immunity mechanisms result in both protection, mediated by Th1 cytokines (interleukin 2, interleukin 12, and gamma interferon [IFN-γ]), and delayed-type hypersensitivity, mediated by chemokines (19). Infection with *M. tuberculosis* results in a delayed-type hypersensitivity reaction to antigens derived from the organism, which is the basis of the TST. Proper use of the TST requires knowledge of the antigen used, the immunologic basis for the reaction to this antigen, the proper technique of administering and reading the test, and the results of epidemiological and clinical experience with the test.

When the material is injected intradermally, a classic delayed hypersensitivity reaction occurs in the infected patient. The initial process of sensitization following infection takes about 6 to 8 weeks, with sensitized T lymphocytes developing in regional lymph nodes and entering the circulation. Restimulation of these lymphocytes by intracutaneous injection of tuberculin results in the indurated skin reaction of a positive result. The induration is due to cellular infiltration mediated by the sensitized lymphocytes. The reaction is maximal at 48 to 72 h and then slowly fades, although it commonly lasts for more than 96 h. Two types of tuberculin preparations have been in use, old tuberculin (OT) and purified protein derivative (PPD).

TUBERCULIN—HISTORICAL PERSPECTIVE

Tuberculin was developed a decade after Robert Koch discovered the tubercle bacillus and also a method of growing it in pure culture in 1882. He came up with this preparation from heat-sterilized cultures of tubercle bacilli that were filtered and concentrated and contained tuberculoproteins. It was initially used and touted as therapeutic. However, the curative value of the preparation was disappointing, but it led to the discovery of tuberculin's diagnostic value. Because the original preparation, known as OT, was an unrefined product with extraneous material present, a positive reaction lacked the sensitivity to be diagnostic of infection with *M. tuberculosis*. Currently, OT is only available in multiple-puncture tests.

Alfred A. Lardizabal and Lee B. Reichman • New Jersey Medical School Global Tuberculosis Institute, University of Medicine and Dentistry of New Jersey, Newark, NJ 07103.

PURIFIED PROTEIN DERIVATIVE

PPD was originally developed by Florence Siebert in 1939 at the Phipps Institute in Philadelphia, PA. It is a precipitate prepared from filtrates of OT with ammonium sulfate or trichloroacetic acid. The reference standard material for all tuberculin is PPD-S (Siebert's lot 49608).

In 1972, the Bureau of Biologics of the Food and Drug Administration mandated that the standard test dose of all Tween-containing PPD tuberculin licensed for use in humans be biologically equivalent to 5 tuberculin units (TU) of PPD-S (12). The definition of tuberculous infection is a positive reaction to 5 TU of PPD (2). Tween 80 is added to the PPD diluent to prevent antigenic material from being adsorbed by glass and plastic containers and syringes, thus preventing decreased potency of the preparation. PPD antigen is administered by multiple-puncture tests and by the intradermal Mantoux test. Multiple-puncture tests (i.e., Tine and Heaf) and PPD strengths of 1 and 250 TU are not accurate and should not be used.

MANTOUX TEST

The Mantoux test is performed by intradermally injecting 0.1 ml of PPD tuberculin (5 TU) into the skin of the volar aspect of the forearm. A single-dose plastic syringe is used with a 26- to 27-gauge needle. The injection is done with the needle bevel upward. A visible wheal 6 to 10 mm in diameter should result. The proper dose is important; the larger the dose, the larger the reaction. Weaker doses produce smaller reactions. The test is read in 48 to 72 h. Test significance depends on the presence or absence of induration. The presence of induration is determined by touch. The diameter of the induration is measured transversely. Erythema is not considered. The size of induration (in millimeters), the antigen strength and lot number, the date of testing, and the date of reading are all recorded.

Adverse reactions to PPD are unusual. Some sensitive individuals may develop local ulceration and necrosis or vesicle formation. Fever and lymphadenopathy may also occur. Aside from local application of petrolatum jelly, no specific therapy is indicated in these instances.

SIGNIFICANCE OF REACTIVITY

The 5-TU dose is used because of its specificity. But tuberculin is a biological product and *M. tuberculosis* shares antigens with other, nontuberculous

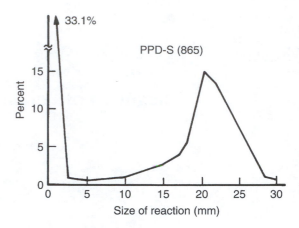

Figure 1. Distribution of reactions to 5 TU of PPD among Alaskans tested in 1962. Reprinted with permission from *Archives of Environmental Health* (13).

mycobacteria, so the 5-TU dose is not completely specific. The use of large doses, such as 250 TU of PPD, would result in an increased number of nonspecific reactions.

Figure 1 (13) shows a bimodal distribution of reactions to 5 TU of PPD among Alaskan Eskimos. In this group, a reaction size of 5 mm results in a clear separation between reactors and nonreactors. In Alaska, reactions above 5 mm also correlate well with the findings in individuals in this population group known to have tuberculous disease. There are no known cross-reacting mycobacteria in Alaska. So, for this population, a reaction size greater than 5 mm of induration instead of 10 mm can be considered positive.

Figure 2 (1) shows the distribution of reactions of 5 TU of PPD in Navy recruits from the state of

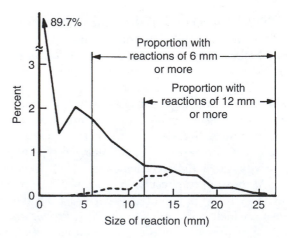

Figure 2. Distribution of reactions to 5 TU of PPD among white Navy recruits from the state of Georgia, with estimate of proportion infected with *M. tuberculosis*. Reprinted with permission from *The Tuberculin Test: Supplement to Diagnostic Standards and Classification of Tuberculosis and Other Mycobacterial Diseases* (1).

Georgia. A situation much different from that in Fig. 1 is shown. There is no clear separation point. In order to clarify this, a frequency distribution curve has been constructed by using 15 mm of induration as the mean. The mirror image of the distribution to the right of 15 mm is placed to the left of the 15-mm mean (dotted line in Fig. 2). It has been found (21) that when 5 TU of PPD is given to patients with cultures positive for *M. tuberculosis*, a symmetrical distribution of about a mean of 16 to 17 mm of induration results. From these data, a 15-mm induration has been suggested for distribution curve construction (3). In Georgia, nontuberculous mycobacteria are found in soil, and cross-reactions to tuberculin tests performed with PPD occur. By constructing the distribution curve, one can assume that the reactions falling between the solid and dotted lines in Fig. 2 are probably due to cross-reactions of nontuberculous mycobacteria. One can also assume that the solid line beyond a 15-mm induration represents true infection and does not included cross-reactions. As demonstrated in Fig. 2, if a 6-mm induration was taken as indicative of positive reaction, almost no cases of true tuberculous infection would be missed, but a large number of reactions, probably due to nontuberculous mycobacteria, would be included. If a 12-mm induration was used as a cutoff point, the number of nontuberculous reactions included would be less, but several cases of true infection would be missed. Therefore, each geographic area and program should determine its own cutoff point for a positive reaction depending on the characteristics of the population, the risk for TB infection, and the prevalence of environmental mycobacteria as exemplified in Fig. 2. Figure 3 illustrates the

distribution of reactors in the New York City metropolitan area, a region with a significantly lower prevalence of nontuberculous mycobacteria.

Other factors are important. Persons in close contact with a bacteriologically positive case of TB or with chest radiographic findings consistent with TB are more likely to experience a PPD reaction that is due to a true tuberculous infection than one due to a cross-reaction. One study of an urban population (23) found that variables such as race, socioeconomic status, age, and sex affected the TST reaction rate as regards infection. More positive reactions occurred in nonwhite ethnic groups, in areas of lower socioeconomic status, in men, and with increasing age.

Currently in the United States, a reaction of more than 5 mm to 5 TU of PPD with the Mantoux test after 48 h is considered positive for those with human immunodeficiency virus (HIV) infection, for those with chest radiographs consistent with old inactive TB, for those with recent, close contact with infectious TB cases, for patients with organ transplants, and for other immunosuppressed patients.

A reaction of more than 10 mm is positive for recent immigrants (i.e., within the last 5 years) from high-prevalence countries; injection drug users; residents and employees of high-risk congregate settings, such as prisons and jails, nursing homes, hospitals, and homeless shelters; mycobacteriology laboratory personnel; those with clinical conditions in which the risk of TB is increased, such as silicosis, diabetes mellitus, chronic renal failure, hematologic and other malignancies, weight loss of more than 10% of ideal body weight, gastrectomy, and jejunoileal bypass; children younger than 4 years of age; and infants,

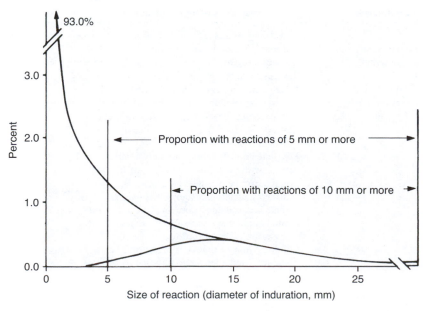

Figure 3. Schema of probable distribution of reactors to 5 TU of PPD in the New York City metropolitan area.

children, and adolescents exposed to adults at high risk.

For all other persons with no risk factors for TB, a reaction of more than 15 mm is considered positive (Table 1) (7).

FALSE-POSITIVE REACTIONS

Inoculation with bacillus Calmette-Guérin (BCG) can be the cause of false-positive tuberculin test results; BCG is a live attenuated mycobacterial strain derived from *Mycobacterium bovis*. Several BCG vaccines are available. The vaccines are derived from the original strain but differ in immunogenicity and reactivity. The tuberculin reaction produced by the BCG vaccine cannot be distinguished from that due to *M. tuberculosis* infection. It is best to manage the patient with a previous BCG vaccination *without regard to the BCG history*, especially because the BCG reaction tends to wane with time. The age at which BCG vaccination is given is important. Tuberculin reactions greater than 10 mm in those vaccinated in infancy should not be attributed to BCG. In persons vaccinated after infancy, positive tuberculin reactions may be due to TB infection or BCG (18). Immunity to tuberculous infection after BCG vaccination is also still seriously in question (25). Infection with various nontuberculous or environmental mycobactria can also cause false-positive reactions. For persons with LTBI and normal immune responsiveness, TST sensitivity approaches 100%. These false-positive reactions result in lower specificity and a low positive predictive value in persons who have a low probability of LTBI. A lower prevalence of TB infection results in higher false-positive reaction, and raising the threshold reaction size that separates positive from negative reactors can improve specificity.

FALSE-NEGATIVE REACTIONS

A negative reaction to the tuberculin test does not rule out tuberculous infection. A negative reaction can be due to true negativity, that is, an individual's not having tuberculous infection. Various technical factors also result in a falsely negative tuberculin test, however. The tuberculin preparation used must be stored properly. Dilutable preparations are no longer used. Despite the use of Tween 80, a loss of potency can occur from denaturation of the preparation due to heat, light, or bacteria.

Poor technique of administration (e.g., too little antigen injected or too deep an injection) can result in a falsely negative reaction. Errors in reading and recording the test can obviously lead to erroneous interpretation.

Various associated conditions can cause a decrease in delayed-type hypersensitivity and cutaneous anergy, resulting in a falsely negative tuberculin test. Conditions associated with anergy include HIV infection, viral infections (e.g., measles or varicella-zoster virus), live virus vaccination, use of immunosuppressive drugs, sarcoidosis, bacterial infections (including

Table 1. Criteria for tuberculin positivity, by risk group[a]

Reaction, ≥5 mm of induration	Reaction, ≥10 mm of induration	Reaction, ≥15 mm of induration
HIV-positive persons	Recent immigrants (i.e., within the last 5 yr) from high-prevalence countries	Persons with no risk factors for TB
Recent contacts of TB case patients	Injection drug users	
Fibrotic changes on chest radiograph consistent with prior TB	Residents and employees[c] of the following high-risk congregate settings: prisons and jails, nursing homes and other long-term facilities for the elderly, hospitals and other health care facilities, residential facilities for patients with AIDS	
Patients with organ transplants and other immunosuppressed patients (receiving the equivalent of ≥15 mg of prednisone/day for 1 mo or more)[b]	Mycobacteriology laboratory personnel	
	Persons with the following clinical conditions that place them at high risk: silicosis, diabetes, mellitus, chronic renal failure, some hematologic disorders (e.g., leukemias and lymphomas), other specific malignancies (e.g., carcinoma of the head or neck)	
	Children younger than 4 yr of age or infants, children, and adolescents exposed to adults at high risk	

[a]Adapted from *Morbidity and Mortality Weekly Report* (5a).
[b]Risk of TB in patients treated with corticosteroids increases with higher dose and longer duration.
[c]For persons who are otherwise at low risk and are tested at the start of employment, a reaction of ≥15 mm of induration is considered positive.

fulminant TB), malignancies (particularly lymphoreticular forms), and malnutrition (25).

HIV infection is particularly important as a cause of cutaneous anergy. About one-third of patients with HIV infection and more than 60% of those with AIDS have a reaction of less than 5 mm to tuberculin despite infection with *M. tuberculosis* (18). Approximately 50% of HIV-infected patients with active TB have negative tuberculin test results, whether a 5- or 10-mm induration is used (6). The usefulness of anergy testing in selecting tuberculin-negative, HIV-infected persons who might benefit from treatment of LTBI has not been demonstrated.

Tuberculin tests indicate infection by the tubercle bacillus. Testing, rather than history, is necessary; however, it has been shown that history is notoriously inaccurate (56%) and that a baseline test is required when a patient enters a new health care delivery situation (22).

BOOSTER EFFECT

Though skin sensitivity usually persists and is lifelong, waning can occur, often with age, resulting in an apparent negative reaction. In such instances reactivity can be accentuated with repeated testing (the booster effect).

The booster effect is only a problem with serial tuberculin testing. With serial testing, some persons show an increase in the size of their reaction. This can occur in all age groups but does increase with age. In a patient whose reaction has waned, the booster effect can result in an apparent conversion of reaction from negative to positive (28). For adults who will be screened periodically (e.g., the yearly testing of medical personnel) a two-step procedure for initial skin testing should be used for the first test. For those for whom results are negative on the initial test, a second test is performed within 1 to 3 weeks. The second test identifies those in whom boosting is occurring (4). If the second test result is positive, the person can be considered infected. If the second test result is negative, the person can be considered uninfected. Any subsequent positive reaction in an individual in whom boosting did not occur initially can be considered a true conversion due to infection.

The booster effect is explained in three clinical situations (Fig. 4). In situation 1, because no repeat testing at the end of 1 week was performed, the change in 1 year from 4 mm of induration to 14 mm may or may not represent true conversion. Situation 2 represents a true conversion (infection), and situation 3 represents the booster effect, ruling out a true conversion.

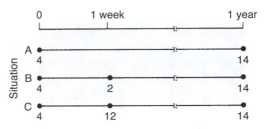

Figure 4. Schematic representation of three booster effect possibilities. (See text for discussion.)

SKIN TEST INDICATIONS—TARGETED TUBERCULIN TESTING

Targeted tuberculin testing for LTBI identifies persons at high risk for TB who would benefit by treatment of LTBI. Persons at high risk for TB either have been infected recently with *M. tuberculosis* or have clinical conditions that are associated with an increased risk of progression of LTBI to active TB. Screening of low-risk persons and testing for administrative purposes should be replaced with targeted testing. With targeted testing, a decision to tuberculin test is a decision to treat. Table 1 summarizes the current CDC recommendations and outlines the various risk groups.

BLOOD ASSAYS FOR *MYCOBACTERIUM TUBERCULOSIS*

The new blood assays to detect *M. tuberculosis* infection are based on the response of antigen-specific memory T cells releasing IFN-γ in response to previously encountered mycobacterial antigens. IFN-γ release assays (IGRAs) measure the cellular immune responses to *M. tuberculosis*-specific antigens, including early-secreted antigenic target 6 (ESAT-6) and culture filtrate protein 10 (CFP-10), antigens encoded in the region of difference (RD1) of the *M. tuberculosis* genome. These proteins are absent from all strains of *M. bovis* BCG and the vast majority of nontuberculous mycobacteria (with the exception of *M. kansasii*, *M. szulgai*, and *M. marinum*) but present in isolates of *M. tuberculosis*. In comparison, the TST uses the mixed, nonspecific PPD, a culture filtrate of tubercle bacilli containing over 200 antigens, which results in its low specificity.

Two IGRA systems using RD1-encoded antigens are currently commercially available for TB detection. One system includes QuantiFERON-TB Gold (QFT-G) and its variant QuantiFERON-TB Gold In-Tube (QFT-GIT) (uses tubes prefilled with antigens) (Cellestis, Victoria, Australia); this system uses whole blood specimens, with an unknown number of leukocytes, to measure IFN-γ released by antigen-activated

T lymphocytes. The other system is the T-SPOT.*TB* (Oxford Immunotec, Oxford, England). It uses the enzyme-linked immunospot (ELISPOT) method, wherein the number of peripheral blood mononuclear cells in the assay is quantified, in order to measure counts of IFN-γ-secreting T cells ("spots") on stimulation by *M. tuberculosis*-specific antigens in microplate wells. The readouts of the two tests are different: QFT-G and QFT-GIT measure the level of IFN-γ in the supernatant of the stimulated whole blood sample using enzyme-linked immunosorbent assay, and T-SPOT.*TB* enumerates individual T cells producing IFN-γ after antigenic stimulation.

These new blood tests have an internal positive control, i.e., a sample well stimulated with a potent nonspecific stimulator of IFN-γ production by T cells. This controls the results of the test for technical errors, such as failure to add viable, functioning cells to the well. The failure of the positive control in the tests provides information that the test's results cannot be reliably interpreted since it may reflect an underlying in vivo immunosuppression, negatively affecting T-cell function in the in vitro stimulation.

TEST PERFORMANCE

Establishing the diagnostic accuracy for LTBI of any test is a major challenge because there is no available "gold standard." As an alternative, some rational approaches based on the epidemiology of TB have been applied. The knowledge that airborne transmission of TB is promoted by close and prolonged contact with an infectious case has been used with the proposition that if a test is a good marker of LTBI, it should correlate closely with the level of exposure. Several studies conducted comparing QFT and TST used in the setting of a contact investigation have results that show these tests to be moderately concordant (5, 17, 26). In comparing the IFN-γ assay to the TST in persons with various levels of risk for *M. tuberculosis* infection, Mazurek et al. (17) showed that the assay was comparable to the TST in its ability to detect LTBI, with an overall agreement of 83%. It was less affected by BCG vaccination, discriminated responses due to nontuberculous mycobacteria, and avoided the variability and subjectivity associated with placing and reading the TST. This test was also used to detect recent infection among contacts in a TB outbreak at a Danish high school. Since a majority of contacts were non-BCG vaccinated, direct comparison between the TST and QFT could be performed. Analysis revealed an excellent agreement between the two tests (94%, kappa value, 0.866) and that

the blood test was not influenced by the vaccination status of the subjects tested (5). Ewer and colleagues investigated a school outbreak that resulted from one infectious index case using the ELISPOT assay and the Heaf test (14). The overall agreement between the two tests was 89%. The ELISPOT assay showed no significant relation to BCG status. By contrast, BCG-vaccinated children were more likely to have higher Heaf grades than unvaccinated children. An isolated positive ELISPOT was associated with exposure, whereas an isolated positive TST result was not. Several studies compared TST and IGRAs with respect to their correlation with exposure to *M. tuberculosis* (5, 14–16, 24). In these studies the RD1-based assays showed stronger positive correlation with increasing intensity of exposure than did the TST.

The sensitivities of IGRAs have been estimated using cases of active TB confirmed by cultures and often excluding HIV-infected individuals. Studies that estimated the specificity of IGRAs were carried out in low-incidence countries with some patients exposed to BCG vaccination and others not. Pai and colleagues (20) in a recent meta-analysis estimated the pooled sensitivity of the QFT studies to be 76% and the sensitivity of T-SPOT.*TB* to be 90%. The pooled specificity for all QFT studies was 98% (99% for QFT among non-BCG-vaccinated populations and 96% for BCG-vaccinated populations). The pooled specificity of T-SPOT.*TB* was 93% (almost all studies included BCG-vaccinated participants). For the TST, the pooled sensitivity estimate was 77%; the specificity in non-BCG-vaccinated persons was 97% but heterogeneous to low and high degrees among BCG-vaccinated participants. From this substantial body of literature, it can be concluded that IGRAs, especially QFT-G and QFT-GIT, have excellent specificity that is unaffected by BCG vaccination. TST has a high specificity among non-BCG-vaccinated individuals. The sensitivity of IGRAs and TST is not consistent across populations, but the T-SPOT.*TB* appears to be more sensitive than QFT or TST. Similar findings were obtained by Diel and colleagues in a meta-analysis they performed in which the TST had a pooled sensitivity of 70%, that of QFT-IT was 81%, and that of T-SPOT. TB was 88%. The specificity of QFT-IT was 99%, compared to 86% for the T-SPOT.*TB* (11). Data on high-risk populations, such as immunocompromised persons and young children, remain limited, and it has been shown that indeterminate results for the IGRAs tend to increase in these groups. In addition, one recent study which evaluated close contacts using both the IGRA (QFT-GIT) and the TST suggested that the IGRA appeared to be a more accurate indicator of the presence of LTBI. It also provided some insight into its predictive value for the development of active TB, since 14.6% of those with a positive QFT-GIT progressed to active TB, compared to only 2.3% among those with a positive TST (10). Questions such as the prognostic ability of these tests to accurately identify individuals with LTBI who are at highest risk for progressing to active TB and the significance of conversions and reversions of these tests over time still need to be clarified.

From the approval by the U.S. Food and Drug Administration (FDA) of QFT-G in May 2005, the U.S. Centers for Disease Control and Prevention (CDC) recommend that "QFT-G may be used in all circumstances in which the TST is currently used, including contact investigations, evaluation of recent immigrants, and sequential testing" with warnings and limitations (8). Updated CDC guidelines for the use of IFN-γ release assays were published in 2010 and state that either the TST or IGRAs (QFT-G, QFT-GIT, T-Spot) may be used as aids in diagnosing *M. tuberculosis* infection. IGRAs are preferred for testing persons who have received BCG (as a vaccine or for cancer therapy) or for testing groups that historically have low rates of returning to have TSTs read. The TST is preferred for testing children aged <5 years. An IGRA or a TST may be used without preference for testing recent contacts of persons with infectious pulmonary TB with considerations for follow-up testing. An IGRA or a TST may also be used without preference for periodic screening of persons who might have occupational exposure to *M. tuberculosis* with considerations for conversions and reversions.

Currently, an IGRA conversion is defined as a change from negative to positive within 2 years without any consideration of the magnitude of the change in TB response (as opposed to the more stringent 10-mm change required for the TST). A more-stringent criterion for conversion using IGRAs has yet to be established. Substantial progress has been made in documenting the utility of IGRAs, but further studies and research determining the value and limitations of IGRAs in situations important to medical care and TB control are needed.

REFERENCES

1. **American Lung Association.** 1974. *The Tuberculin Skin Test: Supplement to Diagnostic Standards and Classification of Tuberculosis and Other Mycobacterial Diseases.* American Lung Association, Washington, DC.
2. **American Thoracic Society.** 1981. Diagnostic standards and classification of tuberculosis and other mycobacterial diseases. *Am. Rev. Respir. Dis.* **123:**343–358.
3. **American Thoracic Society.** 1981. The tuberculin skin test. *Am. Rev. Respir. Dis.* **124:**356–363.
4. **American Thoracic Society.** 1992. Control of tuberculosis in the United States. *Am. Rev. Respir. Dis.* **146:**1623–1633.
5. **Brock, I., K. Weldingh, T. Lillebaek, F. Follmann, and P. Andersen.** 2004. Comparison of a new specific blood test and the skin test in tuberculosis contacts. *Am. J. Respir. Crit. Care Med.* **170:**65–69.
5a.**Centers for Disease Control and Prevention.** 1995. Screening for tuberculosis and tuberculosis infection in high-risk populations: recommendations of the Advisory Council for the Elimination of Tuberculosis. *MMWR Morb. Mortal. Wkly. Rep.* **44(RR-11):**19–34.
6. **Centers for Disease Control and Prevention.** 2000. *Core Curriculum on Tuberculosis,* 4th ed. U.S. Government Printing Office, Washington, DC.
7. **Centers for Disease Control and Prevention.** 2000. Targeted tuberculin testing and treatment of latent tuberculosis infection. *MMWR Morb. Mortal. Wkly. Rep.* **49(RR-6):**1–51.
8. **Centers for Disease Control and Prevention.** 2003. Guidelines for using the QuantiFERON-TB test for diagnosing latent *Mycobacterium tuberculosis* infection. *MMWR Morb. Mortal. Wkly. Rep.* **52(RR02):**15–18.
9. **Centers for Disease Control and Prevention.** 2010. Decrease in reported tuberculosis cases—United States, 2009. *MMWR Morb. Mortal. Wkly. Rep.* **59:**289–294.
10. **Diel, R., R. Loddenkemper, K. Meywald-Walter, S. Niemann, and A. Nienhaus.** 2008. Predictive value of a whole blood IFN-γ assay for the development of active tuberculosis disease after recent infection with *Mycobacterium tuberculosis. Am. J. Respir. Crit. Care Med.* **177:**1164–1170.
11. **Diel, R., R. Loddenkemper, and A. Nienhaus.** 2010. Evidence-based comparison of commercial interferon-γ release assays for detecting active TB. *Chest* doi:10.1378/chest.09-2350.
12. **Edwards, P. Q.** 1972. Tuberculin negative? *N. Engl. J. Med.* **286:**373–374. (Editorial.)
13. **Edwards, P. Q., G. W. Comstock, and C. E. Palmer.** 1968. Contributions of northern population to the understanding of tuberculin sensitivity. *Arch. Environ. Health* **17:**507.
14. **Ewer, K., J. Deeks, L. Alvarez, G. Bryant, S. Waller, P. Andersen, P. Monk, and A. Lalvani.** 2003. Comparison of T-cell based assay with tuberculin skin testing for the diagnosis of *Mycobacterium tuberculosis* infection in a school outbreak. *Lancet* **361:**1168–1173.
15. **Hill, P. C., R. H. Brooks, A. Fox, K. Fielding, D. J. Jeffries, D. Jackson-Sillah, M. D. Lugos, P. K. Owiafe, S. A. Donkor, A. S. Hammond, J. K. Out, T. Corrah, R. A. Adegbola, and K. P. McAdam.** 2004. Large scale evaluation of enzyme-linked immunospot assay and skin test for diagnosis of *Mycobacterium tuberculosis* infection against a gradient of exposure in The Gambia. *Clin. Infect. Dis.* **38:**966–973.
16. **Lalvani, A., A. A. Pathan, H. Durkan, K. A. Wilkinson, A. Whelan, J. J. Deeks, W. H. H. Reece, M. Latif, G. Pasvol, and A. V. Hill.** 2001. Enhanced contact tracing and spatial tracking of *Mycobacterium tuberculosis* infection by enumeration of antigen specific T-cells. *Lancet* **357:**2017–2021.
17. **Mazurek, G. H., P. A. LoBue, C. L. Daley, J. Bernardo, A. A. Lardizabal, W. R. Bishai, M. F. Iademarco, and J. S. Rothel.** 2001. Comparison of a whole-blood interferon γ assay with tuberculin skin testing for detecting latent *Mycobacterium tuberculosis* infection. *JAMA* **286:**1740–1747.
18. **Menzies, R., and B. Vissandjee.** 1992. Effect of Bacille Calmette-Guerin vaccination on tuberculin reactivity. *Am. Rev. Respir. Dis.* **145:**621–625.
19. **Orme, I. M., and A. M. Cooper.** 1999. Cytokine/chemokine cascades in immunity to tuberculosis. *Immunol. Today* **20:**307–312.

20. **Pai, M., A. Zwerling, and D. Menzies.** 2008. Systematic review: T-cell-based assays for the diagnosis of latent tuberculosis infection: an update. *Ann. Intern. Med.* **149:**1–8.
21. **Palmer, C. E., L. B. Edwards, and L. Hopwood.** 1959. Experimental and epidemiologic basis for the interpretation of tuberculin sensitivity. *J. Pediatr.* **55:**413–429.
22. **Reichman, L. B., and R. O'Day.** 1977. The influence of a history of a previous test on the prevalence and size of reaction to tuberculin. *Am. Rev. Respir. Dis.* **115:**737–741.
23. **Reichman, L. B., and R. O'Day.** 1978. Tuberculous infection in a large urban population. *Am. Rev. Respir. Dis.* **117:**705–712.
24. **Richeldi, L., K. Ewer, M. Losi, B. M. Bergamini, P. Roversi, J. Deeks, L. M. Fabbri, and A. Lalvani.** 2004. T-cell based

tracking of multidrug resistant tuberculosis infection after brief exposure. *Am. J. Respir. Crit. Care Med.* **170:**288–295.
25. **Snider, D. E.** 1985. Bacille Calmette-Guerin vaccinations and tuberculin skin tests. *JAMA* **253:**3438–3439.
26. **Streeton, J. A., N. Desem, and S. L. Jones.** 1998. Sensitivity and specificity of a gamma interferon blood test tuberculosis infection. *Int. J. Tuberc. Lung Dis.* **2:**443–450.
27. **Styblo, K.** 1980. Recent advances in epidemiological research in tuberculosis. *Adv. Tuberc. Res.* **20:**1–63.
28. **Thompson, N. J., J. L. Glasroth, D. E. Snider, and L. S. Farer.** 1979. The booster phenomenon in serial tuberculin testing. *Am. Rev. Respir. Dis.* **119:**587–597.

Tuberculosis and Nontuberculous Mycobacterial Infections, 6th ed.
Edited by David Schlossberg
© 2011 ASM Press, Washington, DC

Chapter 6

Treatment of Latent Tuberculosis Infection

CONNIE A. HALEY

The World Health Organization (WHO) estimates that more than 2 billion people, equal to one-third of the world's population, are latently infected with *Mycobacterium tuberculosis* and are at risk of progression to active tuberculosis (TB) without treatment (35, 151). Because most cases of TB disease arise from persons with latent TB infection (LTBI), treatment of such persons is necessary to achieve the ultimate goal of TB elimination (4, 17, 59, 137, 152). In developing countries with high TB incidence rates, however, the spread of *M. tuberculosis* is controlled primarily through identification and treatment of infectious persons; active contact tracing and screening of other high-risk persons for LTBI are rarely implemented due to resource constraints (2, 102, 150, 151). In such areas, immunization with bacillus Calmette-Guérin (BCG) vaccination is used to reduce the morbidity and mortality of TB among young children but is not effective for preventing primary *M. tuberculosis* infection or reactivation from latent infection to active disease later in life (45, 104, 137). In countries with lower TB disease incidence and higher levels of resources, such as the United States, identification and treatment of the large reservoir of persons with LTBI have become important components of TB control and elimination (59, 78, 137). The focus of this chapter is the treatment of persons with LTBI to prevent future development of TB disease. The epidemiology of latent and active TB, BCG vaccination, diagnosis of LTBI, and treatment of children and human immunodeficiency virus (HIV)-infected persons with LTBI are covered in greater detail in other chapters.

LTBI

LTBI is characterized by infection with *M. tuberculosis* without evidence of active TB disease, including no clinical signs or symptoms and a normal chest radiograph. After infection, a person with LTBI develops immune sensitivity to mycobacterial proteins, as demonstrated by a positive intracutaneous tuberculin skin test (TST) or interferon gamma release assay (IGRA) test result (8, 42) (see chapter 5). *M. tuberculosis* bacilli may then quickly multiply, resulting in progressive primary disease. In the majority of persons, however, the host immune response contains active replication and the bacilli remain dormant for many years in a state of clinical latency, with no evidence of active disease. The risk of progression from latent to active TB is highest in the first 2 years after infection, declining thereafter for a lifetime risk of approximately 10% (4, 27, 40, 55, 135). The likelihood of TB reactivation varies based on characteristics of the infected person, including age and underlying medical conditions, with the highest risk found among young children (especially <4 years old), persons exposed in the preceding 1 to 2 years, and those with silicosis, HIV infection, or other immunosuppressive conditions (e.g., organ transplantation, treatment with tumor necrosis factor alpha [TNF-α] inhibitors, etc.) (4, 13, 32, 45, 55, 84, 125, 132). The risk of TB reactivation is significantly reduced by treating LTBI to eradicate asymptomatic infection in order to prevent disease (4).

RISK OF LTBI

The identification and treatment of persons with LTBI constitute an essential component of TB elimination through two fundamental mechanisms (4, 71, 137). The first is the individual clinical benefit conferred through the prevention of morbidity and mortality associated with active TB disease. The second benefit is gained at the population level through the prevention of spread of *M. tuberculosis* infection within the community and the associated

Connie A. Haley • Division of Infectious Diseases and Institute for Global Health, Vanderbilt University Medical Center, Nashville, TN 37203.

reduction in health care spending. In order to accelerate the decline of TB in the United States, the Institute of Medicine has recommended a strategy of targeted tuberculin testing among high-risk groups who would benefit from treatment of LTBI. In 2000, the American Thoracic Society (ATS) and the Centers for Disease Control and Prevention (CDC) published specific guidelines providing evidence-based recommendations for which risk groups should be tested, regimens for LTBI therapy, and strategies for monitoring and adherence during treatment (4). Screening of low-risk groups and testing for administrative purposes are discouraged, and treatment of high-risk persons diagnosed with LTBI is recommended regardless of age unless there are clinical contraindications. Other developed countries follow a similar practice of screening high-risk persons for LTBI and providing treatment when indicated, though both the United Kingdom and Canada continue to include age criteria as a prominent consideration for LTBI treatment (97, 115). To evaluate the potential scope and impact of treatment of LTBI at a population level, the Tuberculosis Epidemiologic Studies Consortium (TBESC) conducted a survey of clinics in the United States (19 sites) and Canada (2 sites) that initiated LTBI treatment for ≥10 patients in 2002. Extrapolating study data to the entire U.S. population and using an estimated 20 to 60% treatment effectiveness and 5% lifetime risk of active TB without treatment, targeted screening and treatment of LTBI likely prevented between 4,000 and 11,000 active TB cases in the United States and was thus effective in reducing the national burden of tuberculosis (133).

In the United States, persons at high risk of TB and LTBI are categorized into two groups: those with increased risk of exposure to *M. tuberculosis* and persons with medical conditions that increase the risk of progression to active TB once infected (4). Groups with increased risk of recent exposure have a high prevalence of LTBI and are thus likely high-yield targets for population-based screening programs as well as for individual screening for latent and active TB. Such groups include immigrants to the United States within the past 5 years from high-prevalence countries, persons in recent contact with person with a case of infectious TB, health care workers with potential exposure to *M. tuberculosis*, persons who inject illicit drugs, and residents and employees of high-risk congregate settings where local epidemiology indicates a high rate of TB disease (e.g., correctional facilities, long-term care facilities, residential centers for patients with AIDS, and homeless shelters) (4). Persons with medical conditions associated with increased risk of progression from latent to active TB should also be evaluated for TB and LTBI and are a priority for treatment if found to be infected. Medical conditions with the highest risk of reactivation of TB include HIV infection, diabetes, silicosis or exposure to silica dust, low body weight, chronic renal failure or hemodialysis, gastrectomy, jejunoileal bypass, cirrhosis of the liver, organ transplantation, anticancer chemotherapy, and other immunosuppressive therapy (e.g., TNF-α antagonists), carcinoma of the head or neck, other neoplasms such as lung cancer, lymphoma and leukemia, and fibrotic changes on chest radiograph film compatible with previous TB (4, 137). The relative risks of reactivation tuberculosis among persons with some of these conditions are included in Table 1. TB exposure risk factors and medical conditions associated with progression from latent to active TB are listed in Table 1 of Chapter 5 according to their specified cut points for a positive TST result. TB control guidelines from both Canada and the United Kingdom include similar

Table 1. Relative risk of reactivation TB among persons with medical conditions that impair immune control of *M. tuberculosis*[a]

Condition	Study	Relative risk (95% CI[b])
Advanced HIV infection	Pablos-Mendez et al. (105)	9.9 (8.7–11.3)[c]
	Moss et al. (93)	9.4 (3.5–25.1)
Old, healed TB	Ferebee (40), Ferebee et al. (41)	5.2 (3.4–8.0)
Chronic renal failure	Pablos-Mendez et al. (105)	2.4 (2.1–2.8)[c]
Infliximab therapy	Keane et al. (67)	2.0 (0.7–5.5)[c]
Poorly controlled diabetes	Pablos-Mendez et al. (105)	1.7 (1.5–2.2)[c]
	Cowie (31)	1.7 (1.3–2.1)[c]
Silicosis	Corbett et al. (30)	1.3 (1.1–1.7)[c]
	Kleinschmidt and Churchyard (68)	1.2 (1.0–1.5)[c]
Underweight (≤10% below normal)	Palmer et al. (107), Edwards et al. (36)	1.6 (1.1–2.2)
Gastrectomy	Thorn et al. (138)	1.4 (1.1–1.9)[c]
	Steiger et al. (131)	1.3 (1.2–1.4)[c]

[a]Table 1 was reprinted from the *New England Journal of Medicine* with permission from the publisher (55).
[b]CI, confidence interval.
[c]The relative risk is estimated, as described in the text (55).

recommendations for targeted screening of high-risk groups, though there are a few minor differences specific to each country (97, 115). Given the limited availability of resources in many countries, the WHO recommends LTBI screening and treatment primarily for HIV-infected persons and pediatric household contacts to infectious persons to provide treatment for persons with LTBI and ensure that active TB is excluded prior to therapy (79, 102, 152, 154). In all countries, a high priority should be given to the identification and treatment of HIV-seropositive individuals infected with *M. tuberculosis*, since HIV infection is the most potent risk factor for the rapid progression of *M. tuberculosis* infection to TB disease and is associated with high TB incidence rates and a greater likelihood of disseminated and extrapulmonary disease (4, 17, 33, 55, 84, 137).

According to current ATS/CDC guidelines, "a decision to test is a decision to treat" (4). For this reason, screening of low-risk persons is discouraged, as the risk-benefit ratio may not favor treatment among persons likely to have a false-negative TST or IGRA result. However, routine administrative screening for LTBI is necessary for low-risk persons at baseline prior to employment at a high-risk worksite such as a hospital, long-term care facility, or correctional facility to enable a distinction between existing and potential future infection (4, 64). In these situations, persons who are not included in any of the preceding risks groups but have evidence of LTBI should also be considered for LTBI therapy to minimize the risk of potential reactivation of active TB in a high-risk setting (4, 64). Local public health programs may also conduct targeted testing and recommend LTBI treatment among other groups defined as high risk based on the incidence of TB, the prevalence of LTBI, and the likelihood of a population-level benefit resulting from such an intervention. This may include medically underserved and low-income minority groups such as U.S.-born Hispanics or African Americans who live or work in a community with a high proportion of persons who have a traditional TB risk factor (4, 137). As an example, six unrelated TB cases (i.e., not exposed to each other) occurred over a 2-year period at a poultry processing facility in rural Tennessee where there was a high prevalence of LTBI and the majority of workers were either U.S.- or foreign-born Hispanics (unpublished data). The Tennessee Department of Health implemented a successful tuberculin testing and treatment program among employees of the plant, which resulted in screening of several thousand employees, diagnosis of three additional persons with active TB, and diagnosis and treatment of 844 persons with LTBI (79% of whom completed treatment).

TREATMENT OF LTBI

Prior to the initiation of treatment, all persons with evidence of LTBI should be evaluated for the presence of pulmonary and extrapulmonary TB disease, including a thorough review for TB symptoms, a clinical examination, and a chest radiograph (4). If the chest radiograph is abnormal or pulmonary symptoms are present, a sputum sample for smear and culture of acid-fast bacilli should also be obtained (3). Once TB has been definitively ruled out, treatment for LTBI should be provided to all infected persons who have not already received an adequate course of therapy (4). Patients with LTBI should be evaluated for preexisting medical conditions that may increase the risk of adverse events during treatment, in particular the risk of hepatotoxicity associated with viral, alcoholic, and drug-induced liver disease, pregnancy (including the postpartum period), regular use of alcohol and other medications with hepatotoxic potential, and previous minor side effects from isoniazid (Fig. 1). As mentioned previously, treatment of LTBI is recommended in the United States regardless of age, though the risk of severe adverse events during therapy (with isoniazid in particular) has been shown to increase with age (4, 43, 86, 98, 155). For all persons, the individual risk-benefit ratio must be considered and additional clinical and laboratory monitoring may be indicated if certain comorbid conditions exist, as is described later in this chapter (Fig. 2) (4, 79). Prior to therapy, patients should also be evaluated for concomitant use of other medications that may cause drug-drug interactions with the LTBI regimen, educated about potential adverse effects of treatment, and counseled regarding the importance of adherence to the recommended course of therapy (4).

The concept of using a single anti-TB agent to prevent active TB originated during the 1950s when Edith Lincoln noted that children hospitalized at Bellevue Hospital in New York City no longer experienced complications of their primary TB following treatment with isoniazid. At her suggestion, the U.S. Public Health Service organized a multiclinic controlled trial among 2,750 children with asymptomatic primary TB or a recent tuberculin conversion (40). Preventive therapy with isoniazid proved to be remarkably effective, producing a 94% reduction in the development of TB during a year of LTBI treatment and a 70% reduction over the following 9-year period (40). Subsequent placebo-controlled trials were conducted to evaluate isoniazid for treatment of infected contacts of TB patients and other persons at high risk (e.g., those with radiographic evidence of prior untreated TB, inmates of mental health institutions, and native Alaskans) (40, 79). Based on

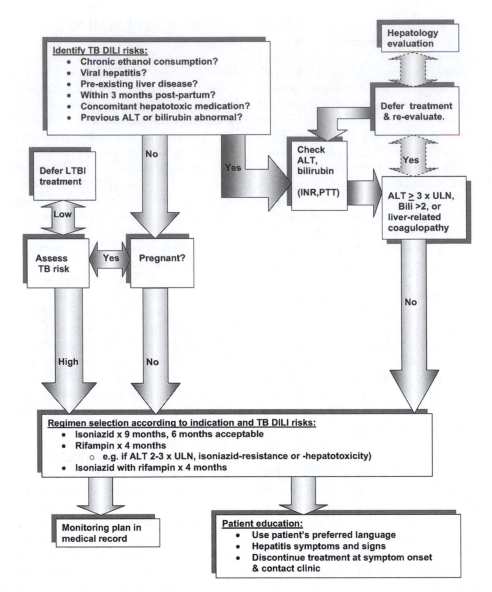

Figure 1. LTBI pretreatment clinical evaluation and counseling. Dotted lines signify management according to physician's discretion. ALT, alanine aminotransferase; INR, international normalized ratio; PTT, partial thromboplastin time. Reprinted with permission of the American Thoracic Society (122).

the results of these early studies, the treatment of LTBI using isoniazid was first recommended by the ATS in 1965 (121). More than four decades after the United States first adopted the treatment of LTBI as a primary strategy to prevent TB disease, isoniazid monotherapy remains the most widely used and only LTBI regimen that has been evaluated in large-scale randomized controlled trials (7, 79). Table 2 includes a list of studies evaluating the efficacy of isoniazid for LTBI treatment.

Despite the potential effectiveness of isoniazid for reducing the incidence of TB, an estimated 90% for adherent patients compared to placebo, treatment completion rates for 6 to 9 months of isoniazid are low, thus substantially reducing the actual benefit of

this regimen (4, 52, 55, 60, 79). Barriers to treatment completion include lack of understanding of the importance of LTBI treatment when symptoms are not present, perceived low risk of progressing from LTBI to TB, concerns regarding the potential risk of toxicity, and the long duration of the therapy (24, 52, 127). In addition, the rate of LTBI treatment initiation is likely suboptimal because providers may not prescribe LTBI when indicated and patients may refuse treatment due to perceptions of either a low risk of reactivation of active TB or a high potential for developing adverse events (55, 56, 79).

Because medication adherence has a significant impact on the effectiveness of LTBI treatment (4, 17, 38, 40), shorter rifampin-based regimens have been

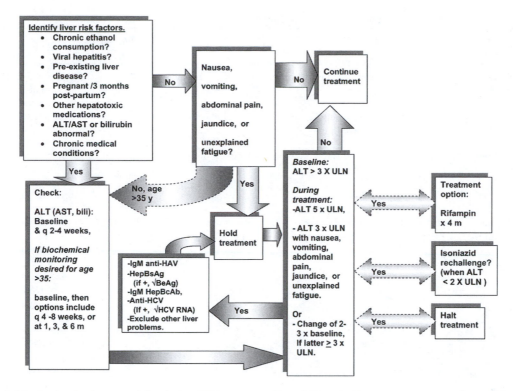

Figure 2. Monitoring for hepatotoxicity during LTBI treatment. Dotted lines signify management according to physician's discretion. ALT, alanine aminotransferase; AST, aspartate aminotransferase; HAV, hepatitis A virus; HCV, hepatitis C virus; HepBsAg, hepatitis B surface antigen. Reprinted with permission of the American Thoracic Society (122).

evaluated for their potential to overcome the low treatment completion rates and perceived risk of toxicity associated with 6 to 9 months of isoniazid (4). Rifamycin antibiotics have greater potency against dormant and semidormant *M. tuberculosis* organisms that characterize latent infection (65, 91). Several studies of short-course rifampin-based LTBI therapy have demonstrated efficacy equal to or greater than that of the longer isoniazid regimen (49, 51, 54, 96). In 2000, ATS/CDC guidelines (also endorsed by the Infectious Diseases Society of America and the American Academy of Pediatrics) provided evidence-based recommendations for the use of two short-course LTBI regimens: rifampin monotherapy for 4 months and a 2-month course of rifampin combined with pyrazinamide (4). An additional 3-month regimen of isoniazid plus rifampin is recommended in Canadian and British TB control guidelines (97, 115). Although earlier studies conducted among HIV-infected persons found that rifampin plus pyrazinamide for 2 months was both safe and effective, subsequent cases of severe and fatal hepatotoxicity were reported when this regimen was widely incorporated into clinical use in the general population (5, 49, 51, 62, 63, 96, 114, 134). In 2003, the CDC and ATS updated the guidelines for LTBI treatment with recommendations against the use of rifampin plus pyrazinamide

for both HIV-seropositive and HIV-seronegative persons (5). Because the safety, tolerability, and adherence rates associated with 4 months of rifampin have been deemed favorable to date, this regimen remains a recommended LTBI regimen for persons who are known to be infected with an isoniazid-resistant *M. tuberculosis* strain and those who are intolerant of isoniazid treatment. Many providers also use the 4-month rifampin regimen for persons assessed as high risk for progression to active TB but who are unlikely to complete a longer (6- to 9-month) course of isoniazid treatment. Clinical trials are currently under way to evaluate the use of rifapentine, a long-acting rifamycin, combined with isoniazid for a once-weekly regimen given only as directly observed therapy for 3 months, and preliminary results appear promising (http://clinicaltrials.gov/ct2/show/NCT00023452). Specific LTBI treatment regimens are described in the text below and summarized in Table 3 according to their effectiveness and level of tolerability.

Isoniazid

More than 20 randomized, placebo-controlled trials of LTBI treatment with isoniazid have been conducted involving more than 100,000 subjects (Table 2) (40, 71, 79, 132). The combined average reduction

Table 2. Placebo-controlled studies of isoniazid efficacy for treatment of LTBI[a]

Study	Yr	Location	Population	Duration of INH[b] (mo)	Reduction in TB rates
Ferebee (40), Mount and Ferebee (94)	1956–1957	United States, multiple sites	Household contacts	12	68% reduction in first 15 mo of follow-up; 60% reduction after 10 yr[c]
Ferebee (40), Mount and Ferebee (94)	1957–1960	United States, multiple sites	Household contacts	12	76% reduction in first 15 mo; 60% reduction after 10 yr[c]
Ferebee (40), Ferebee et al. (41)	1957–1960	United States, multiple sites	Residents of mental institutions	12	88% reduction in first 15 mo; 62% reduction after 10 yr
Comstock et al. (28)	1957–1964	Alaska	Native Alaskans	12	59% reduction after 43–76 mo
International Union Against Tuberculosis Committee on Prophylaxis (60)	Started 1969	Eastern Europe	Person with fibrotic pulmonary lesions (inactive TB)	3, 6, 12	After 5 yr of follow-up in all randomized 21% reduction for 3 mo of INH 65% reduction for 6 mo of INH 75% reduction for 12 mo of INH After 5 yr of follow-up in completer/compliers 30% reduction for 3 mo of INH 69% reduction for 6 mo of INH 93% reduction for 12 mo of INH
Pape et al. (109)	1983–1989	Haiti	HIV-infected persons	12	71% reduction after 60 mo
Whalen et al. (147)	1993–1995	Uganda	HIV-infected persons	6	For TST-positive persons: 67% reduction after 15 mo In anergic persons: no reduction

[a]Reprinted from *Respirology* with permission of the publisher (79).
[b]INH, isoniazid.
[c]Sixty percent reduction for 10-year follow-up was calculated from aggregate results of first two studies listed as reported in references 4, 39, and 115.

in TB reported in these studies was 60% during the period of observation, being somewhat higher during the year of treatment. These results were based on the total study populations treated, regardless of how regularly medication was taken. Among these trials, the five reporting less than 50% effectiveness included one that used small doses of isoniazid, one in which compliance was poor, and one that included patients who had undergone previous isoniazid therapy, a group now known not to benefit from additional treatment (40). When analyses were limited to participants who took their medication for most of the treatment year, efficacy approximated 90% (60). Protection also appears to be long-lasting, being demonstrable nearly 20 years after initiation of treatment (27).

The optimal duration of isoniazid treatment was addressed in a large International Union Against Tuberculosis trial conducted in six Eastern European countries among persons with untreated inactive TB (60). Regimens of daily isoniazid for 3, 6, and 12 months were tested against daily placebo for the same durations. The results of 5 years' observation of the total population showed that treatment for 12 months resulted in a 75% reduction in TB, compared with reductions of 65% in those treated for 6 months and 21% for those treated for only 3 months. When the analysis was restricted to those who took at least 80% of the prescribed regimen, efficacy increased to 93% for the 12-month group but improved only slightly for those treated for 6 and 3 months. In the U.S. Public Health Service trials among household contacts and Alaskan villagers, the optimal duration of treatment appeared to be 9 to 10 months (27, 40, 79, 132) (Fig. 3). In the contact trial, irregular treatment was still effective as long

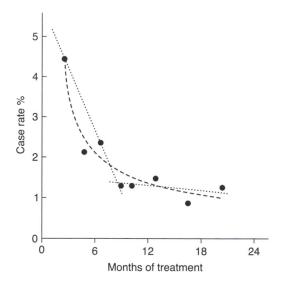

Figure 3. TB case rates in the Bethel Isoniazid Studies population according to the number of months that isoniazid was taken in the combined programs. Dots represent observed values; dashed line, the calculated curve ($y = a + b/x$); and dotted lines, the calculated values based on the first four and the last five observations ($y = a + bx$). Reprinted by permission of the *International Union Against Tuberculosis and Lung Disease* (27).

as 80% of the 12-month dose (i.e., 9 to 10 months) was taken within a reasonable time. Although the effectiveness of 9 months of isoniazid has never been directly compared with a 6- or 12-month regimen, the United States and Canada currently recommend isoniazid given for a treatment duration of 9 months as the preferred option for HIV-negative individuals with LTBI (4, 79, 115). Isoniazid taken for only 6 months is considered acceptable, though less effective, in the United States and Canada if it allows a higher likelihood of treatment completion (4, 29, 79, 115). A 6-month duration of isoniazid treatment is favored in British TB control guidelines and by the WHO (2, 79, 97, 152).

Most of the studies referenced above that evaluated the use of isoniazid monotherapy for LTBI treatment were conducted prior to the 1960s and therefore did not include HIV-seropositive persons. However, a meta-analysis of seven randomized controlled trials from Mexico, Haiti, the United States, Zambia, Uganda, and Kenya conducted between 1985 and 1997 confirmed that isoniazid is more effective than placebo in preventing active TB among HIV-infected persons with a positive TST, reducing the TB incidence by 60 to 80% (13). Some, but not all, of these trials found an association between the use of isoniazid for LTBI treatment in persons with HIV infection and improved survival. The duration of protection provided by a single course of isoniazid preventive

therapy in this population has varied in different settings; a prolonged benefit was apparent in clinical trials done among HIV-seropositive persons in developed and some developing countries, while the effect was lost after 18 to 48 months in clinical studies done in Zambia and Uganda (49, 51, 66, 96, 116). In countries with a prevalence of LTBI of >30%, the WHO recommends the use of isoniazid to prevent TB in persons living with HIV without TB disease, regardless of their TST result, as some studies have shown this practice to reduce the risk of developing TB by 33 to 67% for up to 48 months in high-burden areas (152, 153). In addition, recent evidence has shown that the combined use of isoniazid preventive therapy and antiretroviral therapy among people living with HIV in high-TB-burden countries significantly reduces the incidence of TB (2, 150–153). This strategy is controversial, however, and is largely not implemented at the country level due to resource constraints and difficulty of ruling out TB prior to initiating isoniazid (2). In low-TB-burden countries, routine chemoprophylaxis of HIV-infected persons without known exposure to active TB and no evidence of LTBI (i.e., positive TST or IGRA) is not recommended (4, 97, 115, 137). Although no randomized clinical trial has specifically evaluated the optimal duration of isoniazid among HIV-infected persons with LTBI, 9 months is preferred in the United States and Canada, whereas 6 months is accepted in the United Kingdom and by the WHO (2, 97, 115).

For HIV-seronegative and -seropositive adults, the recommended dose of daily isoniazid is 5 mg/kg of body weight, not to exceed 300 mg. For children, the dose is 10 to 20 mg/kg, not to exceed 300 mg. Isoniazid can also be administered twice weekly, at doses of 15 mg/kg in adults and 20 to 40 mg/kg in children, not to exceed 900 mg in either group. The twice-weekly regimen must be given as directly observed preventive therapy (DOPT). Overall, isoniazid is one of the least toxic of the anti-TB drugs; most of the reactions are mild and transient, including dose-related peripheral neurotoxicity, central nervous system effects (e.g., irritability, dysphoria, seizures, impaired concentration, etc.), hypersensitivity reactions, lupus-like syndrome, and mild gastrointestinal discomfort (Table 4) (4). Neuropathy is more common among persons who are already predisposed due to conditions such as HIV infection, diabetes, renal failure, poor nutrition, and alcoholism, as well as women who are pregnant or breast-feeding. Supplementation with pyridoxine (25 mg/day) is recommended for these persons during treatment with isoniazid (5). Aminotransferase elevations up to five times the upper limit of normal (ULN) occur in 10 to 20% of

Table 3. Regimens for the treatment of LTBI[a]

Regimen	Duration	Administration	Effectiveness	Toxicity requiring drug discontinuation	Current status	Comments
Isoniazid	9 mo	Daily self-administered or twice weekly via DOT	Not studied 6 mo: 65% 12 mo: 75%	Not studied 6 to 12 mo regimens: HIV negative, 2.2–31.3% HIV positive, 0–9.2%	Recommended by ATS, CDC, IDSA, AAP for adults and children	Although the 9-mo regimen has not been evaluated, post hoc analysis suggests optimal effectiveness at 9–10 mo of treatment
Rifampin	4 mo	Daily self-administered	Not studied		Recommended as alternative when patient is unable to take isoniazid due to drug resistance or intolerance	Concern in HIV-positive persons, in whom TB can be difficult to diagnose; if patient has TB, could develop rifampin resistance
Isoniazid + rifampin	3 mo	Daily self-administered	3-mo regimen: HIV negative, 46–50% HIV positive, not studied HIV negative, 41%	HIV negative, 1.9–3.1% HIV positive, not studied HIV negative, 0–5.1%	Fair amount of data on tolerability and effectiveness; used in United Kingdom but not in ATS/CDC recommendations	Probably a good alternative option
Isoniazid + rifapentine	3 mo	Once-weekly via DOT	HIV positive, 60% HIV negative, one small study; similar to rifampin + pyrazinamide	HIV positive, 2.3% HIV negative, 0.5%	Under evaluation: TBTC Study 26, South Africa (JHU)	Shows promise, but more data needed before it can be used outside of clinical trials
Rifampin + pyrazinamide	2 mo	Daily self-administered Twice weekly via DOT	HIV positive, not studied HIV negative, not studied HIV positive, similar to isoniazid	HIV positive, not studied HIV negative, 2.0–17.6% HIV positive, 0–9.5% Hepatitis-associated mortality, 1 per 1,000	Not recommended	High risk of severe hepatotoxicity

Drug	Duration	Administration	Effectiveness	Toxicity	Recommendations	Comments
Isoniazid	9 mo	Daily self-administered or twice weekly via DOT	Not studied 6 mo: 65% 12 mo: 75%	6 to 12 mo regimens: HIV negative, 2.2–31.3% HIV positive, 0–9.2%	Recommended by ATS, CDC, IDSA, AAP for adults and children	Although the 9-mo regimen has not been evaluated, post hoc analysis suggests optimal effectiveness at 9–10 mo of treatment
Rifampin	4 mo	Daily self-administered	Not studied 3-mo regimen: HIV negative, 46–50% HIV positive, not studied		Recommended as alternative when patient is unable to take isoniazid due to drug resistance or intolerance	Concern in HIV-positive persons, in whom TB can be difficult to diagnose; if patient has TB, could develop rifampin resistance
Isoniazid + rifampin	3 mo	Daily self-administered	HIV negative, 41% HIV positive, 60%	HIV negative, 1.9–3.1% HIV positive, not studied HIV negative, 0–5.1% HIV positive, 2.3%	Fair amount of data on tolerability and effectiveness; used in United Kingdom but not in ATS/CDC recommendations	Probably a good alternative option

aReprinted from the *Seminars in Respiratory and Critical Care Medicine* with permission of the publisher (132). AAP, American Academy of Pediatrics; DOT, directly observed therapy; IDSA, Infectious Diseases Society of America; JHU, Johns Hopkins University. See text for references regarding effectiveness and toxicity of the regimens.

Table 4. Adverse effects of LTBI treatment drugs[a]

Drug	Type of adverse events	Frequency (%)	Comments
Isoniazid	Asymptomatic increase in liver enzymes	10–20	An increase in enzyme concentration up to five times the ULN can be acceptable in patients who are free of symptoms if the serum bilirubin concentration is normal. Enzyme levels will usually normalize even if treatment is continued.
	Gastrointestinal intolerance	1–2.8	
	Rash	0–2.1	
	Peripheral neuropathy	<0.2	More likely in subjects with diabetes, chronic renal failure, HIV, alcoholism, or daily alcohol intake. Vitamin B_6 is recommended for such conditions and is also recommended for pregnant and breast-feeding women.
	Hepatitis	0.1–0.15	
	Others	2.5	Adverse side effects commonly lead to drug discontinuation in 11.3%.
Rifampin	Cutaneous reaction	3–6	Pruritus most common (with or without rash), usually self-limited and not considered a hypersensitivity reaction per se. Continued treatment may be possible.
	Hepatitis	0.6	More likely to occur when combined with isoniazid
	Gastrointestinal	2–3	Nausea, anorexia, abdominal pain
	Others	2.8	Orange discoloration of body fluid; can result in permanent stain of soft contact lenses
	Drug interaction	≈100	Increased metabolism of certain drugs, resulting in lower plasma concentrations of methadone, warfarin, oral contraceptives, and phenytoin. Interaction with most protease inhibitors and NNRTIs used in the treatment of HIV infection. Use rifabutin instead.
Pyrazinamide	Hepatitis	2–6	More frequent if combined with rifampin
	Elevated uric acid levels	≈100	Gout is not common.
	Arthralgia		Occurs frequently, unrelated to hyperuricemia

[a]Reprinted from the *International Journal of Tuberculosis and Lung Diseases* with permission of the publisher (71, 89). RMP, rifampin; NNRTI, nonnucleoside reverse transcriptase inhibitor.

persons receiving isoniazid monotherapy, and levels usually return to normal even with continued administration of the drug (122). The side effect of principal concern is drug-induced liver injury (DILI). Although hepatitis was rarely reported in early studies using isoniazid to treat LTBI, the potential for this drug to cause both asymptomatic transaminase elevation and clinically significant hepatitis, including death, was recognized in the late 1960s and 1970s (46, 69, 90, 122). Subsequent studies from the 1970s to 1990s reported much lower rates of isoniazid-related hospitalization and death, which has been attributed to careful patient selection, education, and active monitoring for adverse reactions during treatment (5, 46, 69, 122). More recent larger reviews have reported a rate of significant transaminase elevation of 0.1 to 0.56% (43, 80, 99, 122). A study of over 11,000 patients who started isoniazid preventive therapy between 1989 and 1995 in a Seattle, Washington, public health TB clinic reported very low (0.1%) rates of hepatotoxic reactions (elevated transaminases more than five times the ULN), though the risk did increase with age ($P = 0.02$) (99). Of note, rates of

transaminase elevation could have been underestimated, since routine monitoring of levels was not performed among asymptomatic patients, and rates of clinically significant hepatotoxicity were measured based on all persons initiating treatment rather than on those actually taking medication. A subsequent study conducted in San Diego, California, reported a 0.3% rate of transaminase elevation among 3,788 LTBI patients treated with isoniazid (defined as three times the ULN for symptomatic patients and five times the ULN for asymptomatic persons) (80). Another observational study conducted in Memphis, Tennessee, from 1996 to 2003 reported significant aspartate aminotransferase elevations among 19 of 3,377 LTBI patients taking isoniazid monotherapy, only one of whom was symptomatic (43).

Even in the context of guidelines for improved patient selection and clinical monitoring during therapy (Fig. 1 and 2), significant hepatotoxicity and deaths due to isoniazid DILI have been reported, especially among persons who continued to take the drug after symptoms of hepatitis had appeared. In January 2004, the CDC began a national passive surveillance system to quantify the frequency of severe adverse events associated with isoniazid for LTBI treatment and to characterize the clinical features of affected patients (18). Between 2004 and 2008, 15 adults and 2 children (aged 11 and 14 years) who received isoniazid therapy experienced severe idiosyncratic DILI; 5 required liver transplants (including 1 child), and 5 adults died. These findings, though uncommon, underscore the potential for severe adverse events during isoniazid therapy and emphasize the importance of sustained clinical monitoring throughout LTBI treatment in accordance with ATS/CDC recommendations (Fig. 2) (4, 18, 122). Predictors of DILI during isoniazid therapy include older age and preexisting liver disease, particularly from hepatitis C virus infection, concomitant use of hepatotoxic medications, prior isoniazid-related hepatotoxicity, and regular alcohol consumption (71, 122). The risk of infected persons developing tuberculosis if preventive therapy is not given must be weighed against the potential risk of developing DILI during treatment, and appropriate monitoring must be conducted according to current guidelines (4, 71). For tuberculin reactors with no additional risk factors, a sensitivity analysis suggested that the balance is most strongly in favor of preventive treatment among children and young adults (120). For persons with additional risk factors, the benefit-to-risk ratio is increased at all ages.

In addition to the actual and perceived risk of toxicity associated with isoniazid, the effectiveness of this therapy for preventing active TB among infected persons is significantly limited by poor adherence. Reported treatment completion rates associated with 6 to 9 months of isoniazid are typically around 50% but can be much lower for specific high-risk groups such as inner city residents, jail inmates, homeless persons, and injection drug users (76, 98, 118, 140, 141, 148, 149). Adherence has been improved in some situations using the twice-weekly regimen given as DOPT; however, data regarding the effectiveness of intermittent isoniazid compared to daily treatment are weak (52, 79).

Rifampin Monotherapy

Rifampin-based regimens were first considered promising for shorter LTBI treatment because of the potent bactericidal activity of rifamycins against *Mycobacterium tuberculosis* and findings from animal model studies suggesting that rifampin alone or in combination could be at least as effective as isoniazid monotherapy (34, 65, 74, 118). Now that the use of rifampin plus pyrazinamide is not generally recommended, daily self-administered rifampin monotherapy is widely accepted as an alternative LTBI treatment regimen for persons who are infected with an isoniazid-resistant strain of *M. tuberculosis* and for those who are intolerant of isoniazid (4, 79, 132).

In contrast to the extensive experience evaluating the efficacy of isoniazid for preventing progression to active TB, only one randomized clinical trial has evaluated rifampin monotherapy for patients with LTBI (54). From 1981 to 1987, a cohort of older Chinese men with silicosis and LTBI was randomly assigned to receive either placebo, rifampin for 3 months, isoniazid for 6 months, or isoniazid plus rifampin for 3 months. While all treatment groups had a reduced cumulative incidence of active TB over the 5-year follow-up period compared to the placebo group, rifampin monotherapy was more effective at preventing active TB than were the isoniazid-rifampin group and isoniazid monotherapy regimens (Fig. 4). The

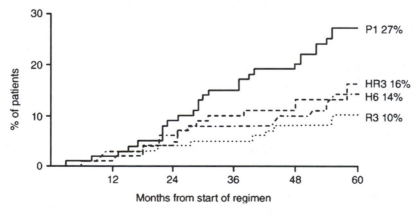

Figure 4. Effectiveness of three regimens for treatment of LTBI in elderly Chinese men with silicosis. Based on 503 patients at 1 year, 474 at 2 years, 418 at 3 years, 367 at 4 years, and 304 at 5 years who received their regimen without known interruption. The *x* axis shows the months from start of the LTBI treatment regimen. The *y* axis shows the percentage of patients who developed TB disease. HR3, isoniazid and rifampin for 3 months; H6, isoniazid for 6 months; Pl, placebo; R3, rifampin for 3 months (79). Reprinted with permission of the American Thoracic Society (54).

effectiveness of 3 months of rifampin compared to placebo was calculated at 50% among persons who completed the 5-year study and at 46% among all persons who initiated treatment (54, 132). Because TB rates were relatively high in this cohort of patients, probably due to their having silicosis, which is a potent facilitator for the progression from LTBI to active TB, experts concluded that the use of 4 months of rifampin would be more prudent than 3 months (4). Several small nonrandomized clinical studies also suggest that the efficacy of 4 months of rifampin is at least equivalent, if not superior, to 6 months of isoniazid (112, 145). In one study of homeless persons who developed a TST conversion during an epidemic of isoniazid-resistant TB, no patients treated with rifampin monotherapy for an average of 6 months developed TB disease, compared to 8.6% of untreated persons (112). In a second observational study, none of the 157 adolescent contacts to an isoniazid-resistant source case who developed skin test conversions after *M. tuberculosis* exposure developed active TB during the 2 years following completion of 6 months of rifampin therapy (145). A large-scale international trial to assess the effectiveness of rifampin monotherapy for 4 months is currently under way (79).

Reported treatment completion rates for 4 months of self-administered rifampin have been consistently high, ranging from 60 to 91% (29, 50, 72, 88, 89, 106). Rifampin also appears to be well tolerated and has been associated with low rates of DILI (50, 54, 88, 106, 112, 122, 145). Two open-label randomized controlled trials conducted in university-based TB clinics in Canada, Brazil, and Saudi Arabia directly compared the rates of both adverse events and treatment completion using 4 months of rifampin compared to 9 months of isoniazid (88, 89). In both studies, treatment of LTBI using the rifampin regimen resulted in better adherence and fewer serious adverse events than with isoniazid. Several observational studies have also demonstrated superior treatment completion rates, good tolerability, and lower rates of hepatotoxicity using 4 months of rifampin compared to 9 months of isoniazid (72, 106, 112, 155).

The most common side effects associated with rifampin include mild cutaneous reactions and gastrointestinal side effects such as nausea, anorexia, and abdominal pain (Table 4) (6). More severe hypersensitivity reactions and severe immunologic reactions such as thrombocytopenia, hemolytic anemia, acute renal failure, and thrombotic thrombocytopenia purpura also occur but are rare. Rifampin interacts with numerous drugs, including warfarin, prednisone, digitoxin, quinidine, ketoconazole, itraconazole, propranolol, clofibrate, sulfonylureas, phenytoin, HIV protease inhibitors, and HIV nonnucleoside reverse transcriptase inhibitors (6, 122). Regular measurements of serum drug concentrations of these medications should therefore be measured during rifampin therapy. Of note, rifamycins universally cause orange discoloration of bodily fluids (sputum, urine, sweat, and tears) and permanently stain soft contacts and clothing.

Rifampin is recommended at a dose of 10 mg/kg for adults, not to exceed 600 mg, for a duration of 4 months. For children, the dose is 10 to 20 mg/kg up to a maximum of 600 mg given daily for 6 months (4, 11). As with isoniazid, it is important to exclude active TB before initiating rifampin monotherapy, particularly in HIV-infected persons (71, 132). There is concern that inadvertent treatment of active TB with rifampin monotherapy can result in the development of resistance to rifampin. However, spontaneous chromosomal mutations of *M. tuberculosis* leading to rifampin resistance are 2 to 3 orders of magnitude less frequent than for isoniazid resistance, and induced resistance has not been demonstrated when isoniazid has been used alone in preventive treatment (40, 79, 118). Nonetheless, particular caution should be used with HIV-infected persons in whom active TB is often difficult to exclude and who may have a larger bacterial burden and thus an increased risk of developing rifampin-resistant TB disease (72, 111, 126, 132). In addition, drug interactions are a significant concern in this population, since rifampin interacts with many antiretrovirals as well as other antimicrobial medications used for other concurrent infections (16, 20, 72). For this reason, isoniazid therapy is the preferred therapy in most situations for LTBI patients with HIV infection (118, 132). When a rifamycin must be used to treat HIV-seropositive patients with LTBI also taking antiretroviral medications, rifabutin can be substituted, though there are no data to support rifabutin-based LTBI therapy (4).

Isoniazid plus Rifampin

While not included in the ATS/CDC guidelines for treatment of LTBI in the United States, the 3-month regimen of isoniazid plus rifampin is recommended in the United Kingdom and Canada (97, 115). A meta-analysis of five randomized trials comprising 1,926 adults from Hong Kong, Spain, and Uganda was conducted in 2005 to determine the equivalence of daily isoniazid plus rifampin for 3 months and isoniazid monotherapy for 6 to 12 months with regard to the development of TB, severe adverse drug reactions, and death (37). During a follow-up period varying from 13 to 37 months, the rates of developing active TB were equivalent for the two regimens. A total of 41 patients (4.2%) who received isoniazid plus rifampin developed TB, compared with 39 patients (4.1%) who received only isoniazid (pooled risk difference, 0%; 95% confidence interval, −1 to 2%). Severe adverse events requiring drug discontinuation were reported with similar frequencies for the two regimens (4.9% for rifampin-isoniazid and 4.8% for isoniazid), and a subanalysis of high-quality trials suggested that the two regimens were equally safe. Mortality rates were also equivalent for the two regimens in the three trials that provided mortality data. Of note, 83% of isoniazid patients in these studies were treated for only 6 months, and less than 11% received treatment for 9 months. In the Hong Kong study evaluating Chinese men with silicosis treated for LTBI, the efficacy of 3 months of isoniazid plus rifampin in preventing active TB was 41% compared to placebo, somewhat less than the efficacy of rifampin monotherapy for 3 months (51%) (54).

The benefits of using a combination of isoniazid and rifampin for 3 months compared to rifampin alone for the same duration are not clear. The effectiveness of combined isoniazid and rifampin therapy has been substantiated in several small trials, although in most of these trials the comparison was to only 6 months of isoniazid (37, 79). In comparison, the efficacy of rifampin monotherapy has only been evaluated in a single randomized controlled trial but is widely presumed to be at least equivalent to that of isoniazid, particularly in light of the higher likelihood of treatment completion, which, in turn, increases effectiveness (54, 72, 118). With regard to potential toxicity, studies evaluating rifampin monotherapy for LTBI treatment have reported lower rates of grade 3 or 4 hepatotoxicity than those obtained with isoniazid monotherapy. Combined isoniazid plus rifampin also has been well tolerated in the few studies conducted to date; similar rates of treatment discontinuation due to adverse drug reactions have been reported for combined therapy and isoniazid monotherapy (54, 79, 103, 129, 132). Of note, however, rifampin has been shown to potentiate the hepatotoxicity of other anti-TB medications, and a meta-analysis evaluating the isoniazid-plus-rifampin combination that included patients with TB disease estimated the rate of symptomatic hepatitis at 2.55%, compared with 1.6% for those treated only with isoniazid (54, 122, 130). These data indicate that the combination of isoniazid plus rifampin may not offer significant benefit over rifampin monotherapy, and the use of two anti-TB agents is more costly than using one drug and has the potential of additive risk for hepatotoxicity (79, 122).

If prescribing combined therapy, the daily doses for isoniazid and rifampin given together are the same as for each drug individually. Canadian TB standards also provide recommendations for the use of isoniazid and rifampin twice weekly under directly observed therapy for 6 months using isoniazid doses of 15 mg/kg for adults and 20 to 30 mg/kg for children, with a maximum dose of 900 mg for all persons, and rifampin doses of 10 mg/kg for adults and 10 to 20 mg/kg for children (maximum of 600 mg) (115). As with monotherapy, intermittent combination LTBI treatment should be given only as DOPT.

Isoniazid plus Rifapentine

A new regimen based on rifapentine, a long-acting rifamycin derivative, is currently being evaluated as a potentially effective and shorter treatment for patients with LTBI. The pharmacokinetic profile of rifapentine has enabled its use in combination with isoniazid for once-weekly administration during the continuation phase of TB treatment of HIV-seronegative persons (11, 146). In HIV-seropositive persons with active TB, once-weekly isoniazid-rifapentine is associated with unacceptably high rates of relapse with rifamycin-resistant *M. tuberculosis*, and it is thus not recommended in this population (10, 136, 143). Murine models of LTBI have demonstrated that weekly isoniazid plus rifapentine is also likely to be effective for preventing reactivation of TB (23, 92). In addition, one small study of household contacts with LTBI found that the incidence rate of developing active TB after completing a course of once-weekly directly observed isoniazid (900 mg) and rifapentine (900 mg) therapy for 3 months was substantially lower (1.46%) than published rates for untreated household contacts (7 to 9%) (124). The Tuberculosis Trials Consortium (TBTC) is currently conducting a large multicenter trial to determine the efficacy of directly observed once-weekly isoniazid-rifapentine (900 mg/900 mg) therapy in preventing active TB among high-risk individuals with LTBI (U.S. Public Health Service Study 26; clinicaltrials .gov/ct2/show/NCT00023452).

The side effects that may occur during treatment with rifapentine are similar to those for rifampin (122). Although the risk of DILI may be increased with use of two potentially hepatotoxic agents (122), isoniazid plus rifapentine was well tolerated in the study of household contacts treated with this regimen, and only 2 of 206 subjects developed grade 3 or 4 hepatotoxicity (122). To date, the safety and tolerability data from TBTC study 26 evaluating weekly isoniazid plus rifapentine appear promising (132). If found to be effective and well tolerated, this regimen will provide a relatively simple rifampin-based LTBI treatment alternative with a high likelihood of completion.

Rifampin plus Pyrazinamide

Earlier studies evaluating the 2-month regimen of rifampin plus pyrazinamide among HIV-infected persons with LTBI demonstrated that this regimen had an effectiveness similar to that of isoniazid and was well tolerated, with a low occurrence of toxicity (4, 79). Based on these data, this regimen was recommended in the targeted tuberculin testing and treatment guidelines issued by the ATS and CDC (4). When rifampin plus pyrazinamide was subsequently used widely in the general population, an unacceptably high risk of severe and fatal hepatotoxicity was recognized and the recommendations for using this regimen for LTBI therapy were withdrawn (5). Toxicity severe enough to require treatment discontinuation ranged from 2.0 to 17.6% in HIV-seronegative persons and 0 to 9.5% in HIV-seropositive persons (79, 132). A survey of state and city TB programs in the United States conducted by the CDC determined that the rate of symptomatic hepatitis was 18.7 per 1,000 persons among 8,087 patients initiating therapy (85). In this survey, the risk of hepatitis-associated death among persons taking rifampin plus pyrazinamide was 10-fold higher than historical isoniazid rates. Another 50 cases of severe liver injury, including 12 deaths, were subsequently reported among persons taking the 2-month rifampin-pyrazinamide regimen (57). Although some clinicians suggest that this regimen can still be used with caution in carefully selected patients and in unusual circumstances where a 2-month treatment duration is much more preferable to 3 to 4 months of rifampin (79), the risk of rifampin plus pyrazinamide far outweighs the benefits in most situations (5, 57, 85, 132).

MONITORING DURING LTBI THERAPY

Drug-induced liver injury can occur with all currently recommended regimens for treatment of LTBI (4, 5, 122). Metabolic idiosyncratic reactions appear to be responsible for most DILI from INH and rifampin monotherapy and for combined isoniazid-rifampin regimens (122). For this reason, routine clinical monitoring (including physical examination) during treatment with isoniazid and other LTBI regimens is indicated for all patients and should be conducted at baseline (Fig. 1) and on a monthly basis (Fig. 2) throughout treatment (4, 122). Providing only a month's supply of medication at each visit facilitates monthly monitoring and provides an opportunity to emphasize the importance of therapy, assess and reinforce medication adherence, and review symptoms of adverse drug effects throughout treatment. It is also important to regularly review patients' medication lists for potential drug-drug interactions and instruct patients to stop therapy and contact their providers if problems occur. Baseline laboratory testing is not recommended except for patients with HIV infection, pregnant women and those within 3 months of delivery, persons with chronic liver disease, and those who use alcohol regularly or are at increased risk of chronic liver disease. Laboratory monitoring, in addition to monthly clinical assessment during therapy, is recommended for patients whose baseline testing is abnormal and other persons at risk for hepatic disease (Fig. 2), although some suggest routine laboratory monitoring for all adult patients (4, 18, 122).

To ensure that the maximal benefit of LTBI therapy is achieved, adherence to treatment should be monitored closely for all patients at the recommended monthly clinical visits (4). While adherence to LTBI treatment was historically based on duration alone and was determined using attendance at monthly clinic visits as a surrogate marker, the current and preferred assessment of treatment completion is to estimate the number of doses taken by each patient in a predefined period (4, 24). For example, completion of 9 months of isoniazid is defined as taking a minimum of 270 daily doses or 76 twice-weekly doses within 12 months. If a 6-month regimen of isoniazid is prescribed, 180 daily doses or 52 twice-weekly doses should be completed in 9 months. For rifampin monotherapy, 120 daily doses taken within 6 months are required. The extended duration for each regimen allows for minor interruptions in therapy.

ADHERENCE TO LTBI THERAPY

Treatment adherence has a substantial impact on the outcome of an individual's LTBI treatment, including the effectiveness for preventing reactivation of TB, complications of both the disease and treatment, and the emergence of potential drug resistance (24, 52, 106). At a community level, low completion rates among patients treated for LTBI result in failure to prevent reactivation of TB and continued risk of *M. tuberculosis* transmission with increased overall health care costs (17, 21, 52, 59, 137). The CDC's Healthy People 2010 objectives for TB elimination include the goals to increase the proportion of infected persons completing a full course of LTBI treatment to 85% for high-risk contacts and to 75% for other high-risk persons (142). Published treatment completion rates, however, consistently fall far short of these benchmarks, particularly those from studies using isoniazid for 6 to 9 months (4, 52, 55, 79, 132).

Furthermore, many persons with LTBI either are not prescribed therapy by their physician or decline recommended treatment (25, 56, 79, 132). The CDC-funded TBESC conducted a randomized retrospective evaluation of clinics prescribing LTBI therapy in the United States and Canada in 2002 (56). This multisite study determined that approximately 17% of persons who were recommended LTBI treatment refused to accept it, and only 47% of those initiating therapy completed the full course. Thus, only a minority (39%) of persons with LTBI eligible for treatment achieved the full benefit of completing therapy to prevent future TB.

Reported completion rates are consistently much higher using short-course rifampin-based therapies (4, 79, 132, 155), and several studies have demonstrated that a shorter duration of treatment is a significant and independent predictor of adherence (50, 56, 75, 106). Among LTBI patients taking rifampin, the favorable tolerability and lower occurrence of severe side effects have also been shown to contribute to enhanced adherence (50, 114, 128, 155). Despite the advantages of adherence, tolerability, and safety associated with rifampin-based treatment, studies have demonstrated a far more frequent clinical use of isoniazid compared to other shorter regimens (55, 56, 75, 133). In the TBESC study of LTBI treatment acceptance and adherence at 68 clinics across the United States and Canada, 84.0% of the 1,994 persons starting therapy were prescribed isoniazid for 9 months and 9.1% were prescribed isoniazid for 6 months. Fewer patients were treated with rifampin monotherapy (4.6%) or the 2-month combination of rifampin and pyrazinamide (0.7%) (56). Anecdotally, the low uptake of rifampin despite the endorsement of national agencies from the United States, Canada, and the United Kingdom is likely due to the lack of established efficacy data using this regimen and concerns for the development of rifampin drug resistance if active TB is inadvertently missed during the pretreatment evaluation (79, 118, 132). Conclusive data demonstrating the long-term efficacy of the shorter rifampin-only and isoniazid-plus-rifampin regimens are needed before they will be more widely utilized in practice. The favorable dosing schedule of the isoniazid-rifapentine regimen (i.e., once-weekly for 12 weeks) will also likely be highly acceptable to both providers and patients if determined to be effective, safe, and associated with high completion rates.

Predicting which individual patients initiating LTBI therapy are likely to need assistance to complete the recommended course may be challenging because adherence is simultaneously affected by multiple factors. In addition to the characteristics of the regimen (e.g., duration and tolerability), individual patient characteristics, socioeconomic factors, the structure and nature of health care services offered, the quality of the patient-provider communication, and the nature of social support that patients receive all contribute to acceptance and completion of LTBI therapy (24). This may explain why studies examining various predictors of adherence to LTBI therapy have reported conflicting findings (Table 5) regarding the association of adherence with sociodemographic characteristics such as age, gender, education, or occupation (52, 79). Low LTBI treatment completion rates have been more consistently reported among certain high-risk groups such as inner-city residents, substance abusers, released jail inmates, homeless persons, and the mentally ill (12, 24, 52, 76, 98, 140, 141, 148, 149). Clinic-based factors such as hours of operation, convenient location, costs, and availability of culturally competent services have also been shown to affect adherence (25, 58, 118). Another important barrier to successful treatment completion is the psychological challenge of understanding the importance of taking medication with potential side effects for prolonged duration in order to treat an asymptomatic condition that may never result in disease (52, 79). Indeed, low perception of the risk of progression from latent to active TB has been demonstrated as a prominent predictor of failure to complete therapy (25, 52, 127). Other knowledge, attitudes, and beliefs have also been associated with patients' willingness to initiate or complete LTBI treatment, in particular a misconception among persons born in TB-endemic countries that BCG vaccine is protective against TB in adults (25). Because foreign-born individuals comprise the majority of patients treated for LTBI in the United States, addressing this and other cultural and behavioral factors that may affect treatment adherence among this population will have a substantial impact on prevention of new TB disease (25, 110, 137).

Various measures have been used to enhance LTBI treatment adherence, but no single intervention has been shown to be consistently effective (52, 79) (Table 5). The use of DOPT has been associated with improved adherence to LTBI therapy in many (but not all) settings, and it is recommended for all intermittent regimens as well as for certain populations at increased risk of nonadherence and subsequent development of active TB, such as children, contacts, and HIV-infected persons (19, 22, 52, 75, 77, 100). DOPT is usually provided or coordinated by the public health department and is most feasible when given in medical clinics, schools, work sites, day care programs, or in homes, particularly when delivered at the same time and site as directly observed therapy

Table 5. Predictors of adherence to LTBI medications[a]

Predictor	Study(ies) showing positive association with adherence	Study showing negative association with adherence
Demographic characteristics		
Age, yr		
>65	Bock et al. (12)	
<35	LoBue and Moser (81)	
Increasing age	Priest et al. (114), Nyamathi et al. (101)	
Sex		
Female	Lavigne et al. (73), LoBue and Moser (81)	
Male	Lobato et al. (76), Tulsky et al. (139)	
Race/ethnicity		
White, Hispanic	LoBue and Moser (81)	
Place of birth		
Foreign-born	Bock et al. (12), LoBue and Moser (81)	
New immigrants (<5 yr)		White et al. (149)
Haiti or Dominican Republic		Parsyan et al. (110)
Patient-related factors		
Recent exposure to TB	Reichler et al. (117)	
Higher education	White et al. (149), Nyamathi et al. (101)	
Substance use		
Injection drug use		Lobato et al. (76)
Excessive alcohol use		LoBue and Moser (81)
Daily alcohol/drug use		Nyamathi et al. (101)
Alcohol use by men		Gilroy et al. (47)
Living conditions		
Homelessness	Nyamathi et al. (101)	LoBue and Moser (81)
Stable housing	Tulsky et al. (139), Tulsksy et al. (140), White et al. (148)	
Marital status		Nyamathi et al. (101)
Health insurance	Nyamathi et al. (101)	
Unemployment		Lardizabal et al. (72), Lobato et al. (76)
Prior BCG vaccination		Shukla et al. (128)
Recent hospitalization		Nyamathi et al. (101)
Importance of treatment completion	Nyamathi et al. (101)	
Intention to adhere	Nyamathi et al. (101)	
Low perceived risk of active disease		Shieh et al. (127)
Social support	Nyamathi et al. (101)	
Treatment characteristics		
Concerns about medication toxicity and side effects		LoBue and Moser (81), Ailinger and Dear (1)
Development of clinical symptoms		Shukla et al. (128), Priest et al. (114)
Fear of venipuncture		Shieh et al. (127)
Concurrent methadone treatment	Batki et al. (9)	Mangura et al. (83)
Concomitant medication use by women		Gilroy et al. (47)

[a]Reprinted from the *International Journal of Tuberculosis and Lung Diseases* with permission of the publisher (52).

for persons with TB disease (19, 52, 75, 118). Despite the benefits of DOPT for ensuring ingestion of medication and facilitating close patient monitoring during treatment, this practice is more costly, requiring additional staff and financial resources, and is thus not widely available (53, 77, 113). Other strategies that have been successfully used to enhance adherence include intensive case management, education programs, peer support, and provision of incentives (e.g., cash, gift cards, coupons, stickers or other rewards for children, etc.) and enablers (e.g., public transportation passes, food, evening clinic hours, fast-track scheduling, etc.). Several studies have shown that case managers attuned to ethnocentric beliefs, patient concerns, and other barriers have been able to improve the acceptance of and adherence to LTBI therapy (24–26, 48, 61). In addition, pill taking at a consistent time during the day, follow-up phone calls to remind patients to continue medication, minimizing clinic wait times, reminder calls before appointments, and tracking adherence to appointments, with rapid rescheduling of missed clinic visits, have been

Table 6. Challenges of treatment adherence and possible solutions in patients with LTBI[a]

Challenges	Examples	Solutions
Access to care	Inconvenient office hours, long waits, lack of privacy, poor physician-patient communication, patient concerns about being scolded for nonadherence	Offer extended hours and reduced waits (e.g., at the end of the day or first thing in the morning). Make sure the physician-patient relationship is supportive by establishing a rapport.
Interpretation of wellness	Lack of understanding about why they are taking medication, the proper treatment duration, or adverse effects Concerns over symptoms	Educate patients on the risks of the disease and benefits of therapy. Be sure to mention potential adverse effects of medication; offer solutions or guidance about when to contact the physician's office.
Financial burden	Loss of time from work Medical expenses associated with treatment visits (e.g., laboratory tests, monitoring)	Work with state and local health departments to determine methods for avoiding additional costs outside of providing free medications.
Attitude, knowledge, and beliefs about treatment	Lack of knowledge about the purpose and effectiveness of therapy Mistrust of traditional medicine, potentially related to cultural beliefs	Discussions should occur in the patient's primary language (this could involve an interpreter), which would help to avoid misunderstandings and assist in identifying potential cultural and religious barriers.
Laws and immigration status	Concerns that the diagnosis may affect immigration status	Make sure that the patient is aware that the diagnosis will not alter the patient's immigration status.
Patient characteristics	Mental health problems, high-risk behaviors, religious beliefs, concern about being labeled "difficult"	Take into account underlying psychiatric or medical conditions (e.g., depression), religious beliefs, or patient concerns that may hinder medication adherence.
Family, community, and household influences	Stigma of disease within the family Community and households limit disclosure and reduce social and economic support	Provide educational materials to the patient, family, and employer to reduce unnecessary stigma or concerns.

[a]Reprinted from the *American Family Physician* with permission of the publisher (58). Information is from reference 95.

employed to encourage treatment acceptance and completion (52, 75, 87). Some of the challenges to treatment adherence and possible solutions for patients with LTBI are described in Table 6 (58).

Most of the adherence strategies, DOPT in particular, are more time-consuming and expensive and thus cannot feasibly be applied to all persons treated (52, 87). However, screening for risk factors for nonadherence at baseline and during therapy can enable the targeted use of such measures when indicated (24, 52, 70, 75, 87). Indeed, one study of LTBI patients treated at an academic medical center TB clinic in Boston, Massachusetts, found that patient views indicative of poor adherence were often evident at the first clinic visit (127), and several studies have demonstrated that poor adherence in the first month of LTBI treatment strongly predicts subsequent loss to follow-up and low likelihood of treatment completion (75, 87, 110, 127). Screening for risk factors for nonadherence at baseline and during the initial month of therapy can thus enable the targeted use of adherence-promoting measures when indicated (24, 52, 70, 75, 87). Adherence may also be facilitated by

the use of shorter LTBI treatment regimens for those with obvious risk factors such as homelessness, substance abuse, and mental illness.

COST-EFFECTIVENESS OF LTBI TREATMENT REGIMENS

Cost-effectiveness is an important consideration for public health programs when determining the most appropriate LTBI treatment regimen to use for targeted testing and LTBI treatment outreach activities. Isoniazid has consistently been found to be a cost-saving strategy compared to no treatment, particularly in populations that are younger and in those at increased risk of progression to active TB once infected (79, 120). More recently, a meta-analysis of published studies was conducted to compare the standard 9-month isoniazid regimen with a shorter, 4-month, rifampin regimen (155). The 4-month rifampin regimen was found to be more cost-effective, with a calculated cost savings of $213 per patient treated ($90/patient without physician fees).

Although the medication cost of isoniazid is much lower than for rifampin, the total cost of treatment is increased due to the additional monitoring and laboratory costs associated with a prolonged treatment period and higher risk of adverse events using isoniazid (88, 155). In another study that used a computerized Markov model to estimate and compare total costs of treatment, quality-adjusted life years gained, and cases of active TB prevented for four LTBI treatment regimens, rifampin was found to be less costly and more effective than both self-administered and directly observed isoniazid regimens over a wide range of estimates for adherence and efficacy. Isoniazid plus rifapentine given as directly observed therapy for 3 months became cost-effective only for patients with the highest risk, such as HIV infection (53).

TREATMENT OF LTBI FOR PERSONS EXPOSED TO DRUG-RESISTANT *MYCOBACTERIUM TUBERCULOSIS* (see also chapter 8)

When there is strong evidence that a person has become infected with a strain of *M. tuberculosis* resistant only to isoniazid, treatment with rifampin for 4 months is recommended (4, 115). As rifampin is the cornerstone of treatment of active TB, it is particularly important to exclude active disease prior to initiating rifampin monotherapy in patients with existing isoniazid resistance to avoid the progression to multidrug-resistant TB (MDR-TB) (i.e., having resistance to both isoniazid and rifampin) (2, 79). Exposure to TB cases with organisms resistant to both isoniazid and rifampin is becoming an increasing threat, particularly among disadvantaged members of society (2). In developed countries, MDR-TB occurs most often among the foreign-born (18). To date, there have been no randomized, controlled trials and few observational studies to assess the most effective regimen for treating contacts exposed to persons with MDR-TB. Thus,

management of persons exposed to MDR-TB must be based largely on clinical and epidemiological judgment, taking into consideration the infectiousness of the case and closeness, intensity, and duration of exposure (14, 115, 144). One prospective cohort study among South African children who were household contacts to an MDR-TB source case demonstrated that LTBI treatment individualized according to the drug susceptibility pattern of the source case was effective compared to no treatment (123). In 1992, the CDC recommended that persons with known exposure to MDR-TB receive LTBI treatment consisting of at least two anti-TB drugs, usually pyrazinamide plus either a fluoroquinolone or ethambutol, depending on the resistance pattern of the organisms from the suspected source case and the patient's ability to tolerate these drugs (14, 19). More recently, updated recommendations from the Francis J. Curry National Tuberculosis Center (San Francisco, CA) introduced the use of monotherapy with either levofloxacin or ofloxacin (44, 79). Table 7 includes treatment options for patients with MDR LTBI that are based on CDC and Francis J. Curry National Tuberculosis Center recommendations (79). Although there is a paucity of clinical experience with the treatment of MDR LTBI, several studies of patients treated with a fluoroquinolone plus pyrazinamide found a high rate of adverse events during treatment, resulting in premature discontinuation in the majority of persons treated (82, 108, 119). Similarly, the use of pyrazinamide plus ethambutol was poorly tolerated and discontinued prior to completion for most persons treated with this MDR LTBI regimen. The most effective duration of treatment for contacts exposed to MDR-TB is unknown, but a 6- to 12-month regimen is recommended at standard dosages, and such persons should be monitored for 2 years after exposure (19). If treatment of persons with LTBI acquired from a source case with MDR-TB is indicated, consultation with or referral to a TB specialist is strongly advised.

Table 7. Treatment of MDR LTBI[a]

Drug resistance pattern of source case isolate	Recommended regimen[b]
INH, RIF	FQN[c] monotherapy or PZA and EMB or FQN and PZA or FQN and EMB
INH, RIF, EMB	FQN monotherapy or FQN and PZA
INH, RIF, PZA	FQN monotherapy or FQN and EMB
INH, RIF, EMB, PZA	FQN monotherapy or FQN and ethionamide
INH, RIF, EMB, PZA, ethionamide	FQN monotherapy or FQN and cycloserine
INH, RIF, PZA, EMB, and FQN	Cycloserine and PAS, PAS and ethionamide, or ethionamide and cycloserine

[a]Reprinted with permission of the *Respirology* publisher (79). EMB, ethambutol; FQN, fluoroquinolone; INH, isoniazid; PAS, *para*-aminosalicylate; PZA, pyrazinamide; RIF, rifampin.
[b]Recommendations are not evidence based; there have been no clinical trials for the use of these regimens in contacts of patients with MDR-TB. Recommendations are based on the expert opinion of the CDC and the Francis J. Curry National Tuberculosis Center (14, 44).
[c]FQN in vitro activity against *M. tuberculosis* strains: moxifloxacin = gatifloxacin > levofloxacin >> ofloxacin > ciprofloxacin. Selection of FQN should take this activity into consideration (more active preferred).

TREATMENT OF LTBI IN PERSONS WITH A NEGATIVE TST OR IGRA

In developed countries such as the United States and Canada, treatment of persons without evidence of LTBI (i.e., positive TST or IGRA result) is recommended only in a few specific circumstances (19, 97, 115). Because children aged <5 years are more susceptible to infection following exposure to *M. tuberculosis* and are more vulnerable to invasive, fatal forms of TB disease, treatment for presumptive *M. tuberculosis* infection (i.e., window prophylaxis) is recommended after TB disease has been excluded if the interval since the last exposure is <8 weeks, even if an initial skin test or IGRA result is negative. If a second LTBI test result is negative 8 to 10 weeks postexposure, treatment should be discontinued. However, if the second result is positive, the full course of treatment for latent *M. tuberculosis* infection should be completed (4, 19).

Similarly, HIV-infected persons, those taking immunosuppressive therapy for organ transplantation, and persons taking TNF-α antagonists are at increased risk of rapidly developing active TB disease once infected. Therefore, after known exposure to *M. tuberculosis*, such persons should complete a full course of LTBI treatment as soon as active TB is ruled out, regardless of the results of the follow-up TST or IGRA even 8 or more weeks after exposure. The risks for TB are less clear for patients who chronically take the equivalent of >15 mg of prednisone per day, and treatment for LTBI should be considered on a case-by-case basis. When determining whether to initiate window period or prophylactic treatment of a potential contact, the contribution of certain factors must be considered, including the extent of disease in the index patient, the duration that the source and the contact are together and their proximity, and local air circulation (19). The public health department can provide consultation regarding the likelihood of clinically significant exposure and whether LTBI treatment is indicated. Of note, isoniazid has not been demonstrated to be effective in preventing TB in skin test-negative HIV-infected persons without known contact to active TB in low-TB-incidence areas and is not recommended (4, 132).

CONCLUSIONS

The WHO Global Plan to Stop TB established a long-term goal of TB elimination, defined as an incidence of <1 per million of the global population, by the year 2050 (150). To achieve this goal, interventions to identify and treat the 2 billion persons living with LTBI worldwide must be combined with current efforts prioritizing the identification and treatment of individuals with active TB (3, 102, 137, 150, 151). Although LTBI treatment has been clearly shown to be effective in preventing future occurrence of TB disease, the effectiveness of this public health measure has been limited by concern for the side effects of treatment (notably hepatotoxicity) (122), poor acceptance of LTBI treatment among health professionals (56, 133), and poor adherence among patients to the lengthy course of therapy (52). Medical providers and public health workers should recognize that there is no one-size-fits-all approach that can be effective for all patients or in all settings; thus, treatment should be individualized. Choosing the most appropriate LTBI regimen, clinical monitoring for potential adverse events, and utilization of adherence-promoting strategies to ensure completion are critical elements for the success of LTBI treatment to prevent additional TB disease.

REFERENCES

1. Ailinger, R. L., and M. R. Dear. 1998. Adherence to tuberculosis preventive therapy among Latino immigrants. *Public Health Nurs.* 15:19–24.

2. Ait-Khaled, N., E. Alarcon, K. Bissell, F. Boillot, J. A. Caminero, C. Y. Chiang, P. Clevenbergh, R. Dlodlo, D. A. Enarson, P. Enarson, O. Ferroussier, P. I. Fujiwara, A. D. Harries, E. Heldal, S. G. Hinderaker, S. J. Kim, C. Lienhardt, H. L. Rieder, I. D. Rusen, A. Trebucq, A. Van Deun, and N. Wilson. 2009. Isoniazid preventive therapy for people living with HIV: public health challenges and implementation issues. *Int. J. Tuberc. Lung Dis.* 13:927–935.

3. American Thoracic Society and Centers for Disease Control and Prevention. 2000. Diagnostic standards and classification of tuberculosis in adults and children. This official statement of the American Thoracic Society and the Centers for Disease Control and Prevention was adopted by the ATS Board of Directors, July 1999. This statement was endorsed by the Council of the Infectious Disease Society of America, September 1999. *Am. J. Respir. Crit. Care Med.* 161:1376–1395.

4. American Thoracic Society and Centers for Disease Control and Prevention. 2000. Targeted tuberculin testing and treatment of latent tuberculosis infection. *Am. J. Respir. Crit. Care Med.* 161:S221–S247.

5. American Thoracic Society and Centers for Disease Control and Prevention. 2003. Update: adverse event data and revised American Thoracic Society/CDC recommendations against the use of rifampin and pyrazinamide for treatment of latent tuberculosis infection—United States, 2003. *MMWR Morb. Mortal. Wkly. Rep.* 52:735–739.

6. American Thoracic Society, Centers for Disease Control and Prevention, and Infectious Diseases Society of America. 2003. Treatment of tuberculosis. *MMWR Recommend. Rep.* 52:1–77.

7. Ashkin, D., J. Julien, M. Lauzardo, and E. Hollender. 2006. Consider rifampin BUT be cautious. *Chest* 130:1638–1640.

8. Barry, C. E., III, H. I. Boshoff, V. Dartois, T. Dick, S. Ehrt, J. Flynn, D. Schnappinger, R. J. Wilkinson, and D. Young. 2009. The spectrum of latent tuberculosis: rethinking the biology and intervention strategies. *Nat. Rev. Microbiol.* 7:845–855.

9. Batki, S. L., V. A. Gruber, J. M. Bradley, M. Bradley, and K. Delucchi. 2002. A controlled trial of methadone treatment combined with directly observed isoniazid for tuberculosis prevention in injection drug users. *Drug Alcohol Depend.* 66:283–293.

10. Benator, D., M. Bhattacharya, L. Bozeman, W. Burman, A. Cantazaro, R. Chaisson, F. Gordin, C. R. Horsburgh, J. Horton, A. Khan, C. Lahart, B. Metchock, C. Pachucki, L. Stanton, A. Vernon, M. E. Villarino, Y. C. Wang, M. Weiner, and S. Weis. 2002. Rifapentine and isoniazid once a week versus rifampicin and isoniazid twice a week for treatment of drug-susceptible pulmonary tuberculosis in HIV-negative patients: a randomised clinical trial. *Lancet* 360:528–534.

11. Blumberg, H. M., W. J. Burman, R. E. Chaisson, C. L. Daley, S. C. Etkind, L. N. Friedman, P. Fujiwara, M. Grzemska, P. C. Hopewell, M. D. Iseman, R. M. Jasmer, V. Koppaka, R. I. Menzies, R. J. O'Brien, R. R. Reves, L. B. Reichman, P. M. Simone, J. R. Starke, and A. A. Vernon. 2003. American Thoracic Society/Centers for Disease Control and Prevention/Infectious Diseases Society of America: treatment of tuberculosis. *Am. J. Respir. Crit. Care Med.* 167:603–662.

12. Bock, N. N., B. S. Metzger, J. R. Tapia, and H. M. Blumberg. 1999. A tuberculin screening and isoniazid preventive therapy program in an inner-city population. *Am. J. Respir. Crit. Care Med.* 159:295–300.

13. Bucher, H. C., L. E. Griffith, G. H. Guyatt, P. Sudre, M. Naef, P. Sendi, and M. Battegay. 1999. Isoniazid prophylaxis for tuberculosis in HIV infection: a meta-analysis of randomized controlled trials. *AIDS* 13:501–507.

14. Centers for Disease Control and Prevention. 1992. Management of persons exposed to multidrug-resistant tuberculosis. *MMWR Recommend. Rep.* 41:61–71.

15. Centers for Disease Control and Prevention. 1995. Screening for tuberculosis and tuberculosis infection in high-risk populations. Recommendations of the Advisory Council for the Elimination of Tuberculosis. *MMWR Recommend. Rep.* 44:19–34.

16. Centers for Disease Control and Prevention. 2007. *Managing Drug Interactions in the Treatment of HIV-Related Tuberculosis.* Centers for Disease Control and Prevention, Atlanta, GA. http://www.cdc.gov/tb/publications/guidelines/TB_HIV_Drugs/default.htm.

17. Centers for Disease Control and Prevention. 1999. Tuberculosis elimination revisited: obstacles, opportunities, and a renewed commitment. Advisory Council for the Elimination of Tuberculosis (ACET). *MMWR Recommend. Rep.* 48:1–13.

18. Centers for Disease Control and Prevention. 2010. Decrease in reported tuberculosis cases—United States, 2009. *MMWR Morb. Mortal. Wkly. Rep.* 59:289–294.

19. Centers for Disease Control and Prevention. 2005. Guidelines for the investigation of contacts of persons with infectious tuberculosis. Recommendations from the National Tuberculosis Controllers Association and CDC. *MMWR Recommend. Rep.* 54:1–47.

20. Centers for Disease Control and Prevention. 2008. Notice to readers: updated guidelines on managing drug interactions in the treatment of HIV-related tuberculosis. *MMWR Morb. Mortal. Wkly. Rep.* 57:98.

21. Centers for Disease Control and Prevention. 2003. Transmission of *Mycobacterium tuberculosis* associated with failed completion of treatment for latent tuberculosis infection—Chickasaw County, Mississippi, June 1999–March 2002. *MMWR Morb. Mortal. Wkly. Rep.* 52:222–224.

22. Chaisson, R. E., G. L. Barnes, J. Hackman, L. Watkinson, L. Kimbrough, S. Metha, S. Cavalcante, and R. D. Moore. 2001. A randomized, controlled trial of interventions to improve adherence to isoniazid therapy to prevent tuberculosis in injection drug users. *Am. J. Med.* 110:610–615.

23. Chapuis, L., B. Ji, C. Truffot-Pernot, R. J. O'Brien, M. C. Raviglione, and J. H. Grosset. 1994. Preventive therapy of tuberculosis with rifapentine in immunocompetent and nude mice. *Am. J. Respir. Crit. Care Med.* 150:1355–1362.

24. Charles P. Felton National Tuberculosis Center. 2005. *Adherence to Treatment for Latent Tuberculosis Infection: a Manual for Health Care Providers.* Charles P. Felton National Tuberculosis Center, New York, NY.

25. Colson, P. W., J. Franks, R. Sondengam, Y. Hirsch-Moverman, and W. El-Sadr. 2010. Tuberculosis knowledge, attitudes, and beliefs in foreign-born and US-born patients with latent tuberculosis infection. *J. Immigr. Minor. Health* 12:859–866.

26. Coly, A., and D. Morisky. 2004. Predicting completion of treatment among foreign-born adolescents treated for latent tuberculosis infection in Los Angeles. *Int. J. Tuberc. Lung Dis.* 8:703–710.

27. Comstock, G. W. 1999. How much isoniazid is needed for prevention of tuberculosis among immunocompetent adults? *Int. J. Tuberc. Lung Dis.* 3:847–850.

28. Comstock, G. W., S. H. Ferebee, and L. M. Hammes. 1967. A controlled trial of community-wide isoniazid prophylaxis in Alaska. *Am. Rev. Respir. Dis.* 95:935–943.

29. Cook, P. P., R. A. Maldonado, C. T. Yarnell, and D. Holbert. 2006. Safety and completion rate of short-course therapy for treatment of latent tuberculosis infection. *Clin. Infect. Dis.* 43:271–275.

30. Corbett, E. L., G. J. Churchyard, T. C. Clayton, B. G. Williams, D. Mulder, R. J. Hayes, and K. M. De Cock. 2000. HIV infection and silicosis: the impact of two potent risk factors on the incidence of mycobacterial disease in South African miners. *AIDS* 14:2759–2768.

31. Cowie, R. L. 1994. The epidemiology of tuberculosis in gold miners with silicosis. *Am. J. Respir. Crit. Care Med.* 150:1460–1462.

32. Cruz, A. T., and J. R. Starke. 2010. Pediatric tuberculosis. *Pediatr. Rev.* 31:13–25; quiz, 25–26.

33. Daley, C. L., P. M. Small, G. F. Schecter, G. K. Schoolnik, R. A. McAdam, W. R. Jacobs, Jr., and P. C. Hopewell. 1992. An outbreak of tuberculosis with accelerated progression among persons infected with the human immunodeficiency virus. An analysis using restriction-fragment-length polymorphisms. *N. Engl. J. Med.* 326:231–235.

34. Dhillon, J., J. M. Dickinson, K. Sole, and D. A. Mitchison. 1996. Preventive chemotherapy of tuberculosis in Cornell model mice with combinations of rifampin, isoniazid, and pyrazinamide. *Antimicrob. Agents Chemother.* 40:552–555.

35. Dye, C., S. Scheele, P. Dolin, V. Pathania, and M. C. Raviglione. 1999. Consensus statement. Global burden of tuberculosis: estimated incidence, prevalence, and mortality by country. WHO Global Surveillance and Monitoring Project. *JAMA* 282:677–686.

36. Edwards, L. B., V. T. Livesay, F. A. Acquaviva, and C. E. Palmer. 1971. Height, weight, tuberculous infection, and tuberculous disease. *Arch. Environ. Health* 22:106–112.

37. Ena, J., and V. Valls. 2005. Short-course therapy with rifampin plus isoniazid, compared with standard therapy with isoniazid, for latent tuberculosis infection: a meta-analysis. *Clin. Infect. Dis.* 40:670–676.

38. Falk, A., and G. F. Fuchs. 1978. Prophylaxis with isoniazid in inactive tuberculosis. A Veterans Administration Cooperative Study XII. *Chest* 73:44–48.

39. Ferebee, S., F. W. Mount, and A. Anastasiades. 1957. Prophylactic effects of isoniazid on primary tuberculosis in children; a preliminary report. *Am. Rev. Tuberc.* 76:942–963.

40. Ferebee, S. H. 1970. Controlled chemoprophylaxis trials in tuberculosis. A general review. *Bibl. Tuberc.* **26:**28–106.

41. Ferebee, S. H., F. W. Mount, F. J. Murray, and V. T. Livesay. 1963. A controlled trial of isoniazid prophylaxis in mental institutions. *Am. Rev. Respir. Dis.* **88:**161–175.

42. Ferrara, G., M. Losi, L. M. Fabbri, G. B. Migliori, L. Richeldi, and L. Casali. 2009. Exploring the immune response against *Mycobacterium tuberculosis* for a better diagnosis of the infection. *Arch. Immunol. Ther. Exp.* (Warsaw) **57:**425–433.

43. Fountain, F. F., E. Tolley, C. R. Chrisman, and T. H. Self. 2005. Isoniazid hepatotoxicity associated with treatment of latent tuberculosis infection: a 7-year evaluation from a public health tuberculosis clinic. *Chest* **128:**116–123.

44. Francis J. Curry National Tuberculosis Center and California Department of Public Health. 2008. *Drug-Resistant Tuberculosis: a Survival Guide for Clinicians.* Francis J. Curry National Tuberculosis Center, San Francisco, CA. http://www.nationaltbcenter.ucsf.edu/drtb.

45. Frothingham, R., J. E. Stout, and C. D. Hamilton. 2005. Current issues in global tuberculosis control. *Int. J. Infect. Dis.* **9:**297–311.

46. Garibaldi, R. A., R. E. Drusin, S. H. Ferebee, and M. B. Gregg. 1972. Isoniazid-associated hepatitis. Report of an outbreak. *Am. Rev. Respir. Dis.* **106:**357–365.

47. Gilroy, S. A., M. A. Rogers, and D. C. Blair. 2000. Treatment of latent tuberculosis infection in patients aged > or = 35 years. *Clin. Infect. Dis.* **31:**826–829.

48. Goldberg, S. V., J. Wallace, J. C. Jackson, C. P. Chaulk, and C. M. Nolan. 2004. Cultural case management of latent tuberculosis infection. *Int. J. Tuberc. Lung Dis.* **8:**76–82.

49. Gordin, F., R. E. Chaisson, J. P. Matts, C. Miller, M. de Lourdes Garcia, R. Hafner, J. L. Valdespino, J. Coberly, M. Schechter, A. J. Klukowicz, M. A. Barry, and R. J. O'Brien for the Terry Beirn Community Programs for Clinical Research on AIDS, the Adult AIDS Clinical Trials Group, the Pan American Health Organization, and the Centers for Disease Control and Prevention Study Group. 2000. Rifampin and pyrazinamide vs isoniazid for prevention of tuberculosis in HIV-infected persons: an international randomized trial. *JAMA* **283:**1445–1450.

50. Haley, C. A., S. Stephan, L. F. Vossel, E. A. Sherfy, K. F. Laserson, and M. A. Kainer. 2008. Successful use of rifampicin for Hispanic foreign-born patients with latent tuberculosis infection. *Int. J. Tuberc. Lung Dis.* **12:**160–167.

51. Halsey, N. A., J. S. Coberly, J. Desormeaux, P. Losikoff, J. Atkinson, L. H. Moulton, M. Contave, M. Johnson, H. Davis, L. Geiter, E. Johnson, R. Huebner, R. Boulos, and R. E. Chaisson. 1998. Randomised trial of isoniazid versus rifampicin and pyrazinamide for prevention of tuberculosis in HIV-1 infection. *Lancet* **351:**786–792.

52. Hirsch-Moverman, Y., A. Daftary, J. Franks, and P. W. Colson. 2008. Adherence to treatment for latent tuberculosis infection: systematic review of studies in the US and Canada. *Int. J. Tuberc. Lung Dis.* **12:**1235–1254.

53. Holland, D. P., G. D. Sanders, C. D. Hamilton, and J. E. Stout. 2009. Costs and cost-effectiveness of four treatment regimens for latent tuberculosis infection. *Am. J. Respir. Crit. Care Med.* **179:**1055–1060.

54. Hong Kong Chest Service, Tuberculosis Research Centre, and Madras/British Medical Research Council. 1992. A double-blind placebo-controlled clinical trial of three antituberculosis chemoprophylaxis regimens in patients with silicosis in Hong Kong. *Am. Rev. Respir. Dis.* **145:**36–41.

55. Horsburgh, C. R., Jr. 2004. Priorities for the treatment of latent tuberculosis infection in the United States. *N. Engl. J. Med.* **350:**2060–2067.

56. Horsburgh, C. R., Jr., S. Goldberg, J. Bethel, S. Chen, P. W. Colson, Y. Hirsch-Moverman, S. Hughes, R. Shrestha-Kuwahara, T. R. Sterling, K. Wall, and P. Weinfurter. 2009. Latent TB infection treatment acceptance and completion in the United States and Canada. *Chest* **137:**401–409.

57. Ijaz, K., J. A. Jereb, L. A. Lambert, W. A. Bower, P. R. Spradling, P. D. McElroy, M. F. Iademarco, T. R. Navin, and K. G. Castro. 2006. Severe or fatal liver injury in 50 patients in the United States taking rifampin and pyrazinamide for latent tuberculosis infection. *Clin. Infect. Dis.* **42:**346–355.

58. Inge, L. D., and J. W. Wilson. 2008. Update on the treatment of tuberculosis. *Am. Fam. Physician* **78:**457–465.

59. Institute of Medicine Committee on the Elimination of Tuberculosis in the United States. 2000. *Ending Neglect: the Elimination of Tuberculosis in the United States.* National Academy Press, Washington, DC.

60. International Union Against Tuberculosis Committee on Prophylaxis. 1982. Efficacy of various durations of isoniazid preventive therapy for tuberculosis: five years of follow-up in the IUAT trial. *Bull. W. H. O.* **60:**555–564.

61. Jackson, J. C., and C. P. Chaulk. 2004. Assessing culture, context, power differences, and psychological development when delivering health care to foreign-born adolescents. *Int. J. Tuberc. Lung Dis.* **8:**687–688.

62. Jasmer, R. M., and C. L. Daley. 2003. Rifampin and pyrazinamide for treatment of latent tuberculosis infection: is it safe? *Am. J. Respir. Crit. Care Med.* **167:**809–810.

63. Jasmer, R. M., J. J. Saukkonen, H. M. Blumberg, C. L. Daley, J. Bernardo, E. Vittinghoff, M. D. King, L. M. Kawamura, and P. C. Hopewell. 2002. Short-course rifampin and pyrazinamide compared with isoniazid for latent tuberculosis infection: a multicenter clinical trial. *Ann. Intern. Med.* **137:**640–647.

64. Jensen, P. A., L. A. Lambert, M. F. Iademarco, and R. Ridzon. 2005. Guidelines for preventing the transmission of *Mycobacterium tuberculosis* in health-care settings, 2005. *MMWR Recommend. Rep.* **54:**1–141.

65. Ji, B., C. Truffot-Pernot, C. Lacroix, M. C. Raviglione, R. J. O'Brien, P. Olliaro, G. Roscigno, and J. Grosset. 1993. Effectiveness of rifampin, rifabutin, and rifapentine for preventive therapy of tuberculosis in mice. *Am. Rev. Respir. Dis.* **148:**1541–1546.

66. Johnson, J. L., A. Okwera, D. L. Hom, H. Mayanja, C. Mutuluuza Kityo, P. Nsubuga, J. G. Nakibali, A. M. Loughlin, H. Yun, P. N. Mugyenyi, A. Vernon, R. D. Mugerwa, J. J. Ellner, and C. C. Whalen. 2001. Duration of efficacy of treatment of latent tuberculosis infection in HIV-infected adults. *AIDS* **15:**2137–2147.

67. Keane, J., S. Gershon, R. P. Wise, E. Mirabile-Levens, J. Kasznica, W. D. Schwieterman, J. N. Siegel, and M. M. Braun. 2001. Tuberculosis associated with infliximab, a tumor necrosis factor alpha-neutralizing agent. *N. Engl. J. Med.* **345:**1098–1104.

68. Kleinschmidt, I., and G. Churchyard. 1997. Variation in incidences of tuberculosis in subgroups of South African gold miners. *Occup. Environ. Med.* **54:**636–641.

69. Kopanoff, D. E., D. E. Snider, Jr., and G. J. Caras. 1978. Isoniazid-related hepatitis: a U.S. Public Health Service cooperative surveillance study. *Am. Rev. Respir. Dis.* **117:**991–1001.

70. Kwara, A., J. S. Herold, J. T. Machan, and E. J. Carter. 2008. Factors associated with failure to complete isoniazid treatment for latent tuberculosis infection in Rhode Island. *Chest* **133:**862–868.

71. Landry, J., and D. Menzies. 2008. Preventive chemotherapy. Where has it got us? Where to go next? *Int. J. Tuberc. Lung Dis.* **12:**1352–1364.

72. Lardizabal, A., M. Passannante, F. Kojakali, C. Hayden, and L. B. Reichman. 2006. Enhancement of treatment completion for latent tuberculosis infection with 4 months of rifampin. *Chest* **130:**1712–1717.

73. Lavigne, M., I. Rocher, C. Steensma, and P. Brassard. 2006. The impact of smoking on adherence to treatment for latent tuberculosis infection. *BMC Public Health* **6:**66.

74. Lecoeur, H. F., C. Truffot-Pernot, and J. H. Grosset. 1989. Experimental short-course preventive therapy of tuberculosis with rifampin and pyrazinamide. *Am. Rev. Respir. Dis.* **140:**1189–1193.

75. Li, J., S. S. Munsiff, T. Tarantino, and M. Dorsinville. 2010. Adherence to treatment of latent tuberculosis infection in a clinical population in New York City. *Int. J. Infect. Dis.* **14:**e292–e297.

76. Lobato, M. N., R. R. Reves, R. M. Jasmer, J. C. Grabau, N. N. Bock, and N. Shang. 2005. Adverse events and treatment completion for latent tuberculosis in jail inmates and homeless persons. *Chest* **127:**1296–1303.

77. Lobato, M. N., S. J. Sun, P. K. Moonan, S. E. Weis, L. Saiman, A. A. Reichard, and K. Feja. 2008. Underuse of effective measures to prevent and manage pediatric tuberculosis in the United States. *Arch. Pediatr. Adolesc. Med.* **162:**426–431.

78. Lobato, M. N., Y. C. Wang, J. E. Becerra, P. M. Simone, and K. G. Castro. 2006. Improved program activities are associated with decreasing tuberculosis incidence in the United States. *Public Health Rep.* **121:**108–115.

79. Lobue, P., and D. Menzies. 2010. Treatment of latent tuberculosis infection: an update. *Respirology* **15:**603–622.

80. LoBue, P. A., and K. S. Moser. 2005. Isoniazid- and rifampin-resistant tuberculosis in San Diego County, California, United States, 1993–2002. *Int. J. Tuberc. Lung Dis.* **9:**501–506.

81. LoBue, P. A., and K. S. Moser. 2003. Use of isoniazid for latent tuberculosis infection in a public health clinic. *Am. J. Respir. Crit. Care Med.* **168:**443–447.

82. Lou, H. X., M. A. Shullo, and T. P. McKaveney. 2002. Limited tolerability of levofloxacin and pyrazinamide for multidrug-resistant tuberculosis prophylaxis in a solid organ transplant population. *Pharmacotherapy* **22:**701–704.

83. Mangura, B. T., M. R. Passannante, and L. B. Reichman. 1997. An incentive in tuberculosis preventive therapy for an inner city population. *Int. J. Tuberc. Lung Dis.* **1:**576–578.

84. Markowitz, N., N. I. Hansen, P. C. Hopewell, J. Glassroth, P. A. Kvale, B. T. Mangura, T. C. Wilcosky, J. M. Wallace, M. J. Rosen, L. B. Reichman, and The Pulmonary Complications of HIV Infection Study Group. 1997. Incidence of tuberculosis in the United States among HIV-infected persons. *Ann. Intern. Med.* **126:**123–132.

85. McElroy, P. D., K. Ijaz, L. A. Lambert, J. A. Jereb, M. F. Iademarco, K. G. Castro, and T. R. Navin. 2005. National survey to measure rates of liver injury, hospitalization, and death associated with rifampin and pyrazinamide for latent tuberculosis infection. *Clin. Infect. Dis.* **41:**1125–1133.

86. McNeill, L., M. Allen, C. Estrada, and P. Cook. 2003. Pyrazinamide and rifampin vs isoniazid for the treatment of latent tuberculosis: improved completion rates but more hepatotoxicity. *Chest* **123:**102–106.

87. Menzies, D., M. J. Dion, D. Francis, I. Parisien, I. Rocher, S. Mannix, and K. Schwartzman. 2005. In closely monitored patients, adherence in the first month predicts completion of therapy for latent tuberculosis infection. *Int. J. Tuberc. Lung Dis.* **9:**1343–1348.

88. Menzies, D., M. J. Dion, B. Rabinovitch, S. Mannix, P. Brassard, and K. Schwartzman. 2004. Treatment completion and costs of a randomized trial of rifampin for 4 months versus isoniazid for 9 months. *Am. J. Respir. Crit. Care Med.* **170:**445–449.

89. Menzies, D., R. Long, A. Trajman, M. J. Dion, J. Yang, H. Al Jahdali, Z. Memish, K. Khan, M. Gardam, V. Hoeppner, A. Benedetti, and K. Schwartzman. 2008. Adverse events with 4 months of rifampin therapy or 9 months of isoniazid therapy for latent tuberculosis infection: a randomized trial. *Ann. Intern. Med.* **149:**689–697.

90. Mitchell, J. R., H. J. Zimmerman, K. G. Ishak, U. P. Thorgeirsson, J. A. Timbrell, W. R. Snodgrass, and S. D. Nelson. 1976. Isoniazid liver injury: clinical spectrum, pathology, and probable pathogenesis. *Ann. Intern. Med.* **84:**181–192.

91. Mitchison, D. A. 1985. The action of antituberculosis drugs in short-course chemotherapy. *Tubercle* **66:**219–225.

92. Miyazaki, E., R. E. Chaisson, and W. R. Bishai. 1999. Analysis of rifapentine for preventive therapy in the Cornell mouse model of latent tuberculosis. *Antimicrob. Agents Chemother.* **43:**2126–2130.

93. Moss, A. R., J. A. Hahn, J. P. Tulsky, C. L. Daley, P. M. Small, and P. C. Hopewell. 2000. Tuberculosis in the homeless. A prospective study. *Am. J. Respir. Crit. Care Med.* **162:**460–464.

94. Mount, F. W., and S. H. Ferebee. 1962. The effect of isoniazid prophylaxis on tuberculosis morbidity among household contacts of previously known cases of tuberculosis. *Am. Rev. Respir. Dis.* **85:**821–827.

95. Munro, S. A., S. A. Lewin, H. J. Smith, M. E. Engel, A. Fretheim, and J. Volmink. 2007. Patient adherence to tuberculosis treatment: a systematic review of qualitative research. *PLoS Med.* **4:**e238.

96. Mwinga, A., M. Hosp, P. Godfrey-Faussett, M. Quigley, P. Mwaba, B. N. Mugala, O. Nyirenda, N. Luo, J. Pobee, A. M. Elliott, K. P. McAdam, and J. D. Porter. 1998. Twice weekly tuberculosis preventive therapy in HIV infection in Zambia. *AIDS* **12:**2447–2457.

97. National Collaborating Centre for Chronic Conditions. 2006. *Tuberculosis: Clinical Diagnosis and Management of Tuberculosis, and Measures for Its Prevention and Control.* Royal College of Physicians, London, United Kingdom.

98. Nolan, C. M. 1999. Community-wide implementation of targeted testing for and treatment of latent tuberculosis infection. *Clin. Infect. Dis.* **29:**880–887.

99. Nolan, C. M., S. V. Goldberg, and S. E. Buskin. 1999. Hepatotoxicity associated with isoniazid preventive therapy: a 7-year survey from a public health tuberculosis clinic. *JAMA* **281:**1014–1018.

100. Nolan, C. M., L. Roll, S. V. Goldberg, and A. M. Elarth. 1997. Directly observed isoniazid preventive therapy for released jail inmates. *Am. J. Respir. Crit. Care Med.* **155:**583–586.

101. Nyamathi, A. M., A. Christiani, P. Nahid, P. Gregerson, and B. Leake. 2006. A randomized controlled trial of two treatment programs for homeless adults with latent tuberculosis infection. *Int. J. Tuberc. Lung Dis.* **10:**775–782.

102. Onozaki, I., and M. Raviglione. Stopping tuberculosis in the 21st century: goals and strategies. *Respirology* **15:**32–43.

103. Ormerod, L. P. 1998. Rifampicin and isoniazid prophylactic chemotherapy for tuberculosis. *Arch. Dis. Child.* **78:**169–171.

104. Ottenhoff, T. H. 2009. Overcoming the global crisis: "yes, we can", but also for TB . . . ? *Eur. J. Immunol.* **39:**2014–2020.

105. Pablos-Mendez, A., J. Blustein, and C. A. Knirsch. 1997. The role of diabetes mellitus in the higher prevalence of tuberculosis among Hispanics. *Am. J. Public Health* **87:**574–579.

106. Page, K. R., F. Sifakis, R. Montes de Oca, W. A. Cronin, M. C. Doherty, L. Federline, S. Bur, T. Walsh, W. Karney, J. Milman,

N. Baruch, A. Adelakun, and S. E. Dorman. 2006. Improved adherence and less toxicity with rifampin vs isoniazid for treatment of latent tuberculosis: a retrospective study. *Arch. Intern. Med.* **166:**1863–1870.

107. Palmer, C. E., S. Jablon, and P. Q. Edwards. 1957. Tuberculosis morbidity of young men in relation to tuberculin sensitivity and body build. *Am. Rev. Tuberc.* **76:**517–539.

108. Papastavros, T., L. R. Dolovich, A. Holbrook, L. Whitehead, and M. Loeb. 2002. Adverse events associated with pyrazinamide and levofloxacin in the treatment of latent multidrug-resistant tuberculosis. *CMAJ* **167:**131–136.

109. Pape, J. W., S. S. Jean, J. L. Ho, A. Hafner, and W. D. Johnson, Jr. 1993. Effect of isoniazid prophylaxis on incidence of active tuberculosis and progression of HIV infection. *Lancet* **342:**268–272.

110. Parsyan, A. E., J. Saukkonen, M. A. Barry, S. Sharnprapai, and C. R. Horsburgh, Jr. 2007. Predictors of failure to complete treatment for latent tuberculosis infection. *J. Infect.* **54:** 262–266.

111. Pepper, T., P. Joseph, C. Mwenya, G. S. McKee, A. Haushalter, A. Carter, J. Warkentin, D. W. Haas, and T. R. Sterling. 2008. Normal chest radiography in pulmonary tuberculosis: implications for obtaining respiratory specimen cultures. *Int. J. Tuberc. Lung Dis.* **12:**397–403.

112. Polesky, A., H. W. Farber, D. J. Gottlieb, H. Park, S. Levinson, J. J. O'Connell, B. McInnis, R. L. Nieves, and J. Bernardo. 1996. Rifampin preventive therapy for tuberculosis in Boston's homeless. *Am. J. Respir. Crit. Care Med.* **154:** 1473–1477.

113. Powell, D. A. 2008. Latent tuberculosis needs attention. *Arch. Pediatr. Adolesc. Med.* **162:**489–490.

114. Priest, D. H., L. F. Vossel, Jr., E. A. Sherfy, D. P. Hoy, and C. A. Haley. 2004. Use of intermittent rifampin and pyrazinamide therapy for latent tuberculosis infection in a targeted tuberculin testing program. *Clin. Infect. Dis.* **39:**1764–1771.

115. Public Health Agency of Canada and Canadian Lung Association. 2007. *Canadian Tuberculosis Standards,* 6th ed. Public Health Agency of Canada and Canadian Lung Association, Ottawa, Canada.

116. Quigley, M. A., A. Mwinga, M. Hosp, I. Lisse, D. Fuchs, J. D. H. Porter, and P. Godfrey-Faussett. 2001. Long-term effect of preventive therapy for tuberculosis in a cohort of HIV-infected Zambian adults. *AIDS* **15:**215–222.

117. Reichler, M. R., R. Reves, S. Bur, J. Ford, V. Thompson, B. Mangura, I. M. Onorato, and S. E. Valway. 2002. Treatment of latent tuberculosis infection in contacts of new tuberculosis cases in the United States. *South. Med. J.* **95:**414–420.

118. Reichman, L. B., A. Lardizabal, and C. H. Hayden. 2004. Considering the role of four months of rifampin in the treatment of latent tuberculosis infection. *Am. J. Respir. Crit. Care Med.* **170:**832–835.

119. Ridzon, R., J. Meador, R. Maxwell, K. Higgins, P. Weismuller, and I. M. Onorato. 1997. Asymptomatic hepatitis in persons who received alternative preventive therapy with pyrazinamide and ofloxacin. *Clin. Infect. Dis.* **24:**1264–1265.

120. Rose, D. N., C. B. Schechter, and A. L. Silver. 1986. The age threshold for isoniazid chemoprophylaxis. A decision analysis for low-risk tuberculin reactors. *JAMA* **256:**2709–2713.

121. Runyon, E. H. 1965. Preventive treatment in tuberculosis: a statement by the Committee on Therapy, American Thoracic Society. *Am. Rev. Respir. Dis.* **91:**297–298.

122. Saukkonen, J. J., D. L. Cohn, R. M. Jasmer, S. Schenker, J. A. Jereb, C. M. Nolan, C. A. Peloquin, F. M. Gordin, D. Nunes, D. B. Strader, J. Bernardo, R. Venkataramanan, and T. R. Sterling. 2006. An official ATS statement: hepatotoxicity of antituberculosis therapy. *Am. J. Respir. Crit. Care Med.* **174:** 935–952.

123. Schaaf, H. S., H. A. Vermeulen, R. P. Gie, N. Beyers, and P. R. Donald. 1999. Evaluation of young children in household contact with adult multidrug-resistant pulmonary tuberculosis cases. *Pediatr. Infect. Dis. J.* **18:**494–500.

124. Schechter, M., R. Zajdenverg, G. Falco, G. L. Barnes, J. C. Faulhaber, J. S. Coberly, R. D. Moore, and R. E. Chaisson. 2006. Weekly rifapentine/isoniazid or daily rifampin/pyrazinamide for latent tuberculosis in household contacts. *Am. J. Respir. Crit. Care Med.* **173:**922–926.

125. Selwyn, P. A., D. Hartel, V. A. Lewis, E. E. Schoenbaum, S. H. Vermund, R. S. Klein, A. T. Walker, and G. H. Friedland. 1989. A prospective study of the risk of tuberculosis among intravenous drug users with human immunodeficiency virus infection. *N. Engl. J. Med.* **320:**545–550.

126. Shafer, R. W., and B. R. Edlin. 1996. Tuberculosis in patients infected with human immunodeficiency virus: perspective on the past decade. *Clin. Infect. Dis.* **22:**683–704.

127. Shieh, F. K., G. Snyder, C. R. Horsburgh, J. Bernardo, C. Murphy, and J. J. Saukkonen. 2006. Predicting non-completion of treatment for latent tuberculous infection: a prospective survey. *Am. J. Respir. Crit. Care Med.* **174:**717–721.

128. Shukla, S. J., D. K. Warren, K. F. Woeltje, C. A. Gruber, and V. J. Fraser. 2002. Factors associated with the treatment of latent tuberculosis infection among health-care workers at a midwestern teaching hospital. *Chest* **122:**1609–1614.

129. Spyridis, N. P., P. G. Spyridis, A. Gelesme, V. Sypsa, M. Valianatou, F. Metsou, D. Gourgiotis, and M. N. Tsolia. 2007. The effectiveness of a 9-month regimen of isoniazid alone versus 3- and 4-month regimens of isoniazid plus rifampin for treatment of latent tuberculosis infection in children: results of an 11-year randomized study. *Clin. Infect. Dis.* **45:**715–722.

130. Steele, M. A., R. F. Burk, and R. M. DesPrez. 1991. Toxic hepatitis with isoniazid and rifampin. A meta-analysis. *Chest* **99:**465–471.

131. Steiger, Z., W. O. Nickel, G. J. Shannon, E. G. Nedwicki, and R. F. Higgins. 1976. Pulmonary tuberculosis after gastric resection. *Am. J. Surg.* **131:**668–671.

132. Sterling, T. R. 2008. New approaches to the treatment of latent tuberculosis. *Semin. Respir. Crit. Care Med.* **29:**532–541.

133. Sterling, T. R., J. Bethel, S. Goldberg, P. Weinfurter, L. Yun, and C. R. Horsburgh. 2006. The scope and impact of treatment of latent tuberculosis infection in the United States and Canada. *Am. J. Respir. Crit. Care Med.* **173:**927–931.

134. Stout, J. E., J. J. Engemann, A. C. Cheng, E. R. Fortenberry, and C. D. Hamilton. 2003. Safety of 2 months of rifampin and pyrazinamide for treatment of latent tuberculosis. *Am. J. Respir. Crit. Care Med.* **167:**824–827.

135. Sutherland, I. 1976. Recent studies in the epidemiology of tuberculosis, based on the risk of being infected with tubercle bacilli. *Adv. Tuberc. Res.* **19:**1–63.

136. Tam, C. M., S. L. Chan, K. M. Kam, E. Sim, D. Staples, K. M. Sole, H. Al-Ghusein, and D. A. Mitchison. 2000. Rifapentine and isoniazid in the continuation phase of a 6-month regimen. Interim report: no activity of isoniazid in the continuation phase. *Int. J. Tuberc. Lung Dis.* **4:**262–267.

137. Taylor, Z., C. M. Nolan, and H. M. Blumberg. 2005. Controlling tuberculosis in the United States. Recommendations from the American Thoracic Society, CDC, and the Infectious Diseases Society of America. *MMWR Recommend. Rep.* **54:** 1–81.

138. Thorn, P. A., V. S. Brookes, and J. A. Waterhouse. 1956. Peptic ulcer, partial gastrectomy, and pulmonary tuberculosis. *Br. Med. J.* **1:**603–608.

139. Tulsky, J. P., J. A. Hahn, H. L. Long, D. B. Chambers, M. J. Robertson, M. A. Chesney, and A. R. Moss. 2004. Can the poor adhere? Incentives for adherence to TB prevention in homeless adults. *Int. J. Tuberc. Lung Dis.* **8**:83–91.

140. Tulsky, J. P., L. Pilote, J. A. Hahn, A. J. Zolopa, M. Burke, M. Chesney, and A. R. Moss. 2000. Adherence to isoniazid prophylaxis in the homeless: a randomized controlled trial. *Arch. Intern. Med.* **160**:697–702.

141. Tulsky, J. P., M. C. White, C. Dawson, T. M. Hoynes, J. Goldenson, and G. Schecter. 1998. Screening for tuberculosis in jail and clinic follow-up after release. *Am. J. Public Health* **88**:223–226.

142. U.S. Department of Health and Human Services. 2000. *Healthy People 2010*, 2nd ed., vol. 2. U.S. Department of Health and Human Services, Washington, DC.

143. Vernon, A., W. Burman, D. Benator, A. Khan, L. Bozeman, and Tuberculosis Trials Consortium. 1999. Acquired rifamycin monoresistance in patients with HIV-related tuberculosis treated with once-weekly rifapentine and isoniazid. *Lancet* **353**:1843–1847.

144. Villarino, M., S. W. Dooley, L. Geiter, K. G. Castro, and D. E. Snider, Jr. 1992. Management of persons exposed to multidrug-resistant tuberculosis. *MMWR Recommend. Rep.* **44**:59–71.

145. Villarino, M. E., R. Ridzon, P. C. Weismuller, M. Elcock, R. M. Maxwell, J. Meador, P. J. Smith, M. L. Carson, and L. J. Geiter. 1997. Rifampin preventive therapy for tuberculosis infection: experience with 157 adolescents. *Am. J. Respir. Crit. Care Med.* **155**:1735–1738.

146. Weiner, M., N. Bock, C. A. Peloquin, W. J. Burman, A. Khan, A. Vernon, Z. Zhao, S. Weis, T. R. Sterling, K. Hayden, and S. Goldberg. 2004. Pharmacokinetics of rifapentine at 600, 900, and 1,200 mg during once-weekly tuberculosis therapy. *Am. J. Respir. Crit. Care Med.* **169**:1191–1197.

147. Whalen, C. C., J. L. Johnson, A. Okwera, D. L. Hom, R. Huebner, P. Mugyenyi, R. D. Mugerwa, and J. J. Ellner for the Uganda-Case Western Reserve University Research Collaboration. 1997. A trial of three regimens to prevent tuberculosis in Ugandan adults infected with the human immunodeficiency virus. *N. Engl. J. Med.* **337**:801–808.

148. White, M. C., J. P. Tulsky, J. Goldenson, C. J. Portillo, M. Kawamura, and E. Menendez. 2002. Randomized controlled trial of interventions to improve follow-up for latent tuberculosis infection after release from jail. *Arch. Intern. Med.* **162**:1044–1050.

149. White, M. C., J. P. Tulsky, E. Menendez, J. Goldenson, and L. M. Kawamura. 2005. Incidence of TB in inmates with latent TB infection: 5-year follow-up. *Am. J. Prev. Med.* **29**:295–301.

150. World Health Organization. 2006. The Global Plan to Stop TB, 2006–2015. Actions for life: towards a world free of tuberculosis. *Int. J. Tuberc. Lung Dis.* **10**:240–241.

151. World Health Organization. 2009. *Global Tuberculosis Control 2009: Epidemiology, Strategy, Financing.* World Health Organization, Geneva, Switzerland.

152. World Health Organization. 2004. *Interim Policy on Collaborative TB/HIV Activities. Stop TB Department and Department of HIV/AIDS.* World Health Organization, Geneva, Switzerland.

153. World Health Organization. 2008. *Three I's Meeting. Intensified Case Finding (ICF), Isoniazid Preventive Therapy (IPT) and TB Infection Control (IC) for People Living with HIV. Report of a Joint World Health Organization HIV/AIDS and TB Department Meeting, 2–4 April, 2008*, p. 1–12. World Health Organization, Geneva, Switzerland.

154. World Health Organization and Centers for Disease Control and Prevention. 2008. *TB/HIV Clinical Manual.* World Health Organization, Geneva, Switzerland.

155. Ziakas, P. D., and E. Mylonakis. 2009. 4 months of rifampin compared with 9 months of isoniazid for the management of latent tuberculosis infection: a meta-analysis and cost-effectiveness study that focuses on compliance and liver toxicity. *Clin. Infect. Dis.* **49**:1883–1889.

Chapter 7

Chemotherapy of Tuberculosis

THOMAS E. DOBBS AND RISA M. WEBB

INTRODUCTION

In this chapter we review the underlying principles of tuberculosis (TB) chemotherapy, medical management, and current treatment recommendations.

BIOLOGY OF TB

TB is caused by members of the *Mycobacterium tuberculosis* complex, with *M. tuberculosis* being responsible for the vast majority of disease. Organisms within this group grow slowly, with generation times of 15 to 20 h. This leads to slow growth on solid culture media, typically 3 to 8 weeks until visible colonies are seen. This low replication rate, a capacity for dormancy, and the currently available treatment options necessitate prolonged treatment courses to ensure the successful eradication of infection.

PRINCIPLES OF TB CHEMOTHERAPY

M. tuberculosis can affect any organ system, but pulmonary disease accounts for the vast majority of active TB cases. In the case of cavitary lung disease, the TB organisms are felt to reside within three distinct populations that can be differentiated by location and growth characteristics (13). The first population resides within an extracellular environment, actively multiplying in the liquid caseous debris of pulmonary cavities. Approximately 10^8 organisms may be present within a typical pulmonary cavity (4). As resistance to antimicrobials in TB occurs through random genetic point mutations, and not from mobile resistance elements, this large population of organisms is the prime location for the natural selection of drug-resistant mycobacteria. A second population consists of slowly growing organisms within macrophages.

There are few organisms within this compartment, but the acidic environment and lack of reproductive activity here limit the utility of many anti-TB agents. A third compartment consists of slowly growing organisms within the solid caseous material. Penetration of drugs into this compartment may be limited by a paucity of blood flow.

To effectively treat active TB, a medication regimen must consist of highly active agents that are capable of reaching the organisms within the various compartments. Additionally, treatment must be continued for sufficient time to ensure the eradication of all viable organisms. Early in the history of anti-TB chemotherapy, the highly effective agent streptomycin (SM) was applied as monotherapy. Although patients would initially improve, subsequent relapse was common due to the development of drug resistance (7, 52). Resistance of *M. tuberculosis* to individual first-line drugs occurs naturally within a given population at a frequency of approximately 1 for every 10^6 to 10^7 organisms, depending upon the drug in question (26). Given the large number of organisms present in cavitary lung disease, monotherapy with any agent can result in a drug-resistant population and subsequent dissemination within the patient. The utilization of multiple effective agents creates a statistical barrier to the development of resistance, since mutations for resistance to any specific drug occur independently.

Current first-line regimens consist of three or four agents that, in concert, can eradicate organisms within all compartments and prevent the development of drug resistance. Rifampin (RIF) is bactericidal against all three populations. Isoniazid (INH) is bactericidal against extracellular and intracellular organisms. Pyrazinamide (PZA) is bactericidal against intracellular organisms and works well in an acidic pH. SM and the aminoglycosides are bactericidal against extracellular organisms. Ethambutol (EMB)

Thomas E. Dobbs • Mississippi State Department of Health, University of Mississippi Medical Center, Jackson, MS 39215.
Risa M. Webb • Department of Infectious Diseases, G.V. "Sonny" Montgomery VA Medical Center, University of Mississippi Medical Center, Mississippi State Department of Health, Jackson, MS 39216.

lacks bactericidal activity and is often used in first-line regimens until drug susceptibility to other agents is ensured (25).

Standard treatment regimens are typically separated into two phases. The initial phase includes the first 8 weeks of treatment. The continuation phase is an additional 4 to 7 months, depending on treatment response. The initial phase of treatment utilizes the potent sterilizing effects of RIF, PZA, and INH to clear live bacilli from sputum in the majority of patients. The combination of INH and RIF in the continuation phase eradicates residual organisms, minimizing relapse of disease.

ADHERENCE TO TREATMENT

Given the propensity for developing resistance and the prolonged treatment regimens required, adherence to therapy is of paramount importance. To this end, directly observed therapy (DOT) is the recommended approach to medication delivery (American Thoracic Society/CDC/Infectious Diseases Society of America) (1). DOT involves the direct administration of medications under the supervision of public health providers or appropriate designees. Medication administration should be strictly monitored to ensure that pills are actually swallowed or are not regurgitated. Effective intermittent dosing regimens (twice or thrice weekly) can facilitate these efforts in the setting of limited public resources. Promoting adherence additionally requires an infrastructure that can assist patients in overcoming barriers, incentivize compliance, and track and locate patients. A legal framework that can protect the community from infectious patients is also a key element.

DRUGS

INH, RIF, PZA, EMB, and SM are the five standard first-line agents. Fluoroquinolones, which have potent bactericidal activity against *M. tuberculosis*, are currently utilized for drug-resistant strains and when first-line agents are not tolerated. See Tables 1, 2, and 3 for additional drug-specific information.

Isoniazid

INH has profound bactericidal activity against actively dividing organisms (16) by interfering with production of the cell wall component mycolic acid (48). INH readily penetrates body tissues and the central nervous system. It is metabolized by the liver and has a half-life of 1 to 3 h, depending on the acetylation status of the individual. It may be dosed daily, twice weekly, or three times weekly (Table 2). It is available in oral and parenteral formulations. There are few drug interactions with INH, but it does increase the levels of phenytoin and carbamazepine, and drug levels should be monitored if either of these is given with INH.

Toxicity

Elevated transaminases, clinical hepatitis, and peripheral neuropathy are among the most common adverse events seen with INH. An elevation in serum aspartate transaminase (AST) and alanine aminotransferase (ALT) of up to five times the upper limit of normal may occur in 10 to 20% of persons receiving INH alone (24), typically returning to normal after cessation of the drug. Clinical hepatitis is a rare but serious adverse event, occurring in <1% of patients on INH. INH-related hepatitis is associated with increasing age (19), alcohol consumption, and chronic hepatitis (44) and is more common when RIF is coadministered (41). Fatal hepatitis is rare, <7 per 100,000 (38), and has been associated with the continuation of INH in the presence of clinical hepatitis (29). Peripheral neuropathy is a dose-related phenomenon, occurring in less than 0.2% of patients (see "Adverse Reactions" below). It is more frequently encountered in patients with coexisting issues such as poor nutritional status, diabetes, human immunodeficiency virus (HIV) infection, renal failure, alcoholism, pregnancy, and breast-feeding. Pyridoxine supplementation of 10 to 50 mg daily is recommended (40), particularly for those with predisposing conditions (1). Pyridoxine at 50 mg biweekly is an option for patients on intermittent dosing regimens. Other, rarely reported adverse events include seizures, rash, hematologic abnormalities, and a lupus-type syndrome.

Rifampin

RIF is a potent bactericidal agent with activity against dividing and semidormant organisms (27). RIF inhibits the DNA-dependent RNA polymerase of *M. tuberculosis*. As an effective sterilizing agent, RIF is a required component of any short-course regimen. RIF has a half-life of 1.5 to 5 h, penetrates most tissues well, and has variable central nervous system penetration. It is available in oral and intravenous formulations. RIF can be dosed daily, twice weekly, or three times weekly (Table 2). It is metabolized by the liver, and by upregulating the cytochrome P-450 oxidase system, it decreases the levels of many other medications. Drug-drug interactions with many antiretroviral agents limit coadministration with RIF, in which

Table 1. Drug characteristics

Drug	Available formulation(s)	Adverse reactions	CNS[a] penetration	Dosing in renal insufficiency	Dosing in hepatic insufficiency	Safety in pregnancy
INH	Oral (50-, 100-, 300-mg tablets and 50-mg/5 ml suspension), intravenous and intramuscular	Hepatitis, rash, peripheral neuropathy, CNS effects	20–100% of serum concns	No change	No change, but use with caution given potential hepatotoxicity	Likely safe[b] Category C
RIF	Oral (150- and 300-mg capsules) and intravenous	Hepatitis, rash, flu-like syndrome, thrombocytopenia	10–20% of serum concns (improved with inflamed meninges)	No change	No change; use with caution	Likely safe Category C
PZA	Oral (500-mg scored and unscored tablets)	Hepatotoxicity, rash, hyperuricemia, photosensitivity, nausea	75–100% of serum concns	Decreased in advanced renal insufficiency (see Table 5)	No change; use with caution	Recommended by WHO
EMB	Oral (100- and 400-mg tablets)	Retrobulbar neuritis, rash (rare)	Poor (inflamed meninges only)	Decreased in advanced renal insufficiency (see Table 5)	No change; can be used safely in patients with liver disease	Likely safe Category C
SM	Intravenous or intramuscular	Nephrotoxicity, ototoxicity, vestibular toxicity, hypokalemia, hypomagnesemia	Poor (improved with inflamed meninges)	Decrease dosage and interval (see Table 5); use with extreme caution	No change	Contraindicated in pregnancy
Ofloxacin	Oral (200-, 300-, and 400-mg tablets)	Tendon rupture, arthralgia, nausea, CNS effects, QTc[c] prolongation	Limited data	Dose adjustment for creatinine clearance of <50 ml/min	Safe	Avoid in pregnancy
Levofloxacin	Oral (250-, 500-, and 750-mg tablets and 25-mg/ml oral suspension) and intravenous	Tendon rupture, arthralgia, nausea, CNS effects, QTc[c] prolongation	16–20% of serum concns	Dose adjustment for creatinine clearance of <50 ml/min	Safe	Avoid in pregnancy
Moxifloxacin	Oral (400-mg tablet) and intravenous	Tendon rupture, arthralgia, nausea, CNS effects, QTc[c] prolongation	Likely good (limited data [18])	Unchanged	Safe; use with caution; rare hepatitis	Avoid in pregnancy
RFB	Oral (150-mg capsule)	Leukopenia, thrombocytopenia, uveitis, rash, hepatitis, arthralgia	Penetrates with inflamed meninges	No change	No change; use with caution	Limited data; use with caution

[a]CNS, central nervous system.
[b]Increased risk of hepatotoxicity with pregnancy. Supplementation with vitamin B$_6$ required due to enhanced nutritional requirements.
[c]QTc, QT Interval Corrected.

Table 2. Dosing of first-line TB drugs[a]

Drug	Daily dose		Twice-weekly dose		Thrice-weekly dose (adults)
	Children	Adults	Children	Adults	
INH	10–15 mg/kg; max, 300 mg	5 mg/kg; max, 300 mg	20–30 mg/kg; max, 900 mg	15 mg/kg; max, 900 mg	15 mg/kg; max, 900 mg
RIF	10–20 mg/kg; max, 600 mg	10 mg/kg; max, 600 mg	10–20 mg/kg; max, 600 mg	10 mg/kg; max, 600 mg	10 mg/kg; max, 600 mg
PZA	15–30 mg/kg; max, 2 g	See Table 3	50 mg/kg; max, 2 g	See Table 3	See Table 3
EMB[b]	15–20 mg/kg; max, 1 g	See Table 3	50 mg/kg; max, 2.5 g	See Table 3	See Table 3
SM	20–40 mg/kg; max, 1 g	15 mg/kg[c]; max, 1 g	20 mg/kg; max, 1.5 g	15 mg/kg[c]; max, 1 g	15 mg/kg[c]; max, 1 g
Ofloxacin	—[d]	600–800 mg daily	—		
Levofloxacin	—	500–1,000 mg daily	—		
Moxifloxacin	—	400 mg daily	—		
RFB		5 mg/kg; max, 300 mg		5 mg/kg; max, 300 mg	5 mg/kg; max, 300 mg

[a]See reference 1. max, maximum.
[b]EMB is not recommended for children too young to reliably monitor for vision changes (less than 8 years old).
[c]A dose of 10 mg/kg (max, 750 mg) for those >59 years old.
[d]—, fluoroquinolones not approved for use in children or pregnant women.

case rifabutin (RFB) is often substituted (see chapter 32). Patients taking oral contraceptives require a different method of birth control while taking rifamycin drugs due to drug interactions. Patients on warfarin require additional monitoring of coagulation studies if RIF is started. An extensive review of all coadministered medications for potential drug-drug interactions must be performed prior to the initiation of RIF.

Toxicity

Hepatotoxicity due to RIF is far less common than that due to INH and occurs more frequently with a cholestatic presentation (35, 41), with elevated bilirubin and alkaline phosphatase. Rash and pruritus may occur in 6% of recipients but is typically transient (47). True hypersensitivity occurs rarely. A separate petechial rash may occur with thrombocytopenia (see below). A flu-like syndrome may occur in <1% of patients on RIF and is typically seen with intermittent (biweekly or thrice weekly) dosing (1). Hematologic reactions are infrequent. RIF-dependent autoimmune thrombocytopenia occurs through antiplatelet antibodies (23) that can improve on cessation of the drug. RIF results in an orange discoloration of body fluids such as urine and tears. This is generally benign but may stain contact lenses and can generate patient anxiety if unexpected (see "Adverse Reactions").

Pyrazinamide

PZA is bactericidal against intracellular organisms residing in an acidic environment (22). PZA exerts its activity through disruption of membrane activity and transport functions (53). It is uniquely effective in eliminating persisting organisms and is used during the first 2 months of treatment to reduce the total length of therapy. The lack of PZA in an anti-TB regimen necessitates a prolongation of treatment to a minimum of 9 months. PZA is available in an oral formulation only. It can be dosed daily, twice weekly, or three times a week (Table 3). PZA has a half-life of 9 to 10 h and is cleared through the kidneys.

Toxicity

Hepatotoxicity is the most important adverse event associated with PZA, occurring in approximately 1% of recipients (9). The risk of hepatotoxicity is not appreciably increased by the coadministration of INH and RIF (39). Elevated uric acid is a commonly encountered phenomenon, does not routinely necessitate drug discontinuation, and is not typically

Table 3. Weight-based dosing for PZA and EMB

Schedule	Dose (mg) at indicated wt (kg)[a]		
	40–55	56–75	76–90
PZA			
Daily	1,000	1,500	2,000[b]
Biweekly	2,000	3,000	4,000[b]
Thrice weekly	1,500	2,500	3,000[b]
EMB			
Daily	800	1,200	1,600[b]
Biweekly	2,000	2,800	4,000[b]
Thrice weekly	1,200	2,000	2,400[b]

[a]Based on estimated lean body mass.
[b]Maximum dose regardless of weight.

Table 4. Alternative treatment regimens in patients intolerant or resistant to INH, RIF, or PZA

Drug absent	INH	PZA	RIF
Treatment options	RIF, PZA, and EMB for 6 mo RIF and EMB for 12 mo (PZA for first 2 mo preferred)	INH, RIF, EMB for 8 wks[a] and followed by INH and RIF for 31 wks[b]	INH, EMB, and a fluoroquinolone for 12–18 mo (PZA initial 2 mo at a minimum)[c]

[a]Daily or 5-days-per-week dosing.
[b]Daily, 5-days-per-week, or intermittent dosing is acceptable. HIV-coinfected patients with CD4 cell counts of <100 cells/μl should receive daily or thrice-weekly treatment.
[c]An aminoglycoside may be included for the initial 2 to 3 months for extensive disease or to shorten treatment to 12 months.

associated with gout symptoms unless individuals have a prior diagnosis of gout (8). Other reported side effects include nausea, vomiting, photosensitivity dermatitis, mild rash (see "Adverse Reactions" below), and nongouty arthralgia. In a standard multidrug TB regimen, PZA is a more likely cause of hepatitis or rash than INH or RIF (51).

Ethambutol

Although bacteriostatic, EMB has proven to be an effective component in certain TB regimens. The primary role of EMB in first-line regimens is to prevent the acquisition of drug resistance while the susceptibility profile of a TB isolate is unknown. It can be used along with RIF and PZA when INH is not tolerated or if an isolate is INH resistant (Table 4). EMB has a half-life of approximately 4 h. It can be dosed daily, twice weekly, or three times weekly (Table 3). EMB is excreted through the kidneys, and dosing adjustments may be required in the setting of renal insufficiency (Table 5). It is available in an oral formulation only.

Toxicity

Optic neuritis is the primary toxicity associated with EMB. It is a dose-related phenomenon that is rare unless the daily dose is greater than 15 mg/kg

Table 5. Dosing with renal dysfunction[a]

Drug	Change in dosing	Recommended dose and frequency[b]
INH	No	300 mg daily or 900 mg thrice weekly
RIF	No	600 mg daily or 600 mg thrice weekly
PZA	Yes	25–35 mg/kg thrice weekly (not daily)
EMB	Yes	15–25 mg/kg thrice weekly (not daily)
Levofloxacin	Yes	750–1,000 mg thrice weekly (not daily)[c]
SM	Yes	12–15 mg/kg biweekly or thrice weekly (not daily)

[a]Adapted from reference 1.
[b]For patients with a creatinine clearance of <30 ml/min or on hemodialysis.
[c]Based on antibacterial data.

of body weight (21). The loss of red-green color discrimination can be an early manifestation. Baseline visual assessments are recommended prior to the initiation of EMB and monthly thereafter. This is particularly important if the dosage exceeds 15 mg/kg daily or if the agent is continued beyond 2 months (1). EMB should be used with caution in young children that cannot be adequately assessed for visual problems. Renal insufficiency is an additional risk factor to the development of optic neuritis with EMB. The detection of visual deterioration while on EMB necessitates discontinuation of the drug. Visual improvement generally follows. Lack of rapid improvement should prompt an ophthalmologic evaluation. Peripheral neuritis and skin eruptions (see "Adverse Reactions" below) are reactions that have been documented rarely.

Streptomycin

SM is an aminoglycoside that exerts its effect on *M. tuberculosis* by disrupting protein synthesis. It is bactericidal against actively growing extracellular organisms. SM is cleared through the kidneys and should be used with caution in patients with renal insufficiency. It is available in parenteral formulations only and can be dosed daily, twice weekly, or three times a week (Table 2). Primary SM resistance is frequently encountered in high-incidence countries, limiting the utility of this agent in those populations.

Toxicity

Toxicity is common in patients receiving SM, occurring in approximately 10% (11). Ototoxicity is the main adverse reaction noted with SM, including vestibular disorders and hearing loss. The risk of toxicity is increased with advancing age, with coadministration of loop diuretics, and when the cumulative dose exceeds 100 g. Significant renal toxicity occurs in about 2% of patients (17). Circumoral paresthesia may occur immediately following administration but is typically benign. Hypokalemia and hypomagnesemia are encountered infrequently.

Alternate Drugs Which May Be Used in First-Line Regimens

Rifabutin

RFB is structurally similar to RIF, has an identical mechanism of action, and is equally active against *M. tuberculosis*. RFB is more lipid soluble, leading to a longer half-life, approximately 45 h. As RFB has less effect on the cytochrome P-450 oxidase system, it can be safely dosed with many agents that are contraindicated with RIF. RFB can be safely used with many antiretroviral regimens (see chapter 32). A review of potential drug-drug interactions should be performed prior to treating patients with RFB.

Hepatitis with RFB occurs with a frequency similar to that with RIF. Leukopenia may occur in 2% of patients (1) and is more common with daily administration than intermittent dosing (12). Other side effects such as uveitis, arthralgias, flu-like syndromes, and rash occur rarely. An orange discoloration of body fluids occurs as with RIF.

Rifapentine

Rifapentine is a rifamycin derivative with activity similar to that of RIF. It has a longer half-life (15 h) and has been evaluated for once-weekly use along with INH in the continuation phase of TB treatment. The role of rifapentine is limited in the treatment of TB, but it may be considered for use in the continuation phase for pan-susceptible pulmonary TB patients with noncavitary disease only if smear conversion occurred in the first 8 weeks of treatment (1, 2). Rifapentine is contraindicated in HIV-infected patients due to the development of RIF resistance (46). The side effects of rifapentine are similar to those encountered with RIF. Rifapentine is also a potent inducer of the cytochrome P-450 system.

Aminoglycosides other than SM

Kanamycin, amikacin, and capreomycin may be used in place of SM when necessary. *M. tuberculosis* strains resistant to SM may be susceptible to other aminoglycosides, but the susceptibility to each agent must be confirmed by resistance testing. Isolates resistant to kanamycin will also be resistant to amikacin. These agents are available in parenteral form only and have side effect profiles similar to that of SM.

Fluoroquinolones

Fluoroquinolones demonstrate potent bactericidal activity against *M. tuberculosis* (28). These agents are critical components of multidrug-resistant TB treatment regimens when susceptible. Fluoroquinolones can also be utilized when first-line agents are held due to intolerance or resistance. The precise role of these agents in first-line treatment is being defined by ongoing research. In the setting of RIF monoresistance or intolerance, a fluoroquinolone is a recommended component of a 12- to 18-month regimen including INH, EMB, and at least 2 months of PZA (1). Moxifloxacin, levofloxacin, and ofloxacin are agents frequently used in this class for the treatment of TB. Moxifloxacin may be the most active agent available based on animal models (31, 34). Fluoroquinolones are available in oral and parenteral formulations. There are no data to support intermittent (twice- or thrice-weekly) dosing of these agents (1).

Adverse events associated with fluoroquinolones include neuropsychiatric disorders, tendon rupture, nausea, and QT prolongation. The use of fluoroquinolones is discouraged in children and pregnant women due to concerns over bone and cartilage development.

Second-Line Agents

Cycloserine, ethionamide, and *p*-aminosalicylic acid agents are available for the treatment of *M. tuberculosis* but have little role in drug-susceptible disease (see chapter 8). These drugs have less activity against *M. tuberculosis* than do first-line agents and have unfavorable side effect profiles.

TREATMENT OF TB

Treatment Regimens

A standard 6-month (26-week) short-course regimen is the preferred treatment of newly diagnosed patients never previously treated for TB. All treatment should be with DOT. This regimen consists of an initial 2-month (8-week) phase of INH, RIF, PZA, and either EMB or SM. EMB or SM should be continued in the initial phase of treatment until susceptibility to INH and RIF is known. EMB, a well-tolerated oral agent, is generally preferred. Following the initial phase, INH and RIF are continued for an additional 4 months (18 weeks). For patients with cavitary pulmonary TB that fail to convert to culture-negative status in the initial phase, the continuation phase should be extended to a total of 7 months (Fig. 1). A continuation phase of once-weekly INH-rifapentine can be used for HIV-negative patients without cavities and negative acid-fast bacillus (AFB) smear status prior to completion of the initial phase (1, 2). All treatment of patients with TB should be done in conjunction with the local health department.

During the initial phase, daily administration is recommended for the first 2 weeks. Thereafter,

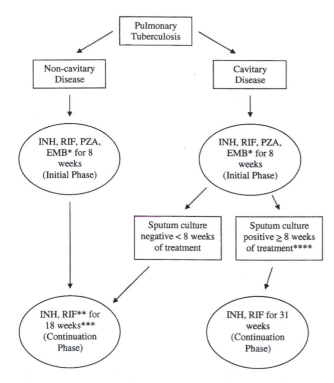

Figure 1. Management of drug-susceptible pulmonary TB. *, EMB may be discontinued if susceptibility to other first-line agents is ensured; **, rifapentene may be an appropriate substitution in HIV-negative patients with noncavitary disease and sputum smear conversion during the initial phase; ***, additional duration of treatment may be considered for delayed clinical or radiographic improvement; ****, delayed culture conversion should prompt consideration of acquired drug resistance, noncompliance, and malabsorption.

Table 6. Preferred first-line treatment regimens[a]

Initial phase		Continuation phase	
Drug	Duration	Drug	Duration
INH RIF PZA EMB[b]	8 wks[c]	INH[d] RIF	18 wks (31 wks for delayed culture conversion—see Fig. 1).
		INH[d] Rifapentene[e]	18 wks (once-weekly dosing)

[a]See reference 1.
[b]EMB may be discontinued if susceptibility to INH, RIF, and PZA is ensured.
[c]Daily or 5-days-per-week dosing is preferable for the first 14 days. Thereafter, twice-weekly or thrice-weekly dosing is acceptable. HIV-coinfected patients with CD4 cell counts of <100 cells/μl should receive daily or thrice-weekly treatment.
[d]Daily, 5-days-per-week, or intermittent dosing is acceptable. HIV-coinfected patients with CD4 cell counts of <100 cells/μl should receive daily or thrice-weekly treatment.
[e]Rifapentene may only be used in HIV-negative patients with noncavitary pulmonary disease and only when culture conversion is achieved in the initial phase.

demonstrating low relapse potential (10). Treatment should consist of INH, RIF, PZA, and EMB (or SM) in the initial phase, followed by INH and RIF for 2 months in the continuation phase (1). At least three adequate sputum specimens must be obtained and more sophisticated techniques, such as bronchoscopy, should be considered when appropriate. Clinical and radiographic data at 2 months should demonstrate improvement attributable to TB treatment.

Monitoring of TB Patients on Treatment

When initiating anti-TB chemotherapy, a medical history and physical exam should be performed along with a CXR and baseline laboratory testing. HIV testing is necessary both to determine the proper treatment schedule and to treat underlying immunodeficiency (see chapter 32). Liver function studies, AST, ALT, bilirubin, and alkaline phosphatase, should be performed to screen for underlying liver abnormalities and to provide a baseline for the detection of adverse drug reactions. An assessment of renal function (serum creatinine) is necessary to determine proper medication dosing. Due to potential hematologic events, a baseline platelet count should be performed as well. An assessment of visual acuity and color discrimination should be performed prior to initiating EMB (1). If SM is used, an assessment of auditory and vestibular function should be performed as a baseline.

During the course of treatment, routine laboratory monitoring of liver function, renal function, and platelets is not required, unless baseline abnormalities are present. Per current American Thoracic Society guidelines, routine monitoring of ALT should be performed on patients who chronically use alcohol,

intermittent dosing on a biweekly or thrice-weekly schedule is a valid option (Table 6). For patients coinfected with HIV, certain intermittent dosing regimens are inappropriate, depending on the CD4 cell count (see chapter 32).

Patients resistant to or intolerant of INH can be treated successfully with other first-line agents. RIF, PZA, and EMB for 6 months is an effective option. An alternative regimen of RIF and EMB for 12 months can also be used, with PZA recommended for the first 2 months. For patients unable to take PZA due to resistance or intolerance, 2 months of INH, RIF, and EMB followed by 7 months of INH and RIF is acceptable. The lack of RIF in a regimen necessitates a prolonged treatment course, from 12 to 18 months depending on the regimen and treatment response (1) (Table 4). The absence of both INH and RIF from a regimen necessitates a prolonged and complex treatment regimen as for multidrug-resistant TB (see chapter 8).

Patients with pulmonary TB based on clinical and radiographic findings, but negative sputum AFB smear and culture, may be candidates for a 4-month total treatment duration based on data have underlying liver disease, have elevated baseline ALT, take other potentially hepatotoxic drugs, are HIV positive, have had prior problems with INH, are pregnant, or are less than 3 months postpartum. Routine liver function monitoring of patients greater than 35 years of age may be warranted as well (36). Regular blood testing is performed by some health departments on all patients as an early indicator of an adverse reaction. Regular symptom assessments for adverse reactions should be performed. For patients on EMB for more than 2 months or on dosages greater than 15 to 20 mg/kg per day, monthly vision testing should be performed. For patients receiving SM, monthly assessments of auditory and vestibular symptoms should be performed.

For patients with pulmonary disease, follow-up CXRs at 2 months of treatment and at the completion of treatment can provide information on treatment response and a new baseline for subsequent imaging, respectively. For culture-negative pulmonary TB, these follow-up CXRs are essential to provide evidence of response to treatment and clinical cure.

Following the microbiological diagnosis of pulmonary TB, subsequent AFB smears and cultures are needed to ensure cure and response to treatment. At a minimum, monthly sputum cultures should be performed until two consecutive negative results are obtained (1). More frequent sputum evaluations (every week or every 2 weeks until culture conversion) are useful to more closely monitor treatment response and to determine the appropriate length of the continuation phase, as negative sputum cultures at less than 2 months of treatment must be documented for the 4-month continuation regimen. Sputum specimens should be attempted initially for extrapulmonary TB cases, as a large proportion (21% of sputum-producing patients) may have positive sputum cultures (32). CXR was found to be a poor predictor of culture positivity.

Treatment Failure

Approximately 95% of patients on appropriate first-line treatment convert to culture-negative status within 3 months. Failure to convert within this time frame should trigger an evaluation of possible causes of a delayed treatment response, including noncompliance, drug resistance, malabsorption (see "Therapeutic Drug Monitoring" below), and laboratory error (contamination). Repeat drug susceptibility testing should be performed on the latest culture isolate. Sensitive molecular assays (20) are also available for the rapid diagnosis of resistance to INH and RIF at specialized centers. Treatment failure is defined as culture positivity after 4 months of appropriate

treatment. If failure is felt to be due to acquired resistance, expert consultation is recommended (see chapter 8). To prevent the development of additional resistance, a single drug should *never* be added to a failing regimen. Although not standardized, the empirical addition of a fluoroquinolone, an injectable agent (SM, amikacin, kanamycin, or capreomycin), and an additional oral agent (*p*-aminosalicylic acid, ethionamide, or cycloserine) may be appropriate when indicated (1).

Relapse

Relapse refers to the recurrence of TB in an individual having completed treatment with evidence of prior cure. This may occur due to lack of sterilization of residual TB organisms and is most likely to occur among patients with extensive disease burden and delayed culture clearance (>2 months on treatment) (5, 14). Relapses typically occur within 6 to 12 months of completing TB treatment. For patients on RIF-based DOT regimens, the relapse organisms typically have the same susceptibility as the initial isolates (15, 26) and standard first-line regimens may be employed. Repeat susceptibility testing should be performed to ensure continued activity of the first-line agents. Relapse should be distinguished from exogenous reinfection, which is well described in high-incidence settings (45) and may be detected through molecular strain typing of the organisms. For patients suspected of drug-resistant strains because of erratic administration, lack of DOT, or other concerns, retreatment should include three new agents that are likely to be active as well (1).

Interruptions in Therapy

Interruptions in therapy may occur during the course of treatment due to other medical illnesses, side effects (see "Adverse Reactions" below), or nonadherence. The impact of treatment interruptions is more profound early in the treatment course, when the disease burden is heavy. In general, if compliance prior to the interruption is ensured, the previous regimen may be reinstituted. If there are concerns about improper administration, two new drugs to which the isolate is known to be sensitive should be added. If a patient is unable to complete the number of doses required for a 6-month regimen in 9 months, the patient should be evaluated for treatment extension or restarting a full course (1). An accepted approach may be found in the New York City Bureau of Tuberculosis Control policies (3) (Fig. 2). If the patient remains culture positive after the treatment interruption, repeat susceptibility testing should be performed.

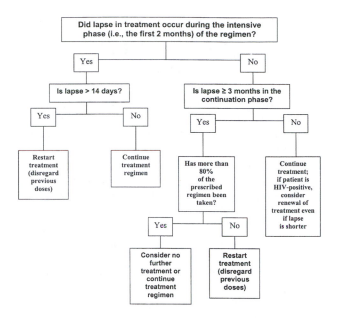

Figure 2. Reinstitution of interrupted or incomplete anti-TB treatment. © 2008 by The City of New York, Department of Health and Mental Hygiene. All rights reserved. (Adapted from *Tuberculosis Clinical Policies and Protocols*, 4th ed. Bureau of Tuberculosis Control, New York City Department of Health and Mental Hygiene, New York, NY, 2008) (3).

Therapeutic Drug Monitoring

Therapeutic monitoring of serum drug concentrations in first-line regimens is not routinely indicated, as these drugs have consistent pharmacokinetics. Furthermore, evidence suggests that diminished levels of INH and RIF are not associated with disease recurrence in the general population (30). Therapeutic drug monitoring may be indicated in several circumstances, such as the following:

1. Lack of appropriate clinical response or culture conversion on treatment with active agents by DOT

2. Suspected malabsorption syndromes

3. Relapse in the setting of an appropriate treatment regimen

4. Use of second-line agents with a narrow therapeutic window and significant toxicities, such as cycloserine and aminoglycosides

5. Treatment of TB disease with limited treatment options (i.e., multidrug-resistant TB), to optimize the regimen

6. Renal insufficiency and associated toxicity concerns (EMB)

For INH, RIF, EMB, and PZA, levels should typically be drawn 2 h after medication administration. Some experts suggest repeat levels 6 h after administration to detect delayed absorption and to determine half-life values. Increased dosing regimens based on drug levels are not standardized, and repeat levels should

be assessed following changes. Barriers to therapeutic drug monitoring include significant costs and the fact that few specialized centers perform testing. Extensive reviews on this topic are available elsewhere (33).

ADVERSE REACTIONS

Gastrointestinal Upset

Gastrointestinal upset is one of the most common complaints of patients taking anti-TB medications. Liver tests should be obtained to ensure that early hepatitis is not occurring. Once hepatitis is ruled out, dosing may be moved to another time of day or given with food to minimize discomfort (1).

Hepatotoxicity

Elevated transaminases during the course of treatment may be due to TB drugs, hepatic adaptation, or an event unrelated to TB treatment (viral hepatitis). Drug-induced liver injury may occur in 2 to 28% of patients on first-line TB drugs (43). Hepatotoxicity, defined as AST >5 times the upper limit of normal or AST >3 times the upper limit of normal along with symptoms of hepatitis, may be due to INH, RIF, or PZA. TB treatment should be held when hepatotoxicity is suspected. Risk factors for drug-induced toxicity include advanced age, female sex, malnutrition, HIV coinfection, and underlying liver disease (43). An elevated bilirubin of >2 times the upper limit of normal is suggestive of more severe disease (49), with jaundice being associated with a >10% mortality rate (54).

Hepatic adaptation is a physiologic adjustment to certain drugs that may cause elevation in transaminases but is not associated with liver injury (6). Asymptomatic AST elevation occurs in approximately 20% of patients on standard first-line treatment (41). Alcohol should not be used, and the concomitant use of other hepatotoxic drugs should be avoided during TB treatment if possible, as they may increase the risk of liver injury.

In the setting of suspected drug-induced liver injury, INH, RIF, and PZA should be held until AST returns to <2 times the upper limit of normal or to baseline levels in those with chronic underlying liver disease (Fig. 3). Patients with extensive disease, meningitis, or HIV may be placed on liver-sparing regimens pending the normalization of liver studies (see "Liver Dysfunction" below). Simultaneous readministration of all drugs leads to recurrent hepatotoxicity in 14 to 24% of cases (37, 42). Current recommendations call for the sequential reintroduction of TB drugs. RIF is the least likely cause of hepatotoxicity

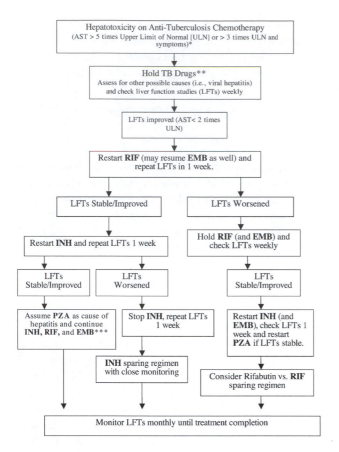

Figure 3. Management of hepatotoxicity. *, if there is a cholestatic pattern, RIF is the likely etiology and RFB may be an appropriate substitute after normalization of liver function tests (LFTs); **, if the patient has extensive disease, meningitis or HIV coinfection or requires a prolonged period off first-line agents, prompt initiation of a nonhepatotoxic regimen such as EMB, SM, and a fluoroquinolone should be pursued; ***, rechallenge with PZA can be considered if hepatitis was not severe.

and should be added first. AST should be repeated in 1 week; if stable, INH should be added to the regimen. Following an additional week, if repeat AST is stable, PZA may be added. If the hepatitis was severe, at this point PZA is the presumed culprit and should be omitted from the regimen. If either RIF or INH is felt to be the inciting agent during the reintroduction, it should be held from the regimen. If the liver injury has a cholestatic pattern (elevated bilirubin and alkaline phosphatase), RIF may be the inciting agent, and RFB may be considered as an alternative. Total treatment length should be based on the final regimen.

Rash

Any of the first-line TB drugs may cause a rash. Mild eruptions can be treated with diphenhydramine or other symptomatic therapy while TB treatment is continued. More severe eruptions, particularly with fever, mucous membrane involvement, or petechia, should prompt discontinuation of all TB drugs. After

the rash has subsided, drugs may be restarted sequentially at 3-day intervals beginning with RIF, then INH, and then either PZA or EMB. If rash recurs, the last agent started should be discontinued. If no rash recurs after the initial three drugs are restarted, the remaining drug is the presumed etiology. Three new agents, including an aminoglycoside and two oral agents, may be initiated if the time to restarting the first-line agents is prolonged or if TB disease is severe. Thrombocytopenia may cause a petechial rash and is typically due to RIF. In such cases RIF should be permanently discontinued and the platelet count monitored until normalized (1).

Peripheral Neuropathy

Peripheral neuropathy due to INH is uncommon, affecting <1% of patients on routine doses. Conditions such as malnutrition, HIV infection, diabetes, renal insufficiency, pregnancy, breast-feeding, and alcohol abuse increase the risk of INH-associated peripheral neuropathy. Pyridoxine supplementation may prevent the onset of neuropathy and should be routinely administered to those at increased risk at a dose of 10 to 50 mg per day (1). Pyridoxine should be administered to patients developing peripheral neuropathy symptoms. Recalcitrant symptoms may require the cessation of INH.

TREATMENT IN SPECIAL CIRCUMSTANCES

Extrapulmonary TB

The drugs used in the standard treatment of pulmonary TB are recommended for all extrapulmonary TB. Six months is considered adequate treatment for most extrapulmonary TB. No recent trials have reviewed treatment duration, but for disease that is slow to respond, treatment may be extended beyond the usual 6 months. Therapy should be extended in meningeal TB to 9 to 12 months. INH and PZA penetrate to the cerebrospinal fluid, reaching levels equivalent to that in the blood. RIF should be included in the treatment, but cerebrospinal fluid penetration may be less than blood levels. Corticosteroids are recommended in pericarditis and meningeal TB (1).

Pediatric TB

Treatment in children is similar to that in adults except for the decreased use of EMB. Unless children have a typical adult presentation with upper lobe disease and cavities, three drugs, INH, RIF, and PZA, are used for the initial phase rather than four, and dosing is weight based. While studies done with children are limited, the bacillary load is often much less than in adults, and the standard 2-month initiation and then 4-month continuation phase are recommended. Medications may need to be crushed and served with other foods or liquids to ensure ingestion. No studies have been completed to fully assess the dosing or crushing of medications to ensure best practices.

TB in Pregnant Women

Congenital TB is considered a far greater risk than treating the pregnant woman with active TB. SM is the only documented teratogenic drug in the primary drug armamentarium and should not be substituted for EMB. Treatment should be started with INH, RIF, and EMB. Although teratogenicity data for PZA are not complete, this agent is recommended for use by the WHO regimen for pregnant women. PZA is not recommended for use in pregnant women in the United States. If PZA is not used, treatment duration should be extended to 9 months.

Women may breast-feed while receiving INH, RIF, and EMB. Doses in breast milk are not adequate to treat the infant. The infant should receive supplemental pyridoxine, though, since the level of INH in breast milk is sufficient to inhibit the availability of this vitamin.

Renal Dysfunction

In patients with renal dysfunction, PZA and EMB dosing should be adjusted. Adjustment is made in the frequency of dosing rather than the dosage (Table 5). For patients on hemodialysis, these drugs should be dosed following hemodialysis treatments. No dosage or interval adjustment is required for INH or RIF. Medications administered daily should be given at the same time each day. Manufacturers' recommendations for fluoroquinolone renal dosing are based not on mycobacterial treatment but, rather, on other bacterial susceptibilities. Serum levels of drugs should be obtained to ensure adequate treatment if any question of adequacy exists.

Liver Dysfunction

Patients with known liver dysfunction can be difficult to treat. INH, RIF, and PZA are all hepatotoxic and can worsen illness in a patient with underlying disease. Additionally, in a patient with advanced disease, laboratory monitoring may not indicate the severity of an adverse reaction. In an infectious patient with advanced liver dysfunction or hepatitis due to first-line drugs, treatment with a nonhepatotoxic regimen is recommended pending resolution of the acute hepatitis or for completion of therapy if the liver dysfunction is severe. EMB, moxifloxacin, and intramuscular SM (or another intravenous aminoglycoside)

can be used pending resolution of the hepatitis. In a patient in whom hepatitis has resolved or liver dysfunction has improved, first-line drugs can be added individually to this regimen. The patient should then be monitored for 7 to 10 days to determine his or her tolerance of the additional drug and additional drugs started back sequentially (see "Adverse Reactions" above). Once sensitivities are available and the patient is tolerant of a standard regimen, the least hepatotoxic regimen can be established.

Malabsorptive Disease

Malabsorptive states require vigilance with drug level testing. Diabetics or other patients with malabsorptive states will likely benefit from drug level testing. Patients may require intramuscular and intravenous treatment regimens until oral absorption can be ensured.

Low-Income and High-Incidence Countries

Management of TB in low-income countries can be challenging due to a lack of resources and an underdeveloped infrastructure. Diagnosis of TB is often based on smear microscopy without culture, and drug susceptibility testing is not routinely available. Current WHO (50) recommendations call for INH, RIF, PZA, and EMB for the initial 2 months of treatment, followed by 4 months of INH and RIF. In areas with a high incidence of INH resistance, INH, RIF, and EMB are recommended for 4 months in the continuation phase. Daily dosing is the preferred means of administration, but thrice-weekly DOT is an acceptable strategy. Fixed-dose combinations of anti-TB agents are recommended to prevent the use of inadequate regimens and monotherapy. Further guidance for the management of TB may be found in the WHO's *Treatment of Tuberculosis: Guidelines*, 4th ed. (50).

TB and HIV Coinfection

The treatment of TB in HIV-infected individuals follows the same principles as for those not infected with HIV. Standard 6-month regimens are similarly effective. Drug-drug interactions, particularly between RIF and antiretroviral agents, complicate the treatment process, with RFB often used in the place of RIF. Biweekly dosing in patients with CD4 counts of <100 cells/µl is contraindicated due to the development of RIF resistance, and rifapentene is contraindicated in HIV-positive patients entirely (1) (see chapter 32).

Acknowledgments. We acknowledge A. Edward Khan and Michael E. Kimerling, authors of this chapter in the previous edition, for guidance on this chapter based on their previous work.

REFERENCES

1. American Thoracic Society, Centers for Disease Control and Prevention, and Infectious Diseases Society of America. 2003. Treatment of tuberculosis. *MMWR Morb. Mortal. Wkly. Rep.* 52(RR11):1–77.

2. Benator, D., M. Bhattacharya, L. Bozeman, W. Burman, A. Cantazaro, R. Chaisson, F. Gordin, C. R. Horsburgh, J. Horton, A. Khan, C. Lahart, B. Metchock, C. Pachucki, L. Stanton, A. Vernon, M. E. Villarino, Y. C. Wang, M. Weiner, and S. Weis. 2002. Rifapentine and isoniazid once a week versus rifampicin and isoniazid twice a week for treatment of drug-susceptible pulmonary tuberculosis in HIV-negative patients: a randomised clinical trial. *Lancet* 360:528–534.

3. Bureau of Tuberculosis Control. 2008. *Clinical Policies and Protocols*, 4th ed., p. 66. Bureau of Tuberculosis Control, New York City Department of Health, New York, NY.

4. Canetti, G. 1965. Present aspects of bacterial resistance in tuberculosis. *Am. Rev. Respir. Dis.* 92:687–703.

5. Catanzaro, A., and R. Horsburgh. 2000. TBTC Study 22: risk factors for relapse with once-weekly isoniazid/rifapentine (HP) in HIV-negative TB patients. *Am. J. Respir. Crit. Care Med.* 161:A252.

6. Chitturi, S., and G. Farrell. 2007. Drug induced liver disease, p. 935–936. *In* E. Schiff, M. Sorrell, and W. Maddrey (ed.), *Schiff's Diseases of the Liver*, 10th ed., vol. I. Lippincott Williams and Wilkins, Philadelphia, PA.

7. Crofton, J., and D. A. Mitchison. 1948. Streptomycin resistance in pulmonary tuberculosis. *Br. Med. J.* 2:1009–1015.

8. Cullen, J. H., L. J. Early, and J. M. Fiore. 1956. The occurrence of hyperuricemia during pyrazinamide-isoniazid therapy. *Am. Rev. Tuberc.* 74:289–292.

9. Døssing, M., J. T. R. Wilcke, D. S. Askgaard, and B. Nybo. 1996. Liver injury during antituberculosis treatment: an 11-year study. *Tuberc. Lung Dis.* 77:335–340.

10. Dutt, A. K., D. Moers, and W. W. Stead. 1989. Smear- and culture-negative pulmonary tuberculosis: four-month short-course chemotherapy. *Am. Rev. Respir. Dis.* 139:867–870.

11. Feldman, W. H. 1954. Streptomycin: some historical aspects of its development as a chemotherapeutic agent in tuberculosis. *Am. Rev. Tuberc.* 89:859–868.

12. Griffith, D. E., B. A. Brown, and R. J. Wallace. 1996. Varying dosages of rifabutin affect white blood cell and platelet counts in human immunodeficiency virus-negative patients who are receiving multidrug regimens for pulmonary *Mycobacterium avium* complex disease. *Clin. Infect. Dis.* 23:1321–1322.

13. Grosset, J. 1980. Bacteriologic basis of short-course chemotherapy for tuberculosis. *Clin. Chest Med.* 1:231–241.

14. Hong Kong Chest Service/British Medical Research Council. 1987. Five-year follow-up of a controlled trial of five 6-month regimens of chemotherapy for tuberculosis. *Am. Rev. Respir. Dis.* 136:1339–1342.

15. Hong Kong Chest Service/British Medical Research Council. 1991. Controlled trial of 2, 4, and 6 months of pyrazinamide in 6-month, three-times weekly regimens for smear-positive pulmonary tuberculosis, including an assessment of a combined preparation of isoniazid, rifampin, and pyrazinamide: results at 30 months. *Am. Rev. Respir. Dis.* 143:700–706.

16. Jindani, A., V. R. Aber, E. A. Edwards, and D. A. Mitchison. 1980. The early bactericidal activity of drugs in patients with pulmonary tuberculosis. *Am. Rev. Respir. Dis.* 121:939–949.

17. Joint Committee on the Study of Streptomycin. 1947. The effects of streptomycin on tuberculosis in man. *JAMA* 135:634–641.

18. Kanellakopoulou, K., A. Pagoulatou, K. Stroumpoulis, M. Vafiadou, H. Kranidioti, H. Giamarellou, and E. J. Giamarellos-Bourboulis. 2008. Pharmacokinetics of moxifloxacin in non-inflamed cerebrospinal fluid of humans: implication for a bactericidal effect. *J. Antimicrob. Chemother.* 61:1328–1331.

19. Kopanoff, D. E., D. E. Snider, and G. J. Caras. 1979. Isoniazid-related hepatitis: a US Public Health Service cooperative surveillance study. *Am. Rev. Respir. Dis.* 117:991–1001.

20. Lacoma, A., N. Garcia-Sierra, C. Prat, J. Ruiz-Manzano, L. Haba, S. Rosés, J. Maldonado, and J. Domínguez. 2008. Geno-Type MTBDRplus assay for molecular detection of rifampin and isoniazid resistance in *Mycobacterium tuberculosis* strains and clinical samples. *J. Clin. Microbiol.* 46:3660–3667.

21. Leibold, J. E. 1966. The ocular toxicity of ethambutol and its relation to dose. *Ann. N. Y. Acad. Sci.* 135:904–909.

22. McDermott, W., and R. Tompsett. 1954. Activation of pyrazinamide and nicotinamide in acid environment in vitro. *Am. Rev. Tuberc.* 70:748.

23. Mehta, Y. S., F. F. Jijina, S. S. Badakere, A. V. Pathare, and D. Mohanty. 1996. Rifampicin-induced immune thrombocytopenia. *Tuberc. Lung Dis.* 77:558–562.

24. Mitchell, J. R., H. J. Zimmerman, K. G. Ishak, U. P. Thorgeirsson, J. A. Timbrell, W. R. Snodgrass, and S. D. Nelson. 1976. Isoniazid liver injury: clinical spectrum, pathology and probable pathogenesis. *Ann. Intern. Med.* 84:181–192.

25. Mitchison, D. 1979. Basic mechanisms of chemotherapy. *Chest* 76:S771–S781.

26. Mitchison, D. A. 1984. Drug resistance in mycobacteria. *Br. Med. Bull.* 40:84–90.

27. Mitchison, D. A. 2000. Role of individual drugs in the chemotherapy of tuberculosis. *Int. J. Tuberc. Lung Dis.* 4:796–806.

28. Moadebi, S., C. K. Harder, M. J. Fitzgerald, K. R. Elwood, and F. Marra. 2007. Fluoroquinolones for the treatment of pulmonary tuberculosis. *Drugs* 67:2077–2099.

29. Moulding, T. S., A. G. Redeker, and G. C. Kanel. 1989. Twenty isoniazid-associated deaths in one state. *Am. Rev. Respir. Dis.* 140:700–705.

30. Narita, M., M. Hisada, B. Thimmappa, J. Stambaugh, E. Ibrahim, E. Hollender, and D. Ashkin. 2001. Tuberculosis recurrence: multivariate analysis of serum levels of tuberculosis drugs, human immunodeficiency virus status, and other risk factors. *Clin. Infect. Dis.* 32:515–517.

31. Nuermberger, E. L., T. Yoshimatsu, S. Tyagi, R. J. O'Brien, A. N. Vernon, R. E. Chaisson, W. R. Bishai, and J. H. Grosset. 2004. Moxifloxacin-containing regimen greatly reduces time to culture conversion in murine tuberculosis. *Am. J. Respir. Crit. Care Med.* 169:421–426.

32. Parimon, T., C. E. Spitters, N. Muangman, J. Euathrongchit, E. Oren, and M. Narita. 2008. Unexpected pulmonary involvement in extrapulmonary tuberculosis patients. *Chest* 134:589–594.

33. Peloquin, C. A. 2002. Therapeutic drug monitoring in the treatment of tuberculosis. *Drugs* 62:2169–2183.

34. Pletz, M. W., A. De Roux, A. Roth, K. H. Neumann, H. Mauch, and H. Lode. 2004. Early bactericidal activity of moxifloxacin in treatment of pulmonary tuberculosis: a prospective, randomized study. *Antimicrob. Agents Chemother.* 48:780–782.

35. Sanders, W. E. J. 1976. Rifampin. *Ann. Intern. Med.* 85:82–86.

36. Saukkonen, J. J., D. L. Cohn, R. M. Jasmer, S. Schenker, J. A. Jereb, C. M. Nolan, C. A. Peloquin, F. M. Gordin, D. Nunes, D. B. Strader, J. Bernardo, R. Venkataramanan, and T. R. Sterling. 2006. An official ATS statement: hepatotoxicity of antituberculosis therapy. *Am. J. Respir. Crit. Care Med.* 174:935–952.

37. Sharma, S. K., R. Singla, P. Sarda, A. Mohan, G. Makharia, A. Jayaswal, V. Sreenivas, and S. Singh. 2010. Safety of 3 different reintroduction regimens of antituberculosis drugs after

development of antituberculosis treatment-induced hepatotoxicity. *Clin. Infect. Dis.* 50:833–839.

38. Snider, D. E., and G. J. Caras. 1992. Isoniazid-associated hepatitis deaths: a review of available information. *Am. Rev. Respir. Dis.* 145:494–497.

39. Snider, D. E., J. Graczyk, E. Bek, and J. Rogowski. 1984. Supervised six-months treatment of newly diagnosed pulmonary tuberculosis using isoniazid, rifampin, and pyrazinamide with and without streptomycin. *Am. Rev. Respir. Dis.* 130:1091–1094.

40. Snider, D. E., Jr. 1980. Pyridoxine supplementation during isoniazid therapy. *Tubercle* 61:191–196.

41. Steele, M. A., R. F. Burk, and R. M. DesPrez. 1991. Toxic hepatitis with isoniazid and rifampin: a meta-analysis. *Chest* 99:465–471.

42. Tahaoğlu, K., G. Ataç, T. Sevim, T. Tärün, O. Yazicioğlu, G. Horzum, I. Gemci, A. Ongel, N. Kapakli, and E. Aksoy. 2001. The management of anti-tuberculosis drug induced hepatotoxicity. *Int. J. Tuberc. Lung Dis.* 5:65–69.

43. Tostmann, A., M. J. Boeree, R. E. Aarnoutse, W. C. M. de Lange, A. J. van der Ven, and R. Dekhuijzen. 2008. Antituberculosis drug-induced hepatotoxicity: concise up-to-date review. *J. Gastroenterol. Hepatol.* 23:192–202.

44. Türktaş, H., M. Unsal, N. Tülek, and O. Orüç. 1994. Hepatotoxicity of antituberculosis therapy (rifampicin, isoniazid and pyrazinamide) or viral hepatitis. *Tuberc. Lung Dis.* 75:58–60.

45. van Rie, A., R. Warren, M. Richardson, T. C. Victor, R. P. Gie, D. A. Enarson, N. Beyers, and P. D. van Helden. 1999. Exogenous reinfection as a cause of recurrent tuberculosis after curative treatment. *N. Engl. J. Med.* 341:1174–1179.

46. Vernon, A., W. Burman, D. Benator, A. Khan, L. Bozeman, and Tuberculosis Trials Consortium. 1999. Acquired rifamycin monoresistance in patients with HIV-related tuberculosis treated with once-weekly rifapentine and isoniazid. *Lancet* 353:1843–1847.

47. Villarino, M. E., R. Ridzon, P. C. Weismuller, M. Elcock, R. M. Maxwell, J. Meador, P. J. Smith, M. L. Carson, and L. J. Geiter. 1997. Rifampin preventive therapy for tuberculosis infection: experience with 157 adolescents. *Am. J. Respir. Crit. Care Med.* 155:1735–1738.

48. Wang, L., and K. Takayama. 1972. Relationship between the uptake of isoniazid and its action on in vivo mycolic acid synthesis in *Mycobacterium tuberculosis. Antimicrob. Agents Chemother.* 2:438–441.

49. Watkins, P., J. Bloom, and C. Hunt. 2009. Biomarkers of acute idiosyncratic hepatocellular injury (AIHI) within clinical trials, p. 42–48. *In* S. Olson, S. Robinson, and R. Giffin (ed.), *Accelerating the Development of Biomarkers for Drug Safety: Workshop Summary. Forum on Drug Discovery, Development, and Translation; Institute of Medicine.* National Academies Press, Washington, DC.

50. World Health Organization. 2010. *Treatment of Tuberculosis: Guidelines,* 4th ed. WHO Press, Geneva, Switzerland.

51. Yee, D., C. Valiquette, M. Pelletier, I. Parisien, I. Rocher, and D. Menzies. 2003. Incidence of serious side effects from first-line antituberculosis drugs among patients treated for active tuberculosis. *Am. J. Respir. Crit. Care Med.* 167:1472–1477.

52. Youman, G. P., E. H. Williston, W. H. Feldman, and C. H. Hinshaw. 1946. Increase in resistance of tubercle bacilli to streptomycin. A preliminary report. *Proc. Mayo Clin.* 21:216.

53. Zhang, Y., M. M. Wade, A. Scorpio, H. Zhang, and Z. Sun. 2003. Mode of action of pyrazinamide: disruption of *Mycobacterium tuberculosis* membrane transport and energetics by pyrazinoic acid. *J. Antimicrob. Chemother.* 52:790–795.

54. Zimmerman, H. J. 1968. The spectrum of hepatotoxicity. *Perspect. Biol. Med.* 12:135–161.

Tuberculosis and Nontuberculous Mycobacterial Infections, 6th ed.
Edited by David Schlossberg
© 2011 ASM Press, Washington, DC

Chapter 8

Therapy of Multidrug-Resistant and Extensively Drug-Resistant Tuberculosis

BARBARA J. SEAWORTH AND ROBERT N. LONGFIELD

OVERVIEW

Multidrug-resistant tuberculosis (MDR-TB), caused by strains resistant to at least isoniazid and rifampin (75), is difficult to treat and requires medications that are expensive, toxic, and less effective. In March 2006 the original definition of extensively drug-resistant TB (XDR-TB) was reported in the CDC's *Morbidity and Mortality Weekly Report* (23). In October of the same year a revised definition was reported (24): TB resistant to isoniazid, rifampin, a second-line injectable drug (kanamycin, amikacin, or capreomycin), and any fluoroquinolone. This new definition was better able to identify a group with poorer outcomes and high mortality rates (124). MDR- and XDR-TB strains are resistant to the most important antituberculous medications required for successful outcomes. The outbreak of MDR-TB in New York City in the 1990s caught the world's attention, as has the more recent outbreak of XDR-TB in KwaZula-Natal Province, South Africa (50, 51).

Epidemiology

TB rates globally are declining, as are the estimates of the number of cases of drug-resistant TB; the World Health Organization (WHO) in 2009 reported an estimated 440,000 cases of MDR-TB, 50,000 cases of XDR-TB, and 150,000 deaths due to MDR-TB (169). This represents a decrease in the estimated number of cases, although laboratory capacity, especially the ability to test second-line drug susceptibility, limits the ability to diagnose MDR- and XDR-TB in many high-burden, low- and moderate-income countries. Fifty-eight countries have now reported at least one case of XDR-TB. Only a small proportion, 7% (<50,000), are diagnosed and appropriately treated by national TB programs (165).

The proportion of MDR cases in the United States has declined slightly. In 2008, the last year for which numbers are available, 107 cases of MDR-TB were reported. There were no reported cases of XDR-TB in 2009 (22). Drug-resistant disease in the United States is more common in individuals who are born in other countries.

Of the estimated 500,000 cases of MDR-TB that emerged in 2007, over 85% were in 27 countries (15 of these were in the European region). The countries with the largest numbers of cases are India (131,000), the People's Republic of China (112, 000), the Russian Federation (43,000), South Africa (16,000), and Bangladesh (15,000) (169). Estimates were based on country reporting and the WHO's fourth report on antituberculous drug resistance in the world (170). This report included drug susceptibility test results on 91,577 patients from 93 settings in 81 countries and 2 special administrative regions of China collected between 2002 and 2007. New information was available from 10 high-burden countries and trend data (three or more data points) from 47 countries. Information was collected only from national laboratories participating in a quality assurance program for first-line drugs and supranational reference laboratories. However, the global incidence is only an estimate of numbers of cases. Information is limited by incomplete reporting from areas such as South Africa due to inadequate laboratory capacity (170). This is especially an issue regarding estimates of XDR-TB, as the diagnosis requires testing for both first- and second-line drugs.

The spread of MDR-TB appears to increase considerably as human immunodeficiency virus (HIV) infection is introduced into areas with established MDR-TB (133). HIV patients may actually serve as a sentinel population among whom the earliest cases of MDR-TB become manifest in a country or region

Barbara J. Seaworth and Robert N. Longfield • Heartland National TB Center, University of Texas Health Science Center, 2303 Southeast Military Drive, San Antonio, TX 78223.

(19). Outbreaks of MDR-TB associated with HIV infection were reported in the 1990s in hospitals and other facilities in New York City (50) and Florida (21). These have had dramatic impacts on global TB control efforts (15). Recently the significant interaction of HIV and TB was highlighted by the report of an outbreak of XDR-TB in a rural hospital in KwaZula-Natal Province, South Africa. The dual epidemics of HIV and TB in the African region pose significant challenges to TB programs. In 2005, 15% of all incident TB cases were coinfected with HIV, with some African countries reporting in 2008 that greater than 60 to 80% of TB cases with known HIV status were coinfected (168).

Outbreaks of MDR- and XDR-TB associated with HIV have developed due to the usual causes related to acquired drug resistance, such as poor adherence and other provider errors, but have been enhanced by amplification of drug resistance due to standardized treatment regimens in the absence of drug susceptibility testing and inadequate drug availability (130). Outbreaks in South Africa have also been associated with significant transmission in facilities and in South Africa within the community as well (18).

MECHANISMS OF DRUG RESISTANCE

Resistance to anti-TB drugs occurs during selective multiplication of drug-resistant mycobacteria which spontaneously emerge. These resistant mutants then are able to flourish and replace the wild-type strains when therapy is inadequate due to either a suboptimal number of medications or low serum drug levels. Molecular epidemiology indicates that MDR-TB strains arise by sequential accumulation of resistance mutations for individual drugs (122). Resistance is not linked between antituberculous drugs. Drug resistance which develops during or after a course of treatment was previously called "acquired drug resistance" but is now referred to as "resistance among previously treated cases" by the WHO. Similarly, drug resistance which develops when there is no history of TB treatment was categorized as "primary drug resistance" but is now called "resistance among new cases." It is often difficult to obtain an accurate history of treatment; however, "new cases" are defined as persons who have never received anti-TB drugs or who have received them for less than 1 month. "Previously treated cases" are persons who have received at least 1 month of therapy (40).

TB treatment errors resulting in inadequate treatment of drug-susceptible disease are the primary cause of MDR-TB in previously treated patients.

Mahmoudi and Iseman (95) found management errors for 28 of 35 (80%) MDR-TB patients between 1989 and 1990. An average of 3.93 errors per patient was noted. The most frequent errors included inadequate primary treatment regimens, the addition of a single drug to a failing treatment regimen, failure to recognize resistance, failure to recognize or ensure adherence, and inappropriate isoniazid monotherapy of TB disease. Treatment errors have been observed more often in patients cared for by private providers, including respiratory physicians (17, 83). Nearly half the patients cared for outside state or city TB control programs received regimens that deviated from guidelines from the CDC and American Thoracic Society, i.e., fewer than four initial drugs despite established local isoniazid resistance above 4% of isolates.

TREATMENT

Second-Line Drugs

Injectable agents: streptomycin, kanamycin, amikacin, and capreomycin

Streptomycin was the first effective drug for TB. Early patient improvement following monotherapy with streptomycin was invariably followed by clinical failure. The peril of sequential monotherapy unfortunately remains a lesson that generations of physicians have had to relearn. Streptomycin was reclassified as a second-line drug in the latest guidelines for treatment of TB of the CDC, American Thoracic Society, and Infectious Diseases Society of America (IDSA) due to the high rate of resistance to this drug, especially in foreign-born persons (4). Streptomycin, amikacin, and kanamycin, which are aminoglycosides, and the closely related polypeptide capreomycin act at the 30S ribosome to inhibit protein synthesis. They demonstrate activity against *Mycobacterium tuberculosis* in vitro and are bactericidal against rapidly growing extracellular mycobacteria, especially those growing in cavitary lesions (64). Due to reduced tissue pH and anaerobic conditions, they are not active against slowly growing organisms in caseous lesions or abscesses (41, 103, 134). Adverse events include ototoxicity, nephrotoxicity, and rare neuromuscular blockade. Aminoglycoside and capreomycin use may be complicated by reductions in serum calcium, magnesium, and potassium (86, 143). Primary resistance to streptomycin is significant in isolates from foreign-born persons. Cross resistance is not seen between streptomycin and amikacin, so unless patients have had prior treatment with either kanamycin or amikacin, these isolates are generally sensitive to amikacin (1). Isolates which are kanamycin resistant are usually resistant to amikacin; however, awareness of kanamycin-resistant but amikacin-susceptible strains has occurred following reports from eastern European countries (84). Inhaled aminoglycosides may increase local drug concentration and nearly eliminate toxicity. Seven of 12 patients with persistently smear- and culture-positive MDR-TB had sputum smear conversion to negative, with this as adjunctive therapy. Successful treatment was documented after inhaled streptomycin was added to a previously failing regimen, and three other successful uses of this therapy have been reported (117). Long-term efficacy is unknown, and this means of administration will not address bacilli in caseous lesions. Adverse events were limited to airway irritability (132).

Fluoroquinolones: Ciprofloxacin, Ofloxacin, Levofloxacin, and Moxifloxacin

There has been considerable experience with the long-term efficacy and safety of fluoroquinolones (10, 76, 92). These drugs are bactericidal against both extracellular rapidly multiplying bacteria and intracellular nonmultiplying bacteria (55). They inhibit bacterial DNA gyrase, an enzyme that is essential for the maintenance of DNA supercoils, which are needed for chromosomal replication (56). The fluoroquinolones penetrate well into tissues (alveolar macrophages), respiratory secretions, and body fluids, with concentrations equal to or higher than those in serum. Central nervous system (CNS) penetration is good, allowing these drugs to be used for tuberculous meningitis (2, 55, 91, 93). The prolonged half-life (5 to 8 h for levofloxacin and 9 to 15 h for moxifloxacin) and significant postantibiotic effect allow once-daily dosing (93). Both of the older fluoroquinolones ciprofloxacin and ofloxacin have been associated with good outcomes in the treatment of drug-susceptible TB (2, 82) and drug-resistant TB (96, 97, 114, 142); however, the WHO no longer recommends ciprofloxacin for MDR-TB due to its relatively weak activity compared to those of the newer fluoroquinolones (166). Moxifloxacin and levofloxacin have lower MIC_{90}s (0.25 and 0.5 to 1 mg/liter) than ciprofloxacin (4 mg/liter) and ofloxacin (2 mg/liter) (54, 55, 123, 129, 131, 155). Furthermore, moxifloxacin has demonstrated early bactericidal activity in sputum that is equivalent to that of rifampin at 2 days and to isoniazid at 5 days (120). Despite the absence of prospective clinical trials using fluoroquinolones for MDR-TB, because of considerable experience with levofloxacin and moxifloxacin, they are regarded as critical to good treatment outcomes (27, 80, 88).

The optimum fluoroquinolone and dose are still unclear, as higher doses of levofloxacin (750 mg to 1,000 mg) have not been evaluated against moxifloxacin dosed at 400 mg or higher. Because these bactericidal agents show concentration-dependent activity as well as time-dependent activity (141, 158), greater exposure of these potent fluoroquinolones will likely translate to greater efficacy. Initial studies were often with levofloxacin at 500 mg, but experience with pushing the dosage to 750 mg daily, which is now the standard dosage of levofloxacin, and to 1,000 mg per day has been well tolerated and produced excellent serum drug levels (118). Moxifloxacin dosed at 400 mg daily has good bactericidal activity (148, 155). In most studies moxifloxacin has the longest serum half-life of the currently available fluoroquinolones; however, a recent study using levofloxacin at 1,000 mg noted half-life ranges of 4 to 16 h for levofloxacin and 4 to 10 h for moxifloxacin (118). These values were somewhat lower than those usually reported in previous studies of moxifloxacin. Moxifloxacin, if pushed to a dose higher than 400 mg, would likely become more efficacious, especially in treatment of XDR-TB when resistance to older fluoroquinolones is present. Studies to identify the optimum dose to enhance efficacy and limit toxicity are needed.

Fluoroquinolone resistance develops as a two-step process, and higher serum levels protect against selection of mutants (38, 65, 100, 118). Resistance to fluoroquinolones develops rapidly when they are used as monotherapy (35, 135). Cross resistance within the class of fluoroquinolones was initially felt to be complete. Recent anecdotal experience of ours and of others noted ofloxacin resistance but susceptibility to the newer agents (108, 171). In contrast, a study of fluoroquinolone susceptibilities in *M. tuberculosis* strains for ofloxacin, moxifloxacin, and gatifloxacin showed that 40 strains shared the same resistance results for the three fluoroquinolones (148). One strain (Asn-533 Thr mutation in *gyrB*) was susceptible to ofloxacin but resistant to moxifloxacin and gatifloxacin (162). Single-fluoroquinolone prescriptions for community-acquired pneumonia in a Canadian study were not associated with development of resistant *M. tuberculosis*, whereas multiple-fluoroquinolone prescriptions were (94). These drugs should always be protected by being given in combination with several other active agents, particularly in cases of suspected or possible *M. tuberculosis* disease (2).

Toxicity with the fluoroquinolone class of drugs most commonly is reported as gastrointestinal upset such as nausea and bloating. Myalgia is relatively common, and, rarely, tendon rupture has been reported (13). Prolongation of the QT interval has been noted in patients taking moxifloxacin but has not been reported for those taking this drug for MDR-TB to our knowledge or in our experience. In 2008 Bayer sent a "Dear Doctor" letter warning physicians about rare but severe hepatological and dermatological adverse events associated with moxifloxacin. In most situations the drug is well tolerated, and the benefits outweigh the risks (158).

Rifabutin

Most reports note that 20 to 30% or more of MDR-TB isolates retain sensitivity to rifabutin (61, 87, 135). Rifabutin is bactericidal, with an MIC for TB less than or equal to 2 µg/ml regarded as susceptible. Although peak serum levels are <1 µg/ml, the drug has excellent activity and penetrates into polymorphonuclear leukocytes, lymphocytes, and macrophages. Tissue levels are significantly higher than serum levels. In the lungs, tissue levels are 5 to 10 times higher than in plasma (85, 110). Rifabutin is used to replace rifampin in drug regimens for persons with HIV to avoid drug interactions with HIV protease inhibitors. Outcomes are similar to those for patients treated with rifampin. The response to rifabutin in patients with MDR-TB is unclear. A controlled trial to study the effect of rifabutin-susceptible isolates in patients with resistance to isoniazid and rifampin has not been done. Most studies have not been able to select a patient group for reliable comparison of results, and some studies do not separate outcomes in patients with initial susceptibility to rifabutin from those with resistance (M. Felton, presented at the American Lung Association and American Thoracic Society Annual Meeting, Las Vegas, NV, 1988; L. Madsen, M. Goble, and M. D. Iseman, presented at the American Lung Association and American Thoracic Society Annual Meeting, Kansas City, MO, 1986). A study of 11 patients with MDR-TB treated with rifabutin and other drugs noted that "two patients had rifabutin-susceptible strains on admission to the study; their temporary responses were among the best and were associated with the emergence of rifabutin resistance, suggesting that rifabutin may have contributed to their response" (70). When laboratory susceptibility to rifabutin is documented, we include it at a dosage of 450 mg daily and aim for a peak serum level at the higher end of the therapeutic range. Hematological toxicity and uveitis may limit use of rifabutin at this dose in patients with HIV infection but have been unusual in HIV-negative patients in our experience. Myalgia is a frequent adverse effect with rifabutin. It can often be managed with analgesics or nonsteroidal anti-inflammatory agents.

Ethionamide

Ethionamide is structurally similar to isoniazid and also appears to inhibit cell wall mycolic acid synthesis. The drug is bactericidal, well absorbed orally, and widely distributed. Ethionamide enhanced the activity of moxifloxacin in a mouse model of MDR-TB, but this has not been shown in humans (44). The most frequent adverse effect is gastrointestinal intolerance, including nausea, epigastric pain, and metallic taste. Significant hepatitis occurs in about 4.3% of patients, but transient abnormalities in liver tests are more common. Hypothyroidism develops in a significant number of patients treated with ethionamide. Replacement of thyroid hormone is required during therapy when this occurs but can often be discontinued after the ethionamide is stopped (146). A study with healthy volunteers indicated that single doses of 500 mg were required to achieve therapeutic serum levels (175). When susceptibilities permit, ethionamide is used as part of multiagent therapy. To reduce intolerance, ethionamide can be started slowly (250 mg daily) and increased to the total daily dose over the first 7 to 10 days of treatment. Treatment is usually given in divided doses totaling 500 to 1,000 mg per day.

Cycloserine

Cycloserine is bacteriostatic for mycobacteria, acting to inhibit cell wall synthesis. It is rapidly absorbed after oral administration and is widely distributed. The most common side effects pertain to the CNS: seizures, psychosis, mania, depression, other emotional disturbances, and drowsiness. Neurotoxicity appears to be dose dependent and is rarely seen if serum drug levels remain below 30 µg/ml. History of a neurologic or psychiatric disorder increases the likelihood of CNS adverse events. When susceptibilities permit, cycloserine is used as a part of multiagent therapy. The usual adult dosage is 750 mg per day, divided into two or three doses. Treatment is usually started at 250 mg twice daily. We recommend that serum levels be determined before increasing the dose of cycloserine further. Adjustment of dose or dosing interval is needed with renal impairment.

para-Aminosalicylic Acid

para-Aminosalicylic acid (PAS) exerts a bacteriostatic effect on *M. tuberculosis* by competitively blocking the conversion of *para*-aminobenzoic acid to folic acid, thereby inhibiting DNA synthesis. PAS is readily absorbed, is extensively protein bound (60 to 70%), and readily diffuses into caseous TB lesions but fails to penetrate noninflamed meninges. Rapidly metabolized by the liver and excreted by the kidneys, PAS must be administered in large, divided oral doses (8 to 12 g/day). Anorexia, nausea, vomiting, and diarrhea are common even with the current formulation of enteric-coated granules. Diarrhea is especially troublesome with the initiation of treatment but often improves after the first weeks of therapy. Many experts recommend starting at a dosage of 4 g daily and increasing over the next 7 to 10 days to the desired daily dose. Most patients will not tolerate doses of >12 g/day. PAS, especially when given with ethionamide, can cause hypothyroidism. Thyroid hormone replacement should be given until the offending medications are discontinued. The associated sodium load may cause fluid retention in susceptible patients. Adjustment of dose or dosing interval is needed with renal impairment.

Clofazimine

Clofazimine is a riminophenazine dye compound used to treat *Mycobacterium leprae* with activity against TB (39). The mechanism of action is unknown but may involve DNA binding. Concentrated in macrophages, clofazimine has proven effective in a murine TB model. Generally well tolerated except for occasional gastrointestinal complaints, the most frequent patient concern is reversible skin darkening due to drug deposition. Clofazimine is now available for MDR-TB treatment in the United States only from the manufacturer (Novartis Pharmaceutical Corporation) under an individual patient investigational new drug.

Linezolid

Linezolid is an oxazolidinone antibacterial agent that blocks ribosomal protein synthesis. It acts by binding to the 50S bacterial ribosomal subunit, which prevents formation of the initiation complex for protein synthesis (14). Linezolid is indicated for the treatment of serious infections caused by resistant gram-positive bacteria. The drug has good in vitro activity against *Mycobacterium tuberculosis*, with modest early bactericidal activity and minimal extended bactericidal activity during days 2 to 7 (37).

Linezolid has been used to treat MDR-TB patients with extensive resistance and XDR-TB due to the limited number of drugs available to treat these patients, even though there are no prospective studies to evaluate outcomes or toxicity. Studies to address this are now in progress. In observational studies the activity of linezolid in multidrug regimens has shown variable effects. Migliori et al. found equivalent results in those receiving and not receiving linezolid but noted that those receiving linezolid had more first- and second-line drug resistance and 4.5 versus 2.3 previous treatment episodes (101). They concluded that linezolid may improve treatment success in the most difficult cases. Others have shown improved outcomes from linezolid in patients with extensive resistance in MDR- and XDR-TB (5, 29, 48, 79, 161) and even when added to a chronically failing regimen as salvage therapy (29). The dosage of linezolid for bacterial infections is 600 mg twice daily, but most have used 600 mg once daily for treatment of TB, in an effort to limit toxicity and cost. Serum drug levels are sufficiently above the MIC with this dosage (37, 101, 113).

Administration of 600 mg daily has not shown significant reduction in toxicity (101). More recently, good outcomes have been reported for small series of patients treated with linezolid at 300 mg daily (81, 172). Most reports show that fairly frequent serious adverse events occur in a significant proportion of patients treated with linezolid and may lead to discontinuation of the drug. These reactions, which are caused by inhibition of mitochondrial protein synthesis (52, 99), include myelosuppression, peripheral and optic neuropathy, and lactic acidosis (8, 52, 99, 101, 125, 136). Peripheral neuropathy has been especially concerning, as it may persist after stopping treatment (8, 11, 47, 109, 161). A California study, however, reported fairly limited toxicity, most of which was reversible after stopping the drug (125, 136). Toxicity is related to duration of therapy. Hematological toxicity may occur in the first weeks to months of therapy, but neurologic toxicity usually occurs after 3 to 4 months. Lactic acidosis occurs during the initial weeks of therapy (5, 8, 109). Linezolid is associated with the serotonin syndrome in up to 25% of patients given selective serotonin reuptake inhibitors or other medications that increase serotonin concentrations in the CNS (9, 33, 109, 152). Patients should also be counseled to avoid foods, dietary supplements, and beverages high in tyramine.

Linezolid is a significant addition to the list of available medications for the treatment of extensively resistant TB; however, it is associated with significant toxicity in most studies, and the optimal dose, long-term efficacy, and tolerability of linezolid and related agents remain to be established.

Imipenem

Limited information regarding the effectiveness of imipenem is available, but it is listed as a third-line agent for treatment of TB by the WHO. Therapeutic efficacy has been reported in TB disease in mice and humans. It is bactericidal but not as potent as isoniazid. In one study, 10 patients who had failed treatment for MDR TB were treated with imipenem. The clinical efficacy was difficult to determine, as the drug was given in combination with aminoglycosides and fluoroquinolones. In selected cases imipenem appeared to have a beneficial effect (25).

Meropenem-Clavulanate

In vitro (only) studies of meropenem, a carbapenem closely related to imipenem, showed potent activity against *M. tuberculosis*, including strains causing MDR-TB, when combined with the beta-lactamase inhibitor clavulanate. The MICs for drug-susceptible and a few MDR isolates were less than 1 μg/ml. The combination of meropenem plus clavulanate sterilized aerobic cultures within 14 days and also inhibited anaerobically grown cultures. Thirteen XDR isolates were inhibited at the same concentrations as for drug-susceptible strains. Clavulanate is not commercially available for parenteral administration, and as this combination must be given parenterally, its use may be limited to patients with extensively resistant disease and few remaining treatment options (73).

Gamma Interferon

Interferon is thought to act by inhibiting mycobacterial growth by the activation of alveolar macrophages and the enhanced production of reactive nitrogen species (68). There have been five limited trials of aerosolized, subcutaneous, or intramuscular recombinant human gamma interferon (IFN-γ) or IFN-α among patients with drug-resistant TB, which demonstrated unsustained minimal to moderate benefit (28). In a study of eight patients with advanced MDR-TB, subcutaneous IFN-γ treatment did not produce clinical, radiologic, microbiological, or immunologic improvement (115). It is likely that other immune-modulating treatments, and potentially therapeutic vaccines, may demonstrate clinical benefit.

Inclusion of Drugs with Established Resistance in Treatment Regimens

The use of high-dose isoniazid, 1,200 to 1,500 mg three times weekly or 1,000 to 1,500 mg daily, in the treatment of MDR-TB can be recommended when there are limited treatment options (4). Available studies demonstrated significant improvement in weight, a trend toward improved sputum smear, and an acceptable toxicity profile (119, 121). Moulding concluded that high-dose isoniazid may be helpful in patients with low-level isoniazid resistance or who

have subpopulations of isoniazid-susceptible mycobacteria. Furthermore, patients in developing countries may benefit because isoniazid is inexpensive (107). Patients with high-level resistance or who have had multiple treatment failures with an isoniazid-containing regimen would not likely benefit from isoniazid, even at high doses (32).

Some clinicians in developing nations with limited laboratory and pharmaceutical support empirically recommend the inclusion of pyrazinamide, despite known resistance, in managing MDR-TB. Since pyrazinamide carries a high potential for serious adverse effects, we endorse its use in treating MDR-TB only with proven susceptibility. This is also the approach recommended by Mitnick et al. based on the Peruvian experience (104).

New Drugs under Development

There has not been a new class of drugs specifically approved for the treatment of TB since rifampin was introduced in 1966. Three new antimicrobials with enhanced activity against *M. tuberculosis* had encouraging results in vitro and in animal studies and are currently in phase II studies. They include R207910, a diarylquinoline compound (also called TMC207), and PA-824 and OPC-67683, two nitroimidazole compounds (7). The inclusion of TMC207 with optimized background therapy for MDR-TB reduced the time to sputum culture conversion to negative compared with placebo (36). Reports of outcomes in the phase II trials for the two additional agents are pending. Two additional compounds are in phase I studies: the pyrrole LL3858 and the diamine SQ 109. Many of the new agents under investigation demonstrate excellent activity against sensitive as well as resistant strains of *M. tuberculosis* (36, 147). If proved safe and effective, the new agents may represent much-needed options for patients with XDR strains and possibly allow shorter treatment regimens for sensitive TB.

TREATMENT OF PATIENTS WITH DRUG-RESISTANT TB (Table 1)

Case Management

We concur with Tiruviluamala and Reichman (153) and Narita et al. (108), who assert that the case management model which is composed of multidisciplinary teams of health care professionals practicing at TB centers of excellence provides the optimal approach for treating patients with MDR- and XDR-TB. Intensive case management is needed during hospitalization and through partnering with local health

Table 1. Treatment regimens for MDR-TB based on drug resistance and extent of disease[a]

Resistance	Recommended regimen (at least five drugs)	Extent/duration of therapy

INH
RIF (rifabutin sensitive)
	Rifabutin, 450 mg daily
	EMB 15 mg/kg daily
	PZA, 20–25 mg/kg daily
	LEVO, 750–1,000 mg daily[b]
	Amikacin or capreomycin[c] 15 mg/kg 5×/week
		Primary or limited
		  Amikacin or capreomycin, 5×/wk until culture conversion and then 3×/week for at least 6 mo
		  Oral drugs for 18 mo
		Extensive
		  Amikacin or capreomycin, 5×/wk for 6 mo and then 3×/week for 6–12 mo
		  Oral drugs for 18–24 mo

INH
RIF
Rifabutin
	Amikacin or capreomycin,[c] 15 mg/kg 5×/week
	LEVO, 750–1,000 mg daily[b]
	PZA, 20–25 mg/kg daily
	EMB, 15 mg/kg daily
	Ethionamide, 500–750 mg daily[d]
	B6, 100 mg daily
		Primary or limited
		  Amikacin or capreomycin, 5×/wk for 4–6 mo and then 3×/week for 6–12 mo
		  Oral drugs for 18–24 mo
		Extensive
		  Amikacin or capreomycin, 5×/wk for 4–6 mo and then 3×/week until culture negative for 12 mo
		  Oral drugs for 24 mo
		  PAS or cycloserine may be added

INH
RIF
Rifabutin
EMB or PZA
	Amikacin or capreomycin,[c] 15 mg/kg 5×/week
	LEVO, 750–1,000 mg daily[b]
	PZA, 20–25 mg/kg daily, or EMB, 15 mg/kg daily
	Ethionamide, 500–750 mg daily[d]
	Cycloserine, 500–750 mg daily and/or[d]
	PAS, 8–12 g q.i.d.[e] daily[f]
	B6, 100 mg daily
		Primary or limited
		  Amikacin or capreomycin, 5×/wk for 4–6 mo and then 3×/week for 6–12 mo
		  PAS or cycloserine should be included in regimen.
		  Oral drugs for 18–24 mo
		Extensive
		  Amikacin or capreomycin, 5×/wk for 6 mo and then 3×/week until culture negative for 12 mo
		  Oral drugs—all five for 24 mo

INH
RIF
Rifabutin
PZA
EMB
	Amikacin or capreomycin,[c] 15 mg/kg 5×/week daily
	LEVO, 750–1,000 mg daily[b]
	Ethionamide, 500–750 mg daily[d]
	PAS, 8–12 g q.i.d. daily[f]
	Cycloserine, 500–750 mg daily[d]
	Linezolid, 600 mg daily[g]
	B6, 100 mg daily
		Primary or limited
		  Amikacin or capreomycin, 5×/wk for 6 mo and then 3×/week until culture negative for 12 mo
		  Oral drugs for 18–24 mo
		Extensive
		  Amikacin or capreomycin, 5×/wk for 6 mo and then 3×/week until culture negative for 12 mo
		  Consider linezolid for extensive disease
		  Oral drugs for 24 mo

INH
RIF
Rifabutin
PZA
EMB
Ethionamide
	Amikacin or capreomycin,[c] 15 mg/kg 5×/week daily
	LEVO, 750–1,000 mg daily[b]
	Cycloserine, 500–750 mg daily[d]
	PAS, 6–8 g daily[f]
	Linezolid, 600 mg daily[g]
		Primary or limited
		  Amikacin or capreomycin, 5×/wk for 6 mo and then 3×/week until culture negative for 12 mo
		  Oral drugs for 24 mo; linezolid should be considered during initial 4–6 mo
		Extensive
		  Amikacin or capreomycin, 5×/wk for 6 mo and then 3×/week until culture negative for 12 mo
		  Linezolid at 600 mg daily essential. Oral drugs should be continued for at least 24 mo.

	Drug/dosage	Schedule
PRE-XDR TB		
INH	LEVO, 750–1,000 mg daily[b]	Primary or limited
RIF	Any first-line drug available	Oral drugs, five or six, if available for 18–24 mo (duration depends on strength of oral drugs)
Rifabutin	PAS, 6–8 g daily[f]	Linezolid for at least 4–6 mo
Amikacin	Cycloserine, 500–750 mg daily[d]	Extensive
Capreomycin/kanamycin	Ethionamide, 500–750 mg daily[d]	Linezolid, 600 mg daily, and five or six oral drugs as available and tolerated
±Others	Linezolid, 600 mg daily[g]	Consider other third-line drugs (see text)
	B₆, 100 mg daily	Continue for at least 24 mo
INH	Use any new fluoroquinolone that may be sensitive	Primary or limited
RIF	Amikacin or capreomycin,[c] 15 mg/kg 5×/week	Amikacin or capreomycin, 5×/wk for 6 mo and then 3×/wk until culture negative for 12 mo
Rifabutin	Any first-line drug available	At least four oral drugs for at least 18 mo, preferably 24 mo
Ofloxacin	Linezolid, 600 mg daily[g]	Extensive
±Others	PAS, 6–8 g daily[f]	Amikacin or capreomycin, 5×/wk for 6 mo and then 3–5×/wk until cultures convert to negative for 12 mo
	Cycloserine, 500–750 mg daily[d]	Oral drugs for 24 mo after culture conversion
	Other line drugs if needed[b]	
XDR-TB		
INH	Use any new fluoroquinolone that is sensitive	Primary or limited
RIF	Use any injectable that may be active	Amikacin (capreomycin or kanamycin), if available, 5×/wk for 6 mo and then 3×/wk until culture negative for 12 mo
Kanamycin and/or amikacin and/or capreomycin	Any first-line drug available	Include linezolid for entire 24 mo
	Linezolid, 600 mg daily	Oral drugs, at least four or five, for 24 mo
Ofloxacin	Ethionamide if available	Extensive
±Others	PAS, 6–8 g daily[f]	Amikacin (capreomycin or kanamycin), if available, 5×/wk for 6 mo and then 3×/wk until culture negative for 12 mo
	Cycloserine, 500–750 mg daily[d]	Include linezolid for entire 24 mo
	Other third-line drugs if needed to have at least five drugs available[b]	Oral drugs, at least four or five, for 24 mo

[a]Treatment should always be in consultation wiht an expert in management of MDR or XDR TB. Extensive disease consists of extensive infiltrates, cavities, or pulmonary destruction. Levofloxacin (LEVO) and all fluoroquinolones should be given 2 h before or after calcium- or magnesium-containing antacid, milk-based food supplements, sucralfate, multivitamins, and iron. Doses of all injectables, ethambutol (EMB), pyrazinamide (PZA), cycloserine, and PAS must be adjusted in patients with chronic renal failure. INH, isoniazid; RIF, rifampin.
[b]We usually prefer LEVO (with a dosage of at least 750 mg daily), but patients with decreased renal failure or those with possible resistance to LEVO should receive moxifloxacin (see text).
[c]Amikacin and capreomycin may be intravenous or intramuscular; capreomycin or streptomycin may be substituted when susceptibility is documented.
[d]Ethionamide and cycloserine can be given in a single daily dose or in two divided doses.
[e]PAS is usually given in two divided doses; most smaller patients (<70 kg) tolerate 6-g doses per day better than 8-g doses.
[f]Consider decrease in dose to 300 mg if toxicity would otherwise cause drug to be stopped.
[g]q.i.d., four times a day.
[h]Use at least five or six drugs.

department nurse case managers following discharge. Case management which is successful includes addressing the patient's social, economic, and additional medical needs (104). Outpatient management has been successful in our experience and even in resource-limited areas, as reported in Peru (104). Despite reports of successful ambulatory MDR treatment, an initial period of hospitalization provides the benefits of limiting community transmission by the index patient, facilitating treatment initiation, and limiting adverse effects. Adverse effects are common and occur with each of the drugs frequently used in the treatment of MDR- and XDR-TB. A recent article from Latvia detailed these effects in 1,027 cases; 807 (79%) experienced at least one adverse event, with a median of three events per case. Nausea (58%), vomiting (39%), and abdominal pain (24%) were reported most often. Other toxicities which were more serious events, such as psychiatric episodes (13%), hepatitis (9%), and renal failure (4%), were relatively frequent. Twenty percent of patients required a change in drug dose due to an adverse event, and 661 (64%) had at least one drug discontinued temporarily or permanently (12).

Treatment of MDR-TB

To date, no second-line regimen has approached the early bactericidal activity and sterilizing ability of isoniazid-rifampin-pyrazinamide in treating sensitive TB (163). Because of this, treatment for MDR-TB must include more drugs and be given for prolonged periods (18 to 24 months or longer). In low-burden countries such as the United States, where access to antituberculous medication is available, individualized treatment regimens are based on the susceptibility of the isolate. Depending on the treatment history and the clinical situation of the patient, an empirical treatment regimen is usually started pending drug susceptibility testing. Rapid access to molecular susceptibility testing enhances the ability to predict an adequate regimen. If the patient has been on treatment at the time drug resistance is identified, repeat drug susceptibility testing on the latest isolate must be done to ensure that if further drug resistance had developed during treatment, this will be identified so that the regimen can be changed appropriately.

Treatment should preferably begin with six but not fewer than four new drugs with proven susceptibility, two of which should be bactericidal (13, 27, 88, 139, 166). A standard approach is to (i) use any first-line drugs to which the isolate remains susceptible even if they have been part of a previously failing regimen, (ii) add an injectable drug, (iii) add a fluoroquinolone (levofloxacin or moxifloxacin), and (iv) choose additional remaining drugs to bring the number of drugs in the regimen to at least five, preferably six, if all susceptibility tests are not yet available. The remaining drugs should be chosen from the weaker second-line oral agents such as ethionamide, cycloserine, and PAS. If there is extensive resistance or a contraindication to some of the first- and second-line drugs, a third-line drug may need to be selected. The agents in this category include linezolid, which has shown some potential in observational studies of XDR; amoxicillin-clavulanic acid; imipenem; clarithromycin; and clofazimine (reserved for M. leprae in most countries).

An aminoglycoside or capreomycin ("injectable") at 15 mg/kg of body weight daily or five times weekly is recommended during the first 4 to 6 months of therapy. We then continue the injectable two or three times weekly for 6 to 12 months of treatment after cultures convert to negative (58, 150). Peak serum drug levels are maintained for amikacin at 25 μg/ml drawn 1 h after an intravenous infusion or 2 h after an intramuscular injection. The oral drugs should be continued for at least 18 to 24 months after sputum cultures convert to negative. Serum drug levels are obtained after the first several weeks and the doses of medications adjusted to achieve optimal serum levels.

The key oral agent is a daily fluoroquinolone, which is continued throughout the treatment course (49, 53, 76, 150). Susceptibility to the fluoroquinolone utilized in the regimen should always be documented. Resistance to the fluoroquinolones, though uncommon, has been reported within a month of initial therapy (149). Most clinical experience exists with levofloxacin. For adults, a dose of 750 to 1,000 mg is usually well tolerated (13, 56). Moxifloxacin, a newer fluoroquinolone, has equivalent or improved activity (54, 60, 129, 131, 154) dosed at 400 mg daily. Experience with pushing the dose is limited, and at a dosage of 400 mg daily, it may not offer much additional benefit over high-dose levofloxacin.

The combination of levofloxacin, ethambutol, and pyrazinamide demonstrated intermediate early bactericidal activity against 12 MDR strains (163). When the isolate is susceptible to pyrazinamide, this drug should be given throughout the treatment course. Susceptibility to rifabutin will be present in 20% or more of rifampin-resistant cases (49, 61). Rifabutin appears to be as effective as rifampin in the treatment of drug-susceptible TB (59, 98), but data on its use in MDR-TB are limited. We include it at a dosage of 450 mg daily whenever susceptibility exists. Tolerance to this dose is usually good in persons without HIV infection. Ethionamide is weakly bactericidal and generally preferred over cycloserine and PAS. Ethionamide, cycloserine, and PAS can all be initiated at low dose and increased over the first 7 to 10 days of treatment. Patients may tolerate these drugs better when doses are escalated and when they are given twice daily in divided doses.

The patient's underlying medical condition and ability to tolerate a given drug should be considered when building a treatment regimen as much as possible without compromising the efficacy of the regimen. For instance, a person with a history of depression, mania, or seizures may be unlikely to tolerate cycloserine, so whenever possible another drug should be chosen. The experience in Peru suggests that depression at the onset of therapy is common and can be managed with the use of an antidepressant (160). In our experience, when depression develops during therapy with cycloserine it is difficult to manage, and medication usually needs to be discontinued. Suicide has been noted for persons suffering from cycloserine-associated depression. Careful attention must be paid during the selection of drug regimens in patients with renal or hepatic dysfunction and drug doses and dosing intervals adjusted accordingly. There are no approved intermittent regimens for MDR-TB, so treatment must be daily for oral medications.

During a treatment course, the patient may improve clinically and even transiently convert sputum cultures to negative. If the resistant mycobacteria multiply, the patient may have a relapse of symptoms and positive cultures. This phenomenon was recognized in the past and referred to as the "the fall and the rise" of TB (166). Without a strong regimen, an initial favorable clinical response does not ensure a successful outcome or justify continuing a weak regimen. Treatment that consists of at least five or six drugs, includes both a fluoroquinolone (76, 150) and an aminoglycoside, and is continued for an adequate duration should have a high degree of success (49, 116). Successful MDR-TB treatment has been associated with prolonged inpatient management, particularly in resource-poor settings and for patients who are medically complex or who lack social support (111). The Partners in Health in Peru report good results using an individually tailored regimen which is based on drug susceptibilities and includes as a foundation of the regimen a quinolone and an aminoglycoside when susceptibility to these agents is documented (43, 104).

The duration of therapy depends on (i) the extent of disease, including the presence of cavitary lesions and pulmonary destruction; (ii) the number of bactericidal drugs included in the treatment regimen which are shown to be effective against the patient's isolate and are tolerated by the patient; (iii) the immune and nutritional status of the patient; and (iv) the patient's clinical, radiographic, and bacteriological responses

to therapy. Open cavitary lesions at the end of treatment for drug-susceptible TB are associated with a greater risk of relapse and presumably would be a risk factor for relapse in MDR- or XDR-TB. The rate of sputum culture conversion has been shown by Holtz et al. to be an important predictor of outcomes (69). Most patients converted their cultures to negative in a median time of 60 days. Treatment outcomes were worse in those who had later conversion times (69). When there is a good regimen, good response, and limited disease, especially if the patient has no history of treatment, therapy can be stopped after 18 months. The injectable drug in these patients may only be needed for 6 months after culture conversion. However, in patients with extensive cavitary disease which is bilateral and has evidence of volume loss and destruction, longer therapy, i.e., at least 12 months of the injectable after conversion of cultures to negative and 24 months of treatment with the oral regimen, is likely to be needed to decrease the incidence of relapse (69, 88, 104, 108). When there is resistance to all first-line drugs as well as ethionamide, even if the isolate is susceptible to a fluoroquinolone and an injectable, treatment will be difficult due to the limited number of oral drugs to support the fluoroquinolone in the second year of treatment. These patients likely would benefit by longer treatment, as options for re-treatment are very limited. This also applies when resistance to either a fluoroquinolone or an injectable is present, which has been termed "pre-XDR TB" by Banerjee et al. (6). The patient's response is also an important determinant of the length of therapy. Treatment often needs to be individualized. This can best be done by working with an expert in the care of MDR-TB.

Many second-line drugs have insufficient data for safety in pregnancy or have been established to be teratogenic. Nonetheless, small case series and our experience have noted favorable maternal and fetal outcomes despite MDR-TB therapy. Women of childbearing potential should be counseled and offered assistance to avoid conception during treatment for MDR-TB (144).

Treatment of XDR-TB

Just as treatment for MDR-TB is largely based on expert opinion and observational studies, so is treatment for XDR-TB. Treatment is even more difficult, as there is less information available to guide providers. It is essential to have both first- and second-line drug susceptibility tests, including tests for all injectable agents, ethionamide, and a newer-generation fluoroquinolone in order to maximize the therapeutic regimen. Treatment should be completely by directly observed therapy (DOT) and guided by an expert in the management of MDR- and XDR-TB.

Treatment of XDR-TB is based on the same principles as is the treatment of MDR-TB. The treatment regimen is built the same way. It is especially important to include any first-line drug to which the isolate remains susceptible. An injectable should always be used if any is identified as effective on second-line drug testing. Resistance is not complete among these three drugs: kanamycin, amikacin, and capreomycin (84). Testing should be done against each, as inclusion of an injectable to which the isolate is susceptible will improve treatment outcomes. If susceptibility to levofloxacin or moxifloxacin is determined, one of these should be used. When susceptibility is pending, moxifloxacin is usually used. Additional second- and third-line drugs should be added to bring the number of drugs in the regimen to at least six. Usually, treatment with both the injectable and the oral drug regimen should be longer and more aggressive, although definite guidelines do not exist (151).

Mitnick et al. reported a cure in 29 of 48 (60.4%) patients with XDR-TB (105). Patients were treated with daily supervised therapy with greater than five drugs which included an injectable drug, a fluoroquinolone, cycloserine, and two or more of the following: clarithromycin, amoxicillin-clavulanate, clofazimine, and rifabutin. No patient received linezolid in this study. Treatment was prolonged, with median durations of injectable for 15.4 months and the oral regimen for 24.9 months. The median time for conversion was 90 days. Treatment of XDR-TB patients in Tomsk, Russia, with greater than five drugs and at least 6 to 9 months of injectable drugs and oral medications for at least 18 months after conversion of the culture to negative was associated with treatment cure or completion in 48.3%. Linezolid was not available to this group of patients.

Linezolid is a critical antituberculous agent for patients with XDR-TB, as it is another bactericidal drug for patients, especially those resistant to all injectables and fluoroquinolones. Improved outcomes have been associated with the use of linezolid (29, 79). The toxicity is significant, and patients must be monitored carefully and the risks and benefits repeatedly reviewed and discussed with the patients. Although it is not uncommon for up to 25% of patients to withdraw from therapy due to linezolid toxicity, giving the drug for as long as it can be tolerated may be critical to achieving a long-term cure.

New antibacterial drugs are desperately needed for care of these patients. None of the newer agents are yet available for treatment. When new agents do come to the market, it will be important to use them wisely. It may be very tempting to utilize new drugs in chronically failing patients. The classic rule of treatment of TB must be remembered—"Never add a single drug to a failing regimen"—in order to protect these new agents.

HIV-Infected Patients with MDR- or XDR-TB

All HIV-infected or otherwise immunocompromised patients with suspected MDR- or XDR-TB must be recognized quickly, assessed for the most likely susceptibility pattern, and started empirically on aggressive combination therapy. Mortality rates have been extraordinarily high in HIV-infected persons with MDR-TB who have delays in initiation of appropriate therapy (50, 51, 151).

XDR-TB is readily transmitted to HIV-coinfected patients, with associated high mortality rates. From January 2005 to March 2006, 52 of 53 HIV patients from KwaZulu-Natal, South Africa, died from XDR-TB, with a median survival time of 16 days after diagnosis (51). This was reminiscent of the MDR-TB outbreak in HIV-infected persons in New York City in the 1990s. When MDR-TB is diagnosed early and patients receive individualized therapy, they can respond with prolonged survival (29, 49, 114, 133, 140). However, most outcomes in HIV-infected persons with XDR-TB have been poor (16).

We recommend an aggressive empirical regimen prior to knowledge of drug sensitivities. Usually six or seven drugs should be used unless there is convincing knowledge of the likely susceptibility. This often means that most, if not all, of the remaining medications to which the person might be susceptible should be prescribed. Rapid molecular assays should be used to quickly identify possible drug resistance and assist with building an empirical regimen pending the results of final drug susceptibility tests. These patients are some of the highest-priority cases for rapid detection of susceptibility via molecular methods. Adverse medication-related events are much more common in HIV-infected patients treated for MDR-TB. Close monitoring clinically and with laboratory tests is needed. The treatment regimen may need to be adjusted on several occasions. It is important to work with an expert in the care of patients with both HIV and MDR-TB to minimize drug toxicity and drug-drug interactions but at the same time ensure an adequate regimen that is not compromised and does not lead to treatment failure and further amplification of drug resistance. Usually treatment should be longer and more aggressive, although definite guidelines do not exist. Many reports detail what has not worked, and experts often treat with the awareness that a slightly longer and more aggressive regimen is preferred to treatment failure and relapse.

MONITORING AND MANAGING MEDICATION TOXICITY

Treatment regimens for MDR-TB include drugs with significant toxicity (Table 2) (137). Patients should be warned to expect some adverse effects but encouraged that once they complete treatment, they may resume normal lives. In our experience, toxicity nearly always becomes less severe and more tolerable as treatment progresses. Exceptions include the auditory or vestibular toxicity with injection medications, which is related to the total dose, usually progresses, and is irreversible. Increasing the dosing interval of the injectable can slow hearing loss and allow continued treatment. Vestibular toxicity, however, usually requires prompt discontinuation of the aminoglycoside or capreomycin. Periodic symptom questionnaires, basic audiometric screens, and simple bedside vestibular function tests assist in monitoring for ototoxicity.

A symptom screen may help identify the onset of drug-related hepatitis; behavioral changes, including psychosis and depression (cycloserine); tendonitis (fluoroquinolones); and visual problems. Medications should be continued whenever possible, as replacements are usually not available and discontinuation of even a single medication may affect regimen effectiveness. Symptomatic treatment or a change in dosing schedule may alleviate nausea and anorexia and should be attempted before discontinuing a medication (58). Significant elevation of liver enzymes, vestibular toxicity, acute renal failure (58), vision loss or uveitis, acute tendonitis or evidence of tendon rupture, seizures, psychosis, and serious depression usually require stopping the responsible medication. Peripheral neuropathy that progresses past grade two usually requires stopping linezolid.

Toxicity monitoring should include at least monthly serum creatinine and assessment of glomerular filtration rate by MDRD calculation (89), or, if significant changes are noted, by a timed urine test for creatinine clearance. Hepatic enzymes and a complete blood count should be done monthly. A significant percentage of patients on ethionamide or PAS develop hypothyroidism after several months of treatment, and patients should have a TSH done at least every 2 to 3 months. Thyroid hormone replacement should be provided when indicated (146) but can often be discontinued after treatment is completed (57). Vision exams and visual symptom screens are important for patients on ethambutol, linezolid, or rifabutin (uveitis) (57, 66). Rare instances of clofazimine visual toxicity have been noted (30, 31).

Radiology

Computerized tomography of the chest has proved an invaluable tool in initial and periodic assessment of MDR-TB cases. Measurable disease serves as an important marker of response to therapy. The chest radiograph should be followed at least twice yearly during therapy and before any major change in therapy. A film should be obtained prior to the end of treatment to evaluate response and to serve as a reference for monitoring the patient.

Drug Susceptibility Testing (see also chapter 4)

Drug susceptibility testing to all four first-line drugs, isoniazid, rifampin, ethambutol, and pyrazinamide, is recommended for all persons diagnosed with TB in the United States (13). The WHO now recommends drug susceptibility testing for all persons with TB (166, 167). Implementation of this recommendation has been slow in many areas lacking laboratory capacity. In areas with high rates of TB, the WHO has recommended rapid identification of rifampin resistance as a marker of MDR-TB using a line probe assay, a rapid molecular method to detect genotypic resistance. The microscopic-observation drug susceptibility assay is a low-cost method of liquid culture and direct drug susceptibility testing which was developed for use in resource-limited countries. It uses a noncommercial laboratory technique that directly inoculates decontaminated patient specimens onto liquid media and then examines the plates using an inverted microscope to detect very early mycobacterial growth. This assay is able to simultaneously identify mycobacterial growth and the presence of drug resistance. It has performed successfully in resource-limited high-burden countries, but questions remain regarding widespread implementation (102, 126). Rapid molecular detection of drug resistance is also a goal of the CDC. The CDC laboratory now accepts cultures of *M. tuberculosis* for rapid detection of isoniazid and rifampin susceptibility and soon will extend testing to ethambutol, pyrazinamide, fluoroquinolones, and injectable drugs. This service is free of charge for appropriate patients who are at risk of drug-resistant TB but needs to be coordinated through the state TB program. Several state public health laboratories also offer rapid molecular testing.

Therapeutic Serum Drug Level Monitoring

The routine use of serum therapeutic drug level monitoring should be considered for all patients with MDR-TB (15, 108). The therapeutic indices of second-line TB medications are narrow. Serum therapeutic

Table 2. Characteristics of second-line drugs for MDR-TB[a]

Drug	Bactericidal	MIC (µg/ml)	Serum drug level (µg/ml)	Dosing	Remarks	Side effects
Streptomycin	Yes	0.25–2.0	25–35	15 mg/kg/day 5–7 days/wk 20–25 mg/kg 2–3 days/wk	Class summary: vestibular screen Baseline audiogram Monitor creatinine Adjust dose and/or interval for renal insufficiency	Ototoxicity—auditory/vestibular (irreversible), renal toxicity, giddiness, perioral numbness, hypersensitivity, pain at injection site (57, 58)
Amikacin	Yes	0.5–1.0	25–35	15 mg–1 kg/day 5–7 days/wk 20–25 mg/kg 2–3 days/wk		Ototoxicity—auditory/vestibular (irreversible), renal toxicity, pain at injection site
Capreomycin	Yes	1.25–2.5	25–35	15 mg/kg/day 5–7 days/wk 20–25 mg/kg 2–3 days/wk		Ototoxicity—auditory/vestibular, hypokalemia, hypocalcemia, hypomagnesemia, pain at injection site Eosinophilia (57, 58)
Levofloxacin	Yes	0.5–1.0	8–12	500–1,000 mg daily (usually 750 mg)	L isomer—all active drug	Class effect: gastrointestinal upset, dizziness, hypersensitivity, photosensitivity, headaches, tendonitis, tendon rupture, insomnia, psychosis, agitation, depression, paranoia, seizures, thrush, hepatitis Sucralfate, antacids with Al, Mg, CaSo₄ or FeSo₄ inhibit absorption, as may enteral supplements (3, 10, 72, 90, 92, 93, 128, 156)
Moxifloxacin	Yes	0.25	4–6	400 mg daily	Good CNS penetration No dose adjustment with renal failure May increase liver enzymes	
Rifabutin	Yes	0.25–0.5	0.3–0.9	450 mg daily	Extensive drug interactions: P-450 induction (less than rifampin) decreases levels of protease inhibitors, methadone, oral contraceptives, diabetic medications, fluconazole, and others: see PDR[b] Concentrates in macrophages.	Decreased white blood count, decreased platelet count, arthralgias, renal impairment, hyperpigmentation, uveitis, discoloration of body fluids, flushing, erythema of the head and trunk, gastrointestinal upset, hepatitis agusia (59, 63, 66, 106)
Ethionamide	Weak	0.3–1.2	1–5	250 mg 2 or 3 times daily or 250 mg a.m./500 mg p.m.	Increase dose gradually; monitor liver function/thyroid function. Increases effect of cycloserine.	Peripheral neuropathy, nausea, vomiting, abdominal pain, hepatitis, hypothyroidism, salivation, metallic taste, giddiness, headache, hypersensitivity, alopecia, gynecomastia, hypotension, impotence, mental disturbance, menstrual irregularity, hypoglycemia, photosensitivity (3, 57, 58, 146)

Drug					Comments	Adverse effects
PAS	No	8.0	20–60 (6 h after dose)	4 g 2 or 3 times daily	Diarrhea improves with time; increase dose gradually over first 7–10 days, mix with acidic juice or applesauce, avoid diphenhydramine	Gastrointestinal upset, diarrhea (self-limiting), hypothyroidism, hypokalemia, hepatitis, thrombocytopenia, increased acidosis in patients with renal failure (57, 58, 146)
Clofazimine	Weak	0.12	0.5–2.0	300 mg daily for 2 mo and then 100 mg daily	Skin problems limited by sunscreen and lubricants	Hyperpigmentation, gastrointestinal complaints, acne flare, retinopathy, ichthyosis, sunburn (3, 30, 31)
Cycloserine	No	N/A[c]	20–35	250 mg 2 times daily or 250 mg a.m./500 p.m.	Avoid in patients with seizures/psychotic disease or ethyl alcohol abuse; check level before increasing dose >500 mg daily. Administer with pyridoxine.	Agitation, psychosis, depression, seizures, dizziness, headache, slurred speech, insomnia (57, 58)
Isoniazid (high dose)	Yes	<5.0	N/A	1,200 mg 3 times weekly	Pyridoxine, 100 mg daily, interacts with phenytoin; only useful if MIC is <5.0 µg/ml	Optic neuritis, positive ANA[d] rash, fever, jaundice, hepatitis, peripheral neuritis, anemia, agranulocytosis, decreased platelets, vasculitis (32)
Linezolid	Yes	0.5–1.0	12–24	600 mg daily; may be able to decrease dosage to 300 mg daily after 4–6 mo	Pyridoxine, 100 mg daily, limits hematological toxicity. Avoid medications and foods that increase serotonin.	Myelosuppression, peripheral and optic neuropathy, lactic acidosis, serotonin syndrome, and gastrointestinal upset

[a]Adapted from references 3, 10, 30–32, 57–59, 63, 66, 72, 90, 92, 93, 106, 128, 146, and 156.
[b]PDR, *Physicians Desk Reference*, 64th ed., 2010 (see each drug in patient's regimen for interaction with rifabutin).
[c]N/A, not available.
[d]ANA, anti-nuclear antibody.

drug level monitoring allows a physician to "push a drug" to exert maximal benefit and still limit toxicity. An attempt should be made to achieve the best ratio of peak serum drug level to MIC. Successful outcomes and prevention of acquired resistance have been achieved by monitoring and adjusting serum fluoroquinolone levels (96, 97, 173). The renal and auditory toxicities associated with injectable agents may be averted by identification of high serum levels and subsequent adjustment of the dose or dosing interval. Cycloserine levels are helpful in order to minimize CNS adverse reactions. Therapeutic monitoring may alert the physician to an unsuspected problem with absorption, patient adherence with treatment, or a drug interaction. Persons with HIV or those at risk for malabsorption should be specifically targeted for therapeutic monitoring.

Surgical Therapy

Persistence of organisms in necrotic lung, poor vascular supply, and resultant limited penetration of medications may lead to treatment failure or relapse. Destroyed pulmonary tissue and old cavitary lesions may be sites for recurrent bacterial or fungal infections (157). Iseman et al. attribute the improved outcomes of patients with MDR-TB treated between 1984 and 1993 at least in part to surgical intervention (74, 76). They and others recommended that surgical intervention be considered for patients with destruction of a lobe or entire lung and those with extensive disease including large or persistent cavities. Another surgical indication is life-threatening or uncontrolled hemoptysis, although bronchial arterial embolization may facilitate control of bleeding. The optimum timing of elective surgical intervention is after 3 to 4 months of therapy and sputum culture conversion to negative. Patients who fail to convert their sputum to negative after 3 to 4 months of intensive therapy may also benefit from surgical intervention (74, 76, 159). Patients should be screened for overall operative risk, likely residual pulmonary function after surgery, and operative risk of devastating broncho-pleural fistula. Therapy should be continued for at least an additional 18 to 24 months after surgery (76, 157). The few experienced centers performing lung resection surgery report infrequent morbidity and mortality (157). However, the reported benefits of resection surgery may be substantially biased by patient selection (62). Residual lung damage is common and extensive in MDR versus susceptible TB cases. Close follow-up of treated cases is warranted to detect and manage relapses, regardless of previous resection surgery (34).

INFECTION CONTROL

Patients with MDR-TB are as infectious as any TB patient (145). Because treatment for latent TB infection (LTBI) is unproven in this group and has been associated with a high rate of adverse effects (72), every effort should be employed to prevent transmission of MDR-TB. Improvement of infection control measures in institutions has been credited with decreasing rates of MDR-TB in urban populations with HIV (49, 164). One study demonstrated a rapid decrease in culture-positive cough aerosols during the first 3 weeks of effective therapy for MDR-TB. Culture-positive aerosols were associated with interruptions in therapy during the previous week ($P = 0.007$) (46). Patients with MDR-TB should be placed individually in engineered negative-pressure isolation rooms. The CDC recommends continuing respiratory isolation throughout the hospital course, even when cultures are negative (78). We require patients with MDR-TB to remain in respiratory isolation at least until they have three separate final negative sputum cultures while adherent with and responding to an optimized regimen. After conversion of cultures to negative, patients should continue to be monitored with monthly sputum cultures. Patients may become sputum culture positive, even after months of negative cultures (58). Decisions about when patients may contact children or immunocompromised individuals are controversial and may need to be individualized following consultation with public health authorities. The issue is often not *if* patients may be discharged but *where* they may be best cared for on an ambulatory basis (138).

In resource-poor settings, limiting inpatient days, improving natural ventilation, cohorting patients in groups of five or less, achieving rapid laboratory identification of resistant cases, and the use of particulate respirators by staff produce the maximum reduction in nosocomial TB transmission. The majority of these benefits can be obtained by relatively low-cost and low-technology improvements to ward and clinic ventilation (77).

PREVENTION

The WHO-recommended directly observed therapy, short course (DOTS), inexpensively treats susceptible TB cases and effectively reduces the emergence of MDR-TB. DOTS is based on the axiom that "you cannot cure multidrug resistant TB as fast as you can create it" (42, 71). The DOTS strategy appears effective for preventing "homegrown" but not "imported" cases of MDR-TB (62). Furthermore, DOTS may serve as a death sentence in countries with a high prevalence of MDR-TB (67). Following Peru's success with ambulatory treatment regimens for MDR-TB, the WHO has since endorsed "DOTS Plus" MDR-TB treatment regimens, but only in countries with well-functioning TB programs (3, 43, 63, 90, 106, 128, 156).

TREATMENT OF LATENT INFECTION POSSIBLY DUE TO MDR-TB (see also chapter 6)

All persons identified as MDR-TB contacts are at risk and should be quickly evaluated for latent infection and active disease. The optimal management of established LTBI is a matter of debate. No regimen has been proved effective, and it is unlikely that a definitive study will be done to guide management. Nevertheless, it is important to monitor all persons with presumed latent MDR-TB for at least 2 years following the exposure. Periodic assessments should include clinical exams and chest radiographs every 3 months for persons with HIV or other immunosuppressing illness and every 6 months for all others (20).

Those who are tuberculin skin test positive, are close contacts of an MDR-TB case, and have no history of a previously positive tuberculin test can be considered for treatment of latent MDR-TB. After discussion of the risks and benefits of treatment, the patient and physician can make a decision regarding LTBI treatment. Management of tuberculin skin test-negative high-risk contacts, especially infants and persons with HIV, varies. Some recommend empirical therapy after active disease is excluded (20). Most clinicians agree that LTBI treatment should be offered to tuberculin skin test-positive, immunosuppressed individuals with documented exposure to MDR-TB. If assessment indicates the likelihood of exposure to drug-susceptible TB, isoniazid therapy may be preferred.

The selection of agents should be guided by the susceptibility profile of the index case. One possible regimen is a combination of pyrazinamide (25 to 30 mg daily) and ethambutol (15 to 25 mg daily). If fluoroquinolone susceptibility is documented, a regimen that combines ofloxacin (800 mg), levofloxacin (750 mg), or moxifloxacin (400 mg) daily with pyrazinamide might be used. A pyrazinamide-fluoroquinolone combination appears to result in enhanced activity within the macrophage (26). The pyrazinamide-based regimens have been associated with high levels of hepatotoxicity (112, 174). A fluoroquinolone also can be combined with ethambutol. Some have recommended quinolone monotherapy, although emergence of resistance is a concern. LTBI treatment is usually prescribed for 6 to 12 months.

CONCLUSION

MDR-TB is a continuing public health problem. Although control of the MDR-TB epidemic has been achieved in New York City, strains of MDR-TB are found in nearly every state. Much of the world faces a growing problem with no immediate solution. The treatment habits and public health policies that have led to the problem persist. Reichman notes that new drug development has been almost nonexistent. The current global interest offers hope that the discovery and development of new anti-TB drugs will accelerate. However, the mere existence and affordability of new drugs for MDR-TB "will not address the main underlying cause of almost all drug resistance, nonadherence of patients and doctors to recommended regimens" (153). He calls for an equal commitment to improving the knowledge and skills of health care workers to use both old and new agents appropriately, so that they may retain their effectiveness for the future (127).

Each year brings new, at-risk immigrants to the United States from all regions of the globe. They bring all the TB problems of their home countries with them. Foreign-born persons will continue to have a major impact on TB control efforts in the next decade and beyond. In the United States, TB elimination programs will need to strengthen the education of caregivers and improve case finding and treatment for MDR-TB. Developing countries need assistance to develop a similar capacity to effectively manage both susceptible and resistant TB. It is estimated that one million persons arrive in the United States each week by plane. A cursory review of resistant TB among the foreign-born should convince even skeptics that global TB programs need our urgent and serious support.

Acknowledgments. We acknowledge Alysia Gibbons for assistance with manuscript preparation and for developing tables, the Texas Department of State Health Services, and nurses and physicians at the Texas Center for Infectious Disease and across the state for their dedicated care of patients with MDR-TB.

REFERENCES

1. **Alangaden, G. J., B. N. Kreiswirth, A. Aouad, M. Khetarpal, F. R. Igno, S. L. Moghazeh, E. K. Manavathu, and S. A. Lerner.** 1998. Mechanism of resistance to amikacin and kanamycin in *Mycobacterium tuberculosis. Antimicrob. Agents Chemother.* **42:**1295–1297.

2. **Alangaden, G. J., and S. A. Lerner.** 1997. The clinical use of fluoroquinolones for the treatment of mycobacterial diseases. *Clin. Infect. Dis.* **25:**1213–1221.

3. **Allen, J. E., T. S. Potter, and K. Hashimoto.** 1995. Drugs that cause photosensitivity. *Med. Lett. Drugs Ther.* **37:**35–36.

4. **American Thoracic Society, Centers for Disease Control and Prevention, and Infectious Diseases Society of America.** 2003. Treatment of tuberculosis. *MMWR Recommend. Rep.* **59:**1–27.

5. Anger, H. A., F. Dworkin, S. Sharma, S. S. Munsiff, D. M. Nilsen, and S. D. Ahuja. 2010. Linezolid use for treatment of multidrug-resistant and extensively drug-resistant tuberculosis, New York City, 2000–06. *J. Antimicrob. Chemother.* 65: 775–783.

6. Banerjee, R., J. Allen, J. Westenhouse, P. Oh, W. Elms, E. Desmond, A. Nitta, S. Royce, and J. Flood. 2008. Extensively drug-resistant tuberculosis in California, 1993–2006. *Clin. Infect. Dis.* 47:450–457.

7. Barry, C. E., III, and M. S. Cheung. 2009. New tactics against tuberculosis. *Sci. Am.* 300:62–69.

8. Beekmann, S. E., D. N. Gilbert, and P. M. Polgreen. 2008. Toxicity of extended courses of linezolid: results of an Infectious Diseases Society of America Emerging Infections Network survey. *Diagn. Microbiol. Infect. Dis.* 62:407–410.

9. Bernard, L., R. Stern, D. Lew, and P. Hoffmeyer. 2003. Serotonin syndrome after concomitant treatment with linezolid and citalopram. *Clin. Infect. Dis.* 36:1197.

10. Berning, S. E., L. Madsen, M. D. Iseman, and C. A. Peloquin. 1995. Long-term safety of ofloxacin and ciprofloxacin in the treatment of mycobacterial infections. *Am. J. Respir. Crit. Care Med.* 151:2006–2009.

11. Bishop, E., S. Melvani, B. P. Howden, P. G. Charles, and M. L. Grayson. 2006. Good clinical outcomes but high rates of adverse reactions during linezolid therapy for serious infections: a proposed protocol for monitoring therapy in complex patients. *Antimicrob. Agents Chemother.* 50:1599–1602.

12. Bloss, E., L. Kuksa, T. H. Holtz, V. Riekstina, V. Skripconoka, S. Kammerer, and V. Leimane. 2010. Adverse events related to multidrug-resistant tuberculosis treatment, Latvia, 2000–2004. *Int. J. Tuberc. Lung Dis.* 14:275–281.

13. Blumberg, H. M., W. J. Burman, R. E. Chaisson, C. L. Daley, S. C. Etkind, L. N. Friedman, P. Fujiwara, M. Grzemska, P. C. Hopewell, M. D. Iseman, R. M. Jasmer, V. Koppaka, R. I. Menzies, R. J. O'Brien, R. R. Reves, L. B. Reichman, P. M. Simone, J. R. Starke, and A. A. Vernon. 2003. American Thoracic Society/Centers for Disease Control and Prevention/Infectious Diseases Society of America: treatment of tuberculosis. *Am. J. Respir. Crit. Care Med.* 167:603–662.

14. Bozdogan, B., and P. C. Appelbaum. 2004. Oxazolidinones: activity, mode of action, and mechanism of resistance. *Int. J. Antimicrob. Agents* 23:113–119.

15. Braden, C. 1997. Commentary: multidrug-resistant tuberculosis. *Infect. Dis. Clin. Pract.* 6:437–440.

16. Burgos, M., L. C. Gonzalez, E. A. Paz, E. Gournis, L. M. Kawamura, G. Schecter, P. C. Hopewell, and C. L. Daley. 2005. Treatment of multidrug-resistant tuberculosis in San Francisco: an outpatient-based approach. *Clin. Infect. Dis.* 40: 968–975.

17. Byrd, R. B., B. R. Horn, D. A. Solomon, G. A. Griggs, and N. J. Wilder. 1977. Treatment of tuberculosis by the nonpulmonary physician. *Ann. Intern. Med.* 86:799–802.

18. Calver, A. D., A. A. Falmer, M. Murray, O. J. Strauss, E. M. Streicher, M. Hanekom, T. Liversage, M. Masibi, P. D. van Helden, R. M. Warren, and T. C. Victor. 2010. Emergence of increased resistance and extensively drug-resistant tuberculosis despite treatment adherence, South Africa. *Emerg. Infect. Dis.* 16:264–271.

19. Campos, P. E., P. G. Suarez, J. Sanchez, D. Zavala, J. Arevalo, E. Ticona, C. M. Nolan, T. M. Hooton, and K. K. Holmes. 2003. Multidrug-resistant *Mycobacterium tuberculosis* in HIV-infected persons, Peru. *Emerg. Infect. Dis.* 9:1571–1578.

20. Centers for Disease Control. 1992. Management of persons exposed to multidrug-resistant tuberculosis. *MMWR Recommend. Rep.* 41:61–71.

21. Centers for Disease Control. 1990. Nosocomial transmission of multidrug-resistant tuberculosis to health-care workers and HIV-infected patients in an urban hospital—Florida. *MMWR Morb. Mortal. Wkly. Rep.* 39:718–722.

22. Centers for Disease Control and Prevention. 2010. Decrease in reported tuberculosis cases—United States, 2009. *MMWR Morb. Mortal. Wkly. Rep.* 59:289–294.

23. Centers for Disease Control and Prevention. 2006. Emergence of *Mycobacterium tuberculosis* with extensive resistance to second-line drugs—worldwide, 2000–2004. *MMWR Morb. Mortal. Wkly. Rep.* 55:301–305.

24. Centers for Disease Control and Prevention. 2006. Notice to readers: revised definition of extensively drug-resistant tuberculosis. *MMWR Morb. Mortal. Wkly. Rep.* 55:1176.

25. Chambers, H. F., J. Turner, G. F. Schecter, M. Kawamura, and P. C. Hopewell. 2005. Imipenem for treatment of tuberculosis in mice and humans. *Antimicrob. Agents Chemother.* 49: 2816–2821.

26. Chan, E. D., and M. D. Iseman. 2002. Current medical treatment for tuberculosis. *BMJ* 325:1282–1286.

27. Chan, E. D., V. Laurel, M. J. Strand, J. F. Chan, M. L. Huynh, M. Goble, and M. D. Iseman. 2004. Treatment and outcome analysis of 205 patients with multidrug-resistant tuberculosis. *Am. J. Respir. Crit. Care Med.* 169:1103–1109.

28. Churchyard, G. J., G. Kaplan, D. Fallows, R. S. Wallis, P. Onyebujoh, and G. A. Rook. 2009. Advances in immunotherapy for tuberculosis treatment. *Clin. Chest Med.* 30:769–782, ix.

29. Condos, R., N. Hadgiangelis, E. Leibert, G. Jacquette, T. Harkin, and W. N. Rom. 2008. Case series report of a linezolid-containing regimen for extensively drug-resistant tuberculosis. *Chest* 134:187–192.

30. Craythorn, J. M., M. Swartz, and D. J. Creel. 1986. Clofazimine-induced bull's-eye retinopathy. *Retina* 6:50–52.

31. Cunningham, C. A., D. N. Friedberg, and R. E. Carr. 1990. Clofazimine-induced generalized retinal degeneration. *Retina* 10:131–134.

32. Cynamon, M. H., Y. Zhang, T. Harpster, S. Cheng, and M. S. DeStefano. 1999. High-dose isoniazid therapy for isoniazid-resistant murine *Mycobacterium tuberculosis* infection. *Antimicrob. Agents Chemother.* 43:2922–2924.

33. Das, P. K., D. I. Warkentin, R. Hewko, and D. L. Forrest. 2008. Serotonin syndrome after concomitant treatment with linezolid and meperidine. *Clin. Infect. Dis.* 46:264–265.

34. de Valliere, S., and R. D. Barker. 2004. Residual lung damage after completion of treatment for multidrug-resistant tuberculosis. *Int. J. Tuberc. Lung Dis.* 8:767–771.

35. Devasia, R. A., A. Blackman, T. Gebretsadik, M. Griffin, A. Shintani, C. May, T. Smith, N. Hooper, F. Maruri, J. Warkentin, E. Mitchel, and T. R. Sterling. 2009. Fluoroquinolone resistance in *Mycobacterium tuberculosis*: the effect of duration and timing of fluoroquinolone exposure. *Am. J. Respir. Crit. Care Med.* 180:365–370.

36. Diacon, A. H., A. Pym, M. Grobusch, R. Patientia, R. Rustomjee, L. Page-Shipp, C. Pistorius, R. Krause, M. Bogoshi, G. Churchyard, A. Venter, J. Allen, J. C. Palomino, T. De Marez, R. P. van Heeswijk, N. Lounis, P. Meyvisch, J. Verbeeck, W. Parys, K. de Beule, K. Andries, and D. F. McNeeley. 2009. The diarylquinoline TMC207 for multidrug-resistant tuberculosis. *N. Engl. J. Med.* 360:2397–2405.

37. Dietze, R., D. J. Hadad, B. McGee, L. P. Molino, E. L. Maciel, C. A. Peloquin, D. F. Johnson, S. M. Debanne, K. Eisenach, W. H. Boom, M. Palaci, and J. L. Johnson. 2008. Early and extended early bactericidal activity of linezolid in pulmonary tuberculosis. *Am. J. Respir. Crit. Care Med.* 178:1180–1185.

38. Dong, Y., C. Xu, X. Zhao, J. Domagala, and K. Drlica. 1998. Fluoroquinolone action against mycobacteria: effects of C-8

substituents on growth, survival, and resistance. *Antimicrob. Agents Chemother.* **42:**2978–2984.

39. du Toit, L. C., V. Pillay, and M. P. Danckwerts. 2006. Tuberculosis chemotherapy: current drug delivery approaches. *Respir. Res.* **7:**118.

40. Dye, C., S. Scheele, P. Dolin, V. Pathania, and M. C. Raviglione. 1999. Consensus statement. Global burden of tuberculosis: estimated incidence, prevalence, and mortality by country. WHO Global Surveillance and Monitoring Project. *JAMA* **282:**677–686.

41. Edson, R. S., and C. L. Terrell. 1999. The aminoglycosides. *Mayo Clin. Proc.* **74:**519–528.

42. Enarson, D. A. 2000. Resistance to antituberculosis medications: hard lessons to learn. *Arch. Intern. Med.* **160:**581–582.

43. Farmer, P., and J. Y. Kim. 1998. Community based approaches to the control of multidrug resistant tuberculosis: introducing "DOTS-plus." *BMJ* **317:**671–674.

44. Fattorini, L., D. Tan, E. Iona, M. Mattei, F. Giannoni, L. Brunori, S. Recchia, and G. Orefici. 2003. Activities of moxifloxacin alone and in combination with other antimicrobial agents against multidrug-resistant *Mycobacterium tuberculosis* infection in BALB/c mice. *Antimicrob. Agents Chemother.* **47:**360–362.

45. Reference deleted.

46. Fennelly, K. P., J. W. Martyny, K. E. Fulton, I. M. Orme, D. M. Cave, and L. B. Heifets. 2004. Cough-generated aerosols of *Mycobacterium tuberculosis*: a new method to study infectiousness. *Am. J. Respir. Crit. Care Med.* **169:**604–609.

47. Ferry, T., B. Ponceau, M. Simon, B. Issartel, P. Petiot, A. Boibieux, F. Biron, C. Chidiac, and D. Peyramond. 2005. Possibly linezolid-induced peripheral and central neurotoxicity: report of four cases. *Infection* **33:**151–154.

48. Fortun, J., P. Martin-Davila, E. Navas, M. J. Perez-Elias, J. Cobo, M. Tato, E. G. De la Pedrosa, E. Gomez-Mampaso, and S. Moreno. 2005. Linezolid for the treatment of multidrug-resistant tuberculosis. *J. Antimicrob. Chemother.* **56:**180–185.

49. Frieden, T. R., L. F. Sherman, K. L. Maw, P. I. Fujiwara, J. T. Crawford, B. Nivin, V. Sharp, D. Hewlett, Jr., K. Brudney, D. Alland, and B. N. Kreisworth. 1996. A multi-institutional outbreak of highly drug-resistant tuberculosis: epidemiology and clinical outcomes. *JAMA* **276:**1229–1235.

50. Frieden, T. R., T. Sterling, A. Pablos-Mendez, J. O. Kilburn, G. M. Cauthen, and S. W. Dooley. 1993. The emergence of drug-resistant tuberculosis in New York City. *N. Engl. J. Med.* **328:**521–526.

51. Gandhi, N. R., A. Moll, A. W. Sturm, R. Pawinski, T. Govender, U. Lalloo, K. Zeller, J. Andrews, and G. Friedland. 2006. Extensively drug-resistant tuberculosis as a cause of death in patients co-infected with tuberculosis and HIV in a rural area of South Africa. *Lancet* **368:**1575–1580.

52. Garrabou, G., A. Soriano, S. Lopez, J. P. Guallar, M. Giralt, F. Villarroya, J. A. Martinez, J. Casademont, F. Cardellach, J. Mensa, and O. Miro. 2007. Reversible inhibition of mitochondrial protein synthesis during linezolid-related hyperlactatemia. *Antimicrob. Agents Chemother.* **51:**962–967.

53. Geerligs, W. A., R. Van Altena, W. C. M. De Lange, D. Van Soolingen, and T. S. Van Der Werf. 2000. Multidrug-resistant tuberculosis: long-term treatment outcome in the Netherlands. *Int. J. Tuberc. Lung Dis.* **4:**758–764.

54. Gillespie, S. H., and O. Billington. 1999. Activity of moxifloxacin against mycobacteria. *J. Antimicrob. Chemother.* **44:**393–395.

55. Gillespie, S. H., and N. Kennedy. 1998. Fluoroquinolones: a new treatment for tuberculosis? *Int. J. Tuberc. Lung Dis.* **2:**265–271.

56. Ginsburg, A. S., J. H. Grosset, and W. R. Bishai. 2003. Fluoroquinolones, tuberculosis, and resistance. *Lancet Infect. Dis.* **3:**432–442.

57. Girling, D. J. 1982. Adverse effects of antituberculosis drugs. *Drugs* **23:**56–74.

58. Goble, M., M. D. Iseman, L. A. Madsen, D. Waite, L. Ackerson, and C. R. Horsburgh, Jr. 1993. Treatment of 171 patients with pulmonary tuberculosis resistant to isoniazid and rifampin. *N. Engl. J. Med.* **328:**527–532.

59. Gonzalez-Montaner, L. J., S. Natal, P. Yongchaiyud, and P. Oliaro. 1994. Rifabutin for the treatment of newly-diagnosed pulmonary tuberculosis: a multinational, randomized, comparative study versus rifampicin. Rifabutin Study Group. *Tuberc. Lung Dis.* **75:**341–347.

60. Gosling, R. D., L. O. Uiso, N. E. Sam, E. Bongard, E. G. Kanduma, M. Nyindo, R. W. Morris, and S. H. Gillespie. 2003. The bactericidal activity of moxifloxacin in patients with pulmonary tuberculosis. *Am. J. Respir. Crit. Care Med.* **168:**1342–1345.

61. Grassi, C., and V. Peona. 1996. Use of rifabutin in the treatment of pulmonary tuberculosis. *Clin. Infect. Dis.* **22**(Suppl. 1):S50–S54.

62. Griffith, D. E. 2004. Treatment of multidrug-resistant tuberculosis: should you try this at home? *Am. J. Respir. Crit. Care Med.* **169:**1082–1083.

63. Griffith, D. E., B. A. Brown, and R. J. Wallace, Jr. 1996. Varying dosages of rifabutin affect white blood cell and platelet counts in human immunodeficiency virus-negative patients who are receiving multidrug regimens for pulmonary *Mycobacterium avium* complex disease. *Clin. Infect. Dis.* **23:**1321–1322.

64. Grosset, J. 1980. Bacteriologic basis of short-course chemotherapy for tuberculosis. *Clin. Chest Med.* **1:**231–241.

65. Gumbo, T., A. Louie, M. R. Deziel, L. M. Parsons, M. Salfinger, and G. L. Drusano. 2004. Selection of a moxifloxacin dose that suppresses drug resistance in *Mycobacterium tuberculosis*, by use of an in vitro pharmacodynamic infection model and mathematical modeling. *J. Infect. Dis.* **190:**1642–1651.

66. Havlir, D., F. Torriani, and M. Dube. 1994. Uveitis associated with rifabutin prophylaxis. *Ann. Intern. Med.* **121:**510–512.

67. Heldal, E., T. Arnadottir, J. R. Cruz, A. Tardencilla, and L. Chacon. 2001. Low failure rate in standardised retreatment of tuberculosis in Nicaragua: patient category, drug resistance and survival of 'chronic' patients. *Int. J. Tuberc. Lung Dis.* **5:**129–136.

68. Holland, S. M., E. M. Eisenstein, D. B. Kuhns, M. L. Turner, T. A. Fleisher, W. Strober, and J. I. Gallin. 1994. Treatment of refractory disseminated nontuberculous mycobacterial infection with interferon gamma. A preliminary report. *N. Engl. J. Med.* **330:**1348–1355.

69. Holtz, T. H., M. Sternberg, S. Kammerer, K. F. Laserson, V. Riekstina, E. Zarovska, V. Skripconoka, C. D. Wells, and V. Leimane. 2006. Time to sputum culture conversion in multidrug-resistant tuberculosis: predictors and relationship to treatment outcome. *Ann. Intern. Med.* **144:**650–659.

70. Hong Kong Chest Service/British Medical Research Council. 1992. A controlled study of rifabutin and an uncontrolled study of ofloxacin in the retreatment of patients with pulmonary tuberculosis resistant to isoniazid, streptomycin and rifampicin. *Tuberc. Lung Dis.* **73:**59–67.

71. Hopewell, P. C. 1999. Global tuberculosis control: an optimist's perspective. *Int. J. Tuberc. Lung Dis.* **3:**270–272.

72. Horn, D. L., D. Hewlett, Jr., C. Alfalla, S. Peterson, and S. M. Opal. 1994. Limited tolerance of ofloxacin and pyrazinamide prophylaxis against tuberculosis. *N. Engl. J. Med.* **330:**1241.

73. Hugonnet, J. E., L. W. Tremblay, H. I. Boshoff, C. E. Barry III, and J. S. Blanchard. 2009. Meropenem-clavulanate is effective

against extensively drug-resistant *Mycobacterium tuberculosis*. *Science* 323:1215–1218.

74. Iseman, M. D. 1999. Treatment and implications of multidrug-resistant tuberculosis for the 21st century. *Chemotherapy* 45(Suppl. 2):34–40.

75. Iseman, M. D. 1993. Treatment of multidrug-resistant tuberculosis. *N. Engl. J. Med.* 329:784–791.

76. Iseman, M. D., L. Madsen, M. Goble, and M. Pomerantz. 1990. Surgical intervention in the treatment of pulmonary disease caused by drug-resistant *Mycobacterium tuberculosis*. *Am. Rev. Respir. Dis.* 141:623–635.

77. Jassal, M., and W. R. Bishai. 2009. Extensively drug-resistant tuberculosis. *Lancet Infect. Dis.* 9:19–30.

78. Jensen, P. A., L. A. Lambert, M. F. Iademarco, and R. Ridzon. 2005. Guidelines for preventing the transmission of *Mycobacterium tuberculosis* in health-care settings, 2005. *MMWR Recommend. Rep.* 54:1–141.

79. Jeon, D. S., D. H. Kim, H. S. Kang, S. H. Hwang, J. H. Min, J. H. Kim, N. M. Sung, M. W. Carroll, and S. K. Park. 2009. Survival and predictors of outcomes in non-HIV-infected patients with extensively drug-resistant tuberculosis. *Int. J. Tuberc. Lung Dis.* 13:594–600.

80. Kliiman, K., and A. Altraja. 2009. Predictors of poor treatment outcome in multi- and extensively drug-resistant pulmonary TB. *Eur. Respir. J.* 33:1085–1094.

81. Koh, W.-J., and T. S. Shim. 2009. Daily 300 mg dose of linezolid for the treatment of intractable multidrug-resistant and extensively drug-resistant tuberculosis—authors' response. *J. Antimicrob. Chemother.* 64:1119–1120.

82. Kohno, S., H. Koga, M. Kaku, S. Maesaki, and K. Hara. 1992. Prospective comparative study of ofloxacin or ethambutol for the treatment of pulmonary tuberculosis. *Chest* 102:1815–1818.

83. Kopanoff, D. E., D. E. Snider, Jr., and M. Johnson. 1988. Recurrent tuberculosis: why do patients develop disease again? A United States Public Health Service cooperative survey. *Am. J. Public Health* 78:30–33.

84. Kruuner, A., P. Jureen, K. Levina, S. Ghebremichael, and S. Hoffner. 2003. Discordant resistance to kanamycin and amikacin in drug-resistant *Mycobacterium tuberculosis*. *Antimicrob. Agents Chemother.* 47:2971–2973.

85. Kunin, C. M. 1996. Antimicrobial activity of rifabutin. *Clin. Infect. Dis.* 22(Suppl. 1):S3–S13; discussion, S13–S14.

86. Law, K. F., and M. Weiden. 1996. *Streptomycin, Other Aminoglycosides, and Capreomycin in Tuberculosis.* Little, Brown and Company, New York, NY.

87. Lee, C. N., T. P. Lin, M. F. Chang, M. V. Jimenez, L. Dolfi, and P. Olliaro. 1996. Rifabutin as salvage therapy for cases of chronic multidrug-resistant pulmonary tuberculosis in Taiwan. *J. Chemother.* 8:137–143.

88. Leimane, V., V. Riekstina, T. H. Holtz, E. Zarovska, V. Skripconoka, L. E. Thorpe, K. F. Laserson, and C. D. Wells. 2005. Clinical outcome of individualised treatment of multidrug-resistant tuberculosis in Latvia: a retrospective cohort study. *Lancet* 365:318–326.

89. Levey, A. S., J. P. Bosch, J. B. Lewis, T. Greene, N. Rogers, and D. Roth for the Modification of Diet in Renal Disease Study Group. 1999. A more accurate method to estimate glomerular filtration rate from serum creatinine: a new prediction equation. *Ann. Intern. Med.* 130:461–470.

90. Lewis, J. R., J. G. Gums, and D. L. Dickensheets. 1999. Levofloxacin-induced bilateral Achilles tendonitis. *Ann. Pharmacother.* 33:792–795.

91. Leysen, D. C., A. Haemers, and S. R. Pattyn. 1989. Mycobacteria and the new quinolones. *Antimicrob. Agents Chemother.* 33:1–5.

92. Lipsky, B. A., and C. A. Baker. 1999. Fluoroquinolone toxicity profiles: a review focusing on newer agents. *Clin. Infect. Dis.* 28:352–364.

93. Lode, H., K. Borner, and P. Koeppe. 1998. Pharmacodynamics of fluoroquinolones. *Clin. Infect. Dis.* 27:33–39.

94. Long, R., H. Chong, V. Hoeppner, H. Shanmuganathan, K. Kowalewska-Grochowska, C. Shandro, J. Manfreda, A. Senthilselvan, A. Elzainy, and T. Marrie. 2009. Empirical treatment of community-acquired pneumonia and the development of fluoroquinolone-resistant tuberculosis. *Clin. Infect. Dis.* 48:1354–1360.

95. Mahmoudi, A., and M. D. Iseman. 1993. Pitfalls in the care of patients with tuberculosis. Common errors and their association with the acquisition of drug resistance. *JAMA* 270(1):65–68.

96. Mangunnegoro, H., and A. Hudoyo. 1999. Efficacy of low-dose ofloxacin in the treatment of multidrug-resistant tuberculosis in Indonesia. *Chemotherapy* 45(Suppl. 2):19–25.

97. Maranetra, K. N. 1999. Quinolones and multidrug-resistant tuberculosis. *Chemotherapy* 45(Suppl. 2):12–18.

98. McGregor, M. M., P. Olliaro, L. Wolmarans, B. Mabuza, M. Bredell, M. K. Felten, and P. B. Fourie. 1996. Efficacy and safety of rifabutin in the treatment of patients with newly diagnosed pulmonary tuberculosis. *Am. J. Respir. Crit. Care Med.* 154:1462–1467.

99. McKee, E. E., M. Ferguson, A. T. Bentley, and T. A. Marks. 2006. Inhibition of mammalian mitochondrial protein synthesis by oxazolidinones. *Antimicrob. Agents Chemother.* 50:2042–2049.

100. Mdluli, K., and Z. Ma. 2007. *Mycobacterium tuberculosis* DNA gyrase as a target for drug discovery. *Infect. Disord. Drug Targets* 7:159–168.

101. Migliori, G. B., B. Eker, M. D. Richardson, G. Sotgiu, J. P. Zellweger, A. Skrahina, J. Ortmann, E. Girardi, H. Hoffmann, G. Besozzi, N. Bevilacqua, D. Kirsten, R. Centis, and C. Lange. 2009. A retrospective TBNET assessment of linezolid safety, tolerability and efficacy in multidrug-resistant tuberculosis. *Eur. Respir. J.* 34:387–393.

102. Minion, J., and M. Pai. 2010. Expanding the role of the microscopic observation drug susceptibility assay in tuberculosis and HIV management. *Clin. Infect. Dis.* 50:997–999.

103. Mitchison, D. A., and J. B. Selkon. 1956. The bactericidal activities of antituberculous drugs. *Am. Rev. Tuberc.* 74:109–116; discussion, 116–123.

104. Mitnick, C., J. Bayona, E. Palacios, S. Shin, J. Furin, F. Alcantara, E. Sanchez, M. Sarria, M. Becerra, M. C. Fawzi, S. Kapiga, D. Neuberg, J. H. Maguire, J. Y. Kim, and P. Farmer. 2003. Community-based therapy for multidrug-resistant tuberculosis in Lima, Peru. *N. Engl. J. Med.* 348:119–128.

105. Mitnick, C. D., S. S. Shin, K. J. Seung, M. L. Rich, S. S. Atwood, J. J. Furin, G. M. Fitzmaurice, F. A. Alcantara Viru, S. C. Appleton, J. N. Bayona, C. A. Bonilla, K. Chalco, S. Choi, M. F. Franke, H. S. Fraser, D. Guerra, R. M. Hurtado, D. Jazayeri, K. Joseph, K. Llaro, L. Mestanza, J. S. Mukherjee, M. Munoz, E. Palacios, E. Sanchez, A. Sloutsky, and M. C. Becerra. 2008. Comprehensive treatment of extensively drug-resistant tuberculosis. *N. Engl. J. Med.* 359:563–574.

106. Morris, J. T., and J. W. Kelly. 1993. Rifabutin-induced ageusia. *Ann. Intern. Med.* 119:171–172.

107. Moulding, T. S. 1981. Should isoniazid be used in retreatment of tuberculosis despite acquired isoniazid resistance? *Am. Rev. Respir. Dis.* 123:262–264.

108. Narita, M., P. Alonso, M. Lauzardo, E. S. Hollender, A. E. Pitchenik, and D. Ashkin. 2001. Treatment experience of multidrug-resistant tuberculosis in Florida, 1994–1997. *Chest* 120:343–348.

109. Narita, M., B. T. Tsuji, and V. L. Yu. 2007. Linezolid-associated peripheral and optic neuropathy, lactic acidosis, and serotonin syndrome. *Pharmacotherapy* 27:1189–1197.

110. O'Brien, R. J., M. A. Lyle, and D. E. Snider, Jr. 1987. Rifabutin (ansamycin LM 427): a new rifamycin-S derivative for the treatment of mycobacterial diseases. *Rev. Infect. Dis.* 9: 519–530.

111. Palmero, D. J., M. Ambroggi, A. Brea, M. De Lucas, A. Fulgenzi, D. Martinez, C. Mosca, R. Musella, M. Natiello, C. Gonzalez, and E. Abbate. 2004. Treatment and follow-up of HIV-negative multidrug-resistant tuberculosis patients in an infectious diseases reference hospital, Buenos Aires, Argentina. *Int. J. Tuberc. Lung Dis.* 8:778–784.

112. Papastavros, T., L. R. Dolovich, A. Holbrook, L. Whitehead, and M. Loeb. 2002. Adverse events associated with pyrazinamide and levofloxacin in the treatment of latent multidrug-resistant tuberculosis. *CMAJ* 167:131–136.

113. Park, I. N., S. B. Hong, Y. M. Oh, M. N. Kim, C. M. Lim, S. D. Lee, Y. Koh, W. S. Kim, D. S. Kim, W. D. Kim, and T. S. Shim. 2006. Efficacy and tolerability of daily-half dose linezolid in patients with intractable multidrug-resistant tuberculosis. *J. Antimicrob. Chemother.* 58:701–704.

114. Park, M. M., A. L. Davis, N. W. Schluger, H. Cohen, and W. N. Rom. 1996. Outcome of MDR-TB patients, 1983–1993. Prolonged survival with appropriate therapy. *Am. J. Respir. Crit. Care Med.* 153:317–324.

115. Park, S. K., S. Cho, I. H. Lee, D. S. Jeon, S. H. Hong, R. A. Smego, Jr., and S. N. Cho. 2007. Subcutaneously administered interferon-gamma for the treatment of multidrug-resistant pulmonary tuberculosis. *Int. J. Infect. Dis.* 11:434–440.

116. Park, S. K., C. T. Kim, and S. D. Song. 1998. Outcome of chemotherapy in 107 patients with pulmonary tuberculosis resistant to isoniazid and rifampin. *Int. J. Tuberc. Lung Dis.* 2:877–884.

117. Parola, P., and P. Brouqui. 2001. Clinical and microbiological efficacy of adjunctive salvage therapy with inhaled aminoglycosides in a patient with refractory cavitary pulmonary tuberculosis. *Clin. Infect. Dis.* 33:1439.

118. Peloquin, C. A., D. J. Hadad, L. P. Molino, M. Palaci, W. H. Boom, R. Dietze, and J. L. Johnson. 2008. Population pharmacokinetics of levofloxacin, gatifloxacin, and moxifloxacin in adults with pulmonary tuberculosis. *Antimicrob. Agents Chemother.* 52:852–857.

119. Petty, T. L., and R. S. Mitchell. 1962. Successful treatment of advanced isoniazid- and streptomycin-resistant pulmonary tuberculosis with ethionamide, pyrazinamide, and isoniazid. *Am. Rev. Respir. Dis.* 86:503–512.

120. Pletz, M. W., A. De Roux, A. Roth, K. H. Neumann, H. Mauch, and H. Lode. 2004. Early bactericidal activity of moxifloxacin in treatment of pulmonary tuberculosis: a prospective, randomized study. *Antimicrob. Agents Chemother.* 48:780–782.

121. Ramasamy, R., A. Reginald, and E. Ganesan. 2000. The use of high-dose isomazid in intermittent regime TB treatment—some preliminary findings. *Trop. Doct.* 30:56.

122. Ramaswamy, S., and J. M. Musser. 1998. Molecular genetic basis of antimicrobial agent resistance in *Mycobacterium tuberculosis*: 1998 update. *Tuberc. Lung Dis.* 79:3–29.

123. Rastogi, N., K. S. Goh, A. Bryskier, and A. Devallois. 1996. In vitro activities of levofloxacin used alone and in combination with first- and second-line antituberculous drugs against *Mycobacterium tuberculosis*. *Antimicrob. Agents Chemother.* 40:1610–1616.

124. Raviglione, M. C., and I. M. Smith. 2007. XDR tuberculosis—implications for global public health. *N. Engl. J. Med.* 356:656–659.

125. Razonable, R. R., D. R. Osmon, and J. M. Steckelberg. 2004. Linezolid therapy for orthopedic infections. *Mayo Clin. Proc.* 79:1137–1144.

126. Reddy, K. P., M. F. Brady, R. H. Gilman, J. Coronel, M. Navincopa, E. Ticona, G. Chavez, E. Sanchez, C. Rojas, L. Solari, J. Valencia, Y. Pinedo, C. Benites, J. S. Friedland, and D. A. Moore. 2010. Microscopic observation drug susceptibility assay for tuberculosis screening before isoniazid preventive therapy in HIV-infected persons. *Clin. Infect. Dis.* 50: 988–996.

127. Reichman, L. B., and A. Fanning. 2001. Drug development for tuberculosis: the missing ingredient. *Lancet* 357:236.

128. Ridzon, R., J. Meador, R. Maxwell, K. Higgins, P. Weismuller, and I. M. Onorato. 1997. Asymptomatic hepatitis in persons who received alternative preventive therapy with pyrazinamide and ofloxacin. *Clin. Infect. Dis.* 24:1264–1265.

129. Rodriguez, J. C., M. Ruiz, A. Climent, and G. Royo. 2001. In vitro activity of four fluoroquinolones against *Mycobacterium tuberculosis*. *Int. J. Antimicrob. Agents* 17:229–231.

130. Rusen, I. D., A. D. Harries, E. Heldal, and C. Mace. 2010. Drug supply shortages in 2010: the inexcusable failure of global tuberculosis control. *Int. J. Tuberc. Lung Dis.* 14: 253–254.

131. Rustomjee, R., C. Lienhardt, T. Kanyok, G. R. Davies, J. Levin, T. Mthiyane, C. Reddy, A. W. Sturm, F. A. Sirgel, J. Allen, D. J. Coleman, B. Fourie, and D. A. Mitchison. 2008. A phase II study of the sterilising activities of ofloxacin, gatifloxacin and moxifloxacin in pulmonary tuberculosis. *Int. J. Tuberc. Lung Dis.* 12:128–138.

132. Sacks, L. V., S. Pendle, D. Orlovic, M. Andre, M. Popara, G. Moore, L. Thonell, and S. Hurwitz. 2001. Adjunctive salvage therapy with inhaled aminoglycosides for patients with persistent smear-positive pulmonary tuberculosis. *Clin. Infect. Dis.* 32:44–49.

133. Salomon, N., and D. C. Perlman. 1999. Editorial response: multidrug-resistant tuberculosis—globally with us for the long haul. *Clin. Infect. Dis.* 29:93–95.

134. Sanders, W. E., Jr., C. Hartwig, N. Schneider, R. Cacciatore, and H. Valdez. 1982. Activity of amikacin against mycobacteria in vitro and in murine tuberculosis. *Tubercle* 63: 201–208.

135. Saribas, Z., T. Kocagoz, A. Alp, and A. Gunalp. 2003. Rapid detection of rifampin resistance in *Mycobacterium tuberculosis* isolates by heteroduplex analysis and determination of rifamycin cross-resistance in rifampin-resistant isolates. *J. Clin. Microbiol.* 41:816–818.

136. Schecter, G. F., C. Scott, L. True, A. Raftery, J. Flood, and S. Mase. 2010. Linezolid in the treatment of multidrug-resistant tuberculosis. *Clin. Infect. Dis.* 50:49–55.

137. Seaworth, B. J. 2004. *Drug-Resistant Tuberculosis: a Survival Guide for Clinicians.* Francis J. Curry National Tuberculosis Center and California Department of Health Services, San Francisco, CA.

138. Sepkowitz, K. A. 2001. Tuberculosis control in the 21st century. *Emerg. Infect. Dis.* 7:259–262.

139. Seung, K. J., K. Joseph, R. Hurtado, M. Rich, S. Shin, J. Furin, F. Leandre, J. Mukherjee, and P. Farmer. 2004. Number of drugs to treat multidrug-resistant tuberculosis. *Am. J. Respir. Crit. Care Med.* 169:1336–1337. (Author's reply, 169:1337.)

140. Seung, K. J., D. B. Omatayo, S. Keshavjee, J. J. Furin, P. E. Farmer, and H. Satti. 2009. Early outcomes of MDR-TB treatment in a high HIV-prevalence setting in Southern Africa. *PLoS One* 4:e7186.

141. Shandil, R. K., R. Jayaram, P. Kaur, S. Gaonkar, B. L. Suresh, B. N. Mahesh, R. Jayashree, V. Nandi, S. Bharath, and V. Balasubramanian. 2007. Moxifloxacin, ofloxacin, sparfloxacin,

and ciprofloxacin against *Mycobacterium tuberculosis*: evaluation of in vitro and pharmacodynamic indices that best predict in vivo efficacy. *Antimicrob. Agents Chemother.* **51:** 576–582.

142. Sharma, S. K., R. Guleria, D. Jain, T. C. Chawla, P. Saha, A. Mohan, and N. K. Jain. 1996. Effect of additional oral ofloxacin administration in the treatment of multidrug-resistant tuberculosis. *Indian J. Chest Dis. Allied Sci.* **38:**73–79.

143. Shin, S., J. Furin, F. Alcantara, A. Hyson, K. Joseph, E. Sanchez, and M. Rich. 2004. Hypokalemia among patients receiving treatment for multidrug-resistant tuberculosis. *Chest* **125:**974–980.

144. Shin, S., D. Guerra, M. Rich, K. J. Seung, J. Mukherjee, K. Joseph, R. Hurtado, F. Alcantara, J. Bayona, C. Bonilla, P. Farmer, and J. Furin. 2003. Treatment of multidrug-resistant tuberculosis during pregnancy: a report of 7 cases. *Clin. Infect. Dis.* **36:**996–1003.

145. Snider, D. E., Jr., G. D. Kelly, G. M. Cauthen, N. J. Thompson, and J. O. Kilburn. 1985. Infection and disease among contacts of tuberculosis cases with drug-resistant and drug-susceptible bacilli. *Am. Rev. Respir. Dis.* **132:**125–132.

146. Soumakis, S. A., D. Berg, and H. W. Harris. 1998. Hypothyroidism in a patient receiving treatment for multidrug-resistant tuberculosis. *Clin. Infect. Dis.* **27:**910–911.

147. Spigelman, M. K. 2007. New tuberculosis therapeutics: a growing pipeline. *J. Infect. Dis.* **196**(Suppl. 1):S28–S34.

148. Stein, G. 2000. The methoxyfluoroquinolones: gatifloxacin and moxifloxacin. *Infect. Med.* **17:**564–570.

149. Sullivan, E. A., B. N. Kreiswirth, L. Palumbo, V. Kapur, J. M. Musser, A. Ebrahimzadeh, and T. R. Frieden. 1995. Emergence of fluoroquinolone-resistant tuberculosis in New York City. *Lancet* **345:**1148–1150.

150. Tahaoglu, K., T. Torun, T. Sevim, G. Atac, A. Kir, L. Karasulu, I. Ozmen, and N. Kapakli. 2001. The treatment of multidrug-resistant tuberculosis in Turkey. *N. Engl. J. Med.* **345:**170–174.

151. Tam, C. M., W. W. Yew, and K. Y. Yuen. 2009. Treatment of multidrug-resistant and extensively drug-resistant tuberculosis: current status and future prospects. *Expert Rev. Clin. Pharmacol.* **2:**405–421.

152. Taylor, J. J., J. W. Wilson, and L. L. Estes. 2006. Linezolid and serotonergic drug interactions: a retrospective survey. *Clin. Infect. Dis.* **43:**180–187.

153. Tiruviluamala, P., and L. B. Reichman. 2002. Tuberculosis. *Annu. Rev. Public Health* **23:**403–426.

154. Tomioka, H. 2000. Prospects for development of new antimycobacterial drugs. *J. Infect. Chemother.* **6:**8–20.

155. Tomioka, H., K. Sato, T. Akaki, H. Kajitani, S. Kawahara, and M. Sakatani. 1999. Comparative in vitro antimicrobial activities of the newly synthesized quinolone HSR-903, sitafloxacin (DU-6859a), gatifloxacin (AM-1155), and levofloxacin against *Mycobacterium tuberculosis* and *Mycobacterium avium* complex. *Antimicrob. Agents Chemother.* **43:**3001–3004.

156. Traeger, S. M., M. F. Bonfiglio, J. A. Wilson, B. R. Martin, and N. A. Nackes. 1995. Seizures associated with ofloxacin therapy. *Clin. Infect. Dis.* **21:**1504–1506.

157. Treasure, R. L., and B. J. Seaworth. 1995. Current role of surgery in *Mycobacterium tuberculosis*. *Ann. Thorac. Surg.* **59:**1405–1407; discussion, 1408–1409.

158. van den Boogaard, J., G. S. Kibiki, E. R. Kisanga, M. J. Boeree, and R. E. Aarnoutse. 2009. New drugs against tuberculosis: problems, progress, and evaluation of agents in clinical development. *Antimicrob. Agents Chemother.* **53:**849–862.

159. van Leuven, M., M. De Groot, K. P. Shean, U. O. von Oppell, and P. A. Willcox. 1997. Pulmonary resection as an adjunct

in the treatment of multiple drug-resistant tuberculosis. *Ann. Thorac. Surg.* **63:**1368–1372; discussion, 1372–1373.

160. Vega, P., A. Sweetland, J. Acha, H. Castillo, D. Guerra, M. C. Smith Fawzi, and S. Shin. 2004. Psychiatric issues in the management of patients with multidrug-resistant tuberculosis. *Int. J. Tuberc. Lung Dis.* **8:**749–759.

161. von der Lippe, B., P. Sandven, and O. Brubakk. 2006. Efficacy and safety of linezolid in multidrug resistant tuberculosis (MDR-TB)—a report of ten cases. *J. Infect.* **52:**92–96.

162. Von Groll, A., A. Martin, P. Jureen, S. Hoffner, P. Vandamme, F. Portaels, J. C. Palomino, and P. A. da Silva. 2009. Fluoroquinolone resistance in *Mycobacterium tuberculosis* and mutations in *gyrA* and *gyrB*. *Antimicrob. Agents Chemother.* **53:**4498–4500.

163. Wallis, R. S., M. Palaci, S. Vinhas, A. G. Hise, F. C. Ribeiro, K. Landen, S. H. Cheon, H. Y. Song, M. Phillips, R. Dietze, and J. J. Ellner. 2001. A whole blood bactericidal assay for tuberculosis. *J. Infect. Dis.* **183:**1300–1303.

164. Wenger, P. N., J. Otten, A. Breeden, D. Orfas, C. M. Beck-Sague, and W. R. Jarvis. 1995. Control of nosocomial transmission of multidrug-resistant *Mycobacterium tuberculosis* among healthcare workers and HIV-infected patients. *Lancet* **345:**235–240.

165. **World Health Organization.** 2009, posting date. *Global Tuberculosis Control: Epidemiology, Planning, Financing.* World Health Organization, Geneva, Switzerland.

166. **World Health Organization.** 2008. *Guidelines for the Programmatic Management of Drug-Resistant Tuberculosis. Emergency Update 2008.* World Health Organization, Geneva, Switzerland.

167. **World Health Organization.** 2008, posting date. *Policy Statement: Molecular Line Probe Assays for Rapid Screening of Patients at Risk of Multi-Drug Resistant Tuberculosis (MDR-TB).* World Health Organization, Geneva, Switzerland.

168. **World Health Organization.** 2009. *The STOP TB Department Newsletter*, November 2009. World Health Organization, Geneva, Switzerland.

169. Reference deleted.

170. **World Health Organization and International Union Against Tuberculosis and Lung Disease.** 2008, posting date. *Anti-Tuberculosis Drug Resistance in the World. Fourth Global Report.* World Health Organization, Geneva, Switzerland.

171. Yew, W. W., C. K. Chan, C. C. Leung, C. H. Chau, C. M. Tam, P. C. Wong, and J. Lee. 2003. Comparative roles of levofloxacin and ofloxacin in the treatment of multidrug-resistant tuberculosis: preliminary results of a retrospective study from Hong Kong. *Chest* **124:**1476–1481.

172. Yew, W. W., K. C. Chang, and C. H. Chau. 2009. What is the optimal dosage of linezolid in treatment of complicated multidrug-resistant tuberculosis? *Eur. Respir. J.* **34:** 1492–1494.

173. Yew, W. W., S. Y. Kwan, W. K. Ma, M. A. Khin, and P. Y. Chau. 1990. In-vitro activity of ofloxacin against *Mycobacterium tuberculosis* and its clinical efficacy in multiply resistant pulmonary tuberculosis. *J. Antimicrob. Chemother.* **26:** 227–236.

174. Younossian, A. B., T. Rochat, J. P. Ketterer, J. Wacker, and J. P. Janssens. 2005. High hepatotoxicity of pyrazinamide and ethambutol for treatment of latent tuberculosis. *Eur. Respir. J.* **26:**462–464.

175. Zhu, M., R. Namdar, J. J. Stambaugh, J. R. Starke, A. E. Bulpitt, S. E. Berning, and C. A. Peloquin. 2002. Population pharmacokinetics of ethionamide in patients with tuberculosis. *Tuberculosis* (Edinburgh) **82:**91–96.

Tuberculosis and Nontuberculous Mycobacterial Infections, 6th ed.
Edited by David Schlossberg
© 2011 ASM Press, Washington, DC

Chapter 9

Role of Surgery in the Diagnosis and Management of Tuberculosis

ALAN D. L. SIHOE AND WING WAI YEW

TB AND THE THORACIC SURGEON

The history of thoracic surgery as a specialty is inseparable from that of the development of tuberculosis (TB) management. Many surgeons would suggest that the very first surgical procedure in the chest was probably performed in the time of the ancient Greeks. Hippocrates himself described a technique of open pleural drainage for empyema thoracis resulting from TB (17). Modern thoracic surgery as clinicians would recognize it today was born soon after the identification of *Mycobacterium tuberculosis* by Koch in the 1880s. When it was realized that the microbe responsible for "consumption" was an obligate aerobe, a variety of collapse therapies were developed in the late 19th and early 20th centuries to kill the organism through oxygen deprivation. These included thoracoplasty, induced pneumothorax, ball plombage, pneumoperitoneum, and phrenic nerve crushing (61). Crucially, most of the basic skills and approaches still used in modern thoracic surgery today were also honed at this time, including the ubiquitous thoracotomy incision. Even minimally invasive thoracic surgery traces its roots to this period, when Jacobaeus introduced the technique of thoracoscopy for pleural biopsy and adhesiolysis in TB patients (28).

By the middle of the 20th century, TB management had become the indication for the majority of thoracic surgical operations. However, the subsequent advent of highly effective antimicrobial drug therapy for TB was a major triumph in modern medicine, and medical therapy rapidly superseded surgery as the mainstay of primary treatment for TB. So comprehensive was this paradigm shift in TB management that the very existence of thoracic surgery as a specialty came under threat. It was only the need to treat surging numbers of lung cancer patients in the latter half of the century that "rescued" thoracic surgery from precipitous decline. Today, general thoracic surgery has expanded tremendously to cover a vast range of diagnostic and therapeutic indications. However, it is fitting that TB has never fully left the long list of diseases managed by the thoracic surgeon.

It can even be said that in recent years, there has been a resurgence of interest in thoracic surgery for TB management. This is mainly the result of three trends. First, far from being eradicated by modern drug therapy, there has actually been an overall increase in the global incidence of TB. This may be due in part to the human immunodeficiency virus epidemic, the increasing survival rate of immunosuppressed patients, and the increased mobility of peoples among regions where TB is endemic. In 2007, it was estimated that the annual worldwide incidence of TB was 9.3 million new cases and that TB accounted for about 1.8 million deaths per year (86). It is suggested that up to a third of the world's population may be infected with *M. tuberculosis*. Although most cases still occur in less developed countries, there has been a noted trend towards an increasing incidence of disease even in the Western world. Second, advances in medical management have achieved remarkable reduction in rates of mortality due to TB which far outstrips the reduction in incidence of new cases. This means that potentially a greater proportion of patients with TB will survive their acute disease and progress to develop chronic sequelae, many of which are only amenable to effective treatment or palliation through thoracic surgery. Third, the world has witnessed the emergence of multidrug-resistant TB (MDR-TB) since the mid-1980s (83). Whereas the underlying bacillary strains may be increasingly resistant to pharmacological therapy, there is emerging evidence that surgery may be effective as an adjunct in curing the disease they cause.

Modern thoracic surgery has risen to the challenge and can now offer effective management of TB with less pain and morbidity than ever before. Significantly, the reduction of surgical trauma through

Alan D. L. Sihoe • Department of Cardiothoracic Surgery, The University of Hong Kong, Queen Mary Hospital, Hong Kong, China.
Wing Wai Yew • Tuberculosis & Chest Unit, Grantham Hospital, Hong Kong, China.

the use of newer minimally invasive thoracic surgical approaches also potentially lowers thresholds for surgical candidacy, allowing more TB patients to receive operative treatment. This chapter aims to provide an overview of the role that modern thoracic surgery can play in diagnosing and managing patients with TB and its sequelae.

THORACIC SURGERY IN TB PATIENTS: BASIC CONSIDERATIONS

When operating on patients with TB, the same fundamental principles and considerations of any thoracic surgical operation still apply. It is worth considering some of these common concepts before proceeding with the detailed discussion of surgery for specific aspects of TB management.

Anesthetic Considerations

The first consideration in any thoracic surgical operation is whether a patient is fit for general anesthesia. Specifically, one must assess whether the patient can tolerate the one-lung ventilation. For most thoracic surgery operations, it is a prerequisite that the lung on the operation site is deflated during surgery to allow for complete exploration of the pleural cavity (71, 94). Fitness for this is most commonly assessed by spirometry and by exclusion of carbon dioxide (CO_2) retention. As a rule of thumb, for major lung resections the requirement is a predicted postoperative forced expiratory volume in 1 min of 40% of the value predicted based on the patient's age, sex, height, and weight. There must also be no CO_2 retention preoperatively. In many patients with TB, there may be considerable heterogeneity in the distribution of disease in the lung parenchyma. If this is the case in a patient with borderline lung function, it is worthwhile considering the proportional contribution to the overall respiration by the part of the lung planned for resection. For example, if a ventilation-perfusion scan shows that the targeted part of the lung is already largely nonfunctional, a surgeon may deem the patient still operable despite marginal spirometry results. A thoracic anesthesiologist's assessment prior to offering surgery is obligatory for all patients.

For less extensive surgery, such as lung biopsy or wedge resections, the requirements may not be as stringent. In selected patients who may not tolerate prolonged one-lung ventilation (and where the anticipated surgery is simple), it may be possible for the surgeon to perform the operation quickly during brief periods of intermittent apnea after general anesthesia is induced. This may be possible, for example, with small wedge excisions or pleural biopsies where no pleural adhesions are anticipated. Limited biopsies via mini-incisions performed under local anesthesia may also be an option for selected patients who cannot tolerate general anesthesia.

Open Thoracotomy

The traditional approach for any thoracic surgery is via a thoracotomy. The patient is placed in a full lateral position with the operation side upwards. The operating table is then "flexed" to widen the rib spaces on the operation side. A traditional full posterolateral thoracotomy begins at the anterior axillary or midaxillary line and extends along the fourth or fifth intercostal space to just below the tip of the scapula. The latissimus dorsi and sometimes the serratus anterior muscles are divided. The ribs are spread apart using surgical retractors, and some surgeons opt to resect or cut a rib to allow better access. The thoracotomy offers excellent exposure of the entire ipsilateral thorax, allowing both direct vision into the chest and bimanual exploration.

However, because of the forceful rib retraction for up to several hours during a major thoracic operation, the thoracotomy is also one of the most painful of all surgical incisions (62). Persistent postthoracotomy pain at 2 months or more after surgery has been estimated to occur in approximately 50 to 70% of patients (23, 62). In 5% of these patients, it has been described as severe and disabling. Over 40% of patients may still have persistent pain a year after surgery. Because of the recognized morbidity that may occur, it is always important for the surgeon to consider whether the impact on a patient's quality of life may outweigh the benefits before offering surgery via open thoracotomy.

For less complicated surgery, such as simple lung biopsy or where there are few pleural adhesions, it is often possible to use a limited thoracotomy—such as an anterior thoracotomy or muscle-sparing lateral thoracotomy. The wound is smaller, and some reports suggest reduced pain compared to traditional posterolateral thoracotomy. However, rib retraction is still used, which may result in some degree of morbidity.

Video-Assisted Thoracic Surgery

Partly as a result of the potential morbidity of open thoracotomy, there has been an inexorable trend worldwide towards using a video-assisted thoracic surgery (VATS) approach for many thoracic operations (94). This is minimally invasive or "keyhole" surgery in the chest. By using a video thoracoscope to visualize inside the thorax, VATS completely forgoes the hurtful rib spreading of open thoracotomy and thereby minimizes surgical access trauma. The established advantages of VATS over open thoracotomy include reduced pain and morbidity, faster recovery, shorter hospital stays, and less postoperative compromise of the patient's respiratory and immune function (32, 40, 42, 43, 58, 59). Importantly, the use of the video thoracoscope provides a 360° complete exploration of the ipsilateral pleural cavity that is potentially superior to that via a limited thoracotomy.

The standard VATS procedure uses three surgical ports of 5 to 15 mm in diameter, through which a video thoracoscope and two surgical instruments can be placed. The patient is placed in a lateral decubitus position with the side of the lesion upwards, and the ports are sited on the lateral chest. Many strategies of port placement have been described previously (71, 94). Generally, for a wedge resection of a lung lesion or a pleural/mediastinal biopsy, a three-port strategy is used with the ports placed according to a baseball diamond pattern (Fig. 1). The surgeon and the assistant holding the video thoracoscope stand on the side of the operating table facing the lesion, and the camera port is placed first at the "home base" position closest to themselves. With the target lesion

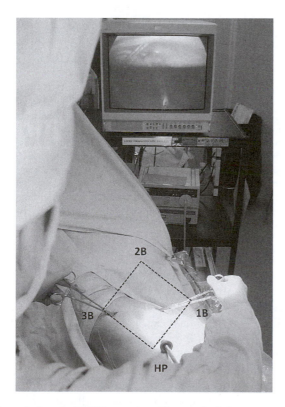

Figure 1. A typical VATS procedure. The standard three-port strategy is used with the ports arranged in a baseball diamond pattern: camera port at the home plate (HP), target lesion at second base (2B), and right and left instrument ports at first (1B) and third (3B) bases, respectively.

visualized to be at the second base of the diamond, the two instrument ports are placed at the first base and third base positions. This allows effective triangulation of the instruments onto the target with minimal "fencing" of the instruments. The important principle is that port sites need not be placed dogmatically according to any specific locations. Instead, the ports should be sited to suit each particular patient, target lesion, and nature of operation.

Ring forceps such as the Rampley sponge-holding forceps are ideal for lung manipulation during VATS, allowing gentle handling of the lung tissue and easy insertion via the ports because of the rounded shape. When locating a target lesion for resection or biopsy, the surgeon relies on both visual inspection and digital palpation. Many lesions in the lung parenchyma show no distinguishing features on the lung surface and must be palpated. If there have been significant pleural adhesions that required releasing—as is common in many TB patients—the lung surface may be particularly scarred afterwards, making visual inspection alone even less reliable. The need for careful digital palpation therefore cannot be overemphasized. Even via the small VATS ports, using a combination of instrument manipulation of the lung and finger exploration, an experienced VATS surgeon can accomplish a digital palpation of the entire lung as thoroughly as via an open thoracotomy in most cases. For deeper lesions that may be more difficult to palpate, one instrument port can be extended to allow insertion of two fingers for a bidigital palpation whereby the lesion can usually be found by rolling between the two fingers.

More recently, "needlescopic" VATS using two or three ports and instruments only 2 to 3 mm wide has also been described (68, 95). Because of the reduction of both wound size and instrument leverage in the intercostal spaces, this approach offers potentially even less pain and morbidity than "conventional" VATS. Needlescopic VATS is a viable option for lung and pleural biopsies and even lung wedge resections (Fig. 2). The reduced surgical access trauma and better cosmesis may lower thresholds for patients to receive surgery.

Few absolute contraindications now exist for the VATS approach. In the past, postinflammatory pleural adhesions between the chest wall and lung—common in TB patients—were considered an indication to convert from a VATS to an open approach. However, for experienced VATS surgeons division of pleural adhesions and even extrapleural dissection are technically feasible. Such cases have therefore become a relative rather than an absolute contraindication for VATS. In experienced hands, conversion to an open procedure is now an infrequent event. It

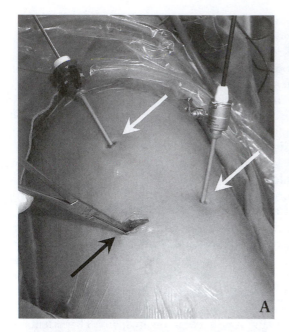

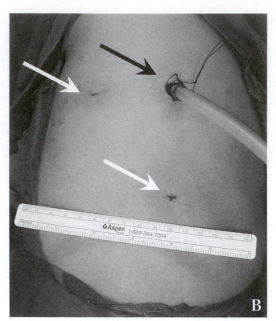

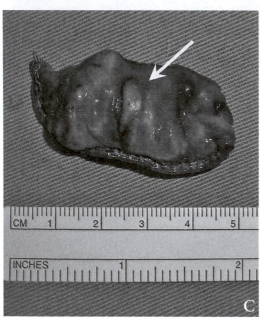

Figure 2. Needlescopic VATS is performed using 3-mm instruments that are little wider than a cocktail stick (A). Here, a lung wedge excision biopsy is performed using two 3-mm ports (white arrows) and one 10-mm port required for delivery of the resected specimen (black arrow). The cosmetic result is satisfactory; the 3-mm ports will be barely visible after healing (B). The excised wedge from this patient is sizeable despite the small wounds, and on cutting open the tissue the discrete target nodular lesion (arrow) is seen resected (C).

was also previously suggested that VATS was mainly suitable for lesions in the peripheral third of the lung. However, experienced VATS surgeons can easily and quickly mobilize the entire lung (such as by releasing adhesions and/or the pulmonary ligament) to allow full access to all parts of the lung, including even medial aspects of all lobes.

Postoperative Care

Following surgery—whether open or VATS—it is customary to place one chest drain. Postoperatively, many surgeons no longer apply suction to the chest drain except where this may promote lung reexpansion after empyema decortication (5, 13). The chest drain is generally removed when over the preceding 24 h there has been no air leak and the drainage is less than 200 ml (though some surgeons accept higher daily outputs).

Although surgeons and anesthetists now use a variety of intraoperative techniques to preempt postsurgical pain (69), some degree of discomfort is inevitable. Postoperatively, a patient is provided with regular oral analgesics. Generally, regular analgesia achieves better pain control than analgesia given only "as required" (57). Also, there has been a trend to reduce reliance on opiates, which can cause adverse side effects such as respiratory depression in a patient who just had chest surgery, impairment of the patient's appetite, and reduction of the patient's ability to mobilize (84). The use of parenteral opiates can be minimized through the use of perioperative regional anesthesia, regular nonopiate oral analgesics, and early chest drain removal.

The objective of analgesia is to enable early mobilization. It is now recognized that early mobilization is conducive to better postoperative recovery and can prevent many complications following surgery (30). After VATS, the patient can generally sit out of bed on the same day and mobilize freely no later than the morning after surgery. Chest physiotherapy and incentive spirometer breathing exercises are also mandatory (with due infection control precautions taken if there are fears of TB transmission in the postoperative period).

SURGERY FOR DIAGNOSIS OF TB

In patients who have clinical manifestations and radiological features that suggest TB and where less invasive investigative modalities have failed to yield a positive diagnosis, surgical biopsy may help to do so.

The first consideration when called upon to diagnose TB through surgery is to identify a potential target site for biopsy. In principle, the target site requiring least surgical access trauma is selected. If palpable lymph nodes in the cervical area are noted, for example, these could be easily biopsied under local anesthesia. If no such easily accessed targets are available and intrathoracic TB involvement is suspected, a thoracic computed tomography (CT) scan remains the most useful tool to look for a target for biopsy. The sites most frequently identified on CT for biopsy include lung parenchyma, mediastinal lymphadenopathy, and pleura. Biopsy of each of these tissues is discussed below. Which site is chosen to be biopsied is primarily determined by the likelihood of positive yield as suggested by the volume and accessibility of affected tissue seen on CT.

Secondary considerations include the patient's suitability for surgery. Requirements for lung function in diagnostic surgery are generally not as stringent as with therapeutic surgery, though candidates for surgery should ideally demonstrate an ability to tolerate one-lung ventilation and/or prolonged anesthesia. Foreseeable obstacles to certain surgical approaches should also be considered. For example, an existing tracheostomy may obstruct mediastinoscopy, or anticipated dense adhesions from previous thoracic surgery or infection may complicate surgical

exploration. It is therefore advisable to adopt a multidisciplinary team approach involving the respiratory physician, the thoracic surgeon, the radiologist, and the anesthetist. The team must identify a suitable target and assess surgical risk prior to embarking on surgery. For patients for whom surgery is potentially hazardous, alternative investigation modalities or even empirical anti-TB treatment may need to be considered.

Lung Parenchyma

No radiological imaging can yet confirm a diagnosis of TB affecting the lung parenchyma. Even modern CT and positron emission tomography have proven too nonspecific. Various modes of nonsurgical pulmonary sampling may also be insufficient for diagnosis. Percutaneous imaging-guided biopsy of suspicious lung lesions yields highly variable rates of positive diagnosis. Published series have suggested rates of positive diagnosis for TB ranging from 80% to as low as 20% (15, 18, 38, 89, 96). Fiber-optic bronchoscopy with bronchoalveolar lavage and/or transbronchial biopsy may give a positive diagnosis in only 30 to 58% of smear-negative TB cases (10, 39, 72). Surgical lung biopsy therefore remains necessary to confirm the diagnosis in a proportion of patients suspected to have TB.

As suggested above, the first consideration is to identify a target site for biopsy. For biopsy of lung parenchyma, the ideal target would be either a discrete mass or a focal area of opacity on CT that is situated at or close to a lung lobe edge or interlobar fissure. Such a location allows a small, simple wedge to be cut out, removing only a small piece of lung (typically several cubic centimeters of tissue), and results in little respiratory impairment for the patient. If radiological changes are more diffuse and no focal target can be identified, a wedge excision can be taken from an area of maximal change that is similarly situated at or close to a lobe edge or interlobar fissure. However, in such situations with diffuse changes there is the potential hazard of a staple or suture line running through inflamed or infected lung parenchyma, raising the risk of staple/suture line air leakage and poor healing.

If all other factors are equal in bilateral disease, some surgeons prefer the right lung for biopsy, as the extra interlobar fissure and lobe edges increase the likelihood of an easy biopsy at a lung lobe edge. It was previously reported that the lingula and right middle lobe made poor biopsy sites, given their alleged propensity for inflammation, scarring, and congestion that can affect histological diagnosis (19). However, others have since found this not to be the case (2), and most surgeons nowadays do not deliberately avoid biopsy at these sites.

Deep-sited lesions situated far from a lobe edge or a fissure typically pose a greater technical challenge for surgical biopsy. If the target lesion is very deep in the lung parenchyma, it is often not possible to remove it without depriving the subtended distal parts of the lung lobe of ventilation and perfusion. To remove such deep lesions, a very large wedge resection (commonly referred to as a hemi-lobectomy) or even an anatomical lobectomy may be required. An alternative is an enucleation procedure using precision electrocautery to spherically excise a lung lesion in a nonanatomical fashion (12). This is an effective procedure in selected patients but may cause potentially greater lung parenchymal trauma than a wedge resection. An enucleation may potentially be associated with a higher risk of air leakage or bleeding. Another problem with small, deep lesions is that they may be technically difficult to locate during surgery. Such lesions are often not visible from the outside of the lung lobe and may be impalpable. It has been estimated that for lesions 10 mm or less in diameter and which are located more than 5 mm beneath the lung surface, the chance of locating the lesion intraoperatively can be as low as 63% (76). In such cases, it is advisable to call upon an experienced interventional radiologist to mark the lesion immediately preoperatively by means of CT-guided placement of a hook wire to facilitate intraoperative detection (55). Because of these technical considerations, the preference is usually for biopsy of superficial lesions rather than deeper ones whenever possible.

The principles of surgery and anesthesia for lung biopsy are as described above. Limited biopsies via a minithoracotomy can be considered for selected patients who cannot tolerate general anesthesia. Otherwise, with general anesthesia and one-lung ventilation, a lung biopsy can be performed via open thoracotomy, conventional VATS, or needlescopic VATS (Fig. 1 and 2). With any approach, a visual and digital exploration is performed of the entire lung, and a representative area of lung tissue is identified for biopsy based on preoperative CT findings and these intraoperative findings.

To take a biopsy sample from the lung parenchyma, the most common method is to sharply excise the target as a wedge between tissue clamps, with suture repair of the cut lung surface. However, wedge excision is usually done nowadays using a surgical staple-resection device which is typically faster and simpler. Typically, about 2 to 3 cm^3 of tissue is sufficient for diagnosis, but this may vary depending on the quality of tissue and individual laboratory requirements. Where possible the line of resection should be sited through relatively normal areas of the line to minimize the risk of staple/suture line air leakage and poor healing. If this is not possible, coverage of the resection line with a pleural flap or surgical sealant (such as fibrin) can be performed in selected cases where such risks are considered high. It is important for the respiratory physician and thoracic surgeon to communicate preoperatively to determine which investigations are required so that adequate but not excessive sizes of lung specimens are removed. For deep lesions, alternatives to a wedge resection include enucleation as described above, or taking a Tru-Cut core biopsy.

For many thoracic surgeons experienced with minimally invasive techniques, the VATS approach is now preferred for most lung biopsies because of the reduced morbidity. With VATS biopsies, most patients are discharged the day after surgery and simpler lung biopsies are now increasingly being performed as day surgery procedures. When it is used for diagnosis of solitary lung lesions, many studies have consistently confirmed that in the hands of experienced VATS surgeons the diagnostic accuracy of VATS can be as high as 95 to 100%, with complication rates of 3 to 6% (45, 53). Because the surgical "footprint" left by a VATS biopsy is nowadays relatively small, surgical lung biopsy should not be considered a last-resort investigation any longer. Instead, VATS biopsy can be considered a viable direct alternative to flexible bronchoscopy or percutaneous needle biopsies in selected patients.

Pleural Effusion

When TB manifests as a pleural effusion, microbiological analysis of the fluid alone may not confirm the diagnosis. Percutaneous biopsy of the parietal pleura is a common strategy used in such patients, but this is essentially a blind procedure. There is generally no effective way of determining whether the pleura at the site of percutaneous puncture is a good site for biopsy. Consequently, pleural biopsy with an Abrams needle gives positive diagnosis in only 50 to 75% of cases (22, 88). With ultrasound guidance, the sensitivity is reportedly improved marginally to 81.8% (36). For cases where diagnosis cannot be achieved by percutaneous biopsy or pleural fluid analysis, surgical exploration can be offered. One advantage of surgery is that if the pleural effusion turns out to be an established stage 2–3 empyema thoracis on exploration, a surgical drainage and decortication procedure can be performed in the same sitting for selected patients (see below).

Patient selection criteria and anesthetic considerations for pleural biopsy are similar to those described above for lung biopsy. Although a limited open thoracotomy incision can be used, pleural biopsy today is usually performed using a minimally invasive VATS approach. Using a 30° angled video thoracoscope, VATS allows potentially better visualization of the lateral chest wall pleura than through an open thoracotomy and hence is usually even more suitable for pleural biopsy. Regardless of the surgical approach used, the first step is to break down loculations or septations due to inflammatory exudates in the pleural space. This allows full drainage of all the pleural fluid and then a thorough inspection of the entire ipsilateral parietal pleura to identify target sites for biopsy. In addition, TB sometimes produces inflammatory exudates and later fibrous peel on the parietal pleura which are readily seen by video thoracoscope. These and any other suspicious areas on the parietal pleura should be generously biopsied by endoscopic biopsy forceps.

The standard three-port VATS strategy described above for lung biopsy can be used for pleural biopsy. As mentioned above, a 30° angled video thoracoscope is preferred. The only caveat is that taking biopsy samples from the lateral chest wall during VATS may sometimes require greater angulation of instruments to reach "upwards" towards the target lesion. This may potentially result in "torquing" at the wounds that can increase pain or paresthesia postoperatively (71). This situation can be avoided or minimized by using curved instruments for biopsy and by siting instrument ports slightly farther away from the target lesion to allow a less acute angle of approach. An alternative is to use a single-port VATS strategy, whereby the biopsy forceps is inserted coaxially with the video thoracoscope, sharing the same port (Fig. 3) (94).

Worldwide experience over the past two decades has shown VATS to be a safe and quick procedure

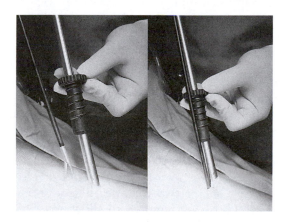

Figure 3. A single-shared-port approach can be used for pleural biopsy with VATS. A biopsy forceps is inserted coaxially with the video thoracoscope, minimizing the number of wounds required.

for diagnosis of pleural pathology in most patients (71, 93). VATS consistently achieves positive diagnosis for indeterminate pleural effusions in 95 to 100% of cases. One meta-analysis of 1,500 cases of indeterminate pleural effusions worldwide confirmed that VATS gave 90% diagnostic accuracy, with only 3% morbidity (48).

The postoperative course for most patients is as described above for lung biopsy. Typically, patients can be safely discharged home within 1 to 2 days of surgery.

One emerging alternative to VATS for indeterminate pleural effusions is "medical" thoracoscopy (or pleuroscopy) under local anesthesia (79, 90). Thoracoscopy is essentially the original procedure pioneered over a century ago by Jacobaeus and is considered the ancestor of modern VATS. Today, the two procedures have diverged so fundamentally that they represent completely different entities, and it is mainly to differentiate between medical thoracoscopy and modern VATS that the latter is no longer referred to as thoracoscopic surgery. With thoracoscopy, a single incision is made in the chest wall through which either a rigid thoracoscope tube or a fiber-optic pleuroscope is advanced into the pleural space. Fluid can be drained from the pleural space and parietal pleural biopsies can be taken via the hollow thoracoscope tube or the working channel of the pleuroscope. Recent reports of the use of semirigid pleuroscopy suggest even more promising diagnostic yields, inclusive of TB pleuritis (41, 52). The key advantage is the avoidance of general anesthesia, making it more suitable as a day case procedure and as an option for patients deemed unsuitable for general anesthesia for VATS. Thoracoscopy may also be potentially cheaper to perform than surgery. However, the lack of one-lung ventilation using local anesthesia means that an inflated or partially inflated lung may obstruct complete exploration of the entire ipsilateral chest. The anxiety and discomfort of the patient (who may have some degree of pneumothorax during the procedure)— plus the possible stress on the operator and nursing staff working on an awake patient—are also sometimes cited as notable disadvantages. At present, further experience is still awaited to establish the definitive role of thoracoscopy in diagnostic algorithms for TB.

Mediastinal Lymphadenopathy

In some TB patients, the only radiologically identifiable targets for biopsy in the chest may be enlarged intrathoracic lymph nodes. When considering lymph node lesions for biopsy, a distinction must be made between hilar nodes and mediastinal nodes in these cases. Hilar lymph nodes correspond to nodal stations 10 to 14 on the standard map for lung cancer lymph node staging adopted by the American Joint Committee on Cancer (AJCC) and the Union Internationale Contre le Cancer (UICC) (Fig. 4) (51). In practice, these nodes are reachable only via thoracotomy or VATS. Where such nodes are enlarged on CT, they also tend to be associated with postinflammatory adhesions in the interlobar fissures and between nodes and adjacent pulmonary vessels. The result is often technically challenging and relatively invasive surgery. Careful consideration should be taken before embarking on biopsies of hilar nodes unless there are other target lesions in the chest which can be biopsied in the same operation.

Mediastinal lymph nodes correspond to nodal stations 1 to 9 on the AJCC-UICC map (Fig. 4). These nodes can be approached transbronchially, via a cervical approach, or via a transthoracic approach. The position and choice of approach for biopsy actually make mediastinal nodes easier to biopsy than hilar nodes (stations 10 to 14) in most cases.

For biopsy of nodal stations 2, 4, 7, and often 10 and 11 on both sides of the chest, perhaps the least invasive approach is by transbronchial needle aspiration (TBNA) via fiber-optic bronchoscopy. This is performed in a similar fashion as conventional fiber-optic bronchoscopy under local or general anesthesia. In experienced hands, TBNA is a safe and effective procedure, with yields reaching 80% or more (3, 6). More recently, endobronchial ultrasonography (EBUS) has emerged as a further advancement or adjunct to TBNA (31, 74). EBUS allows detailed imaging of lymph nodes coupled with color Doppler assessment of the nodal vasculature. The shape, size, and vascular patterns of the nodes can be used to help distinguish between benign or malignant lymph nodes and to guide TBNA with potentially greater safety and accuracy. Nonetheless, as a relatively new technique, the role of EBUS in the investigation of TB remains to be confirmed by future experience. It should be borne in mind, however, that the total volume of tissue sampled by TBNA (traditional or EBUS guided) is substantially smaller than with any of the above surgical procedures. Where TBNA fails to yield a positive diagnosis, more invasive surgical biopsy may be considered.

The traditional surgical approach to the paratracheal lymph nodes in the mediastinum is the cervical mediastinoscopy procedure. Under general anesthesia, a small (2- to 3-cm) incision is made in the anterior neck midline and a rigid mediastinoscope tube can be placed along the pretracheal plane to access nodal stations 1, 2, and 4 on both sides, and often station 7 as well. Entire nodes at each station can be excised intact via the hollow mediastinoscope tube. If these nodal stations are the only preoperatively identified target lesions and there is no need to explore the whole pleural space, mediastinoscopy is often preferable to VATS. This is because mediastinoscopy does not require one-lung ventilation during anesthesia and can be better tolerated by patients with poor lung function. However, cervical mediastinoscopy cannot reach the inferior mediastinal nodal stations. The main contraindication to mediastinoscopy is previous radiotherapy or surgery in the sternal and tracheal area (including tracheostomy), as the resulting scarring can obliterate the pretracheal plane.

Anterior mediastinotomy (often called a Chamberlain's procedure) is an older surgical approach used most commonly on the left side to gain access to the nodal stations 5 and 6, which are not reachable via standard cervical mediastinoscopy. A parasternal, intercostal incision is made (typically through the third intercostal space) and often the internal mammary artery underneath is ligated and divided. In some cases, one or two costal cartilages or a short segment of a rib are removed to allow better access. Anterior mediastinotomy has been largely supplanted by VATS nowadays, which is less traumatic and offers an even better exploration of the thorax. However,

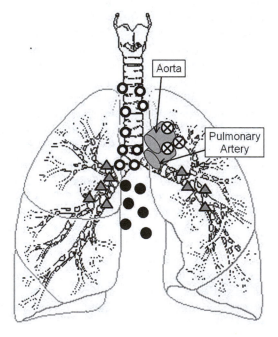

Figure 4. The surgical technique used for thoracic lymph node biopsy depends on the positions of the nodes. Mediastinal nodes corresponding to stations 2, 4, and 7 on the AJCC-UICC map (O) can be biopsied using TBNA, EBUS-guided fine-needle aspiration mediastinoscopy, VATS, or thoracotomy. Aortic nodes of stations 5 and 6 (⊗) are most commonly accessed by left VATS, mediastinotomy, or thoracotomy. Inferior mediastinal nodes of stations 8 and 9 (●) and hilar nodes of stations 10 and 11 (▲) are most commonly accessed by VATS or thoracotomy.

it still has a role to play in selected patients with suspicious nodes in stations 5 and 6 who cannot tolerate the one-lung ventilation required for VATS.

Stations 2, 3, 4, 7, 8, and 9 on the right side and stations 2, 4, 5, 6, 7, 8, and 9 on the left side can be accessed using VATS or, less commonly, open thoracotomy. Either approach allows a complete exploration of the ipsilateral pleural cavity as well as enabling complete removal of an entire mediastinal node in most cases. During a VATS nodal biopsy, the mediastinal pleura over each station is first opened using diathermy or an ultrasonic dissector, and the node is exposed through gentle sharp and blunt dissection. By gripping and lifting the node using a ring forceps, the entire node package can be excised intact with gentle diathermy or an ultrasonic dissector. Although nominally more invasive than both TBNA and even mediastinoscopy, VATS mediastinal lymph node biopsy is often a short, safe procedure which offers greater volume of tissue for investigations than those other approaches. The main limitation of VATS and thoracotomy is that normally only lesions on one side of the chest can be biopsied in one sitting (bilateral VATS is possible but rarely indicated).

SURGICAL LUNG RESECTION FOR PULMONARY TB

Surgery as Adjunctive Treatment of Pulmonary TB

The primary management of TB today is undoubtedly medical, and anti-TB drugs are highly effective in the vast majority of cases. Nonetheless, surgical lung resection as a therapeutic adjunct remains an option for a small, selected proportion of patients with TB. The most commonly reported indications include the treatment of MDR-TB, persistent bacteriologically positive TB despite adequate drug therapy; localized "sequestered" disease (such as a cavitary lesion or destroyed lobe); and infections by some nontuberculous mycobacteria.

The problem of MDR-TB deserves special mention. Currently, MDR-TB is recognized as a serious and growing health problem worldwide (85). For patients for whom anti-TB chemotherapy has been inadequate in curing MDR-TB, adjunctive surgical resection has been advocated (9, 80). Such resection may be effective and feasible where the disease is relatively localized in the lung and the patient has adequate cardiopulmonary reserve. Although there has been no randomized study to address the comparative efficacy of chemotherapy versus combined chemotherapy and surgery in the management of MDR-TB, one recent small series reported significant and durable improvement with surgery and postoperative

first-line chemotherapy in patients with MDR-TB and extensively drug-resistant TB (XDR-TB), perhaps suggesting the independent role of surgery (60). The recent worldwide emergence of XDR-TB, denoting MDR-TB with additional bacillary resistance to fluoroquinolones and second-line injectable drugs, may further increase the potential demand for lung resections in TB patients (37).

The aim of surgical treatment is to remove the predominant pulmonary lesion(s), thereby circumventing difficulty in drug penetration and reducing the mycobacterial burden (25, 67). In recent years, there have been a number of reports of achieving bacteriological cure or improvement in MDR-TB patients using a strategy of pulmonary resection combined with the best available chemotherapy (33, 35, 49, 66, 73, 82). A summary of the results of the most recent case series reporting the use of surgery as an adjunct in the management of MDR-TB is given in Table 1. It has been suggested that factors predictive of poor outcome in surgical resection for MDR-TB include poor lung function, preoperative hemoptysis, low body mass index, primary resistance, resistance to ofloxacin, and cavitary lesions that are not amenable to complete resection (33, 73).

In selecting any TB patient for major lung resection, several principles should be observed. Firstly, there should be a localized target area of TB involvement identified by radiological imaging for surgical resection. A greater anatomic extent or a diffuse, homogeneous distribution of disease as suggested on preoperative CT has been reported to be associated with greater surgical morbidity (87). Secondly, surgery should not be regarded as curative in the absence of appropriate anti-TB medical therapy. It must be ensured that safe and effective antimicrobial drug therapy has been selected for patients receiving surgery and will be available for use before and after surgery to minimize the impact of TB on bronchial stump and wound healing (25). Thirdly, preoperative lung function testing with the necessary precautions is mandatory. Because many TB patients may have compromised respiratory reserves, their risks of developing postoperative respiratory complications may be higher than for other patients undergoing thoracic surgery. A multidisciplinary assessment by the respiratory physician, the thoracic surgeon, and the anesthetist is required to determine if the patient is fit for surgery.

Once the decision is made to proceed with surgery, it is important to realize that this is an elective and not an emergency procedure. Sufficient time should be spent to fully optimize the patient before surgery. Where possible, the patient should ideally receive at least 2 to 3 months of anti-TB drug therapy

Table 1. Summary of selected recent case series reporting lung resection surgery for MDR-TB

Case series (reference)	No. of patients	Avg age (yrs)	Indications for surgery	% Bacteriologically positive at surgery	% Pneumonectomy	% Mortality	% Complications	TB treatment outcome
Kim et al. (2006) (33)	79	29 (median)	Refractory to drug Tx[a] Localized disease	98 (culture)	22	1	23	72% culture negative for final 12 mo of Tx
Kir et al. (2006) (35)	79	38 (mean)	Refractory to drug Tx High risk of relapse	16 (smear)	53	2.5	25	97.5% patients sputum negative postop 1.4% relapse on follow-up
Somocurcio et al. (2007) (73)	121	27 (median)	Refractory to drug Tx Progressive symptoms Localized disease	79 (culture)	22	5	23	73% of patients who were culture positive converted to culture negative postop 63% "cured" at median follow-up of 36 mo
Mohsen et al. (2007) (49)	23	24 (mean)	Refractory to drug Tx High risk of relapse	35 (smear)	48	4	35	100% patients sputum negative postop 4% relapse at 12 mo
Wang et al. (2008) (82)	56	39 (mean)	Progressive symptoms Localized disease	100 (smear)	45	0	25	91% patients sputum negative postop 4% relapse at 30 mo
Shiraishi et al. (2009) (66)	56	46 (mean)	Refractory to drug Tx High risk of relapse Associated empyema	32 (smear)	36	0	16	100% patients sputum negative postop 9% relapse after median follow-up for 39 mo

[a] Tx, treatment.

and be rendered culture negative before the operation (25, 67). This not only reduces the risks of postoperative complications and of transmission of TB to operating theater staff but also reduces the mycobacterial burden impairing bronchial stump and tissue healing. The nutritional status of many TB patients is also often poor, and it is advisable to optimize their nutrition in conjunction with clinical dieticians prior to major surgery. Poor nutrition not only contributes to postoperative complications but also reduces the bulk of chest wall muscles that may be required for use as flaps during surgery.

Resectional surgery for TB typically involves an anatomical lobectomy. In some situations, bilobectomies, pneumonectomies, or sublobar resections may be considered (49). The technique of resection is no different from major lung resection for lung cancer. However, in TB patients dense postinflammatory adhesions are often found around the pulmonary vessels in the lung hilum. In particular, TB-affected lymph nodes can adhere extremely densely onto the hilar vessels. These hilar adhesions often render lung resections in TB patients more difficult and time-consuming than in lung cancer patients.

Traditionally, the surgical approach of choice is a full posterolateral thoracotomy. However, increasingly it is possible to perform such major lung resections via a VATS approach in selected patients. The technique used by one of us (A.D.L.S.) has been previously described in detail (71). For a VATS lobectomy, a three-port strategy is typically used, with one port extended to a 3- to 4-cm-long utility incision to allow extraction of the resected lobe (Fig. 5). Typically, the utility incision is placed in the anterior axillary or midaxillary line in the fourth intercostal space for upper lobectomies and in the fifth intercostal space for middle and lower lobectomies. To

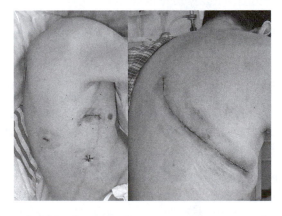

Figure 5. Major lung resections are nowadays commonly performed using a VATS approach (left). The contrast with the traditional posterolateral thoracotomy approach (right) in terms of wound trauma is obvious. Both photos were taken on the first postoperative day.

be defined as a VATS lobectomy, the entire operation must be performed without rib spreading and using purely endoscopic techniques with 100% monitor vision exclusively (64, 77). By eschewing rib spreading altogether, the same operation can be performed with potentially less pain and morbidity than with open thoracotomy. As mentioned above, hilar dissections in TB patients can sometimes be difficult, but with experience even such technically demanding operations can be performed safely using the VATS approach. However, surgeons should have little hesitation in converting to an open procedure should the risk of vascular injury be high.

It is now well established that VATS reduces pain and complication rates and better preserves postoperative respiratory function, immune function, quality of life, and shoulder mobility (32, 40, 42, 43, 59, 71). The upshot of these benefits is that some patients deemed unfit for surgery in the past may now be eligible for curative lung resection surgery. Recent studies indeed suggest that VATS lobectomy can be safely performed in patients with relatively poor lung function or advanced age (20). Selected TB patients previously regarded as marginal candidates for open surgery may therefore benefit from a multidisciplinary assessment involving physicians, thoracic surgeons, and anesthesiologists to consider if VATS surgery is feasible.

Regardless of surgical approach, the operative mortality rate for lung resection in TB in general is typically quoted as less than 5% and the postoperative complication rate at between 9 and 26% (49, 54, 66, 67, 78). This compares with a typical mortality rate of less than 3% for lobectomies for lung cancer (71). The higher risk for lung resections in TB patients reflects the greater technical difficulty when operating on TB patients as described above. Of the complications, postoperative persistent air leakage resulting from release of pleural adhesions is by far the most common, occurring in up to 40% of cases (75). Because of reduced lung compliance in many patients with TB, residual air space is another complication that may occur due to the residual lung inadequately expanding to fill the pleural cavity. It is recognized that in MDR-TB cases, recurrent infections may arise in any residual postoperative air space, and hence the need to prevent the occurrence of this situation is particularly great in these patients. Surgeons should routinely endeavor to minimize this problem using an array of surgical techniques, such as pulmonary release procedures, induced phrenic palsy, pleural tent creation, or pneumoperitoneum induction. Other complications after lung resections in TB patients include empyema thoracis, pneumonia, wound breakdown and fistulation (notoriously associated with TB), respiratory failure, recurrent laryngeal nerve palsy, and others. Acute exacerbations of TB pneumonitis may also occur.

However, the most feared complication after TB surgery is a bronchopleural fistula (BPF). For the thoracic surgeon, a BPF specifically refers to a breakdown of the bronchial stump after surgery. A BPF is more likely to occur after a pneumonectomy than a lobectomy. The reported incidence of BPF in most case series is between 0 and 16%, but it should be borne in mind that the pneumonectomy rates in these series can be as high as 48% (33, 49, 67, 73, 82). The significance of postoperative BPF is that it can quickly lead to a pleural space infection with a high rate of mortality. Once a BPF occurs, it is difficult to treat and may require very radical, debilitating thoracoplasty, muscle flap procedures, or prolonged pleural space decontamination strategies (8). TB patients are at particular risk for BPF given their often poor nutritional status at the time of surgery and the usually already inflamed/infected bronchi. Endobronchial TB in particular has been identified as a risk factor for development of BPF (82). There have therefore been calls for careful preoperative bronchoscopic assessments or even on-table frozen-section analysis of bronchial margins to exclude endobronchial TB, especially in cases of MDR-TB. The technique most commonly applied to reduce the risk of BPF is coverage of the bronchial stump with a flap. Such flaps may be fashioned from pericardial fat, from pleura or pericardium, or from pedicled muscles, including pedicled intercostal muscle flaps or latissimus dorsi flaps. This highlights the need for good nutrition prior to surgery in order to maintain healthy viable muscles should muscle flaps become necessary. The use of surgical sealants for bronchial stump reinforcement to reduce BPF risk after lobectomies is still under investigation.

Postoperatively, patients who are otherwise free of complications have chest drains removed in 2 days and can usually be discharged home in about 7 to 8 days (4 to 5 days if the VATS approach is used). Good nutrition and early mobilization are essential for recovery in TB patients after surgery. If necessary, dietary supplements and even parenteral feeding may be considered. Anti-TB drug therapy is continued following surgery (25), with a longer duration for patients with MDR-TB and XDR-TB.

Overall, the rate of eventual treatment success is quoted to be 75 to 98% (25, 66, 78). Nonetheless, it remains difficult to fully gauge the benefit of surgery given that the sickest patients who most require surgery are paradoxically often the ones who are least physically fit to endure major surgery (9, 80). The fact that many patients receiving surgical treatment often die of other causes means that long-term follow-up data such as 5-year survival are often lacking. Consequently, firm guidelines defining the role of surgery have yet to be established. The risks and benefits of surgical therapy for each potential surgical candidate should therefore always be carefully assessed on a case-by-case basis by a multidisciplinary panel involving experienced respiratory physicians, microbiologists, anesthesiologists, radiologists, physiotherapists, social workers, and dieticians as well as thoracic surgeons.

Surgery for Bronchiectasis

One of the corollaries of highly effective anti-TB drug therapy today is that most patients survive the initial TB episode, and hence more patients remain with complications resulting from their disease. The development of bronchiectasis following TB remains a complication still seen in many Asian countries (including the People's Republic of China). In some patients, the condition may progress and predispose to significant hemoptysis and/or mycetoma formation. Conventionally, management is medical, with symptomatic control of exacerbations and complications as they arise. However, by definition bronchiectasis is irreversible, and there appears to be no reliable medical means to halt its progression. Surgery is therefore occasionally indicated for those patients with severe manifestations, such as hemoptysis and recurrent infections.

Emergency surgical management of massive hemoptysis is dealt with separately below. Elective surgery for hemoptysis is warranted when it affects the patient's quality of life, or where increasing frequency and/or volume of hemoptysis may be heralding the onset of massive hemoptysis. In such cases, resectional surgery may be considered once the site of the bleeding can be identified by bronchoscopy and/or bronchial angiography. Although CT can be used to highlight sites of maximal bronchiectatic change, such changes alone are insufficiently specific to confirm the site of bleed when major irreversible surgery is being contemplated. Once a bleeding site is confirmed, alternative approaches such as bronchial arterial embolization (BAE) should always be considered prior to embarking on surgery. BAE is proven to be effective even for severe hemoptysis and is relatively less invasive than surgery (16, 29). Surgery more reliably halts the bleeding, but given its traumatic and irreversible nature, elective surgery is typically reserved only for patients in whom BAE is ineffective or unavailable.

Recurrent or recalcitrant lung infections are not uncommon in patients with bronchiectasis. Should frequent admissions be required for this, or if the chronic purulent sputum production causes significant impairment to the patient's quality of life, surgery may be considered. Again, it is important to identify a target for resection. Focal bronchiectasis localized to one lobe, a lung abscess, or a mycetoma represents a clear-cut and valid target for resection. In a patient with a lung abscess who is considered to have high risk for surgery, percutaneous insertion of a drainage catheter remains a less traumatic alternative to surgery (21). For mycetomas, intracavitary instillation of an antifungal agent (such as amphotericin B) appears to be a viable alternative to major lung resection in selected patients with poor lung function (27).

Whenever surgery is considered for a patient with bronchiectasis, it is crucial to fully counsel him or her on the implications of surgery. Firstly, this is technically difficult surgery with a relatively high rate of morbidity due to the extremely dense pleural adhesions associated with bronchiectasis. CT evidence of bronchiectatic change is a fairly reliable indicator of significant pleural and hilar adhesions. Secondly, surgery cannot prevent the progress of bronchiectasis in other parts of the lungs, and hence recurrent symptoms after surgery are entirely possible. Thirdly, because surgery results in the irreversible loss of a major part of a lung, it is usually most unlikely that the patient can receive further lung surgery in the future should such symptoms recur or other indications arise. Suitably high thresholds for surgery should therefore be maintained for most bronchiectasis patients, especially young ones who may have many years ahead of them during which the disease may progress.

Once decided upon, surgery is performed as described above for primary treatment of TB. Typically, a lobectomy is performed. However, surgery for bronchiectasis is often even more technically demanding because the chronicity of the disease and the recurrent infections associated with bronchiectasis usually result in extreme degrees of pleural and hilar adhesions. Prolonged surgery, relatively greater blood loss, and persistent postoperative air leakage are relatively common. Also, the remaining unresected lung is usually diseased with loss of compliance. Failure of the stiff lung to reexpand and fill the pleural cavity may result in residual air spaces, which may, in turn, compromise respiration or become infected.

Massive Hemoptysis

Massive hemoptysis can occur in patients with active TB but is more commonly associated with post-TB bronchiectasis. While some degree of blood-stained sputum production is common in many TB or bronchiectasis patients, true massive hemoptysis is, thankfully, infrequent. Massive hemoptysis can be defined as blood loss into the tracheobronchial tree that causes cardiorespiratory compromise or is life threatening (46). Massive hemoptysis is a definite medical emergency that carries a mortality rate of up to 75% if not promptly treated.

In the acute setting, the patient who is coughing up a massive volume of blood must first receive hemodynamic resuscitation and be managed in the intensive care unit. Most patients who die from massive hemoptysis do so because of asphyxiation. Therefore, should any suspicion of respiratory compromise be noted, the patient must be promptly intubated. Ideally, a double-lumen endotracheal tube should be placed by an experienced anesthesiologist. This provides isolation of the left and right lungs, reducing the risk of blood from the hemorrhaging lung flooding the other lung.

Once the patient is adequately stabilized, the most important consideration is to locate the site of bleeding. Considerable controversy surrounds the relative merits of CT scanning, rigid bronchoscopy, and fiber-optic bronchoscopy as the first-line investigation. Regardless of which method is used, promptly determining laterality of the bleeding is vital. Firstly, it allows the patient to be laid in bed with the bleeding side down to protect the nonbleeding lung. Secondly, should a thoracotomy be required, the surgeon will know which side to incise. Thirdly, should urgent BAE be required, the interventional radiologist will know which side to focus on to find the bleeding source, saving precious time.

The options for hemostasis include rigid bronchoscopy, BAE, and emergency surgery. Rigid bronchoscopy under general anesthesia can be offered by the thoracic surgeon. This aims to remove blood and clots from the airways and then achieve hemostasis through localized therapy, such as application of topical adrenaline, surgical sealants, or intrabronchial balloon catheters for tamponade. The advantage of rigid bronchoscopy is that immediate airway control is gained if a patient with active hemoptysis has not already been intubated. However, hemostasis via rigid bronchoscopy is often suboptimal given that the scope only reaches the proximal airways, but the site of bleeding may be very peripheral in the lung. BAE is highly effective in the acute cessation of bleeding, even in severe cases of hemoptysis (16, 29). It is less invasive than emergency surgery and can be repeated if necessary for recurrent episodes. However, the patient must usually be transported to the radiology suite for the procedure, and the process itself may be slow, as the interventional radiologist must carefully explore the bronchial arterial vasculature to locate and adequately embolize the bleeding site. Therefore, BAE may not always be suitable for hemodynamically unstable patients who are losing a large amount of blood.

Emergency surgery is the most invasive option. In the emergency setting, there is no role for a VATS or limited thoracotomy approach. Instead, a full posterolateral thoracotomy is used. In the operating theater, hemodynamic control is established and the patient is intubated and anesthetized. Further fiberoptic bronchoscopy can be performed to reconfirm the site of the bleeding. The lung lobe containing the bleeding site is promptly dissected and resected. However, expeditious surgery is often hindered by the inevitable post-TB adhesions, hemodynamic instability during general anesthesia, and coagulopathy if the patient has had significant blood loss already. Another critical consideration is that for many acutely hemoptysizing patients, lung function tests have usually not been done and it may be impossible to determine if the patient can tolerate major lung resection.

For massive hemoptysis, many surgeons nowadays prefer to achieve acute control of blood loss with BAE first. One can then consider if surgery is indicated later as an early elective procedure after BAE has bought time for more thorough patient assessment to be conducted (29). A recent study has shown that if a "BAE-first" strategy is used whereby BAE is used instead of emergency surgery wherever possible for the first 48 h, in-hospital mortality rates for massive hemoptysis can be significantly reduced (65). Even among patients who ultimately do require surgery, using a BAE-first approach reduced the rate of postoperative complications.

PLEURAL SPACE COMPLICATIONS FROM TB

Empyema Thoracis and Fibrothorax

The pleural space can often be involved in TB. In Hong Kong, around a third of all indeterminate pleural effusions are ultimately found to be secondary to TB (92). As with any parapneumonic effusion, pleural involvement with TB can progress through three recognized phases as defined by the American Thoracic Society: exudative effusion, fibrinopurulent empyema thoracis, and organized fibrothorax (44). Each phase is managed differently. Most early, phase 1 exudative effusions may resolve through control of the underlying infection, with or without simple pleural drainage. However, thoracic surgical intervention is commonly required to manage the later phases.

In phase 2 purulent empyema thoracis, antimicrobial management is often inadequate because of poor drug penetration to the pleural collection (91).

Simple chest drainage is also often ineffective because the pus is thick and the collection may be multiloculated with fibrous septations. Failure to resolve the condition can result in persistent sepsis, development of empyema necessitans, fistulation of the empyema through the skin or into other viscera, and the development of restrictive fibrothorax. Therefore, timely surgical drainage of a phase 2 empyema is crucial to preclude complications.

Patients who survive a phase 2 empyema without drainage may progress to develop a phase 3 organized fibrothorax. In such cases, there is little or no residual pus to drain. Instead, the fibrous exudate has formed a postinflammatory fibrous peel on the lung surface which can often be very thick and extremely adherent. The peel may cause restrictive inhibition of lung expansion. In such cases, surgical decortication is indicated to remove the peel from the lung and chest wall surfaces and restore full lung reexpansion. However, the stripped lung surface is raw and prone to air leakage, and there may be considerable blood loss from stripping of the chest wall. This highlights the need for early surgical intervention in phase 2 purulent empyema to prevent progression to organized phase 3 fibrothorax. The respiratory physician and the thoracic surgeon should work together to identify patients with evolving empyema for prompt surgery and reduce the incidence of such progression (91).

In patients who ultimately do present late to the surgeon, it may paradoxically be advisable to delay surgery further unless the patient is septic or developing complications from the empyema that indicate prompt surgery. For a stable, late-presenting patient, delaying surgery for a few weeks may allow tissue planes to become better defined between fibrous peel and lung surface over time, allowing slightly easier decortication.

Regardless of the phase of pleural disease, preoperative considerations are the same as described above. A CT scan is mandatory for all patients referred for surgery. This is necessary to plan the site of the surgical incision(s) and to locate the major pleural collections to be drained. Effective anti-TB chemotherapy should be administered prior to pleural surgery to reduce the risk of postoperative complications such as pleurocutaneous fistulation along the surgical wounds.

The operation for a phase 2 empyema is a drainage/decortication procedure. The first step is to mechanically break down all the pleural septations, rendering a multiloculated collection into a unilocular pleural space amenable to complete drainage by one or more chest drains. Next, all the empyema is fully drained and the pleural space thoroughly lavaged with antibiotic or antiseptic solution. In many cases, the pleural collection may contain not frank pus but fibrino-exudative "chicken fat" material and sometimes caseous sludge that is characteristic of TB. Finally, fibrous exudates on the chest wall and—most importantly—the lung surface are removed as completely as possible by a process of decortication. The objective is to completely free the lung of tethering by the fibrous deposits, allowing it to fully reexpand and fill the pleural cavity (7). Surgery should only be considered complete if all these have been done. It is important that no significant space is left which may harbor infection.

The operation for a phase 3 fibrothorax is similar. The main difference is that in fibrothorax there is little pus or soft exudates. Instead, as described above, thick fibrous peel on the lung is the predominant feature, and this must be stripped fully to allow lung reexpansion (Fig. 6).

When performing a drainage and decortication procedure, the traditional approach is via open thoracotomy. In recent years, however, VATS has been a viable alternative to open surgery, even for TB empyema (7). Potential advantages of VATS include better clearance of peel at the lateral chest wall, reduced pain, better patient satisfaction and recovery, and lower rates of wound complications. Studies have now confirmed that VATS can be used for decortication of empyema thoracis (including late-phase disease) with equivalent safety and efficacy—as measured by clinical and radiographical improvement—as open thoracotomy (7). With growing experience, some thoracic surgeons now find that even extremely thick and dense organized pleural peel can be fully decorticated using VATS, achieving lung reexpansion as good as with open surgery (Fig. 6). For individual surgeons,

VATS has now become the standard approach used for both purulent empyema and organized fibrothorax, and conversion to open thoracotomy is increasingly rarely required.

Persistent Pleural Space

Despite much progress in thoracic surgery, not every TB patient with pleural space involvement can achieve full lung reexpansion. Sometimes a significant pleural space remains after decortication surgery. In such patients, the underlying TB may have resulted in interstitial fibrosis or damage of the lung, so that its compliance and volume are irreversibly reduced. The lung may not fill the pleural space even after removal of all pleural peel. Some patients experience no further complications or symptoms related to the residual space and can be managed conservatively. In others, however, there may be persistent or recurrent infection in the pleural space that demands surgical intervention.

Historically, the earliest-described intervention for such post-TB residual pleural spaces which become infected is open drainage. This can range from applying a stoma bag over a pleurocutaneous fistula, through open drainage with a corrugated drain, to creation of a window thoracostomy (an Eloesser procedure) (50). Popular in the heyday of TB surgery in the mid-20th century, these operations are much less commonly performed nowadays. They do, however, retain a role for patients who may not tolerate more radical procedures.

If sepsis persists despite drainage as described above, attempts can be made to clean or sterilize an infected pleural space. Several strategies have been

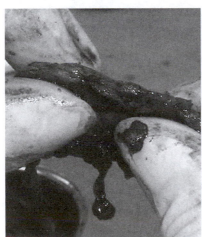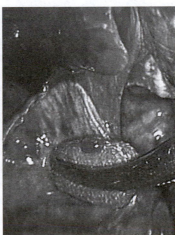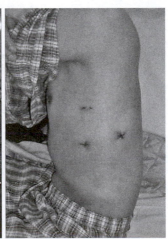

Figure 6. If an empyema thoracis is not promptly drained, it may progress to become a fibrothorax in which a very thick postinflammatory peel (left) can encase the lung. Decortication is required to allow lung reexpansion. Nowadays, complete decortication for even advanced empyema and fibrothorax can be achieved by VATS, which gives excellent intrathoracic visualization (center) and minimal surgical wound trauma (right).

described to do this, such as repeated lavage and/or packing of the pleural space with antiseptics (47). Antiseptic instillations for lavage may be given via an open thoracostomy or via an indwelling chest tube. For some patients, the cleansing of the pleural space is an intermediate step towards subsequent thoracoplasty and/or muscle flap placement. For other patients, the pleural cleansing may represent a definitive procedure, especially if the patient is unfit for more radical surgery and is no longer septic or symptomatic after pleural cleansing.

Where a space persists and remains clinically problematic despite the above measures, surgical obliteration of the pleural space defect can be offered to provide a more definitive "cure." This can be done by a thoracoplasty procedure, by filling the space, or by a combination of both (8, 50). With thoracoplasty, the principle is that if the lung cannot expand out to meet the chest wall, then the chest wall can be pushed in to meet the lung. Many variations exist on how to do this, but the most common strategy involves multiple rib resections to remove the bony "scaffold" propping up the muscular chest wall. The latter can then be pressed inwards onto the lung surface, obliterating the space. This procedure is disfiguring and can result in respiratory compromise, but it is often highly effective in managing the persistent space. The alternative to thoracoplasty is to fill the persistent space with a filler material. Several decades ago, plombage with foreign objects was popular. Today, persistent spaces are most commonly filled by applying a muscle flap (such as latissimus dorsi) into the space in a myoplasty procedure. Thoracoplasty operations are nowadays infrequently performed, as many TB empyemas are managed aggressively and early surgical drainage can preclude progression of the disease.

AIRWAY STENOSIS FOLLOWING ENDOBRONCHIAL TB

In Hong Kong, it has been estimated that up to 18% of patients with pulmonary TB also have central airway involvement by the disease (72). Such involvement of major airways by TB may result in their fibrosis and consequent stricture. This, in turn, can result in significant airway obstruction with impairment of pulmonary function and exercise capacity. In parts of the world where TB is endemic, some patients with respiratory symptoms may be unaware that they have previously contracted TB. Clinicians should remain vigilant when facing patients from such regions with wheeze and dyspnea that do not respond to standard therapy for asthma.

Patients with significant impairment of quality of life or with recurrent lung infections resulting from post-TB airway strictures can be considered for surgical intervention. Investigations for potential surgical candidates should include fiber-optic bronchoscopy and CT scanning. Modern high-resolution CT scanners can produce three-dimensional images of the airways or "virtual bronchoscopy" images reconstructed from the digital scan data (Fig. 7). These high-quality images have proved an invaluable asset in airway assessment but should nonetheless not be regarded as a complete substitute for fiber-optic bronchoscopy. The objective of the imaging is not only to locate the stricture and the degree of narrowing but also to assess the airways and lung distal to the stricture. If all the distal airways are significantly narrowed, for example, dilatation of a more proximal stenosis alone will hardly improve ventilation into that part of the lung. The ideal candidate for intervention should have a short-segment stenosis of the trachea, main bronchi, or lobar bronchi, with relatively patent airways and relatively healthy lung tissue distal to the stenosis. Patients with very long stenotic segments (several centimeters or more) or with stenotic airways extending to the segmental bronchi or beyond are usually not good candidates.

If the lung parenchyma in the part of the lung distal to the stricture is grossly destroyed by TB and bronchiectatic change, relief of the stricture itself may serve only to allow ventilation to essentially nonfunctional lung parenchyma. It may sometimes be more useful to resect that part of the lung rather than intervene in the airways. Such resections may be indicated for recurrent infections in the destroyed part of the lung and are performed as described above for lung parenchymal TB. In patients without need for urgent resections or who may not tolerate such resections, autopneumonectomy or -lobectomy may be allowed to occur. In such cases, the airway stenosis is allowed to occlude ventilation into the grossly destroyed lung, which then collapses and fibroses, hence precluding subsequent infection within without requiring major surgery.

In patients with salvageable lung distal to a stricture and with features favoring intervention as described above, airway intervention can be offered. The "gold standard" for managing most short-segment benign strictures of proximal airways (trachea and main bronchi) remains surgical resection of the stricture with primary reanastomosis, or more complex tracheobronchoplasty operations (70). Though effective, these operations are technically demanding, and the best results are usually seen only with high-volume specialist centers highly experienced in airway

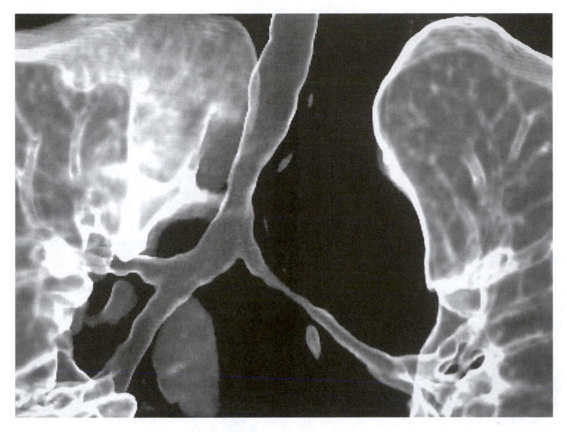

Figure 7. Modern CT scanning—with spectacular three-dimensional reconstruction images of the airways—gives highly detailed images that are invaluable for planning airway interventions. In this image, the site, diameter, and length of a stenotic segment in the left main bronchus can be clearly seen.

surgery. Furthermore, restenosis at anastomotic sites has been reported.

In some centers, airway dilatation with stenting has emerged as an effective and less traumatic alternative (26, 81). The procedure is performed via rigid bronchoscopy with the patient under general anesthesia. Through the rigid bronchoscope tube, the stenotic segment can be progressively dilated by the surgeon using graduated bougie or balloon dilators. Once an adequate airway diameter is achieved, an airway stent can be placed to maintain the airway patency. A well-placed stent not only will maintain airway patency but also may help "mold" the airway to the dilated diameter and probably prevent subsequent restenosis even after eventual stent removal. For technical reasons, it is usually not feasible to dilate and stent airways more distal than the level of the lobar bronchi. It is also technically more difficult to dilate the upper lobe bronchi. This emphasizes the need for accurate CT or bronchoscopy to assess the stenosis prior to intervention.

Airway stents generally fall into the categories of either the self-expandable metallic stents (SEMS) or the silicone stents (70). Although effective, SEMS are regarded by many surgeons as less user-friendly because they are difficult to reposition or remove after placement. There are also concerns over their potential for triggering airway inflammation and other complications (56). Silicone stents are not as rigidly fixed as SEMS in the airway lumen, and rarely has it been reported that they may be coughed out by patients. However, their advantages are that they are easy to place, position, and remove should they be suspected of causing any complications.

Tracheobronchial dilatation plus stenting with silicone stents has already been shown to provide effective and lasting treatment for airway stenosis secondary to TB (63, 81). Almost all patients experience immediate and significant symptomatic improvement after stenting. The degree of such improvement can be up to 7 points on a 10-point visual analog scale (81). After placement, controversy exists over if and when the stent(s) should be removed. Empirically, early pioneers suggested removal after 6 to 12 months. However, more recent reports have shown that silicone stents are well tolerated in patients for up to 5 years (63). Some surgeons now choose to only remove silicone stents should they show dislodgement or complications (such as local mucosal inflammation or plugging by sputum).

Patients receiving rigid bronchoscopy, dilatation, and stenting can generally be discharged home the morning after the procedure. Regular surveillance bronchoscopy may be offered as an outpatient procedure for stented patients following discharge. This serves to exclude both stent migration and intraluminal sputum plugging within the stent.

OTHER SURGICAL ISSUES IN TB PATIENTS

The above sections have outlined the main areas where the thoracic surgeon is most commonly involved in the management of TB. However, given the capacity of *M. tuberculosis* to affect almost any part of the human body, other clinical manifestations may also require the attention of the thoracic surgeon. Secondary spontaneous pneumothorax from the diseased lungs of TB patients is sometimes encountered, but it is managed in the same fashion as other secondary pneumothoraces (4). Mediastinal lymphadenopathy from TB has been reported on rare occasions to cause significant airway compression and compromise in young children. These can be removed or decompressed using a VATS or open surgical approach (24). Cold abscesses in the chest wall are infrequently encountered but can be readily excised or surgically debrided in most cases without undue difficulty (11).

It is also worth noting that TB and lung cancer can coexist in the same patient, especially in regions where TB is endemic. Many lung cancer resections in such regions are therefore performed in patients with confirmed or suspected history of TB. This can pose clinical challenges for the respiratory physician and thoracic surgeon alike in several ways (14). Firstly, when investigating suspicious lung mass lesions, a diagnosis of TB does not automatically exclude the presence of lung cancer. In particular, lung cancer has been reported to occasionally arise within preexisting lung opacities that have resulted from previous TB (the so-called "scar cancers") (1). Secondly, TB can confound the accuracy of noninvasive staging modalities for lung cancer. It is recognized that enlarged lymph nodes on CT or hypermetabolic lesions on positron emission tomography can just as easily represent TB as metastatic deposits (34). This emphasizes the need to involve the surgeon in invasive staging for suspicious lesions in regions where TB is endemic. Thirdly, as mentioned above, previous TB can give rise to significant pleural and hilar adhesions, which can considerably increase the technical difficulty of major lung resections. Given that many patients receiving lobectomy for lung cancer in TB-endemic countries have histories or radiological evidence of previous pulmonary TB, surgical outcomes

for lung cancer surgery may potentially be adversely affected in these countries. How this may affect the results of lung cancer surgery in countries where TB is endemic compared with countries where TB is rare has never been addressed.

CONCLUSIONS

Although the management of bronchopleuropulmonary TB remains mostly medical, thoracic surgery provides unique diagnostic and therapeutic options for selected subgroups of patients. Today, modern thoracic surgery not only offers highly effective treatment of TB and its sequelae but also promises to deliver it with less trauma and morbidity than ever before. The advantage of minimally invasive thoracic surgery is not only its capacity to reduce morbidity for individual patients but also its potential to allow a wider range of TB patients to be considered for effective surgical management.

REFERENCES

1. Ashizawa, K., N. Matsuyama, T. Okimoto, H. Hayashi, T. Takahashi, T. Oka, T. Nagayasu, and K. Hayashi. 2004. Coexistence of lung cancer and tuberculoma in the same lesion: demonstration by high resolution and contrast-enhanced dynamic CT. *Br. J. Radiol.* 77:959–962.
2. Ayed, A. K. 2003. Video-assisted thoracoscopic lung biopsy in the diagnosis of diffuse interstitial lung disease: a prospective study. *J. Cardiovasc. Surg.* 44:115–118.
3. Bilaçeroğlu, S., O. Günel, N. Eriş, U. Cağirici, and A. C. Mehta. 2004. Transbronchial needle aspiration in diagnosing intrathoracic tuberculous lymphadenitis. *Chest* 126:259–267.
4. Blanco-Perez, J., J. Bordón, L. Pinero-Amigo, R. Roca-Serrano, R. Izquierdo, and J. Abal-Arca. 1998. Pneumothorax in active pulmonary tuberculosis: resurgence of an old complication? *Respir. Med.* 92:1269–1273.
5. Cerfolio, R. J., C. Bass, and C. R. Katholi. 2001. Prospective randomized trial compares suction versus water seal for air leaks. *Ann. Thorac. Surg.* 71:1613–1617.
6. Cetinkaya, E., P. Yildiz, F. Kadakal, A. Tekin, F. Soysal, S. Elibol, and V. Yilmaz. 2002. Transbronchial needle aspiration in the diagnosis of intrathoracic lymphadenopathy. *Respiration* 69:335–338.
7. Chan, D. T. L., A. D. L. Sihoe, S. Chan, D. S. F. Tsang, B. Fang, T. W. Lee, and L. C. Cheng. 2007. Surgery for empyema thoracis: is video-assisted thoracic surgery 'better' than thoracotomy? *Ann. Thorac. Surg.* 84:225–231.
8. Chan, E. C. K., T. W. Lee, C. S. H. Ng, I. Y. P. Wan, A. D. L. Sihoe, and A. P. C. Yim. 2002. Closure of postpneumonectomy bronchopleural fistula by means of single, perforator-based, latissimus dorsi muscle flap. *J. Thorac. Cardiovasc. Surg.* 124:1235–1236.
9. Chan, E. D., V. Laurel, M. J. Strand, J. F. Chan, M.-L. N. Huynh, M. Goble, and M. D. Iseman. 2004. Treatment and outcome analysis of 205 patients with multidrug-resistant tuberculosis. *Am. J. Respir. Crit. Care Med.* 169:1103–1109.
10. Charoenratanakul, S., W. Dejsomritrutai, and A. Chaiprasert. 1995. Diagnostic role of fiberoptic bronchoscopy in suspected

smear negative pulmonary tuberculosis. *Respir. Med.* 89:621–623.

11. Cho, K. D., D. G. Cho, M. S. Jo, M. I. Ahn, and C. B. Park. 2006. Current surgical therapy for patients with tuberculous abscess of the chest wall. *Ann. Thorac. Surg.* 81:1220–1226.

12. Cooper, J. D., M. Perelman, T. R. Todd, R. J. Ginsberg, G. A. Patterson, and F. G. Pearson. 1986. Precision cautery excision of pulmonary lesions. *Ann. Thorac. Surg.* 41:51–53.

13. Cummin, A. R., N. L. Wright, and A. E. Joseph. 1991. Suction drainage: a new approach to the treatment of empyema. *Thorax* 46:259–260.

14. Dacosta, N. A., and S. G. Kinare. 1991. Association of lung carcinoma and tuberculosis. *J. Postgrad. Med.* 37:185–189.

15. Das, D. K., C. S. Pant, J. N. Pant, and P. Sodhani. 1995. Transthoracic (percutaneous) fine needle aspiration cytology diagnosis of pulmonary tuberculosis. *Tuberc. Lung Dis.* 76:84–89.

16. Endo, S., S. Otani, N. Saito, T. Hasegawa, Y. Kanai, Y. Sato, and Y. Sohara. 2003. Management of massive hemoptysis in a thoracic surgical unit. *Eur. J. Cardiothorac. Surg.* 23:467–472.

17. Fallon, W. F., Jr. 1994. Post-traumatic empyema. *J. Am. Coll. Surg.* 179:483–492.

18. Ferreirós, J., A. Bustos, S. Merino, E. Castro, M. Dorao, and C. Crespo. 1999. Transthoracic needle aspiration biopsy: value in the diagnosis of mycobacterial lung opacities. *J. Thorac. Imaging* 14:194–200.

19. Gaensler, E. A., and C. B. Carrington. 1980. Open biopsy for chronic diffuse infiltrative lung disease: clinical, roentgenographic, and physiological correlations in 502 patients. *Ann. Thorac. Surg.* 30:411–426.

20. Garzon, J. C., C. S. H. Ng, A. D. L. Sihoe, A. V. Manlulu, R. H. L. Wong, T. W. Lee, and A. P. C. Yim. 2006. Video-assisted thoracic surgery pulmonary resection for lung cancer in patients with poor lung function. *Ann. Thorac. Surg.* 81:1996–2003.

21. Ghaye, B., and R. F. Dondelinger. 2001. Imaging guided thoracic interventions. *Eur. Respir. J.* 17:507–528.

22. Gopi, A., S. M. Madhavan, S. K. Sharma, and S. A. Sahn. 2007. Diagnosis and treatment of tuberculous pleural effusion in 2006. *Chest* 131:880–889.

23. Gotoda, Y., N. Kambara, T. Sakai, Y. Kishi, K. Kodama, and T. Koyama. 2001. The morbidity, time course and predictive factors for persistent post-thoracotomy pain. *Eur. J. Pain* 5:89–96.

24. Hewitson, J. P., and U. O. Von Oppell. 1997. Role of thoracic surgery for childhood tuberculosis. *World J. Surg.* 21:468–474.

25. Iseman, M. D., L. Madsen, M. Goble, and M. Pomerantz. 1990. Surgical intervention in the treatment of pulmonary disease caused by drug-resistant *Mycobacterium tuberculosis*. *Am. Rev. Respir. Dis.* 141:623–625.

26. Iwamoto, Y., T. Miyazawa, N. Kurimoto, Y. Miyazu, A. Ishida, K. Matsuo, and Y. Watanabe. 2004. Interventional bronchoscopy in the management of airway stenosis due to tracheobronchial tuberculosis. *Chest* 126:1344–1352.

27. Jackson, M., C. D. Flower, and J. M. Shneerson. 1993. Treatment of symptomatic pulmonary aspergillomas with intracavitary instillation of amphotericin B through an indwelling catheter. *Thorax* 48:928–930.

28. Jacobaeus, H. C. 1910. Ueber die Möglichkeit die Zystoskopie bei Untersuchungseröserlöhlungenanzuwenden. *Munchen Med. Wochenschr.* 57:2090–2092.

29. Jougon, J., M. Ballester, F. Delcambre, T. MacBride, P. Valat, F. Gomez, F. Laurent, and J. F. Velly. 2002. Massive hemoptysis: what place for medical and surgical treatment. *Eur. J. Cardiothorac. Surg.* 22:345–351.

30. Kaneda, H., Y. Saito, M. Okamoto, T. Maniwa, K. Minami, and H. Imammura. 2007. Early postoperative mobilization

with walking at 4 hours after lobectomy in lung cancer patients. *Gen. Thorac. Cardiovasc. Surg.* 55:493–498.

31. Kanoh, K., T. Miyazawa, N. Kurimoto, Y. Iwamoto, Y. Miyazu, and N. Kohno. 2005. Endobronchial ultrasonography guidance for transbronchial needle aspiration using a double-channel bronchoscope. *Chest* 128:388–393.

32. Kaseda, S., T. Aoki, N. Hangai, and K. Shimizu. 2000. Better pulmonary function and prognosis with video-assisted thoracic surgery than with thoracotomy. *Ann. Thorac. Surg.* 70:1644–1646.

33. Kim, H. J., C. H. Kang, Y. T. Kim, S. W. Sung, J. H. Kim, S. M. Lee, C. G. Yoo, C. T. Lee, Y. W. Kim, S. K. Han, Y. S. Shim, and J. J. Yim. 2006. Prognostic factors for surgical resection in patients with multidrug-resistant tuberculosis. *Eur. Respir. J.* 28:576–580.

34. Kim, Y. K., K. S. Lee, B. T. Kim, J. Y. Choi, H. Kim, O. J. Kwon, Y. M. Shim, C. A. Yi, H. Y. Kim, and M. J. Chung. 2007. Mediastinal nodal staging of nonsmall cell lung cancer using integrated ^{18}F-FDG PET/CT in a tuberculosis-endemic country. *Cancer* 109:1068–1077.

35. Kir, A., I. Inci, T. Torun, A. Atasalihi, and K. Tahaoglu. 2006. Adjuvant resectional surgery improves cure rates in multidrug-resistant tuberculosis. *J. Thorac. Cardiovasc. Surg.* 131:693–696.

36. Koegelenberg, C. F., C. T. Bolliger, J. Theron, G. Walzl, C. A. Wright, M. Louw, and A. H. Diacon. 2010. Direct comparison of the diagnostic yield of ultrasound-assisted Abrams and Tru-Cut needle biopsies for pleural tuberculosis. *Thorax* 65:857–862. [Epub ahead of print.]

37. Kwon, Y. S., Y. H. Kim, G. Y. Suh, M. P. Chung, H. Kim, O. J. Kwon, Y. S. Choi, K. Kim, J. Kim, Y. M. Shim, and W. J. Koh. 2008. Treatment outcomes for HIV-uninfected patients with multidrug-resistant and extensively drug-resistant tuberculosis. *Clin. Infect. Dis.* 47:496–502.

38. Lacasse, Y., E. Wong, G. H. Guyatt, and D. J. Cook. 1999. Transthoracic needle aspiration biopsy for the diagnosis of localized pulmonary lesions: a meta-analysis. *Thorax* 54:884–893.

39. Lai, R. S., S. S. Lee, Y. M. Ting, H. C. Wang, C. C. Lin, and J. Y. Lu. 1996. Diagnostic value of transbronchial lung biopsy under fluoroscopic guidance in solitary pulmonary nodule in an endemic area of tuberculosis. *Respir. Med.* 90:139–143.

40. Landreneau, R. J., M. J. Mack, S. R. Hazelrigg, R. D. Rowling, D. Burke, J. Gavlick, M. K. Perrino, P. S. Ritter, C. M. Bowers, and J. DeFino. 1993. Post-operative pain-related morbidity: video-assisted thoracic surgery versus thoracotomy. *Ann. Thorac. Surg.* 56:1285–1289.

41. Lee, P., A. Hsu, C. Lo, and H. G. Colt. 2007. Prospective evaluation of flex-rigid pleuroscopy for indeterminate pleural effusion: accuracy, safety and outcome. *Respirology* 12:881–886.

42. Li, W. W., R. L. Lee, T. W. Lee, C. S. Ng, A. D. Sihoe, I. Y. Wan, A. A. Arifi, and A. P. Yim. 2003. The impact of thoracic surgical access on early shoulder function: video-assisted thoracic surgery versus posterolateral thoracotomy. *Eur. J. Cardiothorac. Surg.* 23:390–396.

43. Li, W. W. L., T. W. Lee, S. S. Y. Lam, C. S. H. Ng, A. D. L. Sihoe, I. Y. Wan, and A. P. Yim. 2002. Quality of life following lung cancer resection: video-assisted thoracic surgery versus thoracotomy. *Chest* 122:584–589.

44. Light, R. W. 2006. Parapneumonic effusions and empyema. *Proc. Am. Thorac. Soc.* 3:75–80.

45. Mack, M. J., S. R. Hazelrigg, R. J. Landreneau, and T. E. Acuff. 1993. Thoracoscopy for the diagnosis of the indeterminate solitary pulmonary nodule. *Ann. Thorac. Surg.* 56:825–830.

46. Mal, H., I. Rullon, F. Mellot, O. Brugière, C. Sleiman, Y. Menu, and M. Fournier. 1999. Immediate and long-term results of

bronchial artery embolization for life-threatening hemoptysis. *Chest* **115:**996–1001.

47. Mennander, A., J. Laurikka, P. Kuukasjarvi, and M. Tarkka. 2005. Continuous pleural lavage may decrease postoperative morbidity in patients undergoing thoracotomy for stage 2 thoracic empyema. *Eur. J. Cardiothorac. Surg.* **27:**32–34.

48. Menzies, R., and M. Charbonneau. 1991. Thoracoscopy for the diagnosis of pleural disease. *Ann. Intern. Med.* **114:**271–276.

49. Mohsen, T., A. Abou Zeid, and S. Haj-Yahia. 2007. Lobectomy or pneumonectomy for multidrug-resistant pulmonary tuberculosis can be performed with acceptable morbidity and mortality: a seven-year review of a single institution's experience. *J. Thorac. Cardiovasc. Surg.* **134:**194–198.

50. Molnar, T. F. 2007. Current surgical treatment of thoracic empyema in adults. *Eur. J. Cardiothorac. Surg.* **32:**422–430.

51. Mountain, C. F., and C. M. Dressler. 1997. Regional lymph node classification for lung cancer staging. *Chest* **111:**1718–1723.

52. Munavvar, M., M. A. Khan, J. Edwards, Z. Waqaruddin, and J. Mills. 2007. The autoclavable semirigid thoracoscope: the way forward in pleural disease? *Eur. Respir. J.* **29:**571–574.

53. Murasugi, M., T. Onuki, T. Ikeda, M. Kansaki, and S. Nitta. 2001. The role of video-assisted thoracoscopic surgery in the diagnosis of the small peripheral pulmonary nodule. *Surg. Endosc.* **15:**734–736.

54. Naidoo, R. 2007. Active pulmonary tuberculosis: experience with resection in 106 cases. *Asian Cardiovasc. Thorac. Ann.* **15:**134–138.

55. Nakashima, S., A. Watanabe, T. Obama, G. Yamada, H. Takahashi, and T. Higami. 2010. Need for preoperative computed tomography guided localization in video-assisted thoracoscopic surgery pulmonary resections of metastatic pulmonary nodules. *Ann. Thorac. Surg.* **89:**212–219.

56. Nashef, S., C. Dromer, and J. F. Velly. 1992. Expanding wire stents in benign tracheobronchial disease: indications and complications. *Ann. Thorac. Surg.* **52:**937–940.

57. Ng, A., F. Hall, A. Atkinson, K. L. Kong, and A. Hahn. 2000. Bridging the analgesic gap. *Acute Pain* **3:**1–6.

58. Ng, C. S., T. W. Lee, S. Wan, I. Y. Wan, A. D. L. Sihoe, A. A. Arifi, and A. P. C. Yim. 2005. Thoracotomy is associated with significantly more profound suppression in lymphocytes and natural killer cells than video-assisted thoracic surgery following major lung resections for cancer. *J. Investig. Surg.* **18:**81–88.

59. Nomori, H., H. Horio, T. Naruke, and K. Suemasu. 2002. Posterolateral thoracotomy is behind limited thoracotomy and thoracoscopic surgery in terms of postoperative pulmonary function and walking capacity. *Eur. J. Cardiothorac. Surg.* **21:**155–156.

60. Park, S. K., J. H. Kim, H. Kang, J. S. Cho, and R. A. Smego, Jr. 2009. Pulmonary resection combined with isoniazid- and rifampin-based drug therapy for patients with multidrug-resistant and extensively drug-resistant tuberculosis. *Int. J. Infect. Dis.* **13:**170–175.

61. Pomerantz, M., and J. D. Mitchell. 2009. Surgery for the management of *Mycobacterium tuberculosis* and nontuberculous mycobacterial (environmental) infections of the lung, p. 1149–1158. *In* T. W. Shields, J. LoCicero, C. E. Reed, and R. H. Feins (ed.), *General Thoracic Surgery*, 7th ed. Lippincott Williams & Wilkins, Philadelphia, PA.

62. Rogers, M. L., and J. P. Duffy. 2000. Surgical aspects of chronic post-thoracotomy pain. *Eur. J. Cardiothorac. Surg.* **18:**711–716.

63. Schmidt, B., H. Olze, A. C. Borges, M. John, U. Liebers, O. Kaschke, K. Haake, and C. Witt. 2001. Endotracheal balloon

dilatation and stent implantation in benign stenoses. *Ann. Thorac. Surg.* **71:**1630–1634.

64. Shigemura, N., A. Akashi, S. Funaki, T. Nakagiri, M. Inoue, N. Sawabata, H. Shiono, M. Minami, Y. Takeuchi, M. Okumura, and Y. Sawa. 2006. Long-term outcomes after a variety of video-assisted thoracoscopic lobectomy approaches for clinical stage IA lung cancer: a multi-institutional study. *J. Thorac. Cardiovasc. Surg.* **132:**507–512.

65. Shigemura, N., I. Y. Wan, S. C. H. Yu, R. H. Wong, M. K. Y. Hsin, K. H. Thung, T. W. Lee, S. Wan, M. J. Underwood, and A. P. C. Yim. 2009. Multidisciplinary management of life-threatening massive hemoptysis: a 10-year experience. *Ann. Thorac. Surg.* **87:**849–853.

66. Shiraishi, Y., N. Katsuragi, H. Kita, Y. Tominaga, K. Kariatsumari, and T. Onda. 2009. Aggressive surgical treatment of multidrug-resistant tuberculosis. *J. Thorac. Cardiovasc. Surg.* **138:**1180–1184.

67. Shiraishi, Y., Y. Nakajima, N. Katsuragi, M. Kurai, and N. Takahashi. 2004. Resectional surgery combined with chemotherapy remains the treatment of choice for multidrug-resistant tuberculosis. *J. Thorac. Cardiovasc. Surg.* **128:**523–528.

68. Sihoe, A. D. L., C. S. Cheung, H. K. Lai, T. W. Lee, K. H. Thung, and A. P. C. Yim. 2005. Incidence of chest wall paresthesia after needlescopic video-assisted thoracic surgery for palmar hyperhidrosis. *Eur. J. Cardiothorac. Surg.* **27:**313–319.

69. Sihoe, A. D. L., A. V. Manlulu, T. W. Lee, K. H. Thung, and A. P. C. Yim. 2007. Pre-emptive local anesthesia for needlescopic video-assisted thoracic surgery: a randomized controlled trial. *Eur. J. Cardiothorac. Surg.* **31:**103–108.

70. Sihoe, A. D. L., I. Y. P. Wan, and A. P. C. Yim. 2004. Airway stenting for unresectable esophageal cancer. *Surg. Oncol.* **13:**17–25.

71. Sihoe, A. D. L., and A. P. C. Yim. 2008. Video-assisted pulmonary resections, p. 970–988. *In* G. A. Patterson, J. D. Cooper, J. Deslauriers, A. E. M. R. Lerut, J. D. Luketich, T. W. Rice, and F. G. Pearson (ed.), *Thoracic Surgery*, 3rd ed. Elsevier, Philadelphia, PA.

72. So, S. Y., W. K. Lam, and D. Y. Yu. 1982. Rapid diagnosis of suspected pulmonary tuberculosis by fiberoptic bronchoscopy. *Tubercle* **63:**195–200.

73. Somocurcio, J. G., A. Sotomayor, S. Shin, S. Portilla, M. Valcarcel, D. Guerra, and J. Furin. 2007. Surgery for patients with drug-resistant tuberculosis: report of 121 cases receiving community-based treatment in Lima, Peru. *Thorax* **62:**416–421.

74. Steinfort, D. P., M. J. Hew, and L. B. Irving. 4 December 2009, posting date. Bronchoscopic evaluation of the mediastinum using endobronchial ultrasound—a description of the first 216 cases performed at an Australian tertiary hospital. *Intern. Med. J.* doi:10.1111/j.1445-5994.2009.02142.x.

75. Stolz, A. J., J. Schutzner, R. Lischke, J. Simonek, and P. Pafko. 2005. Predictors of prolonged air leak following pulmonary lobectomy. *Eur. J. Cardiothorac. Surg.* **27:**334–336.

76. Suzuki, K., K. Nagai, J. Yoshida, H. Ohmatsu, K. Takahashi, M. Nishimura, and Y. Nishiwaki. 1999. Video assisted thoracoscopic surgery for small indeterminate pulmonary nodules. *Chest* **115:**563.

77. Swanson, S. J., J. E. Herndon, T. A. D'Amico, T. L. Demmy, R. J. McKenna, Jr., M. R. Green, and D. J. Sugarbaker. 2007. Video-assisted thoracic surgery (VATS) lobectomy—report of CALGB 39802: a prospective, multi-institutional feasibility study. *J. Clin. Oncol.* **25:**4993–4997.

78. Takeda, S., H. Maeda, M. Hayakawa, N. Sawabata, and R. Maekura. 2005. Current surgical intervention for pulmonary tuberculosis. *Ann. Thorac. Surg.* **79:**959–963.

79. Tassi, G. F., R. J. O. Davies, and M. Noppen. 2006. Advanced techniques in medical thoracoscopy. *Eur. Respir. J.* **28:**1051–1059.

80. Torun, T., K. Tahaoglu, I. Ozmen, T. Sevim, G. Atac, A. Kir, G. Güngör, Y. Bölükbaşi, and E. Maden. 2007. The role of surgery and fluoroquinolone in the treatment of multidrug-resistant tuberculosis. *Int. J. Tuberc. Lung Dis.* **11:**979–985.

81. Wan, I. Y. P., T. W. Lee, H. C. K. Lam, V. Abdullah, and A. P. C. Yim. 2002. Tracheobronchial stenting for tuberculous airway stenosis. *Chest* **122:**370–374.

82. Wang, H., H. Lin, and G. Jiang. 2008. Pulmonary resection in the treatment of multidrug-resistant tuberculosis: a retrospective study of 56 cases. *Ann. Thorac. Surg.* **86:**1640–1645.

83. Weissberg, D., and Y. Refaely. 2000. The place of surgery in the treatment of re-emerging pulmonary tuberculosis. *Ann. Ital. Chir.* **71:**649–652.

84. Wheeler, M., G. M. Oderda, M. A. Ashburn, and A. G. Lipman. 2002. Adverse events associated with postoperative opioid analgesia: a systematic review. *J. Pain* **3:**159–180.

85. **WHO/IUATLD Global Project on Anti-Tuberculosis Drug Resistance Surveillance, 1999–2002.** 2004. *Anti-Tuberculosis Drug Resistance in the World: Report No. 3.* WHO/CDS/TB/2004.343. World Health Organization, Geneva, Switzerland.

86. **World Health Organization.** 2009. *Global Tuberculosis Control 2009: Epidemiology, Strategy, Financing.* WHO/HTM/TB/2009.411. World Health Organization, Geneva, Switzerland.

87. Wu, M. H., J. M. Chang, T. M. Haung, L. L. Cheng, Y. L. Tseng, M. Y. Lin, and W. W. Lai. 2004. Computed tomographic assessment of the surgical risks associated with fibrocavernous pulmonary tuberculosis. *Surg. Today* **34:**204–208.

88. Yew, W. W., C. Y. Chen, S. Y. Kwan, S. W. Cheung, and G. L. French. 1991. Diagnosis of tuberculous pleural effusion by the detection of tuberculostearic acid in pleural aspirates. *Chest* **100:**1261–1263.

89. Yew, W. W., S. Y. Kwan, P. C. Wong, and K. H. Fu. 1991. Percutaneous transthoracic needle biopsies in the rapid diagnosis of pulmonary tuberculosis. *Lung* **169:**285–289.

90. Yim, A. P. C. 1995. Is flexible fiberoptic pleuroscopy more cost-effective compared with VATS? *Chest* **108:**1179–1180.

91. Yim, A. P. C. 1999. Paradigm shift in empyema management. *Chest* **115:**611–612.

92. Yim, A. P. C., J. K. S. Ho, T. W. Lee, and S. S. Chung. 1995. Thoracoscopic management of pleural effusion revisited. *Aust. N. Z. J. Surg.* **65:**308.

93. Yim, A. P. C., T. W. Lee, M. B. Izzat, and S. Wan. 2001. Place of video-thoracoscopy in thoracic surgical practice. *World J. Surg.* **25:**157–161.

94. Yim, A. P. C., and A. D. L. Sihoe. 2009. VATS as a diagnostic tool, p. 313–323. *In* T. W. Shields, J. LoCicero, C. E. Reed, and R. H. Feins (ed.), *General Thoracic Surgery*, 7th ed. Lippincott Williams & Wilkins, Philadelphia, PA.

95. Yim, A. P. C., A. D. L. Sihoe, T. W. Lee, and A. A. Arifi. 2002. A simple maneuver to detect airleak on-table following 'needle-scopic' VATS. *J. Thorac. Cardiovasc. Surg.* **124:**1029–1030.

96. Yuan, A., P. C. Yang, D. B. Chang, C. J. Yu, L. N. Lee, H. D. Wu, S. H. Kuo, and K. T. Luh. 1993. Ultrasound guided aspiration biopsy for pulmonary tuberculosis with unusual radiographic appearances. *Thorax* **48:**167–170.

Tuberculosis and Nontuberculous Mycobacterial Infections, 6th ed.
Edited by David Schlossberg
© 2011 ASM Press, Washington, DC

Chapter 10

Mycobacterium bovis BCG and New Vaccines against Tuberculosis

TIMOTHY LAHEY AND C. FORDHAM VON REYN

INTRODUCTION

A critical component of global tuberculosis control is the development of more effective immunization strategies. Several tuberculosis vaccines have been shown to reduce the risk of disease and death due to tuberculosis in humans, but only one is used in global immunization programs: *Mycobacterium bovis* bacillus Calmette-Guérin (BCG). BCG is an attenuated live vaccine administered at birth to children in most countries where tuberculosis is endemic. BCG has been the most widely administered vaccine in the world, with an estimated three billion doses administered to date (43). BCG has likely reduced the burden of tuberculosis in many areas, but it has numerous limitations. These limitations, together with the continuation of the global tuberculosis epidemic, have made the development of a more effective vaccine against tuberculosis a major international public health priority (5, 22).

The development of new tuberculosis vaccines has been informed by evolving data on the natural history of tuberculosis, by new data on the immunology of infection with and immunization against *Mycobacterium tuberculosis*, by reanalysis of the role of nontuberculous mycobacteria (NTM) in protection against tuberculosis, by a clearer understanding of the benefits and risks of BCG, and by molecular techniques that have permitted identification of immunodominant antigens of *M. tuberculosis* and new methods of antigen delivery.

GLOBAL TUBERCULOSIS IN THE BCG ERA

Approximately one-third of the world's population is infected with *M. tuberculosis*, with an annual per-person incidence of new infections in the developing world of 1 to 5%. In 2008, there were 9 million new cases of active tuberculosis disease, 11 million prevalent cases of active tuberculosis disease, and 1.8 million deaths attributable to tuberculosis. Most tuberculosis morbidity and mortality occurs in the developing world, with the highest case burdens occurring in India (2.2 million) and China (1.2 million) and the highest tuberculosis incidence rates found in sub-Saharan Africa ($\geq$300/100,000). A major and continuing stimulus for the ongoing tuberculosis epidemic in sub-Saharan Africa and around the world is the human immunodeficiency virus (HIV) epidemic: over 1.4 million tuberculosis cases occurred in people with HIV, and 500,000 died of HIV-associated tuberculosis in 2008 (175). Complicating things still further, in 2008 there were approximately 440,000 cases of multidrug-resistant (MDR) tuberculosis worldwide, and, by early 2010, 58 countries reported at least one case of extensively drug-resistant tuberculosis (176). For these many reasons, improving vaccine-based prevention of tuberculosis disease is a key global health priority.

MANIFESTATIONS OF INFECTION AND DISEASE DUE TO *M. TUBERCULOSIS*: IMPLICATIONS FOR PREVENTIVE IMMUNIZATION

Initial Infection

M. tuberculosis infects humans when humans inhale droplet nuclei containing viable organisms, which reach the alveoli of a nonimmune host. An initial bacteremia distributes organisms to other organ sites and to other areas of the lung. Approximately 10% of infected persons subsequently develop active disease: 5% who develop progressive primary disease within the first 2 years of infection and 5% who develop reactivation disease in the lungs or another organ site years later. The likelihood of developing primary or reactivation tuberculosis varies widely, however, with substantial incidence rates in vulnerable

Timothy Lahey and C. Fordham von Reyn • Section of Infectious Diseases and International Health, Department of Medicine, Dartmouth Medical School, Lebanon, NH 03756.

populations such as children, the elderly, and immunocompromised individuals. The ideal tuberculosis vaccine would prevent both initial tuberculosis infection and primary or reactivation tuberculosis disease in healthy hosts as well as in particularly vulnerable populations.

Tuberculosis in Children

Most new infections and approximately 10% of all cases of disease due to *M. tuberculosis* worldwide occur in children (171). Most infections in neonates result from exposure of the infant to an adult with active pulmonary disease soon after delivery (144). Primary infection in children is often asymptomatic, although approximately 40% of infants and 15% of children under the age of 5 develop active disease within 1 to 2 years of infection. The protean manifestations of childhood tuberculosis, the difficulty in diagnosis, and the high mortality rate are all arguments for a more effective vaccination strategy to prevent tuberculosis in children.

Tuberculosis in Older Children and Adults

After infancy and early childhood, progression of latent infection to active disease is most common in early adulthood (15 to 25 years of age) and in the elderly. While infection in children from ages 5 to 14 years may occur, this age group is relatively resistant to disease progression. Infection after the age of 15 progresses to active disease in 5% in the first 2 years and then in 5% over the remainder of life. Infection after age 35 is less likely to progress to active disease (70) and has a better prognosis. New infection or reinfection in the elderly tends to progress to active disease in a manner similar to that in adolescents and has a high mortality rate (146). The high rate of disease and high mortality rate in the elderly emphasize the importance of a vaccine strategy that produces durable immunity.

Tuberculosis in the Elderly

The risk of reactivation tuberculosis increases with age, likely through waning cellular immunity. Furthermore, the likelihood of institutionalization increases with age, and institutionalization carries with it additional risk of tuberculosis disease likely related to both infirmity and intrainstitutional transmission of tuberculosis. For instance, one Arkansas study showed tuberculosis case rates of 20/100,000 for the general population, 60/100,000 for individuals over age 65 who lived at home, and 234/100,000 for individuals over age 65 who lived in a nursing home (145). In the United States, the incidence of reactivation tuberculosis among the elderly has fallen dramatically, likely due to the disappearance of untreated old tuberculosis (71).

Tuberculosis and HIV Infection

Among the 1.8 million people who died of tuberculosis disease in 2008, approximately 500,000 were HIV infected. Like with other forms of immunodeficiency, the risk of progression from latent tuberculosis infection to active tuberculosis is heightened during HIV infection, to 10% per year. In many HIV-endemic countries, more than 50% of new cases of tuberculosis occur in HIV positives, and this figure reaches 70% in some regions of sub-Saharan Africa (56). Although the tuberculosis risk in HIV positives is due in part to an increased risk of reactivation disease, patients with HIV infection also have a substantial risk of reinfection with *M. tuberculosis* (142). This implies that diminished immune function in HIV infection impairs the relative protection against tuberculosis reinfection that has been observed in healthy subjects (45). The net effect of increased rates of both reactivation and new infection is that in areas of the world where tuberculosis is endemic, it is the most common cause of death in persons with HIV infection (56).

Isoniazid preventive therapy provides potent, if not durable, protection from reactivation tuberculosis among HIV-infected individuals (50, 76, 180), and antiretroviral therapy reduces the risk of tuberculosis by 80% (9, 48). Given the decreased sensitivity of the tuberculin skin test among HIV-infected individuals and the substantial challenge of delivering antiretrovirals in developing countries, improved immunization strategies against tuberculosis are needed for persons with HIV infection.

Tuberculosis in Other Immunocompromised Hosts

Heightened risk of tuberculosis disease is described in multiple immunodeficiency states besides HIV infection. Heritable defects of gamma interferon (IFN-γ) and interleukin 12 signaling are associated with dramatic susceptibility to mycobacterial disease (78), as are multiple acquired immunodeficiency states such as receipt of tumor necrosis factor alpha antagonists and other immunosuppressive therapies (98, 113, 179). Malnutrition has long been recognized to contribute to tuberculosis endemicity in the developing world (26, 110), presumably through an effect on immune function. Obesity has been noted to protect against tuberculosis among persons with HIV infection (55), and yet the immunologic impairment associated with diabetes is increasingly recognized as an important and increasingly prevalent risk factor for tuberculosis (74). The safety and efficacy of any new tuberculosis vaccine will need to be tested in a wide variety of immunodeficiency states.

Tuberculosis in Health Care Providers and Other International Travelers

Health care providers, international outreach workers, and others working in areas where tuberculosis is endemic have a heightened risk for developing tuberculosis compared to the general population in low-prevalence countries (92, 111). Tuberculosis transmission to health care providers and other international travelers poses a health threat to individual travelers and could fuel the global spread of MDR and extensively drug-resistant tuberculosis. As a result, targeted BCG immunization for at-risk travelers to areas where MDR tuberculosis is endemic is being considered for reintroduction into national immunization guidelines in the United States.

SOURCES OF IMMUNE PROTECTION AGAINST TUBERCULOSIS

At least partial immune protection from tuberculosis disease results from prior mycobacterial infection, whether naturally acquired or vaccine induced (Table 1). This observation implies the generation of immune responses to shared mycobacterial antigens, although it is possible that exposure to NTM exerts a nonspecific impact on the immune response to tuberculosis infection. Regardless, the magnitude of this protection is often not quantified and unlikely absolute.

Natural Infection or Disease Due to *M. tuberculosis*

Epidemiological and experimental animal studies indicate that prior infection with tuberculosis confers relative protection against subsequent disease due to reexposure (45, 181). Such protection seems

Table 1. Known sources of protection against tuberculosis in humans

Naturally acquired mycobacterial infection
  M. tuberculosis
  NTM

Vaccine-induced mycobacterial infection
  BCG (live)
  M. microti (live)
  Whole-cell mycobacterial vaccines (inactivated), including
    M. vaccae

to be diminished in the face of cellular immunodeficiency, exemplified by reports of reinfection with new strains of *M. tuberculosis* among patients with untreated HIV infection (142). Recent data from South Africa indicated that both HIV-positive and HIV-negative persons with a first episode of active tuberculosis are at increased risk of a second episode of active tuberculosis (47). This raises the possibility that there are as-yet-unidentified host genetic factors which affect susceptibility to tuberculosis. The fact that reinfection has now been demonstrated in some persons does not contradict the prevailing view that most healthy persons with tuberculosis have some level of protection against reinfection. Nor does it suggest that protective immunization against tuberculosis is not possible. Population-based studies will be required to assess the magnitude of the protective effect of prior infection and its implications for tuberculosis vaccine development.

Natural Infection with NTM

Skin test studies in humans suggest that prior infection with NTM, acquired naturally from exposure to colonized water or soil, confers protection against tuberculosis (38, 44). Experimental data for animals demonstrate that infection with NTM protects against tuberculosis (39, 44). Infection with NTM is common in most regions of the world (163), and infections are usually acquired in childhood (41). In the United States, approximately 40% of adults have positive skin test reactions to NTM of the *Mycobacterium avium* complex (MAC), and most of these adults have negative tuberculin skin tests (164). Naturally acquired NTM infection may produce levels of protection against tuberculosis equal to BCG, and high rates of background infection with NTM in older children and adults have been proposed as an explanation for the lack of efficacy of BCG in some areas of the world (44). Prior mycobacterial infection may also reduce the efficacy of BCG by limiting its replication. Recent data indicate that infection of mice with environmental mycobacteria inhibits BCG replication and induction of a BCG-mediated immune response and impairs the protective effect of BCG after challenge with *M. tuberculosis* (20).

Immunization with Live *Mycobacterium microti*

The Medical Research Council conducted a controlled clinical trial of another live mycobacterial vaccine, *Mycobacterium microti* (the vole bacillus), in 1950. A single dose of *M. microti* was found to have a 5-year efficacy of 84%, equivalent to BCG, in a trial involving 54,239 tuberculin-negative British adolescents (59). These data indicate that antigens other than those derived from *M. tuberculosis* or *M. bovis* may protect humans against tuberculosis. Immunologic techniques were not available to assess mycobacterium-specific cellular immune responses; thus, the in vitro correlates of protection with this vaccine have not been identified.

Immunization with Inactivated Whole-Cell Mycobacterial Vaccines

Inactivated whole-cell mycobacterial vaccines were tested before the widespread acceptance of BCG and were shown to be effective in preventing tuberculosis in humans. Multiple doses were required, and animal studies indicated that the inoculum had to be higher than for BCG since replication did not occur after immunization (172). Jules Freund demonstrated that a multiple-dose series of heat-killed *M. tuberculosis* had an efficacy of 42% against tuberculosis in a controlled clinical trial in the 1930s (118). More than 100,000 Italian children have been immunized with inactivated whole-cell mycobacterial vaccines (including a vaccine that combined *M. tuberculosis*, *M. bovis*, and *M. avium*), and a study with more than 18,000 of these children showed a reduction in the tuberculosis mortality rate from 5% in unimmunized children to 0% in immunized children (172).

MECHANISMS OF IMMUNE CONTROL OF TUBERCULOSIS

Macrophage and T-Cell Containment of Tuberculosis

Cellular immunity is essential to protection from tuberculosis disease. After initial infection and systemic dissemination, *M. tuberculosis* engages with Toll-like receptors 2 and 4 as well as other surface receptors on macrophages, and phagocytosis ensues. The resultant local and systemic cytokine cascade promotes T-cell recruitment to sites of tissue infection. Toll-like receptor activation and signaling by IFN-γ and other Th1 cytokines from T cells and nearby macrophages foster *M. tuberculosis* autophagy (52, 57, 178) as well as the degradation of *M. tuberculosis* by reactive oxygen and nitrogen intermediates within the maturing phagosome (97, 152).

The promotion of intracellular degradation of *M. tuberculosis* within macrophages by Th1 cytokines secreted by CD4$^+$ T cells is considered the most important component of long-term immune defense against tuberculosis disease. This observation is based in part on the observation that major histocompatibility complex (MHC) class I knockout mice are less

susceptible to tuberculosis disease than MHC class II knockouts (112). However, this model has been complicated by the identification of a number of CD4$^+$ T-cell subsets that participate in the immune response to *M. tuberculosis*, including memory T-cell subsets and $\gamma\delta$ T cells, as well as regulatory and Th17 T cells (36, 83, 86, 174), with no data yet regarding the relative contribution of each to immune protection from tuberculosis disease. Furthermore, the contribution of CD8$^+$ T cells to protection against tuberculosis disease is being reconsidered in light of the identification of $\alpha\beta$ T-cell receptor-positive, CD4$^-$, non-MHC class I-restricted T-cell responses to tuberculosis (86), and data from a nonhuman primate model in which susceptibility to tuberculosis was dramatically enhanced after antibody depletion of CD8$^+$ T cells (26a).

Beyond the clear importance of cellular immune responses to immune protection from tuberculosis, tuberculosis-specific antibodies have conferred protection from tuberculosis or reduced CFUs in lungs after tuberculosis challenge in mouse models, either via direct antibody-tuberculosis interactions or via antibody-mediated immune modulation (1). To date, there are no convincing human data supporting a role for antibodies in immune protection from tuberculosis.

Intracellular Persistence of Tuberculosis

The potent and multifaceted macrophage and T-cell immune response to infection with *M. tuberculosis* in healthy human hosts leads to successful containment of tuberculosis as latent disease in 90% of subjects. However, this immune response ultimately fails to eradicate *M. tuberculosis* in 10% of subjects and results in progression to active disease or later reactivation disease. Beyond host immunodeficiency, mechanisms for ongoing *M. tuberculosis* persistence in macrophages include inhibition of phagosomal maturation and lysosomal fusion, and perturbations in calcium and iron homeostasis as well as cellular lipid metabolism (19, 58, 87, 109). The result is an immunologic stalemate in which the coordinated responses of macrophages and T cells foster immune containment of *M. tuberculosis*, but instead of full eradication, long-term intracellular persistence of *M. tuberculosis* results, allowing for later reactivation in the setting of waning cellular immunity.

Antigen Specificity of the Protective Immune Response to Tuberculosis

Amidst an increasingly complicated model of the protective immune response to tuberculosis, our understanding of the antigen specificity of the protective immune response against tuberculosis has evolved as well. Conventional CD4$^+$ T cells clearly target immunodominant antigens such as early secretory antigenic target 6 (ESAT-6) and antigen 85 (Ag85), and data from a guinea pig model and observational studies in humans suggest greater protection from tuberculosis with immune responses targeting multiple compared to single antigens (117; T. Lahey, unpublished data). Furthermore, it is clear that the range of mycobacterial antigens targeted by CD4$^+$ and CD8$^+$ T cells is broad; it includes DosR regulon-encoded proteins (18) and antigens presented to non-classically restricted T cells (77, 95, 96). Furthermore, the immune response to tuberculosis includes CD1-restricted T and NK T cells responding to lipid antigens (159), while γδ T cells target small phosphate-containing nonpeptidic antigens (33, 151).

The increasing complexity of the working model of protective immunity to tuberculosis has had a practical consequence: it is unclear when assessing candidate vaccine immunogenicity which immune responses against which antigens will best correlate with the induction of a protective immune response against tuberculosis.

BCG VACCINE

History

Mycobacterium bovis BCG was developed by Leon Calmette and Camille Guérin, the former a physician, the latter a veterinarian. Beginning in 1902 they passed a strain of *M. bovis* isolated from a cow with tuberculous mastitis in culture every 3 weeks for a total of 230 passages. Beginning in 1913 they inoculated calves and then guinea pigs with the attenuated *M. bovis* strain, with no evidence of infection. They subsequently challenged immunized cows with a wild-type, virulent strain of *M. bovis*, without any resulting evidence of infection. Protection was then demonstrated in pigs, rabbits, and horses. In 1921 the vaccine was first administered orally to humans. The first recipient was a 3-day-old infant whose mother had died of tuberculosis a few hours after giving birth. The grandmother also had advanced tuberculosis and was the child's guardian. In these circumstances, which mimic the current recommendation for use of BCG in the United States by the American Academy of Pediatrics, the infant's risk of developing infection with disseminated disease and/or meningitis was deemed to outweigh the unknown risks of the new vaccine. The child had no ill effects from the vaccine and was raised by the grandmother without developing tuberculosis. Between 1921 and 1924 the vaccine was given to an additional 600

children, without serious complications. Production and vaccination efforts were increased so that approximately 100,000 doses had been administered by 1928, including to Calmette's own grandchildren (133). In 1928 the vaccine was certified as safe by the League of Nations. Soon thereafter, however, 251 children were vaccinated in Lubeck, Germany, with a lot contaminated with virulent *M. tuberculosis*. This resulted in 172 deaths and at least 108 cases of active disease (15).

BCG Strain Variation

Although all strains of BCG originated from the parent BCG strain developed by Calmette and Guérin, this strain was distributed and maintained by different laboratories and subsequently evolved into several genetically distinct strains (14). The first randomized, controlled trial of vaccine efficacy was undertaken by Aronson between 1935 and 1938 (6). In 1947 the World Health Organization (WHO) initiated a tuberculosis control program that included widespread use of BCG. From the mid-1950s until 1997 seed lots of vaccine were established under the direction of the WHO and administered by the Danish State Serum Institute in Copenhagen, Denmark. Responsibility for vaccine manufacture and quality control now rests with the individual manufacturer and with regulatory agencies in the country of production. Four strains (Glaxo, Danish, Pasteur, and Tokyo) account for over 90% of vaccine currently administered (14).

Immune Response to BCG Immunization

In vitro responses

Immunization with BCG induces a mild systemic infection in healthy hosts. Autopsy studies of recently immunized children who died from diverse causes indicate widespread granuloma formation (154). This attenuated mycobacterial infection elicits both cell-mediated and humoral immune responses to mycobacterial antigens. Subjects vaccinated with BCG exhibit lymphocyte proliferation responses to proteins secreted by BCG and *M. tuberculosis* (102, 148). In addition, BCG vaccination results in IFN-γ and other Th1 cytokine responses to whole-cell and secreted antigens (82, 101, 116, 123). More recent studies have shown in addition that BCG vaccination elicits a variety of cytokine responses outside of the Th1 paradigm (89), and that the different populations of memory T cells contribute differentially to the production of different cytokine responses (141). Regarding humoral immune responses elicited by

BCG, both immunoglobulin G and M responses have been demonstrated against purified protein derivative and peptide antigens (17, 67, 131, 158). While cellular immune responses to *M. tuberculosis* whole-cell lysate in BCG-immunized humans correlate with postimmunization tuberculin skin test results and local vaccine reactogenicity (82), no studies of immune responses after BCG vaccination were conducted in the context of clinical trials assessing the protective efficacy of BCG, so it is not clear which immune response can be used as a surrogate for protective immunity (22). As an example, while intradermal immunization is more immunogenic than subcutaneous immunization (82), a randomized trial with 11,680 infants in Cape Town, South Africa, showed that percutaneous and intradermal immunizations with Tokyo 172 BCG provide equivalent protection from tuberculosis disease at 2 years of follow-up (60). It has been shown that immune responses to BCG are impaired in infants with HIV infection (105).

Tuberculin skin test responses

Most tuberculin-negative subjects who are immunized with BCG develop a positive tuberculin skin test several weeks later. This effect wanes with time, and thus it is recommended that tuberculin reactions >10 mm several years after immunization be interpreted as latent infection with *M. tuberculosis* rather than the persistent effect of BCG. However, BCG-induced tuberculin reactions are often larger than 10 mm and can be boosted with repeated tuberculin skin tests. Although it is generally stated that the development of BCG-induced tuberculin sensitivity is not a surrogate for protective immunity against tuberculosis, this issue has not been rigorously studied in a BCG efficacy trial. Further, a volunteer study in the United States showed a correlation between BCG-induced tuberculin sensitivity and contemporary in vitro markers of immune response to BCG (68).

Efficacy of BCG against Tuberculosis

Overview

Although most countries and international bodies have concluded that childhood BCG immunization is effective in the prevention of tuberculosis, this view was never widely accepted in the United States. The controversy is based largely on the variable results of BCG efficacy trials and on different interpretations of these trials. Reexamination of the major prospective trials in light of contemporary knowledge of mycobacterial immunity and an improved understanding of critical trial design issues supports the view that childhood immunization is effective. Retrospective analysis of tuberculosis risk in subjects with and without BCG scars is subject to potential confounding by socioeconomic status (i.e., those without childhood BCG immunization may have come from lower socioeconomic groups and be at an inherently higher risk of tuberculosis) and is not useful in assessing the efficacy of BCG.

Because prior infection with either *M. tuberculosis* or NTM confers protection against tuberculosis comparable to BCG, vaccine efficacy for childhood immunization programs can only be assessed adequately by prospective trials of BCG immunization in mycobacterium-naïve hosts, i.e., newborns. Numerous older trials attempted to screen out older children and adults with preexisting mycobacterial immunity by using intradermal skin tests. However, contemporary in vitro studies demonstrate that many skin test-negative subjects have demonstrable cellular and humoral immune responses to mycobacteria and are therefore not mycobacteria naïve (67, 108, 123, 167; J. Vuola, B. Cole, M. Matee, L. Mtei, C. R. Horsburgh, R. D. Arbeit, K. J. Pallangyo, and C. F. von Reyn, presented at the 42nd Annual Meeting of the Infectious Diseases Society of America, 30 September to 3 October 2004). Accordingly, retrospective studies that compare rates of tuberculosis in subjects with and without BCG scars are subject to potential bias, since absence of immunization might reasonably be expected to correlate with lower socioeconomic status, which is itself a risk factor for disease (13). Thus, efficacy trials should be separated into those conducted with mycobacterium-naïve newborns and those conducted with mycobacterium-experienced older children and adults using newer assays of exposure to mycobacteria.

Trials in mycobacterium-naïve subjects

Four prospective trials have assessed the efficacy of BCG immunization against tuberculosis in newborns and infants (Table 2) (6, 42, 94, 129, 130). Collectively these trials demonstrate efficacies of 73% against disease and 87% against death. An exemplary trial in this group was the randomized, placebo-controlled study conducted in Chicago in the 1930s by Rosenthal et al. (130). Participants were infants less than 3 months of age, and BCG was given by the multiple-puncture technique. Approximately 1,700 subjects were enrolled in each arm and monitored for 12 to 23 years; a vaccine efficacy of 74% was demonstrated. Trials with children have demonstrated that BCG is 86% effective in the prevention of bacteremic disease, including disseminated tuberculosis and tuberculous meningitis (125).

Table 2. Efficacy of BCG against tuberculosis: trials in newborns

Author(s)	Yr	Location	Subjects	No.	% Efficacy (disease)	% Efficacy (death)	Reference
Aronson	1948	Western United States	Newborns (Native Americans)	232	59	100	6
Ferguson and Simes	1949	Montreal	Newborns	609	80	78	42
Rosenthal et al.	1960	Chicago	Newborns	451	74	100	129
Rosenthal et al.	1961	Chicago	Newborns	3,381	72	84	130
Total				4,673	73	87	

Trials in mycobacterium-experienced subjects

Numerous BCG trials have been conducted with older children and adults. Each of these trials is subject to potential bias introduced by including subjects who have already been infected with *M. tuberculosis* (in tuberculosis-endemic regions) or NTM (in most areas of the world). As noted above, contemporary in vitro immunologic techniques suggest that the tuberculin skin tests used to screen out mycobacterium-experienced subjects may not have been sufficiently sensitive to identify preexisting mycobacterial immunity. Thus, negative trials in this category may simply have been an attempt to immunize persons with naturally acquired immunity.

However, some studies with older children and adults demonstrated the protective efficacy of BCG immunization. One example is the large trial conducted between 1935 and 1938 in Native Americans by Aronson (6). This was a randomized, placebo-controlled study of persons ages 0 to 20 years (28% less than age 5) with baseline single and extra-strength tuberculin screening to exclude those with prior mycobacterial exposure. The original study enrolled 3,287 participants. Evaluation at 11 years demonstrated a 75% reduction in radiographically diagnosed tuberculosis, and evaluation at 20 years demonstrated an 82% reduction in mortality. The overall vaccine efficacy was 70%. A recent report provided the longest-term follow-up of any BCG trial: data on 1,998 of 2,963 original participants showed vaccine efficacy of 52% against disease after 50 to 60 years (7).

Another well-designed prospective study conducted among 14- to 15-year-old British school children in the 1950s enrolled over 25,000 subjects in the vaccine and control groups. Baseline screening excluded children with reactions to standard or extra-strength tuberculin. Vaccine efficacy was determined to be 76% over a follow-up period of 15 years (59).

Chingleput, South India, trial

The South India trial deserves special consideration since it was designed as the ultimate randomized, controlled trial to investigate the protective efficacy of BCG against tuberculosis (156; S. Tripahty, presented at the International Union Against Tuberculosis, Singapore, 1986) and is often cited to show that BCG is not effective. The study had the objectives of comparing the efficacies of different BCG strains and doses and assessing the efficacy of BCG in those with and without prior infection (determined by baseline tuberculin skin testing). In fact, the trial was principally a study of the effect of BCG in older children and adults, many of whom were already tuberculin positive and all of whom lived in an area of high leprosy prevalence. The trial was initiated in 1968 and enrolled over 270,000 subjects, but it only enrolled 1,500 (0.6%) aged 0 to 1 month for randomization to vaccine or placebo. Surveillance for tuberculosis was based on a positive chest X ray, and these were only performed at age 5 or above; those with positive X rays had sputum microbiology. Tuberculosis endpoints were said to be positive only if the subject had a positive sputum culture or positive acid-fast bacillus stain, and there were no methods for detecting extrapulmonary tuberculosis. Collectively these endpoint definitions would be very insensitive for detecting tuberculosis in children. Further, surveillance in the overall study was not uniform in all subject groups, and the rate of tuberculosis endpoints was only half the predicted rate. Lastly, when the multivariate analyses were restricted to the subset of 40,342 study subjects without baseline skin test reactions to NTM, BCG immunization was associated with a 32% reduction in the risk of tuberculosis (115). The most reasonable interpretation of this large trial is that BCG vaccination of mycobacterium-experienced older children and adults in India did not lead to reduction in sputum culture-positive pulmonary tuberculosis.

Trials in HIV infection

In spite of the substantial burden of tuberculosis-related morbidity and mortality among people infected with HIV, and the potential for HIV infection to compromise immune responses to BCG vaccination, there are no prospective trials of the efficacy of BCG immunization in the prevention of tuberculosis in persons with HIV infection. Retrospective and case control studies have provided conflicting results, with one study suggesting protection against disseminated tuberculosis (107) and another showing no protection (170). However, since BCG immunization in HIV-infected infants carries a risk of disseminated BCG disease, vaccine should not be administered to infants with known HIV infection (63, 64, 107, 150, 170).

Interpretation of trials

Two meta-analyses have evaluated the major prospective trials of BCG efficacy. A review by Feinstein and colleagues evaluated the methodology of eight community trials with specific reference to susceptibility bias, surveillance bias, and diagnostic testing bias; confidence intervals for reported efficacy were also calculated. The three trials judged to meet strict methodological criteria were the North American Indian, Chicago, and British trials: all showed protective efficacy (Table 3) (29). These three were also the only three with narrow confidence intervals; the remaining five, including those that purported to show negative efficacy, had broad confidence intervals including negative and positive efficacy. The South India trial was not interpreted to have adequate protection against surveillance bias and diagnostic testing bias.

A review by Colditz and colleagues analyzed 14 prospective trials and 12 case control studies, including several that were considered to have inadequate methods by the Feinstein analysis (31, 32). Based on both prospective and case control studies, the Colditz reviewers concluded that the overall protective efficacies of BCG were 50% for tuberculosis disease, 71% for tuberculosis mortality, and 64% for tuberculous meningitis.

Vaccine trial endpoints

Tuberculosis disease endpoints vary considerably in various tuberculosis vaccine trials, ranging from culture confirmation to clinical criteria. Two

prospective BCG trials and one trial of a new TB vaccine used both definite (culture confirmed) and probable (clinical criteria) definitions of tuberculosis. All three showed vaccine efficacy against definite tuberculosis but either lower or absent efficacy against probable tuberculosis (7, 160, 165). This finding has two possible explanations: misclassification of probable cases (unlikely, since criteria are rigorous) or existence of two forms of tuberculosis disease, one of which is more amenable to vaccine-based protection. It is possible that patients with probable or clinical tuberculosis have a paucibacillary form of disease similar to tuberculoid leprosy and already have a vigorous mycobacterial immune response that cannot be improved with immunization.

Prevention of infection

Most studies have evaluated the efficacy of BCG for protection against active tuberculosis disease. Latent infection had not been assessed as an efficacy endpoint when the presence of latent infection could only be assessed by tuberculin skin test (whose utility is limited since BCG itself can sometimes induce a positive tuberculin test). However, since IFN-γ release assays (IGRAs) are not affected by BCG, they can now be used to assess tuberculosis infection risk after immunization. Two studies have now suggested that BCG may reduce the risk of tuberculosis infection after high-risk exposure. In a Turkish study, 979 children with exposure to pulmonary tuberculosis were evaluated for latent tuberculosis infection using a T-cell-based enzyme-linked immunospot assay (143). BCG vaccination was protective for latent tuberculosis infection (odds ratio, 0.60; 95% confidence interval, 0.43 to 0.83). A British study found a similar reduction in risk of tuberculosis infection after a high-risk school exposure (40). Since IGRAs detect immune responses to *M. tuberculosis*-specific antigens, they cannot be used to assess protection against new vaccines that include attenuated or inactivated strains of *M. tuberculosis* or *M. tuberculosis*-specific antigens used in IGRAs.

Table 3. Efficacy of BCG against tuberculosis: trials meeting strict methodologic criteria[a]

Author(s)	Yr	Location	Subjects	No.	% Efficacy (disease)	% Efficacy (death)	Reference
Stein and Aronson	1953	Western United States	Age 0–20 yr (Native Americans)	3,008	67	82	147
Hart and Sutherland	1977	England	Newborns	26,465	76	NA	59
Rosenthal et al.	1961	Chicago	Newborns	3,381	72	84	130
Total				32,854	71	82	

[a]Studies selected based on analysis by Feinstein et al. (29). NA, not applicable.

Variations in BCG Efficacy

Other possible explanations for observed variations in the efficacy of BCG have included differences in potency of various strains, genetic or age differences in target populations, variations in efficacy against different forms of disease, and reduced virulence of some strains of *M. tuberculosis* (31). None of these hypotheses explains the observed variations as well as methodological differences in the trials and/or differences in preexisting mycobacterial immunity.

BCG revaccination

Although a few countries still administer booster doses of BCG to tuberculin-negative children, there is no evidence that revaccination confers additional protection against tuberculosis disease (35, 80, 93, 126) despite the enhancement of IFN-γ responses to mycobacterial antigens (10). Since BCG must replicate to induce immunity (20), it may be that the initial dose of BCG confers a sufficient immune response against the organism to prevent replication of the subsequent dose.

Efficacy of BCG against Other Diseases

M. leprae

Several studies have demonstrated efficacy of 50 to 80% against *M. leprae*, and this effect may be increased with booster doses of BCG (80), although these data are inconsistent (35).

M. ulcerans

BCG is also approximately 50% effective in preventing Buruli ulcer disease due to *M. ulcerans* (140). This includes protection against osteomyelitis, a major complication of *M. ulcerans* infection (120).

MAC

BCG also provides cross protection against childhood lymphadenitis due to MAC (81). Cessation of childhood BCG immunization has been associated with a marked increase in the rate of childhood adenitis due to NTM (127).

Childhood mortality

In addition, BCG immunization of children in developing countries has been associated with reduced all-cause mortality (84, 132). This effect is not specifically attributable to reduction in mortality from tuberculosis and is not fully understood.

Administration of BCG

Aventis Pasteur has withdrawn its license to distribute BCG in the United States for the prevention of tuberculosis, leaving the reconstituted Tice vaccine (Organon) as the sole licensed tuberculosis vaccine in the United States. The Tice vaccine contains a mixture of killed and live bacilli with a range of 37,500 to 3,000,000 CFU per dose (139), and the manufacturer recommends that 0.2 to 0.3 ml of vaccine reconstituted in 1.0 ml of sterile water be administered in the lower deltoid area by the multiple-puncture technique (0.2 to 0.3 ml reconstituted in 2 ml of sterile water for infants less than 1 year of age). The manufacturer's instructions should be consulted. Reconstituted vaccine should be refrigerated and should be protected from exposure to light. Unused vaccine should be discarded after 2 to 4 h and should be treated as infectious waste, as should all equipment used in vaccine preparation and manufacture. Tuberculin skin test conversion usually occurs 6 to 12 weeks after immunization.

Side Effects of BCG

General

Side effects of BCG immunization have been shown to be dependent on the BCG strain, dose, method of administration, and recipient (99). Neonates are more likely to experience complications than older children and adults. Small clusters of increased complication rates have been associated with a change in the strain or method of vaccination. Among strains currently in use, Pasteur and Danish have been associated with the highest rate of side effects. For example, lymphadenitis is more common with the Pasteur strain than with Tokyo or Brazil strain (121). The average amount (CFU) of viable bacilli varies by vaccine strain, and most products also include nonviable bacilli. Intradermal inoculation is associated with a higher rate of local reactions. The multiple-puncture technique has a lower rate of local reactions but is more costly, less precise, more time-consuming, and more technically involved (121). Adverse effects of BCG immunization are summarized in Table 4.

Common and local reactions

The most common side effect of BCG is a local reaction at the site of inoculation characterized by pain, swelling, and erythema. This is seen in 95% of vaccine recipients, typically lasts several weeks, and usually resolves by 3 months without any complication other than scar formation (23). Approximately 75% of

Table 4. Adverse effects of parenteral BCG immunization

Reaction type	Incidence	Comment(s)[a]	Reference(s)
Mild			
Injection site induration, pain, erythema	95%	Essentially all vaccines	23
Ulceration at inoculation site	70%	Varies with strain; increased in neonates	99, 100
Local ulceration/adenopathy	1–2%		100, 121
Serious			
Osteomyelitis	0.01–300/million	Varies with strain	85, 100
Disseminated infection	0.19–1.56/million	Associated with immunocompromised state (CGD, SCID, HIV, etc.)	16, 100, 116

[a]CGD, chronic granulomatous disease; SCID, severe combined immunodeficiency.

vaccinees also experience some myalgia. Seventy percent have ulceration with drainage at the vaccine site. Vaccine site abscess has been reported for 2% of recipients and regional lymphadenitis for 1 to 2% (85, 157).

Among those who develop adenitis, ulceration with drainage is more likely if the lesion develops rapidly and within 2 months after vaccination. Surgery is usually required if fistulas and drainage develop. The role of adjunctive antimycobacterial therapy remains controversial. More indolent and later-developing lesions are best managed with observation alone (25, 49).

Osteomyelitis

Osteomyelitis has been reported at a rate of between 0.01 per million vaccinees in Japan (multiple-puncture technique) and 300 per million in Finland (intradermal technique) (85). Treatment of osteomyelitis is accomplished with isoniazid and rifampin (BCG is resistant to pyrazinamide).

Disseminated disease

Disseminated disease, including fatal outcome, is reported at an overall rate between 0.19 and 1.56 per million vaccinees. Prior to the HIV epidemic, most cases of disseminated BCG occurred in infants with unrecognized severe combined immunodeficiency. Studies conducted in South Africa have documented disseminated BCG rates in the range of 407 to 1,300/100,000 HIV-infected infants (62). However, studies in other regions and with different BCG strains have found lower risk or no risk (8). Treatment is with isoniazid and rifampin (150) (see chapter 41).

Current Use of BCG

Developing countries

BCG is administered routinely to newborns in tuberculosis-endemic countries (149). Vaccine is typically administered over the deltoid or on the forearm. Because BCG is included in the list of recommended childhood immunizations by the WHO, current coverage is >80% in many countries. In countries with endemic HIV infection the World Health Organization recommends testing infants for HIV infection prior to administration of BCG. This recommendation should not be interpreted to cease routine BCG immunization of infants if HIV testing cannot be implemented (62).

Developed countries

BCG is still administered universally at birth in some developed countries and is administered selectively to just high-risk infants in other developed countries such as the United Kingdom, Finland, and Sweden, where the incidence of tuberculosis is falling (128, 134, 149). Selective immunization can strike a reasonable balance between protection and vaccine side effects in countries where the general incidence of tuberculosis is falling but high-risk groups can be identified at birth (61).

BCG has never been administered routinely in the United States but was used more widely before the incidence of tuberculosis reached its current low levels. For example, health care workers were often immunized in the last century, and many physicians and nurses who practiced in that era still have BCG scars (2). Because U.S. policy for the prevention of tuberculosis places a strong emphasis on tuberculin skin testing and treatment of latent infection, and because BCG may interfere with the tuberculin skin test, there has been a strong reluctance to endorse BCG for all potential high-risk groups. Current guidelines from the American Academy of Pediatrics and from the CDC Advisory Committee on Immunization Practices are listed in Table 5. The guidelines recommend BCG for a child who is continually exposed to a person with untreated or ineffectively treated tuberculosis and cannot be given antituberculous therapy. Additionally, BCG is recommended for a child exposed to a person with MDR tuberculosis when the child cannot be removed from contact with

Table 5. Recommendations for BCG use in the United States[a]

Advisory group recommendations
  Children with continuous exposure to a person with contagious
    MDR tuberculosis (and who cannot be removed from
    contact with the person)[b]
  Children with continuous exposure to a person with untreated
    or ineffectively treated pulmonary tuberculosis (and who
    cannot be removed from contact with the person)[b]
  Health care workers exposed to contagious MDR tuberculosis
    in settings where infection control programs have failed to
    prevent transmission[c]
Additional recommendations
  Tuberculin-negative homeless persons (24)
  Infants or tuberculin-negative adults moving to tuberculosis-
    endemic countries
  Health care workers (medical students, physicians, nurses, etc.),
    medical relief workers, missionaries, and others traveling to
    conduct direct patient care activities in tuberculosis-endemic
    countries (30)
Contraindications
  HIV infection or other immunodeficiency (e.g., SCID, DiGeorge
    syndrome)
  Hematologic or generalized malignancy
  Immunosuppression (e.g., TNF blocking agents, chronic steroid
    therapy, alkylating agents, antimetabolites, radiation)
  Positive tuberculin skin test or prior tuberculosis

[a]SCID, severe combined immunodeficiency; TNF, tumor necrosis factor.
[b]See reference 4a.
[c]See reference 25a.

Table 6. Characteristics of BCG

Favorable characteristics
  Newborn immunization reduces risk of disease and death due
    to childhood tuberculosis
  Newborn immunization reduces risk of miliary and meningeal
    tuberculosis
  Newborn immunization reduces risk of childhood
    nontuberculous lymphadenitis, leprosy, and M. ulcerans
    infection
  Low cost
Unfavorable characteristics
  Limited efficacy against reactivation disease
  Limited efficacy in mycobacterium-experienced children and
    adults
  Uncertain efficacy in HIV infection
  Limited duration of efficacy
  Genetic variation in licensed vaccine strains
  Frequency and duration of local vaccine site reactions
  Risk of BCG adenitis or osteomyelitis in healthy recipients
  Risk of disseminated BCG in HIV-infected recipients
  Absence of booster effect
  Requirement for parenteral immunization
  Effect on skin test reaction to tuberculin
  Unknown immune correlate of protection

the index case. These guidelines are sufficiently restrictive that BCG manufacturers have been reluctant to distribute vaccine in the United States. The guidelines do not include other important high-risk groups such as homeless persons in the United States (24), medical relief personnel from low-incidence countries working in tuberculosis-endemic areas (30), and U.S. children moving to tuberculosis-endemic countries. A revision of U.S. guidelines is currently under way and will likely include a recommendation for immunization of health care and medical relief workers working in regions where they may be exposed to MDR tuberculosis. Until then, the predominant use of BCG in the United States is topical installation in the bladder for treatment of bladder cancer (137).

NEW VACCINES AGAINST TUBERCULOSIS

Rationale

The favorable and unfavorable characteristics of BCG are summarized in Table 6. The efficacy of BCG against tuberculosis is high when administered to newborns, but this protection from tuberculosis disease likely wanes into adulthood, and there is likely minimal, if any, protection against reactivation tuberculosis in adults. In addition, BCG boosters are

ineffective (126). There is thus wide consensus that additional tuberculosis vaccine development should focus on identifying a booster vaccine to follow BCG immunization, or on developing a completely novel two-vaccine booster regimen. Although enhanced potency is cited as one goal of new tuberculosis vaccine development, equally important goals include reducing the risk of side effects and improving the duration of protection. Because HIV-associated tuberculosis may now account for more than 50% of global cases of tuberculosis, another important goal is the development of a safe, effective, and durable vaccine strategy for the prevention of HIV-associated tuberculosis (166). Further, new vaccines should be economical, and single-dose vaccines would be preferable to those that require multiple doses. It would also be advantageous to have a vaccine that does not require parenteral immunization (66). Fortunately, the development of IGRAs has made vaccine-mediated interference with tuberculin skin test responses less critical for new tuberculosis vaccine candidates.

Animal Testing

Candidate vaccines are typically screened for immunogenicity and protective efficacy in the mouse model. BCG vaccine is used as a "gold standard" and generally produces a 0.7-log reduction in CFU in the lung after virulent M. tuberculosis challenge (119). However, disease in mice differs in several respects from disease in humans. For example, latent TB does not occur in mice, and thus it is not known whether vaccines which reduce lung CFUs in mice will prevent tuberculosis in humans. There are examples where this model is not predictive. For example, *M. microti* is effective in humans but was found to have only marginal activity in the standard mouse model (119). Recent studies in the mouse model indicate that the immune response to challenge depends on the inoculum: higher inocula produce immune responses resembling immune responses in humans naturally exposed to tuberculosis, reinforcing that extrapolation from the animal model (114).

The guinea pig is more sensitive than the mouse to *M. tuberculosis* infection and demonstrates higher CFUs after challenge and progressive lung pathology. In this model protection can be assessed using the endpoints of survival time and degree of lung pathology (119). Macaques and cynomolgus monkeys can also be used for preclinical evaluation of vaccine candidates and have several advantages over rodent models (disease more closely mimics human tuberculosis, antigen presentation and T-cell receptor repertoire are similar to those in humans, and there has been more relevant safety evaluation), but testing in primates is expensive (91). Regardless of the animal model used, animal model immunogenicity is not certain to correlate with vaccine-mediated protection against tuberculosis disease in humans.

Human Trials

Candidate vaccines are first tested for safety in small numbers of healthy adults, then in children, and subsequently in immunocompromised subjects such as those with HIV infection. Safety trials are conducted in both mycobacterium-naïve and mycobacterium-experienced populations, including subjects with and without prior BCG and subjects from tuberculosis-endemic regions. Safe vaccines then proceed to human immunogenicity (phase II) testing in the same populations. Relevant immune responses are identified above and include polyfunctional and memory responses to a wide range of mycobacterial antigens by $CD4^+$ and $CD8^+$ T cells, antibody responses, and assays of immune cell proliferation. Subsequent phase II studies are designed to determine optimal doses and schedules. Controlled efficacy trials (phase III) then follow. Trials in adult subjects can be targeted to high-risk subjects to reduce sample sizes and follow-up periods (69). Household contacts of tuberculosis cases and persons with early HIV infection would both be suitable. In pediatric and HIV-positive subjects, both pulmonary and bacteremic tuberculosis should be used as endpoints (162).

Vaccine Strategies

Many new candidate tuberculosis vaccines are in various stages of development and testing (90). Each approach has theoretical advantages and disadvantages. Selected vaccines with current or imminent testing in humans are listed in Table 7 and are described below.

Candidate antigens are often selected for use in tuberculosis vaccines because they elicit detectable immune responses among the majority of individuals exposed to tuberculosis, perhaps via enhanced antigen exposure on the surface of infected cells (8). Other antigens have been selected from those to which healthy purified protein derivative-positive donors (i.e., persons who have successfully contained latent infection) respond (4). Leading subunit antigens include *M. tuberculosis* Ag85, ESAT, CFP 10, and Mtb72f. Advantages of subunit vaccine approaches include safety, low reactogenicity, and easy evaluation of vaccine immunogenicity. Potential downsides include the elicitation of immune responses against a narrow antigen repertoire.

Animal studies have demonstrated the efficacy of whole-cell inactivated vaccines, emphasizing the potential importance of multiple antigens, including those derived from cell wall, membrane, and cytosolic components of the organism (3). These findings, and the observation of tuberculosis protection after immunization with BCG or live *M. microti*, have driven the continued use of whole-cell vaccines, like BCG, and the development of novel whole-cell vaccines such as whole inactivated *M. vaccae* (104, 169). A phase III efficacy study of *M. vaccae* conducted among HIV-infected subjects in Tanzania with prior BCG immunization showed that a multiple-dose series was safe and reduced the risk of definite tuberculosis by 39% (165). Whole-cell vaccines may elicit immune responses against a broader repertoire of mycobacterial antigens, but live whole-cell mycobacterial vaccines may have decreased vaccine replication in previously BCG-immunized hosts, thus compromising vaccine immunogenicity.

Recombinant versions of BCG have been engineered to enhance vaccine immunogenicity. Examples include recombinant BCG engineered to overexpress Ag85, or the recombinant BCG Prague strain expressing listeriolysin, which improves antigen presentation by enhancing antigen escape from the phagosome (51). It remains to be seen if the enhanced immunogenicity of newer-generation BCG-based vaccines may come at a cost of exacerbated reactogenicity, and the efficacy of any live vaccine must be weighed against the risk of disseminated vaccine disease in immunocompromised hosts.

Table 7. Selected promising tuberculosis candidate vaccines

Type of vaccine	Vaccine	Description	Supporting evidence	Stage of development	Reference(s)
Priming vaccines					
Whole organism, recombinant, live	rBCG30	Recombinant BCG enhanced by overexpression of Ag 85	Superior to BCG in a guinea pig aerosol challenge model. Elicits humoral and cellular immune responses in guinea pigs, the former correlating with protection. Boosts immune responses to tuberculosis antigens in humans.	Phase I completed	65, 72, 73
	VPM 1002	Recombinant rBCG Prague strain expressing listeriolysin; carries a urease deletion mutation which allows escape from the phagosome and thus improved antigen presentation	Superior to BCG in murine aerosol challenge models	Phase I	51
Booster vaccines					
Whole organism, inactivated	*Mycobacterium vaccae*	NTM infection protects against tuberculosis	Elicits protection from aerosol tuberculosis challenge in mice. Boosts immune responses to vaccine antigen in BCG-immunized humans. Protects against culture-confirmed tuberculosis in phase III randomized placebo-controlled trial in HIV-infected and BCG-immunized adults.	Phase III completed 2008	88a, 165, 168, 169
Viral vector/subunit	Oxford MVA85A/ Virus Aeras-485	Modified vaccinia Ankara vector expressing Ag85A	Intranasal but not intradermal immunization boosts BCG protection from aerosol tuberculosis challenge in mice. Immunization boosts immune responses to vaccine antigen in BCG-immunized humans. Immunization in BCG-primed humans is safe and elicits polyfunctional CD4$^+$ and CD8$^+$ T-cell responses to mycobacterial antigens in humans.	Phase IIb	46, 135, 136, 173
	Crucell Ad35/ Aeras-402	Replication-deficient adenovirus 35 vector expressing Ag85A, Ag85B, and TB10.4	Intranasal or intramuscular administration elicits CD4$^+$ and CD8$^+$ T-cell responses to mycobacterial antigens and protects mice from aerosol tuberculosis challenge. Safe in healthy human subjects.	Phase II	12, 103, 122, 138
Adjuvanted subunit	Mtb72f /AS02A	Combination of Mtb39 cell membrane-associated protein and Mtb32 modified serine protease in the AS02A adjuvant platform	Coadministration with BCG enhances guinea pig protection from aerosol challenge. Administration after BCG affords protection from central nervous system challenge similar to that of BCG alone in a rabbit model. Equivalent to BCG alone in rabbit model. Boosted BCG responses and afforded superior protection in intratracheal tuberculosis challenge compared to BCG in a cynomolgus monkey model.	Phase II	21, 124, 155
Mucosal	NasL3/AM85B conjugate	Intranasal vaccine with man-capped arabinomannan oligosaccharide conjugated to Ag85B in a proprietary adjuvant	Immunogenic in mice and, when used to boost BCG, provides augmented protection from tuberculosis in the spleen but not lungs. Mice immunized with NasL3/AM85B conjugate booster exhibited less lung inflammation and granuloma formation.	Phase I	53, 54

BCG was originally given orally, and given the propensity of mucosal immunization with tuberculosis vaccine candidates to elicit greater immune responses in mucosal sites such as the lungs (11, 27, 66, 75, 88), mucosal immunization regimens remain the subject of ongoing study and candidate vaccine development (79). One candidate mucosal vaccine against tuberculosis is NasL3/AM85B conjugate vaccine. Furthermore, there have been promising immunogenicity and aerosol challenge results in animal models of a lipid-encapsulated oral formulation of BCG (28, 34, 37, 153, 161). It will be important to determine if the efficacy of mucosal immunization against tuberculosis will be compromised by diarrheal illnesses prevalent in areas where tuberculosis is endemic, such as affected the efficacy of oral polio vaccination programs (177).

CONCLUSIONS

BCG is associated with protection from tuberculosis in mycobacterium-naïve hosts but is frequently associated with local side effects and also carries a risk of life-threatening disseminated BCG disease in newborns who have HIV infection. Despite global use of BCG immunization, morbidity and mortality from tuberculosis remain unacceptably high. Multiple new tuberculosis vaccine candidates are now in various stages of development, either to improve upon the safety and immunogenicity of BCG or to boost BCG responses.

Acknowledgment. We thank Jerome Larkin for contributions to an earlier version of this chapter.

REFERENCES

1. Abebe, F., and G. Bjune. 2009. The protective role of antibody responses during *Mycobacterium tuberculosis* infection. *Clin. Exp. Immunol.* 157:235–243.
2. Abruzzi, W. A., Jr., and R. J. Hummel. 1953. Tuberculosis: incidence among American medical students, prevention and control and the use of BCG. *N. Engl. J. Med.* 248:722–729.
3. Agger, E. M., K. Weldingh, A. W. Olsen, I. Rosenkrands, and P. Andersen. 2002. Specific acquired resistance in mice immunized with killed mycobacteria. *Scand. J. Immunol.* 56:443–447.
4. Alderson, M. R., T. Bement, C. H. Day, L. Zhu, D. Molesh, Y. A. Skeiky, R. N. Coler, D. M. Lewinsohn, S. G. Reed, and S. G. Dillon. 2000. Expression cloning of an immunodominant family of *Mycobacterium tuberculosis* antigens using human CD4+ T cells. *J. Exp. Med.* 191:551–559.
4a. American Academy of Pediatrics. 2003. *Report of the Committee on Infectious Diseases.* American Academy of Pediatrics, Elk Grove, IL.
5. Andersen, P. 2001. TB vaccines: progress and problems. *Trends Immunol.* 22:160–168.
6. Aronson, J. D. 1948. Protective vaccination against tuberculosis with special reference to BCG vaccination. *Am. Rev. Tuberc.* 58:255–281.
7. Aronson, N. E., M. Santosham, G. W. Comstock, R. S. Howard, L. H. Moulton, E. R. Rhoades, and L. H. Harrison. 2004. Long-term efficacy of BCG vaccine in American Indians and Alaska Natives: a 60-year follow-up study. *JAMA* 291:2086–2091.
8. Azzopardi, P., C. M. Bennett, S. M. Graham, and T. Duke. 2009. Bacille Calmette-Guerin vaccine-related disease in HIV-infected children: a systematic review. *Int. J. Tuberc. Lung Dis.* 13:1331–1344.
9. Badri, M., W. Wilson, and R. Wood. 2002. Effect of highly active antiretroviral therapy on incidence of tuberculosis in South Africa: a cohort study. *Lancet* 359:2059–2064.
10. Barbosa, T., S. Arruda, B. D. Fernandes, L. P. Carvalho, S. Cardoso, S. Cunha, M. L. Barreto, S. M. Pereira, L. C. Rodrigues, and M. Barral-Netto. 2003. BCG (Bacille of Calmette-Guerin) revaccination leads to improved in vitro IFN-gamma response to mycobacterial antigen independent of tuberculin sensitization in Brazilian school-age children. *Vaccine* 21:2152–2160.
11. Barclay, W. R., W. M. Busey, D. W. Dalgard, R. C. Good, B. W. Janicki, J. E. Kasik, E. Ribi, C. E. Ulrich, and E. Wolinsky. 1973. Protection of monkeys against airborne tuberculosis by aerosol vaccination with Bacillus Calmette-Guerin. *Am. Rev. Respir. Dis.* 107:351–358.
12. Barker, L. F., M. J. Brennan, P. K. Rosenstein, and J. C. Sadoff. 2009. Tuberculosis vaccine research: the impact of immunology. *Curr. Opin. Immunol.* 21:331–338.
13. Barreto, M. L., S. S. Cunha, S. M. Pereira, B. Genser, M. A. Hijjar, M. Yury Ichihara, S. C. de Brito, I. Dourado, A. Cruz, C. Santa'Ana, and L. C. Rodrigues. 2005. Neonatal BCG protection against tuberculosis lasts for 20 years in Brazil. *Int. J. Tuberc. Lung Dis.* 9:1171–1173.
14. Behr, M. A. 2001. Correlation between BCG genomics and protective efficacy. *Scand. J. Infect. Dis.* 33:249–252.
15. Bendiner, E. 1992. Albert Calmette: a vaccine and its vindication. *Hosp. Pract. (Off. Ed.)* 27:113–116, 119–122, 125 passim.
16. Besnard, M., S. Sauvion, C. Offredo, J. Gaudelus, J. L. Gaillard, F. Veber, and S. Blanche. 1993. Bacillus Calmette-Guerin infection after vaccination of human immunodeficiency virus-infected children. *Pediatr. Infect. Dis. J.* 12:993–997.
17. Beyazova, U., S. Rota, C. Cevheroglu, and T. Karsligil. 1995. Humoral immune response in infants after BCG vaccination. *Tuberc. Lung Dis.* 76:248–253.
18. Black, G. F., B. A. Thiel, M. O. Ota, S. K. Parida, R. Adegbola, W. H. Boom, H. M. Dockrell, K. L. Franken, A. H. Friggen, P. C. Hill, M. R. Klein, M. K. Lalor, H. Mayanja, G. Schoolnik, K. Stanley, K. Weldingh, S. H. Kaufmann, G. Walzl, and T. H. Ottenhoff. 2009. Immunogenicity of novel DosR regulon-encoded candidate antigens of *Mycobacterium tuberculosis* in three high-burden populations in Africa. *Clin. Vaccine Immunol.* 16:1203–1212.
19. Boelaert, J. R., S. J. Vandecasteele, R. Appelberg, and V. R. Gordeuk. 2007. The effect of the host's iron status on tuberculosis. *J. Infect. Dis.* 195:1745–1753.
20. Brandt, L., J. F. Cunha, A. W. Olsen, B. Chilima, P. Hirsch, R. Appleberg, and P. Andersen. 2002. Failure of the *Mycobacterium bovis* BCG vaccine: some species of environmental mycobacteria block multiplication of BCG and induction of protective immunity to tuberculosis. *Infect. Immun.* 70:672–678.
21. Brandt, L., Y. A. Skeiky, M. R. Alderson, Y. Lobet, W. Dalemans, O. C. Turner, R. J. Basaraba, A. A. Izzo, T. M. Lasco, P. L. Chapman, S. G. Reed, and I. M. Orme. 2004. The protective

effect of the *Mycobacterium bovis* BCG vaccine is increased by coadministration with the *Mycobacterium tuberculosis* 72-kilodalton fusion polyprotein Mtb72F in *M. tuberculosis*-infected guinea pigs. *Infect. Immun.* **72**:6622–6632.

22. **Brennan, M. J., and U. Fruth.** 2002. Global forum on TB vaccine research and development. World Health Organization, June 7–8, 2001, Geneva. *Tuberculosis* (Edinburgh) **81**:365–368.

23. **Brewer, M. A., K. M. Edwards, P. S. Palmer, and H. P. Hinson.** 1994. Bacille Calmette-Guerin immunization in normal healthy adults. *J. Infect. Dis.* **170**:476–479.

24. **Brewer, T. F., S. J. Heymann, S. M. Krumplitsh, M. E. Wilson, G. A. Colditz, and H. V. Fineberg.** 2001. Strategies to decrease tuberculosis in US homeless populations. *JAMA* **286**:834–842.

25. **Caglayan, S., O. Yegin, K. Kayran, N. Timocin, E. Kasirga, and M. Gun.** 1987. Is medical therapy effective for regional lymphadenitis following BCG vaccination? *Am. J. Dis. Child.* **141**:1213–1214.

25a. **Centers for Disease Control and Prevention.** 1996. The role of BCG vaccine in the prevention and control of tuberculosis in the United States: a joint statement by the Advisory Committee for the Elimination of Tuberculosis and the Advisory Committee on Immunization Practices. *MMWR Morb. Mortal. Wkly. Rep.* **45**:1–18.

26. **Chandra, R. N. P.** 1977. *Nutrition, Immunity and Infection: Mechanisms of Interactions.* Plenum Press, New York, NY.

26a. **Chen, C. Y., D. Huang, R. C. Wang, L. Shen, G. Zeng, S. Yao, Y. Shen, L. Halliday, J. Fortman, M. McAllister, J. Estep, R. Hunt, D. Vasconcelos, G. Du, S. A. Porcelli, M. H. Larsen, W. R. Jacobs, Jr., B. F. Haynes, N. L. Letvin, and Z. W. Chen.** 2009. A critical role for CD8 T cells in a nonhuman primate model of tuberculosis. *PLoS* **5**(4):e1000392.

27. **Chen, L., J. Wang, A. Zganiacz, and Z. Xing.** 2004. Single intranasal mucosal *Mycobacterium bovis* BCG vaccination confers improved protection compared to subcutaneous vaccination against pulmonary tuberculosis. *Infect. Immun.* **72**:238–246.

28. **Clark, S., M. L. Cross, A. Smith, P. Court, J. Vipond, A. Nadian, R. G. Hewinson, H. K. Batchelor, Y. Perrie, A. Williams, F. E. Aldwell, and M. A. Chambers.** 2008. Assessment of different formulations of oral *Mycobacterium bovis* Bacille Calmette-Guerin (BCG) vaccine in rodent models for immunogenicity and protection against aerosol challenge with *M. bovis. Vaccine* **26**:5791–5797.

29. **Clemens, J. D., J. J. Chuong, and A. R. Feinstein.** 1983. The BCG controversy: a methodological and statistical reappraisal. *JAMA* **249**:2362–2369.

30. **Cobelens, F. G., H. van Deutekom, I. Draayer-Jansen, A. C. Schepp-Beelen, P. J. van Gerven, R. P. van Kessel, and M. E. Mensen.** 2000. Risk of infection with *Mycobacterium tuberculosis* in travellers to areas of high tuberculosis endemicity. *Lancet* **356**:461–465.

31. **Colditz, G. A., C. S. Berkey, F. Mosteller, T. F. Brewer, M. E. Wilson, E. Burdick, and H. V. Fineberg.** 1995. The efficacy of bacillus Calmette-Guérin vaccination of newborns and infants in the prevention of tuberculosis: meta-analyses of the published literature. *Pediatrics* **96**:29–35.

32. **Colditz, G. A., T. F. Brewer, C. S. Berkey, M. E. Wilson, E. Burdick, H. V. Fineberg, and F. Mosteller.** 1994. Efficacy of BCG vaccine in the prevention of tuberculosis: meta-analysis of the published literature. *JAMA* **271**:698–702.

33. **Constant, P., F. Davodeau, M. A. Peyrat, Y. Poquet, G. Puzo, M. Bonneville, and J. J. Fournie.** 1994. Stimulation of human gamma delta T cells by nonpeptidic mycobacterial ligands. *Science* **264**:267–270.

34. **Cross, M. L., M. R. Lambeth, Y. Coughlan, and F. E. Aldwell.** 2007. Oral vaccination of mice with lipid-encapsulated *Mycobacterium bovis* BCG: effect of reducing or eliminating BCG load on cell-mediated immunity. *Vaccine* **25**:1297–1303.

35. **Cunha, S. S., N. Alexander, M. L. Barreto, E. S. Pereira, I. Dourado, F. Maroja Mde, Y. Ichihara, S. Brito, S. Pereira, and L. C. Rodrigues.** 2008. BCG revaccination does not protect against leprosy in the Brazilian Amazon: a cluster randomised trial. *PLoS Negl. Trop. Dis.* **2**:e167.

36. **Day, C. L., N. Mkhwanazi, S. Reddy, Z. Mncube, M. van der Stok, P. Klenerman, and B. D. Walker.** 2008. Detection of polyfunctional *Mycobacterium tuberculosis*-specific T cells and association with viral load in HIV-1-infected persons. *J. Infect. Dis.* **197**:990–999.

37. **Dorer, D. E., W. Czepluch, M. R. Lambeth, A. C. Dunn, C. Reitinger, F. E. Aldwell, and A. D. McLellan.** 2007. Lymphatic tracing and T cell responses following oral vaccination with live *Mycobacterium bovis* (BCG). *Cell. Microbiol.* **9**:544–553.

38. **Edwards, L. B., and C. E. Palmer.** 1968. Identification of the tuberculous-infected by skin tests. *Ann. N. Y. Acad. Sci.* **154**:140–148.

39. **Edwards, M. L., J. M. Goodrich, D. Muller, A. Pollack, J. E. Ziegler, and D. W. Smith.** 1982. Infection with *Mycobacterium avium-intracellulare* and the protective effects of Bacille Calmette-Guerin. *J. Infect. Dis.* **145**:733–741.

40. **Eisenhut, M., S. Paranjothy, I. Abubakar, S. Bracebridge, M. Lilley, R. Mulla, K. Lack, D. Chalkley, and M. McEvoy.** 2009. BCG vaccination reduces risk of infection with *Mycobacterium tuberculosis* as detected by gamma interferon release assay. *Vaccine* **27**:6116–6120.

41. **Fairchok, M. P., J. H. Rouse, and S. L. Morris.** 1995. Age-dependent humoral responses of children to mycobacterial antigens. *Clin. Diagn. Lab. Immunol.* **2**:443–447.

42. **Ferguson, R. G., and A. B. Simes.** 1949. BCG vaccination of infant Indians in Saskatchewan. *Tubercle* **30**:5–11.

43. **Fine, P. E., I. A. Carneiro, J. B. Milstien, and C. J. Clements.** 1999. *Issues Relating to the Use of BCG in Immunization Programs: a Discussion Document.* Department of Vaccines and Biologicals, World Health Organization, Geneva, Switzerland.

44. **Fine, P. E. M.** 1995. Variation in protection by BCG: implications of and for heterologous immunity. *Lancet* **346**:1339–1345.

45. **Flahiff, E. W.** 1939. The occurrence of tuberculosis in persons who failed to react to tuberculin, and in persons with positive tuberculin reaction. *Am. J. Epidemiol.* **30**(Section B):69–74.

46. **Forbes, E. K., C. Sander, E. O. Ronan, H. McShane, A. V. Hill, P. C. Beverley, and E. Z. Tchilian.** 2008. Multifunctional, high-level cytokine-producing Th1 cells in the lung, but not spleen, correlate with protection against *Mycobacterium tuberculosis* aerosol challenge in mice. *J. Immunol.* **181**:4955–4964.

47. **Glynn, J. R., J. Murray, A. Bester, G. Nelson, S. Shearer, and P. Sonnenberg.** 2010. High rates of recurrence in HIV-infected and HIV-uninfected patients with tuberculosis. *J. Infect. Dis.* **201**:704–711.

48. **Golub, J. E., V. Saraceni, S. C. Cavalcante, A. G. Pacheco, L. H. Moulton, B. S. King, A. Efron, R. D. Moore, R. E. Chaisson, and B. Durovni.** 2007. The impact of antiretroviral therapy and isoniazid preventive therapy on tuberculosis incidence in HIV-infected patients in Rio de Janeiro, Brazil. *AIDS* **21**:1441–1448.

49. **Goraya, J. S., and V. S. Virdi.** 2001. Treatment of Calmette-Guerin bacillus adenitis: a metaanalysis. *Pediatr. Infect. Dis. J.* **20**:632–634.

50. **Grant, A. D., S. Charalambous, K. L. Fielding, J. H. Day, E. L. Corbett, R. E. Chaisson, K. M. De Cock, R. J. Hayes, and G. J. Churchyard.** 2005. Effect of routine isoniazid preventive therapy on tuberculosis incidence among HIV-infected men in South Africa: a novel randomized incremental recruitment study. *JAMA* **293**:2719–2725.

51. Grode, L., P. Seiler, S. Baumann, J. Hess, V. Brinkmann, A. Nasser Eddine, P. Mann, C. Goosmann, S. Bandermann, D. Smith, G. J. Bancroft, J. M. Reyrat, D. van Soolingen, B. Raupach, and S. H. Kaufmann. 2005. Increased vaccine efficacy against tuberculosis of recombinant *Mycobacterium bovis* bacille Calmette-Guerin mutants that secrete listeriolysin. *J. Clin. Investig.* **115:**2472–2479.

52. Gutierrez, M. G., S. S. Master, S. B. Singh, G. A. Taylor, M. I. Colombo, and V. Deretic. 2004. Autophagy is a defense mechanism inhibiting BCG and *Mycobacterium tuberculosis* survival in infected macrophages. *Cell* **119:**753–766.

53. Haile, M., B. Hamasur, T. Jaxmar, D. Gavier-Widen, M. A. Chambers, B. Sanchez, U. Schroder, G. Kallenius, S. B. Svenson, and A. Pawlowski. 2005. Nasal boost with adjuvanted heat-killed BCG or arabinomannan-protein conjugate improves primary BCG-induced protection in C57BL/6 mice. *Tuberculosis* (Edinburgh) **85:**107–114.

54. Haile, M., U. Schroder, B. Hamasur, A. Pawlowski, T. Jaxmar, G. Kallenius, and S. B. Svenson. 2004. Immunization with heat-killed *Mycobacterium bovis* bacille Calmette-Guerin (BCG) in Eurocine L3 adjuvant protects against tuberculosis. *Vaccine* **22:**1498–1508.

55. Hanrahan, C. F., J. E. Golub, L. Mohapi, N. Tshabangu, T. Modisenyane, R. E. Chaisson, G. E. Gray, J. A. McIntyre, and N. A. Martinson. 2010. BMI and risk of tuberculosis and death: a prospective cohort of HIV-infected adults from South Africa. *AIDS* **24:**1501–1508.

56. Harries, A. D., N. J. Hargreaves, J. Kemp, A. Jindani, D. A. Enarson, D. Maher, and F. M. Salanponi. 2001. Deaths from tuberculosis in sub-Saharan African countries with a high prevalence of HIV-1. *Lancet* **357:**1519–1523.

57. Harris, J., S. A. De Haro, S. S. Master, J. Keane, E. A. Roberts, M. Delgado, and V. Deretic. 2007. T helper 2 cytokines inhibit autophagic control of intracellular *Mycobacterium tuberculosis*. *Immunity* **27:**505–517.

58. Hart, P. D., J. A. Armstrong, C. A. Brown, and P. Draper. 1972. Ultrastructural study of the behavior of macrophages toward parasitic mycobacteria. *Infect. Immun.* **5:**803–807.

59. Hart, P. D., and I. Sutherland. 1977. BCG and vole bacillus vaccines in the prevention of tuberculosis in adolescence and early adult life. *Br. Med. J.* **2:**293–295.

60. Hawkridge, A., M. Hatherill, F. Little, M. A. Goetz, L. Barker, H. Mahomed, J. Sadoff, W. Hanekom, L. Geiter, and G. Hussey. 2008. Efficacy of percutaneous versus intradermal BCG in the prevention of tuberculosis in South African infants: randomised trial. *BMJ* **337:**a2052.

61. Hersh, A. L., M. Tala-Heikkilä, E. Tala, A. N. A. Tosteson, and C. F. von Reyn. 2002. A cost-effectiveness analysis of universal versus selective immunization with *Mycobacterium bovis* bacille Calmette-Guerin in Finland. *Int. J. Tuberc. Lung Dis.* **7:**22–29.

62. Hesseling, A. C., M. F. Cotton, C. Fordham von Reyn, S. M. Graham, R. P. Gie, and G. D. Hussey. 2008. Consensus statement on the revised World Health Organization recommendations for BCG vaccination in HIV-infected infants. *Int. J. Tuberc. Lung Dis.* **12:**1376–1379.

63. Hesseling, A. C., B. J. Marais, R. P. Gie, H. S. Schaaf, P. E. Fine, P. Godfrey-Faussett, and N. Beyers. 2007. The risk of disseminated Bacille Calmette-Guerin (BCG) disease in HIV-infected children. *Vaccine* **25:**14–18.

64. Hesseling, A. C., H. S. Schaaf, W. A. Hanekom, N. Beyers, M. F. Cotton, R. P. Gie, B. J. Marais, P. van Helden, and R. M. Warren. 2003. Danish bacille Calmette-Guerin vaccine-induced disease in human immunodeficiency virus-infected children. *Clin. Infect. Dis.* **37:**1226–1233.

65. Hoft, D. F., A. Blazevic, G. Abate, W. A. Hanekom, G. Kaplan, J. H. Soler, F. Weichold, L. Geiter, J. C. Sadoff, and M. A. Horwitz. 2008. A new recombinant bacille Calmette-Guerin vaccine safely induces significantly enhanced tuberculosis-specific immunity in human volunteers. *J. Infect. Dis.* **198:**1491–1501.

66. Hoft, D. F., R. M. Brown, and R. B. Belshe. 2000. Mucosal Bacille Calmette Guerin vaccination of humans inhibits delayed type hypersensitivity to purified protein derivative but induces mycobacteria-specific interferon gamma responses. *Clin. Infect. Dis.* **30**(Suppl. 3):S217–S222.

67. Hoft, D. F., E. B. Kemp, O. Marinaro, H. Cruz, J. R. Kiyono, J. T. McGhee, T. W. Belisle, J. P. Miller, and R. B. Belshe. 1999. A double-blind, placebo-controlled study of *Mycobacterium*-specific human immune responses induced by intradermal bacille Calmette-Guérin vaccination. *J. Lab. Clin. Med.* **134:**244–252.

68. Hoft, D. F., and J. M. Tennant. 1999. Persistence and boosting of Bacille Calmette-Guérin-induced delayed-type hypersensitivity. *Ann. Intern. Med.* **131:**32–36.

69. Horsburgh, C. R. 2000. A large, simple trial of a tuberculosis vaccine. *Clin. Infect. Dis.* **30**(Suppl. 3):S213–216.

70. Horsburgh, C. R., Jr. 2004. Priorities for the treatment of latent tuberculosis infection in the United States. *N. Engl. J. Med.* **350:**2060–2067.

71. Horsburgh, C. R., Jr., M. O'Donnell, S. Chamblee, J. L. Moreland, J. Johnson, B. J. Marsh, M. Narita, L. S. Johnson, and C. F. von Reyn. 2010. Revisiting rates of reactivation tuberculosis: a population-based approach. *Am. J. Respir. Crit. Care Med.* **182:**420–425.

72. Horwitz, M. A., and G. Harth. 2003. A new vaccine against tuberculosis affords greater survival after challenge than the current vaccine in the guinea pig model of pulmonary tuberculosis. *Infect. Immun.* **71:**1672–1679.

73. Horwitz, M. A., G. Harth, B. J. Dillon, and S. Maslesa-Galic. 2006. Extraordinarily few organisms of a live recombinant BCG vaccine against tuberculosis induce maximal cell-mediated and protective immunity. *Vaccine* **24:**443–451.

74. Jeon, C. Y., and M. B. Murray. 2008. Diabetes mellitus increases the risk of active tuberculosis: a systematic review of 13 observational studies. *PLoS Med.* **5:**e152.

75. Jeyanathan, M., J. Mu, S. McCormick, D. Damjanovic, C. L. Small, C. R. Shaler, K. Kugathasan, and Z. Xing. Murine airway luminal antituberculosis memory CD8 T cells by mucosal immunization are maintained via antigen-driven in situ proliferation, independent of peripheral T cell recruitment. *Am. J. Respir. Crit. Care Med.* **181:**862–872.

76. Johnson, J. L., A. Okwera, D. L. Hom, H. Mayanja, C. Mutuluuza Kityo, P. Nsubuga, J. G. Nakibali, A. M. Loughlin, H. Yun, P. N. Mugyenyi, A. Vernon, R. D. Mugerwa, J. J. Ellner, and C. C. Whalen. 2001. Duration of efficacy of treatment of latent tuberculosis infection in HIV-infected adults. *AIDS* **15:**2137–2147.

77. Joosten, S. A., K. E. van Meijgaarden, P. C. van Weeren, F. Kazi, A. Geluk, N. D. Savage, J. W. Drijfhout, D. R. Flower, W. A. Hanekom, M. R. Klein, and T. H. Ottenhoff. 2010. *Mycobacterium tuberculosis* peptides presented by HLA-E molecules are targets for human CD8 T-cells with cytotoxic as well as regulatory activity. *PLoS Pathog.* **6:**e1000782.

78. Jouanguy, E., F. Altare, S. Lamhamedi, P. Revy, J. F. Emile, M. Newport, M. Levin, S. Blanche, E. Seboun, A. Fischer, J. L. Casanova, E. Jouanguy, F. Altare, S. Lamhamedi, P. Revy, J. F. Emile, M. Newport, M. Levin, S. Blanche, E. Seboun, A. Fischer, and J. L. Casanova. 1996. Interferon-gamma-receptor deficiency in an infant with fatal bacille Calmette-Guerin infection. *N. Engl. J. Med.* **335:**1956–1961.

79. Kallenius, G., A. Pawlowski, P. Brandtzaeg, and S. Svenson. 2007. Should a new tuberculosis vaccine be administered intranasally? *Tuberculosis* (Edinburgh) **87:**257–266.

80. Karonga Trial Prevention Group. 1996. Randomised controlled trial of single BCG, repeated BCG, or combined BCG and killed *Mycobacterium leprae* vaccine for prevention of leprosy and tuberculosis in Malawi. *Lancet* 348:17–24.

81. Katila, M. L., E. Brander, and A. Backman. 1987. Neonatal BCG vaccination and mycobacterial cervical adenitis in childhood. *Tubercle* 68:291–296.

82. Kemp, E. B., R. B. Belshe, and D. F. Hoft. 1996. Immune responses stimulated by percutaneous and intradermal Bacille Calmette-Guerin. *J. Infect. Dis.* 174:113–119.

83. Khader, S. A., J. E. Pearl, K. Sakamoto, L. Gilmartin, G. K. Bell, D. M. Jelley-Gibbs, N. Ghilardi, F. deSauvage, and A. M. Cooper. 2005. IL-23 compensates for the absence of IL-12p70 and is essential for the IL-17 response during tuberculosis but is dispensable for protection and antigen-specific IFN-gamma responses if IL-12p70 is available. *J. Immunol.* 175:788–795.

84. Kristensen, I., P. Aaby, and H. Jensen. 2000. Routine vaccinations and child survival: follow up study in Guinea-Bissau, West Africa. *BMJ* 321:1435–1438.

85. Kröger, L., M. Korppi, E. Brander, H. Kröger, O. Wasz-Höckert, A. Backman, J. Rapola, K. Launiala, and M. Katila. 1995. Osteitis caused by Bacille Calmette-Guérin vaccination: a retrospective analysis of 222 cases. *J. Infect. Dis.* 172:574–576.

86. Kursar, M., M. Koch, H. W. Mittrucker, G. Nouailles, K. Bonhagen, T. Kamradt, and S. H. Kaufmann. 2007. Cutting edge: regulatory T cells prevent efficient clearance of *Mycobacterium tuberculosis*. *J. Immunol.* 178:2661–2665.

87. Kusner, D. J. 2005. Mechanisms of mycobacterial persistence in tuberculosis. *Clin. Immunol.* 114:239–247.

88. Lagranderie, M., A. M. Balazuc, M. Abolhassani, P. Chavarot, M. A. Nahori, F. Thouron, G. Milon, and G. Marchal. 2002. Development of mixed Th1/Th2 type immune response and protection against *Mycobacterium tuberculosis* after rectal or subcutaneous immunization of newborn and adult mice with *Mycobacterium bovis* BCG. *Scand. J. Immunol.* 55:293–303.

88a. Lahey, T., R. D. Arbeit, M. Bakari, C. R. Horsburgh, M. Matee, R. Waddel, L. Mtei, J. M. Vuola, K. Pallangyo, and C. F. von Reyn. 2010. Immunogenicity of a protective whole cell mycobacterial vaccine in HIV-infected adults: a phase III study in Tanzania. *Vaccine* 28:7652–7658.

89. Lalor, M. K., S. G. Smith, S. Floyd, P. Gorak-Stolinska, R. E. Weir, R. Blitz, K. Branson, P. E. Fine, and H. M. Dockrell. 2010. Complex cytokine profiles induced by BCG vaccination in UK infants. *Vaccine* 28:1635–1641.

90. Lambert, P. H., T. Hawkridge, and W. A. Hanekom. 2009. New vaccines against tuberculosis. *Clin. Chest Med.* 30:811–826, x.

91. Langermans, J. A., P. Andersen, D. van Soolingen, R. A. Vervenne, P. A. Frost, T. van der Laan, L. A. van Pinxteren, J. van den Hombergh, S. Kroon, I. Peekel, S. Florquin, and A. W. Thomas. 2001. Divergent effect of bacillus Calmette-Guerin (BCG) vaccination on *Mycobacterium tuberculosis* infection in highly related macaque species: implications for primate models in tuberculosis vaccine research. *Proc. Natl. Acad. Sci. USA* 98:11497–11502.

92. Leroy, H., C. Arvieux, J. Biziragusenyuka, J. M. Chapplain, C. Guiguen, C. Michelet, and P. Tattevin. 2008. A retrospective study of 230 consecutive patients hospitalized for presumed travel-related illness (2000–2006). *Eur. J. Clin. Microbiol. Infect. Dis.* 27:1137–1140.

93. Leung, C. C., C. M. Tam, S. L. Chan, M. Chan-Yeung, C. K. Chan, and K. C. Chang. 2001. Efficacy of the BCG revaccination programme in a cohort given BCG vaccination at birth in Hong Kong. *Int. J. Tuberc. Lung Dis.* 5:717–723.

94. Levine, M. I., and M. F. Sackett. 1948. Results of BCG immunization in New York City. *Am. Rev. Tuberc.* 53:517–532.

95. Lewinsohn, D. A., E. Winata, G. M. Swarbrick, K. E. Tanner, M. S. Cook, M. D. Null, M. E. Cansler, A. Sette, J. Sidney, and D. M. Lewinsohn. 2007. Immunodominant tuberculosis CD8 antigens preferentially restricted by HLA-B. *PLoS Pathog.* 3:1240–1249.

96. Lewinsohn, D. M., A. L. Briden, S. G. Reed, K. H. Grabstein, and M. R. Alderson. 2000. *Mycobacterium tuberculosis*-reactive CD8+ T lymphocytes: the relative contribution of classical versus nonclassical HLA restriction. *J. Immunol.* 165:925–930.

97. Liu, P. T., S. Stenger, H. Li, L. Wenzel, B. H. Tan, S. R. Krutzik, M. T. Ochoa, J. Schauber, K. Wu, C. Meinken, D. L. Kamen, M. Wagner, R. Bals, A. Steinmeyer, U. Zugel, R. L. Gallo, D. Eisenberg, M. Hewison, B. W. Hollis, J. S. Adams, B. R. Bloom, and R. L. Modlin. 2006. Toll-like receptor triggering of a vitamin D-mediated human antimicrobial response. *Science* 311:1770–1773.

98. Lopez de Castilla, D., and N. W. Schluger. 2009. Tuberculosis following solid organ transplantation. *Transpl. Infect. Dis.* 12:106–112.

99. Lotte, A., O. Wasz-Hockert, N. Poisson, N. Dumitrescu, M. Verron, and E. Couvet. 1984. BCG complications. Estimates of the risks among vaccinated subjects and statistical analysis of their main characteristics. *Adv. Tuberc. Res.* 21:107–193.

100. Lotte, A., O. Wasz-Hockert, N. Poisson, H. Engbaek, H. Landmann, U. Quast, B. Andrasofszky, L. Lugosi, I. Vadasz, and P. Mihailescu. 1988. Second IUATLD study on complications induced by intradermal BCG-vaccination. *Bull. Int. Union Tuberc. Lung Dis.* 63:47–59.

101. Lowry, P. W., T. S. Ludwig, J. A. Adams, M. L. Fitzpatrick, S. M. Grant, G. A. Andrle, M. R. Offerdahl, S. Cho, and D. R. Jacobs. 1998. Cellular immune responses to four doses of percutaneous Bacille Calmette-Guérin in healthy adults. *J. Infect. Dis.* 178:138–146.

102. Lowry, P. W., T. S. Ludwig, J. A. Adams, M. L. Fitzpatrick, S. M. Grant, G. A. Andrle, M. R. Offerdahl, S. N. Cho, and D. R. Jacobs, Jr. 1998. Cellular immune responses to four doses of percutaneous bacille Calmette-Guerin in healthy adults. *J. Infect. Dis.* 178:138–146.

103. Magalhaes, I., D. R. Sizemore, R. K. Ahmed, S. Mueller, L. Wehlin, C. Scanga, F. Weichold, G. Schirru, M. G. Pau, J. Goudsmit, S. Kuhlmann-Berenzon, M. Spangberg, J. Andersson, H. Gaines, R. Thorstensson, Y. A. Skeiky, J. Sadoff, and M. Maeurer. 2008. rBCG induces strong antigen-specific T cell responses in rhesus macaques in a prime-boost setting with an adenovirus 35 tuberculosis vaccine vector. *PLoS One* 3:e3790.

104. Manabe, Y. C., C. P. Scott, and W. R. Bishai. 2002. Naturally attenuated, orally administered *Mycobacterium microti* as a tuberculosis vaccine is better than subcutaneous *Mycobacterium bovis* BCG. *Infect. Immun.* 70:1566–1570.

105. Mansoor, N., T. J. Scriba, M. de Kock, M. Tameris, B. Abel, A. Keyser, F. Little, A. Soares, S. Gelderbloem, S. Mlenjeni, L. Denation, A. Hawkridge, W. H. Boom, G. Kaplan, G. D. Hussey, and W. A. Hanekom. 2009. HIV-1 infection in infants severely impairs the immune response induced by Bacille Calmette-Guerin vaccine. *J. Infect. Dis.* 199:982–990.

106. Marchant, A., T. Goetghebuer, M. O. Ota, et al. 1999. Newborns develop a Th1-type immune response to *Mycobacterium bovis* Bacillus Calmette-Guerin vaccination. *J. Immunol.* 163:2249–2255.

107. Marsh, B. J., C. F. von Reyn, J. Edwards, M. A. Ristola, C. Bartholomew, R. J. Brindle, C. F. Gilks, R. W. Waddell, A. N.

Tosteson, R. Peltz, C. H. Sox, R. Frothingham, R. D. Arbeit, and International MAC Study Group. 1997. The risks and benefits of childhood bacille Calmette-Guerin immunization among adults with AIDS. *AIDS* 11:669–672.

108. Matee, M., T. Lahey, J. M. Vuola, L. Mtei, B. F. Cole, M. Bakari, R. D. Arbeit, C. R. Horsburgh, K. Pallangyo, and C. F. von Reyn. 2007. Baseline mycobacterial immune responses in HIV-infected adults primed with bacille Calmette-Guerin during childhood and entering a tuberculosis booster vaccine trial. *J. Infect. Dis.* 195:118–123.

109. McKinney, J. D., K. Honer zu Bentrup, E. J. Munoz-Elias, A. Miczak, B. Chen, W. T. Chan, D. Swenson, J. C. Sacchettini, W. R. Jacobs, Jr., and D. G. Russell. 2000. Persistence of *Mycobacterium tuberculosis* in macrophages and mice requires the glyoxylate shunt enzyme isocitrate lyase. *Nature* 406:735–738.

110. McMurray, D. N. 1981. Cellular immune changes in undernourished children. *Prog. Clin. Biol. Res.* 67:305–318.

111. Modi, S., A. M. Buff, C. J. Lawson, D. Rodriguez, H. L. Kirking, H. Lipman, and D. B. Fishbein. 2009. Reporting patterns and characteristics of tuberculosis among international travelers, United States, June 2006 to May 2008. *Clin. Infect. Dis.* 49:885–891.

112. Mogues, T., M. E. Goodrich, L. Ryan, R. LaCourse, and R. J. North. 2001. The relative importance of T cell subsets in immunity and immunopathology of airborne *Mycobacterium tuberculosis* infection in mice. *J. Exp. Med.* 193:271–280.

113. Mohan, A. K., T. R. Cote, J. A. Block, A. M. Manadan, J. N. Siegel, and M. M. Braun. 2004. Tuberculosis following the use of etanercept, a tumor necrosis factor inhibitor. *Clin. Infect. Dis.* 39:295–299.

114. Morais Fonseca, D., R. S. Rosada, M. Oliveira e Paula, P. F. Wowk, L. H. Franco, E. G. Soares, C. L. Silva, and V. L. Deperon Bonato. 2010. Experimental tuberculosis: designing a better model to test vaccines against tuberculosis. *Tuberculosis* (Edinburgh) 90:135–142.

115. Narayanan, P. R. 2006. Influence of sex, age & nontuberculous infection at intake on the efficacy of BCG: re-analysis of 15-year data from a double-blind randomized control trial in South India. *Indian J. Med. Res.* 123:119–124.

116. Ninane, J., A. Grymonprez, G. Burtonboy, A. Francois, and G. Cornu. 1988. Disseminated BCG in HIV infection. *Arch. Dis. Child.* 63:1268–1269.

117. Olsen, A. W., A. Williams, L. M. Okkels, G. Hatch, and P. Andersen. 2004. Protective effect of a tuberculosis subunit vaccine based on a fusion of antigen 85B and ESAT-6 in the aerosol guinea pig model. *Infect. Immun.* 72:6148–6150.

118. Opie, E. L., E. W. Flahiff, and H. H. Smith. 1939. Protective inoculation against human tuberculosis with heat-killed tubercle bacilli. *Am. J. Hyg.* 29:155–164.

119. Orme, I. M., D. N. McMurray, and J. T. Belisle. 2001. Tuberculosis vaccine development: recent progress. *Trends Microbiol.* 9:115–118.

120. Portaels, F., J. Aguiar, M. Debacker, A. Guedenon, C. Steunou, C. Zinsou, and W. M. Meyers. 2004. *Mycobacterium bovis* BCG vaccination as prophylaxis against *Mycobacterium ulcerans* osteomyelitis in Buruli ulcer disease. *Infect. Immun.* 72:62–65.

121. Praveen, K. N., M. F. Smikle, P. Prabhakar, D. Pande, B. Johnson, and D. Ashley. 1990. Outbreak of Bacillus Calmette-Guerin-associated lymphadenitis and abscesses in Jamaican children. *Pediatr. Infect. Dis. J.* 9:890–893.

122. Radosevic, K., C. W. Wieland, A. Rodriguez, G. J. Weverling, R. Mintardjo, G. Gillissen, R. Vogels, Y. A. Skeiky, D. M. Hone, J. C. Sadoff, T. van der Poll, M. Havenga, and J. Goudsmit. 2007. Protective immune responses to a recombinant adenovirus type 35 tuberculosis vaccine in two mouse strains: CD4 and CD8 T-cell epitope mapping and role of gamma interferon. *Infect. Immun.* 75:4105–4115.

123. Ravn, P., H. Boesen, and B. K. Pedersen. 1997. Human T cell responses induced by vaccination with *Mycobacterium bovis* Bacillus Calmette-Guerin. *J. Immunol.* 158:1949–1955.

124. Reed, S. G., R. N. Coler, W. Dalemans, E. V. Tan, E. C. DeLa Cruz, R. J. Basaraba, I. M. Orme, Y. A. Skeiky, M. R. Alderson, K. D. Cowgill, J. P. Prieels, R. M. Abalos, M. C. Dubois, J. Cohen, P. Mettens, and Y. Lobet. 2009. Defined tuberculosis vaccine, Mtb72F/AS02A, evidence of protection in cynomolgus monkeys. *Proc. Natl. Acad. Sci. USA* 106:2301–2306.

125. Rodrigues, L. C., V. K. Diwan, and J. G. Wheeler. 1993. Protective effect of BCG against tuberculosis meningitis and miliary tuberculosis: a meta-analysis. *Int. J. Epidemiol.* 22:1154–1158.

126. Rodrigues, L. C., S. M. Pereira, S. S. Cunha, B. Genser, M. Y. Ichihara, S. C. de Brito, M. A. Hijjar, I. Dourado, A. A. Cruz, C. Sant'Anna, A. L. Bierrenbach, and M. L. Barreto. 2005. Effect of BCG revaccination on incidence of tuberculosis in school-aged children in Brazil: the BCG-REVAC cluster-randomised trial. *Lancet* 366:1290–1295.

127. Romanus, V., H. H. Hallander, P. Wahlen, A. M. Olinder-Nielsen, P. H. W. Magnusson, and I. Juhlin. 1995. Atypical mycobacteria in extrapulmonary disease among children. Incidence in Sweden from 1969 to 1990, related to changing BCG-vaccination coverage. *Tuber. Lung Dis.* 76:300–310.

128. Romanus, V., A. Svensson, and H. O. Hallander. 1992. The impact of changing BCG coverage on tuberculosis incidence in Swedish born children between 1969 and 1989. *Tubercle* 73:150–161.

129. Rosenthal, S. R., E. Loewinsohn, M. L. Graham, D. Liveright, M. G. Thorne, and V. Johnson. 1960. BCG vaccination in tuberculous households. *Am. Rev. Respir. Dis.* 84:690–704.

130. Rosenthal, S. R., E. Loewinsohn, M. L. Graham, D. Liveright, M. G. Thorne, V. Johnson, and H. C. Batson. 1961. BCG vaccination against tuberculosis in Chicago: a twenty year study statistically analyzed. *Pediatrics* 28:622–641.

131. Rota, S., U. Beyazova, T. Karsligil, and C. Cevheroglu. 1994. Humoral immune response against antigen 60 in BCG-vaccinated infants. *Eur. J. Epidemiol.* 10:713–718.

132. Roth, A., H. Jensen, M. L. Garly, Q. Djana, C. L. Martins, M. Sodemann, A. Rodrigues, and P. Aaby. 2004. Low birth weight infants and Calmette-Guerin bacillus vaccination at birth: community study from Guinea-Bissau. *Pediatr. Infect. Dis. J.* 23:544–550.

133. Sakula, A. 1983. BCG: who were Calmette and Guerin? *Thorax* 38:806–812.

134. Salo, E. P. 2006. BCG in Finland: changing from a universal to a selected programme. *Eur. Surveill.* 11:18–20.

135. Sander, C. R., A. A. Pathan, N. E. Beveridge, I. Poulton, A. Minassian, N. Alder, J. Van Wijgerden, A. V. Hill, F. V. Gleeson, R. J. Davies, G. Pasvol, and H. McShane. 2009. Safety and immunogenicity of a new tuberculosis vaccine, MVA85A, in *Mycobacterium tuberculosis*-infected individuals. *Am. J. Respir. Crit. Care Med.* 179:724–733.

136. Scriba, T. J., M. Tameris, N. Mansoor, E. Smit, L. van der Merwe, F. Isaacs, A. Keyser, S. Moyo, N. Brittain, A. Lawrie, S. Gelderbloem, A. Veldsman, M. Hatherill, A. Hawkridge, A. V. Hill, G. D. Hussey, H. Mahomed, H. McShane, and W. A. Hanekom. 2010. Modified vaccinia Ankara-expressing Ag85A, a novel tuberculosis vaccine, is safe in adolescents and children, and induces polyfunctional CD4+ T cells. *Eur. J. Immunol.* 40:279–290.

137. Shelley, M. D., T. J. Wilt, J. Court, B. Coles, H. Kynaston, and M. D. Mason. 2004. Intravesical bacillus Calmette-Guerin is superior to mitomycin C in reducing tumour recurrence in high-risk superficial bladder cancer: a meta-analysis of randomized trials. *BJU Int.* **93:**485–490.

138. Skeiky, Y. A., and J. C. Sadoff. 2006. Advances in tuberculosis vaccine strategies. *Nat. Rev. Microbiol.* **4:**469–476.

139. Smith, K. C., and J. R. Starke. 1999. Bacille Calmette Guerin vaccine, p. 121. *In* S. A. Plotkin and W. A. Orenstein (ed.), *Vaccines.* W. B. Saunders, Philadelphia, PA.

140. Smith, P. G., W. D. Revill, E. Lukwago, and Y. P. Rykushin. 1977. The protective effect of BCG against *Mycobacterium ulcerans* disease: a controlled trial in an endemic area of Uganda. *Trans. R. Soc. Trop. Med. Hyg.* **70:**449–457.

141. Soares, A. P., T. J. Scriba, S. Joseph, R. Harbacheuski, R. A. Murray, S. J. Gelderbloem, A. Hawkridge, G. D. Hussey, H. Maecker, G. Kaplan, and W. A. Hanekom. 2008. Bacillus Calmette-Guerin vaccination of human newborns induces T cells with complex cytokine and phenotypic profiles. *J. Immunol.* **180:**3569–3577.

142. Sonnenberg, P., J. Murray, J. R. Glynn, S. Shearer, B. Kambashi, and P. Godfrey-Faussett. 2001. HIV-1 and recurrence, relapse, and reinfection of tuberculosis after cure: a cohort study in South African mineworkers. *Lancet* **358:**1687–1693.

143. Soysal, A., K. A. Millington, M. Bakir, D. Dosanjh, Y. Aslan, J. J. Deeks, S. Efe, I. Staveley, K. Ewer, and A. Lalvani. 2005. Effect of BCG vaccination on risk of *Mycobacterium tuberculosis* infection in children with household tuberculosis contact: a prospective community-based study. *Lancet* **366:**1443–1451.

144. Starke, J. R. 2001. Transmission of *Mycobacterium tuberculosis* to and from children and adolescents. *Semin. Pediatr. Infect. Dis.* **12:**115.

145. Stead, W. W., and A. K. Dutt. 1989. Tuberculosis in the elderly. *Semin. Respir. Infect.* **4:**189–197.

146. Stead, W. W., J. P. Lofgren, E. Warren, and C. Thomas. 1985. Tuberculosis as an endemic and nosocomial infection among the elderly in nursing homes. *N. Engl. J. Med.* **312:**1483–1487.

147. Stein, S. C., and J. D. Aronson. 1953. The occurrence of pulmonary lesions in BCG vaccinated and unvacccinated persons. *Am. Rev. Tuberc.* **68:**692–712.

148. Surekha Rani, H., V. Vijaya Lakshmi, G. Sumanlatha, and K. J. Murthy. 2005. Cell-mediated immune responses in children towards secreted proteins of *Mycobacterium bovis* BCG. *Tuberculosis* (Edinburgh) **85:**89–93.

149. Tala, E., V. Romanus, and M. Tala-Heikkilä. 1997. Bacille Calmette-Guérin vaccination in the 21st century. *Eur. Respir. Mon.* **4:**327–353.

150. Talbot, E. A., M. D. Perkins, S. F. Silva, and R. Frothingham. 1997. Disseminated bacille Calmette-Guerin disease after vaccination: case report and review. *Clin. Infect. Dis.* **24:**1139–1146.

151. Tanaka, Y., C. T. Morita, E. Nieves, M. B. Brenner, and B. R. Bloom. 1995. Natural and synthetic non-peptide antigens recognized by human gamma delta T cells. *Nature* **375:**155–158.

152. Thoma-Uszynski, S., S. Stenger, O. Takeuchi, M. T. Ochoa, M. Engele, P. A. Sieling, P. F. Barnes, M. Rollinghoff, P. L. Bolcskei, M. Wagner, S. Akira, M. V. Norgard, J. T. Belisle, P. J. Godowski, B. R. Bloom, and R. L. Modlin. 2001. Induction of direct antimicrobial activity through mammalian Toll-like receptors. *Science* **291:**1544–1547.

153. Tompkins, D. M., D. S. Ramsey, M. L. Cross, F. E. Aldwell, G. W. de Lisle, and B. M. Buddle. 2009. Oral vaccination reduces the incidence of tuberculosis in free-living brushtail possums. *Proc. Biol. Sci.* **276:**2987–2995.

154. Trevenen, C. L., and R. D. Pagtakhan. 1982. Disseminated tuberculoid lesions in infants following BCG vaccination. *Can. Med. Assoc. J.* **127:**502–504.

155. Tsenova, L., R. Harbacheuski, A. L. Moreira, E. Ellison, W. Dalemans, M. R. Alderson, B. Mathema, S. G. Reed, Y. A. Skeiky, and G. Kaplan. 2006. Evaluation of the Mtb72F polyprotein vaccine in a rabbit model of tuberculous meningitis. *Infect. Immun.* **74:**2392–2401.

156. Tuberculosis Prevention Trial, Madras. 1980. Trial of BCG vaccines in South India for tuberculosis prevention. *Indian J. Med. Res.* **72**(Suppl.):1–74.

157. Turnbull, F. M., P. B. McIntyre, H. M. Achat, H. Wang, R. Stapledon, M. Gold, and M. A. Burgess. 2002. National study of adverse reactions after vaccination with Bacille Calmette-Guerin. *Clin. Infect. Dis.* **34:**447–453.

158. Turneer, M., J. P. Van Vooren, J. Nyabenda, F. Legros, A. Lecomte, J. Thiriaux, E. Serruys, and J. C. Yernault. 1988. The humoral immune response after BCG vaccination in humans: consequences for the serodiagnosis of tuberculosis. *Eur. Respir. J.* **1:**589–593.

159. Ulrichs, T., D. B. Moody, E. Grant, S. H. Kaufmann, and S. A. Porcelli. 2003. T-cell responses to CD1-presented lipid antigens in humans with *Mycobacterium tuberculosis* infection. *Infect. Immun.* **71:**3076–3087.

160. Vandiviere, H. M., M. Dworski, I. G. Melvin, K. A. Watson, and J. Begley. 1973. Efficacy of bacillus Calmette-Guerin and isoniazid-resistant bacillus Calmette-Guerin with and without isoniazid chemoprophylaxis from day of vaccination. II. Field trial in man. *Am. Rev. Respir. Dis.* **108:**301–313.

161. Vipond, J., M. L. Cross, M. R. Lambeth, S. Clark, F. E. Aldwell, and A. Williams. 2008. Immunogenicity of orally-delivered lipid-formulated BCG vaccines and protection against *Mycobacterium tuberculosis* infection. *Microbes Infect.* **10:**1577–1581.

162. von Reyn, C. F. 1999. The significance of bacteremic tuberculosis among persons with HIV infection in developing countries. *AIDS* **13:**2193–2195.

163. von Reyn, C. F., T. W. Barber, R. D. Arbeit, C. H. Sox, G. T. O'Connor, R. J. Brindle, C. F. Gilks, K. Hakkarainen, A. Ranki, C. Bartholomew, A. N. A. Tosteson, and M. Magnusson. 1993. Evidence of previous infection with *M. avium* among healthy subjects: an international study of dominant mycobacterial skin test reactions. *J. Infect. Dis.* **168:**1553–1558.

164. von Reyn, C. F., C. R. Horsburgh, K. N. Olivier, P. F. Barnes, R. Waddell, C. Warren, S. Tvaroha, A. S. Jaeger, A. D. Lein, R. Alexander, D. J. Weber, and A. N. Tosteson. 2001. Skin test reactions to *Mycobacterium tuberculosis* purified protein derivative and *Mycobacterium avium* sensitin among health care workers and medical students in the United States. *Int. J. Tuberc. Lung Dis.* **5:**1122–1128.

165. von Reyn, C. F., L. Mtei, R. D. Arbeit, R. Waddell, B. Cole, T. Mackenzie, M. Matee, M. Bakari, S. Tvaroha, L. V. Adams, C. R. Horsburgh, and K. Pallangyo. 2010. Prevention of tuberculosis in Bacille Calmette-Guerin-primed, HIV-infected adults boosted with an inactivated whole-cell mycobacterial vaccine. *AIDS* **24:**675–685.

166. von Reyn, C. F., and J. Vuola. 2002. New vaccines for the prevention of tuberculosis. *Clin. Infect. Dis.* **35:**465–474.

167. von Reyn, C. F., P. Williams, H. Lederman, J. A. McCutchan, S. L. Koletar, R. L. Murphy, S. E. Cohn, T. Evans, A. E. Heald, D. Colquhoun, E. L. Bassily, and J. S. Currier. 2001. Skin test reactivity and cellular immune responses to *Mycobacterium*

avium sensitin in AIDS patients at risk for disseminated *M. avium* infection. *Clin. Diagn. Lab. Immunol.* 8:1277–1278.

168. Vuola, J. M., M. A. Ristola, B. Cole, A. Jarviluoma, S. Tvaroha, T. Ronkko, O. Rautio, R. D. Arbeit, and C. F. Reyn. 2003. Immunogenicity of an inactivated mycobacterial vaccine for the prevention of HIV-associated tuberculosis: a randomized, controlled trial. *AIDS* 17:2351–2355.

169. Waddell, R. D., C. Chintu, A. D. Lein, A. Zumla, M. R. Karagas, K. S. Baboo, J. D. F. Habbema, A. N. A. Tosteson, P. Morin, S. Tvaroha, R. D. Arbeit, A. Mwinga, and C. F. von Reyn. 2000. Safety and immunogenicity of a five-dose series of inactivated *Mycobacterium vaccae* vaccination for the prevention of HIV-associated tuberculosis. *Clin. Infect. Dis.* 30(Suppl. 3):S309–S315.

170. Waddell, R. D., K. Lishimpi, C. F. von Reyn, C. Chintu, K. S. Baboo, B. Kreiswirth, E. Talbot, M. R. Karagas, and Dartmouth/UCLMS/UNZA Collaborative Study Group. 2001. Bacteremia due to *Mycobacterium tuberculosis* or *M. bovis*, Bacille Calmette-Guerin (BCG) among HIV-positive children and adults in Zambia. *AIDS* 15:55–60.

171. Walls, T., and D. Shingadia. 2004. Global epidemiology of paediatric tuberculosis. *J. Infect.* 48:13–22.

172. Weiss, D. W. 1959. Vaccination against tuberculosis with non-living vaccines. I. The problem and its historical background. *Am. Rev. Respir. Dis.* 80:676–688.

173. Whelan, K. T., A. A. Pathan, C. R. Sander, H. A. Fletcher, I. Poulton, N. C. Alder, A. V. Hill, and H. McShane. 2009. Safety and immunogenicity of boosting BCG vaccinated subjects with BCG: comparison with boosting with a new TB vaccine, MVA85A. *PLoS One* 4:e5934.

174. Wilkinson, K. A., R. Seldon, G. Meintjes, M. X. Rangaka, W. A. Hanekom, G. Maartens, and R. J. Wilkinson. 2009. Dissection of regenerating T-cell responses against tuberculosis in HIV-infected adults sensitized by *Mycobacterium tuberculosis*. *Am. J. Respir. Crit. Care Med.* 180:674–683.

175. World Health Organization. 2009. *Global Tuberculosis Control: a Short Update to the 2009 Report*. World Health Organization, Geneva, Switzerland.

176. World Health Organization. 2010. *Multidrug and Extensively Drug-Resistant TB (M/XDR-TB): 2010 Global Report on Surveillance and Response*. World Health Organization, Geneva, Switzerland.

177. World Health Organization Collaborative Study Group on Oral Poliovirus Vaccine. 1995. Factors affecting the immunogenicity of oral poliovirus vaccine: a prospective evaluation in Brazil and the Gambia. *J. Infect. Dis.* 171:1097–1106.

178. Xu, Y., C. Jagannath, X. D. Liu, A. Sharafkhaneh, K. E. Kolodziejska, and N. T. Eissa. 2007. Toll-like receptor 4 is a sensor for autophagy associated with innate immunity. *Immunity* 27:135–144.

179. Yuen, K. Y., and P. C. Woo. 2002. Tuberculosis in blood and marrow transplant recipients. *Hematol. Oncol.* 20:51–62.

180. Zar, H. J., M. F. Cotton, S. Strauss, J. Karpakis, G. Hussey, H. S. Schaaf, H. Rabie, and C. J. Lombard. 2007. Effect of isoniazid prophylaxis on mortality and incidence of tuberculosis in children with HIV: randomised controlled trial. *BMJ* 334:136.

181. Ziegler, J. E., M. L. Edwards, and D. W. Smith. 1985. Exogenous reinfection in experimental airborne tuberculosis. *Tubercle* 66:121–128.

Chapter 11

Tuberculosis—a World Health Organization Perspective

MARCOS A. ESPINAL AND MARIO C. RAVIGLIONE

INTRODUCTION

More than 15 years after the World Health Organization (WHO) declared tuberculosis (TB) a global emergency (79), the disease remains one of the major causes of human suffering and deaths, and a pandemic of devastating proportions. Yet great progress has been made in the fight against TB in the last 15 years, and renewed efforts, spearheaded by WHO and the Stop TB Partnership's numerous partners, justify a great deal of hope that TB may be eventually contained and eliminated as a public health problem by 2050, the target adopted by the international community (Table 1) (22). However, new challenges such as the appearance of extensively drug-resistant TB (XDR-TB), the coepidemic of TB and human immunodeficiency virus (HIV), an increasingly weak and underfinanced health system in many poor settings, the lack of access to proper care, and the growing concern about the linkage of TB to socioeconomic determinants of ill health threaten to worsen the pandemic and set back the achievements of the last decade. A new comprehensive approach to fight TB, the Stop TB Strategy (Table 2) (60, 90), was introduced by the WHO in 2006 to build on and enhance DOTS (an acronym derived from "directly observed treatment, short course"), the prior strategy (85) that was extensively promoted since the declaration by the WHO of TB as a global emergency in 1993. DOTS-based programs across the world treated successfully a total of 49 million TB patients and averted about 5 million deaths between 1995 and 2009 (P. Glaziou, K. Floyd, E. Korenromp, B. Sismanidis, A. Bierrenbach, B. Williams, R. Atun, and M. Raviglione, unpublished data). One of the main goals was the interruption of transmission of *Mycobacterium tuberculosis* through early detection using sputum smear microscopy and the cure of infectious TB cases through short-course chemotherapy (SCC). DOTS, however, was not sufficient any longer to face new challenges, and some essential elements of control of TB had to be emphasized, including the concept of universal access to care for all TB patients, the engagement of nonstate and private for-profit practitioners, and the participation of civil society in TB control efforts. In addition, DOTS was not designed to address properly the threats of the HIV and multidrug-resistant TB (MDR-TB). There was, therefore, the need to strengthen DOTS in order to sustain the gains, accelerate action, and address all new challenges. The Stop TB Strategy sets out a series of objectives and components that sustain existing achievements, underpin efforts to strengthen health care systems, boost research and development, alleviate poverty, and promote human rights.

In the last edition of this book, this chapter focused mainly on the importance of new approaches to improving the extent and effectiveness of implementation of the five elements of the DOTS strategy. In this edition, this chapter describes progress and challenges in implementing the Stop TB Strategy, built around DOTS, through the Global Plan to Stop TB 2006–2015. The global burden of TB is also presented in terms of incidence, prevalence, mortality, HIV-related TB, and drug-resistant TB, specially MDR-TB and XDR-TB. The chapter also reviews progress towards the achievement of the 2015 TB-related Millennium Development Goals (MDG) and the Stop TB Partnership targets of halving prevalence and mortality compared to 1990 levels.

REVIEW OF THE GLOBAL TB EPIDEMIC

TB is ranked among the leading 10 causes of death worldwide, and most of its burden, expressed as disability-adjusted life years, is due to early deaths of young adults (92). TB is also one of the oldest epidemics humankind has endured and a reflection of our own failure in alleviating poverty as a whole. This section summarizes the current status of the global TB epidemic in terms of morbidity, mortality, and economic burden.

Marcos Espinal and Mario Raviglione • Stop TB Partnership, World Health Organization, Geneva, Switzerland.

Table 1. Goals, targets, and indicators for TB control

MDG 6: combat HIV/AIDS, malaria, and other diseases
  Target 6c: halt and begin to reverse the incidence of malaria and other major diseases
  Indicator 6.9: incidence, prevalence, and death rates associated with TB
  Indicator 6.10: proportion of TB cases detected and cured under DOTS
Stop TB Partnership targets
  By 2015: global burden of TB (per-capita prevalence and death rates) halved compared with baseline of 1990
  By 2050: global incidence of active TB less than 1 case per million population per year

TB Morbidity and Mortality

The most important long-term goal of TB control is elimination of TB as a public health problem. Progress towards such a goal is measured by means of three key indicators: incidence, prevalence, and mortality. Incidence is very challenging to measure because of the rarity of the disease and the intrinsic difficulties in detecting all cases. In low-TB-incidence, high-income countries, routine surveillance through systematic case reporting may allow a satisfactory assessment of true incidence. This is not the case in the vast majority of middle- and low-income countries with a high incidence of TB, where detection of cases and reporting are not entirely effective, and therefore, information collected through routine surveillance may not reflect the magnitude of the real incidence of TB. In recent years, however, our knowledge of the estimated incidence of TB has matured substantially as a result of improved case notifications, advanced statistical analysis, increasing numbers of disease prevalence surveys, availability of vital registrations, and improved expertise and knowledge through the WHO Global Task Force on TB Impact Measurement (24).

Since 1995, the WHO has put in place a global surveillance and monitoring system that allows assessment of progress in implementation of the six different components of the Stop TB Strategy (19, 59). In 2009 this information system became a web-based online system that was successfully used by 198 of 204 countries and territories to report their data. The reporting countries represented more than 99% of the world's population. Furthermore, the WHO publishes estimates of the incidence of TB at country, regional, and global levels annually, in addition to reporting official case notifications, to account for some of the limitations of the data reported by countries and attempt to better estimate the global burden of disease. In 2008 there were an estimated 9.4 million incident cases (139 cases per 100,000 population) worldwide, of which 3.6 million were among women (96). There were also 11 million prevalent cases of TB (164 cases per 100,000 population). The WHO South-East Asia and African regions accounted for 3.2 million and 2.8

Table 2. The Stop TB strategy

1. Pursue high-quality DOTS expansion and enhancement.
   a. Secure political commitment with adequate and sustained financing.
   b. Ensure early case detection and diagnosis through quality-assured bacteriology.
   c. Provide standardized treatment with supervision and patient support.
   d. Ensure effective drug supply and management.
   e. Monitor and evaluate performance and impact.

2. Address TB/HIV, MDR-TB, and the needs of poor and vulnerable populations.
   a. Scale up collaborative TB/HIV activities.
   b. Scale up prevention and management of MDR-TB.
   c. Address the needs of TB contacts and of poor and vulnerable populations.

3. Contribute to health care system strengthening based on primary health care.
   a. Help improve health policies, human resource development, financing, supplies, service delivery, and information.
   b. Strengthen infection control in health services, other congregate settings, and households.
   c. Upgrade laboratory networks and implement the Practical Approach to Lung Health.
   d. Adapt successful approaches from other fields and sectors, and foster action on the social determinants of health.

4. Engage all care providers.
   a. Involve all public, voluntary, corporate, and private providers through PPM approaches.
   b. Promote use of the International Standards for Tuberculosis Care.

5. Empower people with TB and communities through partnership.
   a. Pursue advocacy, communication, and social mobilization.
   b. Foster community participation in TB care and prevention and health promotion.
   c. Promote use of the Patients' Charter for Tuberculosis Care.

6. Enable and promote research.
   a. Conduct program-based operational research.
   b. Advocate for and participate in research to develop new diagnostics, drugs, and vaccines.

Table 3. Summary of TB estimates in 2008 by WHO region[a]

| Parameter | Data for the following WHO region (population, in millions): | | | | | | |
	AFR (804)	AMR (919)	EMR (584)	EUR (889)	SEAR (1,760)	WPR (1,788)	Global (6,746)
New cases of TB, all forms							
No. of incident cases (thousands)	2,828	281	674	425	3,213	1,946	9,369
Incidence rate (per 100,000)	351	31	115	48	182	109	139
Change in incidence rate (%/yr)	3.9	−3.7	−0.5	−0.8	−0.1	−1.0	1.1
HIV prevalence in all cases (%)	38	13	2.2	5.6	5.7	2.3	15
No. of estimated MDR-TB cases in 2007 (in thousands)	76	10	23	92	174	135	510
Estimated % of all TB cases with MDR-TB	2.4	3.2	3.8	17	4.8	6.3	4.9
New smear-positive TB cases							
No. of incident cases (thousands)	1,300	160	280	130	1,500	950	4,300
Incident rate SS$^+$ TB (per 100,000)	160	17	49	15	84	53	64
Deaths from TB							
Deaths from TB (thousands), excluding HIV	385	29	115	55	477	261	1,324
Deaths from TB (per 100,000), excluding HIV	48	3.2	19.7	6.3	27	14.7	20
Deaths from TB in HIV-positive adults (thousands)	414	12	5	7	65	16	520

[a]Data are from references 95 and 96. AFR, Africa; AMR, Americas; EMR, Eastern Mediterranean; EUR, Europe; SEAR, South-East Asia; WPR, Western Pacific; SS$^+$, sputum smear positive. The WHO African Region comprises sub-Saharan Africa and Algeria. The remaining north African countries are included in the WHO Eastern Mediterranean region. Adults mentioned were between 15 and 49 years old.

million new cases, respectively (Table 3). India (1.9 million), China (1.3 million), and 20 other countries accounted for 80% of the 9.4 million new cases. Figures 1 and 2 show estimated TB incidence numbers and rates by country. Of the 9.4 million estimated new TB cases, 5.7 million were officially notified by national TB programs (NTP) (Table 4). Three WHO regions, Africa, South-East Asia, and the Western Pacific, reported 83% of the cases. In 2008, there were an estimated 1.3 million deaths (20 deaths per 100,000 population) among HIV-negative incident cases of TB, including 0.5 million deaths among women. The South-East Asia and Africa regions were the top contributors of deaths, with about 477,000 and 385,000 deaths, respectively (Table 3) (96). An additional 0.5 million deaths occurred among patients with incident TB cases who were HIV positive. Thus, the total number of deaths due to TB can be estimated at 1.8 million worldwide in 2008.

Table 4. TB case notifications and rates by WHO region, 2008[a]

WHO region	No. of cases notified (new cases and relapses)	Rate (per 100,000 population)
Africa	1,329,581	165
Americas	218,249	24
Eastern Mediterranean	392,633	67
Europe	336,443	38
South-East Asia	2,078,238	118
Western Pacific	1,363,479	76
Global	5,718,623	85

[a]From *Global Tuberculosis Control. Surveillance, Planning, Financing* (96).

The global TB burden remains grave for several reasons: (i) poverty and the widening gap between the rich and poor in various populations (e.g., developing countries in general, inner-city populations in developed countries, and migratory populations), (ii) previous long-term neglect of TB control (inadequate case detection, diagnosis, and cure), (iii) changing demographics (increasing world population and changing age structure), (iv) the emergence of the HIV/AIDS epidemic and drug-resistant TB, (v) other social and economic determinants favoring TB (tobacco use, diabetes, alcohol abuse, and undernutrition), and (vi) changing patterns in the genetics of *Mycobacterium tuberculosis* (strain fitness variability and different polymorphisms affecting susceptibility).

HIV-Related TB

The AIDS pandemic has fueled TB in populations where there is an overlap between those infected with HIV and those infected with *Mycobacterium tuberculosis*. An extensive body of literature documenting the extent to which HIV is fueling the TB epidemic in countries with high HIV prevalence is now available (11, 12). The incidence rate ratio of TB among people living with HIV in countries with high HIV prevalence is at least 20, compared to people not infected with HIV (95). Persons infected with HIV who subsequently become infected with *Mycobacterium tuberculosis* have an extraordinarily high risk of developing active TB within a short period, transitioning from primary infection to disease in a matter

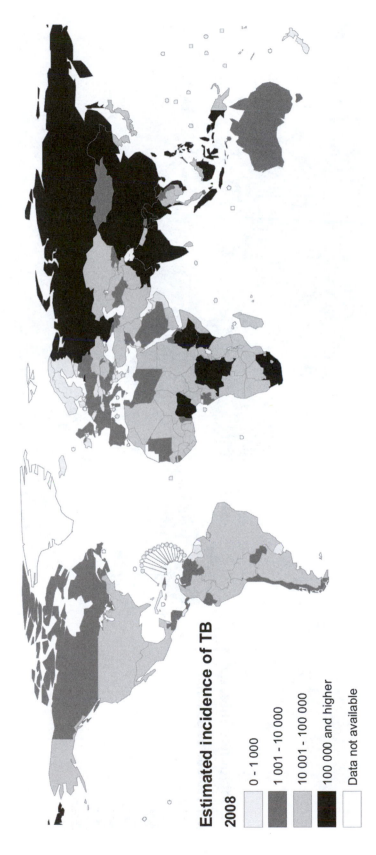

Figure 1. Estimated TB incident cases, 2008.

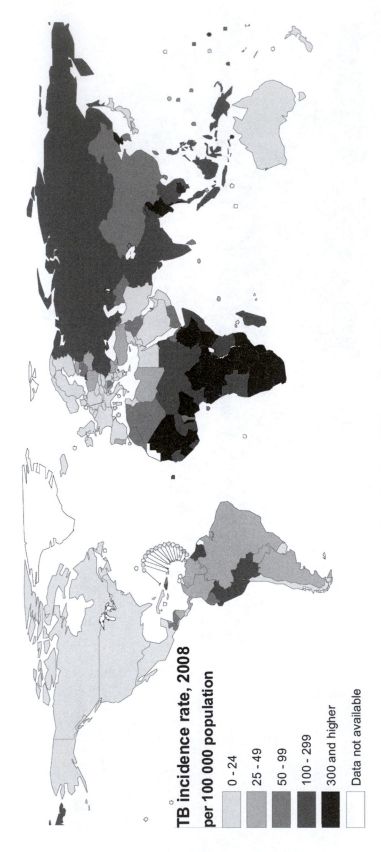

Figure 2. Estimated TB incident rates, 2008.

of weeks (14, 16). Untreated HIV infection leads to progressive immunodeficiency and increased susceptibility to some infectious diseases, including TB. As a result, the risk of developing TB increases with worsening immunosuppression. This situation results in marked increases of TB morbidity and mortality, unless specific interventions to reduce the burden of HIV on TB are in place.

In 2008, as new information became available, it was possible for the WHO to revise estimates regarding the number of HIV-positive TB cases and deaths for that year and for prior years. Table 3 shows the breakdown of global estimates of the burden of HIV-related TB by world region. Globally, of the 9.4 million incident cases in 2008, an estimated 1.4 million (15%) were infected with HIV (96). Of these HIV-positive cases, 78% were in sub-Saharan Africa and 13% were in South-East Asia. Of the 2.8 million incident TB cases in Africa, 38% were among people infected with HIV; the next highest rate was in the Americas, where 13% of the estimated 281,000 persons with incident TB cases were living with HIV. The proportion of new TB cases infected with HIV in the remaining regions was below 5%. In 2008, there were 500,000 TB deaths among people living with HIV, equivalent to 37% of all TB deaths.

Regarding the 22 high-burden countries, China, Bangladesh, Pakistan, and the Philippines had HIV prevalence among incident TB cases of less than 2% (Fig. 3). On the other hand, Kenya, Mozambique, South Africa, Tanzania, Uganda, and Zimbabwe had an HIV prevalence among incident TB cases of more than 40%, which confirms the overwhelming combined effect of these two epidemics in sub-Saharan Africa. In the period from 1990 to 2004, the annual increase in TB incidence in African countries with high HIV prevalence ran parallel to the change in HIV prevalence in the general population. With the stabilization of HIV prevalence rates in the general population around 2000, the annual increase in TB incidence also began to slow down and eventually peaked in 2004.

The halting of the increase of TB incidence in Africa brings hope that the coepidemic in this continent, and in the end the TB epidemic worldwide, can be reversed. However, there is still a long way to go for Africa, as TB and HIV programs will need to coordinate their efforts to make TB incidence decline in a sustained manner. Full scale-up of collaborative activities (86, 89) between the HIV and TB national programs aiming to reduce the burden of HIV among people infected with *Mycobacterium tuberculosis* and vice versa will be critical to accelerate TB control in the region.

Multidrug-Resistant Tuberculosis

Since 1994 the WHO has been monitoring prevalence and trends of drug-resistant TB using standardized methods (97). Five global reports have been published with information from a total of 114 countries (2, 28, 57, 99, 102). National routine surveillance systems are in place in about 42 countries, while ad hoc or periodic surveys have been conducted in the remaining countries. MDR-TB is defined as TB with resistance to, at least, the two most potent first-line drugs, isoniazid and rifampin. XDR-TB is defined as MDR-TB plus additional resistance to second-line drugs, namely, at least, any of the fluoroquinolones and any of the three injectables (amikacin, kanamycin, and capreomycin). The prevalence of MDR among new cases of TB has ranged from 0 to 28% across different settings in the 15 years of the Global Project on Anti-tuberculosis Drug Resistance Surveillance (99). High prevalence of MDR-TB has been identified in certain areas of the world, including the new countries of the former Soviet Union and some provinces of China.

While identification of several hot spots for MDR-TB has been possible over the years, the data available, being often based on a single survey, do not allow a precise estimate of the trend of MDR-TB in the world. Most countries still do not conduct routine drug susceptibility testing in all TB patients. In addition, the great majority of countries for which data are available have conducted only two or three surveys. These limitations restrict our capacity to confidently conclude on trends of MDR-TB. There is, however, encouraging evidence suggesting that drug-resistant TB can be controlled if proper measures are in place. Data from the Orel and Tomsk oblasts, in the Russian Federation, show decreasing trends in the absolute numbers and rates of MDR-TB after reaching peaks in 2004 and 2006, respectively (99). This is likely due to the implementation of sound TB control policies, in line with Stop TB Strategy, including efforts to stop the production of new drug-resistant cases through the implementation of DOTS and to diagnose as early as possible and manage effectively existing drug-resistant TB cases, thus interrupting transmission. Likewise, since the late 1990s, two Baltic countries—Estonia and Latvia—have shown decreasing trends in the annual number of notified new and relapse TB cases, while the proportion of MDR-TB has stabilized. As a result, the number of MDR-TB cases has decreased substantially in the last decade. Some other countries for which time trends are available, such as the United States and Hong Kong, have shown consistent declines in the number

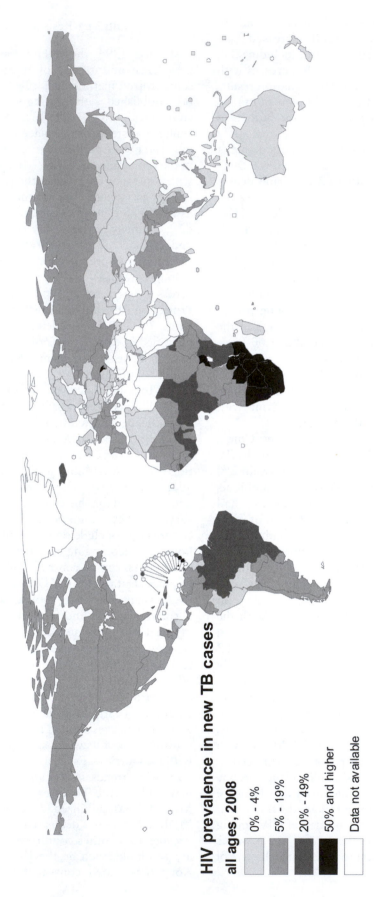

Figure 3. Estimated HIV prevalence in new TB cases, 2008.

HIV prevalence in new TB cases

all ages, 2008

- 0% - 4%
- 5% - 19%
- 20% - 49%
- 50% and higher
- Data not available

and prevalence of MDR-TB cases, although the burden in these two settings has always been low.

In addition to MDR-TB, several reports of resistance to second-line anti-TB drugs have recently emerged (32, 63, 64). As of March 2010, 58 countries have reported to the WHO at least one case of XDR-TB. Combined data from 50 countries and territories suggest that 5.4% of all MDR-TB cases have already evolved towards XDR-TB (99). Resistance to second-line drugs is a serious challenge, as currently there are only a very few promising new compounds in the research and development pipeline.

Estimates on the global magnitude of MDR-TB are published periodically, to account for the lack of data in various settings and the uncertainty surrounding the limited information available from prevalence surveys (21, 103). In 2008 there were about 510,000 estimated cases of MDR-TB (Table 3): 85% of them were in 27 countries, including 15 in the former Soviet Union and Eastern Europe. India (100,000 cases), China (99,000 cases), Russia (38,000), and South Africa (16,000) are the top high-MDR-TB-burden countries. Estimates on XDR-TB are quite uncertain, due to lack of information in many settings, but a rough estimate suggests that about 25,000 cases of XDR-TB are emerging annually (http://www .who.int/tb/features_archive/world_tb_day_2010/ mdrfactsheet15mar10_19h00.pdf).

The frequency of MDR-TB in some areas of the world, the looming threat of XDR-TB, and the lack of long-term trend data in most middle- and low-income countries are clear warnings that further improvement of surveillance of drug-resistant TB should be a top priority. This will help to understand better the magnitude of the problem, epidemiological trends, and the potential influence on TB control efforts.

Economic Burden of TB

Illness attributable to TB places a great burden on those affected by the disease, their families, and their communities. The great majority of people who die from TB are between 15 and 49 years of age. The loss of working-age, economically productive adults has an impact on households' well-being. Beside the microeconomic consequences, it affects negatively national economies through the direct loss of productivity and by reducing households' investments in activities with less certain or longer-term payoffs, such as education or infrastructure. The economic costs of TB fall into two categories: (i) indirect costs to society, the community, and the patient's family through lost production and (ii) direct costs to the health care services and to the patient and the patient's family

(83). The largest indirect cost of TB for a patient is income lost by being too sick to work. Studies suggest that, on average, 3 to 4 months of work time is lost, resulting in average lost potential earnings of 20 to 40% of the annual household income (42, 58). Others have suggested even higher losses. A study in China suggested that the opportunity cost of not working due to TB accounted for 91% of the average annual household income (40). For the families of those who die from the disease, there is the further loss of about 15 years of income because of the premature death of the TB sufferer. Regarding direct costs, the substantial nontreatment costs borne by TB patients and their families are often greater than the costs of treatment borne by the health care sector.

The cost of treating TB also can be significant. Mean household spending on TB can account for as much as 8 to 20% of annual household income, varying by region (62). Households deal with the costs of illness and death through different sorts of strategies, including the selling of assets and removal of children from school. In the short run these actions may help to cope with the disease and its consequences, but in the long term they will exercise a very negative impact and prove catastrophic for the community. Selling assets, for instance, can reduce a household's economic prospects. Removing children from school can seriously undermine their health, education, and future prospects.

Recently the World Bank estimated the economic benefit of sustaining strong TB control programs. Full implementation of the Stop TB Strategy's interventions suggested in the Global Plan to Stop TB may well yield huge economic gains (44). Significant benefits to the implementation of sustained DOTS and the Global Plan's interventions relative to a baseline of no strategy were detected. The economic burden of TB between 2006 and 2015 for the 22 high-burden countries (HBCs) was estimated to be about $3.4 trillion (U.S. dollars) under no DOTS. Implementing the Global Plan initiatives in these countries would result in an estimated economic gain of around $1.9 trillion. In sub-Saharan Africa the economic burden of TB deaths was estimated at $519 billion in a scenario with no DOTS, of which $418 billion was attributable to the burden in countries with a high level of HIV coinfection. The benefit of moving from no DOTS to the scenario of the Global Plan initiatives, including sustained DOTS, was estimated at $218 billion. The benefits of implementing the Global Plan in Africa, taking into account HIV coinfection, thus exceeded the costs by a 10:1 margin relative to the no-TB-control baseline. In other words, investing in TB control may yield gains that are 10 times higher than the investments themselves.

EVOLUTION OF TB CONTROL: FROM CHEMOTHERAPY TO DOTS AND TO THE STOP TB STRATEGY

Since the development and introduction of anti-TB drugs in the late 1940s, control of TB has evolved by way of different strategies. The positive spin is that such evolution has built on different models, all interconnected to each other. The "Edinburg approach" developed by Sir John Crofton in the early 1950s, based on the administration of triple-combination 18-month chemotherapy and intensive follow-up of the patient, was the first public health attempt to tackle the epidemic in the postchemotherapeutic era (61). Combination of anti-TB drugs was soon demonstrated to result in high cure rates and low risk of relapse and creation of drug resistance (13). The addition of well-structured case finding to this model served as the basis for the "Styblo approach." Crafted in the 1970s by Karel Styblo, this model assumed the use of existing health care facilities at the primary level where cases are suspected and detected and the administration of effective SCC to people with the disease under supervision for at least 2 months (69). The model also included a proper drug supply system and, importantly, a new way of monitoring programs based on recording of cases and their treatment outcomes and quarterly reports by the lowest administrative units in the country. At the same time, in 1974, the 14th WHO Expert Committee on Tuberculosis formulated four principles which were later the basis of TB control. The NTP must be integrated into general health services, within the Ministry of Health facilities; countrywide; permanent, because of the nature and chronicity of the disease; and adapted to the needs of the people, with TB services being as close to the community as possible (77).

The 1990s, under the renewed leadership of the WHO, saw the advent of the DOTS strategy and its five critical elements derived from the model used by Styblo in a few countries, mainly in Africa: political commitment; provision of standardized SCC under proper case management conditions, including directly observed therapy; bacteriological diagnosis; effective drug supply and management; and monitoring and evaluation of cases and outcomes of treatment (85). Following the 1991 World Health Assembly (WHA) resolution recognizing TB as a major global public health problem (78) and the 1993 declaration of TB as a global emergency (79), the WHO started the promotion of the implementation and expansion of DOTS as the internationally recommended TB control strategy. As part of the 1991 resolution, two global targets for TB control were established—detection of 70% of new smear-positive cases and cure

of 85% of such cases by the year 2000. Modeling exercises had in fact suggested that if at least 70% of cases are detected and 85% of those are cured, and in the absence of HIV infection, TB incidence rate should eventually fall at around 5 to 10% per year (3, 18, 70).

Despite the intense work of the WHO to ensure that member states adopted DOTS, by 1998 it was clear that the year 2000 targets would not be met on time. WHO then convened an ad hoc committee to review barriers to progress and make recommendations to strengthen implementation of DOTS and accelerate impact (80). This ad hoc committee recommended the establishment of a global alliance—subsequently named the Stop TB Initiative—that was launched in October 1998 to ensure a wide inclusive participation of different stakeholders and to pursue the placement of the fight against TB in the political and development agendas of world leaders (67). The ad hoc committee also recommended a ministerial conference that was held in Amsterdam, The Netherlands, in March 2000 to call for renewed political commitment (81) and a strategic focus on the 22 highest-burden countries. In 2000, the WHA decided to postpone the target date to 2005 (82). In February 2001, in Bellagio, Italy, and following the Amsterdam Declaration compiled at the meeting in that city, the Stop TB Initiative evolved into the Stop TB Partnership, a global movement to accelerate social and political action to stop TB.

Throughout its expansion, the implementation of DOTS was threatened by the emergence of the HIV epidemic and the proliferation of drug resistance. It was clear that the HIV epidemic was fueling TB in settings with high HIV prevalence (11) and that SCC was ineffective against MDR-TB (29). The WHO and partners decided to work on complementary policies and strategies to address these important threats to TB control. These included the development of collaborative activities against TB and HIV for implementation by both disease control programs (86, 89) and the design and testing of strategies to manage MDR-TB, originally known as "DOTS-plus for MDR-TB" (27, 84). Expansion of access to diagnosis and treatment through community TB care and approaches aimed at engaging all care providers—state and nonstate—in DOTS implementation were assertively pursued. Innovative mechanisms such as the Green Light Committee (GLC) and the Global Drug Facility were established in 2000 and 2001, respectively, to improve access to quality-assured, affordable first- and second-line anti-TB drugs in resource-poor settings (36, 37, 50, 66). The Stop TB Partnership launched its first Global Plan in October 2001 at its first Partners Forum in Washington, DC.

The recommendations of a second ad hoc committee convened by the WHO in 2003 (88) served as the basis of what became later the new strategy to comprehensively tackle TB—the Stop TB Strategy (60) (Table 2). This strategy, which builds on DOTS, includes a response to all major challenges of today and promotes the notion of the best standards of care for all people with TB. It also underpins the Stop TB Partnership Global Plan to Stop TB (49, 68), launched in 2006. The second version of the Global Plan addresses each major challenge, providing the rationale for interventions, estimation of their potential impact, and costs and financial gaps. It contributes regional scenarios and the strategic plans of the seven working groups of the Stop TB Partnership. It is the business plan of all partners to implement the actions and interventions needed to achieve the Stop TB Partnership's targets for 2015 and the MDG related to TB. It also includes the assessments of financial needs for new tools, such as diagnostics, drugs, and vaccines. In 2010 the Stop TB Partnership decided to revise the Global Plan, as it was the midpoint to 2015, including its epidemiological and financial scenarios towards 2015. Overall, between 2011 and 2015, on average around $8 billion to $9 billion per annum will be necessary to achieve the targets established within the MDG and by the Stop TB Partnership and to introduce the necessary new tools to set the path for TB elimination.

CURRENT STATUS OF TB CONTROL: IMPACT, ACHIEVEMENTS, AND CHALLENGES

This section summarizes the most recent assessment of the status of global TB control as set out in the 2009 updated WHO report, which reports progress in implementing the components of the Stop TB Strategy through the Global Plan to Stop TB (95, 96).

Component 1: DOTS

TB case detection

In 2008 5.7 million cases of TB (new and relapse cases) were notified to the WHO by national authorities (Table 4) (96). These included 2.6 million new smear-positive cases, 2.0 million new smear-negative cases, and 0.8 million new extrapulmonary cases. Practically all TB cases (99%) notified were reported to the WHO by DOTS-based programs. Sixty-two percent of the estimated new smear-positive cases were detected in 2008, which is still below the 70% target set in 1991 by the WHA and the 71% milestone set in the Global Plan to Stop TB. Case detection is

one of the greatest challenges that national TB control programs are currently facing. Variations in the rate of detection of new smear-positive TB cases ranged from 47% in the African region to 78% in the American and European regions. The South-East Asia and Western Pacific regions are estimated to have detected 68 and 70% of the cases, respectively.

The case detection rate is calculated as the number of notified cases of TB in 1 year divided by the number of estimated incident cases of TB in the same year and is expressed as a percentage. In recent years, the availability of improved data and refined expert opinion have shown that in many countries previous estimates of case detection rates were not as accurate as previously thought. The difficulties in estimating the real incidence of disease makes the case detection rate a measure subject to flaws and unexpected variations. Still the best available data and estimates suggest that globally the case detection rate for smear-positive TB cases experienced remarkable progress since the introduction of DOTS in 1995. It increased slowly from 35% in 1995 to 40% in 2000 and then to a more substantial increase from 40 to 57% between 2001 and 2005, reaching 62% in 2008 (96). India and China, the top two HBCs, have been at the forefront of such acceleration thanks to a remarkable expansion of proper TB control practices. India increased the detection of cases from 34% in 1995 to 64% in 2008. China increased the detection of cases from 20% in 1995 to 72% in 2008. Notwithstanding the impressive achievements by India and China, detection of TB cases continues to be a major challenge, and several HBCs, including Ethiopia, Nigeria, Myanmar, Mozambique, and Zimbabwe, still detect less than half of their estimated TB cases. Furthermore, since 2006 the case detection rate has slowed down considerably, to the point that between 2007 and 2008 there has been stagnation. Globally 38% of the estimated infectious cases are not notified if detected or are not detected at all. Those diagnosed and not notified are also likely to receive substandard care not in agreement with international recommendations.

In light of the principles of universal health care coverage and access, the WHO and the Stop TB Partnership will continue helping countries to improve detection of cases and their care. This will be done through the introduction of new diagnostic tools that can facilitate diagnosis and innovative approaches, such as public-private mix (PPM), that should ensure engagement of all providers towards better care for all. A recently created facility to fund innovative approaches to increase case detection named TB Reach and promoted by the Stop TB Partnership will finance programs to achieve these aims.

Treatment success

The cure rate is reported by each country through cohort analysis (of treatment outcomes of registered patients). Since practices vary considerably among countries in documenting negative sputum smears on completion of treatment, for practical purposes patients cured plus those who complete treatment are grouped together and considered as treatment success. Global treatment success for new smear-positive cases in the 2007 cohort was 87% on average (96). This is a major achievement for TB control; for the first time the treatment success rate has clearly exceeded the old WHA global target of 85%. Figure 4 shows treatment outcomes for the six WHO regions. The Eastern Mediterranean (88%), Western Pacific (92%), and South-East Asia (88%) regions exceeded the treatment success target as well. The Global Drug Facility has extensively contributed to reach the 85% treatment success global target by providing more than 16 million first-line drug treatments against TB, via grants and direct procurement, to more than 80 countries worldwide in the last 10 years. While great progress was made in the remaining regions, more work needs to be done in order to ensure the highest possible treatment success. Fatal outcomes were most common in Africa, where a higher fraction of cases are HIV positive, and Europe, where a higher fraction of cases occur among the elderly and those with MDR-TB.

Among the 22 HBCs, 13 have exceeded the 85% treatment success target. While this is progress, one must realize that figures on treatment success are limited only to the cases detected and notified. Those not detected or those not notified and perhaps improperly managed outside of the state sector may contribute to continued transmission in society. This may explain the lack of observed impact in many settings reporting high cure rates. Therefore, countries with low case detection must focus on ensuring maximum diagnosis and full access to treatment in order to reach the impact targets related to incidence, prevalence, and mortality.

The current first-line drug treatment regimen for TB is highly efficacious. However, it is no secret that adherence to therapy is a major challenge and sometimes logistically difficult. There is also a great need to shorten substantially the current treatment regimen with the purpose of improving adherence. Efforts are currently under way via promising controlled clinical trials (34, 46).

Incidence, prevalence, and mortality

Between 1990 and 2004 the incidence of TB was increasing, largely due to the upsurge of TB cases in Eastern Europe and sub-Saharan Africa. In Eastern Europe increased transmission occurred as a result of the socioeconomic crisis that followed the collapse of the Soviet Union and outdated TB control practices. In sub-Saharan Africa the rising of TB cases was related to the rapid dissemination of HIV infection. In 2004, the global epidemic peaked at 143 per 100,000 population and started to decline. Currently the global TB incidence rate per capita is falling very slowly, at an estimated 0.7% per year (96). This decline is much inferior to the expected reduction of 5 to 10% annually suggested by previous models (3, 18, 70). In fact, the absolute number of new TB cases

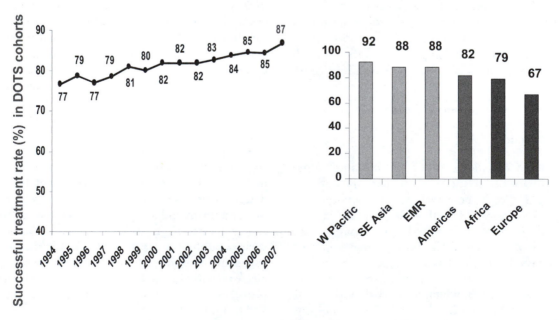

Figure 4. Treatment success globally and by WHO region.

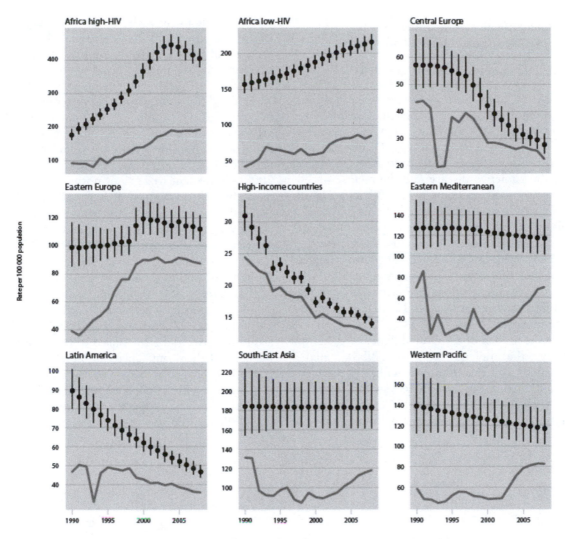

Figure 5. Trends in estimated incidence rates (black) and notification rates (gray) in nine subregions, 1990 to 2008.

is still increasing as the per-capita gains are offset by the growth of the world population (96). Eight of the nine epidemiological subregions (Fig. 5) for which the WHO evaluates such tendencies show declining trends, from less than 1% per year in South-East Asia to around 4% per year in Latin America. The only region in which the incidence rate per capita of TB is still increasing comprises African countries with a low prevalence of HIV.

At the country level, there is good evidence suggesting that the proper implementation of TB control according to recommended guidelines makes incidence decline. Peru, for example, after introducing DOTS in 1991 saw an average annual rate of decline in TB incidence of 6.5% per year between 1992 and 2000 (71). In Morocco, the incidence of pulmonary TB in children aged 0 to 4 years fell at a rate of 8% annually between 1996 and 2005, suggesting that the risk of infection, i.e., the transmission of infection by *Mycobacterium tuberculosis*, was also falling (23).

The halving of prevalence by 2015 with regard to 1990 levels remains on track in several regions of the world. The available data suggest that the target has been already reached in Europe, Latin America, and the Western Pacific (96). Africa is the only region not on track to halve prevalence by 2015. At the country level, China has reported a 32% reduction between 1991 and 2000 in the prevalence of smear-positive TB in the areas where DOTS was under implementation (8). Similarly, in Indonesia a national prevalence survey suggested that the prevalence of smear-positive TB was threefold lower than in previous years following introduction and expansion of DOTS (65).

Mortality rates are also declining, but the halving of mortality rates globally by 2015 will be a major challenge due to the impact of the TB/HIV epidemic in Africa. However, Europe, Latin America, and the Western Pacific region have already reached the mortality target (96).

Component 2: Addressing TB/HIV, MDR-TB, and Other Challenges

Scale-up of collaborative TB/HIV activities

HIV/AIDS and TB are so closely connected that they are often referred to as coepidemics or dual epidemics. HIV affects the immune system and increases the likelihood of people developing TB disease (14, 16). HIV promotes both the progression of latent TB infection to active disease and the relapse of TB in previously treated patients (11). TB is considered the leading cause of death in people living with HIV, particularly in sub-Saharan Africa (12). Control of HIV-related TB depends on collaboration between TB and HIV programs to implement preventive and treatment interventions against TB and against HIV (86, 89). These interventions are critical to control and prevent similar emergence of TB/HIV in other regions of the world.

Since the launch of the Global Plan and the Stop TB Strategy, the implementation of TB/HIV collaborative activities at the country level has progressed considerably. Countries have acted swiftly, and encouraging results are emerging (96). For instance, the number of countries that had a national policy to screen people living with HIV for TB increased from 27 in 2005 to 52 in 2008. Fifty of these countries are part of the 63 priority countries that bear 97% of estimated HIV-positive cases worldwide. Globally, there were 50 countries in which 75% of TB patients were tested for, and informed about, their HIV status in 2008 (96). The number of TB patients with known HIV status increased from 21,806 patients across 9 countries in 2002 (less than 1% of notified TB cases) to almost 1.4 million patients across 135 countries in 2008—equivalent to 22% of notified TB cases, a remarkable achievement in such a short period (Fig. 6). Similarly, the provision of co-trimoxazole preventive therapy against other fatal bacterial infections and antiretroviral therapy for HIV-positive TB patients has increased significantly in the last few years, although still slightly behind the milestones set in the Global Plan.

Progress in activities towards reducing the burden of TB among HIV-positive people globally has been less impressive, and efforts need to be strengthened to further roll them out. This will largely depend upon HIV/AIDS programs becoming more involved than they are today in the implementation of life-saving interventions for the people they care for. Between 2007 and 2008 the provision of isoniazid preventive therapy

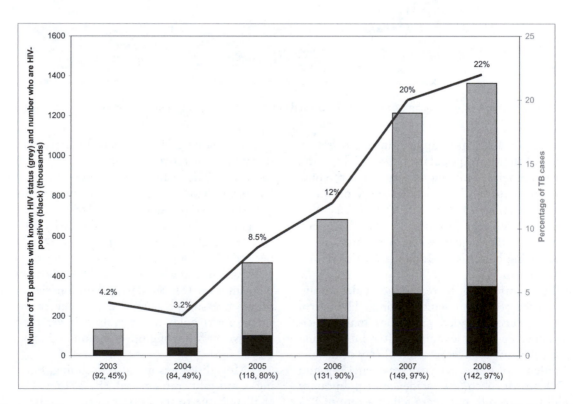

Figure 6. HIV testing for TB patients, 2003 to 2008. Shown are numbers (bars) and percentages (line) of notified new and retreatment TB cases for which the HIV status (HIV positivity in black) of the patient was recorded in the TB register. The numbers under the bars are the numbers of countries reporting data, followed by the percentages of total estimated HIV-positive TB cases accounted for by reporting countries.

to people living with HIV doubled from below 30,000 in 2007 to above 50,000 in 2008 (96). Furthermore, the number of HIV-positive cases screened for TB doubled from 0.6 million to 1.4 million in the same period (96). However, both these figures represent still a small achievement, considering that the estimated total number of people living with HIV globally is around 34 million. As a response, in 2008 WHO and partners started to promote the "three I's," a package of three key interventions to reduce the impact of TB on people living with HIV—isoniazid preventive therapy, intensified case finding for active TB, and infection control in congregate and clinical settings (38). The three I's should be a central part of HIV care and treatment. The success of antiretroviral therapy scale-up, with the potential to prevent a large number of TB cases among people living with HIV, will very much depend on the successful rollout of the three I's.

Scale-up of prevention and management of MDR-TB

Mathematical modeling has estimated that approximately 70% of prevalent, infectious MDR-TB cases should be detected and treated each year, and at least 80% of these cases should be cured, in order to prevent outbreaks of MDR-TB (20). An approach (27, 84, 94) for piloting the management of MDR-TB in resource-limited settings was launched in 1999 and, through the GLC, it has been proven to be effective, feasible, and cost-effective. Later, the pilot

model was expanded from a limited project focus towards a wider programmatic approach that needs to be part of any national plan to control TB. Thus, it became an integral part of the Global Plan to Stop TB, with a modest target of some 800,000 cases of MDR-TB to be detected and treated cumulatively between 2006 and 2015. The description of XDR-TB in 2006 prompted the WHO and the Stop TB Partnership to update the Global Plan to Stop TB. Thus, the new "Global MDR-TB & XDR-TB Response Plan" included a revision of the target for patients to be treated—up from 800,000 to 1.6 million—and set a new target for universal access and an operational plan for the global response (91). Despite these efforts, management of MDR-TB is still disappointingly limited. The number of new patients diagnosed with MDR-TB in 2008 and reported to the WHO was 30,000, a small increase with regard to the 18,000 cases notified in 2005. Similarly, enrollment of MDR-TB cases on treatment according to recommended guidelines remains very limited, although it is gradually increasing. By the end of 2009, a cumulative 19,000 patients with MDR-TB were reported to be under treatment, and the total number of patients that the GLC approved for treatment was just over 63,000 (Fig. 7) (99).

The gap between GLC approval and enrollment at the country level proves that national programs encounter at times insurmountable bottlenecks in handling MDR-TB, starting with a lack of diagnostic capacity. To address this and other constraints

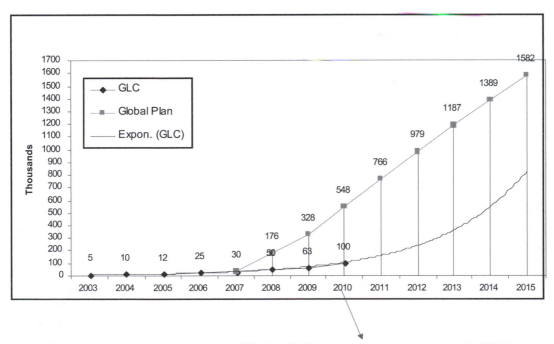

100,000 treatments are estimated to be approved in 2010, about 80,000 treatments have been approved as of April 2010

Figure 7. Gap between GLC-approved treatments and revised Global Plan, 2006 to 2015.

impeding scale-up, a ministerial meeting of the 27 high-MDR-TB-burden countries was held in April 2009 in Beijing, China. There, countries committed to speed up action against MDR-TB and XDR-TB. The meeting was followed by a resolution of the WHA (98) in which WHO member states were urged to achieve universal access to diagnosis and treatment of MDR-TB and XDR-TB. Several countries have responded to the WHA resolution by updating their policies and national plans to scale up prevention and management of MDR-TB and XDR-TB. These plans include raising the laboratory capacity required to meet the diagnostic demands of drug-resistant and HIV-associated TB and the adoption of new and rapid technologies (liquid culture media, rapid *M. tuberculosis* identification, and molecular line probe assays) recently endorsed by the WHO. A major multipartner initiative (the EXPAND-TB Project) targeting 27 key countries, promoted by the WHO, the Foundation for New Innovative Diagnostics (FIND), and the international drug-purchasing facility UNITAID under the umbrella of the Stop TB Partnership, will introduce new and rapid diagnostic technologies within appropriate laboratory services through 2013.

The management of MDR-TB is more complex and requires many more resources than the management of drug-susceptible TB. Funding through the Global Fund to fight AIDS, TB, and Malaria and UNITAID has increased in recent years, making the prospects to improve cure and survival of affected patients a real possibility. But funding is only one piece of the puzzle. Capacity at the country level is limited. Diagnosis is today feasible only in some countries, and treatment with second-line drugs is long, cumbersome, and linked to severe side effects. In addition, while second-line drugs can today be accessed even in poor settings through the GLC thanks to its concessionary price policy (36, 37), and despite the availability of new suppliers, results of treatment are modest. The latest treatment outcomes reported to the WHO from 71 settings approved by the GLC show a 64% cure rate (99). These results are in line with previous available evidence showing the difficulties in managing and curing MDR-TB (54, 56, 72) with current tools. This suggests that new, more potent, and less toxic drugs are urgently necessary to face the challenge.

Component 3: Contributing to Health Care System Strengthening Based on Primary Health Care

TB control must rely on well-functioning health care systems that are available and accessible to the poorest people in need. A well-trained and qualified human workforce, high-quality commodities (e.g., drugs, diagnostics, vaccines, and laboratory supplies),

adequate health infrastructure, sound public health policies, stewardship, and financial commitment all form the foundations of health care systems, but they are also essential elements of TB control. While the concept to keep a small dedicated team at a central level to oversee progress and ensure that policies are implemented is critical, it is important to realize that TB care and control need to be integrated within primary health care. All 22 HBCs and 83% of all others reported to the WHO in 2007 that TB control services were delivered through primary care facilities (95). Likewise, most laboratories (80% of countries) performing sputum smear microcopy are fully integrated into general laboratory services (95).

There is increasing evidence that TB control programs contribute to strengthening health care systems. In the last few years countries have paid attention to the need to align workforce planning and development with wider plans for human resources for health. The latest reports to the WHO suggest that in 2007 training related to TB control was increasingly part of the basic curriculum of doctors (141 countries), nurses (133 countries), and laboratory technicians (135 countries) (95). In addition, planning, budgeting, and financing for TB control are becoming increasingly aligned with larger planning and financial frameworks such as sector-wide approaches, medium-term expenditure frameworks, and national health plans. One area that needs stronger support is infection control to reduce transmission of *Mycobacterium tuberculosis* within clinical settings, especially where HIV is frequent. This includes TB-specific measures but also actions relevant to other airborne infectious diseases.

TB is one of the many issues underfunded and overwhelmed health care systems have to cope with, such as HIV/AIDS, diabetes, malnutrition, tobacco use, and alcohol problems. Evidence suggests that these problems are determinants of TB (45, 52). In addition, migration, urbanization, poverty, population growth, and aging are also associated with the rise of TB (25). Tackling some of these social and economic determinants will definitely help to control TB, but the greatest contribution to the potential elimination of TB may rely on the wider political and development agenda of countries. Moreover, ensuring and fostering access to health care by those who need it most, the poorest, is the necessary step towards the goal of universal access to TB care. For instance, the vast majority of TB cases affect the poor, who in many middle- and low-income countries lack health insurance and social protection, thus incurring catastrophic expenditures when affected by TB. Financial reforms yielding protection of all potential users of the health services is conducive to increased access and benefit tremendously TB control. The establishment in Mexico of the "System of Social Protection in Health," which introduced financial rules for public health, community-based services, and personal health care through the also new "popular health insurance," has been a landmark to provide access to health care to more than 50 million uninsured Mexican citizens (31). This reform offers free access at the point of delivery to a set of interventions, including TB care. More importantly, the poorest 20% of families are exempt from contribution, which is essential to the aspiration of universal access to care. Engagement of civil society and community empowerment will also be critical to ensure that people use health care systems accordingly and that the prospect of controlling and eliminating TB is realized.

Component 4: Engaging All Care Providers in TB Control

People with TB in many instances do not seek care in the public health care system. Evidence shows that in many countries and especially those with a high burden of TB, significant proportions of people with symptoms of TB often present to a variety of care providers not associated with organized national efforts to control TB (75). These providers range widely and include, for example, traditional healers in Malawi, pharmacies in Cambodia, village doctors in Bangladesh, general hospitals in the Philippines and China, and private practitioners in India and Pakistan (26, 74). Furthermore, health institutions belonging to the public, private, corporate, or voluntary sectors are often not linked to the NTP and do not follow its standards. Depending on the setting, this is true for different branches of health facilities under the ministry of health (7) or for other government health facilities not under the ministry of health. Engaging private practitioners in the provision of TB care using the international standards for TB care and recommended guidelines is therefore crucial to ensure universal access to quality care (39, 101).

Progress on component 4 of the Stop TB Strategy is encouraging. As of 2009 all HBCs had explicit policies facilitating productive engagement of relevant private and public care providers in TB control, and many had produced specific guidelines for the purpose. Funding via the Global Fund to fight AIDS, TB, and Malaria has been catalytic of PPM at the country level. As of 2008, 58 out of the 93 active proposals approved for funding included PPM components in their grants. Several countries have demonstrated that PPM for TB care and control not only is feasible and effective in increasing case detection and improving cure rates but also is cost-effective, is scalable, and

affords financial protection to the poor. Encouraged by demonstration in numerous pilot projects that PPM can increase case detection by over 20% (43, 53), the revised NTP of India has currently engaged 273 public and private medical colleges. Around 22,000 private practitioners have been trained, and 1,500 private and public hospitals, 150 corporate institutions, and 2,500 nongovernmental organizations have been involved in TB care and control. The medical colleges alone, a third of which are private, examined around 570,000 TB suspects and diagnosed 85,457 sputum smear-positive TB cases, 45,666 sputum smear-negative cases, and 71,531 extrapulmonary TB cases (51). Similarly, remarkable results have been obtained in Bangladesh as well, where more than 18,000 village doctors in rural areas have been engaged in TB control. It is estimated that more than 60% of 24,000 cases notified in 2007 received treatment from village doctors (96). China's public-public mix strategy of setting up collaboration between TB dispensaries implementing the national program and general hospitals, facilitated by a web-based disease control notification system that includes TB, helped the country meet the global targets, with the hospitals contributing about 30% sputum smear-positive cases in 2008 (100). In the Philippines, almost 50,000 TB cases have been managed through a PPM initiative since 2003 (96). The nonstate care providers were the major contributors to TB case referrals in Syria, Jordan, Iraq, and Iran in 2009, with the private for-profit sector alone contributing about 50, 32, 23, and 25% referrals, respectively (100). An aggregate figure for the private sector in Pakistan contributing 13% cases in 2008 conceals the fact that in Karachi alone, the largest city of the country, about 50% of the 14,000 cases detected were contributed by private practitioners engaged through a social franchising program by a nongovernmental organization (NGO) (95). In Nairobi, Kenya, over 10% of TB cases are managed under DOTS by private chest physicians (6). In 2008, the National Health Insurance System of Mexico reported 23% of all TB cases, while 12% were reported by public and private institutions not under the purview of the NTP.

Precise measurement of the global contribution of the fourth component of the Stop TB Strategy is fraught with challenges, such as inadequate recording and reporting systems, diversity of care providers, and the wide spectrum of their contributions to TB care and control, from simply referring TB suspects or undertaking direct observation of therapy only to complete case management. PPM should be seen and promoted as an approach to comprehensive TB control across all the components of the Stop TB Strategy, including TB/HIV and MDR-TB, rather than a single set of precisely measurable interventions.

Component 5: Empowering People with TB and Communities through Partnerships

TB is not only a biomedical problem but also a complex socioeconomic issue requiring broad societal engagement. Communities have played an important role in TB control in developed countries (4). They are also essential to the demand for, and the delivery of, TB care in middle- and low-income countries (48). Two key roles include (i) support to patients in ensuring adherence to treatment (47) and (ii) voicing demand for quality TB care. Pilot projects in several different settings have shown that engagement of the community in TB control is feasible, effective, affordable, and cost-effective in ensuring a satisfactory cure rate (33, 87). Local nongovernmental organizations are also crucial to mobilize people and organize action. Available guidelines (93) describe the essential steps needed to implement sound community involvement initiatives, underscoring the basic principle that people should not be passive beneficiaries of health care services but, rather, coresponsible for their personal health and that of their community. Community TB care is on the agenda of an increasing number of countries, as proven by the inclusion of such principle in national TB control plans and funding proposals.

Advocacy, communication, and social mobilization (ACSM) is a set of coordinated activities that support all components of the Stop TB Strategy by addressing the human and social dimensions of TB. More countries are shifting from ad hoc projects on ACSM to strategic and systematic planning and implementation based on needs (95). In 2009 12 of the 22 HBCs reported having incorporated ACSM into their national plans, compared with just 5 HBCs in 2005. Similarly, 14 HBCs reported having conducted or having plans to conduct knowledge, attitude, and practice surveys or similar research to guide development of targeted ACSM plans. A diverse and active network of ACSM partners under the umbrella of the Stop TB Partnership's DOTS Expansion Working Group has identified gaps and challenges at the country level and jointly produced ACSM tools (http://www.stoptb.org/countries/acsm/resources/tools.asp) aimed at simplifying implementation.

Progress made in empowering communities through local partnership can be also seen through the growing network of global and national partners. The Stop TB Partnership has seen its number of committed partners increase from 7 founding partners in 2001 to close to 1,200 partner organizations or individuals as of the end of 2009. The majority of the partners (more than 750) are civil society organizations. Up to 2009, 32 national partnering initiatives had been established, indicating better collaboration between all

country level stakeholders to build on each of their competencies and to share resources, risks, and responsibilities to attain a common goal. The Stop TB Partnership created the Challenge Facility for Civil Society (CFCS) in 2007 (http://www.stoptb.org/global/awards/cfcs/). It is a mechanism to make the voices of vulnerable communities heard by local politicians as well as to support innovative community-led projects to be scaled up. More than 45 NGOs in 23 countries have been funded by the CFCS so far. In addition, concerted efforts to empower people with TB have resulted in increased local TB activism. A tool to equip patients and advocates is the patients' charter for TB care (http://www.stoptb.org/assets/documents/resources/publications/acsm/istc_charter.pdf), which outlines the rights and responsibilities of people with TB. At the 3rd Stop TB Partners' Forum, held in March 2009 in Rio de Janeiro, Brazil, advocates from around the world drafted and issued the Rio Communities' Declaration (http://www.stoptb.org/events/meetings/partners_forum/2009/) urging governments, donors, global policy makers, researchers, and fellow civil society activists to act with a sense of urgency, involve all stakeholders in the response to TB and, most importantly, ensure a rights-based response that meets the needs of the most marginalized.

This encouraging progress and the attention being placed on ACSM now need to be fully assessed, looking at the effectiveness of these local initiatives in helping countries move forward in TB control and in raising the necessary political commitment and awareness.

Component 6: Enabling and Promoting Research

Scientific research has been essential to shape TB control policies and strategies throughout history. The discovery of *Mycobacterium tuberculosis* by Robert Koch in 1882, the introduction and subsequent trials of the only TB vaccine known today in the 1920s, the discovery of the anti-TB drugs starting in the 1940s, the numerous clinical trials on combined chemotherapy in the 1970s that led to today's SCC, the concept of direct observation of therapy, and the completion of the genome sequence are some of the finest examples of how biomedical and health research has driven the course of the TB epidemic (5, 10, 15). There is no doubt that in the last 100 years, an extensive wealth of knowledge on TB has been generated through research, with some historical landmarks leading to the assignment of Nobel Prizes to TB researchers (http://nobelprize.org/educational_games/medicine/tuberculosis/readmore.html).

The introduction of some of these remarkable breakthroughs, however, made the international community fall into complacency, believing that the days of TB research were over and there was no need to invest further in it. TB was on the decline in the industrialized world, and the scientific community became interested in other pressing problems. In recent times, the intensity of the research response has been truly remarkable. For instance, in the case of HIV/AIDS, the disease was described in 1981, HIV discovered in 1983, HIV testing introduced in 1985, and the first drug developed by 1987. Subsequently, the drug research pipeline has produced generations of antiretroviral medicines in as little time as 20 years. In marked contrast, no new anti-TB drug has been developed since 1971, when rifampin was introduced into clinical treatment.

In the last 30 years of the past century the attention on TB relied mostly on control efforts with *Mycobacterium bovis* BCG, SCC, and the very old diagnostic tools. The advent of major global threats in the 1990s (including TB/HIV and MDR-TB), the slow advance in TB case detection, and the operational complexities inherent to the implementation of TB control were all catalytic events for the international community to rethink the role of TB research. It was clear that the tools in use were not going to make the required drive to hope for the elimination of TB. A new paradigm was in order. The sequencing of the *Mycobacterium tuberculosis* genome in 1998 was probably the turning point for the realization that the development of new tools against TB could be within reach (10), as new frontiers were to open in the field of basic TB research. The first decade of the 21st century saw an influx of renewed efforts to scale up research in TB. The launch of several public-private development partnerships for new vaccines, drugs, and diagnostics for TB were important steps in the pursuit of new tools (41, 46, 76). The creation of three Stop TB Partnership R&D working groups to speed up such efforts and the launch of the 1st and 2nd Global Plan to Stop TB in 2001 and 2006, respectively, were also critical to further advance the scientific research agenda. The Global Plan strongly advocates for the development and introduction of new tools against TB. In addition to these efforts, the last decade also saw an influx of several research agendas on specific issues related to TB (9, 17, 30, 55).

To further boost efforts, in 2006 the Coordinating Board of the Stop TB Partnership agreed to undertake a research mapping exercise and landscape analysis (http://stoptb.org/assets/documents/about/cb/meetings/11/2.06-01.1%20Decisions%20Points%20Abuja,%20Nigeria%2024-25%20April%202006.pdf). The Board suggested the need for an overarching research plan for TB connected to strategic targets and for how basic research should be included in the Partnership Framework. It was the birth of the Stop TB Partnership TB Research Movement (http://stoptb.org/global/research/). The main objective of the TB Research Movement is to engage the full range of researchers, donors, TB program managers, and affected communities. This is to be done in a collaborative and concerted strategic effort to increase the scope, scale, and speed of TB research, ensuring that research needs are addressed and opportunities prioritized. The movement aims to support the development of an innovative international research agenda covering all critical aspects of the research spectrum—from the discovery and development of new tools to development of novel control strategies aimed at effective introduction of new tools into practice. The development of this research agenda will be critical to the transformation needed to pave the way towards the goal of TB elimination by 2050.

There is now hope thanks to the progress achieved over the last decade in the development of new tools for TB control. In diagnostics, a major recent breakthrough now under implementation in resource-limited settings has been the introduction of molecular line probe assays for the rapid detection of MDR-TB. Another tool capable of diagnosing resistant forms of TB in 2 h will soon be available (76). The pipeline of new TB drugs has increased, with 38 compounds in preclinical and clinical development, including five novel candidates in phase I and II clinical trials (34, 46). Eleven vaccine candidates have entered clinical trials, of which several are in phase II trials (41). Global TB research and development financing increased from $363 million in 2005 to $510 million in 2008, a rise of 43%. This is, however, far lower than what is required to sustain development and delivery of more effective tools to control and eliminate TB (73).

Recent modeling exercises suggest that the combined use of new tools may be able to cut the estimated incidence of TB down by 71% by 2050 (1). While such modeling implies that achievement of the elimination target may not be reached even with such tools, the prospect of reducing the burden of TB by almost three-quarters is definitely something worth pursuing. Furthermore, having the vision to eliminate TB even before 2050 should not be impossible, if we accelerate research efforts and introduce tools that could really make the difference in preventing, detecting, and curing TB faster. A point-of-care rapid test, a weekly treatment regimen for drug-susceptible TB, and a replacement for BCG should not be futile ambitions but achievable goals. History has shown that if humanity wants, humanity will break through. It should not be forgotten that reaching the moon was an impossibility until the moon was reached.

CONCLUDING REMARKS

The global progress in implementation of the Stop TB strategy via the Global Plan to Stop TB and progress in the development of new and improved TB control tools (drugs, diagnostics, and vaccines) indicate some cause for optimism regarding future prospects for controlling the global TB epidemic. However, still several factors mitigate prospects for improved TB control, including the spread of HIV, MDR-TB, and XDR-TB; demographic changes; socioeconomic determinants; and increasing poverty.

Despite a substantial increase in external aid flows for TB control to developing countries over the past decade, TB control globally is still underfunded. Data reported to the WHO from 118 countries that account for 94% of the total number of TB cases globally suggest that funding for TB control has grown from $2.7 billion in 2006 to $4.1 billion in 2010 (Fig. 8) (96). National governments account for 86% of such funding, while the remainder of funding is provided by donors, including the Global Fund to Fight AIDS, TB and Malaria. The gap between the funding reported in these countries in 2010 and the funding requirements for these countries according to the Global Plan to Stop TB 2006–2015 (96) is $2.1 billion. Most of the extra funding needed is for drug-resistant TB and TB/HIV control activities. Closing this financial gap is paramount to enable universal access to effective TB care in line with the six components of the Stop TB strategy. All concerned with TB control and poverty reduction must help mobilize the political will necessary to ensure adequate funds to implement effective programs that can be sustained for several decades.

The development of new tools for TB control, including a more effective vaccine, better diagnostic tests, and improved preventive and therapeutic approaches, holds out the prospect of rapid progress in the fight against TB and its eventual elimination by 2050. Already several new diagnostic tests are being rolled out in the field, including rapid diagnostics for MDR-TB. Hopefully new treatment regimens and vaccines will be as well available and introduced in the next few years. In the meantime, the challenge in maximizing the impact of currently available methods of diagnosis and treatment lies in implementing the Stop TB strategy as effectively and as widely as possible. The achievement and further sustainability of the Stop TB Partnership targets and the MDGs related to TB by 2015 are the greatest challenges countries are facing in order to set the path for elimination of TB. Not reaching such goals will be tremendously devastating for humanity. We cannot afford to lose the momentum.

Acknowledgments. Thanks go to Mukund Uplekar and Young Ae Chu for very useful suggestions and comments and Charalampos Sismanidis for useful help with part of the data.

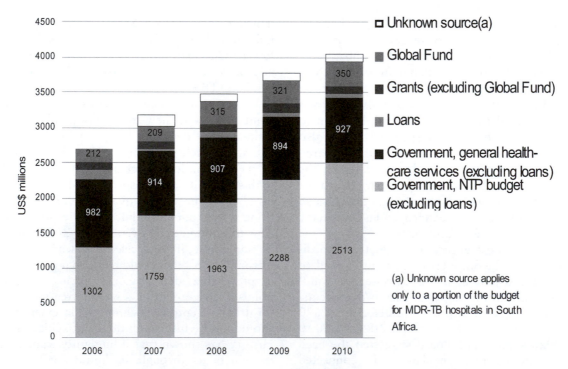

Figure 8. Funding for TB control by source of funding for 22 HBCs and 96 other countries, 2006 to 2010.

REFERENCES

1. Abu-Raddad, L. J., L. Sabatelli, J. T. Achterberg, J. D. Sugimoto, I. M. Longini, Jr., C. Dye, and M. E. Halloran. 2009. Epidemiological benefits of more effective tuberculosis vaccines, drugs and diagnostics. *Proc. Natl. Acad. Sci. USA* 106: 13980–13985.

2. Aziz, M. A., A. Wright, A. Laszlo, A. D. Muynck, F. Portaels, A. V. Deun, C. Wells, P. Nunn, L. Blanc, and M. Raviglione. 2006. Epidemiology of antituberculosis drug resistance (the Global Project on Anti-tuberculosis Drug Resistance Surveillance): an updated analysis. *Lancet* 368:2142–2154.

3. Borgdorff, M. W., K. Floyd, and J. F. Broekmans. 2002. Interventions to reduce tuberculosis mortality and transmission in low- and middle-income countries. *Bull. W. H. O.* 80: 217–227.

4. Broekmans, J. F., G. B. Migliori, H. L. Rieder, J. Lees, P. Ruutu, R. Loddenkemper, and M. C. Raviglione. 2002. European framework for tuberculosis control and elimination in countries with a low incidence: recommendations of the World Health Organization (WHO), International Union Against Tuberculosis and Lung Disease (IUATLD), and Royal Netherlands Tuberculosis Association (KNCV) Working Group. *Eur. Respir. J.* 19:765–775.

5. Chaisson, R., and M. Harrington. 2009. How research can help control of tuberculosis. *Int. J. Tuberc. Lung Dis.* 13: 558–568.

6. Chakaya, J., M. Uplekar, J. Mansoer, A. Kutwa, G. Karanja, V. Ombeka, D. Muthama, P. Kimuu, J. Odhiambo, H. Njiru, D. Kibuga, and J. Sitienei. 2008. Public-private mix for control of tuberculosis and TB-HIV in Nairobi, Kenya: outcomes, opportunities and obstacles. *Int. J. Tuberc. Lung Dis.* 12:1274–1278.

7. Chen, X., F. Zhao, H. Duanmu, L. Wan, L. Wang, X. Du, and D. P. Chin. The DOTS strategy in China: results and lessons after 10 years. *Bull. W. H. O.* 80:430–436.

8. China Tuberculosis Control Collaboration. 2004. The effect of tuberculosis control in China. *Lancet* 364:417–422.

9. Cobelens, F. G. J., E. Heldal, M. E. Kimerling, C. D. Mitnick, L. J. Podewils, R. Ramachandran, H. L. Rieder, K. Weyer, and M. Zignol, on behalf of the Working Group on MDR-TB of the Stop TB Partnership. 2008. Scaling up programmatic management of drug-resistant tuberculosis: a prioritized research agenda. *PLoS Med.* 5:e150. doi:10.1371/journal.pmed.0050150.

10. Cole, S. T., R. Brosch, J. Parkhill, T. Garnier, C. Churcher, D. Harris, S. V. Gordon, K. Eiglmeier, S. Gas, C. E. Barry, F. Tekaia, K. Badcock, D. Basham, D. Brown, T. Chillingworth, R. Connor, R. Davies, K. Devlin, T. Feltwell, S. Gentles, N. Hamlin, S. Holroyd, T. Hornsby, K. Jagels, A. Krogh, J. McLean, S. Moule, L. Murphy, K. Oliver, J. Osborne, M. A. Quail, M. A. Rajandream, J. Rogers, S. Rutter, K. Seeger, J. Skelton, R. Squares, S. Squares, J. E. Sulston, K. Taylor, S. Whitehead, and B. G. Barrell. 1998. Deciphering the biology of *Mycobacterium tuberculosis* from the complete genome sequence. *Nature* 393:537–544.

11. Corbett, E. L., C. J. Watt, N. Walker, D. Maher, B. G. Williams, M. C. Raviglione, and C. Dye. 2003. The growing burden of tuberculosis: global trends and interactions with the HIV epidemic. *Arch. Intern. Med.* 163:1009–1021.

12. Corbett, E. L., B. Marston, G. J. Churchyard, and K. M. De Cock. 2006. Tuberculosis in sub-Saharan Africa: opportunities, challenges, and change in the era of antiretroviral treatment. *Lancet* 367:926–937.

13. Crofton, J. 1960. Tuberculosis undefeated. *Br. Med. J.* 2: 679–687.

14. Daley, C., P. Small, G. Schecter, G. K. Schoolnik, R. A. McAdam, W. R. Jacobs, and P. C. Hopewell. 1992. An outbreak of tuberculosis with accelerated progression among persons with the human immunodeficiency virus: an analysis using restriction-fragment-length polymorphism. *N. Engl. J. Med.* 326:231–235.

15. Daniel, T. M. 2009. The history of tuberculosis: past, present, and challenges for the future, p. 1–7. *In* H. S. Schaaf and A. Zumla (ed.), *Tuberculosis: a Comprehensive Clinical Reference*. Saunders Elsevier, London, United Kingdom.

16. Di Perri, G., M. Cruciani, M. C. Danzi, R. Luzzati, G. De Checchi, M. Malena, S. Pizzighella, R. Mazzi, M. Solbiati, and E. Concia. 1989. Nosocomial epidemic of active tuberculosis among HIV-infected patients. *Lancet* ii:1502–1504.

17. Donald, P. R., D. Maher, and D. Qazi. 2007. A research agenda to promote the management of childhood tuberculosis within national tuberculosis programmes. *Int. J. Tuberc. Lung Dis.* 11:370–380.

18. Dye, C., G. P. Garnett, K. Sleeman, and B. G. Williams. 1998. Prospects for worldwide tuberculosis control under the WHO DOTS strategy. Directly observed short-course therapy. *Lancet* 352:1886–1891.

19. Dye, C., S. Scheele, P. Dolin, V. Pathania, and M. C. Raviglione. 1999. Global burden of tuberculosis: estimated incidence, prevalence and mortality by country. *JAMA* 282:677–686.

20. Dye, C., and B. G. Williams. 2000. Criteria for the control of drug-resistant tuberculosis. *Proc. Natl. Acad. Sci. USA* 97: 8180–8185.

21. Dye, C., M. A. Espinal, C. Watt, C. Mbiaga, and B. G. Williams. 2002. Worldwide incidence of multidrug-resistant tuberculosis. *J. Infect. Dis.* 185:1197–1202.

22. Dye, C., D. Maher, D. Weil, M. Espinal, and M. Raviglione. 2006. Targets for tuberculosis control. *Int. J. Tuberc. Lung Dis.* 10:460–462.

23. Dye, C., S. Ottmani, L. Laasri, and N. Bencheikh. 2007. The decline of tuberculosis epidemics under chemotherapy: a case study in Morocco. *Int. J. Tuberc. Lung Dis.* 11:1225–1231.

24. Dye, C., A. Bassili, A. L. Bierrenbach, J. F. Broekmans, V. K. Chadha, P. Glaziou, P. G. Gopi, M. Hosseini, S. J. Kim, D. Manissero, I. Onozaki, H. L. Rieder, S. Scheele, F. van Leth, M. van der Werf, and B. G. Williams. 2008. Measuring tuberculosis burden, trends, and the impact of control programmes. *Lancet Infect. Dis.* 8:233–243.

25. Dye, C., and B. G. Williams. 2010. The new population dynamics and control of tuberculosis. *Science* 328:856–861.

26. Elzinga, G., M. C. Raviglione, and D. Maher. 2004. Scale up: meeting targets in global tuberculosis control. *Lancet* 363: 814–819.

27. Espinal, M. A., C. Dye, M. Raviglione, and A. Kochi. 1999. Rational 'DOTS-Plus' for the control of MDR-TB. *Int. J. Tuberc. Lung Dis.* 3:561–563.

28. Espinal, M. A., A. Laszlo, L. Simonsen, F. Boulahbal, S. J. Kim, A. Reniero, S. Hoffner, H. L. Rieder, N. Binkin, C. Dye, R. Williams, and M. C. Raviglione. 2001. Global trends in resistance to antituberculosis drugs. *N. Engl. J. Med.* 344:1294–1303.

29. Espinal, M. A., S. J. Kim, P. G. Suarez, K. M. Kam, A. G. Khomenko, G. B. Migliori, J. Baéz, A. Kochi, C. Dye, and M. C. Raviglione. 2000. Standard short-course chemotherapy for drug-resistant tuberculosis: treatment outcome in 6 countries. *JAMA* 283:2537–2545.

30. Fauci, A. S., and NIAID Tuberculosis Working Group. 2008. Multi-drug resistant and extensively drug-resistant tuberculosis: the National Institute of Allergy and Infectious Diseases research agenda and recommendations for priority research. *J. Infect. Dis.* 197:1493–1498.

31. Frenk, J. 2006. Bridging the divide: global lessons from evidence-based health policy in Mexico. *Lancet* 368:954–961.

32. Gandhi, N. R., A. Moll, A. W. Sturm, R. Pawinski, T. Govender, U. Lalloo, K. Zeller, J. Andrews, and G. Friedland. 2006.

Extensively drug-resistant tuberculosis as a cause of death in patients co-infected with tuberculosis and HIV in a rural area of South Africa. *Lancet* **368:**1575–1580.

33. Gargioni, G. 2009. Role of communities in tuberculosis care and prevention, p. 660–667. *In* H. S. Schaaf and A. Zumla (ed.), *Tuberculosis: a Comprehensive Clinical Reference.* Saunders Elsevier, London, United Kingdom.

34. Ginsberg, A. M. 2008. Emerging drugs for active tuberculosis. *Semin. Respir. Crit. Care Med.* **29:**552–559.

35. Reference deleted.

36. Gupta, R., J. Y. Kim, M. A. Espinal, J. M. Caudron, B. Pecoul, P. Farmer, and M. C. Raviglione. 2001. Responding to market failure in tuberculosis control. *Science* **293:**1049–1051.

37. Gupta, R., J. P. Cegielski, M. A. Espinal, M. Henkens, J. Y. Kim, C. S. Lambregts-Van Weezenbeek, J. W. Lee, M. C. Raviglione, P. G. Suarez, and F. Varaine. 2002. Increasing transparency in partnerships for health—introducing the Green Light Committee. *Trop. Med. Int. Health* **7:**970–976.

38. Harries, A. D., R. Zachariah, E. L. Corbett, S. D. Lawn, E. T. Santos-Filho, R. Chimzizi, M. Harrington, D. Maher, B. G. Williams, and K. M. De Cock. 2010. The HIV-associated tuberculosis epidemic—when will we act? *Lancet* **375:**43–56.

39. Hopewell, P. C., M. Pai, D. Maher, M. Uplekar, and M. C. Raviglione. 2006. International standards for tuberculosis care. *Lancet Infect. Dis.* **11:**710–725.

40. Jackson, S., A. C. Sleigh, G.-J. Wang, and X.-L. Liu. 2006. Poverty and the economic effects of TB in rural China. *Int. J. Tuberc. Lung Dis.* **10:**1104–1110.

41. Kaufmann, S. H. E., G. Hussey, and P. H. Lambert. 2010. New vaccines for tuberculosis. *Lancet* **375:**85–94.

42. Kik, S. V., S. P. J. Olthof, J. T. N. de Vries, D. Menzies, N. Kincler, J. van Loenhout-Rooyakkers, C. Burdo, and S. Verver. 2009. Direct and indirect costs of tuberculosis among immigrant patients in the Netherlands. *BMC Public Health* **9:**283–287.

43. Kumar, M. K., P. K. Dewan, P. K. Nair, T. R. Frieden, S. Sahu, F. Wares, K. Laserson, C. Wells, R. Granich, and L. S. Chauhan. 2005. Improved tuberculosis case detection through public-private partnership and laboratory-based surveillance, Kannur District, Kerala, India, 2001–2002. *Int. J. Tuberc. Lung Dis.* **9:**870–876.

44. Laxminarayan, R., E. Y. Klein, S. Darley, and O. Adeyi. 2009. Global investment in TB control: economic benefits. *Health Affairs* **28:**W730–W742.

45. Lonnroth, K., E. Jaramillo, B. G. Williams, C. Dye, and M. Raviglione. 2009. Drivers of tuberculosis epidemics: the role of risk factors and social determinants. *Soc. Sci. Med.* **68:**2240–2246.

46. Ma, Z., and C. Lienhardt. 2009. Towards an optimized therapy for tuberculosis? Drugs in clinical trials and in preclinical development. *Clin. Chest Med.* **30:**755–768.

47. Maher, D., J. L. C. van Gorkom, P. C. F. M. Gondrie, and M. Raviglione. 1999. Community contribution to tuberculosis care in high tuberculosis prevalence countries: past, present and future. *Int. J. Tuberc. Lung Dis.* **3:**762–768.

48. Maher, D. 2003. The role of the community in the control of tuberculosis. *Tuberculosis* **83:**177–182.

49. Maher, D., C. Dye, K. Floyd, A. Pantoja, K. Lonnroth, A. Reid, E. Nathanson, T. Pennas, U. Fruth, J. Cunningham, H. Ignatius, M. C. Raviglione, I. Koek, and M. Espinal. 2007. Planning to improve global health: the next decade of tuberculosis control. *Bull. W. H. O.* **85:**341–347.

50. Matiru, R., and T. Ryan. 2007. The Global Drug Facility: a unique, holistic, and pioneering approach to drug procurement and management. *Bull. W. H. O.* **85:**348–353.

51. Ministry of Health and Family Welfare. 2010. *TB India 2010: RNTCP Status Report.* Central TB Division, New Delhi, India.

52. Murray, M. 2009. Epidemiology of TB, p. 23–59. *In* M. C. Raviglione (ed.), *Tuberculosis: the Essentials,* 4th ed. Informa Healthcare, New York, NY.

53. Murthy, K. J. R., T. R. Frieden, A. Yazdani, and P. Hreshikesh. 2001. Public-private partnership in tuberculosis control: experience in Hyderabad, India. *Int. J. Tuberc. Lung Dis.* **5:**354–359.

54. Nathanson, E., C. Lambregts-van Weezenbeek, M. L. Rich, R. Gupta, J. Bayona, K. Blöndal, J. A. Caminero, P. J. Cegielski, M. Danilovits, M. A. Espinal, V. Hollo, E. Jaramillo, V. Leimane, C. D. Mitnick, J. S. Mukherjee, P. Nunn, A. Pasechnikov, T. Tupasi, C. Wells, and M. C. Raviglione. 2006. Multidrug-resistant tuberculosis management in resource-limited settings. *Emerg. Infect. Dis.* **12:**1389–1397.

55. Nunn, P., A. Harries, P. Godfrey-Faussett, R. Gupta, D. Maher, and M. Raviglione. 2002. The research agenda for improving health policy, systems performance, and service delivery for tuberculosis control: a WHO perspective. *Bull. W. H. O.* **80:**471–476.

56. Orenstein, E. W., S. Basu, N. S. Shah, J. R. Andrews, G. H. Friedland, A. P. Moll, N. R. Gandhi, and A. P. Galvani. 2009. Treatment outcomes among patients with multidrug-resistant tuberculosis: systematic review and meta-analysis. *Lancet Infect. Dis.* **9:**153–161.

57. Pablos-Mendes, A., M. C. Raviglione, A. Laszlo, N. Binkin, H. L. Rieder, F. Bustreo, D. L. Cohn, C. S. B. Lambregts-van Weezenbeek, S. J. Kim, P. Chaulet, and P. Nunn. 1998. Global surveillance for antituberculosis-drug resistance, 1994–1997. *N. Engl. J. Med.* **338:**1641–1649. (Erratum, *N. Engl. J. Med.* **339:**139.)

58. Rajeswari, R., R. Balasubramanian, M. Muniyandi, S. Geetharamani, X. Thresa, and P. Venkatesan. 1999. Socio-economic impact of tuberculosis on patients and family in India. *Int. J. Tuberc. Lung Dis.* **3:**869–877.

59. Raviglione, M., C. Dye, S. Schmidt, and A. Kochi. 1997. Assessment of worldwide tuberculosis control. *Lancet* **350:**624–629.

60. Raviglione, M., and M. W. Uplekar. 2006. WHO's new Stop TB Strategy. *Lancet* **367:**952–955.

61. Ross, J. D., N. W. Horne, I. W. B. Grant, and J. W. Crofton. 1958. Hospital treatment of pulmonary tuberculosis. *Br. Med. J.* **1:**237–242.

62. Russell, S. 2004. The economic burden of illness for households in developing countries: a review of studies focusing on malaria, tuberculosis, and human immunodeficiency virus/acquired immunodeficiency syndrome. *Am. J. Trop. Med. Hyg.* **71**(2 Suppl.):147–155.

63. Shah, N. S., A. Wright, G. H. Bai, L. Barrera, F. Boulahbal, N. Martín-Casabona, F. Drobniewski, C. Gilpin, M. Havelková, R. Lepe, R. Lumb, B. Metchock, F. Portaels, M. F. Rodrigues, S. Rüsch-Gerdes, A. V. Deun, A. Vincent, K. Laserson, C. Wells, and J. P. Cegielski. 2007. Worldwide emergence of extensively drug-resistant tuberculosis. *Emerg. Infect. Dis.* **13:**380–387.

64. Shah, N. S., R. Pratt, L. Armstrong, V. Robison, K. G. Castro, and J. P. Cegielski. 2008. Extensively drug-resistant tuberculosis in the United States, 1993–2007. *JAMA* **300:**2153–2160.

65. Soemantri, S., F. P. Senewe, D. H. Tjandrarini, R. Day, C. Basri, D. Manissero, F. Mehta, and C. Dye. 2007. Three-fold reduction in the prevalence of tuberculosis over 25 years in Indonesia. *Int. J. Tuberc. Lung Dis.* **11:**398–407.

66. Stop TB Initiative. 2001. *Global TB Drug Facility—Prospectus. World Health Organization.* WHO/CDS/STB/2001.10a. World Health Organization, Geneva, Switzerland.

67. **Stop TB Partnership.** 2001. *Annual Report 2001.* WHO/CDS/STB/2002.17. World Health Organization, Geneva, Switzerland.

68. **Stop TB Partnership and World Health Organization.** 2006. *The Global Plan to Stop TB, 2006–2015.* WHO/HTM/STB/2006.35. World Health Organization, Geneva, Switzerland.

69. **Styblo, K.** 1989. Overview and epidemiological assessment of the current global tuberculosis situation with an emphasis on control in developing countries. *Rev. Infect. Dis.* **11**(Suppl. 2):339–346.

70. **Styblo, K., and J. R. Bumgarner.** 1991. *Tuberculosis Can Be Controlled with Existing Technologies: Evidence.* Tuberculosis, Surveillance Research Unit, International Union Against Tuberculosis and Lung Disease, Paris, France.

71. **Suarez, P. G., C. J. Watt, E. Alarcón, J. Portocarrero, D. Zavala, R. Canales, F. Luelmo, M. A. Espinal, and C. Dye.** 2001. The dynamics of tuberculosis in response to 10 years of intensive control effort in Peru. *J. Infect. Dis.* **184**:473–478.

72. **Suarez, P. G., K. Floyd, J. Portocarrero, E. Alarcón, E. Rapiti, G. Ramos, C. Bonilla, I. Sabogal, I. Aranda, C. Dye, M. Raviglione, and M. A. Espinal.** 2002. Feasibility and cost-effectiveness of standardised second-line drug treatment for chronic tuberculosis patients: a national cohort study in Peru. *Lancet* **359**:1980–1989.

73. **Treatment Action Group.** 2009. *Tuberculosis Research and Development: a Critical Analysis.* Treatment Action Group, New York, NY.

74. **Uplekar, M., S. Juvekar, S. Morankar, S. Rangan, and P. Nunn.** 1998. Tuberculosis patients and practitioners in private clinics in India. *Int. J. Tuberc. Lung Dis.* **2**:324–329.

75. **Uplekar, M., V. Pathania, and M. Raviglione.** 2001. Private practitioners and public health: weak links in tuberculosis control. *Lancet* **358**:912–916.

76. **Wallis, R. S., M. Pai, D. Menzies, T. M. Doherty, G. Walzl, M. D. Perkins, and A. Zumla.** 2010. Biomarkers and diagnostics for tuberculosis: progress, needs, and translation into practice. *Lancet* **375**:57–74.

77. **World Health Organization.** 1974. *Expert Committee on Tuberculosis: Ninth Report.* Technical report series 552. World Health Organization, Geneva, Switzerland.

78. **World Health Organization.** 1991. *Forty-Fourth World Health Assembly. Resolutions and Decisions. Resolution WHA 44.8.* WHA44/1991/REC/1. World Health Organization, Geneva, Switzerland.

79. **World Health Organization.** 1994. *47th World Health Assembly: Provisional Agenda Item 19. Tuberculosis Programme— Progress Report by the Director-General.* WHA47/1994/A47/12. World Health Organization, Geneva, Switzerland.

80. **World Health Organization.** 1998. *Global Tuberculosis Programme. Report of the Ad Hoc Committee on the Tuberculosis Epidemic. London, 17–19 March 1998.* WHO/TB/98.245. World Health Organization, Geneva, Switzerland.

81. **World Health Organization.** 2000. *Stop TB Initiative. Amsterdam, 22–24 March 2000— "Tuberculosis and Sustainable Development." Report of a Conference.* WHO/CDS/STB/2000.6. World Health Organization, Geneva, Switzerland.

82. **World Health Organization.** 2000. *Fifty-Third World Health Assembly. Resolutions and Decisions. Resolution WHA 53.1.* World Health Organization, Geneva, Switzerland.

83. **World Health Organization.** 2000. *The Economic Impacts of Tuberculosis. The Stop TB Initiative 2000 Series.* WHO/CDS/STB/2000.5. World Health Organization, Geneva, Switzerland.

84. **World Health Organization.** 2000. *Guidelines for Establishing DOTS-Plus Pilot Projects for the Management of Multidrug-Resistant Tuberculosis.* WHO/CDS/TB/2000.279. World Health Organization, Geneva, Switzerland.

85. **World Health Organization.** 2002. *An Expanded DOTS Framework for Effective Tuberculosis Control.* WHO/CDS/TB/2002.297. World Health Organization, Geneva, Switzerland.

86. **World Health Organization.** 2002. *A Strategic Framework To Decrease the Burden of TB/HIV.* WHO/CDS/TB/2002.296. World Health Organization, Geneva, Switzerland.

87. **World Health Organization.** 2003. *Community Contribution to TB Care: Practice and Policy.* WHO/CDS/TB/2003.312. World Health Organization, Geneva, Switzerland.

88. **World Health Organization.** 2004. *Report on the Meeting of the Second Ad Hoc Committee on the TB Epidemic. Montreux, Switzerland, 18–19 September 2003. Recommendations to Stop TB Partners.* WHO/HTM/STB/2004.28. World Health Organization, Geneva, Switzerland.

89. **World Health Organization.** 2004. *Interim Policy on Collaborative TB/HIV Activities.* WHO/HTM/TB/2004.330. World Health Organization, Geneva, Switzerland.

90. **World Health Organization.** 2006. *The Stop TB Strategy: Building On and Enhancing DOTS To Meet the Millennium Development Goals.* WHO/HTM/TB/2006.368. World Health Organization, Geneva, Switzerland.

91. **World Health Organization.** 2007. *The Global MDR-TB and XDR-TB Response Plan 2007–2008.* WHO/HTM/TB/2007.387. World Health Organization, Geneva, Switzerland.

92. **World Health Organization.** 2008. *The Global Burden of Disease: 2004 Update.* World Health Organization, Geneva, Switzerland.

93. **World Health Organization.** 2008. *Community Involvement in Tuberculosis Care and Prevention: Towards Partnerships for Health. Guiding Principles and Recommendations Based on a WHO Review.* WHO/HTM/TB/2008.397. World Health Organization, Geneva, Switzerland.

94. **World Health Organization.** 2008. *Guidelines for the Programmatic Management of Drug-Resistant Tuberculosis. Emergency Update 2008.* WHO/HTM/TB.2008.402. World Health Organization, Geneva, Switzerland.

95. **World Health Organization.** 2009. *Global Tuberculosis Control: Epidemiology, Strategy, Financing.* WHO/HTM/TB/2009.411. World Health Organization, Geneva, Switzerland.

96. **World Health Organization.** 2009. *Global Tuberculosis Control. A Short Update to the 2009 Report.* WHO/HTM/TB/2009.426. World Health Organization, Geneva, Switzerland.

97. **World Health Organization.** 2009. *Guidelines for Surveillance of Drug Resistance in Tuberculosis,* 4th ed. WHO/HTM/STB.2009.422. World Health Organization, Geneva, Switzerland.

98. **World Health Organization.** 2009. *Sixty-Second World Health Assembly. Resolutions and Decisions. Resolution WHA 62.15.* World Health Organization, Geneva, Switzerland.

99. **World Health Organization.** 2010. *Multidrug and Extensively Drug Resistant TB (M/XDR-TB). 2010 Global Report on Surveillance and Response.* WHO/HTM/TB/2010.3. World Health Organization, Geneva, Switzerland.

100. **World Health Organization.** 2010. *Public-Private Mix for TB Care and Control. Report of the Sixth Meeting of the Subgroup on Public-Private Mix for TB Care and Control.* WHO/HTM/TB/2010.5. World Health Organization, Geneva, Switzerland.

101. **World Health Organization and International Labour Office.** 2003. *Guidelines for Workplace TB Control Activities.* WHO/CDS/TB/2003.323. World Health Organization, Geneva, Switzerland.

102. **Wright, A., M. Zignol, A. V. Deun, D. Falzon, S. R. Gerdes, K. Feldman, S. Hoffner, F. Drobniewski, L. Barrera, D. V. Soolingen, F. Boulabhal, C. N. Paramasivan, K. M. Kam, S. Mitarai, P. Nunn, and M. Raviglione.** 2009. Epidemiology of antituberculosis drug resistance 2002–07: an updated analysis of the Global Project on Anti-Tuberculosis Drug Resistance Surveillance. *Lancet* **373:**1861–1873.

103. **Zignol, M., M. S. Hosseini, A. Wright, C. L.Weezenbeek, P. Nunn, C. J. Watt, B. G. Williams, and C. Dye.** 2006. Global incidence of multidrug-resistant tuberculosis. *J. Infect. Dis.* **194:**479–485.

Chapter 12

Tuberculosis in Enclosed Populations

SORANA SEGAL-MAURER

INTRODUCTION

The 1990s saw a dramatic resurgence in cases of tuberculosis (TB), especially nosocomial and multidrug-resistant tuberculosis (MDR-TB). Reports from congregate settings emphasized the increased transmission of TB in closed or indoor environments, particularly among high-risk hosts. Factors that contributed to outbreaks of TB in hospitals, prisons, shelters, and long-term care facilities (LTCFs) in the early 1990s included the decay in public health infrastructure, the rise of human immunodeficiency virus (HIV) coinfection, the increase in the number of homeless and destitute persons, health care workers' (HCWs) decreased vigilance, and few existing adequate isolation facilities. The resulting major public health efforts to upgrade facilities in hospitals and jails, provide directly observed treatment (DOT), and educate HCWs and the public all led to a dramatic decrease in new TB cases (especially MDR-TB) from 10.5 cases per 100,000 in 1992 to 3.8 cases per 100,000 in 2009 (30). The 2009 rate showed the greatest single-year decrease ever recorded and was the lowest recorded rate since national TB surveillance began in 1953 (30). In spite of a decrease in nosocomial transmission of TB and MDR-TB, there is an increase in TB among foreign-born people, immigrants from areas of endemicity, migrant workers, and residents of homeless shelters, with continued spread to susceptible persons in local communities (13, 30). This new wave is fueled by the global HIV epidemic, ease of worldwide mobility, changing economic milieu, and continued global ravages of TB. Continued vigilance and support and implementation of local, national, and international programs remain paramount for control of TB.

This chapter reviews the factors involved in the transmission of TB in various congregate settings and the methods employed for curtailment and prevention. The focus is on implementation of infection control practices for the safety of susceptible persons, residents, patients, and HCWs.

EPIDEMIOLOGY OF TRANSMISSION

The probability of transmission of *Mycobacterium tuberculosis* depends on the concentration of infectious droplet nuclei in the air, the duration of exposure to these particles, and the closeness of contact with infectious persons (69). Infection is best transmitted in overcrowded environments and confined spaces where poor ventilation or air recirculation permits the accumulation of infectious particles (69). Numerous non-health care, community-based outbreaks of TB have been described to occur in schools, offices and workplaces, neighborhood bars, ships, and airplanes (35, 58). All outbreaks were characterized by highly infectious persons in proximity to those susceptible in enclosed, poorly ventilated environments.

OUTBREAKS OF THE 1990S—"THE PROBLEM"

Prior to 1990, nosocomial outbreaks of TB in the United States were relatively few, propagated slowly among patients, and rarely involved MDR-TB strains (47). Health care personnel who were infected as a result of these exposures demonstrated close and prolonged contact with patients with either unrecognized TB or TB in the initial phases of treatment. In many reports, specific aerosol-producing medical procedures, such as bronchoscopy, endotracheal intubation, wound manipulation, respiratory tract manipulation, or autopsy, were associated with transmission. Patient-to-patient transmission of TB was uncommon.

Sorana Segal-Maurer • Division of Infectious Diseases, New York Hospital Queens, Flushing, NY 11355, and Weill Cornell Medical College, New York, NY 10065.

During the 1990s, by contrast, nosocomial spread of TB occurred as multiple institutional outbreaks that propagated rapidly and involved MDR-TB strains. In New York City alone, 57 medical facilities (including the medical examiner's office) and 2 correctional facilities reported outbreaks with MDR-TB (66, 67). Many outbreaks involved strain "W," a strain of *M. tuberculosis* resistant to more than six anti-TB medications. During the period from 1990 to 1993, it was seen in one-third of New York City's MDR-TB cases and in one-fourth of all U.S. MDR-TB cases, with cure rates of 50 to 60% (in contrast to 95 to 97% for drug-susceptible TB) (27). Attack rates were highest among U.S.-born, HIV-coinfected patients and among HCWs caring for them. Molecular epidemiology indicated that over 40% of TB cases were a result of recent transmission rather than reactivation of latent disease (2, 89).

Although no longer present in health care or congregate settings, the "W" strain is still seen sporadically in the community among patients with contact to prior infected patients, released inmates, or HCWs (67). Current U.S. surveillance for either MDR-TB or extensively drug-resistant TB (XDR-TB) demonstrated 107 cases of MDR-TB for 2008, with the most common risk factor being foreign birth (77.6% of MDR-TB cases) and a history of having had TB (4.3%), a marked change from the outbreaks of the early 1990s, which occurred mainly among the U.S.-born population (30). As a result of implementation of the 1992 CDC Action Plan for Control of XDR-TB, the reported annual incidence of MDR-TB in the United States declined from 485 cases in 1993 to 119 cases in 2007, representing a 75% decrease (27). As of March 2010, there are no new cases of XDR-TB reported for 2009 in the United States (27).

We now recognize that HIV infection increases the risk of progression from latent TB infection to active TB disease and increases the possibility of atypical presentation (with delays in diagnosis), as well as more rapid clinical progression (5, 8, 15, 31, 42, 65, 79). The highly infectious nature of these patients was elegantly demonstrated in a study where all the air from a negative-pressure HIV-TB ward was exhausted over guinea pigs housed in an airborne-study facility (36). One-half of exposed guinea pigs developed TB, with 90% of TB transmission occurring from several inadequately treated MDR-TB patients (three were highly infectious, producing 226, 52, and 40 airborne infectious units or quanta per hour). This explains, in part, the increased prevalence of nosocomial outbreaks in areas where patients with HIV coinfection work, receive care, or reside and the need for added awareness following early outbreaks. Improved TB surveillance and control and increased

HIV testing have led to a decrease in outbreak situations. Among persons with TB with a known HIV test result during 2009, 10.2% were coinfected with HIV, a marked improvement from the prior 25% rate of known coinfection seen in the early 1990s (30).

Acute Care Facilities

Nosocomial spread of TB in the early 1990s has been described extensively (5, 15, 24, 42, 49, 56, 91). These outbreaks were characterized by HIV coinfection prevalence greater than 80%, a median of 8 weeks from the time of diagnosis to death (average, 4 to 16 weeks), and a mortality rate in excess of 70%. Temporal clustering of clinical cases and distinct anti-TB medication susceptibility patterns led to the eventual recognition of distinct outbreaks. In most instances, patients were housed on dedicated HIV wards or attended HIV clinics (5, 15, 42). Numerous HCWs were infected, and a number developed active disease.

Factors that contributed to patient and HCW infection are listed in Table 1. Common to each outbreak were the failures to isolate patients early and to maintain isolation pending clinical improvement or diagnosis. Laboratory delays, infection control lapses, and facility shortcomings all contributed to spread of MDR-TB among patients and staff. The period between specimen collection and the identification of *M. tuberculosis* (6 weeks) and completion of susceptibility testing (up to 12 weeks) frequently occurred after the patient's death. Since the presence of

Table 1. Factors contributing to nosocomial outbreaks of MDR-TB, 1990s[a]

Source or patient factors
  Increased homelessness
  HIV
    Advanced disease (i.e., end-stage AIDS)
    Atypical presentation of *M. tuberculosis*
    Attendance in a dedicated HIV clinic
    Housing in HIV congregate setting
  Previous hospitalization, especially prior exposure (on the same ward) to infectious MDR-TB patient
  Aerosolized pentamidine treatment

Infection control factors
  Low clinical suspicion (leading to delayed recognition)
  Cohorting of patients
  Problems with isolation of infectious patients
    Delayed institution of isolation
    Premature discontinuation of isolation
    Inadequate isolation facilities
    Lack of enforcement of strict isolation policies
  Slow laboratory turnaround time for AFB smears, culture, and susceptibility results
  Delayed initiation of effective treatment regimens (undiagnosed MDR-TB), resulting in prolonged period of infectiousness

[a]Data adapted from references 5, 8, and 24.

resistant organisms was not recognized quickly, patients remained on inadequate anti-TB regimens for prolonged periods, and many persons were removed from isolation while still infectious (15, 42).

Nosocomial transmission of TB declined sharply following the issuance and widespread implementation of the Centers for Disease Control and Prevention (CDC) guidelines in 1994, which focused on risk assessment, appropriate isolation, rapid laboratory testing, DOT programs administered by departments of health, and an improvement in the health infrastructure (24). Advances in HIV antiretroviral therapy improved patients' health and decreased their hospitalization, thereby reducing a highly susceptible population. In addition, the concern over bioterrorism, new strains of influenza virus, and severe acute respiratory syndrome (SARS) increased our awareness regarding airborne infections (9). In spite of this, isolated outbreaks still occurred due to breaches in infection control and HCWs' low index of suspicion (22). Even during SARS screening efforts in Taiwan, HCWs with active TB were identified (23). Vigilance and administrative controls remain the most important methods to prevent nosocomial outbreaks.

The CDC updated its health care guidelines for the control of TB in 2005 "to maintain momentum and expertise needed to avert another TB resurgence" (24). Compared to the previous guidelines, which were aimed primarily at hospital-based facilities, the 2005 guidelines were expanded to address a broader concept. "Setting" was chosen rather than "facility" in order to expand the scope of potential places for which these guidelines apply (24). "Setting" implies any relationship (physical or organizational, inpatient or outpatient, and health care or non-health care areas) in which HCWs might share air space with persons with TB disease or in which HCWs might be in contact with TB clinical specimens. Thus, a single facility may have several "setting" types (24). Also, the airborne infection isolation (AII) room was defined and specific recommendations were made as to its use (24).

Correctional Facilities

According to the U.S. Bureau of Justice Statistics, over 7.3 million people were on probation, in jail or in prison, or on parole at the end of 2008, representing 3.2% of all U.S. adult residents or 1 in every 31 adults (12). Up to 25% of U.S. inmates have latent TB infection (LTBI), and the incidence of active TB infection among inmates is 6 to 10 times that in the nonincarcerated population (6). HIV infection, which is the strongest risk factor for progression from LTBI to active disease, is 10 to 20 times more prevalent among the incarcerated population than among the nonincarcerated. TB transmission from inmates to employees, visitors, volunteers, and other inmates has been documented (6).

During the outbreaks of the early 1990s, the incidence of TB among prisoners was 10-fold greater than that in the general U.S. population (25). This was the result of 11 outbreaks of TB (most with MDR-TB) occurring in prisons in eight states from 1985 to 1992 (25, 97). Over 171 inmates with TB were diagnosed in the New York State prison system alone from 1990 to 1991. Approximately one-third of them had MDR-TB, and 97% were HIV coinfected (97). Infectious inmates were transferred through a number of correctional facilities and local hospitals for medical care prior to diagnosis of TB. One-third of inmates who were exposed converted their tuberculin skin test (TST) (one-half after close contact with index patients), as did a number of HCWs and patients at local hospitals (97). Federal and state systems reported a 25% prevalence of TB infection, increased TST conversions, and an HIV coinfection rate of more than 10% among inmates incarcerated from 1990 to 1995 (25, 97).

Factors that contributed to these correctional facility TB outbreaks included the rise in HIV coinfection with rapid progression of disease, low index of suspicion for TB and delays in diagnosis, the increase in MDR-TB with extensive resistance to empirical anti-TB regimens, overcrowding, poor ventilation and inadequate isolation facilities, and failure to adhere to recognized standards for prevention, screening, and containment (Table 2). The transmission of *M. tuberculosis* within jails and prisons increased spread

Table 2. Factors contributing to TB outbreaks in correctional facilities, 1990s[a]

National drug control strategy with incarceration of illegal substance-using persons
Increase in HIV-positive or HIV-at-risk inmates (primarily due to intravenous substance use)
Overcrowding of facilities
Security (not health care) as prime objective in policy and edifice design
Increasing rates in communities
Nosocomial spread in acute care facilities to and from transferred inmates
Diagnostic failures (clinical and laboratory delays)
Inter-correctional facility transfer of infectious inmates
Inadequate TST screening and loss to follow-up
Noncompliance with therapy and prophylactic therapy
Long or multiple incarcerations
Lack of adequate AII facilities
Loss to follow-up (i.e., transfer to health care facilities with return to other correctional facilities, release without appropriate department of health follow-up)

[a]Data adapted from references 25, 38, and 97.

to the nonincarcerated population, including visitors, surrounding communities, and homeless shelters (6, 25, 71). Reports document extensive spread to local communities and international settings of MDR-TB strains found in Eastern European correctional facilities facilitated by discharged inmates and/or their families and visitors (63).

Studies document correlation between length of incarceration and positive TST response, indicating that transmission occurs in these facilities (25). At least three factors contribute to the high rate of TB in correctional and detention facilities. First, disparate numbers of incarcerated persons are at high risk for *M. tuberculosis* infection (e.g., users of illicit substances, persons of low socioeconomic status, and persons with HIV infection). These persons often have not received standard public health interventions or nonemergency medical care before incarceration. Second, the physical structure of the facilities contributes to disease transmission, as facilities often provide close living quarters, might have inadequate ventilation, and can be overcrowded. Third, movement of inmates into and out of overcrowded and inadequately ventilated facilities, coupled with existing TB-related risk factors of the inmates, makes correctional and detention facilities a high-risk environment for the transmission of TB and makes implementation of TB control measures particularly difficult (25). Furthermore, inmates are often abruptly summoned for court appearances and are summarily transferred or released (6).

Homeless Shelters, Single-Resident Occupancy (SRO) Hotels, and Other Facilities

Approximately 1.6 million persons used an emergency shelter or a transitional housing program during the 12-month period between 1 October 2007 and 30 September 2008 (71). This number suggests that 1 in every 190 persons in the United States used the shelter system at some point in that period (71). In 2008, more than two-thirds of all sheltered homeless people were located in principal cities. Between 2007 and 2008, there was an increase in the number of sheltered homeless individuals who were in institutional settings (e.g., prisons, jails, or inpatient facilities) the night before they became homeless (71).

In 1993, the CDC requested health departments to indicate the proportion of homelessness among annually reported TB cases (43). The proportion of TB cases associated with homelessness was approximately 6.1 to 6.7% from 1994 to 2003, the first full decade of national TB surveillance that included this assessment (43). Foreign-born cases of TB were found among 18% of homeless persons, compared to

Table 3. Factors contributing to TB outbreaks in shelters and SRO hotels, 1990s[a]

Human factors
  Increasing age of occupants
  Socioeconomic factors (poverty, stress, and malnutrition)
  Substance use (intravenous drug use and alcoholism)
  HIV coinfection
  Mental illness
  Transient nature of homeless persons
  History of prior incarceration, hospitalization, or contact with others with such history

Facility factors
  Close living quarters in open areas
  Increasing length of stay (>24 mo)
  Inadequate ventilation

Infection control factors
  Inability to identify contacts due to nature of transient status or fear of incarceration
  Poor medical screening and health care

[a]Data adapted from references 10, 43, 53, 65, 70, and 102.

44% among nonhomeless. At the time of TB diagnosis, more homeless than nonhomeless persons were incarcerated (9% versus 3%). In the past, the degree of "homelessness" was linked to risk of acquisition of TB, with persons sleeping in a shelter or on the street less likely to acquire TB than those sleeping in an SRO hotel or a rehabilitation program (4). Factors leading to TB outbreaks among homeless persons are listed in Table 3.

Homeless persons with TB had a higher prevalence of substance use than did nonhomeless persons (54% alcohol abuse, 29.5% noninjected drug use, and 14% injected drug use) (40, 70). Sputum smear-positive disease is twofold more prevalent among HIV-negative substance users than nonusers but not more likely to be drug resistant (43, 70, 76). Patients who abused substances were twofold more likely to be involved in a county-level genotype cluster of TB suggesting ongoing or recent transmission (70). International reports of TB among homeless substance users demonstrate a similarly high rate of transmission to contacts (35).

One-third of homeless persons with TB who are tested for HIV have coinfection, adding to their risk for disease progression (43). The association among homelessness, TB, and HIV infection is well described and was recently demonstrated in a longitudinal study of the homeless in San Francisco, California (65). The authors found the evolution of TB cases and their HIV-coinfected contacts to be highly related (a finding not present among nonhomeless), confirming the hypothesis that the dynamics of HIV and TB are significantly intertwined and that HIV is likely a key factor in the sustenance of TB transmission among the San Francisco homeless.

TST screening and initiating and completing treatment for LTBI in individuals with unstable housing are difficult tasks. Homeless persons are frequently reluctant to answer screening questions related to symptoms or past TB infection for fear that they may be denied a benefit (such as a shelter bed or substance use treatment) or be compelled to enter coercive treatment. Although numerous persons are potentially exposed in shelter outbreaks, their transient and migratory lifestyles hinder the ability to identify and follow up contacts (53, 102). Even when contacts were identified during outbreaks, less than half of those who began LTBI treatment actually completed a full course (102).

Long-Term Care Facilities

As the result of the strengthening of TB control programs nationwide, a decline in the overall number of reported TB cases in the United States has been observed within the last 10 years. Despite these declines in absolute numbers, the elderly continue to account for a disproportionate share of the cases and constitute a large reservoir of LTBI (28). The risk of reactivation increases as immunologic status declines with age (16, 19, 24, 30, 78, 90, 98). For 2008, the incidence of active TB among persons over the age of 65 was 2,500 per 100,000 persons (compared to 4,911 for ages 40 to 64 and 3,266 for ages 25 to 39) (28).

Evidence suggests that the institutionalized elderly are at a greater risk for reactivation of latent TB and for the acquisition of new TB infection than are their community-dwelling counterparts (104). During the 1990s, positive TST reactions occurred in a third of persons entering LTCFs (especially after two-step testing was implemented) (19, 68). Many persons older than 64 years of age with active TB live in an LTCF or nursing home at the time of diagnosis (46). In addition, 20% of LTCF residents developed active TB as a result of a recent exposure, with spread to other patients, employees, and visitors (16, 48). In Germany, 12% of TB outbreaks were concentrated in nursing homes according to a recent German electronic surveillance system report for infectious diseases during 2004 and 2005 (51). In spite of the recognized importance of beginning and completing a course of LTBI treatment, employees and residents have a threefold risk of failing to complete a course (44).

Although the majority of TB in older persons presents as pulmonary reactivation, a quarter of persons present with atypical symptoms of extrapulmonary or disseminated disease, making diagnosis more challenging and prolonging the period of potential exposure to others (78). The high number of cases

Table 4. Risk factors for spread of *Mycobacterium tuberculosis* in LTCFs, 1990s[a]

Source or patient factors
  Elderly
  High prevalence of TST positivity (and increased risk of recrudescence)
  Comorbid medical conditions increasing the risk of reactivation or of exogenous reinfection
  Waning of immunity to prior infection
  Unsuspected disease (frequently confused with carcinoma or bacterial infection)
  Prolonged exposure (frequently over 12 mo)
  Frequent atypical chest radiograph appearance of TB

Facility and infection control factors
  Congregate surroundings/close contact
  Few or no isolation facilities
  Variable compliance with annual TST programs
  Inadequate education concerning infection and transmission
  Inadequate use of prophylactic therapy

[a]Data adapted from references 16 and 68.

diagnosed at autopsy among the elderly suggests that this condition often remains unrecognized (104).

LTCFs caring for the handicapped, mentally ill, and developmentally disabled also reported TB outbreaks (52). These were facilitated by prolonged contagiousness due to delay in diagnosis of the source, difficulty in medical examination or communication with impaired or psychotic patients, crowded or communal living conditions, and lack of isolation facilities. Factors contributing to transmission of TB in LTCFs appear in Table 4.

Foreign-Born Persons

Persons who are foreign-born living in the United States frequently live in extended-family and/or overcrowded situations and then come into contact with susceptible persons (72). Within urban areas, the rate of overcrowding is the highest in central cities. Among the foreign-born, overcrowding appears most prevalent among the Hispanic population, with the number of overcrowded Hispanic households more than doubling from 1985 to 2005 (72).

In 2009, The TB rate in foreign-born persons was nearly 11 times higher than in U.S.-born persons (30). TB rates among Hispanics and blacks were nearly eight times higher than among non-Hispanic whites, and rates among Asians were nearly 23 times higher than among non-Hispanic whites. In 2009, four countries accounted for 50.1% of TB cases in foreign-born persons: Mexico, the Philippines, India, and Vietnam (30). Among XDR-TB cases in California, 83% of cases involved foreign-born patients, and 43% were diagnosed in patients within 6 months after arrival in the United States. Mexico was the most common country of origin (3). History of travel to or deportation from the United States and incarceration were independently associated with a reported lifetime diagnosis of TB among injection drug users in Tijuana from 2006 and 2007 (34). Although it is generally assumed that TB in immigrants is the result of importation of infection, recent reports indicate recent transmission among immigrant communities and from them to resident populations (14, 60, 92).

Data for overseas screening for TB in U.S.-bound immigrants and refugees from 1999 through 2005 reveals prevalence rates of over 900 cases per 100,000 for smear-negative TB among immigrants and over 1,000 cases per 100,000 among refugees (55). The rates for LTBI (abnormal chest radiographs in asymptomatic persons) ranged from over 800 to over 2,800 per 100,000 persons among immigrants and refugees, respectively. Active pulmonary TB (acid-fast bacillus [AFB] smear positive) was diagnosed in the United States in 7.0% of immigrants and refugees with an overseas diagnosis of smear-negative TB and in 1.6% of those with an overseas diagnosis of inactive TB (55).

Over 150 TB cases are identified annually among Immigration and Naturalization Service (INS) detainees in processing centers and contract detention facilities. Data for 2001 to 2002 indicate that the prevalence of culture-confirmed TB reported from eight of these centers was approximately 67 cases per 100,000 INS detainees, 12 times the overall U.S. incidence of 5.6 cases in 2001 and 2.5 times the rate for the U.S. foreign-born population (21). The average length of TB treatment in a center was 22 days before release or deportation. From January 2000 to March 2001, CURE-TB reported that 25% of TB patients deported to Latin America with known follow-up eventually returned to the United States, with additional reports of new drug-resistant TB which was not present initially (21). These persons frequently pass through correctional facilities, increasing exposure of inmates and workers, legal personnel, and, following deportation, persons in the native country. INS policies require that before transfer or deportation, detainees with TB disease receive treatment until they become noncontagious, even if a treatment course is not completed fully, falling short of the Advisory Council for the Elimination of Tuberculosis recommendations for the postdetention completion of TB treatment for persons deported or released from the custody of the INS (21).

Migrant workers and those frequently crossing borders are often lost to follow-up and are unable to participate in contact tracing (92). Most cases of TB are reported from Florida, Texas, and California, with increased numbers of cases seen in migrant farm workers (MFWs). These were more likely to be among male, foreign-born, or Hispanic (most from Mexico) and to have a history of alcohol abuse and homelessness than were non-MFWs (83). HIV status was poorly reported, with results available for only 28% of MFW and 33% of non-MFW cases (82, 83). Of the MFWs tested, 28% were HIV infected, whereas 34% of non-MFWs were HIV infected. Twenty percent of MFWs move or are lost to follow-up before completing therapy (83).

Congregate Travel

The International Civil Aviation Organization has forecast that there will be more than 2.5 billion air passengers per year by 2015. Findings to date document a small risk of transmission of any infectious disease aboard aircraft. However, transmission probably occurs more frequently than reported, since many diseases have an incubation period longer than the duration of air travel. Of the airborne and droplet-borne diseases that are potentially transmissible aboard aircraft, the most important are TB, influenza, SARS, meningococcal disease, and measles (58, 100). In view of the worldwide increase in cases of TB, MDR-TB, and XDR-TB, international authorities are more vigilant about congregate travel (27).

From 1992 to 1994, the CDC conducted seven contact investigations involving a crew member and six passengers. The number of potentially exposed passengers and cabin crew exceeded 2,600 on a total of 191 flights involving nine different types of aircraft (100). All index patients were highly infectious (one patient with confirmed laryngeal TB). Two passengers, who were flying to the United States for medical care, knew that they had active TB at the time of their flights but did not inform the airline of their disease. In the other five cases, TB was diagnosed after the flights (100). In only two of the investigations was there evidence to suggest transmission of TB: one from a cabin crew member to other crew members (linked to over 12 h of exposure) and another from a passenger to other passengers (linked to close proximity for over 8 h).

In recent years, MDR-TB has become an increasingly important public health problem in many countries, exacerbated by the emergence of XDR-TB (59). An investigation in 2007 involved the unapproved travel of a person with documented pulmonary MDR-TB (but AFB smear negative, clinically asymptomatic, and without TST conversion among close contacts). Fortunately, there were no reported TST conversions among airline passengers or crew.

While screening for TB is usually mandatory for immigrants and refugees, the overwhelming majority of passengers flying on commercial aircraft do not fall into any category for which screening is a requirement (100). Investigations of possible TB transmission aboard commercial aircraft are usually initiated several weeks to months after the flight, and passengers are often difficult to locate (100).

IMPACT ON HCWs

Globally, the prevalence of LTBI among HCWs can be as high 54% (50, 95). Estimates of the annual risk of LTBI ranges from 0.5 to 14.3%, and the annual incidence of TB in HCWs ranges from 69 to 5,780 per 100,000 in countries with middle and lower income levels (50). The attributable risk for TB disease among these HCWs, compared to the risk in the general population, ranges from 25 to 5,361 per 100,000 per year. A higher risk of acquiring *M. tuberculosis* infection is associated with certain work locations (inpatient TB facility, laboratory, internal medicine, and emergency facilities) and occupational categories (radiology technicians, patient attendants, nurses, ward attendants, paramedics, and clinical officers) (50).

The baseline prevalence of positive TSTs among U.S. HCWs is reported to be as low as 1.4% to as high as 18% (and over 50% during the early 1990s) (62, 77, 86, 99). While HCW ethnicity, socioeconomic status, and location of residence may play a role in community transmission of TB to HCWs, TST reaction prevalence rates among HCWs are 10 to 100 times greater than those in the general population and are explained by occupational exposure (62). Although frequent and prolonged exposure is necessary to produce disease in HCWs, studies have demonstrated relatively short but close contact with a highly infectious patient or involvement with aerosol-producing procedures to be a source of widespread infection (62, 81).

During nosocomial outbreaks of the 1990s, TST conversion occurred in over three-quarters of exposed HCWs. The risk was eightfold greater for exposed than nonexposed HCWs, with higher disease rates and increased mortality rates among HIV-coinfected HCWs (62, 103). Spread of TB from HCWs to others (coworkers and patients) occurred infrequently (103). Although the prevalence of TST conversions among HCWs decreased after the peak of the TB epidemic in the early 1990s (26.4 to 3.9%), the conversion rate among HCWs in high-risk occupational settings for TB exposure continues to be greater than that among HCWs in low-risk settings (32, 77, 99).

Despite the general decline in TB rates in recent years in the United States, a marked geographic variation in TB case rates persists (30). Four states (California, Florida, New York, and Texas) reported more than 500 cases of active TB each for 2009. Combined, these four states accounted for half of all TB cases in 2009. HCWs in these states are at particular increased risk of encountering patients with active TB. In addition, a proportion of HCWs working in the United States come from or have traveled to areas of the world with high endemic risk for TB.

CURTAILMENT AND PREVENTION— "THE SOLUTION"

TB reemerged in the United States at a time when compliance with existing guidelines for prevention of nosocomial spread of TB was not strictly enforced. In most cases, outbreaks were curtailed with implementation of established infection control practices, increased diagnostic and therapeutic aggressiveness, and establishment of an active TST surveillance program, all prior to any environmental or personal protective equipment (PPE) changes (i.e., masks or respirators) (24). Administrative measures alone at one hospital in New York City led to a marked decrease in TST conversion rates among HCWs, from 17 to 5%, a decrease to the same rate of conversion as seen among controls (56). In many instances, the contribution of PPE use to curtailing outbreaks was not directly measurable, since use was not uniform and different PPE models were chosen (24). Also, many facilities implemented a number of changes simultaneously, and individual contributions could not be assessed (24, 56).

In response to the MDR-TB outbreaks in hospitals and correctional facilities from 1988 to 1991, the CDC convened a Federal TB Task Force with representatives from multiple U.S. agencies. In June 1992, the Federal TB Task Force published an action plan that provided a framework for response and specific action steps for state and local health departments and federal agencies. These action steps were grouped into nine categories: (i) surveillance and epidemiology, (ii) laboratory diagnosis, (iii) patient management, (iv) screening and preventive therapy, (v) infection control, (vi) outbreak control, (vii) program evaluation, (viii) information dissemination/training and education, and (ix) research. Emergency federal funding was appropriated to allow the Federal TB Task Force and state and local health departments to implement certain parts of the plan. In addition, multiple organizations and institutions, national and international, were recruited to improve research and to implement findings (27). The CDC also published TB control guidelines to address particular settings or groups of people, including acute care facilities, correctional facilities, homeless persons, LTCFs, migrant workers, and air travel (16–19, 24–27).

The most recent (2005) CDC guidelines for health care facilities were designed for broad application in various settings and facilities (both in- and outpatient) where health care is delivered and where patients with TB would be encountered (24). New components of the updated guidelines included an explicit discussion of risk assessment, description of hierarchy of TB controls, the applicability to numerous settings, detailed explanations for environmental and PPE modalities, and the availability of worksheets to aid in creating an appropriate TB infection control program (24). The hierarchy of TB controls remained (i) administrative controls with guidelines for programs in patient care (education, diagnosis, isolation, and treatment) and HCW safety (education, TST, and LTBI treatment), (ii) environmental controls (improvement in ventilation and decontamination of air and equipment), and (iii) use of PPE (selection, education, and fit testing).

Annual (or periodic) risk assessment was made the cornerstone of a TB infection control program. Determining the risk level (prevalence, incidence, and risk of acquisition of TB infection to ascertain the risk of nosocomial spread of TB) determines the extent to which other TB control measures need to be implemented. The three potential TB screening risk classifications include low risk, medium risk, and potential ongoing transmission. The document provides ample descriptions and examples so that personnel at each facility may decide the appropriate applicable risk category. Low risk is applied to settings (or HCWs or clinical specimens) in which persons with TB disease are unlikely to be encountered, and, therefore, exposure to *M. tuberculosis* is unlikely (24). Medium risk is applied to settings where there exists the possibility of exposure to *M. tuberculosis*. Potential ongoing transmission is a temporary classification and is applied to any setting (or group of HCWs) when there is documented person-to-person transmission of *M. tuberculosis* within the previous 12 months (24). All classifications require ongoing risk assessment, including review of local community epidemiology (with the aid of local departments of health), review of the facility's previous 5 years of suspected and/or confirmed cases, and evaluation of HCWs, requiring inclusion in a TB screening program (24).

Administrative Controls

Surveillance (gathering and timely analysis of data), education, and clinical suspicion remain primary to TB infection control. To limit the risk of nosocomial spread, persons considered at risk for active TB need to be placed in AII and must remain there until laboratory and clinical data can eliminate the possibility of TB or the risk of contagion. Additionally, use of PPE is required to protect HCWs. Rapid diagnosis and empirical (and appropriate) anti-TB therapy (after adequate samples are obtained for culture) are additional factors in decreasing the potential for spread. TST screening of patients, inmates, residents, and HCWs and the use of LTBI treatment add to an effective TB infection control program.

LTBI screening

Guidelines for LTBI screening are published and are discussed in detail in chapter 5 (19, 24, 29). During the outbreaks of the 1990s, many facilities based their HCW TST program upon perceived risk and, as a result, did not always have a reliable baseline to document conversions following exposures (24). The CDC health care guidelines of 2005 address increased HCW risk for exposure when caring for particular populations, including foreign-born persons (with arrival to the United States within 5 years from areas with high incidence of TB), frequent travelers to areas of high incidence, residents of congregate settings, medically underserved populations, and children and adolescents in contact with high-risk adults. The frequency of performing TST depends on the results of baseline testing and risk classification for exposure (24).

In spite of documented risk, not all HCWs who experience TST conversion agree to receive or complete a full course of LTBI treatment. Employees at health care facilities have been shown to be more likely to decline, whereas those in contact with a known patient with TB were less likely to decline (44). Unfortunately, some infected employees who do not comply with LTBI treatment have gone on to develop TB and to expose others (42, 56, 103).

The CDC encourages use of a two-step TST program for all new HCWs (especially for those from areas where bacillus Calmette-Guérin [BCG] vaccination is administered and/or infections with other mycobacteria are endemic). Although the cost of implementing and maintaining an LTBI program in hospitals and health departments can be significant, the benefit of monitoring conversions and early intervention well outweighs the cost (24). The newer gamma interferon release assays (IGRAs) can be used in place of the traditional TST when deemed appropriate (i.e., contact investigations, evaluation of recent immigrants, serial-testing surveillance programs for infection control, in the setting of previous BCG vaccination, and when boosting is not desired). New guidelines exist for use of these tests (29). A number of studies have suggested that IGRAs may be a more reliable marker of LTBI than TST and of utility in the setting of HCW BCG vaccination (1, 73, 74, 81, 99). However, some studies suggest that IGRAs may pick up only those HCWs at greatest risk for reactivation or those exposed for prolonged periods (29, 77). For the elderly, there is potential benefit for the use of IGRAs to detect recent or reactivation disease, since TST does not discriminate between recent TB infection and LTBI (39).

Acute care facilities

Key elements in reducing nosocomial outbreaks are case recognition and a high index of suspicion for the myriad of clinical presentations of TB. Special considerations should be made for the unusual manifestations of TB in the elderly (frequently mistaken for aspiration pneumonia or carcinoma) and in HIV-coinfected persons. In one facility, an outbreak was curtailed with isolation of all HIV-infected patients with abnormal chest radiograph results (7). Unfortunately, some degree of overisolation will continue to occur. Not every (non-HIV-infected) person with pulmonary complaints or symptoms can or should be isolated (especially during seasonal increases in viral and bacterial respiratory infections). For patients unlikely to have TB, isolation may be discontinued after an alternative diagnosis has been made or three negative AFB sputum smears are obtained (8 to 24 h apart) (24).

Recent studies analyzed the value of three AFB smears prior to discontinuation of respiratory isolation for patients suspected of TB disease (33, 88). Fewer than three AFB specimens may be sufficient to discontinue isolation in low-prevalence areas and in nonoutbreak situations (33, 88). However, further data are needed prior to changing current recommendations. The length of time required for a TB patient to become noninfectious after initiating TB therapy also varies considerably. Airborne isolation should be discontinued only when the patient is receiving effective therapy for 2 weeks, is improving clinically, and has had three consecutive negative AFB smears from specimens collected 8 to 24 h apart (24). Although smear-negative TB patients are less likely to transmit TB, the rate is not low enough to discontinue isolation and place patients in the general hospital population. Table 5 lists some criteria for establishing as well as discontinuing airborne isolation for potentially infectious patients.

In 1992, the New York City Department of Health (NYCDOH) implemented a number of administrative controls in their chest clinics to reduce the risk of exposure from potentially infectious patients

Table 5. Criteria for *M. tuberculosis* airborne isolation[a]

Criteria for initiation of isolation
  Persons with HIV coinfection with respiratory or constitutional symptoms and/or abnormal chest radiograph
  Persons from geographic areas characterized by high TB incidence presenting with clinical symptoms consistent with TB
  Persons with the following:
    Unexplained systemic symptoms *or* respiratory illness without response to adequate/broad antimicrobial therapy within 72 h
    History of TB or TST positive with respiratory symptoms and/or abnormal chest radiograph
    History of contact with institution with prior outbreak of MDR-TB and respiratory symptoms and/or abnormal radiograph
    Undergoing treatment for TB with unknown compliance or with documented persistent sputum AFB positivity

Criteria for continuation of isolation
  Sputum smear AFB negative without alternative diagnosis and persistent symptoms while undergoing further workup
  Empirical anti-TB therapy begun without evidence of clinical and/or radiographic improvement
  Persistently AFB smear positive in spite of clinical improvement and unable to discharge to appropriate home setting

Criteria for discontinuation of isolation
  Three consecutive negative AFB smears[b] *and* clinical, AFB smear, and radiographic improvement on empirical anti-TB therapy *or* alternative diagnosis made or improvement with institution of non-anti-TB treatment (i.e., improvement with antibacterial agents or diagnosis of noninfectious etiology of radiographic or clinical symptoms)

[a]Data adapted from reference 24.
[b]Each of the three sputum specimens should be collected in 8- to 24-h intervals and at least one specimen should be an early-morning specimen (patients are potentially released from airborne precautions in 2 days).

(32). These included earlier morning appointments scheduled at times when the clinic would be empty, immediate triage with reduced waiting time, the use of PPE by patients and staff, and physical separation from other patients through the use of a separate waiting area.

Correctional facilities

Three major factors are emphasized in a TB infection control program: screening (identification of persons with LTBI and TB), containment (prompt isolation of contagious persons and appropriate use of airborne precautions), and assessment (swift performance of contact investigations and successful completion of treatment for LTBI and TB) (6). New guidelines exist for control of TB control in correctional settings as well as screening and treating LTBI and TB (24, 25, 38). Medical settings within correctional facilities are required to conform to TB infection control program components similar to those applicable to acute care facilities (24).

New inmates require complete screening prior to admission to the general corrections population. Initial TB screening of inmates includes a detailed history regarding active symptoms, TST (and/or IGRA) and HIV status, and chest radiographs (25, 38). Screening with both TST and chest radiographs has been shown to be superior to screening with TST alone among short-term-incarcerated persons and among HIV-infected persons exhibiting cutaneous anergy. The new Federal Bureau of Prisoners guidelines recommends two-step TST for all foreign-born inmates who have not been tested in the previous 12 months and for anyone who has received BCG vaccine (38). All inmates with a TST of 5 mm or greater are required to have a chest radiograph. While not currently in use within the Bureau of Prisons, QuantiFERON-G will be reevaluated for future use. For inmates entering the Bureau of Prisons, prior documentation of QuantiFERON-G results (positive or negative) is considered evidence of the presence or absence of LTBI (38).

Significant progress has been made in administrative and structural changes of most facilities, allowing immediate inmate placement in an AII room (24). Inmates require transfer to other facilities or hospitals if appropriate isolation facilities are not available locally. Criteria for continuing and discontinuing isolation have been delineated in recent guidelines (three negative AFB sputum smear results and a minimum 2-week treatment with a four-drug regimen and accompanying signs of clinical improvement, etc.) (38). Patients with TB disease who have negative AFB sputum smears can still be infectious and should not be released to an area in which patients with immunocompromising conditions are housed (in spite of otherwise meeting criteria for release from airborne precautions) (25). Patients with active TB should not be transported or released without the approval of the responsible physician (6).

Increased vigilance, cooperation among correctional facilities, and communication with local departments of health significantly decreased numbers of TB cases and new conversions among inmates (24, 25, 38). Unlike previously, when compliance with isoniazid therapy was variable (approximately 60% among state and federal inmates and 35% among city and county inmates), compliance levels have risen significantly due to a better understanding of the need to prevent further disease. Local departments of health continue to provide DOT and directly observed preventive therapy for a majority of inmates after institutional discharge, and routine use of the National TB Controller Association Inter-Jurisdictional Tuberculosis Notification form is required (38).

Homeless shelters, SRO hotels, and other facilities

The highest priority of TB control is surveillance (detection, evaluation, and reporting) of active TB and completion of an appropriate course of treatment (17, 24). The second priority is screening for LTBI, especially among high-risk groups (HIV-coinfected persons, those with chronic medical conditions, active substance users, etc.). The association between HIV and homelessness is well described (61, 65, 71). Offering rapid HIV testing in shelters or congregate facilities may be a significant intervention to a transient population.

In the early 1990s, over 90% of a New York City homeless cohort with newly diagnosed TB was lost to follow-up or failed to complete therapy (10). One-quarter were readmitted within the first year after discharge with active TB, and of these, the majority were lost to follow-up on the second discharge. In spite of this, a national survey of health departments during the following years demonstrated a significant improvement in TB management (in spite of newer CDC guidelines for TB among the homeless since 1992) (17). In more recent years, health departments managed over 80% of TB cases in homeless persons and DOT was used for 86% of them and was associated with timely completion of therapy (43). A retrospective study of trends in LTBI and TB rates among homeless persons in shelters in New York City from 1992 to 2006 revealed a decrease in TB case rates from 1,502/100,000 population to 0. This was shown in spite of a 31% LTBI rate in 2006, demonstrating the value of timely identification and DOT among the homeless (61).

Mass TST and chest radiograph screening has not proven to be effective in identifying all cases among contacts of homeless persons due to their transient and migratory patterns (53, 61). An additional tool implemented by the NYCDOH to identify contacts has been to search the TB registry, which identifies patient clusters by address of residence (53). Applying a calculated "homelessness score" to focus contact identification efforts on locations frequented by homeless patients and the average amount of time spent at these locations during the infectious period may increase success in contact tracing. Use of genotyping techniques has made tracing contacts easier and has added to traditional methods in identifying outbreaks (11, 61). Incentives such as food, housing, vouchers, and financial rewards have been used with some success to aid compliance with completing LTBI treatment (17, 96). Short-term incarceration (less than 30 days) can be used for those where DOT alone is not successful and is sometimes continued for the whole duration of the TB treatment course (25, 38).

LTCFs

Guidelines for nursing homes and other LTCFs include the same components of surveillance and record keeping (TST of residents and employees at baseline, intervals, and following exposures), containment of active cases, LTBI treatment of exposed persons (residents and employees, regardless of age), and education of residents and employees (16, 19, 24, 78). Unusual or atypical presentation of TB may occur, and emphasis is placed on identification of active cases and referral to a setting where they can be evaluated and managed (if deemed infectious and the LTCF does not have the appropriate TB environmental and PPE controls in place) (24, 78).

New recommendations for home-based and outreach services are available (24). Certain patients can be instructed to remain at home until they are determined not to have TB or to be noninfectious. For HCWs entering the homes of patients with suspected or confirmed TB disease, it is recommended to have increased ventilation (open windows, etc.) and for the HCWs to use PPE (i.e., N95 disposable respirators).

Foreign-born persons, migrant workers, and travelers

The Federal TB Task Force established by the CDC in the early 1990s, in conjunction with multiple national and international agencies (U.S. Agency for International Development, the Division of Immigration Health Services, Green Light Committee, etc.), developed and implemented a number of programs aimed at promoting continuity of care, worldwide access to medications for MDR-TB, better communication about "no-fly" lists, and ensuring completion of appropriate therapy in order to curtail the spread of MDR- and XDR-TB among foreign-born persons, migrant workers, and travelers from areas of endemicity (27). In addition, in 2007, the CDC issued revised technical instructions for TB screening and treatment among persons applying for immigration to the United States to help address the persistent presence of TB among foreign-born persons. The revision included instructions for more comprehensive diagnostic testing among applicants, the administration of DOT overseas before entry into the United States, and targeted TST (before entry into the United States) of children from high-incidence countries and contacts of persons known to have TB (30). Data for overseas screening for TB in U.S.-bound immigrants and refugees from 1999 through 2005 support the efficacy of overseas screening for TB with added follow-up evaluation after arrival in the United States as a high-yield intervention that could reduce the number of TB cases among foreign-born persons in the United States (27, 55).

The World Health Organization (WHO) published guidelines in 1998 addressing infectious disease risk associated with air travel (100). "No Fly" restrictions are applied in the setting of sputum AFB smear positivity and/or culture positivity and clinical symptoms of TB (i.e., cough at the time of the flight) and (i) not receiving adequate TB treatment, (ii) receiving adequate TB treatment for less than 2 weeks, or (iii) receiving adequate TB treatment for more than 2 weeks but with no evidence of response (e.g., no clinical improvement or no documentation of sputum conversion from AFB smear positivity to AFB smear negativity). The person should not fly if he or she has documented MDR-TB and (i) is not receiving adequate treatment or (ii) is receiving adequate treatment for any length of time but with no evidence of culture conversion. Informing close contacts is indicated if the total flight duration exceeds 8 h. Informing passengers and crew should be limited to flights that took place during the 3 months before notification of the TB case to the health authorities (100).

In June 2007, federal agencies developed a public health Do Not Board list, enabling domestic and international public health officials to request that persons with communicable diseases who meet specific criteria and pose a serious threat to the public be restricted from boarding commercial aircraft departing from or arriving to the United States (26). The public health Do Not Board list is managed by the CDC and the U.S. Department of Homeland Security. From June 2007 to May 2008, there were requests for 33 persons with communicable diseases not to fly (26). The proportion of active TB disease reports leading to a federal travel restriction increased from 6.8% in 2006 to 2007 to 15.4% in 2007 to 2008 (64).

The newer IGRAs may have a role in the future in place of the traditional TST in the evaluation of recent immigrants or in the setting of previous BCG vaccination, which is seen frequently in persons arriving from areas where TB is endemic (29). Improved outreach programs may help with migrant workers in obtaining consistent follow-up.

Environmental Controls

Although source control is the optimal way to avoid exposure to TB, it is only possible when TB is suspected and infectious droplets are minimized (limit cough-inducing procedures, cover mouth, etc.). However, unsuspected and undiagnosed cases of infectious TB disease are believed to represent a substantial proportion of the current risk to HCWs (24). Conditions which increase the spread of TB include limited or poor ventilation, increased numbers of susceptible persons in proximity to infectious persons, and procedures and/or clinical disease that increases the discharge of infectious droplets (24, 69, 84). Adjunct modalities to decreasing the risk are collectively referred to as environmental controls. These refer to engineering modalities for removal or disinfection of air containing *M. tuberculosis*, including ventilation of a given space measured in air changes per hour (ACH), directional airflow and pressurization (laminar and negative or positive pressure), air mixing, air filtration, and air disinfection (24, 69, 84). The CDC published several guidelines for environmental control of TB in the past two decades, with the most recent (and exhaustive) in 2005 (24). Recent CDC guidelines delineate the exact requirements for appropriate environmental controls and emphasize the need to consult with experts who can give specific advice on ventilation system design, selection, installation, and maintenance for every setting (24). These recommendations take into account the need to address newer and older building design as well as nonfixed patient delivery areas. Extremely detailed worksheets to aid in decision making are included.

Ventilation

Attention to ventilation has increased recently due to SARS and H5N1 outbreaks (54). There is strong and sufficient evidence to demonstrate the association between ventilation, air movements in buildings, and the transmission or spread of infectious diseases (i.e., measles, TB, chicken pox, influenza, smallpox, and SARS). To date, there are insufficient data to specify minimum ventilation requirements (54).

In resource-limited settings, protective measures such as negative-pressure isolation rooms are difficult to implement. Natural ventilation measures (high ceilings, large windows, many doors, etc.) frequently abound and may offer a low-cost alternative. A recent study compared several hospitals built during various years with various capabilities for natural or mechanical ventilation (37). Infection risk was measured using the Wells-Riley model of airborne infection. Opening windows and doors provided a median ventilation of 28 ACH, more than double that of mechanically ventilated negative-pressure rooms (ventilated at the 12 ACH recommended for high-risk areas) and 18 times that with windows and doors closed ($P < 0.001$). Natural ventilation of facilities built more than 50 years ago was greater than natural ventilation of more modern buildings (40 versus 17 ACH; $P < 0.001$). Even within the lowest quartile of

wind speeds, natural ventilation exceeded mechanical ($P < 0.001$). The Wells-Riley airborne infection model predicted that in mechanically ventilated rooms, 39% of susceptible individuals would become infected following 24 h of exposure to untreated TB patients. This infection rate compared with 33% in modern and 11% in pre-1950 naturally ventilated facilities with windows and doors open (37).

Designated AII rooms require the following: ventilation of 12 or more ACH for new construction after 2001 and 6 or more ACH for construction before 2001 (a minimum of 2 ACH should be outdoor air); negative pressure (use of anterooms is preferred); direct external exhaust is preferred (25 ft or more from air intake vents, 6 ft above ground, or 3 ft above roof levels), but if recirculation is unavoidable, then air is first passed through a HEPA filter (24). Although mechanical ventilation is universally available in modern buildings and generally adaptable to current needs, it is most effective in smaller areas, such as individual patient rooms. Attempting to retrofit older buildings to comply with the appropriate ACH, direct outdoor exhaust, and negative pressure differential can be a daunting experience requiring significant investment of capital and resources. As a result, the new CDC guidelines offer the ability to increase the airflow to 12 ACH either by adjusting the existing ventilation system or by using air-cleaning methods (i.e., portable HEPA filter-containing units or UV germicidal irradiation [UVGI] systems) to increase the "equivalent" ACH (24). Recommendations are also made for special care areas (operating rooms, autopsy suites, outpatient areas, etc.).

UV Germicidal Irradiation

UVGI is the least well understood of the three approaches to air disinfection despite its use for over 70 years. Although there are good laboratory data supporting the germicidal activity against a number of virulent bacteria, viruses, and mycobacteria (including *M. tuberculosis*), there are few recent field trials showing that it can prevent TB transmission in populations (24, 69, 84). However, due to extensive clinical and anecdotal experiences, UVGI has been recommended as a supplement or adjunct to other TB infection control and ventilation measures in settings in which the killing or inactivation of *M. tuberculosis* is essential. UVGI is considered supplemental to and not a substitute for ventilation and is not considered a substitute for HEPA filtration if air is required to be recirculated (24).

UVGI lamps can be placed in ducts, fixed or portable room air recirculation units, or upper-air irradiation systems. UVGI has been implemented successfully in large areas where ventilation alone is insufficient to cleanse stagnant air pockets (69). Upper-air UVGI may minimize the spread of *M. tuberculosis*, especially from unsuspected patient sources, provided that the appropriate air mixing can occur. Additional recent studies performed with mannequins "aerosolizing" mycobacteria in isolation rooms found a linear relationship between UV irradiation and germicidal efficacy (101). However, efficacy dropped drastically (from 89 to 9%) when air humidity was raised above 75%, when ventilation mixing fans were turned off, and when wintertime ventilation conditions were established (101). More recently, UVGI has been studied as a possible adjuvant to diminish airborne infections associated with bioterrorism (9).

A historical limitation to widespread use of UVGI has been HCWs' apprehension of eye and skin toxicity. UVGI placed in enclosed ducts, in wall-mounted metal boxes with fans, or in wall-mounted devices with upward-directed louvers can address this concern. Additional locations for placement include on the wall near the ceiling or suspended from the ceiling. Guidelines exist for placement, use, and maintenance of UVGI devices (24).

Air Filtration

Air filtration has been a long-practiced modality in industrial settings for removal of airborne contaminants (84). Air filtration via HEPA filters can supplement other recommended ventilation measures by providing a minimum removal efficiency of 99.97% of particles 0.3 μm or larger in diameter. Although there exist few data concerning *M. tuberculosis*, experience with *Aspergillus* outbreaks on oncology wards has affirmed HEPA filtration capacity and efficiency (24). The efficacy of HEPA filters is closely related to having a well-functioning ventilation system that is able to move air past them and to the adequacy of prefilters which, when placed upstream, significantly extend the life of HEPA filters by removing larger debris. HEPA filters can be used to clean air before it is (i) exhausted to the outside, (ii) recirculated to other areas of a health care setting, or (iii) recirculated in an AII room. Their use in systems that recirculate air back into the general ventilation system from AII rooms and treatment rooms should be avoided (24).

HEPA filters can also be used for air recirculation when contained in portable air cleaners (many of which also contain UVGI) (24). Use of these units is considered either when a room has no general ventilation system or when the existing system cannot provide adequate ACH. As with placement of HEPA filters in ventilation ducts, the effectiveness of portable HEPA filter units depends on the ability to circulate as much of the air in the room as possible through the HEPA filter. Depending on the space configuration (and location of air vents, furniture, etc.), the units could be potentially hampered by intake of air at the site of discharge, short-circuiting air cleaning. Furthermore, patients and HCWs sometimes turn off these units due to their perception that the noise and heat generated by the fans interfere with health care delivery. As a result, special attention must be paid to ensure their proper and continuous functioning. Also, filters must be monitored for quality and cleanliness, with scheduled changes as designated by manufacturers (24).

In addition to administrative changes implemented in 1992, the NYCDOH implemented a number of environmental changes in its chest clinics to minimize exposure to potentially infectious patients (32). Separate waiting areas were dedicated to high-risk patients and UVGI was installed in all moderate- to high-risk areas, including patient waiting areas, examination rooms, and areas where sputum induction was performed. Sputum induction booths were fitted with HEPA filtration systems for external air exhaust, and the rooms that contained the booths were maintained under negative pressure and had a minimum of 50 ACH. As demonstrated by the NYCDOH environmental interventions, ventilation was maximized in smaller areas, where control of airflow is easier to manage, and HEPA filters were installed for cleansing of exhaust air. UVGI was used in large congregate spaces (such as waiting rooms), where control of airflow is not easily accomplished, and in high-risk areas, such as examination rooms, as an adjuvant to ventilation. Lastly, PPE was used by staff caring for these patients.

Acute care facilities

Facilities with respiratory isolation rooms in compliance with early 1990 CDC guidelines (and with a census of at least six TB patients) were associated with significantly lower rates of TST conversions among HCWs than those not employing such measures, even though outbreaks with transmission still occurred due to insufficient administrative controls (41). However, when all controls were put into effect, further outbreaks were curtailed (24). By the late 1990s, nationwide increases in appropriate airborne isolation (from 63 to 100% of the facilities) and appropriate PPE use (from 60 to 90% of facilities) led to significant decreases in further outbreaks and HCW TST conversion rates (57). Lapses occurred when at-risk patients were not identified and, therefore, not placed in appropriate AII and PPE was not used (94).

Environmental changes posed a significant constraint on many facilities, since efforts in reduction of energy expenditure and cost forced many facilities to recirculate air, seal windows to prevent heat loss, and operate the ventilation system in cycles rather than continuously. Retrofitting existing rooms, creation of anterooms, and creation of negative pressure led to varied compliance with ventilation and negative pressure in a number of facilities from 1992 to 1998. Over one-quarter of facilities that performed daily smoke testing of isolation rooms reported a discrepancy with measurements of automated monitoring devices (75). Use of UVGI and portable HEPA devices allowed for greater compliance, and facilities found regularly scheduled maintenance to be more cost-effective than installation of intricate alarm systems (24).

Specific recommendations are detailed for numerous health care settings (24). For inpatient settings, emphasis is on use of AII and adjunctive UVGI and/ or portable HEPA devices when AII is not possible. For "problem" areas where there is the likelihood of failure of administrative controls or increased risk of aerosol-generating procedures (emergency and ambulatory care areas, bronchoscopy suites, mycobacterial laboratories, morgues, etc.), addition of UVGI (contained in either louvered or enclosed metallic boxes with fans) and/or portable HEPA filters are reasonable modalities to interrupt TB transmission (24). In addition, the large spaces of emergency and ambulatory care waiting areas experience increased traffic and erratic air mixing which can overwhelm ventilation systems. UVGI (and/or portable HEPA filters) should be considered after a risk assessment is performed. Signs for patients to cover their mouths while coughing along with providing tissues and surgical masks can significantly decrease the spread of droplet nuclei (24).

Previously, inadequate ventilation and creation of aerosols during postmortem examinations and processing of tissue or mycobacteriology samples led to transmission of TB to susceptible HCWs (62). Better education, increased ventilation, use of UVGI, and strict use of PPE have all helped to reduce TB exposures among pathologists and other laboratory or morgue personnel. Frequent testing of ventilation and hood operation are crucial in mycobacteriology and pathology areas (85).

Correctional facilities

Immediately upon arrival, all new inmates should be screened for symptoms, and any inmate with symptoms suggestive of TB should be placed in an AII room and evaluated promptly for TB (25, 38). At least one AII room should be available in any correctional facility. Inmates with suspected or confirmed TB should be placed in an AII room or transferred immediately to a facility that has one. Inmates with suspected or confirmed TB who require transport outside an AII room for medically essential procedures should wear a surgical mask during transport, if possible. Anyone accompanying these inmates requires use of PPE (24, 25, 38).

Specific environmental control recommendations conform to those for health care facilities (24, 25). Following a risk assessment, UVGI (ceiling or wall fixtures or within ventilation ducts) can supplement ventilation in high-risk, overcrowded areas such as holding and communal areas. Medical settings contained within correctional facilities need to conform to the same environmental and respiratory program recommendations as apply to acute care facilities (24). The number of AII rooms needed is based on the risk assessment for the setting (24, 25, 38).

Homeless shelters, SRO hotels, and other facilities

Installation of UVGI can reduce the risk of transmission of TB in shelters where large and open communal areas exist to serve transient residents who may not adhere to accepted TB surveillance programs (17, 69). Financial support for shelters is meager and does not accommodate retrofitting of ventilation systems in older buildings. Adherence to strict administrative controls with strong programs in identifying and treating LTBI among residents is crucial to prevent outbreaks in shelters.

LTCFs

LTCFs were not designed with infection control as a primary objective. Few or no isolation rooms exist, and ventilation systems are for occupant comfort rather than disease transmission control. Implementation of administrative controls (including symptom screening) is of primary importance. The decision to implement environmental and respiratory protection programs (creation of isolation rooms, changes in ventilation and exhaust, implementation of HEPA and/or UVGI, PPE, etc.) is based upon individual facility TB risk assessment (24). Residents with suspected or confirmed TB should not stay in LTCFs unless adequate environmental and respiratory programs are in place.

Foreign-Born Persons, Migrant Workers, and Travelers

Administrative controls and international involvement in attempts to control spread of TB are ongoing. The risk of air travel centers around suboptimal ventilation as well as the close proximity of infected and susceptible persons. An influenza outbreak was facilitated by an interruption of outside air during a 3-hour ground delay (100). At cruising altitude, outside ambient air is virtually free of microorganisms and the recirculated cabin air has to pass through multiple filters of progressively decreasing pore sizes (including HEPA filters) before reentering the passenger cabin. In addition, the rate of recirculation is high enough to reduce bacterial concentrations following a cough or a sneeze within 3 min (100). However, as stated above, the recognition of persons at risk, "do not fly" lists, and ensuring adequate access and completion of TB and LTBI treatment on an international scale have all contributed to limiting the spread of TB during travel.

Personal Protective Equipment

Administrative and environmental controls minimize the number of areas in which exposure to TB might occur and reduce, but do not eliminate, the risk in the few areas in which exposures can still occur (e.g., AII rooms and rooms where cough-inducing or aerosol-generating procedures are performed). Because persons entering these areas might be exposed to airborne M. tuberculosis, the third level of the hierarchy is the use of respiratory protective equipment (PPE) (24). In the United Kingdom, unlike the United States, negative-pressure isolation rooms and PPE use are recommended only for patients with suspected MDR-TB or where aerosol-generating procedures occur (45). Observational studies and mathematical modeling suggest that all measures are required for effective prevention, as MDR-TB may not always be apparent on admission (45).

In response to the increased HCW exposures to TB (and especially MDR-TB), the Occupational and Safety and Health Administration published standards for occupational exposure to TB requiring use of respirators as PPE (24). Respirators are distinct from ordinary surgical masks. Respirators are designed to prevent inhalation of particulate air contaminants, including infectious droplet nuclei, whereas surgical masks protect the operating field from the wearer. Thus, filtration media and face seal are extremely important on respirators. Unlike environmental control, PPE use requires active implementation and the foresight that there is a risk at hand. The CDC and Occupational and Safety and Health Administration directives were put into place at a time when health care facilities were attempting to implement long-needed engineering changes, and the PPE mandate was initially perceived as an added hardship requiring diversion of limited health care dollars.

In 1995, the National Institute for Occupational Safety and Health revised categories of particulate filter respirators, and the N95 particulate filter respirator (95% efficiency for filtering particles of 1 μm or less; Technol, Fort Worth, TX) was implemented for HCW PPE (24). Once trapped by the N95 respirator, M. tuberculosis droplet nuclei are unlikely to reaerosolize (80). A summary of applicable respirators and their uses appears in recent CDC guidelines, and options are provided for HCWs whose facial features (especially facial hair) make it impractical to wear the N95 respirator or who require other options based on use (24). Because fit and face seal are crucial to appropriate use (and expected protection with) N95 respirators, annual fit testing is recommended (or sooner if there is a change in facial features) (24). Indications for use of PPE appear in recent guidelines and include use when entering an AII room, during any cough- or aerosol-producing procedures, and whenever environmental controls are deemed insufficient (during patient transport, during urgent surgical or dental procedures, etc.). Disposable respirators can be functional for a significant period and can be reused by the same HCW. Reuse is limited by hygiene, damage, breathing resistance, and manufacturer instructions (24). Implementation of PPE programs overcame initial obstacles and has become an integral component of successful TB control programs.

Limiting droplet nuclei at the source (i.e., patients) is considered an effective source of control by all experts. Therefore, tissues or surgical masks should be used routinely for patients, especially when coughing. It is important to reiterate that prior nosocomial outbreaks were frequently curtailed through rigorous implementation of established infection control practices. In the instances where several modalities were employed simultaneously, the value of individual components in curtailing the outbreak could not be ascertained (24).

Other Methods of HCW Protection

In the United States, BCG vaccination (see chapter 10) is not recommended routinely for anyone, including HCWs or children (24). Its use was considered at the peak of TB outbreaks due to the extensive occupational exposure to TB (and especially to MDR-TB) (20). Cohort studies suggest that rates of TB may be substantially lower among HCWs who receive the BCG vaccine than among those who remain unvaccinated, and efficacy appears to increase with risk of exposure (69 to 85%) (87). A national policy on use of BCG has not been endorsed in this country for multiple reasons, including (i) overall low risk of acquiring TB, (ii) difficulty interpreting TST in light of BCG vaccination (although IGRAs may still be considered useful), (iii) incomplete vaccine protection, and (iv) inability to administer vaccine to HIV-infected or immunosuppressed persons (24).

CONCLUSIONS

Recent nosocomial spread of TB serves as a reminder of the importance of adequate clinical, diagnostic, and infection control practices. Clinicians must maintain a high index of suspicion for TB. The least expensive and most cost-effective intervention is an institutional administrative TB control program. Even those institutions with limited resources for implementation of all environmental changes can implement surveillance, isolation, empirical therapy, and rapid diagnostic plans. Adjuvant environmental control programs can reduce transmission of TB from unsuspected sources. Airborne isolation policies must be enforced and PPE used in indicated situations. Current CDC guidelines offer specific TB infection control program recommendations for numerous settings and emphasize basing components on periodic individual and local risk assessment (24). In addition, transfer of patients with TB to and from acute care facilities can occur when they are no longer infectious or when appropriate isolation is arranged. Guidelines exist for discharging these patients into the general community (24).

Facilities providing care for persons with TB must continue to foster close relationships with local, state, and federal programs for the control of this disease. Local and state departments of health have made significant impact on the control of TB with DOT, yielding decreases in hospitalization rates (93). Continuing challenges are continued increased vigilance in health care settings for TB; local, national, and international focus on management of TB and LTBI among foreign-born persons; community reintegration of discharged inmates, homeless persons, or hospitalized patients with recently identified TB; and continued enforcement and support of DOT programs.

CDC surveillance for TB in 2009 revealed a rate of 3.8 cases per 100,000 population, which remains higher than the final goal of less than 1 case per 1,000,000 population by 2010 (24). In spite of a decade of decline in numbers of TB cases, recent data mark incremental declines in annual numbers, with specific focus increasing on foreign-born sources and a need to approach TB on a global level in order to control local spread. The role of newer techniques for immediate clinical diagnosis, susceptibility testing, epidemiological analyses, and quality control is increasing. TB is a disease on the rise and with changing targets. Our focus on its importance cannot waver.

REFERENCES

1. **Abdalhamid, J., S. H. Hinrichs, J. L. Garrett, J. M. O'Neill, K. M. Hansen-Cain, A. A. Armbrust, and P. C. Iwen.** 23 June 2010. Utilization of the QuantiFeron-TB Gold test in a two-step process with the tuberculin skin test to evaluate health care workers for latent tuberculosis. *J. Clin. Microbiol.* **48:** 2955–2956. [Epub ahead of print.]
2. **Alland, D., G. E. Kalkut, A. R. Moss, et al.** 1994. Transmission of tuberculosis in New York City: an analysis by DNA fingerprinting and conventional epidemiologic methods. *N. Engl. J. Med.* **330:**1710–1716.
3. **Banerjee, R., J. Allen, J. Westenhouse, P. Oh, W. Elms, E. Desmond, A. Nitta, S. Royce, and J. Flood.** 2008. Extensively drug-resistant tuberculosis in California, 1993–2006. *Clin. Infect. Dis.* **47:**450–457.
4. **Barnes, P. F., Z. Yang, S. Preston-Martin, et al.** 1997. Patterns of tuberculosis transmission in central Los Angeles. *JAMA* **278:**1159–1163.
5. **Beck-Sagué, C., S. W. Dooley, M. D. Hutton, et al.** 1992. Hospital outbreak of multidrug-resistant *Mycobacterium tuberculosis* infections: factors in transmission to staff and HIV-infected patients. *JAMA* **268:**1280–1286.
6. **Bick, J. A.** 2007. Infection control in jails and prisons. *Clin. Infect. Dis.* **45:**1047–1055.
7. **Blumberg, H. M., D. L. Watkins, J. D. Berschling, et al.** 1995. Preventing the nosocomial transmission of tuberculosis. *Ann. Intern. Med.* **122:**658–663.
8. **Bock, N., and L. B. Reichman.** 2004. Tuberculosis and HIV/AIDS: epidemiological and clinical aspects (world perspective). *Semin. Respir. Crit. Care Med.* **25:**337–344.
9. **Brickner, P. W., R. L. Vincent, M. First, et al.** 2003. The application of ultraviolet germicidal irradiation to control transmission of airborne disease: bioterrorism countermeasure. *Public Health Rep.* **118:**99–118.
10. **Brudney, K., and J. Dobkin.** 1991. Resurgent tuberculosis in New York City: human immunodeficiency virus, homelessness, and the decline of tuberculosis control programs. *Am. Rev. Respir. Dis.* **144:**745–749.
11. **Buff, A. M., L. E. Sosa, A. J. Hoopes, D. Buxton-Morris, T. B. Condren, J. L. Hadler, M. B. Haddad, P. K. Moonan, and M. N. Lobato.** 2009. Two tuberculosis genotyping clusters, one preventable outbreak. *Public Health Rep.* **124:**490–494.
12. **Bureau of Justice Statistics.** 2010. *Prison Inmates at Midyear 2009—Statistical Tables.* Office of Justice Statistics, U.S. Department of Justice. http://bjs.ojp.usdoj.gov/index.cfm?ty=pbse&sid=38. Accessed 21 July 2010.
13. **Burzynski, J., and N. W. Schluger.** 2008. The epidemiology of tuberculosis in the United States. *Semin. Respir. Crit. Care Med.* **29:**492–498.
14. **Cain, K. P., S. R. Benoit, C. A. Winston, and W. R. MacKenzie.** 2008. Tuberculosis among foreign-born persons in the United States. *JAMA* **300:**405–412.
15. **Castro, K. G.** 1995. Tuberculosis as an opportunistic disease in persons infected with human immunodeficiency virus. *Clin. Infect. Dis.* **21**(Suppl. 1):S66–S71.
16. **Centers for Disease Control.** 1990. Prevention and control of tuberculosis in facilities providing long-term care to the

elderly: recommendations of the Advisory Committee for the Elimination of Tuberculosis. *MMWR Morb. Mortal. Wkly. Rep.* 39(RR-10):7–20.

17. **Centers for Disease Control.** 1992. Prevention and control of tuberculosis among homeless persons: recommendations of the Advisory Council for the Elimination of Tuberculosis. *MMWR Morb. Mortal. Wkly. Rep.* 41(RR-5):13–23.

18. **Centers for Disease Control.** 1992. Prevention and control of tuberculosis in migrant farm workers: recommendations of the Advisory Council for the Elimination of Tuberculosis. *MMWR Morb. Mortal. Wkly. Rep.* 41(RR-10):1–15.

19. **Centers for Disease Control and Prevention.** 1995. Screening for tuberculosis and tuberculosis infection in high-risk populations: recommendations of the Advisory Council for the Elimination of Tuberculosis. *MMWR Morb. Mortal. Wkly. Rep.* 44(RR-11):18–34.

20. **Centers for Disease Control and Prevention.** 1996. The role of BCG vaccine in the prevention and control of tuberculosis in the United States: a joint statement by the Advisory Council for the Elimination of Tuberculosis and the Advisory Committee on Immunization Practices. *MMWR Morb. Mortal. Wkly. Rep.* 45(RR-4):1–18.

21. **Centers for Disease Control and Prevention.** 2003. Post-detention completion of tuberculosis treatment for persons deported or released from the custody of the Immigration and Naturalization Service—United States, 2003. *MMWR Morb. Mortal. Wkly. Rep.* 52:438–441.

22. **Centers for Disease Control and Prevention.** 2004. Tuberculosis outbreak in a community hospital—District of Columbia, 2002. *MMWR Morb. Mortal. Wkly. Rep.* 53:214–216.

23. **Centers for Disease Control and Prevention.** 2004. Nosocomial transmission of *Mycobacterium tuberculosis* found through screening for severe acute respiratory syndrome—Taipei, Taiwan, 2003. *MMWR Morb. Mortal. Wkly. Rep.* 53:321–322.

24. **Centers for Disease Control and Prevention.** 2005. Guidelines for preventing the transmission of *Mycobacterium tuberculosis* in health-care settings, 2005. *MMWR Morb. Mortal. Wkly. Rep.* 54(RR-17):1–147.

25. **Centers for Disease Control and Prevention.** 2006. Prevention and control of tuberculosis in correctional and detention facilities: recommendations from CDC. *MMWR Morb. Mortal. Wkly. Rep.* 55(RR-9):1–54.

26. **Centers for Disease Control and Prevention.** 2008. Federal air travel restrictions for public health purposes—United States, June 2007–May 2008. *MMWR Morb. Mortal. Wkly. Rep.* 57:1009–1012.

27. **Centers for Disease Control and Prevention.** 2009. Plan to combat extensively drug-resistant tuberculosis: recommendations of the Federal Tuberculosis Task Force. *MMWR Morb. Mortal. Wkly. Rep.* 59(RR-3):1–46.

28. **Centers for Disease Control and Prevention.** 2010. Summary of notifiable diseases—United States, 2008. *MMWR Morb. Mortal. Wkly. Rep.* 57:1–98.

29. **Centers for Disease Control and Prevention.** 2010. Updated guidelines for using interferon gamma release assays to detect *Mycobacterium tuberculosis* infection—United States, 2010. *MMWR Morb. Mortal. Wkly. Rep.* 59(RR-5):1–25.

30. **Centers for Disease Control and Prevention.** 2010. Decrease in reported tuberculosis cases—United States, 2009. *MMWR Morb. Mortal. Wkly. Rep.* 59:289–294.

31. **Churchyard, G. J., and E. Wardell.** 2007. Tuberculosis and HIV coinfection: current state of knowledge and research priorities. *J. Infect. Dis.* 196(Suppl. 1):S1–S3.

32. **Cook, S., K. L. Maw, S. S. Munsiff, et al.** 2003. Prevalence of tuberculin skin test positivity and conversions among healthcare workers in New York City during 1994 to 2001. *Infect. Control Hosp. Epidemiol.* 24:807–813.

33. **Craft, D. W., M. C. Jones, C. N. Blanchet, et al.** 2000. Value of examining three acid-fast bacillus sputum smears for removal of patients suspected of having tuberculosis from the "airborne precautions" category. *J. Clin. Microbiol.* 38:4285–4287.

34. **Deiss, R., R. S. Garfein, R. Lozada, J. L. Burgos, K. C. Brouwer, K. S. Moser, M. L. Zuniga, T. C. Rodwell, V. D. Ojeda, and S. A. Strathdee.** 2009. Influences of cross-border mobility on tuberculosis diagnoses and treatment interruption among injection drug users in Tijuana, Mexico. *Am. J. Public Health* 99:1491–1495.

35. **Diel, R., K. Meywald-Walter, R. Gottschalk, S. Rüsch-Gerdes, and S. Niemann.** 2004. Ongoing outbreak of tuberculosis in a low-incidence community: a molecular-epidemiological evaluation. *Int. J. Tuberc. Lung Dis.* 8:855–861.

36. **Escombe, A. R., D. A. Moore, R. H. Gilman, W. Pan, M. Navincopa, E. Ticona, C. Martínez, L. Caviedes, P. Sheen, A. Gonzalez, C. J. Noakes, J. S. Friedland, and C. A. Evans.** 2008. The infectiousness of tuberculosis patients coinfected with HIV. *PLoS Med.* 30:e188.

37. **Escombe, A. R., C. C. Oeser, R. H. Gilman, M. Navincopa, E. Ticona, W. Pan, C. Martínez, J. Chacaltana, R. Rodríguez, D. A. Moore, J. S. Friedland, and C. A. Evans.** 2007. Natural ventilation for the prevention of airborne contagion. *PLoS Med.* 4:e68.

38. **Federal Bureau of Prisons.** 2010. *Clinical Practice Guidelines: Management of Tuberculosis. January 2010.* Federal Bureau of Prisons, Washington, DC. http://www.bop.gov/news/medresources.jsp. Accessed 21 July 2010.

39. **Ferrara, G., M. Losi, R. D'Amico, R. Cagarelli, A. M. Pezzi, M. Meacci, B. Meccugni, I. Marchetti-Dori, F. Rumpianesi, P. Roversi, L. Casali, L. M. Fabbri, and L. Richeldi.** 2009. Interferon-gamma-release assays detect recent tuberculosis reinfection in elderly contacts. *Int. J. Immunopathol. Pharmacol.* 22:669–677.

40. **Fok, A., Y. Numata, M. Schulzer, and M. J. FitzGerald.** 2008. Risk factors for clustering of tuberculosis cases: a systematic review of population-based molecular epidemiology studies. *Int. J. Tuberc. Lung Dis.* 12:480–492.

41. **Fridkin, S. K., L. Manangan, E. Bolyard, et al.** 1995. SHEA-CDC TB survey, part I: status of TB infection control programs at member hospitals, 1989–1992. *Infect. Control Hosp. Epidemiol.* 16:129–134.

42. **Frieden, T. R., L. F. Sherman, K. L. Maw, et al.** 1996. A multiinstitutional outbreak of highly drug-resistant tuberculosis: epidemiology and clinical outcomes. *JAMA* 276:1229–1235.

43. **Haddad, M. B., T. W. Wilson, K. Ijaz, S. M. Marks, and M. Moore.** 2005. Tuberculosis and homelessness in the United States, 1994–2003. *JAMA* 293:2762–2766.

44. **Horsburgh, C. R., Jr., S. Goldberg, J. Bethel, S. Chen, P. W. Colson, Y. Hirsch Moverman, S. Hughes, R. Shrestha-Kuwahara, T. R. Sterling, K. Wall, and P. Weinfurter.** 2010. Tuberculosis Epidemiologic Studies Consortium. Latent TB infection treatment acceptance and completion in the United States and Canada. *Chest* 137:401–409.

45. **Humphreys, H.** 2007. Control and prevention of healthcare-associated tuberculosis: the role of respiratory isolation and personal respiratory protection. *J. Hosp. Infect.* 66:1–5.

46. **Hutton, M. D., G. M. Cauthen, and A. B. Bloch.** 1993. Results of a 29-state survey of tuberculosis in nursing homes and correctional facilities. *Public Health Rep.* 108:305–314.

47. **Hutton, M. D., S. W. Dooley, and G. M. Cauthen.** 1992. *Nosocomial TB transmission: characteristics of source-patients in reported outbreaks, 1970–1991. First World Congress on Tuberculosis, November 15–18, 1992, Rockville, MD.*

48. Ijaz, K., J. A. Dillaha, Z. Yang, M. D. Cave, and J. H. Bates. 2002. Unrecognized tuberculosis in a nursing home causing death with spread to the community. *J. Am. Geriatr. Soc.* 50: 1213–1218.

49. Jarvis, W. R. 1995. Nosocomial transmission of multidrug-resistant *Mycobacterium tuberculosis*. *Am. J. Infect. Control* 23:146–151.

50. Joshi, R., A. L. Reingold, D. Menzies, and M. Pai. 2006. Tuberculosis among health-care workers in low- and middle-income countries: a systematic review. *PLoS Med.* 3:2376–2391.

51. Krause, G., D. Altmann, D. Faensen, K. Proten, J. Benzler, T. Pfoch, A. Ammon, M. H. Kramer, and H. Claus. 2007. SurvNet electronic surveillance system for infectious disease outbreaks, Germany. *Emerg. Infect. Dis.* 13:1548–1555.

52. Lemaitre, N., W. Sougakoff, D. Coetmeur, et al. 1996. Nosocomial transmission of tuberculosis among mentally-handicapped patients in a long-term care facility. *Tuber. Lung Dis.* 77:531–536.

53. Li, J., C. R. Driver, S. S. Munsiff, and P. I. Fujiwara. 2003. Finding contacts of homeless tuberculosis patients in New York City. *Int. J. Tuberc. Lung Dis.* 7:S397–S404.

54. Li, Y., G. M. Leung, J. W. Tang, X. Yang, C. Y. Chao, J. Z. Lin, J. W. Lu, P. V. Nielsen, J. Niu, H. Qian, A. C. Sleigh, H. J. Su, J. Sundell, T. W. Wong, and P. L. Yuen. 2007. Role of ventilation in airborne transmission of infectious agents in the built environment—a multidisciplinary systematic review. *Indoor Air* 17:2–18.

55. Liu, Y., M. S. Weinberg, L. S. Ortega, J. A. Painter, and S. A. Maloney. 2009. Overseas screening for tuberculosis in U.S.-bound immigrants and refugees. *N. Engl. J. Med.* 360:2406–2415.

56. Maloney, S. A., M. L. Pearson, M. T. Gordon, et al. 1995. Efficacy of control measures in preventing nosocomial transmission of multidrug-resistant tuberculosis to patients and health care workers. *Ann. Intern. Med.* 122:90–95.

57. Manangan, L. P., C. L. Bennett, N. Tablan, et al. 2000. Nosocomial tuberculosis prevention measures among two groups of US hospitals, 1992 to 1996. *Chest* 117:380–384.

58. Mangili, A., and M. A. Gendreau. 2005. Transmission of infectious diseases during commercial air travel. *Lancet* 365: 989–996.

59. Martinez, L., L. Blanc, P. Nunn, and M. Raviglione. 2008. Tuberculosis and air travel: WHO guidance in the era of drug-resistant TB. *Travel Med. Infect. Dis.* 6:177–181.

60. Martínez-Lirola, M., N. Alonso-Rodriguez, M. L. Sánchez, M. Herranz, S. Andrés, T. Peñafiel, M. C. Rogado, T. Cabezas, J. Martínez, M. A. Lucerna, M. Rodríguez, M. C. Bonillo, E. Bouza, and D. García de Viedma. 2008. Advanced survey of tuberculosis transmission in a complex socioepidemiologic scenario with a high proportion of cases in immigrants. *Clin. Infect. Dis.* 47:8–14.

61. McAdam, J. M., S. J. Bucher, P. W. Brickner, R. L. Vincent, and S. Lascher. 2009. Latent tuberculosis and active tuberculosis disease rates among the homeless, New York, New York, USA, 1992–2006. *Emerg. Infect. Dis.* 15:1109–1111.

62. Menzies, D., A. Fanning, L. Yuan, et al. 1995. Tuberculosis among health care workers. *N. Engl. J. Med.* 332:92–98.

63. Migliori, G. B., and R. Centis. 2002. Problems to control TB in eastern Europe and consequences in low incidence countries. *Monaldi Arch. Chest Dis.* 57:285–290.

64. Modi, S., A. M. Buff, C. J. Lawson, D. Rodriguez, H. L. Kirking, H. Lipman, and D. B. Fishbein. 2009. Reporting patterns and characteristics of tuberculosis among international travelers, United States, June 2006 to May 2008. *Clin. Infect. Dis.* 49:885–891.

65. Mohtashemi, M., and L. M. Kawamura. 2010. Empirical evidence for synchrony in the evolution of TB cases and HIV+

contacts among the San Francisco homeless. *PLoS One* 5: e8851.

66. Moss, A. R., D. Alland, E. Telzak, et al. 1997. A city-wide outbreak of a multiple-drug-resistant strain of *Mycobacterium tuberculosis* in New York. *Int. J. Tuberc. Lung Dis.* 1:115–121.

67. Munsiff, S. S., B. Nivin, G. Sacajiu, et al. 2003. Persistence of a highly resistant strain of tuberculosis in New York City during 1990–1999. *J. Infect. Dis.* 188:356–363.

68. Naglie, G., M. McArthur, A. Simor, et al. 1995. Tuberculosis surveillance practices in long-term care institutions. *Infect. Control Hosp. Epidemiol.* 16:148–151.

69. Nardell, E. A. 2003. Environmental infection control of tuberculosis. *Semin. Respir. Infect.* 18:307–319.

70. Oeltmann, J. E., S. Kammerer, E. S. Pevzner, and P. K. Moonan. 2009. Tuberculosis and substance abuse in the United States, 1997–2006. *Arch. Intern. Med.* 169:189–197.

71. **Office of Community Planning and Development.** 9 July 2010. *The 2008 Annual Homeless Assessment Report to Congress.* U.S. Department of Housing and Urban Development, Washington, DC. http://www.hudre.info/documents/4thHomeless AssessmentReport.pdf. Accessed 21 July 2010.

72. **Office of Policy Department and Research, U.S. Department of Housing and Urban Development.** September 2007. *Measuring Overcrowding in Housing.* U.S. Department of Housing and Urban Development, Washington, DC. http://www .huduser.org/publications/pdf/Measuring_Overcrowding_in_ Hsg.pdf. Accessed 26 July 2010.

73. **Pai, M., R. Joshi, S. Dogra, D. K. Mendiratta, P. Narang, S. Kalantri, A. L. Reingold, J. M. Colford, Jr., L. W. Riley, and D. Menzies.** 2006. Serial testing of healthcare workers for tuberculosis using interferon assay. *Am. J. Respir. Crit. Care Med.* 174:349–355.

74. **Pai, M., A. Zwerling, and D. Menzies.** 2008. Systematic review: T-cell-based assays for the diagnosis of latent tuberculosis infection: an update. *Ann. Intern. Med.* 149:177–184.

75. **Pavelchak, N., K. Cummings, R. Stricof, et al.** 2001. Negative-pressure monitoring of tuberculosis isolation rooms within New York State Hospitals. *Infect. Control Hosp. Epidemiol.* 22:518–519.

76. **Peto, H. M., R. H. Pratt, T. A. Harrington, P. A. LoBue, and L. R. Armstrong.** 2009. Epidemiology of extrapulmonary tuberculosis in the United States, 1993–2006. *Clin. Infect. Dis.* 49:1350–1357.

77. **Pollock, N. R., A. Campos-Neto, S. Kashino, D. Napolitano, S. M. Behar, D. Shin, A. Sloutsky, S. Joshi, J. Guillet, M. Wong, and E. Nardell.** 2008. Discordant QuantiFERON-TB Gold test results among US healthcare workers with increased risk of latent tuberculosis infection: a problem or solution? *Infect. Control Hosp. Epidemiol.* 29:878–886.

78. **Rajagopalan, S., and T. T. Yoshikawa.** 2000. Tuberculosis in long-term-care facilities. *Infect. Control Hosp. Epidemiol.* 21: 611–615.

79. **Reichler, M. R., S. Bur, R. Reves, et al.** 2003. Results of testing for human immunodeficiency virus infection among recent contacts of infectious tuberculosis cases in the United States. *Int. J. Tuberc. Lung Dis.* 7:S471–S478.

80. **Reponen, T. A., Z. Wang, K. Willeke, et al.** 1999. Survival of mycobacteria on N95 personal respirators. *Infect. Control Hosp. Epidemiol.* 20:237–241.

81. **Ringshausen, F. C., S. Schlosser, A. Nienhaus, A. Schablon, G. Schultze-Werninghaus, and G. Rohde.** 2009. In-hospital contact investigation among healthcare workers after exposure to smear-negative tuberculosis. *J. Occup. Med. Toxicol.* 4:11–22.

82. **Schneider, E., K. F. Laserson, C. D. Wells, and M. Moore.** 2004. Tuberculosis along the United States-Mexico border, 1993–2001. *Rev Panam. Salud Publica* 16:23–34.

83. Schulte, J. M., S. E. Valway, E. McCray, and I. M. Onorato. 2001. Tuberculosis cases reported among migrant farm workers in the United States, 1993–97. *J. Health Care Poor Underserved* **12:**311–322.

84. Segal-Maurer, S., and G. E. Kalkut. 1994. Environmental control of tuberculosis: continuing controversy. *Clin. Infect. Dis.* **19:**299–308.

85. Segal-Maurer, S., B. N. Kreiswirth, J. M. Burns, et al. 1998. *Mycobacterium tuberculosis* specimen contamination revisited: the role of laboratory environmental control in a pseudo-outbreak. *Infect. Control Hosp. Epidemiol.* **19:**101–105.

86. Sepkowitz, K. A. 1995. AIDS, tuberculosis, and the health care worker. *Clin. Infect. Dis.* **20:**232–242.

87. Sepkowitz, K. A. 1994. Tuberculosis and the health care worker: a historical perspective. *Ann. Intern. Med.* **120:**71–79.

88. Siddiqui, A. H., T. M. Perl, M. Conlon, et al. 2002. Preventing nosocomial transmission of pulmonary tuberculosis: when may isolation be discontinued for patients with suspected tuberculosis? *Infect. Control Hosp. Epidemiol.* **23:**141–144.

89. Small, P. M., P. C. Hopewell, S. P. Singh, et al. 1994. The epidemiology of tuberculosis in San Francisco: a population-based study using conventional and molecular methods. *N. Engl. J. Med.* **330:**1703–1709.

90. Strausbaugh, L. J., S. R. Sukumar, and C. L. Joseph. 2003. Infectious disease outbreaks in nursing homes: an unappreciated hazard for frail elderly persons. *Clin. Infect. Dis.* **36:**870–876.

91. Stroud, L. A., J. I. Tokars, M. H. Grieco, et al. 1995. Evaluation of infection control measures in preventing the nosocomial transmission of multidrug-resistant *Mycobacterium tuberculosis* in a New York City hospital. *Infect. Control Hosp. Epidemiol.* **16:**141–147.

92. Tardin, A., D. M. Dominicé, B. Ninet, and J. P. Janssens. 2009. Tuberculosis cluster in an immigrant community: case identification issues and a transcultural perspective. *Trop. Med. Int. Health* **14:**995–1002.

93. Terry, M. B., M. Desvarieux, and M. Short. 2002. Temporal trends in tuberculosis hospitalization rates before and after implementation of directly observed therapy: New York City, 1988–1995. *Infect. Control Hosp. Epidemiol.* **23:**221–223.

94. Tokars, J. I., G. F. McKinley, J. Otten, et al. 2001. Use and efficacy of tuberculosis infection control practices at hospitals with previous outbreaks of multidrug-resistant tuberculosis. *Infect. Control Hosp. Epidemiol.* **22:**449–455.

95. Torres Costa, J., R. Silva, R. Sa, M. J. Cardoso, and A. Nienhau. 2010. Results of five-year systematic screening for latent tuberculosis infection in healthcare workers in Portugal. *J. Occup. Med. Toxicol.* **5:**22. doi:10.1186/1745-6673-5-22.

96. Tulsky, J. P., J. A. Hahn, H. L. Long, et al. 2004. Can the poor adhere? Incentives for adherence to TB prevention in homeless adults. *Int. J. Tuberc. Lung Dis.* **8:**83–91.

97. Valway, S. E., R. B. Greifinger, M. Papania, et al. 1994. Multidrug-resistant tuberculosis in the New York State prison system, 1990–1991. *J. Infect. Dis.* **170:**151–156.

98. Van den Brande, P. 2005. Revised guidelines for the diagnosis and control of tuberculosis: impact on management in the elderly. *Drug Aging* **22:**663–686.

99. Welbel, S. F., A. L. French, P. Bush, D. DeGuzman, and R. Weinstein. 2009. Protecting healthcare workers from tuberculosis: a 10-year experience. *Am. J. Infect. Control* **37:**668–673.

100. World Health Organization. 2006. *Tuberculosis and Air Travel: Guidelines for Prevention and Control*, 2nd ed. World Health Organization, Geneva, Switzerland.

101. Xu, P., J. Peccia, P. Fabiana, et al. 2003. Efficacy of ultraviolet germicidal irradiation of upper-room air in inactivating airborne bacterial spores and mycobacteria in full-scale studies. *Atmosph. Environ.* **37:**405–419.

102. Yun, L. W. H., R. R. Reves, M. R. Reichler, et al. 2003. Outcomes of contact investigation among homeless persons with infectious tuberculosis. *Int. J. Tuberc. Lung Dis.* **7:**S405–S411.

103. Zaza, S., H. M. Blumberg, C. Beck-Sagué, et al. 1995. Nosocomial transmission of *Mycobacterium tuberculosis*: role of health care workers in outbreak propagation. *J. Infect. Dis.* **172:**1542–1549.

104. Zevallos, M., and J. E. Justman. 2003. Tuberculosis in the elderly. *Clin. Geriatr. Med.* **19:**121–138.

Tuberculosis and Nontuberculous Mycobacterial Infections, 6th ed.
Edited by David Schlossberg
© 2011 ASM Press, Washington, DC

Chapter 13

Role of the Health Department— Legal and Public Health Considerations

MELISA THOMBLEY, KASHEF IJAZ, BEVERLY METCHOCK, AND PHILIP LOBUE

Tuberculosis is an archetypical public health disease. Tuberculosis is caused by an infectious organism, spread through a common vehicle, the air, and public health measures are essential for control of the disease. There are three priority strategies for tuberculosis prevention and control in the United States: (i) identifying and treating persons who have tuberculosis disease; (ii) finding persons exposed to infectious tuberculosis patients, evaluating them for *Mycobacterium tuberculosis* infection and disease, and providing subsequent treatment, if appropriate; and (iii) screening populations at high risk for latent tuberculosis infection (LTBI) and progression to tuberculosis disease to identify infected persons and provide treatment to prevent progression to disease (2).

Although prevention and control of tuberculosis in the United States are primarily the responsibility of state and local tuberculosis control programs, rarely are these activities implemented solely by the health department. Patients with tuberculosis disease are usually diagnosed and often treated by private providers. Contacts to infectious cases may also be evaluated and treated by their private physicians or other community providers. Private providers, as well as non-health department community or governmental entities, also screen and treat individuals at high risk for LTBI. However, the health department is responsible for coordination and oversight of these activities to ensure that objectives related to tuberculosis prevention and control are achieved.

The Advisory Council for the Elimination of Tuberculosis (ACET) identified seven core components of public health tuberculosis control programs (2):

- Conducting overall planning and development of policy
- Identifying persons who have clinically active tuberculosis

- Managing persons who have or who are suspected of having disease
- Identifying and managing persons infected with *Mycobacterium tuberculosis*
- Providing laboratory and diagnostic services
- Collecting and analyzing data
- Providing training and education

This chapter describes the role of the health department in the context of these core components. This discussion is primarily applicable to tuberculosis prevention and control programs in the United States.

HISTORICAL AND EPIDEMIOLOGICAL CONTEXT OF TUBERCULOSIS CONTROL

Public health control measures for tuberculosis have mirrored the knowledge and availability of treatment options. Prior to the discovery of the tubercle bacillus by Koch, there were few public health measures to control tuberculosis, although morbidity and mortality data were collected by some jurisdictions. Following the discovery of the tubercle bacillus and the advent of the sanatorium movement, the primary public health measure became the isolation of infectious persons in sanatoria. Hospitalization in sanatoria was intended for treatment initially, but it soon evolved into a control measure as well with the forced hospitalization of some patients (37). However, the availability of beds never met the demand. In 1945, the United States had 450 tuberculosis hospitals with 79,000 beds, despite having many more reported incident cases. With the advent of effective chemotherapy, hospitalization duration declined as the adoption of outpatient treatment of tuberculosis became the standard. In the 1960s and early 1970s, the previous lack of availability was reversed, with many beds in tuberculosis hospitals remaining empty,

Melisa Thombley, Kashef Ijaz, Beverly Metchock, and Philip LoBue • Division of Tuberculosis Elimination, Centers for Disease Control and Prevention, Mail Stop E-10, 1600 Clifton Road, Atlanta, GA 30333.

resulting in the eventual closure of the tuberculosis hospitals. Hospitalization is now reserved for acute care, although forced confinement continues for a small number of recalcitrant patients (10, 29, 50, 57).

Tuberculosis incidence and mortality began declining in the United States prior to the widespread use of sanatoria and well before the advent of effective chemotherapy (31). National statistics, which have been kept since 1953, demonstrate a steady decline in disease from 1953 to 1985. In 1953, there were 83,304 incident cases reported, and in 1985, there were 22,201 incident cases reported (15). As cases of tuberculosis declined to historical lows in the United States, the public health infrastructure for control also declined, as categorical federal funding ended and local funding was shifted to other priorities (2). Reported incident tuberculosis cases increased from 22,768 cases in 1986 to 26,673 cases in 1992. This increase coincided with the onset of the human immunodeficiency virus (HIV) epidemic, with tuberculosis in HIV-infected persons contributing to the increase (2). Other factors associated with the increase in tuberculosis included nosocomial and institutional transmission of M. *tuberculosis* and increased cases occurring in foreign-born persons who immigrated from countries with high rates of tuberculosis (2). Following the resurgence of tuberculosis, federal resources for tuberculosis prevention and control were substantially increased. These resources were directed to improve surveillance, increase the capacity of public health laboratories, and increase the number of tuberculosis patients treated with directly observed therapy (DOT) (1). As a result, the incidence of tuberculosis steadily declined from 1993 through 2009; in 2009, a historical low of 11,545 incident cases of tuberculosis was reported in the United States (16).

The complexity of tuberculosis control and the challenges facing elimination of tuberculosis have, however, not diminished. In 2009, more than 50% of cases reported in the United States occurred in persons born in other countries (16). A local tuberculosis control program may now have individuals from several different countries with tuberculosis disease in their jurisdiction. Therefore, the program must provide interpreter services, be responsive to the cultural issues of their patients, and provide patient education to persons who may have different perceptions than health department staff and providers regarding tuberculosis disease and treatment. Along the U.S.-Mexico border, persons with tuberculosis travel back and forth, complicating treatment of their tuberculosis and the identification and follow-up of contacts (59). Persons diagnosed and beginning treatment in Mexico may travel to the United States to continue and complete treatment, a burden of prevalent cases

not included in incident case reports. Coinfection with HIV occurs in 6% of patients reported with tuberculosis (16). This complicates treatment options because of drug-drug interactions between highly active antiretroviral therapy and antituberculous medications (36). Outbreaks in low-incidence areas often overwhelm local tuberculosis control program staff, resulting in increased transmission and morbidity from tuberculosis. Although rates of drug-resistant tuberculosis, particularly multidrug-resistant (MDR) tuberculosis, have declined since 1993, these cases continue to complicate treatment and prevention efforts (16). Currently approximately 1% of tuberculosis cases are MDR, with nearly 80% of MDR cases occurring in foreign-born persons (16). All of these factors complicate efforts to control and eventually eliminate tuberculosis in the United States.

ORGANIZATION OF PUBLIC HEALTH TUBERCULOSIS CONTROL PROGRAMS

Tuberculosis control in the United States is the legal responsibility of the state and local governments (2, 9). Most of the activities of tuberculosis control, such as surveillance, case management, and contact investigation, are conducted by the local (city, county, or district) health departments with oversight by the state tuberculosis control program. Medical care for patients with tuberculosis disease or LTBI is often provided by the health department; however, in many areas of the United States, medical care is provided by private, community physicians who may have an established relationship with the local tuberculosis control program. Regardless of where the medical care is provided, local tuberculosis control programs continue to have responsibility for supervision of care and ensuring that patients complete treatment for their disease.

State tuberculosis control programs generally provide funding and technical support to local programs. State programs also compile and report surveillance data, as do large local programs. State programs may assist local programs with investigations of outbreaks. Some state programs also conduct operational and epidemiological research related to tuberculosis control either by themselves or in collaboration with an academic institution. Public health laboratories are generally part of the state program, although large cities, counties, or jurisdictions may also have public health laboratories. State tuberculosis programs are responsible for interactions with other state government entities that may have a role in tuberculosis control, such as correctional facilities, college or universities, and homeless shelters.

The Centers for Disease Control and Prevention (CDC) is primarily responsible for the federal public health aspects of tuberculosis control (9). This includes providing funding for state and local tuberculosis programs, providing technical assistance to programs, compiling and reporting surveillance data, providing support and investigating outbreaks of tuberculosis, and funding and conducting operational, epidemiological, clinical, and basic and applied laboratory studies relevant to programmatic tuberculosis control activities. The CDC provides funding through cooperative agreements to 68 project areas, including 50 states, 10 large cities, and 8 U.S. jurisdictions and territories. In 1992, during the tuberculosis resurgence in the United States, the federal funding for tuberculosis prevention and control activities provided via the cooperative agreement mechanism increased substantially in response to a dramatic rise in tuberculosis cases. Funding levels were based on the resurgence of tuberculosis and emergence of MDR tuberculosis in the late 1980s and early 1990s, with the greatest amount of additional funding going to those large cities hardest hit by the epidemic. Since that time, the epidemiology of tuberculosis in the United States has evolved, however, while the funding amounts have remained static and purchasing power has decreased due to inflation.

In 2005, the CDC's Division of Tuberculosis Elimination (DTBE), in consultation with the National Tuberculosis Controllers Association (NTCA), developed a funding formula to redistribute funds based on epidemiological needs across tuberculosis programs in the country. The funding formula is based on consistently reported tuberculosis surveillance data by the states using the National Tuberculosis Surveillance System. Currently, the allocation of tuberculosis funding is done using the tuberculosis funding formula. In 2009, the funding formula was updated along with an increase in the amount of redistribution of funds. The fiscal year 2010 formula for the prevention and control component includes an increase in the funding redistribution to 45% based on averaged tuberculosis data reported to the CDC for 2004 to 2008. The formula consists of the following specific variables and corresponding weights:

- Incident cases, 30%
- U.S.-born minorities and foreign-born persons, 35%
- Persons coinfected with HIV, 5%
- Persons with MDR tuberculosis, 5%
- Substance abusers, 5%
- Homeless, 5%
- Persons with smear- or culture-positive pulmonary tuberculosis, 15%

As part of providing technical assistance to the tuberculosis programs, the CDC provides funding to support four Regional Training and Medical Consultation Centers (RTMCCs). These centers are regionally assigned to cover all 50 states and the U.S. territories. They are responsible for providing (i) training and technical assistance on various aspects of tuberculosis control for state and local health department staff to build human resource capacity and (ii) medical consultations for treatment related to tuberculosis cases. Additionally, these centers develop tuberculosis educational materials and products.

The majority of CDC-funded epidemiological and clinical research is conducted through either the Tuberculosis Epidemiologic Studies Consortium (TBESC) or the Tuberculosis Trials Consortium (TBTC). The TBESC was established in 2001 and is currently comprised of 16 domestic sites. Each of these sites has established partnerships between an academic institution and a tuberculosis control program. The consortium jointly conducts programmatically relevant epidemiological, behavioral, economic, laboratory, and operations research on various aspects of tuberculosis control. The TBTC has a rich lineage that can be traced back to 1960, when the (U.S. Public Health Service) Tuberculosis Division was transferred to the CDC. The TBTC is primarily engaged in conducting clinical trials and diagnostics research. It currently has a network of 29 clinical sites worldwide, which conduct research that expands clinical and epidemiological knowledge of tuberculosis and facilitates the diagnosis, clinical management, and prevention of tuberculosis infection and disease.

LEGAL BASIS FOR PUBLIC HEALTH AUTHORITY

Federal and International Authority To Control Tuberculosis

To ensure optimal coordination with appropriate federal public health officials or entities, state and local health officials should understand the circumstances where federal legal authority to control tuberculosis may be used. This authority includes the U.S. Constitution, statutes, regulations, and Executive Orders. The U.S. Constitution, Article I, Section 8, implicitly provides limited public health authority under the clauses granting to the federal government the power to tax and spend and the power to regulate commerce "with foreign Nations, and among the several States, and with the Indian Tribes" (commonly referred to as the Commerce Clause) (61).

The Commerce Clause is the legal foundation for section 361 of the Public Health Service Act, authorizing the Secretary of Health and Human Services to make and enforce regulations to prevent the entry and spread of communicable diseases from foreign countries into the United States and between states (60). The Secretary delegated this authority to the CDC. Under the Public Health Service Act, communicable diseases for which federal isolation and quarantine are authorized are limited to those diseases specifically enumerated by the President of the United States through Executive Order. (An executive order is issued by or on behalf of the President and is usually intended to direct or instruct the actions of executive agencies or government officials or to set policies for the executive branch to follow.)

Executive Order 13375, signed by the President on 1 April 2005, amended Executive Order 13295, to add novel influenza with the potential to cause a pandemic to the existing list comprising the following communicable diseases: cholera, diphtheria, plague, smallpox, yellow fever, viral hemorrhagic fevers, severe acute respiratory syndrome, and infectious tuberculosis.

Under its regulatory authority to prevent the introduction and spread of communicable diseases, the CDC is authorized to detain, medically examine, and conditionally release persons arriving into the United States who are suspected of having one of the communicable diseases listed in Executive Order 13375, including infectious tuberculosis (26). Further, the CDC has the authority, though it rarely exercises it, to quarantine, isolate, or place persons under surveillance who have infectious tuberculosis and are arriving into the United States or are moving between states (26). Under section 361 of the Public Health Services Act, the CDC may only apprehend and examine persons moving between states who are reasonably believed to be infected with a specified communicable disease in its qualifying stage, defined as the communicable stage of the disease or a precommunicable stage if the disease would be likely to cause a public health emergency if transmitted to other individuals. If such persons are found to be infected, then the CDC may detain them as reasonably necessary.

A related mechanism for preventing transmission of tuberculosis is the public health Do Not Board (DNB) list developed and managed by the CDC in cooperation with the Department of Homeland Security (DHS). The public health DNB list may be employed to prevent individuals who meet specific criteria and pose a serious threat to the public from boarding a commercial aircraft departing from or arriving into the United States. International officials and U.S. government agencies, state and local health officials, and health care providers may submit a request (to the CDC Emergency Operations Center, regional CDC Quarantine Station, or relevant state or local public

health department) for placement of a person's name on the DNB list. Upon receipt of such a request, the CDC determines whether a person (i) likely is contagious with a communicable disease that would constitute a serious public health threat should the person be permitted to board a flight; (ii) is unaware of or likely to be nonadherent to public health recommendations, including treatment; and (iii) likely will attempt to board a commercial aircraft (14).

If the CDC determines that a person who is the subject of the DNB list request meets these criteria, the person's name is added to this federal air travel restriction list by the DHS, and airlines are instructed not to issue the individual a boarding pass for any commercial flight departing from or arriving into the United States. Use of the DNB list is intended to supplement existing disease control measures that may be implemented by international or domestic health authorities. With respect to tuberculosis, criteria have been developed to determine when a person with suspected or confirmed pulmonary tuberculosis poses a serious public health threat, prompting placement on the public health DNB list. These criteria include an assessment of infectiousness, "based on clinical, radiographic, and mycobacteriologic response (e.g., sputum smear microscopy and culture results)" (14). Individuals with suspected or confirmed MDR or extensively drug-resistant tuberculosis are subject to more stringent criteria, based on World Health Organization (WHO) guidelines for tuberculosis and air travel. These criteria include the requirement of a negative culture result prior to removal from the list.

The United States is also responsible for adhering to the requirements set forth in the revised International Health Regulations (IHR), promulgated by the WHO in 2005 and entered into force in 2007. The United States is one of 194 countries (193 WHO Member States, plus Taiwan) that are bound by the IHR, an international agreement related to prevention of and response to the international spread of disease. Under the IHR, the United States (and other parties to the agreement) must notify the WHO of (i) all events which may constitute a public health emergency of international concern within its territory and (ii) to the extent practicable, public health risks identified outside its territory that may cause international disease spread as manifested by exported or imported human cases, vectors which carry infection or contamination, or goods that are contaminated (66). {A public health emergency of international concern is defined as "an extraordinary event which is determined, as provided in [the IHR] (i) to constitute a public health risk to other States through the international spread of disease and (ii) to potentially require a coordinated international response." Multiple factors determine when or if a person with tuberculosis would require notification under the IHR: (i) the potential for an international public health concern, (ii) the seriousness of the event's public health impact, (iii) the unusual or unexpected nature of the event, (iv) whether there is a significant risk of international disease spread, and (v) whether there is a significant risk of international travel or trade restrictions.}

State Authority To Control Tuberculosis

States retain primary authority over public health through the Tenth Amendment to the U.S. Constitution. (The Tenth Amendment reads as follows. "The powers not delegated to the United States by the Constitution, nor prohibited by it to the States, are reserved to the States respectively, or to the people. U.S. Constitution, 10th Amendment.") They exercise "police power" to protect the public's health; police power is defined as power exercised by the states to enact legislation and regulations to protect the public health, welfare, and morals and to promote the common good. State health departments are responsible for implementation to control the spread of infectious disease, including tuberculosis. This power creates responsibilities, and state and local public health officials must respect the limits of police power. States may also delegate police power to local governments. For example, the California Constitution states that "a county or city may make and enforce within its limits all local, police, sanitary, and other ordinances and regulations not in conflict with general laws" (11).

The following laws serve to control the spread of tuberculosis: (i) statutes, which are laws enacted by state legislatures (localities similarly pass ordinances, but these laws must be consistent with state legal authorities) (typically, the city council passes ordinances, but in many jurisdictions ordinances related to health or public health are passed by county boards of health or the equivalent); (ii) regulations, which are laws promulgated by state agencies—they generally have the force of law and are usually more detailed than statutes; and (iii) case law, which consists of decisions by judges interpreting laws, with binding precedent created by appellate courts.

With considerable variation from state to state, statutory and regulatory provisions may address the following areas of tuberculosis control and prevention: case identification, management of tuberculosis cases, and other protections (1). Case identification laws include reporting laws and screening laws. Tuberculosis is a reportable disease in all 50 states, but there is significant variation concerning required reporters, reporting time frame, and required content of reports (1). In some states, such as Iowa and Nebraska, penalties are imposed for failure to report tuberculosis cases as required by law (34, 48). Requirements can also include a duty to report nonadherent patients or other special circumstances (e.g., drug susceptibility test results or HIV status). Screening is usually required of populations at high risk of exposure to tuberculosis, such as health care workers and jail inmates, and may be a prerequisite for certain types of employment (e.g., grade school teachers and employees in day care facilities).

The majority of state tuberculosis control provisions concern aspects of tuberculosis case management, including, but not limited to, identification of tuberculosis cases (examination and contact investigations), provision of treatment (DOT and adherence to a treatment plan), treatment facilities, financing treatment, emergency detention, isolation (home isolation or isolation at a health or other appropriate facility), commitment, social distancing measures (exclusion from the workplace or school), and penalties for nonadherent patients. State and local health officials employ an incremental approach to implementing disease control measures, beginning with the least restrictive measure necessary to address the specific facts and circumstances of a case. Long-term commitment in a health or other appropriate facility is a significant restriction of individual liberty and due process is required, with periodic review of the court order imposing such confinement (constitutional provisions, including due process, are more fully discussed below). Finally, "other protections" accorded by statutes or regulations might address privacy and confidentiality, religious exemptions for tuberculosis treatment, specific due process procedures, and antidiscrimination provisions.

State and local public health officials must administer state tuberculosis control laws in conformance with constitutional requirements. Relevant provisions may include the First, Fourth, Eighth, and Fourteenth Amendments to the U.S. Constitution (the First, Fourth, and Eighth Amendments apply to the States through the Fourteenth Amendment) and similar state constitutional provisions (Table 1). The First Amendment states that "Congress shall make no law respecting an establishment of religion, or prohibiting the free exercise thereof" (62). An individual's right to free exercise of religion is not violated if the law is neutral and of general applicability. Many states provide religious exemptions for compulsory treatment for tuberculosis, in deference to the First Amendment, state constitutional provisions, or other legal or policy considerations. The Fourth Amendment prohibits the government from conducting unreasonable searches and seizures. Courts evaluate the reasonableness of a search by weighing the intrusion into individual privacy against the government's need for information. In the context of tuberculosis control, courts have held that a tuberculin skin test

Table 1. Selected cases involving relevant constitutional provisions

Case	Constitutional issue	Facts	Holding
Greene v. Edwards 263 S.E.2d 661 (W.Va. 1980)	14th Amendment, procedural due process clause	Appellant was involuntarily committed to a West Virginia hospital for active tuberculosis. He received notice of the commitment hearing but was not informed of the right to counsel. An attorney was appointed for him during the hearing, but the trial court proceeded without allowing the patient and his attorney to consult privately. Appellant filed a writ of habeas corpus, challenging the constitutionality of the statute.	Court held that the W.V. Tuberculosis Control Act must afford the same protections granted to those involuntarily committed for mental illness, including (i) adequate written notice detailing the grounds and underlying facts on which commitment is sought; (ii) right to counsel; (iii) right to be present, to cross-examine, and to confront witnesses; (iv) standard of proof that is clear and cogent, and convincing evidence; and (v) right to a transcript of the proceeding for appeal purposes.
McCormick v. Stalder 105 F.3d 1059 (5th Cir. 1997)	8th Amendment	Appellant tested positive for tuberculosis in prison and, in accordance with prison policy, was required to receive treatment for LTBI. If inmates are nonadherent, the policy provides that they can be isolated until the degree to which isolation is necessary is determined. Appellant claimed his 8th Amendment rights were violated because he submitted to medication to avoid isolation, he was not warned of side effects, and his consent to treatment was never obtained.	Court held that appellant's 8th Amendment rights were not violated. Appellant failed to show that prison medical officials were "deliberately indifferent to his serious medical needs." Note: This case concerns medical care and the rights of prisoners, involving a lower constitutional standard and minimal liberty interests compared to tuberculosis control efforts in the general population.
Newark v. J.S. 652 A.2d 265 (N.J. 1993)	14th Amendment, substantive due process clause	J.S. was being treated for active tuberculosis in a city hospital when he sought to leave against medical advice. City authorities called an emergency commitment hearing, based on J.S.'s active tuberculosis status, homelessness, and history of nonadherence. The judge granted the emergency order, and the city then sought a final order for commitment while the patient was being treated for active tuberculosis.	The court weighed the city's compelling interest of protecting its citizenry from disease against the fundamental liberty interest of being free from confinement. The court found that involuntary hospitalization was the least restrictive means to ensure prevention of the spread of tuberculosis in this case, because the patient was homeless and neither the patient nor his attorney proposed an alternate, less restrictive setting to be isolated from the public while receiving treatment for tuberculosis.
State v. Armstrong 239 P2d 545 (Wash. 1952)	1st Amendment, free exercise clause	University of Washington board of regents promulgated a regulation requiring all students to submit to chest X-ray examination prior to registration. The appellant requested an exemption from the examination, citing religious views.	Court held in favor of the board of regents, arguing that the regulation is preventive in nature—"Its primary concern is not for the possibly infected student, but is for those jeopardized by contact with such an individual." Court weighed the public health interest of students and university employees against the 1st Amendment interest of individual student. "Infringement of appellant's rights is a necessary consequence of a practical attempt to avoid the danger."
Washington v. Cambra 165 F.3d 920 (Cal. 1998)	4th Amendment	A California state prison had a policy that required two tuberculosis tests for each prisoner—one when the prisoner is admitted to the facility and a second after 12 wks. Prison officials administered the second tuberculosis test against appellant's (a prisoner) will. Appellant alleged that the prison officials violated his 4th Amendment rights against unreasonable search and seizure.	Summary judgment in favor of the prison officials affirmed. While the tuberculosis test is considered a 4th Amendment search, the prison's tuberculosis testing policy was reasonably related to the legitimate goal of detecting and containing tuberculosis.

(TST) required by a government entity is considered a search under the Fourth Amendment. The Eighth Amendment prohibits the infliction of cruel and unusual punishment and may be raised, for example, by jail inmates contesting tuberculosis control measures, such as testing, isolation, or treatment.

The Fourteenth Amendment prohibits states from depriving any person of life, liberty, or property without due process of law, and due process has been a frequent subject of state court challenges to tuberculosis control measures. "Substantive due process" requires the government to have adequate justification for implementing laws or taking other official actions that affect life, liberty, or property. The greater the liberty interest at stake, the more substantial the government justification must be. "Procedural due process" requires the government to use fair and reasonable procedures when contemplating action that will restrain a person's liberty. Notice and an opportunity to be heard are among the most fundamental procedures that must be made available. State and local public health departments must work with their legal counsel to ensure that their actions comport with constitutional provisions and their jurisdiction's legal authorities to prevent and control tuberculosis.

Interjurisdictional Agreements

Many states do not have appropriate facilities to treat patients with tuberculosis who need long-term inpatient treatment. For these states, consideration should be given to developing agreements with other states that have appropriate medical facilities and are willing to accept tuberculosis patients for care and treatment. While mutual aid agreements or memoranda of understanding have often been developed and used in the emergency preparedness context, such agreements may be effective for the voluntary or involuntary transfer of tuberculosis patients to out-of-state facilities.

For example, New Mexico does not have a secure medical facility in which to detain and treat nonadherent patients with tuberculosis. As an alternative to possibly detaining the nonadherent patient in a correctional facility, the New Mexico Department of Health negotiated with the Texas Department of State Health Services and ultimately entered into a Memorandum of Agreement (hereafter referred to simply as an Agreement) in 2007 for the purpose of providing

> New Mexico residents who are diagnosed with active TB, are non-adherent in taking their medications, and are under court order, access to the Texas Center for Infectious Diseases (TCID) so that they can be confined in order to ensure that the prescribed treatment regimen is completed and to prevent transmission of the disease (49)

The terms of the Agreement specify that the New Mexico Department of Health is responsible for coordinating transportation of patients to and from the Texas Center for Infectious Disease and for paying all costs of hospitalization and treatment of patients at a fixed rate.

As an alternative to case-by-case decision making, states without appropriate medical facilities in which to treat patients who need long-term inpatient treatment (whether voluntary or involuntary) may want to consider entering into standing agreements with states possessing appropriate facilities. Legal counsel to state and local health departments should be consulted throughout the process of initiating, negotiating, executing, and implementing agreements.

CONDUCTING OVERALL PLANNING AND DEVELOPMENT OF POLICY

Rational planning for tuberculosis program activities begins with an analysis of current data with close attention to recent trends. Morbidity trends (total cases and case rates) provide a general indication of future resource requirements. Not only do they provide insight into the amount of resources necessary for the management of tuberculosis patients but also they help to predict resources needed for contact investigation and tuberculin testing and LTBI treatment, since the numbers of contact investigations conducted and persons with LTBI tend to be proportional to tuberculosis morbidity.

The next level of analysis should focus on epidemiological trends, specifically the distribution of tuberculosis morbidity in the population served by the health department. Although general associations between tuberculosis and certain risk groups have been well documented (e.g., HIV infected, homeless, foreign-born, and racial and ethnic minorities), the relative importance of these risk groups varies based on location. Therefore, analysis of morbidity trends among these groups at the state and local levels is crucial to planning activities and interventions. This type of analysis also informs the tuberculosis program with respect to the needs for outreach to specific communities and hiring employees with suitable cultural and linguistic competencies.

Formal program evaluation is a critical process that contributes to both planning and accountability. In program evaluation, measurable indicators of program performance are created, and objectives are set for each indicator. This allows the program to determine if it is achieving its goals. CDC has developed a framework for program evaluation of public health practices (17). The CDC framework is based on four principles: utility, i.e., ensuring that the user's information needs are satisfied; feasibility, i.e., ensuring that the evaluation is viable and pragmatic; propriety, i.e., ensuring that the evaluation is ethical; and accuracy, i.e., ensuring that the evaluation produces findings that are considered correct. The framework includes six steps:

- Engage stakeholders.
- Describe the program.
- Focus the evaluation design.
- Gather credible evidence.
- Justify conclusions.
- Ensure use and share lessons learned.

Use of this methodology allows detailed examination of various aspects of a tuberculosis program. The program can determine which aspects are successful and which are in need of improvement. For those that need improvement, action steps can be designed and implemented to address shortcomings. Program evaluation should be a continual, iterative process.

Using this framework, in 2006, the development of National Tuberculosis Indicators Project (NTIP) was launched. NTIP is a web-based system that enables the use of regularly reported tuberculosis surveillance data to measure program performance. The stakeholders for initiating the development of this system included representatives of state and local health departments, the NTCA, and the CDC. Fifteen categories of national tuberculosis program objectives highlighting priority activities and outcomes (Table 2) were selected. The algorithms for calculating the indicators for these objectives were designed through this process. The year 2015 targets were derived from recent results of programs ranked at the 90th percentile for the respective performance indicators. Data for 12 of the 15 categories of objectives come from three current national surveillance systems: the National Tuberculosis Surveillance System (case reports, diagnosis, and management), the Aggregate Reports for Program Evaluation (contact investigations), and the Electronic Disease Notification System (immigrant and refugee health screening after U.S. arrival). The NTIP was launched with 11 reports for 10 categories of objectives in March 2009. Data related to refugees and immigrants are expected to be incorporated in the future. Officials at all 68 tuberculosis control programs (50 states, 10 large cities, and 8 U.S.-affiliated jurisdictions and territories) receiving federal tuberculosis cooperative agreement funds have online access to their own NTIP reports and the national summary (32).

Table 2. National tuberculosis program objective categories

No.	Category
1	Completion of treatment
2	Tuberculosis case rates
	U.S.-born persons
	Foreign-born persons
	U.S.-born non-Hispanic blacks
	Children younger than 5 yrs of age
3	Contact investigation
	Contact elicitation
	Evaluation
	Treatment initiation
	Treatment completion
4	Laboratory reporting
	Turnaround time
	Drug susceptibility test results
5	Treatment initiation
6	Sputum culture conversion
7	Data reporting
	Report of verified cases of tuberculosis
	Aggregate reports of program evaluation
	Electronic disease notification system
8	Recommended initial therapy
9	Universal genotyping
10	Known HIV status
11	Evaluation of immigrants and refugees
	Evaluation initiation
	Evaluation completion
	Treatment initiation
	Treatment completion
12	Sputum culture reported
13	Program evaluation
14	Human resource development plan
15	Training focal point

Some tuberculosis programs have also created sets of indicators to provide an overall assessment of their performance at the local and state levels (54). A good example of tuberculosis program evaluation using the CDC framework has been reported by the Massachusetts Department of Public Health (41). Massachusetts applied the CDC framework to tuberculosis contact investigation in five city health departments. Stakeholders of the evaluation were engaged. Models describing the components of contact investigation at the state and local level were created, and self-evaluation tools were developed. Based on this experience, Massachusetts plans to apply the evaluation process statewide and use the findings to target areas that need improvement.

In order to develop capacity for conducting effective program evaluations at the state and local levels, the CDC in collaboration with state and local tuberculosis controllers and representatives from the NTCA and ACET convened a strategic planning meeting in fall 2008. The purpose of the meeting was to develop a strategic plan for conducting effective program evaluations and build local capacity for the next 5 years. The strategic plan called for establishing a Tuberculosis Program Evaluation Network (TB-PEN). The first annual conference of TB-PEN was held in summer 2009. The goal of TB-PEN is to build capacity for tuberculosis program evaluation activities in state and local tuberculosis programs and increase the number of programs that are evaluating their program activities through the following means:

- Engaging tuberculosis control professionals to monitor and evaluate tuberculosis control activities
- Providing expertise and technical assistance for conducting tuberculosis program evaluation
- Identifying and communicating effective program evaluations

The TB-PEN has a network of designated tuberculosis evaluation focal points in each tuberculosis control program. These focal points serve as the trainers and experts to help provide technical assistance and build program evaluation capacity within their state and local tuberculosis control programs. Additionally, the TB-PEN comprises five specific teams to provide technical assistance, help develop evaluation tools, provide training, help with implementation of evaluation process and recommendations, and facilitate communication of results of these findings.

IDENTIFYING PERSONS WHO HAVE CLINICALLY ACTIVE TUBERCULOSIS

The first priority of tuberculosis control in the United States is detection and treatment of patients with active tuberculosis. Discovery of a previously undiagnosed tuberculosis patient triggers several interventions that interrupt transmission. These include placing the patient in respiratory isolation if contagious, starting the patient on tuberculosis treatment, and conducting a contact investigation. Health departments seek to be notified of patients with tuberculosis as early as possible and use active and passive methods of case finding to achieve this goal.

Active case finding occurs through contact and outbreak investigations and screening of high-risk populations. The purpose of contact investigation is to find persons recently infected with tuberculosis. Although most recently infected individuals will have LTBI, approximately 1 to 2% of contacts evaluated will be diagnosed with active tuberculosis (35). When several tuberculosis cases are linked through traditional or molecular epidemiological methods, this may constitute an outbreak. Because an outbreak indicates significant ongoing transmission, more intensive methods may be used to ensure that all cases

in the outbreak have been discovered. This may include screening with chest radiographs (CXRs) and sputum sampling regardless of TST or interferon gamma release assay (IGRA) results or symptoms. Because these tests incur considerable additional cost, their use in the initial phase of screening has usually been restricted to large outbreaks or those involving congregate settings or very high-risk populations (e.g., those in homeless shelters or prisons and HIV-infected persons) (40).

Screening of high-risk populations generally begins with targeted testing for LTBI. As with contact investigation, most persons found to be infected with tuberculosis have LTBI, but occasionally individuals with active tuberculosis are also identified (55). The health department may also work with congregate facilities with high rates of active disease to conduct active case finding using CXR screening. Several of these screening programs have been successful in early case detection (6, 52).

Passive case finding consists of accepting reports of tuberculosis suspects and patients from community medical providers. In all U.S. states, reporting of tuberculosis patients is required by law (1). While patients found through the passive reporting system frequently have advanced disease, this passive case-finding mechanism remains important because it allows mobilization of health department services, including monitoring of respiratory isolation, case management, DOT, and contact investigation, that help to prevent further transmission. In addition, this surveillance activity makes possible the collection of epidemiological data, facilitating the examination of tuberculosis trends at the local, state, and national levels. By examining these trends, tuberculosis programs are able to utilize resources more effectively.

EVALUATION OF IMMIGRANTS

In the United States, the percentage of tuberculosis cases in foreign-born persons has been increasing, rising from 30% in 1993 to 59% in 2009. This reflects a slower decline in the incidence rate for the foreign-born population than for the U.S.-born population. In 2007, the rate for the foreign-born population was 10.2 times greater than for the U.S.-born population. More than half of the 6,854 foreign-born cases in 2009 were reported to occur in persons from four countries: Mexico (1,598), the Philippines (806), India (533), and Vietnam (526) (16). With the majority of tuberculosis cases in the United States occurring among individuals born outside the country, the link between immigration and overseas screening for tuberculosis has become increasingly important. One effort taken by the CDC to reduce this burden has been to strengthen the overseas medical examination for tuberculosis in people seeking an immigrant visa.

Each year, approximately 400,000 immigrants and 80,000 refugees enter the United States from overseas locations (63). Before entry into the United States, these applicants are required to undergo medical screening for any disease of public health significance, referred to as an inadmissible condition, which includes infectious tuberculosis. The CDC's Division of Global Migration and Quarantine (DGMQ) has regulatory authority to define communicable diseases of public health significance and requirements of the scope of the medical examination. The DGMQ provides guidance through technical instructions (TI) to physicians who are responsible for conducting the medical exam (12, 27).

Physicians who perform the required medical screening throughout the world are called panel physicians, contracted to the U.S. Department of State to serve in this capacity. Immigrants pay for the cost of their required screening, while the Bureau of Populations, Refugees, and Migration, Department of State, funds the screening of refugees.

The DGMQ provides technical oversight of the medical screening and designates teams who perform on-site visits using standardized evaluation tools. For tuberculosis, the DGMQ also identifies or helps develop tuberculosis laboratory and DOT facilities.

The DTBE provides subject matter expertise to the DGMQ for the tuberculosis portion of the required medical examination. This expertise has included consultation on various aspects of the screening algorithm used to detect tuberculosis and manage patients who are diagnosed with tuberculosis during the screening process. In turn, the DTBE has consulted with various groups for technical review of this work, including the ACET and NTCA.

TI for Tuberculosis (TB TI) were first issued in 1991 (Fig. 1). These instructions required a CXR for applicants who were 15 years of age or older. Applicants with a CXR suggestive of tuberculosis had to provide three sputum specimens, which underwent microscopy for acid-fast bacilli (AFB). Applicants with at least one positive sputum smear were required to postpone travel to the United States and undergo treatment for tuberculosis disease until sputum smears were negative. Medical clearance was valid for 12 months for applicants with a CXR with no evidence of active tuberculosis disease and 6 months for applicants with an abnormal CXR suggestive of tuberculosis but with sputum smears negative for AFB (12).

The 1991 screening protocol was able to identify many people with infectious tuberculosis. However, the 2005 experience of resettling Hmong refugees from Wat Tham Krabok, Thailand, to the United States underscored the importance of modernizing the 1991 TB TI (13). The Hmong resettlement and a study among immigrants in Vietnam demonstrated the failure of the 1991 TB TI to detect smear-negative, culture-positive cases of tuberculosis disease (42). In

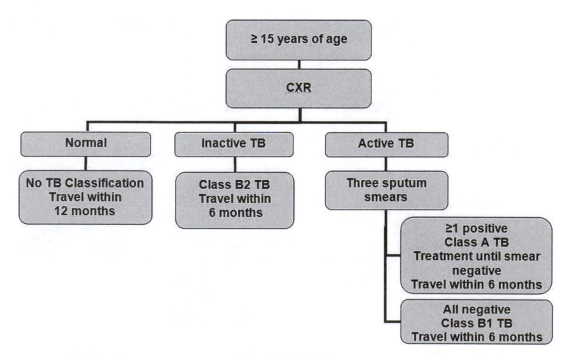

Figure 1. 1991 TB TI.

the Hmong resettlement, a significant fraction of the undetected overseas cases were MDR tuberculosis (13). Additional studies have demonstrated the challenges of preventing importation of tuberculosis disease (8, 64, 65). The U.S. tuberculosis community had recommended updating the 1991 TB TI, with consideration given toward incorporating mycobacterial cultures and TST into the algorithm and developing classifications for applicants suspected of having LTBI (19, 20, 28, 33). The emergence of extensively drug-resistant tuberculosis further reinforced the importance of an overseas screening system for U.S. immigration applicants that can detect and adequately treat tuberculosis disease in the immigrant's country of origin (21).

In 2007, the CDC published revised instructions for overseas medical screening of applicants for U.S. immigration to better detect and treat tuberculosis disease and improve risk stratification of applicants (22). While the instructions in effect since 1991 specified that applicants or refugees 15 years of age and older receive a CXR to identify active tuberculosis disease, further evaluation of tuberculosis suspects included only smear microscopy. In addition, the evaluation of children less than 15 years of age was limited to symptom review. The 2007 TI (Fig. 2) included several features to enhance tuberculosis case detection: (i) applicants 2 to 14 years of age living in countries with a WHO-estimated tuberculosis incidence rate of more than 20 cases per 100,000 population should have a TST, and if the TST result is 5 mm

or greater, a CXR should be performed; (ii) sputum smears and culture for *M. tuberculosis* are required for applicants with a CXR suggestive of tuberculosis disease, with drug susceptibility testing required on positive isolates; and (iii) applicants with smear-positive or culture-positive tuberculosis must receive therapy according to the American Thoracic Society, CDC, and Infectious Diseases Society of America tuberculosis treatment guidelines delivered as DOT.

A key recommendation by the ACET was to perform intensive review of each immigrant and refugee screening program to evaluate the implementation of the 2007 TB TI. The objectives for each evaluation are twofold: (i) to provide recommendations to the organizations responsible for screening, diagnosis, and treatment of tuberculosis in refugees and immigrants migrating to the United States and (ii) to provide recommendations to the CDC's DGMQ and DTBE to improve the effectiveness and feasibility of the new instructions.

Evaluations conducted to date of refugee and immigrant tuberculosis screening and treatment programs in Thailand, Philippines, and Nepal have provided clear evidence that culture for *M. tuberculosis* and drug susceptibility testing add immense value. In addition, U.S. surveillance data show a reduction in imported tuberculosis disease from these countries as a result of the 2007 TI. The evaluations have also contributed key recommendations to the CDC regarding further improvements of the TI to be incorporated in the next release.

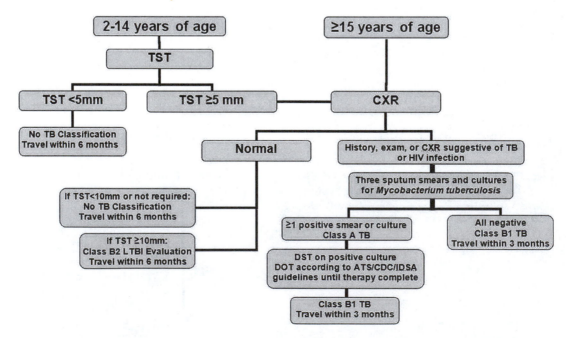

Figure 2. 2007 TI for tuberculosis screening and treatment for applicants in countries with WHO-estimated tuberculosis incidence rates of ≥20 cases per 100,000 population.

MANAGING PERSONS WHO HAVE OR ARE SUSPECTED OF HAVING DISEASE

After a patient with tuberculosis has been reported to the health department, it is the responsibility of the health department, in conjunction with the patient's medical provider (if the provider is not the health department), to ensure that the patient completes an adequate treatment regimen (4). In this context, case management involves accessing and employing the medical and social resources needed to shepherd a patient through completion of treatment.

The first task of the case manager is to make certain that the patient has a medical provider who will assume responsibility for the patient's tuberculosis treatment. The case manager should also oversee the administration of DOT, making it as convenient as possible for the patient while closely monitoring adherence. Monitoring for adverse effects and response to treatment (e.g., collection of follow-up sputum samples) should be performed, with any problems being promptly reported to the patient's medical provider.

In addition to oversight of medical care, it is also important to assist the patient to overcome social barriers that may impede adherence to treatment (24). Being ill with tuberculosis can impose significant financial hardship due to inability to work and due to costs of medical care that may not be covered by the health department (e.g., hospitalization). Patients may be eligible for medical and financial benefits such as Medicaid, Medicare, or disability insurance. The case manager should help the patient access social services to obtain these benefits and direct the patient to other governmental or nongovernmental community-based programs that can assist with housing, food, and transportation if needed (Table 3) (4, 38).

Culture and language present other potential barriers to adherence. It is preferable that culturally and linguistically competent staff be used to provide medical care and education (24). If not available, it is essential to have ready access to interpreters. In addition, all education materials should be appropriate for the culture, language, and reading level of the patient.

The final responsibility of the case manager is to review the treatment record before the case is closed to the health department. The case manager should ensure that an adequate number of doses of medication have been taken within the recommended duration and that the patient has had a good response to therapy indicative of cure. If these criteria have not been met, the case manager should confer with the tuberculosis controller and the patient's medical provider to determine the appropriate course of action.

Table 3. Possible components of a multifaceted, patient-centered treatment strategy[a]

Enablers: interventions to assist the patient in completing therapy
- Transportation vouchers
- Child care
- Convenient clinic hours and locations
- Clinic personnel who speak the languages of the populations served
- Reminder systems and follow-up of missed appointments
- Social service assistance (referrals for substance abuse treatment and counseling, housing, and other services)
- Outreach workers (bilingual/bicultural as needed; can provide many services related to maintaining patient adherence, including provision of DOT, follow-up on missed appointments, monthly monitoring, transportation, sputum collection, social service assistance, and educational reinforcement)
- Integration of care for tuberculosis with care for other conditions

Incentives: interventions to motivate the patient, tailored to individual patient wishes and needs and, thus, meaningful to the patient
- Food stamps or snacks and meals
- Restaurant coupons
- Assistance in finding or provision of housing
- Clothing or other personal products
- Books
- Stipends
- Patient contract

[a]Reproduced from the work of the American Thoracic Society, CDC, and Infectious Diseases Society of America (4).

MEDICAL CONSULTATION

As tuberculosis cases have decreased in the United States, so have the number of medical providers with experience in treating tuberculosis patients (33). For this reason, the only local or statewide clinical expertise may reside within the public health department. Therefore, it is often necessary that health department physicians and nurses be available to provide medical consultation on diagnostic and treatment issues. Frequently, this service can be provided via telephone or e-mail. In some areas, medical providers can refer patients to a health department tuberculosis clinic for a more formal consultation. However, even health departments may no longer possess expertise in treating tuberculosis if they are in low-incidence areas. To address this need and increase access to expert medical consultation, since 2005 the CDC has funded RTMCCs to provide coverage throughout the United States. Currently four centers located in New Jersey, Florida, Texas, and California (Fig. 3) are each responsible for providing medical consultation services to an assigned region. The RTMCCs are staffed by nationally recognized tuberculosis experts, and consultations are available by telephone or e-mail.

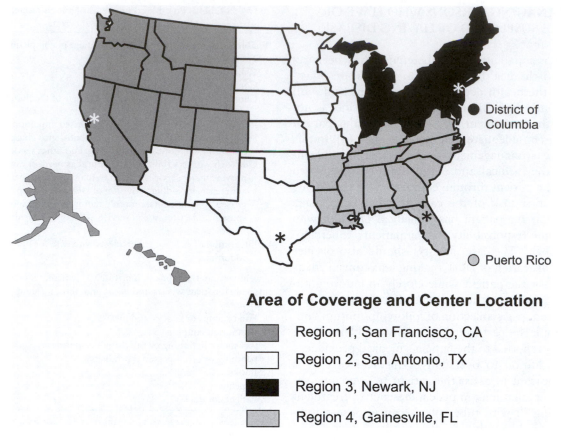

Area of Coverage and Center Location

Region 1, San Francisco, CA

Region 2, San Antonio, TX

Region 3, Newark, NJ

Region 4, Gainesville, FL

Figure 3. RTMCCs: areas of coverage.

The RTMCC medical consultants work closely with state and local tuberculosis programs in their region to ensure that critical public health activities related to tuberculosis patients are addressed.

INTERJURISDICTIONAL REFERRALS

Ensuring completion of treatment for all patients is critical in achieving and maintaining tuberculosis control. When patients move from one health department jurisdiction to another, making certain that they complete treatment becomes more difficult. According to one study, patients who move are five times more likely to default (25). This underscores the necessity of close cooperation and coordination between tuberculosis control programs when caring for mobile patients if optimal outcomes are to be attained.

To deal with the complexities of managing tuberculosis patients relocating while on therapy, the NTCA has developed a system for interjurisdictional referrals. A brief protocol can be downloaded from their website (http://www.ntca-tb.org). A form for transferring pertinent information about tuberculosis patients from the discharging health department to the receiving health department can also be found on the website. Information collected on the form includes identifying, demographic, clinical, laboratory, and treatment data. In addition, the form allows for exchange of information related to contact investigation and patients being treated for LTBI. When the discharging jurisdiction has reported the patient as a case to the CDC, it is also responsible for reporting the treatment outcome. Therefore, the receiving jurisdiction should provide follow-up information on transferred patients to the discharging jurisdiction. A form and instructions for providing interjurisdictional follow-up are also available on the NTCA website.

The NTCA system is primarily meant for interstate referrals. For intrastate referrals, it is best for local health departments to contact their state tuberculosis control program. Some states, such as California, have existing intrastate interjurisdictional referral systems that are similar to the one implemented by the NTCA.

Occasionally tuberculosis programs may need to exchange information regarding tuberculosis patients with tuberculosis programs in other countries. The

Cure-TB binational referral program, which is managed by the County of San Diego's Tuberculosis Control Program (http://www.sandiegotbcontrol.org), assists with managing tuberculosis patients moving to or from Mexico. For assistance in exchanging information about patients moving to or from countries other than Mexico, it is recommended that health departments contact the International Research and Programs Branch of the DTBE.

IDENTIFYING AND MANAGING PERSONS INFECTED WITH *M. TUBERCULOSIS*

Investigation of Contacts to Infectious Tuberculosis Cases

Contact investigations are an essential function of tuberculosis control in the United States and have been identified as a priority strategy for prevention and control of tuberculosis (2). Among close contacts, approximately 1 to 2% will have tuberculosis disease and 31 to 36% will have LTBI (43, 53). Up to 5% of contacts with newly acquired LTBI will develop tuberculosis within 2 years of infection (30). Contact investigations are therefore an effective method for active case finding and identifying persons with LTBI who are also at a high risk of developing tuberculosis disease. State and local public health agencies are responsible for ensuring that contact investigations are effectively conducted and that all exposed contacts are identified, evaluated for tuberculosis infection and disease, and appropriately treated. Consequently, 90% of contact investigations in the United States are performed by public health departments (33).

Targeted Testing and Treatment of LTBI

The number of persons in the United States with LTBI is currently estimated at 8.9 million to 14.0 million (7). To continue progress toward the elimination of tuberculosis in the United States, public health programs must devise effective strategies to address the challenge of preventing tuberculosis in this population of infected persons. Guidelines on targeted testing and treatment of LTBI have been published and revised (3, 18). Those guidelines include recommendations for diagnosis and treatment of LTBI, as well as recommendations for identifying persons and groups to target for testing.

The health department has several potential roles in testing and treatment of persons with LTBI. Health departments may evaluate and treat persons who have been referred to the health department following diagnosis of LTBI by community providers. The health department may also test persons who are

required to document that they are free from tuberculosis because of existing state and local regulations. This group may include food handlers, teachers, or students. Since these two activities are not necessarily targeted towards populations at risk for tuberculosis infection, their impact and effectiveness tend to be limited at best and counterproductive at worst in that resources may be diverted from higher-priority tuberculosis control and prevention activities.

Greater impact can be achieved by targeting populations at greater risk for LTBI and at greater risk for progression to tuberculosis if infected. The health department can do this by providing technical assistance and collaborating with persons, facilities, or agencies providing health care services to populations at risk or by implementing targeted testing and treatment programs in high-risk populations. Health departments must regularly evaluate the effectiveness and impact of their targeted testing activities to ensure that resources are appropriately allocated. Ineffective practices, such as testing low-risk populations, should be discontinued.

For decades, the TST was the only available tool for diagnosing LTBI. However, in 2001 the Food and Drug Administration (FDA) approved the first alternative test for the diagnosis of latent tuberculosis infection, an IGRA named QuantiFERON-TB (45). Since that time, three more IGRAs have been approved by the FDA (51). All are based on the same principle that peripheral blood lymphocytes sensitized by *M. tuberculosis* infection will produce gamma interferon when subsequently exposed to *M. tuberculosis* antigens. Advantages of these tests include the need for only one patient visit (as opposed to two for TST), use of specific *M. tuberculosis* antigens that are not found in bacillus Calmette-Guérin (BCG) or most nontuberculous mycobacteria, and objective measurement of gamma interferon release (as opposed to the more subjective measurement of induration for TST). While the CDC has stated that IGRAs can be used in any instance for which TST is used, a number of questions about IGRAs remain (44). Foremost among these is the likelihood of progressing to tuberculosis disease based on IGRA test results compared with TST.

Similarly, for many years treatment of LTBI has primarily been limited to a single drug, isoniazid. While isoniazid has been demonstrated to be highly efficacious in the prevention of progression to tuberculosis disease in persons with LTBI, the drug's effectiveness is limited by the need for a prolonged course of treatment and hepatotoxicity. Completion rates for a 6- to 9-month course of isoniazid are 50 to 60% at best (39). A 4-month course of rifampin, which is currently recommended as an acceptable alternative to isoniazid, appears to be better tolerated, with higher completion rates (46, 47). However, this regimen has never been actually demonstrated to be efficacious, and recommendation for its use was based on extrapolation of findings of studies using multidrug rifampin-containing regimens for tuberculosis disease and LTBI. A 2-month regimen of rifampin and pyrazinamide was initially found to be promising but is no longer recommended because of excessive hepatotoxicity (18). A 3-month, once-weekly regimen of isoniazid and rifapentine is currently being evaluated in clinical trials (58).

PROVIDING LABORATORY AND DIAGNOSTIC SERVICES

Public health tuberculosis control programs are responsible for ensuring that suitable laboratory and diagnostic services are available for tuberculosis suspects and patients. The most important component is the availability of accurate and rapid mycobacteriology laboratory services, since the laboratory is an essential part of the diagnosis, treatment, prevention, and control of tuberculosis (56). Core public health mycobacteriology services include fluorescent acid-fast microscopy, liquid culture, identification of *M. tuberculosis* complex isolates using rapid methods, and testing of *M. tuberculosis* complex isolates for susceptibility to first-line drugs used for treatment by rapid methods (5). Public health laboratories should also develop systems to facilitate specimen transport and ensure rapid reporting of results to TB control as well as the community health care providers and laboratories they serve.

In addition to core services, public health laboratories should provide or ensure availability of nucleic acid amplification to detect *M. tuberculosis* complex directly in clinical specimens, when clinically indicated for patients for whom a diagnosis of tuberculosis is being considered but has not yet been established, and for whom the test result would alter case management or tuberculosis control activities (23). It is necessary for public health laboratories to work with tuberculosis program partners to establish policies ensuring the appropriate utilization and interpretation of nucleic acid amplification (5). Public health laboratories that do not perform second-line drug susceptibility testing should have protocols in place for rapid referral of *M. tuberculosis* complex isolates to a reference laboratory as soon as rifampin resistance, or resistance to any two first-line drugs, is suspected.

Although IGRAs are currently not considered a core service of public health tuberculosis laboratories (5), many public health laboratories perform these tests. Laboratories and tuberculosis control programs should collaborate to determine the need for IGRA in their jurisdiction.

The health department should also ensure that outpatient and inpatient facilities involved in the diagnosis and treatment of tuberculosis have access to chest radiology services, including interpretation. Prompt reporting of CXR findings is essential to providing care to tuberculosis suspects and patients. HIV counseling, testing, and referral must be readily available also. Finally, facilities providing tuberculosis treatments should provide adequate laboratory and diagnostic services to monitor patients for adverse reactions to treatment.

COLLECTING AND ANALYZING DATA

Public health programs cannot function effectively without rapid and accurate disease surveillance systems. The critical first step in maintaining effective surveillance is prompt tuberculosis case reporting. A vital element of this process is reporting of positive test results from laboratories to the health department. Reporting from physicians, hospitals, and other community health care providers also plays a crucial role. The health department should institute both passive and active case finding to facilitate case reporting. Active case finding includes routine communication with infection control practitioners in hospitals, correctional facilities, and other facilities that diagnose tuberculosis. The health department should create a tuberculosis registry and have the capacity for the electronic storage of records with updated information on all current and suspect tuberculosis cases. Data collection should include all information necessary to ensure the appropriate follow-up of tuberculosis suspects and patients and for compiling local, state, and national surveillance reports. All clinically relevant information, including diagnostic laboratory results, drug susceptibility testing results, and treatment regimens, should be included in the registry. Ideally, the health department should also collect and store data on contacts and persons tested for LTBI. Sufficient safeguards to ensure the quality of the data and to protect the confidentiality of the records should be instituted.

Tuberculosis control programs should analyze the data collected to monitor morbidity trends, determine the demographic characteristics of their patient population, monitor drug resistance rates, and determine the outcomes of treatment. Additional analyses should be done on the effectiveness and outcomes of contact investigations and LTBI targeted testing and treatment programs. These analyses should be used to assess program performance and progress toward achieving locally and nationally established program objectives. Planning for use of resources and implementation of interventions should be based on the results of the analysis of surveillance and program data. Annual reports of local tuberculosis morbidity rates and trends should be prepared and distributed to community providers and organizations, professional societies, and leaders.

An important component of data collection by the local health department is the prompt and complete reporting of tuberculosis cases to state tuberculosis control programs, with the states forwarding the reports to the CDC. These data are essential for state and national planning, assessment, and resource allocation.

PROVIDING TRAINING AND EDUCATION

The primary training responsibility of state and local health departments is training the health department staff directly involved in tuberculosis prevention and control activities. Health department staff need ongoing training and education to remain current on treatment, patient management, and programmatic issues. As new guidelines for tuberculosis treatment, prevention, and control are published, staff need updates and related training. New staff members need intensive training to become adept at their job and gain general knowledge regarding tuberculosis transmission, infection, and disease, as well as develop proficiency in infection control procedures.

A secondary responsibility is education of the external community to ensure that community providers and clinicians have the knowledge and skills to appropriately diagnose and treat tuberculosis. Health care planners and policy makers should be educated on the continuing need to control and eliminate tuberculosis in their jurisdictions. Institutions, such as hospitals, correctional facilities, nursing homes, and homeless shelters, should be instructed on the need to maintain vigilance and adequate infection control practices to prevent the transmission of tuberculosis within their facilities. Tuberculosis control programs must work diligently with community groups, minority organizations, professional societies, and medical and nursing schools to meet the training and education needs of the community.

The TB Education and Training Network was formed in 2000 to bring TB professionals together to network, share resources, and build education and training skills. Membership includes representatives from TB programs, correctional facilities, hospitals, nursing homes, federal agencies, universities, the American Lung Association, RTMCCs, and other U.S. and international organizations interested in TB education and training issues.

Goals of this network include furthering TB education and training by the following:

- Building, strengthening, and maintaining collaboration
- Providing a mechanism for sharing resources to avoid duplication
- Developing, improving, and maintaining access to resources
- Providing updated information about TB courses and training initiatives
- Assisting members in skill building

CONCLUSION

With the continued decline in tuberculosis incidence in the United States, programs must confront the decline in resources available for tuberculosis control and the decline in knowledge and skills among community providers and their own staff regarding the diagnosis, treatment, and control of tuberculosis. At the same time, outbreaks of tuberculosis resulting from delayed diagnosis of persons with infectious tuberculosis will continue to occur and can easily overwhelm the capacity of small public health programs to respond. New paradigms of public health response to tuberculosis, such as strengthening laboratory networks and regionalization of programs, will be necessary to meet the needs of low-incidence areas.

If current trends in the epidemiology of tuberculosis persist, tuberculosis in the United States will eventually be a disease of persons born in other countries. This will continue to challenge public health programs as they struggle to control tuberculosis in patient populations with diverse languages, cultures, and understandings of and beliefs about tuberculosis. Many programs have already adapted to this changing epidemiology of tuberculosis. Ultimately, control and elimination of tuberculosis in the United States will depend not only on the efforts of the state and local health departments and community providers but also on the success of international efforts.

In *Ending Neglect: the Elimination of Tuberculosis in the United States*, the Institute of Medicine recommended that the United States maintain control of tuberculosis while adjusting control measures to declining incidence of disease and while also accelerating the rate of decline of tuberculosis (33). This fundamental challenge for tuberculosis public health programs will define their efforts and activities in the coming years.

REFERENCES

1. Advisory Council for the Elimination of Tuberculosis. 1993. Tuberculosis control laws—United States, 1993. Recommendations of the Advisory Council for the Elimination of Tuberculosis (ACET). *MMWR Recommend. Rep.* **42:**1–28.

2. Advisory Council for the Elimination of Tuberculosis. 1995. Essential components of a tuberculosis prevention and control program. Recommendations of the Advisory Council for the Elimination of Tuberculosis. *MMWR Recommend. Rep.* **44:**1–16.

3. American Thoracic Society and Centers for Disease Control and Prevention. 2000. Targeted tuberculin testing and treatment of latent tuberculosis infection. *MMWR Recommend. Rep.* **49:**1–51.

4. American Thoracic Society, Centers for Disease Control and Prevention, and Infectious Diseases Society of America. 2003. Treatment of tuberculosis. *MMWR Recommend. Rep.* **52:**1–77.

5. Association of Public Health Laboratories. 2009. *Core TB Laboratory Services for Public Health Laboratories.* Association of Public Health Laboratories, Silver Spring, MD.

6. Barry, M. A., C. Wall, L. Shirley, J. Bernardo, P. Schwingl, E. Brigandi, and G. A. Lamb. 1986. Tuberculosis screening in Boston's homeless shelters. *Public Health Rep.* **101:**487–494.

7. Bennett, D. E., J. M. Courval, I. Onorato, T. Agerton, J. D. Gibson, L. Lambert, G. M. McQuillan, B. Lewis, T. R. Navin, and K. G. Castro. 2008. Prevalence of tuberculosis infection in the United States population: the national health and nutrition examination survey, 1999–2000. *Am. J. Respir. Crit. Care Med.* **177:**348–355.

8. Binkin, N. J., P. L. Zuber, C. D. Wells, M. A. Tipple, and K. G. Castro. 1996. Overseas screening for tuberculosis in immigrants and refugees to the United States: current status. *Clin. Infect. Dis.* **23:**1226–1232.

9. Binkin, N. J., A. A. Vernon, P. M. Simone, E. McCray, B. I. Miller, C. W. Schieffelbein, and K. G. Castro. 1999. Tuberculosis prevention and control activities in the United States: an overview of the organization of tuberculosis services. *Int. J. Tuberc. Lung Dis.* **3:**663–674.

10. Burman, W. J., D. L. Cohn, C. A. Rietmeijer, F. N. Judson, J. A. Sbarbaro, and R. R. Reves. 1997. Short-term incarceration for the management of noncompliance with tuberculosis treatment. *Chest* **112:**57–62.

11. California Constitution, article 11, sec. 7.

12. Centers for Disease Control. 1991. *Technical Instructions for Medical Examination of Aliens, 1991.* Centers for Disease Control, Atlanta, GA. http://www.cdc.gov/immigrantrefugee health/exams/ti/index.html.

13. Centers for Disease Control and Prevention. 2005. Multi-drug resistant tuberculosis in Hmong refugees resettling from Thailand to the United States, 2004–2005. *MMWR Morb. Mortal. Wkly. Rep.* **30:**741–744.

14. Centers for Disease Control and Prevention. 2008. Federal air travel restrictions for public health purposes—United States. *MMWR Morb. Mortal. Wkly. Rep.* **57:**1009–1012.

15. Centers for Disease Control and Prevention. 2003. *Reported Tuberculosis in the United States, 2002.* Centers for Disease Control and Prevention, U.S. Department of Health and Human Services, Atlanta, GA.

16. Centers for Disease Control and Prevention. 2010. *Reported Tuberculosis in the United States, 2009.* Centers for Disease Control and Prevention, U.S. Department of Health and Human Services, Atlanta, GA.

17. Centers for Disease Control and Prevention. 1999. Framework for program evaluation in public health. *MMWR Recommend. Rep.* **48:**1–40.

18. Centers for Disease Control and Prevention. 2003. Update: adverse event data and revised American Thoracic Society/CDC recommendations against the use of rifampin and pyrazinamide for treatment of latent tuberculosis infection—United States, 2003. *MMWR Morb. Mortal. Wkly. Rep.* **52:**735–739.

19. Centers for Disease Control and Prevention. 2002. *CDC's Response to Ending Neglect: the Elimination of Tuberculosis in the United States.* Centers for Disease Control and Prevention, U.S. Department of Health and Human Services, Atlanta, GA.

20. Centers for Disease Control and Prevention. 2005. Controlling tuberculosis in the United States: recommendations from the American Thoracic Society, CDC, and the Infectious Diseases Society of America. *MMWR Morb. Mortal. Wkly. Rep.* **54:**1–81.

21. Centers for Disease Control and Prevention. 2006. Emergence of *Mycobacterium tuberculosis* with extensive resistance to second-line drugs—worldwide, 2000–2004. *MMWR Morb. Mortal. Wkly. Rep.* **55:**301–305.

22. Centers for Disease Control and Prevention. 2009. *CDC Immigration Requirements: Technical Instructions for Tuberculosis Screening and Treatment Using Cultures and Directly Observed Therapy.* Centers for Disease Control and Prevention, Atlanta, GA.

23. Centers for Disease Control and Prevention. 2009. Updated guidelines for the use of nucleic acid amplification tests in the diagnosis of tuberculosis. *MMWR Morb. Mortal. Wkly. Rep.* **58:**7–10.

24. Chaulk, C. P., and V. A. Kazandjian. 1998. Directly observed therapy for treatment completion of pulmonary tuberculosis: Consensus Statement of the Public Health Tuberculosis Guidelines Panel. *JAMA* **279:**943–948.

25. Cummings, K. C., J. Mohle-Boetani, S. E. Royce, and D. P. Chin. 1998. Movement of tuberculosis patients and the failure to complete antituberculosis treatment. *Am. J. Respir. Crit. Care Med.* **157:**1249–1252.

26. Federal Register. 2003. Control of communicable diseases, interim final rule. *Fed. Regist.* **68:**17558–17560.

27. Federal Register. 2008. Medical examination of aliens—revisions to medical screening process, interim final rule with comment period. *Fed. Regist.* **73:**58047–58056.

28. The Federal Tuberculosis Task Force. 2003. *Federal Tuberculosis Task Force Plan in Response to the Institute of Medicine Report, Ending Neglect: the Elimination of Tuberculosis in the United States.* Centers for Disease Control and Prevention, U.S. Department of Health and Human Services, Atlanta, GA.

29. Feldman, G., P. Srivastava, E. Eden, and T. R. Frieden. 1997. Detention until cure as a last resort: New York City's experience with involuntary in-hospital civil detention of persistently nonadherent tuberculosis patients. *Semin. Respir. Crit. Care Med.* **18:**493–501.

30. Ferebee, S. H. 1970. Controlled chemoprophylaxis trials in tuberculosis. A general review. *Bibl. Tuberc.* **26:**28–106.

31. Horsburgh, C. R., M. Moore, and K. G. Castro. 2004. Epidemiology of tuberculosis in the United States, p. 31–45. *In* W. N. Rom and S. M. Garay (ed.), *Tuberculosis.* Williams and Wilkins, Philadelphia, PA.

32. Hughes, S., D. Sodt, K. Young, J. Jereb, B. Pratt, T. Navin, K. Ijaz, and A. Khan. 2010. Monitoring tuberculosis control programmatic activities in the United States—the National Tuberculosis Indicator Project (NTIP). *MMWR Morb. Mortal. Wkly. Rep.* **59:**295–298.

33. Institute of Medicine. 2000. *Ending Neglect: the Elimination of Tuberculosis in the United States.* National Academy Press, Washington, DC.

34. Iowa Code sec. 139A.25, 2008.

35. Jereb, J., S. C. Etkind, O. T. Joglar, M. Moore, and Z. Taylor. 2003. Tuberculosis contact investigations: outcomes in selected areas of the United States, 1999. *Int. J. Tuberc. Lung Dis.* **7:**S384–S390.

36. Kaplan, J. E., C. Benson, K. H. Holmes, J. T. Brooks, A. Pau, and H. Masur. 2009. Guidelines for prevention and treatment of opportunistic infections in HIV-infected adults and adolescents: recommendations from CDC, the National Institutes of Health, and the HIV Medicine Association of the Infectious Diseases Society of America. *MMWR Recommend. Rep.* **58:**1–207.

37. Lerner, B. H. 1999. Catching patients: tuberculosis and detention in the 1990s. *Chest* **115:**236–241.

38. LoBue, P. A., R. Cass, D. Lobo, K. Moser, and A. Catanzaro. 1999. Development of housing programs to aid in the treatment of tuberculosis in homeless individuals: a pilot study. *Chest* **115:**218–223.

39. LoBue, P. A., and K. S. Moser. 2003. Use of isoniazid for latent tuberculosis infection in a public health clinic. *Am. J. Respir. Crit. Care Med.* **168:**443–447.

40. Lofy, K. H., P. D. McElroy, L. Lake, L. S. Cowan, L. A. Diem, S. V. Goldberg, G. A. Cangelosi, S. P. Tribble, M. D. Cave, and M. Narita. 2006. Outbreak of tuberculosis in a homeless population involving multiple sites of transmission. *Int. J. Tuberc. Lung Dis.* **10:**683–689.

41. Logan, S., J. Boutotte, M. Wilce, and S. Etkind. 2003. Using the CDC framework for program evaluation in public health to assess tuberculosis contact investigation programs. *Int. J. Tuberc. Lung Dis.* **7:**S375–S383.

42. Maloney, S. A., K. L. Fielding, K. F. Laserson, W. Jones, T. N. Nguyen, Q. A. Dang, H. P. Nguyen, A. T. Nguyen, T. C. Duong, T. C. Vo, M. F. Seawright, T. O'Rourke, X. L. Truong, T. N. Nguyen, N. Binkin, and M. S. Cetron. 2006. Assessing the performance of overseas tuberculosis screening programs: a study among U.S.-bound immigrants in Vietnam. *Arch. Intern. Med.* **166:**234–240.

43. Marks, S. M., Z. Taylor, N. L. Qualls, R. J. Shrestha-Kuwahara, M. A. Wilce, and C. H. Nguyen. 2000. Outcomes of contact investigations of infectious tuberculosis patients. *Am. J. Respir. Crit. Care Med.* **162:**2033–2038.

44. Mazurek, G. H., J. Jereb, A. Vernon, P. LoBue, S. Goldberg, and K. G. Castro. 2010. Updated guidelines for using interferon gamma release assays to detect *Mycobacterium tuberculosis* infection, United States. *MMWR Recommend. Rep.* **59:**1–25.

45. Mazurek, G. H., and M. E. Villarino. 2003. Guidelines for using the QuantiFERON-TB test for diagnosing latent *Mycobacterium tuberculosis* infection. *MMWR Recommend. Rep.* **52:**15–18.

46. Menzies, D., M. J. Dion, B. Rabinovitch, S. Mannix, P. Brassard, and K. Schwartzman. 2004. Treatment completion and costs of a randomized trial of rifampin for 4 months versus isoniazid for 9 months. *Am. J. Respir. Crit Care Med.* **170:**445–449.

47. Menzies, D., R. Long, A. Trajman, M. J. Dion, J. Yang, J. H. Al, Z. Memish, K. Khan, M. Gardam, V. Hoeppner, A. Benedetti, and K. Schwartzman. 2008. Adverse events with 4 months of rifampin therapy or 9 months of isoniazid therapy for latent tuberculosis infection: a randomized trial. *Ann. Intern. Med.* **149:**689–697.

48. Nebraska Revised Statutes Annotated, sec. 71-503, 2009.

49. New Mexico Department of Heath and Texas Department of State Health Services. 2007. *Memorandum of Agreement between New Mexico Department of Health and Texas Department of State Health Services.* Centers for Disease Control and Prevention, Atlanta, GA. http://www2a.cdc.gov/phlp/docs/NM_TX_TB.pdf.

50. Oscherwitz, T., J. P. Tulsky, S. Roger, S. Sciortino, A. Alpers, S. Royce, and B. Lo. 1997. Detention of persistently nonadherent patients with tuberculosis. *JAMA* **278:**843–846.

51. Pai, M., A. Zwerling, and D. Menzies. 2008. Systematic review: T-cell-based assays for the diagnosis of latent tuberculosis infection: an update. *Ann. Intern. Med.* **149:**177–184.

52. Puisis, M., J. Feinglass, E. Lidow, and M. Mansour. 1996. Radiographic screening for tuberculosis in a large urban county jail. *Public Health Rep.* **111:**330–334.

53. Reichler, M. R., R. Reves, S. Bur, V. Thompson, B. T. Mangura, J. Ford, S. E. Valway, and I. M. Onorato. 2002. Evaluation of investigations conducted to detect and prevent transmission of tuberculosis. *JAMA* **287:**991–995.

54. Rodrigo, T., J. A. Cayla, H. Galdos-Tanguis, P. García de Olalla, M. T. Brugal, and J. M. Jansa. 2001. Proposing indicators for evaluation of tuberculosis control programmes in large cities based on the experience of Barcelona. *Int. J. Tuberc. Lung Dis.* **5:**432–440.

55. Saunders, D. L., D. M. Olive, S. B. Wallace, D. Lacy, R. Leyba, and N. E. Kendig. 2001. Tuberculosis screening in the federal prison system: an opportunity to treat and prevent tuberculosis in foreign-born populations. *Public Health Rep.* **116:**210–218.

56. Shinnick, T. M., M. F. Iademarco, and J. C. Ridderhof. 2005. National plan for reliable tuberculosis laboratory services using a systems approach. Recommendations from CDC and the Association of Public Health Laboratories Task Force on Tuberculosis Laboratory Services. *MMWR Recommend. Rep.* **54:**1–12.

57. Singleton, L., M. Turner, R. Haskal, S. Etkind, M. Tricarico, and E. Nardell. 1997. Long-term hospitalization for tuberculosis control. Experience with a medical-psychosocial inpatient unit. *JAMA* **278:**838–842.

58. Sterling, T. R. 2008. New approaches to the treatment of latent tuberculosis. *Semin. Respir. Crit. Care Med.* **29:**532–541.

59. Tuberculosis Along the U.S.-Mexico Border Work Group and Centers for Disease Control and Prevention. 2001. Preventing and controlling tuberculosis along the U.S.-Mexico border. *MMWR Recommend. Rep.* **50:**1–27.

60. 42 U.S. Code section 264.

61. U.S. Constitution, art. I, sec. 8.

62. U.S. Constitution, First Amendment.

63. U.S. Department of Homeland Security. 2005. *Yearbook of Immigration Statistics, 2005.* U.S. Government Printing Office, Washington, DC.

64. Weis, S. E., P. K. Moonan, J. M. Pogoda, L. Turk, B. King, S. Freeman-Thompson, and G. Burgess. 2001. Tuberculosis in the foreign-born population of Tarrant County, Texas by immigration status. *Am. J. Respir. Crit. Care Med.* **164:**953–957.

65. Wells, C. D., P. L. Zuber, C. M. Nolan, N. J. Binkin, and S. V. Goldberg. 1997. Tuberculosis prevention among foreign-born persons in Seattle-King County, Washington. *Am. J. Respir. Crit. Care Med.* **156**(2 Pt. 1):573–577.

66. World Health Organization. 2005. *International Health Regulations (2005)*, 2nd ed. World Health Organization, Geneva, Switzerland. http://www.who.int/ihr/9789241596664/en/index.html.

II. CLINICAL SYNDROMES

Tuberculosis and Nontuberculous Mycobacterial Infections, 6th ed.
Edited by David Schlossberg
© 2011 ASM Press, Washington, DC

Chapter 14

Pulmonary Tuberculosis

MARY ELIZABETH KREIDER AND MILTON D. ROSSMAN

INTRODUCTION

The lung is the most commonly affected organ in tuberculosis (TB) infection in the immunocompetent host, with estimates of lung involvement in subjects with active tuberculosis of 80 to 87% (3, 15). Estimates of lung involvement are similar in immunocompromised hosts, such as those with human immunodeficiency virus (HIV) infection, with studies from the 1980s to 1990s suggesting that the rates of pulmonary involvement were on the order of 70 to 92% (40, 48, 49). However, these individuals are also more likely to have extrapulmonary disease as well (47).

The lung is the portal of entry in the majority of cases of TB (18, 37). The first contact with the organism results in few or no clinical symptoms or signs. Ordinarily, the tubercle bacillus sets up a localized infection in the periphery of the lung, where it has been deposited by inhalation. Body defenses appear to have little effect on the organism until the time of development of tuberculin hypersensitivity (4 to 6 weeks). At this time, mild fever and malaise develop, and occasionally other hypersensitivity manifestations are noted.

In the majority of patients, no additional evidence of TB develops, and the process is contained by local and systemic defenses. Since the primary pulmonary focus is usually subpleural, rupture into the pleural space may result, with the development of a tuberculous pleurisy with effusion. This is usually accompanied by the classic but nonspecific symptoms of pleurisy. Local spread to the hilar lymph nodes is a common occurrence, and from there the disease spreads to other areas of the body. It is this hematogenous dissemination of the organism that results in the pulmonary and extrapulmonary foci that are responsible for the major clinical manifestations of TB. Radiographically, spread is manifested by enlargement of the lymph nodes, with later calcification of both the lymph nodes and the parenchymal lesion. This is the classic Ghon's complex and is suggestive not only of an old tuberculous infection but also of diseases such as histoplasmosis. Progressive (reactivation) tuberculosis usually develops after a period of dormancy and arises from the sites of hematogenous dissemination (10).

Thus, the first infection with TB frequently is clinically insignificant and unrecognized. In the majority of patients, the disease stays dormant either indefinitely or for many years, and when a breakdown occurs, it may be secondary to a decrease in body immunity (Table 1).

CLINICAL PRESENTATION

Symptoms and Signs

Pulmonary TB frequently develops without any striking clinical evidence of disease. However, since the disease has a wide spectrum of manifestations ranging from skin positivity with negative X rays to far-advanced tuberculosis, a variety of clinical presentations may also occur. Ordinarily, until the disease is moderately or far advanced, as shown by changes on the roentgenogram, symptoms are minimal and often attributable to other causes, such as excessive smoking, hard work, pregnancy, or other conditions.

Symptoms may be divided into two categories: constitutional and pulmonary. The frequency of these symptoms differs according to whether the patient has primary tuberculosis or reactivation TB. Subjects with primary TB are much more likely to be asymptomatic or minimally symptomatic. See Table 2 for a list of the most common symptoms and their relative frequencies in representative case series of both primary and reactivation TB. The constitutional symptom most frequently seen is fever, low grade at the onset but becoming quite marked if the disease progresses. Characteristically, the fever develops

Mary Elizabeth Kreider and Milton D. Rossman • Pulmonary and Critical Care Section, Hospital of the University of Pennsylvania, Philadelphia, PA 19104-4283.

Table 1. Increased susceptibility to TB

Nonspecific decrease in resistance
  Adolescence
  Senescence
  Malnutrition
  Postgastrectomy state
  Diabetes mellitus

Decrease in resistance due to hormonal effects
  Pregnancy
  Therapy with adrenocortical steroids

Decrease in local resistance
  Silicosis

Decrease in specific immunity
  Lymphomas
  Uremia
  Immunosuppressive therapy
  Sarcoidosis
  Live virus vaccination
  HIV infection

in the late afternoon and may not be accompanied by pronounced symptoms. With defervescence, usually during sleep, sweating occurs—the classic "night sweats." Other signs of toxemia, such as malaise, irritability, weakness, unusual fatigue, headache, and weight loss, may be present. With the development of caseation necrosis and concomitant liquefaction of the caseation, the patient will usually notice cough and sputum, often associated with mild hemoptysis. Chest pain may be localized and pleuritic. Shortness of breath usually indicates extensive disease with widespread involvement of the lung and parenchyma or some form of tracheobronchial obstruction and therefore usually occurs late in the course of the disease.

Physical examination of the chest is ordinarily of minimal help early in the disease. At this stage, the principal finding over areas of infiltration is one of fine rales detected on deep inspiration followed by full expiration and a hard, terminal cough—the so-called posttussive rales. This sign is found particularly in the apexes of the lungs, where reactivation disease has its onset in a large majority of patients. As the disease progresses, more extensive findings are present, corresponding to the areas of involvement

Table 2. Clinical symptoms of patients presenting with active TB[a]

| Symptom | % of patients affected | |
	Primary	Reactivation
Cough	23–37	42
Fever	18–42	37–79
Weight loss	NR	7–24
Hemoptysis	8	9

[a]Estimates based on several studies (3, 8, 9, 28, 32). NR, not reported.

and type of pathology. Allergic manifestations may occur, usually developing at the time of onset of infection. These include erythema nodosum and phlyctenular conjunctivitis. Erythema induratum (22), involvement of the lower leg and foot with redness, swelling, and necrosis, probably represents a combination of local subcutaneous bacterial infection with an allergic response and should not be confused with erythema nodosum, the latter considered to be due to circulating immune complexes with resultant localized vascular damage. Initially, erythema nodosum occurs in the dependent portion of the body and, if the reaction is severe, may be followed by a more disseminated process.

Laboratory Examination

Routine laboratory examinations are rarely helpful in establishing or suggesting the diagnosis (34). A mild normochromic normocytic anemia may be present in chronic tuberculosis. The white blood cell count is often normal, and counts over $20,000/\mu l$ would suggest another infectious process; however, a leukemoid reaction may occasionally occur in miliary TB, but not in TB confined to the chest. Although a "left shift" in the differential white blood cell count can occur in advanced disease, these changes are neither specific nor useful. Other nonspecific tests that may be elevated in active TB include the sedimentation rate, α_2-globulins, and gamma globulin. The finding of pyuria without bacteria by Gram's stain is suggestive of renal involvement. Liver enzymes (transaminases and alkaline phosphatase) may occasionally be elevated prior to treatment. However, this finding is usually due to concomitant liver disease secondary to other problems such as alcoholism rather than to tuberculous involvement. Since the drugs used in the treatment of TB are often associated with hepatotoxicity, it is important to quantitate any hepatic abnormalities prior to treatment (17). On rare occasions, the serum sodium may be depressed owing to inappropriate secretion of antidiuretic hormone. This occurs only in advanced pulmonary TB.

A positive delayed hypersensitivity reaction to tuberculin (as discussed in chapter 5) indicates only the occurrence of a prior primary infection (24).

CHEST RADIOGRAPHY

The chest radiograph is the single most useful study for suggesting the diagnosis of TB. The appearance of the radiograph differs in primary (Fig. 1 to 3) and reactivation TB (16). In the past primary TB was seen mostly in children and reactivation TB in adults.

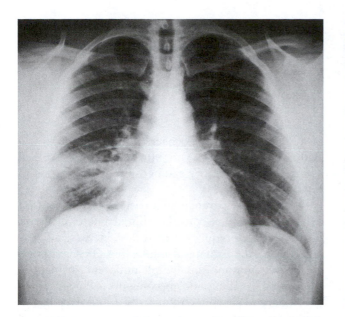

Figure 1. Primary TB in an adult. Shown is a right lower-lobe infiltrate with bilateral hilar adenopathy.

However, primary TB can occur at any age (especially in low-incidence countries), and HIV-infected persons may present with atypical patterns; consequently, some radiologists prefer a radiologic classification (1) that is descriptive (i.e., lymph node, air space parenchymal, tuberculoma, miliary, cavitary, pleural, and fibrosis and destruction).

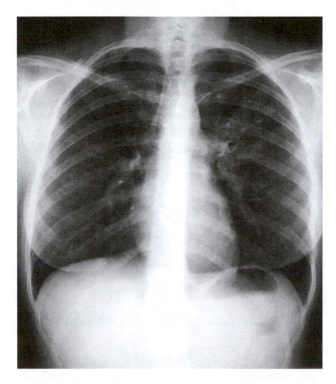

Figure 2. Left upper-lobe TB. Shown is a typical fibronodular pattern of reactivation TB with linear densities extending to the left hilum.

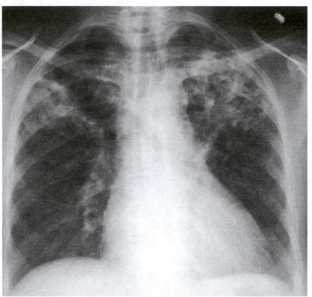

A

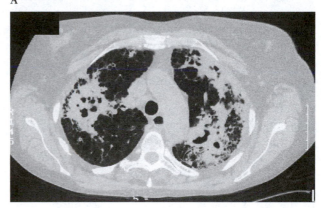

B

Figure 3. Late changes of upper-lobe TB. (A) Posterior-anterior chest radiograph with volume loss of the right upper lobe is indicated by the elevated minor fissure. Small cavities are not clearly seen, but there is endobronchial spread to the superior segment of the right lower lobe, suggesting cavitary formation. (B) A computerized axial tomography scan of the same patient that clearly demonstrates extensive bilateral cavitary disease.

Primary TB

As opposed to reactivation TB, which usually involves the superior and dorsal segments, in primary TB parenchymal involvement can happen in any segment of the lung (53). In the primary infection there is only a slight predilection for the upper lobes; also, anterior as well as posterior segments can be involved. The air space consolidation appears as a homogeneous density with ill-defined borders (Fig. 1), and cavitation is rare except in malnourished or other immunocompromised patients. Miliary involvement at the onset is seen in less than 3% of cases; these are most commonly in children under 2 to 3 years of age, but it can also be seen in adults (Fig. 4).

Hilar or paratracheal lymph node enlargement is a characteristic finding in primary TB. In 15% of the cases, bilateral hilar adenopathy may be present. More commonly, the adenopathy is unilateral. Unilateral hilar adenopathy and unilateral hilar and paratracheal adenopathy are equally common. Massive hilar adenopathy may herald a complicated course.

Atelectasis with an obstructive pneumonia may result from bronchial compression by inflamed lymph nodes or from a caseous lymph node that ruptures into a bronchus. Obstructive "emphysema" or a localized hyperinflated segment at times precedes atelectasis. The most common segments involved are the anterior segment of the right upper lobe or the medial segment of the right middle lobe. Right-sided collapse is twice as common as left-sided collapse. Residual bronchiectatic changes may persist after the obstruction has cleared.

An isolated pleural effusion of mild to moderate degree may be the only manifestation of primary TB. However, the most common radiographic appearance of primary TB is a normal radiograph.

Reactivation TB

Although reactivation TB may involve any lung segment, the characteristic distribution usually suggests the disease. In 95% of localized pulmonary TB, the lesions are present in the apical or posterior segment of the upper lobes or the superior segment of the lower lobes (Fig. 3 and 4). The anterior segment of the upper lobe is almost never the only manifest area of involvement (41). Although some radiologists attempt to describe the activity of a lesion on the basis of its radiographic appearance, the documentation

Table 3. Criteria for activity in pulmonary TB

Symptoms
Change in roentgenogram
Evidence of cavitation
Positive sputum by smear or culture
Response to therapeutic trial

of activity is best left to bacteriological and clinical evaluation (Table 3). Too often a lesion described as inactive or stable by radiography will progress to symptomatic TB.

The typical parenchymal pattern of reactivation TB is of an air space consolidation in a patchy or confluent nature. Frequently there are increased linear densities to the ipsilateral hilum (Fig. 3). Cavitation is not uncommon, and lymph node enlargement is rarely seen. As the lesions become more chronic, they become more sharply circumscribed and irregular in contour. Fibrosis leads to volume loss in the involved lung. The combination of patchy pneumonitis, fibrosis, and calcification is always suggestive of chronic granulomatous disease, usually TB.

The cavities that develop in TB are characterized by a moderately thick wall, a smooth inner surface, and the lack of an air-fluid level (Fig. 3). Cavitation is frequently associated with endobronchial spread of disease. Radiographically, it appears as multiple small acinar shadows.

Chest CT Findings in Pulmonary TB

Computed tomography (CT) scans allow practitioners to examine both the pulmonary parenchyma and the lymph nodes in greater detail than can be done with plain chest X ray alone. The chest CT for

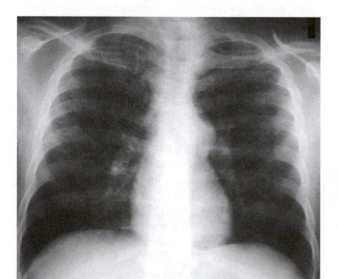

A

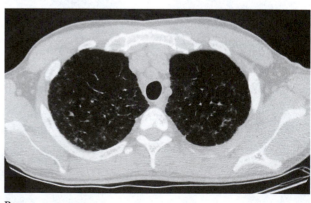

B

Figure 4. Miliary TB. (A) Characteristic diffuse small nodules are seen in the posterior-anterior radiograph. (B) A computerized axial tomography scan of the lung in the same subject demonstrates the diffuse small nodular disease.

patients with primary TB typically demonstrates lobar consolidation in association with mediastinal or hilar adenopathy. The consolidation is usually well defined, dense, homogenous, and confined to a segment or lobe. Small cavities may be appreciated on the CT that were not seen on plain chest X ray (Fig. 3). In reactivation TB one can see centrilobular nodules or branching linear structures ("tree in bud") with or without bronchial wall thickening, lobular consolidation, cavity formation, bronchiectasis, and/or fibrotic changes (23, 31). Controversy exists over whether CT scans can reliably distinguish active TB from latent infection, with several authors arguing that findings such as the tree in bud and/or areas of centrilobular nodules predict active disease (23, 31).

DIAGNOSIS

The diagnosis of TB often can be very difficult. Some of the problems that occur are listed in Table 4. A firm diagnosis of TB requires bacteriological confirmation. It is important to remember that a positive acid-fast smear is not specific for *Mycobacterium tuberculosis*. Other mycobacteria, both saprophytes and potential pathogens, can be acid fast. Thus, culture of *M. tuberculosis* is the only absolute way of confirming the diagnosis.

Freshly expectorated sputum is the best sample to stain and culture for *M. tuberculosis*. Sputum samples 24 h old are frequently overgrown with members of the mouth microbiota and are much less useful. If the patient is not spontaneously producing sputum, induced sputum is the next best specimen for study. It can be obtained by having the patient breathe an aerosol of isotonic or hypertonic saline for 5 to 15 min. If the patient cannot cooperate to give a spontaneous sputum sample, a gastric aspirate to obtain swallowed sputum may be useful. This sample must be obtained in the morning before the patient arises or eats.

For the majority of patients, the above procedures will be successful in obtaining positive material for culture. Smears of gastric contents for acid-fast bacilli (AFB) are of limited value because of the presence of nontuberculous ingested AFB. In a few

Table 4. Diagnostic difficulties

Lack of organisms for culture
Slow growth of TB culture
Chest X-ray findings absent or misinterpreted
Biopsy material may not be specific
Decreased tuberculin sensitivity
Symptoms and signs of TB easily attributed to a preexisting disease

cases, one may have to resort to bronchoscopy. For 41 patients proven to have TB, cultures of specimens, taken during fiber-optic bronchoscopy, were positive in 39 cases (52). Stainable mycobacteria were seen in 14 of the cases, and in 8 cases granulomas were seen on biopsy. Similar results have been obtained in another study of 22 patients with proven mycobacterial disease and negative smears prior to bronchoscopy (12). The local anesthetics used during fiber-optic bronchoscopy may be lethal to *M. tuberculosis*, so specimens for culture should be obtained using a minimal amount of anesthesia. However, irritation of the bronchial tree during the fiber-optic bronchoscopy procedure will frequently leave the patient with a productive cough. Thus, collection of the postbronchoscopy sputum can provide another valuable source of diagnostic material. In nine (13%) of the above cases, the postbronchoscopy sputum was the only source of positive material.

In 2008, as reported to the Centers for Disease Control and Prevention (7), 46% of pulmonary cases of TB were smear positive, 43% were negative, and 11% were not done or unknown. Sputum culture was positive in 69%, negative in 19%, and unknown in 12% of cases. Thus, in a significant number of cases, the diagnosis of TB had been made in the absence of bacteriological confirmation. In these cases, the diagnosis was made by a combination of a positive skin test, a compatible chest radiograph, and a therapeutic trial.

Differential Diagnosis

Since TB today is a disease frequently present in older individuals, one major differential diagnosis is usually between TB and carcinoma of the lung. An important concept to remember is that carcinoma may cause a focus of TB to spread; thus, carcinoma of the lung and TB may be present simultaneously. In cases with the simultaneous presentation of carcinoma and TB, the diagnosis of TB frequently is made first, and the diagnosis of carcinoma is delayed for several months. Thus, if radiograph and clinical findings suggest carcinoma but the sputum has AFB, further procedures to diagnose carcinoma may still be indicated. Isolated involvement of the anterior segment of the upper lobe, isolated lower-lobe involvement, or the presence of irregular cavities would suggest carcinoma, and further diagnostic workup may be indicated despite AFB in the sputum smear.

Any type of infectious or granulomatous disease may be radiologically identical to TB. Three broad categories must be distinguished: fungi (histoplasmosis, coccidioidomycosis, and blastomycosis), bacteria (*Pseudomonas pseudomallei*), and atypical mycobacteria (mainly *Mycobacterium kansasii* and *Mycobacterium intracellulare*). Culture of the organism from the patient's sputum is the best way to differentiate these diseases, although serum titers of antibody to fungi are also valuable.

Common bacterial pneumonias are usually easily differentiated from TB. The localized alveolar infiltrate on the chest radiograph and the prompt response to antibiotic therapy usually differentiate bacterial pneumonia from TB. When in doubt, treatment for bacterial pneumonia should be given first and TB therapy withheld until adequate sputum samples have been obtained and the response to antibiotics has been determined. Lung abscesses can usually be differentiated from tuberculous cavities by (i) prominent air-fluid level, (ii) more common lower-lobe distribution, and (iii) clinical findings (associated with seizures, alcoholism, dental caries, etc.).

TB AND AIDS

HIV infection increases the risks of reactivation of latent TB and progression of active disease and predisposes to atypical presentations of TB in patients with more advanced immunosuppression (2, 11, 46). The global burden of HIV-associated TB is astounding. The World Health Organization estimates that of the 9.4 million new cases of TB worldwide in 2008, 13 to 16% were HIV associated and that there were approximately 0.5 million HIV-TB deaths (54). These deaths represent 23% of the estimated 2 million deaths from HIV/AIDS in 2007 (30). Sub-Saharan Africa accounts for a disproportionate percentage of these HIV-TB cases, approximately 78% of them (54).

Several important differences have emerged about the clinical presentation of subjects with TB with and without HIV infection. Patients with HIV infection are more likely to present with disseminated disease. Additionally, they tend to have an increased number and severity of symptoms and have a more rapid progression to death unless treatment is begun (48).

Radiographic findings of TB in HIV-infected patients have been found to correlate with the degree of immunosuppression due to HIV itself (40). Lower CD4 counts (i.e., <200/mm^3) are associated more often with hilar and mediastinal lymphadenopathy, while higher CD4 counts are more frequently associated with cavitation. Additionally, some studies have suggested that HIV-infected subjects are more likely to have nonapical infiltrates, pleural effusions, and miliary infiltrates (47). In addition, patients with more advanced immunosuppression are more likely to have disseminated disease (14).

For patients with HIV infection but without the manifestations of AIDS, the tuberculin skin test is positive in 50 to 80% of patients with TB. Once an individual has developed AIDS, the tuberculin skin test is less likely to be positive, but reactivity may still be seen in as many as 30 to 50% of patients. Active TB should be considered for any HIV-infected patient with a tuberculin skin test greater than 5 mm of induration.

In addition, HIV infection can lead to a paucibacillary disease which can decrease the sensitivity of the acid-fast sputum smear test (14). This reduced yield of diagnostic testing can lead to a delay in diagnosis, which can further increase the mortality rate of the disease (21).

Treatment of the HIV disease with antiretroviral therapy (ART) may lead to a phenomenon of an almost hyperinflammatory state due to the reconstitution of a functional immune system (see chapter 34). This reconstitution can lead to unusual clinical presentations of infections due to an exuberant response to newly recognized antigens by the now functional immune system. This syndrome, named immune reconstitution inflammatory syndrome (IRIS), can occur in response to almost any coinfection but is most commonly seen with TB (30). With TB IRIS can be seen either as a paradoxical worsening of TB symptoms in an otherwise improving patient as ART is started or as an unmasking of previous subclinical TB infection. Symptoms typically include shortness of breath, cough, fever, and lymphadenopathy. Chest radiographs can also demonstrate worsening infiltrates, increasing lymphadenopathy, and/or effusions (25). The risk of IRIS is greatest within the first few weeks of ART and if the ART is started within the first 3 months of TB treatment (30). Fortunately, the rate of mortality from IRIS is low and typically symptomatic therapy is all that is required; both the ART and TB treatment are continued (25).

TB IN THE ELDERLY

As the population ages, increasing attention has been paid to how disease behaves differently in the elderly. Some studies now suggest not only that increasing age is a risk factor for the development of active TB (50) but also that the disease itself may present differently in the elderly, making it harder to recognize and therefore diagnose. A representative study examining the presentation differences in the elderly prospectively examined 93 consecutive patients over the age of 60 admitted with pulmonary TB to a hospital in South Africa (38). Among these patients "atypical" radiographic findings were the norm rather than the exception. For instance, only 7% had purely apical infiltrates, while 48% had middle and lower lung zones only, and 46% had mixed infiltrates between upper and lower lung fields. A pleural reaction was common (46%) and cavities were not (33%), with half of those seen in the lower and middle lung fields. In addition, the investigators found that systemic abnormalities of routine blood work were common, including anemia (66%), elevated erythrocyte sedimentation rates (90%), hyponatremia (60%), and hypoalbuminemia (83%). However, not all studies have confirmed these differences (29). One meta-analysis of 12 studies of TB found that the elderly were less likely to have symptoms such as fever, sweating, hemoptysis, and cavitary lung disease. They were more likely to have dyspnea and significant comorbidities (39). In this study, the only difference seen in radiographic patterns between young adults and the elderly was an increased incidence of miliary disease in the older population. This difficulty in making the correct diagnosis may lead to a delay in diagnosis and an increased attributable morbidity and mortality. In fact, one study found that increasing age was associated with an increasing risk of the TB not being diagnosed until autopsy (44). Another prospective cohort study of patients diagnosed with TB at a hospital in Spain from 1995 to 2004 found that 34% of the patients were aged 65 or greater (45). This older group was then compared to the younger patients and found to have a greater amount of extrapulmonary and disseminated TB (50% versus 26%). As noted in those prior studies, cavitation was less frequent and sputum smears were less frequently positive. Importantly, they also found that the older group had more toxicity from the TB therapy (22% versus 9%) and a greater 30-day mortality rate (18% versus 2%). They further analyzed a group older than 80 and found that their mortality rate was higher yet (30-day mortality rate for those >80 with TB, 42%, versus 11% for those >80 without TB). However, this mortality rate difference disappeared when patients who had TB diagnosed at autopsy or those who died within 72 h of admission were excluded, suggesting that the excessive mortality was largely due to late and/or missed diagnosis.

TB IN PATIENTS TAKING TNF INHIBITORS

Tumor necrosis factor alpha (TNF-α) is a cytokine which acts as a central mediator of inflammation and immune regulation. Inhibition of TNF-α is now used for the treatment of several diseases, including rheumatoid arthritis, Crohn's disease, juvenile rheumatoid arthritis, ankylosing spondylitis, and psoriatric arthritis. Three main anti-TNF agents are currently approved by the FDA: infliximab, a chimeric (human and murine) monoclonal antibody against TNF-α that is administered intravenously; etanercept, a TNF-α antagonist which acts by binding to the Fc region of human immunoglobulin G and is administered subcutaneously; and adalimumab, a human anti-TNF monoclonal antibody which is also administered subcutaneously (43).

All TNF-α antagonists have the potential to predispose patients to granulomatous infections (26). However, the monoclonal antibodies, infliximab and adalimumab, carry the greatest risk due to their induction of complement-mediated cell lysis. If, for example, lysis of a macrophage involved in the formation of a granuloma occurs, this could destabilize the granuloma, resulting in dissemination of the infection. Indeed, one case of TB was seen in preapproval clinical trials of infliximab (35). After FDA approval of infliximab in 1998, an increasing frequency of TB infections was noted in postmarketing surveillance. In one study, 70 reported cases of TB after the initiation of infliximab therapy were analyzed (27). Forty-eight of the patients developed TB after three or fewer infusions, with a median interval of 12 weeks. Forty had extrapulmonary disease, and 17 had disseminated TB. Of these 70 patients, 12 died, and at least four of these deaths were thought to be directly related to TB infection. During the same period, only nine cases of TB during the treatment with etanercept were reported to the FDA. However, by 2002, 25 cases of TB in patients receiving etanercept were described. A total of 52% of these, or 13, had extrapulmonary disease, and 1 patient died secondary to the infection. Several TB cases attributed to high-dose adalimumab therapy have now also been reported.

A Spanish study analyzed the annual incidence rate in 1,540 patients treated with infliximab or etanercept at multiple participating centers compared to the background rate as well as to the rate in a cohort of patients with rheumatoid arthritis not treated with such agents (19). Seventeen cases of TB were identified in patients treated with infliximab. A significantly increased risk of TB was seen, with a relative risk of 90.1 (95% confidence interval, 58.8 to 146.0) compared to the background rate in the Spanish population in 2000. The relative risk of TB in patients with rheumatoid arthritis treated with infliximab compared to patients not treated with infliximab was 10.9 (95% confidence interval, 16.2 to 24.8) in the same year.

Several important points have been learned from these reports. TNF-α antagonists do increase the incidence of active TB. Patients who develop TB on TNF-α antagonist therapy usually do so after only

2 to 3 months of therapy and have more extrapulmonary and disseminated disease than do immunocompetent, HIV-negative patients. This may reflect
either a delay in the diagnosis of TB or atypical presentations of TB in this subgroup of patients. Current
recommendations include screening all patients with
skin testing for TB and treatment of any latent TB
(more than 5 mm of induration on purified protein
derivative) prior to initiation of TNF-α antagonist
therapy (19, 26).

PLEURAL EFFUSIONS DUE TO TB

Pleural effusion is a relatively uncommon manifestation, particularly of primary TB, occurring in
only 4% of clinical cases in the United States (4),
though it may be more common in other parts of the
world. Tuberculous pleural effusions are usually due
to rupture of a subpleural focus of TB. This release
is then followed by a T-cell-mediated hypersensitivity
response with marked inflammation (42). The effusions in TB are typically unilateral and mild to moderate in extent. Accompanying parenchymal changes
on chest X ray are uncommon, but CT scans demonstrate these changes more frequently (40 to 85%)
(42). The natural course of a tuberculous pleural effusion is to gradually resorb and frequently disappear
completely or with minimal changes on the chest radiograph, even without anti-TB therapy. However,
since approximately half of untreated patients will go
on to develop more overt disease in the future, it is
necessary to correctly diagnose and treat individuals
with TB pleural effusions (42).

There are several studies that can be performed
on pleural fluid to help make the diagnosis of pleural
TB. Chemistries including pleural fluid protein may
be most useful for differentiating tuberculous effusions from transudates (33). Almost without fail, the
pleural fluid protein in TB will be greater than 4 g/
dl (exudate), whereas it is most unusual for congestive heart failure fluid to have protein levels this high
(transudate). The differentiation of carcinomatous
from tuberculous effusions is more difficult. Both
may appear exudative with high levels of lactic dehydrogenase and protein in the pleural fluid. A low
pleural fluid glucose (less than 30 mg/dl) is common
in TB and rare in carcinoma. In addition, the profile
of cells within the fluid may be helpful. In tuberculous effusions, the differential count of the cells in
the pleural fluid usually contains few mesothelial cells
(5%). Tuberculous effusions can be differentiated
from bacterial effusions, since bacterial effusions usually contain a predominance of neutrophils, whereas
tuberculous effusions are predominantly lymphocytic

(55). However, early in the course of tuberculous effusions, neutrophils may be seen.

A Gram stain of the pleural fluid and a culture of
the fluid, sputum, and blood will usually establish the
etiologic agent of bacterial effusions. However, AFB
stains of pleural fluid are positive in less than 5% of
cases of tuberculous pleuritis (51). AFB culture also
has a low sensitivity (positive 24 to 58% of the time)
(51). While the newer gamma interferon-based assays
of tuberculin sensitivity can be applied to pleural fluid
cells, their use has not proven helpful (51). When patients have a positive 5-tuberculin unit tuberculin test
(greater than 10 mm of induration), their effusions
should be presumed to be tuberculous until proven
otherwise. If a patient has an undiagnosed exudative
effusion and a negative tuberculin test, the tuberculin test should be repeated within 2 weeks, since it
is not uncommon for patients with tuberculous effusions to have an initially negative tuberculin test (5,
24). Closed pleural biopsies have increased sensitivity
in the diagnosis of pleural TB compared to culture,
approximately 80% with histologic examination and
up to 90% when the tissue is also sent for culture
(42). Obtaining biopsy samples under direct visualization improves the accuracy to virtually 100% (13).

A multitude of newer tests are being developed
to try to improve the diagnosis of tuberculous pleural
effusions. In general these tests may be nonspecific
markers of increased immune response (adenosine
deaminase [ADA], gamma interferon, neopterin, etc.)
or may try to assess a more specific marker of response (T-cell-based gamma interferon release assays,
antibody detection, etc.) or direct detection of the
mycobacterial presence (DNA amplification testing).
To date, the best data for any of these tests exist for
ADA.

ADA testing is relatively inexpensive and easy to
perform on pleural effusions. ADA is an enzyme that
is predominantly produced by T cells, macrophages,
and neutrophils. The most widely accepted cutoff
value for this test is 40 U/liter. Higher levels are associated with a greater chance that the patient has
tuberculous pleuritis. Empyema can lead to similarly
high ADA levels and thus must be clinically distinguished. Parapneumonic effusions can also have elevated ADA levels, though only about 30% of the time
will they be greater than the cutoff value of 40 (42).
The performance characteristics of the ADA test have
been studied in many populations. One meta-analysis
of 31 studies found a pooled sensitivity of 92% and
a pooled specificity of 89% (20). Based on this, the
authors concluded that in low- and intermediate-TB-
incidence settings, the negative predictive value was
such that a negative ADA test was sufficient to exclude the diagnosis without further evaluation, while

a positive test in that setting would still require additional investigation (i.e., biopsy). In a high-prevalence area a positive test would be sufficient to make the diagnosis.

Due to the limitations of individual tests for accurately diagnosing TB pleurisy, many authors have suggested that scoring systems that combine numerous clinical and laboratory values may be more effective than any single test. One representative model used four variables to predict tuberculous effusion, including an ADA greater than 40 U/liter, age less than 35, fever, and a pleural fluid red blood cell count less than 5×10^9/liter (42). A high score derived from this model had a sensitivity of 95% and a specificity of 94% for differentiating TB from malignant effusions. While few of these models have been validated in other populations, it seems likely that a combination of testing will perform better than considering any one fluid characteristic in isolation.

ACTIVITY

Table 3 lists criteria for activity in TB. Since TB is a chronic disease with multiple exacerbations and remissions, it is important to determine if the disease is "healed," quiescent, or progressive. Decisions concerning infectiousness and the need for chemotherapy depend on this evaluation. The bases for these decisions are (i) clinical signs of infection (fever, weight loss, cough, sputum, etc.), (ii) progressive X-ray changes, and (iii) a positive sputum smear or culture. An improving X-ray study is also presumed to represent prior active TB. In the appropriate setting, the presence of any one of these findings is an indication for full therapy.

Therapy for pulmonary or pleural TB is discussed in chapter 7. Corticosteroids are used as an adjunct to specific chemotherapy only in the most severe cases of active pulmonary TB. In the patient who is in danger of dying from TB, corticosteroids can be lifesaving by causing a rapid defervescence, symptomatic improvement, and weight gain. However, the routine use of corticosteroids has been shown to have no effect on the late effects of pulmonary or pleural TB.

COMPLICATIONS

Although a relatively uncommon complication of tuberculous infection, the development of a pneumothorax requires rapid attention. One of the postulated theories of etiology is the rupture of a cavity that then connects the tracheobronchial tree with the pleural space, creating a bronchopleural fistula. In this occurrence, contamination of the pleural space with caseous material results in spread of the infection to the pleura and should be corrected immediately because of the tendency to produce pleural fibrosis with expansion failure.

A second possible mechanism is the development of a submucosal bronchiolar lesion with air trapping in an acinus or subsegment that causes the development of a bleb. Rupture of this bleb allows air to enter the pleural space, but often without tuberculous infection of the pleura. However, both occurrences should be treated with rapid expansion of the lungs by tube suction to avoid the possibility of further infection and fibrosis of the pleura with trapping of the lung. A bronchopleural fistula may persist after these episodes of pneumothorax and, especially if untreated, often results in major problems owing to the tuberculous infection complicated by secondary invaders ("mixed" empyema).

Minor endobronchial disease is a common occurrence in TB but usually involves the distal bronchi. Resected lung specimens frequently show either ulceration or stenosis of the draining bronchioles or bronchi. Bronchial stenosis of significance may occur in the major bronchi but is rare. At times, it results from involvement of the central lymph nodes draining into the lobar bronchi with caseation, ulceration, and fibrosis. Since fibrosis due to TB tends to contract and aggravate the stenosis, resection of the involved lung segment may be required after chemotherapy has produced inactivity of the acute inflammatory reaction.

The same endobronchial processes may result in bronchiectasis due to destruction of the bronchial wall. This usually is distal and frequently is in the upper lobes. So-called "dry" bronchiectasis (without sputum) often is the result of prior pulmonary TB and may manifest chiefly as low-grade hemoptysis.

Empyema due to TB may result uncommonly from a primary infection with an associated tuberculous pleural effusion. However, the latter usually clears; empyema is more common later in the disease and is associated with debility and loss of resistance to infection (Fig. 5). It is usually a part of a progressive, extensive parenchymal infection with caseation and cavitation, the presumed sources for pleural contamination. In contrast to tuberculous pleurisy, which does not require surgery, tuberculous empyema is usually accompanied by a thick pleural peal and requires surgical drainage or decortication (Fig. 5) in addition to anti-TB therapy.

After treatment of extensive TB, the patient is often left with open, healed cavities as well as with areas of bronchiectasis. Colonization of these areas

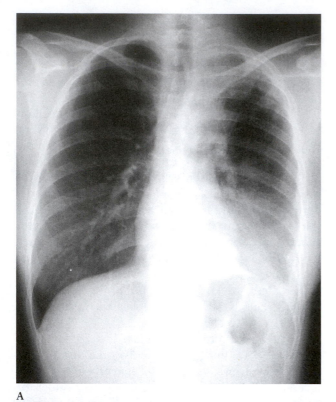

A

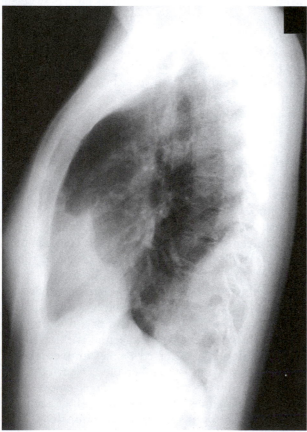

B

Figure 5. Tuberculous empyema. Shown are posterior-anterior (A) and lateral (B) chest radiographs demonstrating a left lower-lobe effusion.

may occur with a variety of infectious agents. Members of the usual ororespiratory microbiota may produce the syndrome of "wet" bronchiectasis, i.e., with sputum production. Other mycobacteria may be recovered during the development of inactivity and were at one time considered to be a sign of healing. The presence of other pathogenic mycobacteria brings up the possibility of a dual infection, especially when found early in the disease.

Aspergillus species are common in badly damaged lung areas, especially those that are cavitary. In England, a prospective study (6) revealed that 25% of clinically healed TB patients who had residual cavities developed positive precipitins to *Aspergillus* species and 11% had demonstrable cavitary "balls," presumed to be aspergillomas or "fungus balls." Three years later, these numbers had risen to 34 and 17%, respectively. This high incidence may be due in part to the increased incidence of *Aspergillus* noted in the United Kingdom, both in the environment and as an infective agent, probably as a result of the more humid environment.

Massive hemorrhage, a dramatic event occurring in advanced cases of TB, is frequently terminal. Mild hemoptysis itself is very common in acute infection and not infrequently calls the attention of an otherwise unconcerned patient to the presence of serious disease. Rupture of a mycotic aneurysm of a branch of the pulmonary or bronchial artery (Rasmussen's aneurysm) has been well publicized as a cause of death; an aspergilloma may also be associated with severe and fatal hemorrhage. However, less well-defined major hemorrhages may also occur. Resection of the involved area has been the most widely used method of control; unhappily, many patients die before this can be accomplished, and often (as in the case of aspergillomas) the areas are multiple, thus not lending themselves to excisional therapy. The extensive disease found in these patients often contraindicates surgery, since functional lung tissue necessary for survival must often be removed along with the diseased area at the time of surgery.

During the acute infectious phase of the disease, two interesting complications have been reported: the syndrome of inappropriate antidiuretic hormone excretion (SIADH) and a reset osmostat (36). Both manifest by abnormally low sodium. However, the former is associated with all of the clinical and renal abnormalities associated with SIADH. A reset osmostat is characterized by decreased serum osmolality without clinical symptoms and the obligatory renal salt wasting found in SIADH. Both conditions disappear with control of the infection; however, they should be differentiated from each other since SIADH requires metabolic control (see chapter 28).

REFERENCES

1. Andronikou, S., F. M. Vanhoenacker, and A. I. Backer. 2009. Advances in imaging chest tuberculosis: blurring of differences between children and adults. *Clin. Chest Med.* 30:717–744.

2. Antonucci, G., E. Girardi, M. C. Raviglione, and G. Ippolito for the Gruppo Italiano di Studio Tubercolosi e AIDS (GISTA). 1995. Risk factors for tuberculosis in HIV-infected persons. A prospective cohort study. *JAMA* 274:143–148.

3. Arango, L., A. W. Brewin, and J. F. Murray. 1973. The spectrum of tuberculosis as currently seen in a metropolitan hospital. *Am. Rev. Respir. Dis.* 108:805–812.

4. Baumann, M. H., R. Nolan, M. Petrini, Y. C. Lee, R. W. Light, and E. Schneider. 2007. Pleural tuberculosis in the United States: incidence and drug resistance. *Chest* 131:1125–1132.

5. Berger, H. W., and E. Mejei. 1973. Tuberculous pleurisy. *Chest* 63:88–92.

6. British Thoracic and Tuberculosis Association Research Council. 1970. Aspergilloma and residual tuberculous cavities—the results of a survey. *Tubercle* 51:227–245.

7. Centers for Disease Control and Prevention. 2009. *Reported Tuberculosis in the United States, 2008.* Centers for Disease Control and Prevention, U.S. Department of Health and Human Services, Atlanta, GA.

8. Choyke, P. L., H. D. Sostman, A. M. Curtis, C. E. Ravin, J. T. T. Chen, J. D. Godwin, and C. H. Putman. 1983. Adult-onset pulmonary tuberculosis. *Radiology* 148:357–362.

9. Chung, D. K. 1969. Hyponatremia in untreated active pulmonary tuberculosis. *Am. Rev. Respir. Dis.* 99:595–597.

10. Comstock, G. W., V. T. Livesay, and S. F. Woolpert. 1974. The prognosis of a positive tuberculin reaction in childhood and adolescence. *Am. J. Epidemiol.* 99:131–138.

11. Daley, C., P. Small, G. F. Schecter, G. K. Schoolnik, R. A. McAdam, W. R. Jacobs, Jr., and P. C. Hopewell. 1992. An outbreak of tuberculosis with accelerated progression among persons infected with the human immunodeficiency virus. An analysis using restriction-fragment-length polymorphisms. *N. Engl. J. Med.* 326:231–235.

12. Danek, S. J., and J. S. Bower. 1979. Diagnosis of pulmonary tuberculosis by flexible fiberoptic bronchoscopy. *Am. Rev. Respir. Dis.* 119:677–679.

13. Diacon, A. H., B. W. Van de Wal, C. Wyser, J. P. Smedema, J. Bezuidenhout, C. T. Bolliger, and G. Walzl. 2003. Diagnostic tools in tuberculous pleurisy: a direct comparative study. *Eur. Respir. J.* 22:589–591.

14. El-Sadr, W. M., and S. J. Tsiouris. 2008. HIV-associated tuberculosis: diagnostic and treatment challenges. *Semin. Respir. Crit. Care Med.* 29:525–531.

15. Farer, L., A. Lowell, and M. Meador. 1979. Extrapulmonary tuberculosis in the United States. *Am. J. Epidemiol.* 109:205–217.

16. Fraser, R. G., and J. A. P. Pare. 1977. Diagnosis of diseases of the chest. W. B. Saunders, Philadelphia, PA.

17. Garibaldi, R. A., R. E. Drusin, S. H. Ferebee, and M. B. Gregg. 1972. Isoniazid-associated hepatitis. Report of an outbreak. *Am. Rev. Respir. Dis.* 106:357–365.

18. Glassroth, J., A. G. Robbins, and D. E. Snider. 1980. Tuberculosis in the 1980's. *N. Engl. J. Med.* 302:1441–1450.

19. Gómez-Reino, J. J., L. Carmona, V. R. Valverde, E. M. Mola, and M. D. Montero, on behalf of the BIOBADASER Group. 2003. Treatment of rheumatoid arthritis with tumor necrosis factor inhibitors may predispose to significant increase in tuberculosis risk: a multicenter active-surveillance report. *Arthritis Rheum.* 48:2122–2127.

20. Greco, S., E. Girardi, R. Masciangelo, G. B. Capoccetta, and C. Saltini. 2003. Adenosine deaminase and interferon gamma measurements for the diagnosis of tuberculous pleurisy: a meta-analysis. *Int. J. Tuberc. Lung Dis.* 7:777–786.

21. Hargreaves, N. J., O. Kadzakumanja, C. J. Whitty, F. M. Salaniponi, A. D. Harries, and S. B. Squire. 2001. 'Smear-negative' pulmonary tuberculosis in a DOTS programme: poor outcomes in an area of high HIV seroprevalence. *Int. J. Tuberc. Lung Dis.* 5:847–854.

22. Hassoun, P. M., K. E. Shepherd, T. J. Flotte, and H. Kazemi. 1988. Erythema induratum and active pulmonary tuberculosis. *Am. J. Med.* 84:784–785.

23. Hatipoglu, O. N., M. M. Manisali, E. S. Ucan, P. Balci, A. Akkoclu, O. Akpinar, C. Karlikaya, and C. Yuksel. 1996. High resolution computed tomographic findings in pulmonary tuberculosis. *Thorax* 51:397–402.

24. Holden, M., M. R. Dubin, and P. H. Diamond. 1971. Frequency of negative intermediate-strength tuberculin sensitivity in patients with active tuberculosis. *N. Engl. J. Med.* 285:1506–1509.

25. Hull, M. W., P. Phillips, and J. S. Montaner. 2008. Changing global epidemiology of pulmonary manifestations of HIV/AIDS. *Chest* 134:1287–1298.

26. Jackson, J. M. 2007. TNF-alpha inhibitors. *Dermatol. Ther.* 20:251–264.

27. Keane, J., S. Gershon, R. P. Wise, E. Mirabile-Levens, J. Kasznica, W. D. Schwieterman, J. N. Siegel, and M. M. Braun. 2001. Tuberculosis associated with infliximab, a tumor necrosis factor alpha-neutralizing agent. *N. Engl. J. Med.* 345:1098–1104.

28. Kiblawi, S. S. O., S. J. Jay, R. B. Stonehill, and J. Norton. 1981. Fever responses of patients on therapy for pulmonary tuberculosis. *Am. Rev. Respir. Dis.* 123:20–24.

29. Korzeniewska-Kosela, M., J. Krysl, N. L. Muller, W. Black, E. Allen, and J. M. Fitzgerald. 1994. Tuberculosis in young adults and the elderly: a prospective comparison study. *Chest* 106:28–32.

30. Lawn, S. D., and G. Churchyard. 2009. Epidemiology of HIV-associated tuberculosis. *Curr. Opin. HIV AIDS* 4:325–333.

31. Lee, K. S., J. W. Hwang, M. P. Chung, J. Kim, and O. J. Kwon. 1996. Utility of CT in the evaluation of pulmonary tuberculosis in patients without AIDS. *Chest* 110:977–984.

32. Leung, A. N., N. L. Muller, P. R. Pineda, and J. M. FitzGerald. 1992. Primary tuberculosis in childhood: radiographic manifestations. *Radiology* 182:87–91.

33. Light, R. W., M. I. MacGregor, P. C. Luchsinger, and W. C. Ball, Jr. 1972. Pleural effusions. The diagnostic separation of transudates and exudates. *Ann. Intern. Med.* 77:507–513.

34. MacGregor, R. R. 1975. A year's experience with tuberculosis in a private urban teaching hospital in the post-sanatorium era. *Am. J. Med.* 58:221–228.

35. Maini, R., E. W. St. Clair, F. Breedveld, D. Furst, J. Kalden, M. Weisman, J. Smolen, P. Emery, G. Harriman, M. Feldmann, and P. Lipsky for the ATTRACT Study Group. 1999. Infliximab (chimeric anti-tumour necrosis factor αmonoclonal antibody) versus placebo in rheumatoid arthritis patients receiving concomitant methotrexate: a randomised phase III trial. *Lancet* 354:1932–1939.

36. Mayock, R. L., and M. Goldberg. 1964. *Metabolic Considerations in Disease of the Respiratory System. Diseases of Metabolism.* W. B. Saunders, Philadelphia, PA.

37. Mayock, R. L., and R. R. MacGregor. 1976. Diagnosis, prevention and early therapy of tuberculosis. *Dis. Month* 22:1–6.

38. Morris, C. D. W. 1989. The radiography, haematology and biochemistry of pulmonary tuberculosis in the aged. *Q. J. Med.* 266:529–535.

39. Perez-Guzman, C., M. Vargas, A. Torres-Cruz, and H. Villarreal-Velarde. 1999. Does aging modify pulmonary tuberculosis? A meta-analytical review. *Chest* **116**:961–967.

40. Perlman, D. C., W. M. El-Sadr, E. T. Nelson, J. P. Matts, E. E. Telzak, N. Salomon, K. Chirgwin, and R. Hafner. 1997. Variation in chest radiographic patterns in pulmonary tuberculosis patients by degree of human immunodeficiency virus-related immunosuppression. *Clin. Infect. Dis.* **25**:242–246.

41. Poppius, H., and K. Thomander. 1957. Segmentary distribution of cavities. A radiologic study of 500 consecutive cases of cavernous pulmonary tuberculosis. *Ann. Med. Intern. Fenn.* **46**:113.

42. Porcel, J. M. 2009. Tuberculous pleural effusion. *Lung* **187**: 263–270.

43. Ramos-Casals, M., P. Brito-Zerón, S. Muñoz, N. Soria, D. Galiana, L. Bertolaccini, M. J. Cuadrado, and M. A. Khamashta. 2007. Autoimmune diseases induced by TNF-targeted therapies: analysis of 233 cases. *Medicine* (Baltimore) **86**:242–251.

44. Rieder, H. L., G. D. Kelly, A. B. Bloch, G. M. Cauthen, and D. E. Snider, Jr. 1991. Tuberculosis diagnosed at death in the United States. *Chest* **100**:678–681.

45. Salvadó, M., C. Garcia-Vidal, P. Vázquez, M. Riera, M. Rodríguez-Carballeira, J. Martínez-Lacasa, E. Cuchi, and J. Garau. 2010. Mortality of tuberculosis in very old people. *J. Am. Geriatr. Soc.* **58**:18–22.

46. Selwyn, P. A., D. Hartel, V. A. Lewis, E. E. Schoenbaum, S. H. Vermund, R. S. Klein, A. T. Walker, and G. H. Friedland. 1989. A prospective study of the risk of tuberculosis among intravenous drug abusers with human immunodeficiency virus infection. *N. Engl. J. Med.* **320**:545–550.

47. Shafer, R. W., and B. R. Edlin. 1996. Tuberculosis in patients infected with human immunodeficiency virus: perspective on the past decade. *Clin. Infect. Dis.* **22**:683–704.

48. Shafer, R. W., D. S. Kim, J. P. Weiss, and J. M. Quale. 1991. Extrapulmonary tuberculosis in patients with human immunodeficiency virus infection. *Medicine* **70**:384–397.

49. Small, P., G. F. Schechter, P. C. Goodman, M. A. Sande, R. E. Chaisson, and P. C. Hopewell. 1991. Treatment of tuberculosis in patients with advanced human immunodeficiency virus infection. *N. Engl. J. Med.* **324**:289–294.

50. Stead, W. W., and J. P. Lofgren. 1983. Does the risk of tuberculosis infection increase in old age? *J. Infect. Dis.* **147**:951–955.

51. Trajman, A., M. Pai, K. Dheda, R. van Zyl Smit, A. A. Zwerling, R. Joshi, S. Kalantri, P. Daley, and D. Menzies. 2008. Novel tests for diagnosing tuberculous pleural effusion: what works and what does not? *Eur. Respir. J.* **31**:1098–1106.

52. Wallace, J. M., A. L. Deutsch, J. H. Harrell, and K. M. Moser. 1981. Bronchoscopy and transbronchial biopsy in evaluation of patients with suspected active tuberculosis. *Am. J. Med.* **70**: 1189–1194.

53. Weber, A. L., K. T. Bird, and W. L. Janower. 1968. Primary tuberculosis in childhood with particular emphasis on changes affecting the tracheobronchial tree. *Am. J. Roentgenol.* **10**: 123–132.

54. World Health Organization. 2009. *Global Tuberculosis Control: a Short Update to the 2009 Report*. World Health Organization, Geneva, Switzerland.

55. Yam, L. T. 1972. Diagnostic significance of lymphocytes in pleural effusions. *Am. Rev. Respir. Dis.* **105**:458–460.

Tuberculosis and Nontuberculous Mycobacterial Infections, 6th ed.
Edited by David Schlossberg
© 2011 ASM Press, Washington, DC

Chapter 15

Upper Respiratory Tract Tuberculosis

SURINDER K. JINDAL AND RITESH AGARWAL

Over the last four decades, the incidence of extrapulmonary tuberculosis (EPTB) as a percentage of the total TB cases has gradually risen (38). Upper respiratory tract TB is one of the rare forms of EPTB. In the prechemotherapeutic era, patients with active pulmonary TB often developed laryngeal, otological, nasal, paranasal, and pharyngeal involvement and deteriorated progressively. However, with the advent of effective antituberculous drugs, the incidence came down significantly.

The upper respiratory tract is the portal of entry of all inhaled matter in the lungs. It also constitutes the first line of defense against the inhalational insults. Tubercular involvement of the upper respiratory tract is not surprising, as inhalation is the most common and important route of mycobacterial infection. On the other hand, it is the relative rarity of upper respiratory tract TB which is somewhat puzzling. Possibly, the continuous airflow and the smooth mucosal lining do not allow the mycobacteria to settle down in the respiratory tract, except for the entrapment areas, such as the larynx.

Almost all parts of the upper respiratory tract from the nose to the vocal cords and larynx can get involved, although the frequency of involvement may vary to a great degree. Patients with TB of different components of the upper respiratory tract may first report to a general physician, an otorhinolaryngologist, or a pulmonologist. Chest physicians, who also handle TB in the developing countries, are frequently confronted with and consulted for upper respiratory tract TB. Factually speaking, TB of upper respiratory tract should be considered and handled on par with that of the lungs.

Symptoms and signs of upper respiratory tract TB depend upon the site of organ involvement (Table 1). Concurrent pulmonary involvement is frequent. Systemic manifestations such as fever and weight loss are uncommon but may occasionally be seen, especially in the presence of involvement of lungs and/or other organs. Nodules or ulcerative lesions are seen on morphological examination. Endoscopic examination is required for mucosal lesions. Most of these lesions are initially missed as nontuberculous infections or are malignant in nature. Diagnosis of TB is suspected on an epidemiological basis in high-prevalence countries or on failure to respond to routine treatment. Smear and/or histopathological examinations help in establishing the final etiological diagnosis.

Tuberculous involvement of upper respiratory tract was seen in less than 2% of TB admissions in the past (78). More recently, however, there has been an increase in the incidence and a change in the spectrum of upper respiratory tract TB (64, 72). This is especially so in patients infected with human immunodeficiency virus (HIV) or on other immunosuppressive therapies (30, 42). For example, of the 538 EPTB cases (28.6%) in a total of 1,878 enrollees, the risk for EPTB in HIV-seropositive patients in a multivariate model was high; African American ethnicity was an independent risk factor for EPTB (30). TB of the upper respiratory tract is also a common cause of cervical lymph node enlargement (4, 54, 64, 66). Any presence of lymph nodes in the neck calls for careful search for a lesion in the upper respiratory tract and vice versa. In a recent series of 17 cases of TB of the nasopharynx from Hong Kong, cervical lymphadenopathy was present in 59% of patients (102). Similarly, in Thailand, the most common site of TB in the head and neck involved the cervical lymph nodes and the nasopharynx (93). In addition, pulmonary lesions are present in about 20% of adults and about 50 to 60% of children (40, 75, 82, 99).

NASAL TB

TB of the nose and paranasal sinuses is an uncommonly reported but a well-described entity in otorhinolaryngology practice (53, 95). In 1997, only

Surinder K. Jindal and Ritesh Agarwal • Department of Pulmonary Medicine, Postgraduate Institute of Medical Education & Research, Sector 12, Chandigarh-160012, India.

Table 1. Common symptoms and signs of upper respiratory tract TB

Location	Symptom(s) or sign(s)
Nose	Nasal discharge/obstruction
	Epistaxis, pain
	External nodule, ulcer (lupus vulgaris), or deformity
	Mucosal ulcer(s)
	Septal perforation
Oral cavity	Ulcers—painless/painful on tongue or buccal or pharyngeal mucosa
	Localized swelling
	Tonsillar infiltration/ulcer
	Sore throat, dysphagia, white patches
	Secondary otitis media—otorrhea
Larynx	Hoarseness
	Odynophagia, dysphagia
	Mucosal ulcers, localized swelling, abscess
	Epiglottic swelling/mass
	Upper airway obstruction—rare

35 cases were identified in a search of the English language medical literature of the last 95 years (13). Several other reports of isolated cases have, however, appeared after 1997, mostly from the developing countries (36, 52, 70, 73). Series of several cases have been reported from India, Pakistan, and Hong Kong, many of which showed no evidence of concomitant pulmonary TB (50, 67, 68, 102). Its reemergence as a major health problem in the United States was attributed to HIV infection, homelessness, and deterioration of the social infrastructure (13). Maxillary sinuses are commonly involved in nasal TB. Very rarely, involvement of other sinuses has been described. TB of sphenoid sinuses established on magnetic resonance imaging and endoscopic biopsy was recently reported in two children (84).

Clinical Features

Patients with nasal TB commonly present with nasal obstruction and purulent rhinorrhea. Epistaxis is another important manifestation (9, 19). Lupus vulgaris, a slowly growing, indolent ulcerative lesion caused by *Mycobacterium tuberculosis*, may affect the nasal vestibule, the septum, and the alae. Occasionally, lupus vulgaris with papulonecrotic TB is reported (81). External deformity may result in about one-third of patients. Physical examination may reveal pallor of the nasal mucosa with multiple minute apple jelly nodules on diascopy. Perforation of septal cartilage can occur. TB can also manifest as a polypoidal lesion in the nasal cavity (12, 69). Sinonasal TB can invade the surrounding bones and result in osteomyelitis and abscess formation (41). Intracranial extension can cause neurological manifestations such as epilepsy and optic neuritis (9, 20). In a series of 18 cases of intrasellar tuberculomas, 6 had involvement

of sphenoid sinus (83). Cervical lymph node enlargement is present in about 30% of patients.

Most of these clinical manifestations can be seen in other diseases involving the nose, such as fungal infections, leprosy, syphilis, and malignancies. Septal perforations have been reported for patients on inhalational corticosteroids, for those with allergic bronchopulmonary aspergillosis, and following chronic exposures to metal fumes in welders (21, 56). Granulomatous involvement of the nose and the sinuses can occur in several other conditions (35). Wegener's granulomatosis, fungal infections, midline granulomatous disease, and leprosy are some such examples. Radiotherapy administered for undifferentiated carcinoma can also cause granulomatous inflammation which in many instances is attributable to TB (18). Differential diagnosis is achieved on histological and microbiological parameters. Confirmation of diagnosis is made on mycobacterial culture, since the acid-fast bacilli (AFB) on smear examination may occasionally represent *Mycobacterium leprae*, an important cause of nasal involvement in zones of endemicity. Mycobacteria were detected on PCR of nasal swabs from 6 of 16 smear-positive TB patients and 1 of 10 household contacts (105). However, the sensitivity and specificity of PCR on nasal swabs in clinical diagnosis of nasal TB are not known. Although *Mycobacterium tuberculosis* is the most common organism, other mycobacteria have, rarely, been implicated. *Mycobacterium africanum* had been isolated in a case of cutaneous TB with nasal sinus invasion, nasal perforation, and bilateral nodular scleritis (8).

Nasal TB responds to standard antituberculous therapy as for pulmonary TB (see chapter 7). Surgical interventions may occasionally be required.

ORAL CAVITY AND PHARYNX

The oral cavity is a rare site of TB involvement. Infection of the oral cavity is associated with poor dental hygiene and other causes which result in mucosal injury. Most patients have concomitant pulmonary TB, and the lesions are believed to result from the infected sputum being coughed out (26). Infection can also be acquired by the hematogenous route. The tongue is the most common site of involvement. Almost any part of the tongue, such as the tip, the borders, dorsum, and base, may be involved. Several isolated cases of lingual TB have been reported in the recent past (3, 6, 15, 39, 63). Very rarely, TB of the lips has been described (22, 37, 47). Similar to TB of the nose, many of these cases are seen in patients with HIV infection (6, 17, 34, 65). Other sites in the oral cavity include the floor of the mouth, soft palate, tonsils, anterior pillars of fauces, and uvula.

Clinical Features

The lesions can manifest as ulcers or nodules which can be either single or multiple anywhere in the mouth. The lesions are usually well circumscribed and painful but can also be irregular, simulating malignant ulcers. Sometimes the lesions are painless. The draining lymph nodes in the neck may also be palpable.

TB of the pharynx can be ulcerative of the lupus vulgaris type or secondary to pulmonary involvement (so-called miliary TB of the pharynx). The nasopharynx is the most common site of pharyngeal involvement (52, 62, 70). Symptoms of nasopharyngeal TB include nasal obstruction, rhinorrhea, and nasal twang of voice, while physical findings may be limited to adenoid hypertrophy without any distinguishing features. Several atypical presentations have been described. Snoring which disappeared after antituberculous therapy was the only complaint reported for a 58-year-old patient (2). Presentation with neck pain and hearing loss was reported recently for a 25-year-old individual (108). Two different patterns of nasopharyngeal TB can be identified on magnetic resonance imaging—the pattern of a discrete polypoidal mass in the adenoids and the pattern of a more diffuse soft tissue thickening of one or two walls of the nasopharynx (51). Extension outside the confines of the nasopharynx was not seen (51). Most infections are primary, and less than 20% demonstrate pulmonary involvement. Postradiation granulomatous inflammation in patients with nasopharyngeal carcinoma should be suspected as occult tubercular infection and diligently investigated (18).

Oropharyngeal TB is likely to manifest with symptoms of sore throat (5, 16). Commonly, there is simultaneous involvement of the larynx causing severe dysphagia and odynophagia (16). Local hyperemia and irregularity of the mucosa, erythematous papules, and swelling of the cheek have been described in different case reports (14, 33, 61). Cervical lymphadenopathy is frequently present. Similarly, cutaneous lupus vulgaris and scrofuloderma may also be seen.

Tonsils constitute another important site of involvement with TB. Again, the involvement may occur in isolation or along with TB of the larynx and the lungs. Tonsillar TB was common in the era of unpasteurized milk and was acquired by drinking milk infected with *Mycobacterium bovis*. It may manifest with features of sore throat, lymphadenopathy, dysphagia, ulceration, masses, and white patches (92, 94, 106). Pharyngeal TB can also spread to the middle ear through the eustachian tube (31). Tympanic membrane perforations (especially multiple), painless otorrhea, and hearing loss may result. Preauricular lymph node enlargement and postauricular fistula are considered pathognomonic of tubercular otitis media. Occasionally, TB might complicate a malignant lesion in this region (74). Physical examination includes unilateral tonsillar enlargement, ulcerations, and fibrosis of the tonsils. Incisional biopsy confirms the diagnosis based on histopathological findings and the identification of AFB. Patients tend to respond quickly to antituberculous chemotherapy; if no response is seen in 2 weeks, the diagnosis should be questioned.

TB of the salivary glands occurs as a result of infection of the oral cavity or secondary to pulmonary TB. Primary sialitis may occur but is rare. Although parotid involvement is the most common, submandibular glands may also be involved (49, 55). The clinical presentation can be either acute or chronic. Most patients present with only parotidomegaly and no other systemic manifestations. In a few case reports, the diagnosis was not suspected until histopathological evidence was obtained (25, 43). When suspected, however, diagnosis can be made by fine-needle aspiration cytology (49). The diagnosis can also be suggested preoperatively by the contrast-enhanced computed tomography (CECT) appearance. The presence of thick-walled rim-enhancing lesions with a central lucency on CECT should suggest the diagnosis. Filling defects with or without thin walls are nonspecific findings and are seen in tumors and other inflammatory processes. In an appropriate clinical setting, thick-walled round rim-enhancing lesions with a central lucency are characteristic of TB (10).

Diagnosis of most forms of extralaryngeal upper respiratory tract TB is difficult and requires biopsy procedures. In a series of 16 cases of TB with involvement of the oral cavity and/or pharynx (8 cases), ear (4), salivary glands (2), nose (1), and frontal sinuses (1), the average duration of symptoms was 11.5 months and biopsy was required in all; the purified protein derivative skin test was also positive in 15 of 16 patients (86).

Treatment for all these patients consists of antituberculous chemotherapy and is generally favorable (86). Surgical intervention should be avoided (66).

TB OF THE LARYNX

The larynx is the most vital part of the upper respiratory tract. It can be involved in different infective, neoplastic, granulomatous, and other conditions. TB is perhaps the most common cause of granulomatous disease of the larynx (11, 87, 104). The clinical presentation of tubercular laryngitis has changed significantly from what it was before the advent of chemotherapy (Table 2) (60), and nowadays, it more closely resembles a laryngeal carcinoma than

Table 2. Changes in clinical spectrum of laryngeal TB, pre- and postchemotherapeutic eras

Parameter	Prechemotherapeutic era	Postchemotherapeutic era
Occurrence	Common	Uncommon
	15–37% of patients with pulmonary TB	Less than 1% of cases
Age	<40 yrs	5th to 6th decade
Constitutional symptoms	Prominent	Less common
Pulmonary involvement	Severe	Advanced disease less common
Lesions	Multiple	Solitary (usually)
	Ulcerative	Hypertrophic
Predilection for postlaryngeal involvement	Yes	No predilection for any laryngeal sites
Pseudotumor form	Uncommon	Common

any other laryngeal illness (23, 90). In the prechemotherapy era, it was a common complication of active cavitary pulmonary disease, occurring in about one-third of cases (59). Presently, it is reported in 1 to 2% of cases (78, 101). The primary infection can involve any part of the larynx, while the previously described direct mode of spread from the lungs predominantly involved the posterior larynx. In some series, almost all patients with laryngeal TB were reported to have some evidence of pulmonary TB and many would demonstrate sputum smear positivity for AFB (79). In the postchemotherapy era, laryngeal TB, especially in the low-prevalence countries, generally occurs as an isolated manifestation (46, 60, 85, 89, 91, 98).

Laryngeal involvement is especially common in patients with immunodeficiency such as HIV infection (80). In a series of 45 patients with upper aerodigestive tract TB, 16 had laryngeal and 23 nasopharyngeal TB; 4 of 26 patients had positive serological tests for HIV infection (93). Similarly, laryngeal TB has been described in other diseases. In a review of 283 patients with systemic lupus erythematosus in Korea, TB was documented for 15 patients, 1 of whom had laryngeal involvement (109). Two cases of laryngeal TB were reported to occur in renal transplant patients; both responded promptly to antituberculous therapy (96). Occasionally, patients on glucocorticoids can develop laryngeal TB. For example, a patient with Addison's disease on glucocorticoids and another on inhaled steroid therapy are reported to have developed tubercular infection (24, 103).

Clinical Features and Diagnosis

There has been a shift in the age and sex distributions of laryngeal TB in the last three or four decades (1, 85). It is now more common in the older age groups and is more common in males than females (57, 59). Above 50 years of age, the male predominance is even more marked. Besides the patients with immunosuppressive states, such as HIV infection, it is also more frequent in individuals of poor constitution and health, especially those who are alcoholics and undernourished (24, 71, 80, 93, 96, 109). Consumption of tobacco is also identified as a risk factor (71).

The presence of laryngeal symptoms is generally quite bothersome and brings the patient to the physician early in the course of disease. The most common symptom is hoarseness of voice, present in over 90% of patients (85, 104). Cough, dysphagia, odynophagia, pain in the throat, and referred pain in the ear are also common (87, 101). Laryngeal involvement can present as an emergency situation with severe upper airway obstruction resulting from edema and granulomatous involvement of the laryngeal mucosa (32, 89). Stridor may be present because of the presence of granulation tissue at the level of the glottis, subglottic stenosis, and vocal cord paralysis secondary to mediastinal lymphadenopathy (89). Involvement of the posterior larynx was thought to result from pooling of infected saliva in the recumbent position, although not all reports have shown this predilection for posterior laryngeal involvement, and some experience has emphasized anterior vocal cord involvement; hypertrophic lesions are seen more commonly than ulcerative lesions (Fig. 1). Occasionally, there is isolated involvement of the epiglottic, supraglottic,

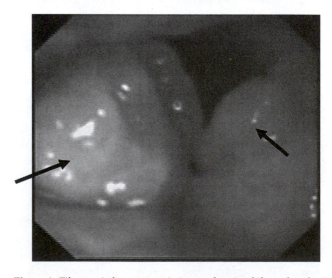

Figure 1. Fiber-optic laryngoscopic image showing bilateral nodular masses above the level of vocal cords. Biopsy from these masses confirmed TB.

or subglottic region (28, 32, 76). Solitary lesions are four times more frequent than multiple lesions.

The clinical picture in patients with underlying HIV infection and AIDS is somewhat different, posing greater difficulties in diagnosis (88). Systemic features such as fever, night sweats, and weight loss are common. Multiple-agent infections are also more frequent. Laryngeal TB, especially the nodular presentation, sometimes with abscess formation, may be difficult to differentiate from cancer on physical examination (32, 58). A good lateral X ray of the neck and CT can help (Fig. 2) (7, 48). In an occasional case

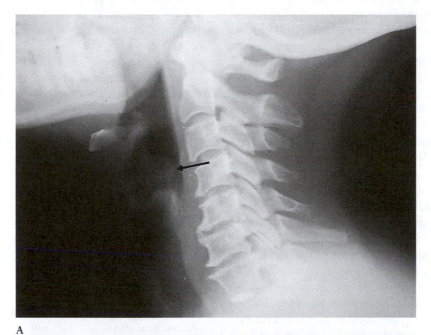

A

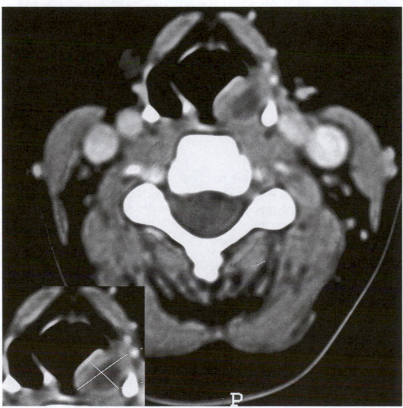

B

Figure 2. Roentgenogram soft tissue (A) and CT scan (B) of the neck showing well-defined tubercular abscess in the left aryepiglottic fold obliterating the left piriform fossa.

F-18 fluorodeoxyglucose positron emission tomography/CT is employed to detect systemic TB presenting as an epiglottic mass (27). Although appearances of laryngeal TB are not specific on CT appearances, the possibility should be raised when there is bilateral involvement, thickening of the free margin of the epiglottis, and preservation of the preepiglottic and paralaryngeal spaces even in the presence of extensive mucosal involvement (48). Any nonspecific chronic laryngitis of poor evolution should lead to a suspicion of laryngeal TB (71). Cartilage destruction is more common in malignancies but may occasionally result from TB (45). Bacterial and fungal infections, Wegener's granulomatosis, sarcoidosis, and malignancies need to be considered in the differential diagnosis.

Histopathological examination is required for a definite diagnosis. Sputum microscopy is positive for 20% of patients with laryngeal TB. A laryngeal swab smear positive for mycobacteria should not be considered diagnostic of laryngeal TB, because it is frequently positive for patients with pulmonary TB, especially children. In a study of 116 children with suspected pulmonary TB, mycobacteria were seen on either smear examination or culture for one-third of 51 patients for whom laryngeal swabs were examined (97). Direct laryngoscopic examination with biopsy provides the most conclusive evidence for diagnosis. The sample should be sent for both histopathological examination and culture. It is the presence of mycobacteria on culture of a biopsy specimen which provides the conclusive etiological evidence of TB. However, in clinical practice, histological demonstration of epithelioid cell caseating granulomas is considered enough to initiate antituberculous therapy.

Treatment and Outcome

The laryngeal lesions of TB respond quickly to standard antituberculous regimens within weeks. The larynx is reported to return to its normal appearance in 18 weeks on average (101). Voice outcomes improve after antituberculous treatment in most patients (107). Sometimes, vocal cord immobility due to fibrosis and adhesion may produce permanent hoarseness in a minority of patients (29, 59). Occasionally, the disease may remain undiagnosed and untreated for long periods, which would result in significant damage. Coexistence of laryngeal TB and carcinoma is reported in 1 to 2% of cases (44). In such patients, antituberculous drugs should be given for at least 3 to 6 weeks before treatment for laryngeal carcinoma is initiated.

Treatment includes antituberculous chemotherapy for at least 6 months, modified on the basis of culture and sensitivity reports in cases of suspected drug resistance. Laryngeal TB generally responds well to multiple-drug antituberculous chemotherapy (77). Surgical intervention such as tracheostomy, partial or complete laryngectomy, or laryngo-tracheoplasty may be required for some patients with abscess formation and progressive disease unresponsive to medical therapy. Airway obstruction, although rare, even in fulminant cases may require tracheostomy for relief (100).

In conclusion, TB should be kept in the differential diagnosis of upper airway diseases and/or cervical lymphadenopathy whenever a patient presents with insidious onset of symptoms, ulcerative or granulomatous lesions, and failure of response to therapy for more common lesions. Classic clinical features may not always be present. Early diagnosis and treatment are essential to prevent long-term complications.

REFERENCES

1. Agarwal, P., and A. S. Bais. 1998. A clinical and videostroboscopic evaluation of laryngeal tuberculosis. *J. Laryngol. Otol.* **112:**45–48.
2. Aktan, B., E. Selimoglu, H. Ucuncu, and Y. Sutbeyaz. 2002. Primary nasopharyngeal tuberculosis in a patient with the complaint of snoring. *J. Laryngol. Otol.* **116:**301–303.
3. Aktogu, S., F. N. Eris, Z. A. Dinc, and G. Tibet. 2000. Tuberculosis of the tongue secondary to pulmonary tuberculosis. *Monaldi Arch. Chest Dis.* **55:**287–288.
4. Al-Serhani, A. M. 2001. Mycobacterial infection of the head and neck: presentation and diagnosis. *Laryngoscope* **111:**2012–2016.
5. Al-Serhani, A. M., and K. Al-Mazrou. 2001. Pharyngeal tuberculosis. *Am. J. Otolaryngol.* **22:**236–240.
6. Anil, S., A. N. Ellepola, L. P. Samaranayake, and V. T. Beena. 2000. Tuberculous ulcer of the tongue as presenting feature of pulmonary tuberculosis and HIV infection. *Gen. Dent.* **48:**458–461.
7. Bailey, C. M. and P. C. Windle-Taylor. 1981. Tuberculous laryngitis: a series of 37 patients. *Laryngoscope* **91:**93–100.
8. Baril, L., E. Caumes, C. Truffot-Pernot, F. Bricaire, J. Grosset, and M. Gentilini. 1995. Tuberculosis caused by *Mycobacterium africanum* associated with involvement of the upper and lower respiratory tract, skin, and mucosa. *Clin. Infect. Dis.* **21:**653–655.
9. Batra, K., N. Chaudhary, G. Motwani, and A. K. Rai. 2002. An unusual case of primary nasal tuberculosis with epistaxis and epilepsy. *Ear Nose Throat J.* **81:**842–844.
10. Bhargava, S., D. J. Watmough, F. A. Chisti, and S. A. Sathar. 1996. Case report: tuberculosis of the parotid gland—diagnosis by CT. *Br. J. Radiol.* **69:**1181–1183.
11. Bhat, V. K., P. Latha, D. Upadhya, and J. Hegde. 2009. Clinicopathological review of tubercular laryngitis in 32 cases of pulmonary Kochs. *Am. J. Otolaryngol.* **30:**327–330.
12. Blanco Aparicio, M., H. Verea-Hernando, and F. Pombo. 1995. Tuberculosis of the nasal fossa manifested by a polypoid mass. *J. Otolaryngol.* **24:**317–318.
13. Butt, A. A. 1997. Nasal tuberculosis in the 20th century. *Am. J. Med. Sci.* **313:**332–335.

14. Cakan, A., Z. Mutlu, A. Ozsoz, A. E. Erbaycu, T. Unal, and B. O. Koyuncu. 2001. Tuberculosis of oral mucosa. *Monaldi Arch. Chest Dis.* **56:**315–317.

15. Carnelio, S., and G. Rodrigues. 2002. Primary lingual tuberculosis: a case report with review of literature. *J. Oral Sci.* **44:**55–57.

16. Caylan, R., and K. Aydin. 2002. Oropharyngeal tuberculosis causing severe odynophagia and dysphagia. *Eur. Arch. Otorhinolaryngol.* **259:**229–230.

17. Ceballos-Salobrena, A., J. M. Aguirre-Urizar, and J. V. Bagan-Sebastian. 1996. Oral manifestations associated with human immunodeficiency virus infection in a Spanish population. *J. Oral Pathol. Med.* **25:**523–526.

18. Chan, A. B., T. K. Ma, B. K. Yu, A. D. King, F. N. Ho, and G. M. Tse. 2004. Nasopharyngeal granulomatous inflammation and tuberculosis complicating undifferentiated carcinoma. *Otolaryngol. Head Neck Surg.* **130:**125–130.

19. Choi, Y. C., Y. S. Park, E. J. Jeon, and S. H. Song. 2000. The disappeared disease: tuberculosis of the nasal septum. *Rhinology* **38:**90–92.

20. Das, J. C., K. Singh, P. Sharma, and R. Singla. 2003. Tuberculous osteomyelitis and optic neuritis. *Ophthalmic Surg. Lasers Imaging* **34:**409–412.

21. Deepak, D., C. Panjabi, S. Gudwani, N. Chaudhary, and A. Shah. 2001. Nasal septal perforation in a patient with allergic bronchopulmonary aspergillosis and rhinitis on long term corticosteroids. *Asian Pac. J. Allergy Immunol.* **19:**287–290.

22. Dixit, R., S. Sharma, and P. Nuwal. 2008. Tuberculosis of oral cavity. *Indian J. Tuberc.* **55:**51–53.

23. Edizer, D. T., E. Karaman, H. Mercan, Y. Alimoglu, T. Esen, and H. Cansiz. 2010. Primary tuberculosis involving epiglottis: a rare case report. *Dysphagia* **25:**258–260.

24. Egeli, E., F. Oghan, M. Alper, U. Harputluoglu, and I. Bulut. 2003. Epiglottic tuberculosis in a patient treated with steroids for Addison's disease. *Tohoku J. Exp. Med.* **201:**119–125.

25. el-Hakim, I. E., and J. D. Langdon. 1989. Unusual presentation of tuberculosis of the head and neck region. Report of three cases. *Int. J. Oral Maxillofac. Surg.* **18:**194–196.

26. Eng, H. L., S. Y. Lu, C. H. Yang, and W. J. Chen. 1996. Oral tuberculosis. *Oral Surg. Oral Med. Oral Pathol. Oral Radiol. Endod.* **81:**415–420.

27. Fernandez, P., M. Guyot, E. Lazaro, J. F. Viallard, M. Allard, and D. Ducassou. 2007. Systemic tuberculosis presenting as an epiglottic mass detected on F-18 FDG PET/CT. *Clin. Nucl. Med.* **32:**719–724.

28. Galli, J., C. Nardi, A. M. Contucci, G. Cadoni, L. Lauriola, and M. Fantoni. 2002. Atypical isolated epiglottic tuberculosis: a case report and a review of the literature. *Am. J. Otolaryngol.* **23:**237–240.

29. Getson, W. R., and Y. W. Park. 1992. Pathologic quiz case 2. Laryngeal tuberculosis. *Arch. Otolaryngol. Head Neck Surg.* **118:**878–879, 881.

30. Gonzalez, O. Y., G. Adams, L. D. Teeter, T. T. Bui, J. M. Musser, and E. A. Graviss. 2003. Extra-pulmonary manifestations in a large metropolitan area with a low incidence of tuberculosis. *Int. J. Tuberc. Lung Dis.* **7:**1178–1185.

31. Greenfield, B. J., S. H. Selesnick, L. Fisher, R. F. Ward, C. P. Kimmelman, and W. G. Harrison. 1995. Aural tuberculosis. *Am. J. Otol.* **16:**175–182.

32. Gupta, R., S. Fotedar, P. Sansanwal, S. P. Yadav, A. Gupta, K. B. Gupta, and K. Saini. 2008. Obstructing mass lesion of epiglottis: it can be tubercular. *Indian J. Tuberc.* **55:**100–103.

33. Hajioff, D., M. H. Snow, H. Thaker, and J. A. Wilson. 1999. Primary tuberculosis of the posterior oropharyngeal wall. *J. Laryngol. Otol.* **113:**1029–1030.

34. Hale, R. G., and D. I. Tucker. 2008. Head and neck manifestations of tuberculosis. *Oral Maxillofac. Surg. Clin. N. Am.* **20:**635–642.

35. Hughes, R. G., and A. Drake-Lee. 2001. Nasal manifestations of granulomatous disease. *Hosp. Med.* **62:**417–421.

36. Hup, A. K., T. Haitjema, and G. de Kuijper. 2001. Primary nasal tuberculosis. *Rhinology* **39:**47–48.

37. Ilyas, S. E., F. F. Chen, T. A. Hodgson, P. M. Speight, C. J. Lacey, and S. R. Porter. 2002. Labial tuberculosis: a unique cause of lip swelling complicating HIV infection. *HIV Med.* **3:**283–286.

38. Iseman, M. D. 2000. Extrapulmonary tuberculosis in adults, p. 145–198. *In* M. D. Iseman (ed.), *A Clinician's Guide to Tuberculosis.* Lippincott Williams & Wilkins, Philadelphia, PA.

39. Iype, E. M., K. Ramdas, M. Pandey, K. Jayasree, G. Thomas, P. Sebastian, and M. K. Nair. 2001. Primary tuberculosis of the tongue: report of three cases. *Br. J. Oral Maxillofac. Surg.* **39:**402–403.

40. Jha, B. C., A. Dass, N. M. Nagarkar, R. Gupta, and S. Singhal. 2001. Cervical tuberculous lymphadenopathy: changing clinical pattern and concepts in management. *Postgrad. Med. J.* **77:**185–187.

41. Jha, D., R. C. Deka, and M. C. Sharma. 2002. Tuberculosis of the maxillary sinus manifesting as a facial abscess. *Ear Nose Throat J.* **81:**102–104.

42. Kandiloros, D. C., T. P. Nikolopoulos, E. A. Ferekidis, A. Tsangaroulakis, J. E. Yiotakis, D. Davilis, and G. K. Adamopoulos. 1997. Laryngeal tuberculosis at the end of the 20th century. *J. Laryngol. Otol.* **111:**619–621.

43. Kant, R., R. P. Sahi, N. N. Mahendra, P. K. Agarwal, and R. Shankhdhar. 1977. Primary tuberculosis of the parotid gland. *J. Indian Med. Assoc.* **68:**212.

44. Kaplan, M. H., D. Armstrong, and P. Rosen. 1974. Tuberculosis complicating neoplastic disease. A review of 201 cases. *Cancer* **33:**850–858.

45. Kenmochi, M., T. Ohashi, H. Nishino, S. Sato, Y. Tanaka, I. Koizuka, and T. Shinagawa. 2003. A case report of difficult diagnosis in the patient with advanced laryngeal tuberculosis. *Auris Nasus Larynx* **30**(Suppl.):S131–S134.

46. Kilgore, T. L., and D. W. Jenkins. 1983. Laryngeal tuberculosis. *Chest* **83:**139–141.

47. Kilic, A., U. Gul, M. Gonul, S. Soylu, S. K. Cakmak, and M. Demiriz. 2009. Orificial tuberculosis of the lip: a case report and review of the literature. *Int. J. Dermatol.* **48:**178–180.

48. Kim, M. D., D. I. Kim, H. Y. Yune, B. H. Lee, K. J. Sung, T. S. Chung, and S. Y. Kim. 1997. CT findings of laryngeal tuberculosis: comparison to laryngeal carcinoma. *J. Comput. Assist. Tomogr.* **21:**29–34.

49. Kim, Y. H., W. J. Jeong, K. Y. Jung, M. W. Sung, K. H. Kim, and C. S. Kim. 2005. Diagnosis of major salivary gland tuberculosis: experience of eight cases and review of the literature. *Acta Otolaryngol.* **125:**1318–1322.

50. Kim, Y. M., A. Y. Kim, Y. H. Park, D. H. Kim, and K. S. Rha. 2007. Eight cases of nasal tuberculosis. *Otolaryngol. Head Neck Surg.* **137:**500–504.

51. King, A. D., A. T. Ahuja, G. M. Tse, A. C. van Hasselt, and A. B. Chan. 2003. MR imaging features of nasopharyngeal tuberculosis: report of three cases and literature review. *Am. J. Neuroradiol.* **24:**279–282.

52. Koktener, A. 2001. Nasopharyngeal tuberculosis. *Eur. J. Radiol.* **39:**186–187.

53. Kukreja, H. K., B. S. Sacha, and K. C. Joshi. 1977. Tuberculosis of maxillary sinus. *Indian J. Otolaryngol.* **29:**27–28.

54. Kumar, A. 2009. Lymph node tuberculosis, p. 397–409. *In* S. K. Sharma and A. Mohan (ed.), *Tuberculosis.* Jaypee Publishers, New Delhi, India.

55. Kumar, S., and A. Dev. 1990. Primary tuberculosis of bilateral submandibular salivary glands. *Indian J. Otolaryngol.* **42**:69–70.

56. Lee, C. R., C. I. Yoo, J. Lee, and S. K. Kang. 2002. Nasal septum perforation of welders. *Ind. Health* **40**:286–289.

57. Levenson, M. J., M. Ingerman, C. Grimes, and W. F. Robbett. 1984. Laryngeal tuberculosis: review of twenty cases. *Laryngoscope* **94**:1094–1097.

58. Lim, J. Y., K. M. Kim, E. C. Choi, Y. H. Kim, H. S. Kim, and H. S. Choi. 2006. Current clinical propensity of laryngeal tuberculosis: review of 60 cases. *Eur. Arch. Otorhinolaryngol.* **263**:838–842.

59. Lindell, M. M., Jr., B. S. Jing, and S. Wallace. 1977. Laryngeal tuberculosis. *Am. J. Roentgenol.* **129**:677–680.

60. Ling, L., S. H. Zhou, and S. Q. Wang. 2010. Changing trends in the clinical features of laryngeal tuberculosis: a report of 19 cases. *Int. J. Infect. Dis.* **14**:e230–e235.

61. Magina, S., C. Lisboa, C. Resende, F. Azevedo, F. Amado, V. Cardoso, F. Almeida, and J. Mesquita-Guimaraes. 2003. Tuberculosis in a child presenting as asymptomatic oropharyngeal and laryngeal lesions. *Pediatr. Dermatol.* **20**:429–431.

62. Mair, I. W., and T. A. Johannessen. 1970. Nasopharyngeal tuberculosis. *Arch. Otolaryngol.* **92**:392–393.

63. Memon, G. A., and I. A. Khushk. 2003. Primary tuberculosis of tongue. *J. Coll. Physicians Surg. Pak.* **13**:604–605.

64. Menon, K., C. Bem, D. Gouldesbrough, and D. R. Strachan. 2007. A clinical review of 128 cases of head and neck tuberculosis presenting over a 10-year period in Bradford, UK. *J. Laryngol. Otol.* **121**:362–368.

65. Miziara, I. D. 2005. Tuberculosis affecting the oral cavity in Brazilian HIV-infected patients. *Oral Surg. Oral Med. Oral Pathol. Oral Radiol. Endod.* **100**:179–182.

66. Munck, K., and A. H. Mandpe. 2003. Mycobacterial infections of the head and neck. *Otolaryngol. Clin. N. Am.* **36**:569–576.

67. Nalini, B., and S. Vinayak. 2006. Tuberculosis in ear, nose, and throat practice: its presentation and diagnosis. *Am. J. Otolaryngol.* **27**:39–45.

68. Nawaz, G., and M. R. Khan. 2004. Primary sinonasal tuberculosis in north-west Pakistan. *J. Coll. Physicians Surg. Pak.* **14**:221–224.

69. Nayar, R. C., J. Al Kaabi, and K. Ghorpade. 2004. Primary nasal tuberculosis: a case report. *Ear Nose Throat J.* **83**:188–191.

70. Percodani, J., F. Braun, P. Arrue, E. Yardeni, M. Murris-Espin, E. Serrano, and J. J. Pessey. 1999. Nasopharyngeal tuberculosis. *J. Laryngol. Otol.* **113**:928–931.

71. Porras Alonso, E., A. Martin Mateos, J. Perez-Requena, and E. Avalos Serrano. 2002. Laryngeal tuberculosis. *Rev. Laryngol. Otol. Rhinol. (Bordeaux)* **123**:47–48.

72. Prasad, K. C., S. Sreedharan, Y. Chakravarthy, and S. C. Prasad. 2007. Tuberculosis in the head and neck: experience in India. *J. Laryngol. Otol.* **121**:979–985.

73. Purohit, S. D., and R. C. Gupta. 1997. Primary tuberculosis of nose. *Indian J. Chest Dis. Allied Sci.* **39**:63–64.

74. Raman, R., and A. Bakthavizian. 1981. Tuberculosis associated with malignancy of the nasopharynx. *Indian J. Otolaryngol.* **33**:149–150.

75. Raviglione, M. C., D. E. Snider, Jr., and A. Kochi. 1995. Global epidemiology of tuberculosis. Morbidity and mortality of a worldwide epidemic. *JAMA* **273**:220–226.

76. Richter, B., M. Fradis, G. Kohler, and G. J. Ridder. 2001. Epiglottic tuberculosis: differential diagnosis and treatment. Case report and review of the literature. *Ann. Otol. Rhinol. Laryngol.* **110**:197–201.

77. Riley, E. C., and D. E. Amundson. 1992. Laryngeal tuberculosis revisited. *Am. Fam. Physician* **46**:759–762.

78. Rohwedder, J. J. 1974. Upper respiratory tract tuberculosis. Sixteen cases in a general hospital. *Ann. Intern. Med.* **80**:708–713.

79. Rupa, V., and T. S. Bhanu. 1989. Laryngeal tuberculosis in the eighties—an Indian experience. *J. Laryngol. Otol.* **103**:864–868.

80. Schmid, D., R. Fretz, H. W. Kuo, R. Rumetshofer, S. Meusburger, E. Magnet, G. Hurbe, A. Indra, W. Ruppitsch, A. T. Pietzka, and F. Allerberger. 2008. An outbreak of multidrug-resistant tuberculosis among refugees in Austria, 2005–2006. *Int. J. Tuberc. Lung Dis.* **12**:1190–1195.

81. Senol, M., A. Ozcan, A. Aydin, Y. Karincaoglu, S. Sasmaz, and S. Sener. 2000. Disseminated lupus vulgaris and papulonecrotic tuberculid: case report. *Pediatr. Dermatol.* **17**:133–135.

82. Seth, V., S. K. Kabra, Y. Jain, O. P. Semwal, S. Mukhopadhyaya, and R. L. Jensen. 1995. Tubercular lymphadenitis: clinical manifestations. *Indian J. Pediatr.* **62**:565–570.

83. Sharma, M. C., R. Arora, A. K. Mahapatra, P. Sarat-Chandra, S. B. Gaikwad, and C. Sarkar. 2000. Intrasellar tuberculoma—an enigmatic pituitary infection: a series of 18 cases. *Clin. Neurol. Neurosurg.* **102**:72–77.

84. Sharma, S. C., and P. Baruah. 2003. Sphenoid sinus tuberculosis in children—a rare entity. *Int. J. Pediatr. Otorhinolaryngol.* **67**:399–401.

85. Shin, J. E., S. Y. Nam, S. J. Yoo, and and S. Y. Kim. 2000. Changing trends in clinical manifestations of laryngeal tuberculosis. *Laryngoscope* **110**:1950–1953.

86. Sierra, C., J. Fortun, C. Barros, E. Melcon, E. Condes, J. Cobo, C. Perez-Martinez, J. Ruiz-Galiana, A. Martinez-Vidal, and F. Alvarez. 2000. Extra-laryngeal head and neck tuberculosis. *Clin. Microbiol. Infect.* **6**:644–648.

87. Silva, L., E. Damrose, F. Bairao, M. L. Nina, J. C. Junior, and H. O. Costa. 2008. Infectious granulomatous laryngitis: a retrospective study of 24 cases. *Eur. Arch. Otorhinolaryngol.* **265**:675–680.

88. Singh, B., A. N. Balwally, M. Nash, G. Har-El, and F. E. Lucente. 1996. Laryngeal tuberculosis in HIV-infected patients: a difficult diagnosis. *Laryngoscope* **106**:1238–1240.

89. Smallman, L. A., D. R. Clark, C. H. Raine, D. W. Proops, and P. M. Shenoi. 1987. The presentation of laryngeal tuberculosis. *Clin. Otolaryngol. Allied Sci.* **12**:221–225.

90. Smulders, Y. E., B. J. De Bondt, M. Lacko, J. A. Hodge, and K. W. Kross. 2009. Laryngeal tuberculosis presenting as a supraglottic carcinoma: a case report and review of the literature. *J. Med. Case Rep.* **3**:9288.

91. Soda, A., H. Rubio, M. Salazar, J. Ganem, D. Berlanga, and A. Sanchez. 1989. Tuberculosis of the larynx: clinical aspects in 19 patients. *Laryngoscope* **99**:1147–1150.

92. Srirompotong, S., and K. Yimtae. 2002. Clinical aspects of tonsillar tuberculosis. *Southeast Asian J. Trop. Med. Public Health* **33**:147–150.

93. Srirompotong, S., and K. Yimtae. 2003. Tuberculosis in the upper aerodigestive tract and human immunodeficiency virus coinfections. *J. Otolaryngol.* **32**:230–233.

94. Sutbeyaz, Y., H. Ucuncu, R. Murat Karasen, and C. Gundogdu. 2000. The association of secondary tonsillar and laryngeal tuberculosis: a case report and literature review. *Auris Nasus Larynx* **27**:371–374.

95. Tas, A., R. Yagiz, M. Kocyigit, and A. R. Karasalihoglu. 2009. Primary nasopharyngeal tuberculosis. *Kulak Burun Bogaz Ihtis. Derg.* **19**:109–111.

96. Tato, A. M., J. Pascual, L. Orofino, G. Fernandez-Juarez, J. Martinez-San-Millan, L. Fogue, F. Liano, and J. Ortuno. 1998.

Laryngeal tuberculosis in renal allograft patients. *Am. J. Kidney Dis.* **31**:701–705.

97. Thakur, A., J. B. Coulter, K. Zutshi, H. K. Pande, M. Sharma, A. Banerjee, K. Richardson, and C. A. Hart. 1999. Laryngeal swabs for diagnosing tuberculosis. *Ann. Trop. Paediatr.* **19:** 333–336.

98. Thaller, S. R., J. R. Gross, B. Z. Pilch, and M. L. Goodman. 1987. Laryngeal tuberculosis as manifested in the decades 1963–1983. *Laryngoscope* **97**:848–850.

99. Thompson, M. M., M. J. Underwood, R. D. Sayers, K. A. Dookeran, and P. R. Bell. 1992. Peripheral tuberculous lymphadenopathy: a review of 67 cases. *Br. J. Surg.* **79**:763–764.

100. Tong, M. C., and C. A. van Hasselt. 1993. Tuberculous laryngitis. *Otolaryngol. Head Neck Surg.* **109**:965–966.

101. Topak, M., C. Oysu, K. Yelken, A. Sahin-Yilmaz, and M. Kulekci. 2008. Laryngeal involvement in patients with active pulmonary tuberculosis. *Eur. Arch. Otorhinolaryngol.* **265:** 327–330.

102. Tse, G. M., T. K. Ma, A. B. Chan, F. N. Ho, A. D. King, K. S. Fung, and A. T. Ahuja. 2003. Tuberculosis of the nasopharynx: a rare entity revisited. *Laryngoscope* **113**:737–740.

103. Wang, B. Y., M. J. Amolat, P. Woo, and M. Brandwein-Gensler. 2008. Atypical mycobacteriosis of the larynx: an unusual clinical presentation secondary to steroids inhalation. *Ann. Diagn. Pathol.* **12**:426–429.

104. Wang, C. C., C. C. Lin, C. P. Wang, S. A. Liu, and R. S. Jiang. 2007. Laryngeal tuberculosis: a review of 26 cases. *Otolaryngol. Head Neck Surg.* **137**:582–588.

105. Warndorff, D. K., J. R. Glynn, P. E. Fine, S. Jamil, M. Y. de Wit, M. M. Munthali, N. G. Stoker, and P. R. Klatser. 1996. Polymerase chain reaction of nasal swabs from tuberculosis patients and their contacts. *Int. J. Lepr. Other Mycobacter. Dis.* **64**:404–408.

106. Yamamoto, K., F. Iwata, A. Nakamura, Y. Iwashima, T. Miyaki, H. Yamada, M. Kurachi, Y. Sato, K. Tsukada, T. Takeuchi, T. Joh, Y. Yokoyama, and M. Itoh. 2002. Tonsillar tuberculosis associated with pulmonary and laryngeal foci. *Intern. Med.* **41**:664–666.

107. Yelken, K., M. Guven, M. Topak, E. Gultekin, and F. Turan. 2008. Effects of antituberculosis treatment on self assessment, perceptual analysis and acoustic analysis of voice quality in laryngeal tuberculosis patients. *J. Laryngol. Otol.* **122:** 378–382.

108. Yoruk, O., V. Fidan, and Y. Sutbeyaz. 2009. Hearing loss unusually caused by tubercular retropharyngeal abscess. *J. Craniofac. Surg.* **20**:955–957.

109. Yun, J. E., S. W. Lee, T. H. Kim, J. B. Jun, S. Jung, S. C. Bae, T. Y. Kim, and D. H. Yoo. 2002. The incidence and clinical characteristics of *Mycobacterium tuberculosis* infection among systemic lupus erythematosus and rheumatoid arthritis patients in Korea. *Clin. Exp. Rheumatol.* **20**:127–132.

Tuberculosis and Nontuberculous Mycobacterial Infections, 6th ed.
Edited by David Schlossberg
© 2011 ASM Press, Washington, DC

Chapter 16

Tuberculous Otomastoiditis

GEORGE A. PANKEY

Tuberculous otitis media and tuberculous mastoiditis occur together as a single disease process and are referred to herein as tuberculous otomastoiditis. One year after the isolation of the tubercle bacillus by Koch in 1882, the organism was cultured from a middle-ear lesion. Otologic tuberculosis has been relegated to the status of "other" in the list of localizations of tuberculosis by the American Thoracic Society in their *Diagnostic Standards and Classification of Tuberculosis and Other Mycobacterial Diseases, 1981* (1). Presumably, it was given this status because tuberculosis of the ear is extremely uncommon in the United States (11 cases reported from 1990 through 2003) (4). However, there are still occasional patients who have chronically draining ears due to *Mycobacterium tuberculosis* (7). In addition, the incidence of tuberculosis is high in the refugee population, especially those from Indochina (1,138 cases/100,000 refugees on arrival and 407/100,000 refugees per year thereafter) (3). These sources of patients with tuberculosis as well as those associated with human immunodeficiency virus infection will undoubtedly spawn other cases of tuberculous otomastoiditis; therefore, a brief summary of the problem is justified.

INCIDENCE

Most of the medical literature on tuberculous otomastoiditis is from Europe and Asia, where the disease is more prevalent. Between 1967 and 1979, 4,000 biological specimens of the middle ear were examined in Tübingen, Germany. Tuberculosis was found in 14 (0.1%), the youngest patient being 10 months and the oldest 69 years (11). In a review of patients at Massachusetts General Hospital and the Massachusetts Eye and Ear Infirmary from 1962 through 1984, there were four cases of tuberculous otomastoiditis out of 6,310 cases of chronic otitis media and out of 1,850 cases of tuberculosis (15). Vaamonde et al. diagnosed 10 cases from 1996

to 2002 in Spain (19). A recent study from Turkey found tuberculous otomastoiditis in 11 of 32 (34%) patients with tuberculous meningitis (18). Laryngitis and otitis media remain the most frequent ear, nose, and throat diseases of tuberculous origin (14).

PATHOGENESIS AND PATHOLOGY

Tuberculosis of the middle ear may be a primary infection in the area of the shorter and large-bored eustachian tube in neonates who have aspirated infected amniotic fluid or in older patients who have ingested and regurgitated tuberculous materials such as contaminated milk. Most cases occur secondarily, however, when organisms are coughed into the nasopharynx from pulmonary lesions or as the result of hematogenous spread. Preauricular or anterior cervical lymphadenopathy and facial nerve paralysis occur infrequently but are more likely with tuberculous than other types of bacterial otitis media.

Pathologically, the disease always involves the mucosa first, with extensive edema, infiltration by round and giant cells, granuloma formation, and, finally, caseation. Histopathology may be altered in immunocompromised patients. Thickening of the tympanic membrane is followed by perforation with associated destruction of the ossicles and purulent discharge. Secondarily, the periosteum becomes involved, followed months later by bone necrosis with resultant complications that are similar to those occurring with other infections of the middle ear and mastoid. The labyrinth appears to be at greatest risk in adults, and the facial nerve and meninges are the greatest risk areas in children (12). Hearing loss with a large neurosensory component is frequent in all patients.

DIAGNOSIS

The history and physical findings in both primary and secondary tuberculous otomastoiditis are

George A. Pankey • Infectious Diseases Research, Ochsner Clinic Foundation, 1514 Jefferson Highway, New Orleans, LA 70121.

frequently nonspecific. Smoler and colleagues (17) believe that in secondary tuberculous otomastoiditis the classic findings of chronic ear infection (otorrhea, absence of pain, and profound hearing loss) are never well defined because of suprainfection with other bacteria. An exception is damage to the facial nerve, paralysis of which is usually associated with tuberculosis. Tympanic membranes are often extensively damaged, with one or more perforations. Older patients may complain of tinnitus and "funny noises" (16).

Tuberculous otomastoiditis has to be considered in the differential diagnosis of chronic otitis media in tuberculous patients as well as in those who have no evidence of tuberculosis elsewhere and whose otorrhea does not improve with the usual medical treatment. A history of tuberculosis in a family member should arouse suspicion and lead to confirmatory studies. Tuberculous otomastoiditis may be masked by suprainfection with other bacteria as well as by systemic antituberculous therapy. Skin testing for tuberculosis in children and adults with chronic otorrhea should be mandatory, although results may be falsely negative (13). Gamma interferon release assays have been reported to be more sensitive and specific in diagnosing extrapulmonary tuberculosis (8). The diagnosis of tuberculous otomastoiditis is considered confirmed by culture of *M. tuberculosis* from the local discharge or biopsy sample. However, the diagnosis can be assumed if pulmonary tuberculosis is confirmed to be associated with chronic otomastoiditis in the absence of other pathogens. Positive acid-fast staining (auramine and Ziehl-Neelsen) of otorrhea is strongly suggestive. Nucleic acid amplification techniques (PCR) may be useful for patients for whom acid-fast stains are negative (6). Histopathological study of tissue as well as improvement following specific antituberculous therapy may support the diagnosis.

Primary tuberculosis of the middle ear is most difficult to diagnose. The tympanic membrane before perforation is swollen, yellowish, and hyperemic. Perforation follows in the untreated patient, and multiple perforations follow in 20 to 30%. In tuberculous otomastoiditis of both the primary and secondary types, abnormalities on X-ray films of the mastoid are less common than with other types of chronic otomastoiditis, but a computed tomography scan showing soft tissue filling the entire tympanum and mastoid air cells and cortical bone destruction without evidence of cholesteatoma is suggestive of tuberculous otomastoiditis (5). Propagation to the inner ear may occur in older children and adults when the disease is subacute and is manifested by slowly progressive hearing loss (initially of the high tones) as a result of cochlear destruction. Extension and hematogenous dissemination from tuberculous otomastoiditis are rare, as evidenced by the frequent chronicity of the disease for many years without such spread (19). The dura mater usually resists direct extension to the brain; however, tuberculous meningitis is definitely associated with chronic tuberculous otomastoiditis (2, 10, 18).

The frequencies of signs and symptoms in patients with tuberculous otomastoiditis before and after 1953 are shown in Table 1.

Differential diagnosis is broad, including histoplasmosis, North American blastomycosis, South American blastomycosis, syphilis, midline granulomas (lethal), Wegener's granulomatosis, sarcoidosis, histocytosis X, eosinophilic granuloma, nocardiosis, necrotizing external otitis, lymphoma, nontuberculous mycobacterial infection, and cholesteatoma.

Table 1. Frequencies of signs and symptoms in patients with tuberculous otomastoiditis[a]

Symptom or sign	No. (%) of patients with indicated feature reported in:			
	Pre-1953	Post-1953–1986	2004[c]	2006
Otorrhea	103 (82)	93 (92)	10 (100)	
Loss of hearing	18 (62)[b]	78 (90)[c]	10 (100)	
Ear pain	10 (0.08)	24 (6.2)	3 (30)	7 (13.2)
Perforations	27 (21)	71 (70)	9 (90)	
Granulations	22 (30)[d]	64 (63)	5 (50)	
Facial palsy	37 (30)	16 (16)	1 (10)	5 (9.6)
Aural polyp	4 (3.2)	13 (13)	1 (10)	
Preauricular lymph node	68 (54)	2 (0.02)	1 (10)	
Tinnitus			4 (40)	

[a]Note that fever, cough, weight loss, night sweats, and periauricular fistulae occurred in <1% of cases both before and after 1953. The percentages are based on the study population as described by Skolink et al. (15). Data came from references 5, 15, and 19.
[b]Ninety-six additional cases were excluded because of lack of adequate documentation.
[c]Fourteen additional cases were excluded because of lack of adequate documentation.
[d]Fifteen additional cases were excluded because of lack of adequate documentation.

TREATMENT

Once the diagnosis of tuberculous otomastoiditis is made, the combined talents of the primary care physician, an ear, nose, and throat surgeon, and an infectious disease specialist are required for optimum therapy. Isoniazid plus rifampin is the preferred antituberculous therapy, with pyrazinamide added for the first 2 months. Ethambutol is also usually given until resistant *M. tuberculosis* is ruled out. Final therapy is based on in vitro susceptibility studies. There have now been at least 12 cases of tuberculous otomastoiditis treated with short-course therapy with favorable responses. Ten were treated with isoniazid, rifampin, and pyrazinamide for 2 months, followed by 4 months (8 patients) or 7 months (2 patients) of isoniazid plus rifampin. Two other patients (1a) received isoniazid, rifampin, ethambutol, and pyrazinamide for 9 months. There are not enough cases of tuberculous otomastoiditis to conduct any treatment trials, but based on reported data most patients should be treated medically for 6 to 9 months.

In addition to obtaining tissue for diagnosis, the surgeon may have a role in therapy by removing a nidus of infected debris. Complications mandating surgical approach include facial nerve paralysis, subperiosteal abscess, labyrinthitis, persistent postauricular fistula, and extension of infection into the central nervous system (9). After therapy is completed, reconstructive procedures may improve hearing in certain patients.

REFERENCES

1. **American Thoracic Society.** 1981. Diagnostic standards and classification of tuberculosis and other mycobacterial diseases, 14th ed. *Am. Rev. Respir. Dis.* **123:**343–358.

1a. **Awan, M. S., and I. Salahuddin.** 2002. Tuberculous otitis media: two case reports and literature review. *Ear Nose Throat J.* **81:**792–794.

2. **Cawthon, T., R. H. Cox, and G. A. Pankey.** 1978. Tuberculous otitis media with complications. *South. Med. J.* **71:**602–604.

3. **Centers for Disease Control.** 1981. Tuberculosis among Indochinese refugees—an update. *MMWR Morb. Mortal. Wkly. Rep.* **30:**603–606.

4. **Chirch, L. M., K. Ahmad, W. Spinner, V. E. Jimenez, S. V. Donelan, and E. Smouha.** 2005. Tuberculous otitis media: report of 2 cases on Long Island, N.Y., and a review of all cases reported in the United States from 1990 through 2003. *Ear Nose Throat J.* **84:**488–497.

5. **Cho, Y. S., H. S. Lee, S. W. Kim, K. H. Chung, D. K. Lee, W. J. Koh, and M. G. Kim.** 2006. Tuberculous otitis media: a clinical and radiologic analysis of 52 patients. *Laryngoscope* **116:**921–927.

6. **Garcovich, A., L. Romano, A. Zampetti, S. Garcovich, F. Ardito, B. Posteraro, M. Sanguinetti, and G. Fadda.** 2004. Tumour-like ear lesion due to *Mycobacterium tuberculosis* diagnosed by polymerase chain reaction-reverse hybridization. *Br. J. Dermatol.* **150:**370–371.

7. **Kirsch, C. M., J. H. Wehner, W. A. Jensen, F. T. Kagawa, and A. C. Campagna.** 1995. Tuberculous otitis media. *South. Med. J.* **88:**363–366.

8. **Kobashi, Y., K. Mouri, S. Yagi, Y. Obase, N. Miyashita, and M. Oka.** 2009. Clinical utility of a T cell-based assay in the diagnosis of extrapulmonary tuberculosis. *Respirology* **14:**276–281.

9. **Lucente, F. E., G. W. Tobias, S. C. Parisier, and P. M. Som.** 1978. Tuberculous otitis media. *Laryngoscope* **88:**1107–1116.

10. **Mongkolrattanothai, K., R. Oram, M. Redleaf, J. Bova, and J. A. Englund.** 2003. Tuberculous otitis media with mastoiditis and central nervous system involvement. *Pediatr. Infect. Dis. J.* **22:**453–456.

11. **Plester, D., A. Pusalkar, and E. Steinbach.** 1980. Middle ear tuberculosis. *J. Laryngol. Otol.* **94:**1415–1421.

12. **Rice, D. H.** 1977. Pathologic quiz case 2. *Arch. Otolaryngol.* **103:**112–115.

13. **Saltzman, S. J., and R. D. Feigin.** 1971. Tuberculous otitis media and mastoiditis. *J. Pediatr.* **79:**1004–1006.

14. **Sellars, S. L., and A. B. Seid.** 1973. Aural tuberculosis in childhood. *S. Afr. Med. J.* **47:**216–218.

15. **Skolnik, P. R., J. B. Nadol, Jr., and A. S. Baker.** 1986. Tuberculosis of the middle ear: review of the literature with an instructive case report. *Rev. Infect. Dis.* **8:**403–410.

16. **Smith, M. H. D., J. R. Starke, and J. R. Marquis.** 1992. Tuberculosis and other mycobacterial infections, p. 1339. *In* R. D. Feigin and J. D. Cherry (ed.), *Textbook of Pediatric Infectious Diseases*, 3rd ed., vol. 1. W. B. Saunders, Philadelphia, PA.

17. **Smoler, J., S. L. Pinto, G. Vivar, and J. L. Ramirez.** 1969. Tuberculous otitis media. *Laryngoscope* **79:**488–493.

18. **Sonmez, G., V. Turhan, M. G. Senol, E. Ozturk, H. O. Sildiroglu, and H. Mutlu.** 2008. Relationship between tuberculous otomastoiditis and tuberculous meningitis. *J. Laryngol. Otol.* **122:**893–897.

19. **Vaamonde, P., C. Castro, N. García-Soto, T. Labella, and A. Lozano.** 2004. Tuberculous otitis media: a significant diagnostic challenge. *Otolaryngol. Head Neck Surg.* **130:**759–766.

Tuberculosis and Nontuberculous Mycobacterial Infections, 6th ed.
Edited by David Schlossberg
© 2011 ASM Press, Washington, DC

Chapter 17

Ocular Tuberculosis

Daniel M. Albert, Matthew J. Thompson, and Robert J. Peralta

HISTORICAL CONSIDERATIONS

Maitre-Jan (55) is often credited with publishing the earliest description of ocular tuberculosis (1707). Major contributions to the understanding of the disease mechanism were not made until the latter part of the 19th century. In 1855, Eduard von Jaeger first described the ophthalmoscopic appearance of choroidal tubercles (93). Cohnheim, in 1867 (20), showed that choroidal tubercles were similar microscopically to tubercles found elsewhere in the body and postulated that ocular involvement was a metastatic manifestation of systemic infection. In addition, Cohnheim was able to produce similar lesions in guinea pigs by injecting them with tuberculous material. In 1882, Koch identified the tubercle bacillus as the causative agent (49), and 1 year later Julius von Michael identified the organism in the eye (94).

INCIDENCE

The reported incidence of ocular involvement varies considerably, depending on the criteria used for diagnosis and the population sampled. Early medical writers considered the infection rare. However, the diagnosis was usually reserved for patients with obvious clinical tubercles. In 1890, Terson (89) reported two cases of tuberculous iritis in a population of 30,000 patients with ocular disease. In patients with known systemic tuberculosis, the incidence of ocular involvement is, as expected, much higher (27, 36, 38). A study reported in 1967 found an incidence of ocular tuberculosis of 1.4% in 10,524 patients at a tuberculosis sanitarium (27). In this group, 74 patients had uveal involvement; 54 had scleral or corneal involvement, including three cases of corneal ulcers; and 12 patients showed disseminated retinitis. Rarer manifestations were retinal periphlebitis (seven cases), phlyctenular

conjunctivitis (six cases), and tuberculosis of the optic nerve (one case). This study illustrates the variety of ocular tissues that can be affected by tuberculosis.

In a more recent series, Rosen et al., in 1990, reported 12 patients with intraocular tuberculosis, 9 of whom presented with retinal vasculitis, 2 with choroidal tubercles, and 1 with chronic anterior uveitis (78). In a prospective study from Spain, Bouza et al. examined 100 randomly selected patients from a population of 300 patients with proven systemic tuberculosis (14). Ocular involvement was diagnosed in 18 patients (18%). Choroidal involvement was present in all but one of these, and retinal involvement was found in 6 patients. Involvement of the anterior segment, sclera, and orbit were noted in single cases. There was an association between miliary tuberculosis and ocular involvement but no association between human immunodeficiency virus (HIV) positivity and ocular tuberculosis (14). Ocular involvement was associated with decreased visual acuity and other ocular symptoms.

A prospective study from Malawi, Africa, reported 3 patients with choroidal granulomas (2.8%) among 109 patients presenting with fever and tuberculosis (8). In patients presenting with uveitis in India, 0.6% of cases were felt to be caused by tuberculosis (9). In a prospective case series in Japan, 20.6% of 126 patients with uveitis had a positive tuberculosis skin test, and 7.9% were believed to have intraocular tuberculosis (62). In Saudi Arabia, tuberculosis was thought to be the cause in 10.5% of cases of uveitis seen in a major ophthalmic referral center (44). In patients presenting with uveitis in Boston between 1982 and 1992, tuberculosis caused this disease in 0.6% of cases (77). These studies reflect the wide variation in the reported incidence of ocular tuberculosis in differing populations and at various time periods.

Recently, a retrospective study by Babu et al. examined 766 consecutive patients coinfected with

Daniel M. Albert and Robert J. Peralta • Department of Ophthalmology and Visual Sciences, University of Wisconsin School of Medicine and Public Health, Madison, WI 53792. **Matthew J. Thompson** • Tower Clock Eye Center, 1087 West Mason Street, Green Bay, WI 54303.

tuberculosis and HIV/AIDS in southern India (6). Ocular tuberculosis was found in 15 patients (19 eyes, 2.0%), the largest cohort in the reported literature. The most common presentation was choroidal tuberculoma (10 cases), followed by subretinal abscess (7), panophthalmitis (1), and a conjunctival mass (1). Three of the seven cases of subretinal abscess progressed to panophthalmitis, a phenomenon rarely encountered in immunocompetent patients. While the previously cited work of Bouza et al. found no association between ocular tuberculosis and HIV/AIDS (14), these findings suggest that coinfection may lead to worse outcomes.

BASIC MECHANISMS OF INFECTION

The eye can become infected with tuberculosis through several different mechanisms.

1. The most common form of ocular involvement is from hematogenous spread. The uveal tract (i.e., the iris, ciliary body, and choroid) is the coat of the eye most frequently involved, presumably because of its high vascular content.

2. Primary exogenous infection of the eye, while unusual, can occur in the lids or in the conjunctiva. Other external tissues less commonly infected include the cornea, sclera, and lacrimal sac.

3. Secondary infection of the eye may occur by direct extension from surrounding tissues or by contamination with the patient's own sputum.

4. Additionally, some forms of ocular tuberculosis, such as phlyctenular disease and Eales' disease, are thought to be the result of a hypersensitivity reaction. Attempts to establish an animal model for phlyctenular disease have led to various results (35, 80, 90).

Rich's law states that the extent of a tuberculous lesion is directly proportional to the number and virulence of the bacilli as well as the degree of hypersensitivity of the infected tissue (75). It is inversely proportional to the host's native and acquired resistance to the organism. Alan Woods was the first to utilize Rich's law to divide ocular tuberculosis into four distinct categories (95). Woods' four categories can be summarized as follows.

1. Foreign body-like reaction (e.g., miliary tubercles of the iris and choroid)
2. Acute circumscribed inflammation that may recur if the patient's resistance decreases (e.g., sclerokeratitis or Eales' disease)
3. Chronic inflammation with multiple recurrences (e.g., ciliary body tuberculoma)
4. Acute, rapidly spreading inflammation with necrosis, caseation, and occasionally a ruptured globe (tuberculous panophthalmitis)

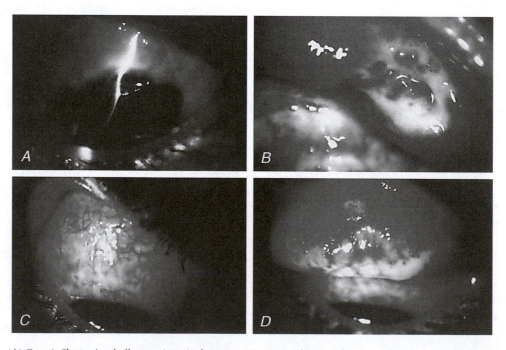

Figure 1. (A) Case 1. Shown is a bulbar conjunctival mass contiguous with a peripheral corneal ulcer with 80% stromal thinning. (B) Everted upper eyelid shows diffuse papillary reaction with tarsal necrosis laterally. (C) Case 2. Downgaze shows ulcerated bulbar conjunctiva. (D) Everted upper eyelid shows diffuse velvety appearance, with cheesy white areas of necrosis involving the upper tarsal border. Reprinted with permission from the *Archives of Ophthalmology* (31). Copyright 2003 American Medical Association. All rights reserved.

EXTERNAL DISEASE

Tuberculosis can involve the lid, conjunctiva, cornea, and sclera. Tuberculous lid disease is rarely an isolated ocular finding, but it can manifest as an acute abscess (96) (a "cold abscess") or as a soft fluctuant mass without acute inflammation, a form that usually occurs in children (59). The skin of the lids may also display lupus vulgaris, the most common form of cutaneous tuberculosis, characterized by reddish-brown nodules that blanch to an "apple jelly" color when pressure is applied (26, 78). Primary infection of the conjunctiva has been reported (17, 31), although it

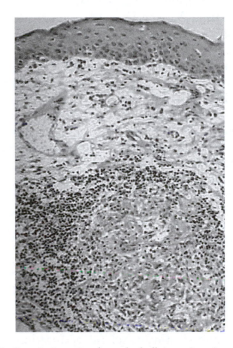

Figure 2. Case 1. A section from the bulbar conjunctiva shows an intact epithelium with discrete epithelioid cell granuloma in the deeper stroma, rimmed by lymphocytes (hematoxylin-eosin; original magnification, ×250). Reprinted with permission from the *Archives of Ophthalmology* (31). Copyright 2003 American Medical Association. All rights reserved.

is unusual in developed countries. Patients usually present with ocular redness, discomfort, mucopurulent discharge, and lid edema. There is often an accompanying marked lymphadenitis (more common in the secondary form), which is absent in most other types of bacterial and allergic conjunctivitis and is less prominent in viral conjunctivitis. Typically, primary tuberculous conjunctivitis is a chronic disease that may lead to scarring of the involved tissue. The young are more susceptible to this form of tuberculosis than are the elderly. Diagnosis usually requires a high degree of clinical suspicion and positive identification of the organism with traditional acid-fast bacillus (AFB) stains or PCR on either a conjunctival smear or a biopsy sample (21, 46) (Fig. 1 to 3).

Corneal involvement can have the appearance of either phlyctenular keratoconjunctivitis or an interstitial keratitis. In phlyctenular keratoconjunctivitis, a small nodule is first noted at the limbus. The nodule generally migrates centrally, "dragging" superficial vessels along. Initially the overlying epithelium is intact, but it often erodes, leading to an epithelial defect. The presentation includes photophobia, foreign-body sensation, redness, and tearing. The severity of symptoms usually corresponds to the degree of corneal involvement (Fig. 4). As previously noted, phlyctenular disease is believed to be a hypersensitivity reaction to a mycobacterial protein. Phlyctenulosis appears to be associated with a positive tuberculin skin test (73). It is, however, rare among patients with proven systemic tuberculosis (27). Attempts have been made to reproduce phlyctenular disease in animal models, with mixed success (35, 80, 90). In confirmed tuberculosis cases, treatment consists of systemic antituberculous chemotherapy in conjunction with topical steroids. Cycloplegia substantially relieves ocular discomfort, and topical antibiotics may be used as prophylaxis against secondary bacterial superinfection if epithelial defects are present.

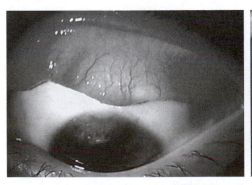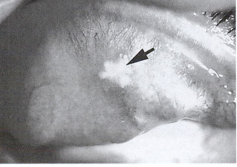

Figure 3. (A) Case 1. At 1-year follow-up, the left eye shows a superior vascularized corneal scar with normal-appearing bulbar and tarsal conjunctiva. (B) Case 2. At 3-month follow-up, the everted right upper eyelid shows a residual area of necrosis (arrow) with mild persistent papillary reaction. Reprinted with permission from the *Archives of Ophthalmology* (31). Copyright 2003 American Medical Association. All rights reserved.

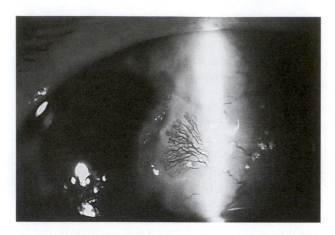

Figure 4. Slit lamp picture of the left cornea showing a peripheral corneal ulcer and a heavily vascularized nodule. Reprinted with permission from the *Archives of Ophthalmology* (33a). Copyright 2000 American Medical Association. All rights reserved.

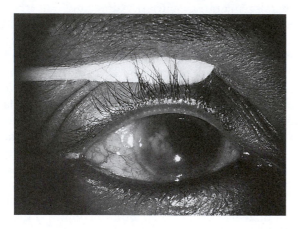

Figure 5. Clinical appearance of a right eye shows mild conjunctival vasodilation and numerous confluent, temporal, tan iris nodules. Reprinted with permission from the *Archives of Ophthalmology* (79). Copyright 1998 American Medical Association. All rights reserved.

Interstitial keratitis is a term used to describe inflammation and vascularization of the corneal stroma without endothelial or epithelial involvement. Tuberculous interstitial keratitis is characteristically unilateral and is seen clinically as a sectoral, peripheral stromal infiltrate with vascularization. Treatment consists of systemic as well as topical antituberculosis chemotherapy and cycloplegia. As in the case with phlyctenular keratoconjunctivitis, mycobacterial proteins are postulated as antigens that induce a corneal hypersensitivity reaction (87).

Tuberculous scleritis is rare but should be considered in patients who are unresponsive to the usual anti-inflammatory therapy for scleritis. Bloomfield and associates (13) reported a case of tuberculous scleritis in an 82-year-old female with extensive pulmonary tuberculosis. This type of scleritis usually presents as a localized area of dark red discoloration of the sclera with chronic granulomatous inflammation and caseous necrosis. Nanda and coworkers (65) discussed a case of an 81-year-old male with culture-proven scleral tuberculosis. The patient initially presented with a scleral ulcer that worsened after initiation of oral prednisone (a medication often used for necrotizing scleritis). Examination of scrapings of the ulcer subsequently revealed numerous AFB. The patient responded rapidly to topical amikacin and the combination of oral rifampin and isoniazid (Fig. 5 and 6). Kesen and colleagues reported a case of a 54-year-old female with multidrug-resistant tuberculosis, pulmonary involvement, and nodular scleritis. Cultures and AFB stains of tissue sections and bodily fluids, including bronchoalveolar lavage fluid, were negative. Despite treatment, scleral perforation ensued. Following enucleation, PCR of the sclera was positive for tuberculosis (47).

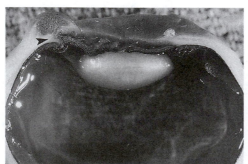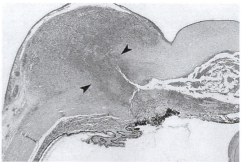

Figure 6. (Left) Gross appearance of the enucleated right eye. Note the scleral necrosis and the perilimbal scleral rupture (arrowhead) located interiorly. The limbal conjunctiva covers a dome-shaped, brown mass. (Right) Histopathological appearance of the enucleated right eye with a subconjunctival necrotic and inflammatory mass. There is necrosis of the iris, and the anterior chamber contains necrotic debris (arrowheads) (hematoxylin-eosin; original magnification, ×5). Reprinted with permission from the *Archives of Ophthalmology* (79). Copyright 1998 American Medical Association. All rights reserved.

UVEITIS

Until well into the 20th century, many cases of uveitis were attributed to presumed tuberculosis. It was gradually appreciated, however, that brucellosis, sarcoidosis, toxoplasmosis, and other infections can also cause uveitis with a similar clinical picture. Moreover, it was realized that uveitis in a tuberculosis patient may not be the direct result of an acid-fast infection. Accordingly, the apparent incidence of tuberculosis as the etiology of uveitis at the Wilmer Institute fell from 79% in 1944 to 22% in 1953 (95). The incidence of uveitis caused by tuberculosis at the Massachusetts Eye and Ear Infirmary from 1982 through 1992 was reported to be 0.6% (77). In parts of the world where the prevalence of tuberculosis infection is higher in the general population, uveitis is still more likely to be attributed to tuberculosis. In patients presenting with uveitis in India, 0.6% of cases were felt to be caused by tuberculosis (9). In a prospective case series in Japan, 20.6% of 126 patients with uveitis had a positive tuberculin skin test, and 7.9% were felt to have intraocular tuberculosis (62). As previously noted, in Saudi Arabia, tuberculosis was stated to be the cause in 10.5% of uveitis cases seen in referral centers (44).

Tuberculous uveitis is classically a chronic granulomatous disease and is often accompanied by other ocular manifestations of chronic granulomatous inflammation, such as mutton fat keratic precipitates (collections of inflammatory cells and macrophages) on the posterior aspect of the cornea as well as iris nodules. A nongranulomatous uveitis also occurs in tuberculosis, usually manifesting as small white keratic precipitates and an absence of iris nodules (1). In both granulomatous and nongranulomatous inflammation, there is inflammation of the anterior segment, and inflammatory cells and flare (the slit lamp manifestation of protein in the aqueous humor) can be seen in the anterior chamber. Uveitis can also manifest as simple iritis, the clinical signs of which are limited to cells and flare in the anterior chamber, or as iridocyclitis with involvement of the ciliary body. Iridocyclitis occurs clinically with inflammatory cells in the ciliary body and anterior vitreous and is associated with ciliary body pain and ciliary vasodilation. Alternatively, the inflammation may involve primarily the posterior part of the uvea (choroids), leading to choroiditis, the most common manifestation of ocular tuberculosis.

CHOROIDITIS

Choroidal tubercles are usually multiple. In one of two reported cases of tuberculous choroiditis

associated with AIDS, the posterior pole was riddled with "innumerable" tubercles (12), whereas in the second case only two tubercles were seen (22). The tubercles may appear as white, gray, or yellow lesions with indistinct borders and may be accompanied by hemorrhages, exudates, or surrounding edema. Their size varies from about 0.5 to 3.0 mm in diameter, which may be estimated at the time of examination by comparing the extent of the lesions to the size of the optic disc, which is about 1.5 mm in diameter. Choroidal tubercles are usually found in the posterior pole and, when present, should be distinctly seen on careful examination with the direct ophthalmoscope (Fig. 7).

Paton (70) described the sudden appearance of choroidal tubercles in a patient 4 days after admission. The lesions were not observed on previous examinations, illustrating the potential need for repeated careful fundus examinations to demonstrate choroidal tubercles. In one series, only a single case of choroidal tubercles had been observed clinically in 63 autopsy cases with acute miliary tuberculosis (18). The authors suggested that this low incidence was the result of inadequate ophthalmoscopic examinations. Another study found a 60% incidence of choroidal tubercles (43). To permit an adequate examination, all pupils were dilated, the small children studied were sedated, and the average time devoted to each fundus examination in a child was 30 min.

Choroidal tubercles should always be looked for on funduscopic examination when a patient is suspected to have tuberculosis or has a fever of unknown origin. The finding of choroidal tubercles is specific and allows the early institution of antituberculosis therapy even before the diagnosis is confirmed by positive sputum specimens. Although it has been claimed that choroidal tubercles occur only in terminally ill patients with miliary tuberculosis or tuberculous meningitis (70), the literature indicates that they can occur in a variety of clinical circumstances. Illingsworth and Wright (43) reported the occurrence of choroidal tubercles in very young children with acute miliary tuberculosis. A case was described in which miliary tubercles were associated with optic neuropathy but without other systemic lesions (56). Massaro and colleagues (57) emphasized that tubercles occasionally occur in patients with pulmonary tuberculosis without evidence of miliary tuberculosis. Mehta and associates found choroidal tubercles in 34.6% of 52 patients with neurotuberculosis, diagnosed by the presence of intracranial granulomas or tuberculous meningitis (60). About half of these patients with neurotuberculosis had systemic involvement. The odds ratio for the presence of systemic tuberculosis with choroidal tubercles was 5.6

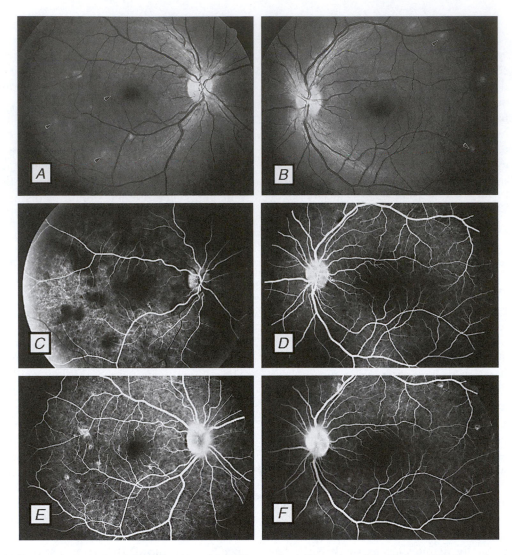

Figure 7. Fundus photographs of the right (A) and left (B) eyes show bilateral, multifocal choroiditis (arrowheads). Serial fluorescein angiographic photographs (C to F) show early blocking hypofluorescence and late-staining hyperfluorescence corresponding to areas of choroidal infiltrate, as well as mild, late leakage from the optic nerve heads in each eye. Reprinted with permission from the *Archives of Ophthalmology* (39). Copyright 1998 American Medical Association. All rights reserved.

to 1, providing further evidence that choroidal tubercles may be one of the earliest signs of disseminated disease. There have been reports of other manifestations of tuberculous infection of the choroid, including multifocal choroiditis (39) and serpiginous-like choroiditis (40).

Several cases of tuberculous choroiditis in patients with AIDS and systemic tuberculosis have been reported (64, 72). The choroidal tubercles in three patients were discovered after the initiation of systemic antituberculous chemotherapy when they were considered to be in a healing stage (72). One patient with central nervous system tuberculosis and tuberculous choroiditis improved dramatically after initiation of triple antituberculous therapy. The cerebrospinal fluid findings returned to normal, and visual acuity improved from 20/200 to 20/20 (60).

It has been suggested that ocular tuberculosis may occur more often in immunocompromised patients. In a study of eyes from the autopsies of AIDS patients, however, intraocular tuberculosis was found in 2 eyes of 235 patients (63). Additionally, Babu and colleagues found ocular tuberculosis present in only 1.95% of patients with HIV/AIDS (15 of 766 consecutive cases) (6). Although HIV is an important risk factor for having systemic tuberculosis, the likelihood of ocular involvement being present does not appear to be related to the HIV status of the patient (14).

Before the advent of chemotherapy, the prognosis for patients with choroidal tubercles was uniformly poor. However, the prognosis is much improved with the rapid use of systemic antituberculous agents. No specific local therapy is needed. Many of these lesions regress completely, with minimal residual damage (25,

57, 67). Other lesions heal with focal chorioretinal scars. An exception to this rule may be tuberculous choroiditis in the setting of AIDS: the ocular changes have been reported to progress in spite of vigorous antituberculous chemotherapy (22). Reports of acquired resistance of mycobacteria are increasing (86), and such resistance may be caused by several mechanisms. In the case reported by Snider and coworkers (86), "resistance" was thought to be the result of incomplete antibiotic treatment and occurred after 8 months of isoniazid and rifampin therapy.

CHOROIDAL TUBERCULOMAS

Whereas choroidal tubercles are generally small and multiple, tuberculomas are usually larger lesions (up to 7 mm in diameter) and solitary. They are typically better defined and have less surrounding edema than tubercles (Fig. 8 to 12). Tuberculomas have a

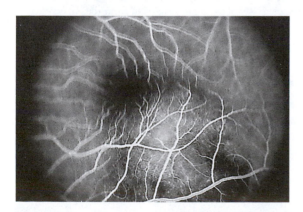

Figure 8. B-scan ultrasonogram of the left eye showing an acoustically dense choroidal lesion with no choroidal excavation. Reprinted with permission from the *Archives of Ophthalmology* (56a). Copyright 2000 American Medical Association. All rights reserved.

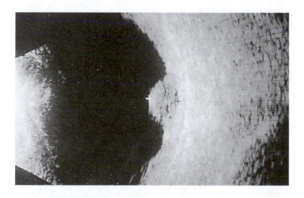

Figure 9. Fluorescein angiogram in the early venous phase showing early blockage at the edges of the lesion and early hyperfluorescence within the central aspect of the choroidal lesion; the overlying retinal vessels are normal and in focus. The other retinal vessels are not in focus secondary to the thickness of the lesion. Reprinted with permission from the *Archives of Ophthalmology* (56a). Copyright 2000 American Medical Association. All rights reserved.

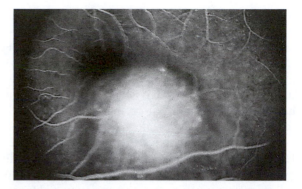

Figure 10. Fluorescein angiogram in the late phase revealing late staining of the choroidal lesion. Reprinted with permission from the *Archives of Ophthalmology* (56a). Copyright 2000 American Medical Association. All rights reserved.

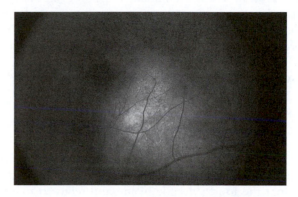

Figure 11. Fundus photograph showing a white choroidal lesion causing the fovea to be ectopic. Reprinted with permission from the *Archives of Ophthalmology* (56a). Copyright 2000 American Medical Association. All rights reserved.

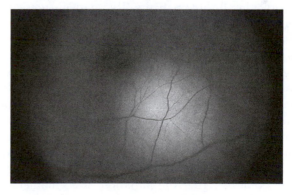

Figure 12. Fundus photograph of the left eye showing resolution of the choroidal tubercle with retinal pigment epithelium stippling within the resolving choroidal tubercle. Reprinted with permission from the *Archives of Ophthalmology* (56a). Copyright 2000 American Medical Association. All rights reserved.

predilection for the foveal and perifoveal area. Large tubercles have been confused with metastatic tumors, leading to unnecessary enucleation (83). Tuberculomas of the uveal tract tend to occur in young adults and have a chronic course with symptoms persisting over months to years (66). Affected patients often have a history of old, healed pulmonary tuberculosis, although sometimes the presumed diagnosis of choroidal tuberculosis may lead to the subsequent diagnosis and treatment of pulmonary tuberculosis (45).

Fluorescein angiography in patients with choroidal tuberculosis shows early hyperfluorescence with choroidal leakage, normal or slightly dilated overlying retinal vessels, late leakage, and, in some cases, associated serous neurosensory retinal detachment (16, 45, 53). Fluorescein angiography is useful in differentiating among choroidal hemangiomas, foreign bodies, metastatic tumors, and melanoma. Fluorescein angiography cannot distinguish between tuberculosis and other granulomatous inflammations such as sarcoid. Serial fluorescein angiography may also be useful to assess the patient's responses to therapy (16). Ultrasound has also been found to be useful in the diagnosis of choroidal tuberculomas (14). The prognosis for resolution of the lesion is usually good with systemic treatment, but if the macular region is involved, visual loss may be permanent (37).

CILIARY BODY TUBERCULOMA

Ciliary body tuberculoma is a rare but aggressive form of uveal tuberculosis. It occurs most frequently before the fourth decade of life and tends to follow a chronic, smoldering course with intermittent recurrences. Ni and associates (66) reported three cases that were enucleated at the Shanghai First Hospital. Results of the purified protein derivative (PPD) test were positive in all three patients. Two patients presented with painless loss of vision and a 1-month to 5-year history of intraocular inflammation. All patients were in generally good health, and only one patient had signs of systemic tuberculosis on examination. There was evidence of granulomatous anterior uveitis in all three patients. On histopathological examination, the eyes showed inflammatory infiltrates of the iris consisting of plasma cells, monocytes, lymphocytes, and typical caseous granulomas in the ciliary body. The authors reported that the fellow eyes of two patients did well after the initiation of chemotherapy; the third patient was lost to follow-up.

TUBERCULOUS RETINITIS

Tuberculosis of the retina most commonly results from the direct extension from the underlying uvea but may also be caused by hematogenous spread. Retinal lesions may take the form of either focal tubercles or diffuse retinitis. The clinical features include vitreous opacification, gray-white retinal

lesions (87), and, rarely, an isolated vasculitis (84) or retinal vascular tumor (51).

Neovascularization and peripheral capillary occlusion have been described in cases of choroiditis, chorioretinitis, and retinal vasculitis (Fig. 13 to 15) (19, 42, 78). A combination of systemic treatment and retinal photocoagulation has been advocated for treatment of retinal neovascularization related to tuberculosis (42, 78).

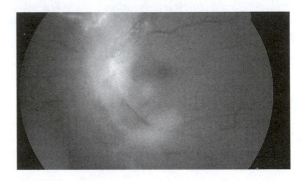

Figure 13. Retinitis and retinal neovascularization obscuring a clear view of the optic disc in a fundus photograph. Reprinted with permission from the *Archives of Ophthalmology* (82a). Copyright 1998 American Medical Association. All rights reserved.

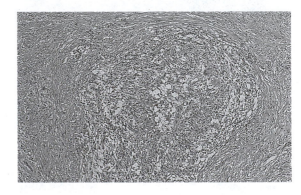

Figure 14. Noncaseating granuloma from a transvitreal biopsy specimen. Reprinted with permission from the *Archives of Ophthalmology* (82a). Copyright 1998 American Medical Association. All rights reserved.

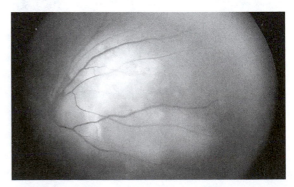

Figure 15. Left fundus photograph illustrating optic disc new vessels with choroidal mass nasally. Reprinted with permission from the *Archives of Ophthalmology* (82a). Copyright 1998 American Medical Association. All rights reserved.

Fountain and Werner (32) described a case of central retinal vein occlusion associated with active pulmonary tuberculosis. Fundus examination revealed engorged and tortuous retinal veins, sheathing of retinal vessels, and dot and blot hemorrhages in the posterior pole, as well as the typical gray-white retinal lesions.

Eales' disease, a poorly understood form of retinal perivasculitis, has sometimes been linked to tuberculosis (30, 95). The disease predominately affects the peripheral retina and is most common in young and otherwise healthy adults (10). Patients with Eales' disease often present with a sudden painless decrease in vision secondary to a vitreous hemorrhage. After the vitreous hemorrhage clears, perivascular exudates and hemorrhages are visible along the retinal vessels. The vasculitis can progress to venous thrombosis, neovascularization, glial tissue proliferation, and eventual tractional retinal detachment. There have been reports of patients with Eales' disease who have had PCR examination of vitreous fluid and epiretinal membrane tissue that was positive for *Mycobacterium tuberculosis* DNA, which supports the contention that tuberculosis is causative for Eales' disease (10, 54). Positive cultures of *M. tuberculosis* could not be successfully grown from any of these samples, suggesting that nonviable organisms in Eales' disease may incite a hypersensitivity reaction (41).

TUBERCULOUS PANOPHTHALMITIS

Acute tuberculous panophthalmitis usually occurs in children or severely ill adults with evidence of systemic tuberculosis. The duration of ocular involvement and of symptoms is relatively short (1 to 2 months). Presentation includes painless, progressive visual loss, decreased ocular motility, corneal cloudiness, signs of granulomatous ocular inflammation, and low intraocular pressure. Perforation of the globe can occur, usually at a site near the equator. Predisposing factors for systemic spread to the eye include poor nutrition, chronic illness, and intravenous drug abuse (45, 66).

There have been reports of tuberculous panophthalmitis and endophthalmitis masquerading as ocular tumors (23, 24). A case of tuberculous panophthalmitis has been described to occur in a woman with systemic lupus erythematosus. She initially presented with a serous retinal detachment that progressed to panophthalmitis with no light perception and glaucoma. Tuberculosis was diagnosed in a patient after enucleation, with recurring postoperative orbital abscesses which improved after administration of systemic antituberculous therapy (3).

ORBITAL TUBERCULOSIS

Tuberculosis of the orbit is extremely rare in the United States and Europe. A review of the literature revealed only five cases reported in the Western literature over the past 50 years (48). Three cases were associated with pulmonary tuberculosis (74, 85, 88), one with tuberculous sinusitis, and one with tuberculous pericarditis (48). Four of the five cases presented with ocular symptoms which included pain and proptosis (48), lid swelling (85), and intermittent periorbital swelling associated with headache and epistaxis (88). In one case, proptosis was an incidental finding in a patient who presented with fatigue, dry cough, and fever (48). Among other clinical findings in the five cases were decreased vision and visual field abnormalities, chemosis, Marcus Gunn pupil, epiphora, increased orbital resistance to retropulsion, and an orbital mass visualized on computerized tomography. Diagnosis was confirmed in four cases by orbital tissue biopsy and culture. In four cases, the orbital masses were monitored with computed tomography and observed to resolve over the 3 months to 6 months following the initiation of systemic antituberculous chemotherapy; one case was treated with additional surgery.

A case of orbital tuberculosis in a 37-year-old American man (74) manifested with a recurring orbital abscess that was not responding to repeated drainage and broad-spectrum antibiotic therapy and steroids. Tuberculosis was diagnosed by histopathological examination of an orbital biopsy sample obtained 1 month after initial presentation.

In India, where tuberculosis is endemic, cases of orbital tuberculosis are more common. In one report, three cases of isolated presumed orbital tuberculoma in children were described. The patients presented with painful proptosis, low-grade fever, lid swelling, mechanical ptosis, and decreased vision. In all three cases, tuberculous mycobacteria were found in orbital fine-needle aspiration specimens. Symptoms improved with systemic antituberculous therapy (28, 58). There have also been reports from Europe of a Somalian child with an orbital tuberculosis abscess and a woman presenting with dacryoadenitis secondary to tuberculosis (76, 91).

DIAGNOSIS

Before the introduction of PCR technology, a definitive diagnosis of ocular tuberculosis was often elusive because it required the demonstration of the *Mycobacterium tuberculosis* bacilli in ocular tissues or secretions by microscopy or culture. Opportunities for culture and biopsy may arise in cases of eyelid, orbital, or corneal involvement. The majority of cases, however, show intraocular involvement wherein a biopsy is not practical. Aqueous and vitreous paracentesis has generally failed to yield positive bacterial cultures (95). In addition to the difficulty of isolating the organism, the extreme variability of ocular manifestations makes routine clinical diagnosis difficult. Finally, the similarity to the presentation of other granulomatous inflammations adds to the diagnostic challenge. As a result, the vast majority of cases with a clinical diagnosis of ocular tuberculosis but without a definitive laboratory diagnosis should more correctly be labeled "presumed ocular tuberculosis."

Woods (95) outlines a thorough diagnostic approach to suspected ocular tuberculosis. Because the majority of ocular cases are associated with systemic findings, a complete history (including exposures and systemic symptoms), physical examination, sputum smear and culture, PPD test, and chest radiography should be performed. Other possible causes of granulomatous inflammation, such as syphilis, brucellosis, toxoplasmosis, *Toxocara* infection, and sarcoid, must be ruled out by history, examination, and appropriate serologic testing.

An initial workup that yields negative results should not eliminate tuberculosis from the differential diagnosis. Abrams and Schlaegel point out that the chest radiograph showed no active or inactive evidence of tuberculosis in 17 of 18 cases of tuberculous uveitis. They caution against requiring a strongly positive PPD response to make the diagnosis of ocular tuberculosis (2). The PPD is less likely to be reactive in immunosuppressed patients. These authors report that of 18 patients with presumed tuberculous uveitis (based on history, physical examination, tests to rule out other etiologies, tuberculin skin test, and the isoniazid therapeutic test) who were tested with intermediate-strength (5 tuberculin units) PPD, only 9 experienced at least 5 mm of induration, 5 experienced no reactivity at all, and 4 had erythema only. The 5 with no reaction to the intermediate PPD were retested with the second-strength PPD (250 tuberculin units). Only two patients experienced more than 5 mm of reaction. All of the reported cases improved clinically with an isoniazid therapeutic test (3 weeks of 300 mg of isoniazid per day) and remained inflammation free, without relapse, during 1 year of antituberculous treatment. An isoniazid therapeutic trial was recommended for patients with uveitis in whom tuberculosis was the suspected etiology on the basis of either history or a positive reaction to an intermediate-strength PPD test. An isoniazid test result is considered positive if there is "dramatic improvement" in 1 to 3 weeks of

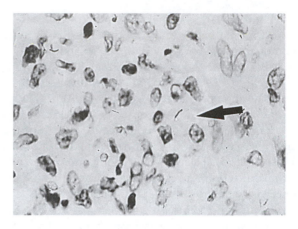

Figure 16. Acid-fast stain of a conjunctival biopsy specimen shows acid-fast positive rods (arrow) within epithelioid histiocytes.

therapy. This trial, however, may be falsely negative in patients with AIDS or in cases of drug-resistant disease (Fig. 16).

With the development of diagnostic molecular biology techniques, diagnosis based on detection of mycobacterial DNA via PCR has become the method of choice. There have also been reports of testing for tuberculosis antigens via enzyme-linked immunosorbent assay, such as the cord factor antigen (81). PCR yields results much faster than mycobacterial cultures, which can require several weeks for a positive result. Detection of mycobacterial DNA has been successful with a variety of nonocular tissues (71). In the past decade, there have been several reports of PCR being used to detect tuberculosis in a host of ocular tissues, including eyelid skin, conjunctiva, aqueous and vitreous humor, fixed choroidal tissue, subretinal fluid, and epiretinal membranes (5, 10, 11, 15, 29, 47, 54, 82). In one recent case from the Illinois Eye and Ear Infirmary, the diagnosis of ocular tuberculosis was made by PCR following negative cultures and AFB stains of bodily fluids and tissues (47). Additionally, a case control study of 22 patients with known tuberculosis uveitis demonstrated a 77.2% sensitivity and 92.1% specificity ($P = 0.022$) for nested PCR in the detection of *Mycobacterium tuberculosis* in aqueous and vitreous aspirates (68). While further investigations are still needed to determine the sensitivity and specificity of PCR and enzyme-linked immunosorbent assay testing for tuberculosis in ocular tissues, these techniques have added a valuable alternative for the diagnosis of intraocular tuberculosis infection.

Gamma interferon release assay (IGRA) is a new blood-based diagnostic test for active tuberculosis infection. IGRA has demonstrated a sensitivity comparable or superior to that of the tuberculin skin test (TST) in the immunocompetent, a more robust response than TST in the immunocompromised (those infected with HIV, those on immunosuppressive drug therapy, the elderly, and those on dialysis), and potential as a possible marker of treatment response (61). In a retrospective cohort study, Ang and associates (4) found that IGRA was more specific but less sensitive than TST in the diagnosis of tuberculous uveitis. These findings suggest that the two tests should still be interpreted together.

TREATMENT

Once the diagnosis of ocular tuberculosis is made, systemic antituberculous therapy should be initiated at once. Systemic treatment is successful in the vast majority of cases, with subsequent resolution of symptoms, inflammation, and often an improvement in visual acuity to near premorbid levels. However, cases are reported in which traditional therapies fail to resolve the ocular infection. In one case, a choroidal tuberculoma did not respond to chemotherapy, and the eye eventually became blind and painful, necessitating enucleation (53). Blodi and colleagues (12) reported that choroidal tuberculosis rapidly progressed despite treatment in an HIV-positive patient. The increasing prevalence of acquired drug resistance of mycobacteria in response to incomplete chemotherapy should also be kept in mind with patients not responding to conventional antituberculous therapy.

Any patient with a clinical picture highly suspicious for ocular tuberculosis should be treated with a multidrug regimen of proven efficacy. Because pulmonary infection and other foci of infection may coexist, primary treatment should always be systemic. Ocular penetration of these drugs varies, and additional topical treatment may be useful in patients with external disease.

Topical ointment and subconjunctival injection of isoniazid can lead to adequate intraocular drug levels, especially in the anterior segment. Parenteral administration, however, causes higher vitreous drug levels that make this route of administration the method of choice in posterior intraocular tuberculosis (50).

Topically administered streptomycin is absorbed by the corneal stroma and penetrates the aqueous at high levels, but only in the presence of an epithelial defect. Parenteral administration of high doses can lead to detectable levels in all ocular tissues (52). Intravitreal injection is more successful in generating therapeutic intraocular levels, but high doses may lead to retinal damage (34).

Rifampin administered orally attained an aqueous concentration of 2 to 9% of its level in serum, which may be a therapeutic level against some organisms (69). Studies regarding the ocular penetration of pyrazinamide have not yet been published.

It should be noted that ethambutol, one of the staples of antituberculous pharmacotherapy, has significant ocular toxicity (33). Toxicity is dose related and rarely seen with a daily dose under 15 mg/kg of body weight. One to two percent of patients on a daily dose of 25 mg/kg or more experience significant ocular effects, most commonly optic neuritis. This toxicity can occur in axial and periaxial forms. Axial optical neuritis is associated with macular degeneration that manifests with decreased central visual acuity and decreased green color perception. Periaxial optic neuritis leads to paracentral scotomas (visual field defects) with normal visual acuity and color perception. Other side effects include photophobia, extraocular muscle paresis, and toxic amblyopia. Symptoms of optic neuritis are most often abrupt and begin 3 to 6 months after the onset of ethambutol therapy.

All patients to be started on ethambutol should undergo a baseline ophthalmic examination including visual acuity, color vision, and visual fields (33). Patients should be examined every 2 to 4 weeks when dosages greater than 15 mg/kg/day are used and every 3 to 6 months for lower doses. The patient should be given a vision card and instructed to stop the ethambutol and seek an ophthalmic examination immediately if there is a decrease in visual acuity. Most symptoms resolve over a period of 3 to 12 months, but cases with permanent vision loss have been reported. If the vision does not improve after 10 to 15 weeks of drug discontinuation, treatment with parenteral hydroxocobalamin, 40 mg daily over a 10- to 28-week period, should be considered.

The role of laser therapy in the treatment of ocular tuberculosis has yet to be defined. Balashevich (7) has used argon laser photocoagulation on tuberculous chorioretinitis lesions near the fovea and concluded that such treatment results in better visual acuity than conventional treatment does. Jabbour and associates (45) reported, however, that a subretinal granuloma-like lesion had grown outside previously placed photocoagulation scars. Gur and colleagues (42) and Rosen and coworkers (78) reported on the successful use of sector photocoagulation for the treatment of subretinal neovascularization in a case of chorioretinitis. Laser therapy should never be used as primary treatment without systemic antituberculosis chemotherapy. Furthermore, treatment should be delayed until the diagnosis is established and the response to chemotherapy is confirmed in order to avoid further confusion of the clinical picture and course.

Recently, a new potential target for treatment has been identified. From studies of *Mycobacterium marinum* in zebrafish, Volkman and associates have identified early secreted antigenic target 6 (ESAT-6), a protein secreted by mycobacteria that induces production of matrix metalloproteinase 9 (MMP9) in epithelial cells (92). MMP9 acts as a trophic factor for macrophages. As the original infected macrophage dies, phagocytosis by the newly recruited macrophages leads to their subsequent infection, resulting in exponential bacterial growth and granuloma proliferation. Interruption of MMP9 function resulted in attenuated bacterial growth and granuloma formation in the animal model and shows promise as a novel antituberculosis treatment strategy for humans.

Acknowledgments. We gratefully acknowledge the contributions of Pascal D. Imesch and Ellen J. Dehm in previous editions of this chapter.

REFERENCES

1. Abrams, A. B., and T. F. Schlaegel. 1982. The role of the isoniazid therapeutic test in tuberculosis uveitis. *Am. J. Ophthalmol.* **94:**511–515.
2. Abrams, A. B., and T. F. Schlaegel. 1983. The tuberculin test in the diagnosis of tuberculosis uveitis. *Am. J. Ophthalmol.* **96:**295–298.
3. Anders, N., and G. Wollensack. 1995. Ocular tuberculosis in systemic lupus erythematosus and immunosuppressive therapy. *Klin. Monatsblaetter Augenheilkunde* **204:**368–371.
4. Ang, M., H. M. Htoon, and S. P. Chee. 2009. Diagnosis of tuberculosis uveitis: clinical application of an interferon-gamma release assay. *Ophthalmology* **116:**1391–1396.
5. Arora, S. K., V. Gupta, A. Gupta, P. Bambery, G. S. Kapoor, and S. Sehgal. 1999. Diagnostic efficacy of polymerase chain reaction in granulomatous uveitis. *Tuber. Lung Dis.* **79:**229–233.
6. Babu, R. B., S. Sudharshan, N. Kumarasamy, L. Therese, and J. Biswas. 2006. Ocular tuberculosis in acquired immunodeficiency syndrome. *Am. J. Ophthalmol.* **142:**413–418.
7. Balashevich, L. I. 1984. Argon laser-coagulation in focal chorioretinitis. *Oftalmologia* **7:**414–416.
8. Beare, N. A., J. G. Kublin, D. K. Lewis, M. J. Schijffelen, R. P. Peters, G. Joaki, J. Kumwenda, and E. E. Zijlstra. 2002. Ocular disease in patients with tuberculosis and HIV presenting with fever in Africa. *Br. J. Ophthalmol.* **86:**1076–1079.
9. Biswas, J., S. Narain, D. Das, and S. K. Ganesh. 1996-1997. Pattern of uveitis in a referral uveitis clinic in India. *Int. Ophthalmol.* **20:**223–228.
10. Biswas, J., L. Therese, and H. N. Madhavan. 1999. Use of polymerase chain reaction in detection of *Mycobacterium tuberculosis* complex DNA from vitreous sample of Eales' disease. *Br. J. Ophthalmol.* **83:**994.
11. Biswas, J., S. K. Kumar, S. Rupauliha, S. Misra, I. Bharadwaj, and L. Therese. 2002. Detection of *Mycobacterium tuberculosis* by nested polymerase chain reaction in a case of subconjunctival tuberculosis. *Cornea* **21:**123–125.
12. Blodi, B. A., N. W. Johnson, and W. M. McLeish. 1989. Presumed choroidal tuberculosis in a human immunodeficiency virus infected host. *Am. J. Ophthalmol.* **103:**605–607.
13. Bloomfield, S. E., B. Mondino, and G. F. Gray. 1976. Scleral tuberculosis. *Arch. Ophthalmol.* **94:**954–956.
14. Bouza, E., P. Merino, P. Munoz, C. Sanchez-Carillo, J. Yanez, and C. Cortes. 1997. Ocular tuberculosis: a prospective study in a general hospital. *Medicine* **76:**53–61.
15. Bowyer, J. D., P. D. Gormley, R. Seth, R. N. Downes, and J. Lowe. 1999. Choroidal tuberculosis diagnosed by polymerase chain reaction. A clinicopathologic case report. *Ophthalmology* **106:**290–294.
16. Cangemi, F. E., A. H. Friedman, and R. Josephberg. 1980. Tuberculoma of the choroid. *Ophthalmology* **84:**252–258.
17. Chandler, A. C., and D. Locatcher-Khorazo. 1964. Primary tuberculosis of the conjunctiva. *Arch. Ophthalmol.* **71:**202–205.
18. Chapman, C. B., and C. M. Whorton. 1946. Acute generalized miliary tuberculosis in adults. *N. Engl. J. Med.* **235:**239–248.
19. Chung, Y., T. Yeh, S. Sheu, and J. H. Liu. 1989. Macular subretinal neovascularization in choroidal tuberculosis. *Ann. Ophthalmol.* **21:**225–229.
20. Cohnheim, J. 1867. Ueber tuberkulose der choroiden. *Virchows Arch. (Pathol. Anat.)* **39:**49–69.
21. Cook, C. D., and M. Hainsworth. 1990. Tuberculosis of the conjunctiva occurring in association with a neighbouring lupus vulgaris lesion. *Br. J. Ophthalmol.* **74:**315–316.
22. Croxatto, J. O., C. Mestre, S. Puente, and G. Gonzalez. 1986. Nonreactive tuberculosis in a patient with acquired immune deficiency syndrome. *Am. J. Ophthalmol.* **102:**659–660.
23. Darrell, R. M. 1967. Acute tuberculosis panophthalmitis. *Arch. Ophthalmol.* **78:**51–54.
24. Demirci, H., C. L. Shields, J. A. Shields, and R. C. Eagle, Jr. 2004. Ocular tuberculosis masquerading as ocular tumors. *Surv. Ophthalmol.* **49:**78–89.
25. Dollfus, M. A. 1949. Fundus lesions in tuberculosis meningitis and miliary pulmonary tuberculosis treated with streptomycin. *Am. J. Ophthalmol.* **32:**821–824.
26. Domonkos, A. N., H. L. Arnold, and R. B. Odom. 1982. *Andrews' Diseases of the Skin, Clinical Dermatology,* 7th ed. W. B. Saunders, Philadelphia, PA.
27. Donahue, H. C. 1967. Ophthalmic experience in a tuberculosis sanatorium. *Am. J. Ophthalmol.* **64:**742–748.
28. D'Souza, P., R. Garg, R. S. Dhaliwal, R. Jain, and M. Jain. 1994. Orbital-tuberculosis [sic]. *Int. Ophthalmol.* **18:**149–152.
29. El-Ghatit, A. M., S. M. El-Deriny, A. A. Mahmoud, and A. S. Ashi. 1999. Presumed periorbital lupus vulgaris with ocular extension. *Ophthalmology* **106:**1990–1993.
30. Eliot, A. 1954. Recurrent intraocular hemorrhage in young adults. *Trans. Am. Ophthalmic Soc.* **52:**811–875.
31. Fernandes, M., G. K. Vemuganti, G. Pasricha, A. K. Bansal, and V. S. Sangwan. 2003. Unilateral tuberculous conjunctivitis with tarsal necrosis. *Arch. Ophthalmol.* **121:**1475–1478.
32. Fountain, J. A., and R. B. Werner. 1984. Tuberculous retinal vasculitis. *Retina* **4:**48–50.
33. Fraundelder, F. T. 1989. *Drug-Induced Ocular Side Effects and Drug Interactions,* 3rd ed. Lea & Febiger, Philadelphia, PA.
33a. Frueh, B. E., O. Dubuis, P. Imesch, M. Böhnke, and T. Bodmer. 2000. *Mycobacterium szulgai* keratitis. *Arch. Ophthalmol.* **118:**1123–1124.
34. Gardiner, P. A., I. C. Michaelson, E. J. W. Rees, and J. M. Robson. 1948. Intravitreous streptomycin: its toxicity and diffusion. *Br. J. Ophthalmol.* **32:**449–456.
35. Gibson, W. S. 1918. The etiology of phlyctenular conjunctivitis. *Am. J. Dis. Child.* **15:**81–115.
36. Glover, L. P. 1930. Some eye observations in tuberculosis patients at the State Sanatorium, Cresson, Pennsylvania. *Am. J. Ophthalmol.* **13:**411–412.
37. Goldberg, M. F. 1982. Presumed tuberculous maculopathy. *Retina* **2:**47–50.
38. Goldenberg, M., and N. D. Fabricant. 1909. The eye in the tuberculous patient. *Trans. Sect. Ophthalmol. Am. Med. Assoc.* **135.**
39. Grewal, A., R. Y. Kim, and E. T. Cunningham, Jr. 1998. Miliary tuberculosis. *Arch. Ophthalmol.* **116:**953–954.

40. **Gupta, V., A. Gupta, S. Arora, P. Bambery, M. R. Dogra, and A. Agarwal.** 2003. Presumed tubercular serpiginouslike chorioiditis: clinical presentations and management. *Ophthalmology* **110:**1744–1749.

41. **Gupta, V., A. Gupta, and N. A. Rao.** 2007. Intraocular tuberculosis—an update. *Surv. Ophthalmol.* **52:**561–587.

42. **Gur, S., B. Z. Silverstone, R. Zylberman, and D. Berson.** 1987. Chorioretinitis and extrapulmonary tuberculosis. *Ann. Ophthalmol.* **19:**112–115.

43. **Illingsworth, R. S., and T. Wright.** 1948. Tubercles of the choroid. *Br. Med. J.* **2:**365–368.

44. **Islam, S. M., and K. F. Tabbara.** 2002. Causes of uveitis at The Eye Center in Saudi Arabia: a retrospective review. *Ophthalmic Epidemiol.* **9:**239–249.

45. **Jabbour, N. M., B. Farris, and C. L. Trempe.** 1985. A case of pulmonary tuberculosis presenting with a choroidal tuberculoma. *Ophthalmology* **92:**834–837.

46. **Jennings, A., M. Bilous, P. Asimakis, and A. J. Maloof.** 2006. *Mycobacterium tuberculosis* presenting as chronic red eye. *Cornea* **25:**1118–1120.

47. **Kesen, M., D. P. Edward, N. A. Rao, J. Sugar, H. H. Tessler, and D. A. Goldstein.** 2009. Atypical infectious nodular scleritis. *Arch. Ophthalmol.* **127:**1079–1080.

48. **Khalil, M., S. Lindley, and E. Matouk.** 1985. Tuberculosis of the orbit. *Ophthalmology* **92:**1624–1627.

49. **Koch, R.** 1882. Die Aetiologe der Tuberculose. *Berliner Klin. Wochenschr.* **15:**221–230.

50. **Kratka, W. H.** 1955. Isoniazid and ocular tuberculosis: an evaluation of experimental and clinical studies. *Arch. Ophthalmol.* **54:**330–344.

51. **Leng, T., A. C. Schefler, and T. G. Murray.** 2009. Retinal vascular tumor and peripheral retinal vasculitis in the setting of systemic tuberculosis. *Ophthalmic Surg. Lasers Imaging* **40:**409–412.

52. **Leopold, I. H., and A. Nichold.** 1946. Intraocular penetration of streptomycin following systemic and local administration. *Arch. Ophthalmol.* **35:**33–38.

53. **Lyon, C. E., B. S. Crimson, and R. L. Peiffer.** 1985. Clinicopathological correlation of a solitary choroidal tuberculoma. *Ophthalmology* **92:**845–850.

54. **Madhavan, H. N., K. L. Therese, P. Gunisha, U. Jayanthi, and J. Biswas.** 2000. Polymerase chain reaction for detection of *Mycobacterium tuberculosis* in epiretinal membrane in Eales' disease. *Investig. Ophthalmol. Vis. Sci.* **41:**822–825.

55. **Maitre-Jan, A.** 1707. *Traite des maladies de l'oeil et des remedes propres pour leur guerison. Enrichy de plusieurs experiences de physique.* Jacques le Febvre, Troyes, France.

56. **Mansour, A. M., and R. Haymond.** 1990. Choroidal tuberculomas without evidence of extraocular tuberculosis. *Albrecht von Graefe's Arch. Clin. Exp. Ophthalmol.* **228:**382–385.

56a. **Mason, J. O.** 2000. Treatment of large macular choroidal tubercle improves vision. *Arch. Ophthalmol.* **118:**1136–1137.

57. **Massaro, D., S. Katz, and M. Sachs.** 1964. Choroidal tubercles. *Ann. Intern. Med.* **60:**231–241.

58. **Maurya, O. P. S., R. Patel, V. Thakur, and R. Singh.** 1990. Tuberculoma of the orbit—a case report. *Indian J. Ophthalmol.* **38:**191–192.

59. **Mehta, D. K.** 1989. Bilateral tubercular lid abscess—a case report. *Indian J. Ophthalmol.* **37:**98.

60. **Mehta, S., V. Chauhan, S. Hastak, P. Jiadani, and P. Dalal.** 2006. Choroidal tubercles in neurotuberculosis: prevalence and significance. *Ocul. Immunol. Inflamm.* **14:**341–345.

61. **Mori, T.** 2009. Usefulness of interferon-gamma release assays for diagnosing TB infection and problems with these assays. *J. Infect. Chemother.* **15:**143–155.

62. **Morimura, Y., A. A. Okada, S. Kawahara, Y. Miyamoto, S. Kawai, A. Hirakata, and T. Hida.** 2002. Tuberculin skin testing in uveitis patients and treatment of presumed intraocular tuberculosis in Japan. *Ophthalmology* **109:**851–857.

63. **Morinelli, E. N., R. U. Dugel, R. Riffenburg, and H. M. Byron.** 1993. Infectious multifocal choroiditis in patients with acquired immunodeficiency syndrome. *Ophthalmology* **100:**1014–1021.

64. **Muccioli, C., and R. Belfort.** 1995. Presumed ocular and central nervous system tuberculosis in a patient with acquired immunodeficiency syndrome. *Am. J. Ophthalmol.* **121:**217–219.

65. **Nanda, M., S. C. Pflugfelder, and S. Holland.** 1989. *Mycobacterium tuberculosis* scleritis. *Am. J. Ophthalmol.* **108:**736–737.

66. **Ni, C., J. J. Papale, and N. L. Robinson.** 1982. Uveal tuberculosis. *Int. Ophthalmol. Clin.* **22:**103–124.

67. **Olazabal, F.** 1967. Choroidal tubercles. *JAMA* **200:**374–377.

68. **Ortega-Larrocea, G., M. Bobadilla del Valle, A. Ponce de Leon, and J. Siguentes Osornio.** 2003. Nested polymerase chain reaction for *Mycobacterium tuberculosis* DNA detection in aqueous and vitreous of patients with uveitis. *Arch. Med. Res.* **34:**116–119.

69. **Outman, W. R., R. E. Levitz, D. A. Hill, and C. H. Nightingale.** 1992. Intraocular penetration of rifampin in humans. *Antimicrob. Agents Chemother.* **36:**1575–1576.

70. **Paton, R. T.** 1932. The clinical significance of choroidal tubercles. *Ann. Intern. Med.* **5:**997–999.

71. **Peneau, A., D. Moinard, I. Berard, O. Pascal, and J. P. Moisan.** 1992. Detection of mycobacteria using the polymerase chain reaction. *Eur. J. Clin. Microbiol. Infect. Dis.* **11:**270–271.

72. **Perez Blazquez, E., M. Montero Rodriguez, and J. Mendez Ramos.** 1994. Tuberculous choroiditis and acquired immunodeficiency syndrome. *Ann. Ophthalmol.* **26:**50–54.

73. **Philip, R. N., G. W. Comstock, and J. H. Shelton.** 1965. Phlyctenular keratoconjunctivitis among Eskimos in Southwestern Alaska. *Am. Rev. Respir. Dis.* **91:**171–187.

74. **Pilai, S., T. J. Malone, and J. C. Abad.** 1995. Orbital tuberculosis. *Ophthalmic Plastic Reconstruct. Surg.* **11:**27–31.

75. **Rich, A., and H. McCordock.** 1929. An enquiry concerning the role of allergy, immunity and other factors of importance in the pathogenesis of human tuberculosis. *Bull. Johns Hopkins Hosp.* **44:**273.

76. **Roberts, B. N., and C. M. Lane.** 1997. Orbital tuberculosis. *Eye* **11:**138–139.

77. **Rodriguez, A., M. Calonge, M. Pedroza-Seres, Y. A. Akova, E. M. Messmer, D. J. D'Amico, and C. S. Foster.** 1996. Referral patterns of uveitis in a tertiary eye care center. *Arch. Ophthalmol.* **114:**593–599.

78. **Rosen, P. H., D. J. Spalton, and E. M. Graham.** 1990. Intraocular tuberculosis. *Eye* **4:**486–492.

79. **Rosenbaum, P. S., J. N. Mbekeani, and Y. Kress.** 1998. Atypical mycobacterial panophthalmitis seen with iris nodules. *Arch. Ophthalmol.* **116:**1524–1527.

80. **Rosenhauch, E.** 1910. Ueber das Verhaeltnis phlyctaenularer Augenentzuendungen zu Tuberkulose. *Albert von Graefes Arch. Ophthalmol.* **76:**370–396.

81. **Sakai, J., S. Matsuzawa, M. Usui, and I. Yano.** 2001. New diagnostic approach for ocular tuberculosis by ELISA using the cord factor as antigen. *Br. J. Ophthalmol.* **85:**130–133.

82. **Salman, A., P. Parmar, M. Rajamohan, P. A. Thomas, and N. Jesudasan.** 2003. Subretinal fluid analysis in the diagnosis of choroidal tuberculosis. *Retina* **23:**796–799.

82a. **Sarvananthan, N., M. Wiselka, and K. Bibby.** 1998. Intraocular tuberculosis without detectable systemic infection. *Arch. Ophthalmol.* **116:**1386–1388.

83. **Seward, D. N. L.** 1973. Tuberculoma of the ciliary body. *Med. J. Aust.* **1:**297–298.

84. Shah, S. M., R. S. Howard, N. J. C. Sarkjes, and E. M. Graham. 1988. Tuberculosis presenting as retinal vasculitis. *J. R. Soc. Med.* **81:**232–233.

85. Sheridan, P. H., J. B. Edman, and S. E. Starr. 1981. Tuberculosis presenting as an orbital mass. *Pediatrics* **67:**847–875.

86. Snider, D. E., Jr., G. M. Cauthen, L. S. Farer, G. D. Kelly, J. O. Kilburn, R. C. Good, and S. W. Dooley. 1991. Drug-resistant tuberculosis. *Am. Rev. Respir. Dis.* **144:**732. (Letter.)

87. Spencer, W. H. 1996. *Ophthalmic Pathology: an Atlas and Textbook*, vol. 1. W. B. Saunders, Philadelphia, PA.

88. Spoor, T. C., and S. A. Harding. 1981. Orbital tuberculosis. *Am. J. Ophthalmol.* **91:**644–647.

89. Terson, A. 1890. Tuberculose oculaire: Excision d'un tubercule de l'iris suivi de succes. *Arch. Ophthalmol.* **10:**7–14.

90. Thygeson, P. 1962. Phlyctenulosis: attempts to produce an experimental model with BCG. *Investig. Ophthalmol. Vis. Sci.* **1:**262–266.

91. van Assen, S., and J. A. Lutterman. 2002. Tuberculous dacryoadenitis: a rare manifestation of tuberculosis. *Neth. J. Med.* **60:**327–329.

92. Volkman, H. E., T. C. Pozos, J. Zheng, J. M. Davis, J. F. Rawls, and L. Ramakrishnan. 2010. Tuberculosis granuloma induction via interaction of a bacterial secreted protein with host epithelium. *Science* **327:**466–469.

93. von Jaeger, E. 1855. Über choroidealtuberkel. *Desterr. Ztschr. Pract. Heilke.* **1:**9–10.

94. von Michel, J. 1881. Über iris und iritis. *Albrecht von Graefe's Arch. Klin. Exp. Ophthalmol.* **27:**171–282.

95. Woods, A. C. 1961. *Endogenous Uveitis*. Williams & Wilkins, Baltimore, MD.

96. Zoric, L. D., D. L. Zoric, and D. M. Zoric. 1996. Bilateral tuberculosis abscesses on the face (eyelids) of a child. *Am. J. Ophthalmol.* **121:**717–718.

Chapter 18

Central Nervous System Tuberculosis

JOHN M. LEONARD

INTRODUCTION

Central nervous system (CNS) tuberculosis (TB) is among the least common yet most devastating forms of human mycobacterial infection. Conceptually, clinical CNS infection is seen to comprise three categories of illness: subacute or chronic meningitis, intracranial tuberculoma, and spinal tuberculous arachnoiditis. All three forms are seen with about equal frequencies in high-prevalence regions of the world where postprimary, extrapulmonary clinical infection is encountered commonly among children and young adults (3). Meningitis syndrome predominates in low-prevalence countries such as the United States and in Europe, where extrapulmonary TB is encountered primarily in older adults with reactivation disease. The natural history of tuberculous meningitis (TBM) is that of insidious onset and subacute progression, prone to rapid acceleration once neurologic deficits supervene, leading to stupor, coma, and, finally, death within 5 to 8 weeks of the onset of illness. Consequently, in order to achieve a favorable therapeutic outcome it is important to begin treatment promptly, empirically during the early stages of illness, relying on clinical suspicion and a presumptive diagnosis rather than awaiting laboratory confirmation. Of necessity, this requires some knowledge of the causes and clinical features of granulomatous meningitis, the pathology that subserves the neurologic manifestations of disease, and the expected radiographic and laboratory (chiefly cerebrospinal fluid [CSF]) findings.

EPIDEMIOLOGY

With regard to TB in general, it is estimated that one-third of the world's population has been infected with *Mycobacterium tuberculosis* and that approximately 15 million persons have active clinical disease. About 9 million new cases and 1.5 million to 2 million deaths occur in the world each year (15). Incidence rates of TB vary widely from country to country in relation to the prevalence of cavitary pulmonary disease and poor socioeconomic conditions. In the United States, where the incidence of TB has declined gradually over the past two decades, 12,904 new cases were reported in 2008, an incidence rate of 4.2 cases per 100,000 persons (14). The proportion of new cases is higher among foreign-born persons residing in the United States (20 cases per 100,000) than among native-born individuals (2 cases per 100,000). Pulmonary TB accounts for 70% of the total, isolated extrapulmonary cases 20%, and combined extrapulmonary and active pulmonary disease the remaining 10%.

Clinical CNS TB occurs in 1 to 2% of all patients with active TB and accounts for about 8% of all extrapulmonary cases of the infection reported to occur in immunocompetent individuals. While the incidence of pulmonary TB in the United States has declined steadily in recent decades, the number of reported cases of CNS infection has changed little, about 180 to 200 per year, and the case fatality rate remains high, at 15 to 40%, despite effective antituberculous chemotherapy (13, 46).

MENINGITIS

Pathogenesis

The sequence of events that leads to clinical neurologic illness begins with the hematogenous dissemination of *Mycobacterium tuberculosis* (bacillemia) that follows primary pulmonary infection or late reactivation TB elsewhere in the body. However, unlike the pathogenesis of pyogenic bacterial meningitis, this bacteremia does not breach the blood-brain barrier to produce an immediate invasion of the meninges and subarachnoid space. Instead, during this

John M. Leonard • Department of Medicine—Infectious Disease, Vanderbilt University Medical Center, 1161 21st Avenue South—A 2200 MCN, Nashville, TN 37232-2582.

bacillemic phase sparse numbers of bacilli are scattered throughout the substance of the brain, meninges, and adjacent tissues, leading to the formation of multiple small granulomatous foci of various sizes and degrees of encapsulation (tubercles). The continued proliferation and coalescence of tubercles result in larger caseous foci. Such lesions, if located adjacent to the ependyma or pia, may subsequently rupture into the subarachnoid space, producing meningitis. This conceptual understanding of the pathogenesis of TBM is derived from the observations of Rich and McCordock, who performed meticulous autopsy examinations of TBM patients dying at the Johns Hopkins Hospital during the early part of the last century (45). In 77 of the 82 cases studied, an older, active caseous focus communicating with the subarachnoid space or ventricles was found in the substance of the brain, meninges, or adjacent bone. While the number, character, and location of granulomas within the CNS were variable, the discharging caseous lesion ("Rich focus") was most commonly situated in the brain or meninges and only rarely in bone or spinal cord. Thus, the chance distribution and progression of a suitably located subependymal or subpial tubercle are the critical events in the subsequent development of TBM.

It follows that the propensity of a lesion to produce meningitis will be determined by its proximity to the surface of the brain, the rapidity of progression, and the rate at which encapsulation follows acquired immune resistance. Moreover, the low-grade, incessant bacillemia associated with progressive disseminated TB greatly increases the likelihood that a juxtaependymal tubercle will be established and from this critical location break through to infect the subarachnoid space (50). CNS TB arises in this manner under conditions of sustained postprimary bacillemia, as in very young (children < 3 years) and the malnourished, and from the failure to sustain immune control of dormant foci (tubercles) within the brain or other tissues of the body, as in the elderly and other adults on immunosuppressive medication or infected with human immunodeficiency virus (HIV).

Although tuberculous CNS infection may be seen as a complication of clinically apparent progressive miliary disease, most adults develop TBM from less apparent or entirely hidden foci of chronic organ TB. Reactivation of latent TB outside the CNS may result in intermittent or chronic progressive bacillemia, producing subependymal tubercles which remain quiescent for months or years, yet harboring bacilli and having the potential to destabilize as a result of local changes in the brain or a decline in host cellular immunity. Aging, use of immunosuppressive drugs, lymphoma, alcoholism, and HIV/AIDS are among the factors known to facilitate progression to the syndrome of "late generalized tuberculosis." In an excellent clinical pathological analysis of 100 patients with this syndrome, careful postmortem examination revealed meningeal involvement in 54% of cases studied (51).

A significant subset of adults with TBM has no clinically evident extracranial infection or apparent defects in host immunity. In the occasional patient, the history of antecedent head and neck trauma suggests that Rich foci within the brain may be destabilized by physical factors as well.

Pathology

Regardless of where the Rich focus is located, the rupture of tubercular protein into the subarachnoid space initiates an intense, cytokine-mediated inflammatory reaction that comes to be most marked at the base of the brain. The resultant pathological changes take three principal forms that, in turn, account for the defining clinical features of the disease: a proliferative basal arachnoiditis, vasculitis, and hydrocephalus (19, 45). Within a matter of days a proliferative, basal arachnoiditis produces a thick, gelatinous exudate extending from the pons to the optic chiasm. In time, the process comes to resemble a fibrous mass that encases and compromises the function of nearby cranial nerves (CNs), most commonly CNs VI, III, and IV.

Arteries and veins traversing the region are caught up in the inflammatory process, resulting in a vasculitis that extends within the substance of the brain itself. Initially, direct invasion of the vessel wall by mycobacteria, or secondary extension of adjacent inflammation, leads to an intense polymorphonuclear reaction within the adventitia, followed by infiltration of lymphocytes, plasma cells, and macrophages. Progressive destruction of the adventitia and disruption of elastic fibers allow the inflammatory process to reach the intima; eventually, fibrinoid degeneration within small arteries and veins leads to aneurysms, thrombi, and focal hemorrhages (24). Multiple lesions are common, and a variety of stroke syndromes result from spasm, thrombosis, or hemorrhage (16). Most commonly involved are branches of the middle cerebral artery and perforating vessels to the basal ganglia, pons, thalamus, and internal capsule. Intracranial vasculitis is found commonly in those dying from TBM and is the major cause of severe neurologic deficits in those who survive. In an autopsy series, phlebitis and various degrees of arteritis were found in 22 of 27 cases studied; of these, 8 patients had an obstructive tuberculous thrombophlebitis with hemorrhagic cerebral infarction (42).

Extension of the inflammatory process to the basal cisterns may impede CSF circulation and absorption, leading to communicating hydrocephalus. This is seen in the majority of cases in which symptoms have been present for 3 weeks or more (7). Obstructive hydrocephalus, arising from edema of the midbrain or a localized brain stem granuloma that occludes the aqueduct, is encountered less often.

Clinical Presentation

Common symptoms and signs

The usual patient with TBM presents with a subacute, progressive febrile illness that passes through three discernible phases. Illness begins with a prodrome of malaise, lassitude, low-grade fever, and intermittent headache, sometimes a vague discomfort in the neck or back, and subtle personality change. In 2 to 3 weeks, a more well-defined meningitic phase emerges as the patient experiences protracted headache, meningismus, vomiting, mild confusion, and various degrees of CN palsy and long-tract signs (26, 31, 32). At this stage the pace of illness may accelerate rapidly to the paralytic phase: delirium followed by stupor and coma, seizures, multiple CN deficits, hemiparesis, and hemiplegia. In the untreated case, death commonly occurs within 5 to 8 weeks of the onset of illness. In children, headache is less common, while irritability, restlessness, anorexia, and protracted vomiting are prominent symptoms, especially in the very young (22). Seizures are more common in children and apt to occur in the early stage of illness. Table 1 lists common symptoms and signs at presentation, and the frequency reported, in 195 patients compiled from four recent clinical series in separate countries of the Western world (31, 32, 43, 61).

Atypical presentations

Uncommonly, patients will present without the characteristic prodrome and subacute progression described above. In the occasional adult, TBM takes the form of a slowly progressive dementia over many months, marked by personality change, social withdrawal, and memory deficits. Others may present with an acute, rapidly progressive meningitis syndrome indistinguishable from pyogenic bacterial infection. At times focal neurologic deficits (CN palsies, hemiparesis, and seizures) or symptoms of hydrocephalus (headache, papilledema, diplopia, and visual disturbance) precede signs of meningitis. There is described for children, and occasionally adults, an "encephalitic" presentation with stupor, coma, and convulsions with neither meningitis signs nor significant CSF abnormalities (59).

Clinical staging and prognosis

For purposes of prognosis and therapy it is useful to categorize patients into clinical stages according to the degree of illness at presentation. Stage 1 comprises patients who are conscious and rational, with or without meningismus but having no focal neurologic signs or evident hydrocephalus; stage 2 patients exhibit lethargy and confusion and may have mild focal neurologic signs such as CN palsy and hemiparesis; and stage 3 patients exhibit signs of advanced disease such as stupor, coma, seizures, multiple CN palsies, and dense hemiplegia (31). The prognosis for treated TBM is greatly influenced by the clinical stage at which treatment is initiated.

TBM and HIV infection

All forms of extrapulmonary disease occur with greater than expected frequency in HIV patients with active TB (11). Among 52 AIDS patients diagnosed with TB over a 3-year period, 10 had CNS disease manifested by meningitis, tuberculoma, or cerebral abscess (8). In another study of 455 HIV patients with TB, 10% developed meningitis, compared to only 2% of a matched HIV-negative cohort with TB (4). Moreover, HIV-positive patients accounted for 59% of TBM cases seen during the study period. Apart from intracerebral tuberculomas, which are seen more frequently in HIV patients with CNS TB, coinfection with HIV does not appear to alter the clinical manifestations, CSF findings, or response to therapy (20, 30).

Diagnosis

Once the diagnosis is considered in a patient with compatible clinical features and suspicious laboratory abnormalities, a rapid, thorough assessment for supporting evidence should be conducted,

Table 1. Presenting symptoms and signs of TBM[a]

Symptom/sign(s)	Frequency reported (%)
Fever	20–70
Headache	25–70
Meningeal irritation	35–90
Lethargy/drowsiness	25–30
Vomiting	30–70
Confusion/delirium	30–65
Focal neurologic signs	25–40
CN palsy	20–35
Hemiparesis	5–30

[a]See references 31, 32, 43, and 61.

followed by the decision of whether to begin empirical treatment. Careful attention to the past medical record, epidemiological setting, and general physical examination may reveal important information. A strong family history of TB and history of head trauma in recent months are helpful clues. Recent past exposure to persons with active TB is apt to be present in cases involving children and in adults with impaired cellular immunity. In urban areas, the association of extrapulmonary TB with underlying conditions such as alcoholism, injection drug use, poverty, and other conditions or therapies that impair cellular immune function add urgency to the consideration. Signs of active infection elsewhere in the body are not infrequent and when present provide the most reliable basis for the presumptive diagnosis in patients presenting with meningeal TB. A careful, thorough examination may reveal choroidal tubercles on the retina (9) or splenomegaly in patients with active disseminated infection or lymphadenopathy, bone and joint lesions, or scrotal mass and draining fistula in patients with focal extrapulmonary disease.

Routine studies

The chest X ray should be examined carefully for hilar adenopathy, interstitial miliary pattern, and parenchymal infiltrate or apical scarring. Such abnormalities are present in the majority of childhood cases and about 50% of adults. Routine blood counts and chemistries are of little value except as they reveal evidence of chronic disease and disseminated infection. Mild anemia and leukocytosis are common. The hyponatremia of inappropriate secretion of antidiuretic hormone has been described in a minority of cases with miliary TB complicated by meningitis (52). Skin testing for tuberculin hypersensitivity is useful, especially in children; however, a negative skin test occurs with such frequency in all forms of active extrapulmonary TB as to be of no use in excluding the diagnosis.

CSF examination and culture

The key to the diagnosis in most instances rests with the proper interpretation of the spinal fluid cellular characteristics and chemistries (the CSF formula) combined with the demonstration of mycobacteria in the CSF by stained smear or culture. At lumbar puncture the opening pressure is usually elevated. The fluid is clear or has a "ground glass" appearance, and a delicate web-like clot often forms at the top. Typically, the CSF formula shows a mononuclear pleocytosis accompanied by high protein and low glucose concentrations (29). The total cell count is between 100 and 500/mm^3 in the majority, less than 100 cells/mm^3

in 15%, and between 500 and 1,500 cells/mm^3 in 20% of cases. Early in the course of illness the cellular reaction may be atypical, with few cells, a mixed pleocytosis, or a transient polymorphonuclear predominance which, on subsequent examinations, evolves in the direction of the expected lymphocytic response (34). The CSF protein concentration is in the range of 100 to 500 mg/dl in most patients, under 100 mg/dl in 25%, and greater than 500 mg/dl in about 10% of reported cases. An extremely high protein concentration, in the range of 2 to 6 g/dl, is indicative of subarachnoid block and carries a poor prognosis. The CSF glucose concentration is abnormally low, less than 45 mg/dl, in 80% of cases; given that the patient will usually have a subacute or chronic meningitis presentation, this feature constitutes strong evidence of a granulomatous infection of the CNS.

The demonstration of M. tuberculosis by stained smear and culture establishes the specific diagnosis. Cultures are positive in about 75% of cases but require 3 to 6 weeks for detectable growth. Consequently, the demonstration of acid-fast bacilli (AFB) by stained smear of CSF sediment remains the most rapid means of reaching an early diagnosis. The sensitivity of both the AFB smear and culture is variable, influenced in part by the selection and volume of the specimen submitted by the clinician and the diligence applied to the process by laboratory personnel. Moreover, there is value in submitting multiple CSF specimens from repeated lumbar punctures. In the series reported by Kennedy and Fallon, the yields on smear and culture were 37% (smear) and 56% (culture) based upon the first CSF specimen submitted, but increased to 87 and 83%, respectively, when up to three additional specimens were examined (31). Importantly, in 30% of cases the diagnosis was made from CSF obtained 1 to 3 days after therapy had been initiated. In another study involving 132 adult patients, designed specifically to evaluate the effectiveness of careful microbiological technique, a positive smear was established for 58% and the yield on culture was 71%. The combined sensitivity of smear and culture was 82% (55). Based on these observations, it is recommended that a minimum of three serial CSF samples be obtained for smear and culture, submitting a 10-ml aliquot of the last fluid removed at lumbar puncture. It is not necessary to defer antituberculous therapy, as the yield remains good for a few days after treatment is started.

Molecular diagnostic techniques

The nucleic acid-based amplification technique, based on PCR, is a new and effective method for the rapid detection of specific bacterial DNA in clinical specimens (10, 28). However, the reliability of PCR testing for *M. tuberculosis* DNA in CSF is not well established, primarily because of variability in sensitivity and specificity across multiple laboratories. In a comparison study of seven participating laboratories, the sensitivity varied widely and the rate of false-positive tests ranged from 3 to 20% (38). More recently, a meta-analysis of nucleic acid-based amplification techniques for TB meningitis showed a high pooled specificity, 98%, but the pooled sensitivity was low, at 56% (41). When clinical suspicion warrants empirical therapy for CNS TB, and initial stains for AFB are negative, CSF specimens should be submitted for PCR testing, bearing in mind that a negative result neither excludes the diagnosis nor provides a basis for discontinuing therapy.

Neuroradiological evaluation

The application of computed tomography (CT) and magnetic resonance imaging (MRI) has greatly facilitated the assessment and management of patients with CNS TB (5, 35, 36, 47). These imaging studies are useful for defining the presence and extent of basal arachnoiditis, cerebral edema and infarction, and the presence and course of hydrocephalus (Fig. 1 and 2). In two early, sizable community-based series, CT scanning demonstrated hydrocephalus in

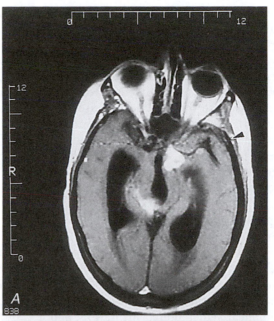

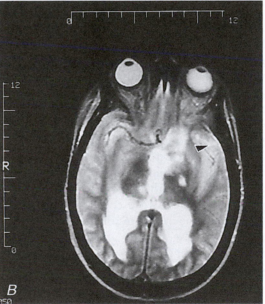

Figure 2. MRI of the same patient as for Fig. 1. (A) After contrast enhancement, showing two dense, bilateral inflammatory masses (tuberculomas) in the region of the thalamus; (B) T-2 weighted image showing inflammatory edema and possible ischemic changes of vasculitis in the basal region of the temporal lobe (arrowhead).

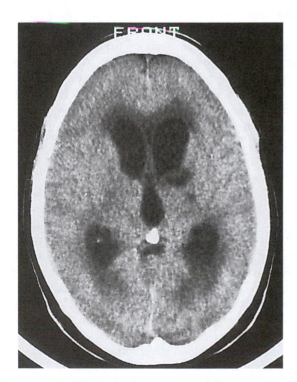

Figure 1. Computerized axial tomogram for a patient with TBM. Note the enlarged ventricles and effacement of sulci, indicating raised intracranial pressure.

75% of patients, basal meningeal enhancement in 38%, cerebral infarcts in 15 to 30%, and tuberculomas in 5 to 10% (7, 40). A number of useful clinical observations can be derived from a review of selected neuroimaging studies reported over the past two decades (7, 33, 40). In a patient with compatible clinical features, CT evidence of basal enhancement combined with any degree of hydrocephalus is strongly suggestive of TBM. If the CT scan is normal at the time therapy is initiated, the prognosis for complete recovery on therapy is excellent. Hydrocephalus combined with marked basal enhancement is indicative of advanced disease and carries a poor prognosis. Marked basal enhancement correlates well with the presence of vasculitis and, therefore, the risk for basal ganglion infarction. MRI is superior to CT for evaluating children and is the preferred modality for defining lesions of the brain stem, midbrain, and basal ganglia in patients of all ages (5, 39, 48).

Differential diagnosis

In most cases the differential diagnosis is that of the patient with classic features of the granulomatous meningitis syndrome—a subacute inflammatory condition of the CNS marked by fever, headache, meningeal signs, altered mentation, and a CSF formula showing a lymphocytic pleocytosis, lowered glucose concentration, and high protein content. Table 2 lists the other principal infections that may manifest in this fashion, along with noninfectious conditions that may mimic certain of these features. Cryptococcal meningitis is the major consideration because it is the most common, along with the other deep-seated fungal infections listed. The syndrome may also be encountered in patients with parameningeal suppurative foci complicating endocarditis, sphenoid sinusitis, and brain abscess. At times TBM can be confused with herpes simplex and mumps encephalitis when the presentation is that of fever, rapid neurologic deterioration, and mild lowering of the CSF glucose. Careful attention to such details as the overall length of illness, meningeal signs, degree of protein elevation, and specific CT/MRI abnormalities will be most helpful in differentiating herpes encephalitis from tuberculous CNS infection. The other diagnoses listed are of importance, as they should cause the clinician to consider the possibility of TBM in any patient suspected of having one of these conditions.

Table 2. Differential diagnosis of TBM

Fungal meningitis (cryptococcosis, histoplasmosis, blastomycosis, coccidioidomycosis)
Neurobrucellosis
Neurosyphilis
Neuroborreliosis
Focal parameningeal infection (sphenoid sinusitis, endocarditis, brain abscess)
CNS toxoplasmosis
Partially treated bacterial meningitis
Neoplastic meningitis (lymphoma, carcinoma)

TUBERCULOMA

Tuberculomas are conglomerate caseous foci in the brain that develop from deep-seated tubercles acquired during a recent or remote disseminated bacillemia. Centrally located, active lesions may reach considerable size without producing meningitis (18, 45). When the host response to infection is poor, this process may result in focal cerebritis and frank abscess formation. More commonly, the lesions coalesce to form caseous granulomas with fibrous encapsulation (tuberculoma). The advent of CT and MRI brain imaging has disclosed that clinically silent single or multiple CNS granulomata occur rather commonly in patients with TBM and in those with miliary TB without meningitis. On CT the characteristic appearance is a nodular enhancing lesion with a central hypodense region; on MRI the early focal cerebritis stage is marked by edema and ill-defined enhancement, the later mature stage by central hypointensity and peripheral enhancement on T-2 weighted images (60, 63, 64). These lesions usually disappear on therapy, without incident. There are occasional reports of clinically significant, transient tuberculomas appearing during the early course of antituberculous therapy (54).

Clinical Tuberculoma

Tuberculoma manifesting as a clinically evident mass lesion of the brain is distinctly uncommon in the West, but in India, the near East, and parts of Asia it is reported to account for 20 to 30% of all intracranial tumors (58). The usual patient is a child or young adult who presents with headache, seizure, progressive hemiplegia, and/or signs of raised intracranial pressure. Most have neither symptoms of systemic infection nor signs of meningitis (2, 3, 25, 58). While the presumptive diagnosis can be made on the basis of clinical and epidemiological considerations, or by needle biopsy, CT scanning with contrast enhancement has proven to be a major advance in the diagnosis and management of these cases. CT is especially useful for assessing the presence of cerebral edema and the risk of brain stem herniation, and for monitoring the response to medical therapy (25). Early surgical intervention, except perhaps for diagnostic needle biopsy, is to be avoided, as it may precipitate severe meningitis (25, 53). Conservative medical management is effective for most cases; surgery is reserved for cases in which critically located lesions have produced obstructive hydrocephalus or compression of the brain stem (25, 58). Corticosteroids are helpful where cerebral edema out of proportion to the mass effect is producing altered mental status or focal neurologic deficits.

SPINAL TUBERCULOUS ARACHNOIDITIS

Arachnoiditis or tuberculoma can arise at any level of the spinal cord in association with the breakdown of a Rich focus within the cord or meninges, or by extension from an adjacent area of spondylitis (34). The resulting inflammatory reaction is usually confined locally and progresses gradually over weeks to months, producing a partial or complete encasement of the cord by a gelatinous or fibrous mass (18). Patients usually present with some combination of nerve root and cord compression signs secondary to impingement by the advancing arachnoiditis. Clinical manifestations are predominately neurologic rather than infectious, are protean in nature, and take the form of an ascending or transverse radiculomyelopathy of variable pace at single or multiple levels (62). Symptoms include pain, hyperesthesia, or paresthesia in the distribution of the nerve root; lower motor neuron paralysis; and bladder or rectal sphincter incontinence. Localized vasculitis may result in thrombosis of the anterior spinal artery and infarction of the cord. All forms of tuberculous arachnoiditis commonly produce subarachnoid block characterized by unusually high CSF protein levels, regardless of whether there is a cellular pleocytosis. The diagnosis of spinal TB arachnoiditis should be considered in a patient with any combination of the following clinical and laboratory features: subacute onset of spinal or nerve root pain, rapidly ascending transverse myelopathy or multilevel myelopathy, increased CSF protein concentration and cell count, signs of arachnoiditis or epidural space infection by MRI, and evidence of TB elsewhere in the body (34, 44). Tissue biopsy for histopathology stains and culture is required for diagnosis. Progression from an initial spinal syndrome to frank TBM occurs in some patients late in the course.

TREATMENT

Antituberculous Therapy

As has been emphasized, the first principle of antituberculous therapy is that it should be initiated on the basis of strong clinical suspicion rather than delayed until proof of the diagnosis has been obtained. The prognosis is good when treatment is begun before the development of focal neurologic signs and altered state of consciousness. Accordingly, the risks of delay, even for only a few days, are greater than those of unnecessary drug treatment so long as one persists in the effort to confirm the diagnosis. There are no randomized trials to establish the optimal drug combination, dose, and duration of treatment for TBM. The principles governing the therapy for TBM are those derived in relation to the management of pulmonary TB (37). The purpose of using combination drug regimens is to enhance the bactericidal effect, cover the possibility of some degree of primary drug resistance, and reduce the likelihood of emerging resistance on therapy. A brief description of the major first-line drugs is given below.

Isoniazid (INH) diffuses readily into the CSF, achieving concentrations severalfold higher than that required for bactericidal activity (21). The daily dose for children is 10 g/kg, and that for adults is 300 mg. Pyridoxine, 25 or 50 mg daily, should be given concurrently so as to avoid the neurologic complications associated with INH-induced pyridoxine deficiency. A parenteral form of INH is available if needed.

Rifampin (RIF) is active early against rapidly dividing organisms and achieves reliable CSF concentrations in the presence of meningeal inflammation. This drug is active against semidormant bacilli, which may be an advantage in achieving late resolution of infectious foci in the CNS and elsewhere in the body. The daily dose in children and adults is 10 mg/kg to a maximum dose of 600 mg. An intravenous formulation is available from the manufacturer on a "compassionate-use" basis.

Pyrazinamide (PZA) penetrates readily into the CSF and is highly active against intracellular organisms. Therapeutic efficacy is enhanced when this agent is used in combination with INH and RIF, but the dose and duration are limited by the propensity to cause hepatotoxicity. At a dose of 25 to 35 mg/kg, and limited to no more than 2 months, the combination is safe and effective (12). For children the daily dose is 15 to 20 mg/kg. For adults, the dose is determined by weight: 40 to 60 kg, 1,000 mg; 56 to 75 kg, 1,500 mg; and 76 to 90 kg, 2,000 mg.

Ethambutol (EMB) is a weak drug that achieves moderately effective CSF concentrations. Its major toxicity is optic neuritis, which developed at a rate of 3% or more when patients were treated with 25 mg/kg. This complication is rare at the current recommended dose of 15 mg/kg; however, it is advisable to monitor patients monthly by following visual acuity, red-green color vision, and visual fields (17).

Recommended Regimen

For the usual drug-sensitive infection, published guidelines call for an initial intensive phase of four-drug therapy with INH, RIF, PZA, and either EMB or streptomycin, administered for 2 months. This is followed by a continuation phase with two drugs, usually INH and RIF, for 7 to 10 months more (1). If PZA is omitted or not tolerated, the duration of treatment should be extended to 18 months.

Risk factors for drug-resistant infection include prior treatment with antituberculous drugs, exposure to persons with known resistant TB, homelessness, and acquisition of primary infection in high-prevalence regions of the world. The impact of drug resistance on outcome is variable, depending on whether the isolate is resistant to INH, to RIF, or to both (56). The second-line drugs ethionamide and cycloserine penetrate well into the CSF and are useful. Novel approaches to the management of drug-resistant TBM, using newer aminoglycosides and fluoroquinolones, have been reported (6).

Adjunctive Corticosteroids

Despite uncertainty regarding the efficacy, and whether the benefit outweighs the risk, patients with TBM have routinely been treated with corticosteroids in an effort to reduce inflammation, limit damage to the CNS, and thus improve outcome. Early clinical studies bearing on this issue are flawed because of the study design, the limited number of cases, and the failure to carefully stratify patients by severity of illness and specific neurologic manifestations. There is at present, however, a growing number of carefully designed, controlled studies from clinical centers around the world showing that adjunctive steroid therapy is beneficial for children and adults with TBM (23, 27, 49, 57).

In a prospective trial, 141 children with TBM were randomized to receive either prednisone or placebo for 4 weeks (49). Prednisone therapy increased the rate of resolution of basal exudate and tuberculomas and improved survival and subsequent measures of intellectual development. A randomized, double-blind trial in Vietnam compared dexamethasone with placebo (tapered dose over 6 to 8 weeks) in 545 patients older than 14 years of age (57). The mortality rate was reduced significantly in the treated group (32%, versus 41%). The benefit was greatest for patients in clinical stage 1 (17%, versus 30%). No mortality benefit was seen in patients in stage 3 or in the 98 patients coinfected with HIV. A follow-up survey conducted by questionnaire at 9 months failed to demonstrate a reduction in residual neurologic deficits and disability.

Adjunctive corticosteroid therapy is recommended for all patients with convincing clinical evidence of CNS TB, the possible exception being adults with mild stage 1 disease. Complications for which corticosteroids are thought to be most beneficial are increased intracranial pressure, cerebral edema, and spinal block. Specific indications based on urgent warning signs are as follows: progression from one clinical stage to the next at or before the start of antituberculous therapy, CT evidence of marked basal enhancement (high risk for vascular complications), moderate or advancing hydrocephalus, spinal block or incipient block (CSF protein above 500 mg/dl), and intracerebral tuberculoma when edema is out of proportion to the mass effect and there are neurologic signs (altered mentation or focal deficits). Either dexamethasone or prednisone may be used. When using dexamethasone the dose is 8 mg daily for children weighing less than 25 kg and 12 mg/day for adults and children weighing more than 25 kg. When using prednisone the dose is 2 to 4 mg/kg daily for children and 60 mg/day for adults. The duration is 3 weeks at the initial dose, followed by a gradual tapering over the next 3 to 4 weeks.

Response and Outcome

The clinical outcome for treated TBM is influenced by age, duration of illness, and extent of arachnoiditis and vasculitis. The clinical stage at the time therapy is initiated also greatly affects both mortality and incidence of subsequent neurologic sequelae (31, 32). This was illustrated in the series of 52 cases reported by Kennedy and Fallon (31). When therapy was begun before patients had progressed beyond clinical stage 1 or early stage 2 disease, the mortality rate was less than 10% and residual neurologic deficits minimal. Of the 11 patients in stage 3 at the time of treatment, 6 died or suffered severe neurologic sequelae. The incidence of residual neurologic deficits after treatment of TBM varied from 10 to 30% in recent series (26, 31, 59, 61). Late sequelae include CN palsies, gait disturbance, hemiplegia, blindness, deafness, learning disabilities, dementia, and various syndromes of hypothalamic and pituitary dysfunction.

REFERENCES

1. **American Thoracic Society, Centers for Disease Control and Prevention, and Infectious Diseases Society of America.** 2003. Treatment of tuberculosis. *MMWR Recommend. Rep.* 52:1–77.

2. **Bagga, A., V. Kalra, and O. P. Ghai.** 1988. Intracranial tuberculoma: evaluation and treatment. *Clin. Pediatr.* 27:487–490.

3. **Behemuka, M., and J. H. Murungi.** 1989. Tuberculosis of the nervous system: a clinical, radiological and pathological study of 39 consecutive cases in Riyadh, South Arabia. *J. Neurol. Sci.* 90:67–76.

4. **Berenguer, J., S. Moreno, F. Laguna, T. Vicente, M. Adrados, A. Ortega, J. Gonzalez-LaHoz, and E. Bouza.** 1992. Tuberculous meningitis in patients infected with the human immunodeficiency virus. *N. Engl. J. Med.* 326:668–672.

5. **Bernaerts, A., F. M. Vanhoenacker, P. M. Parizel, J. W. Van Goethem, R. Van Altena, A. Laridon, J. De Roeck, V. Coeman, and A. M. De Schepper.** 2003. Tuberculosis of the central ner-

vous system: overview of neuroradiological findings. *Eur. Radiol.* **13:**1876–1890.

6. Berning, S. E., T. A. Cherry, and M. D. Iseman. 2001. Novel treatment of meningitis caused by multidrug-resistant *Mycobacterium tuberculosis* with intrathecal levofloxacin and amikacin: case report. *Clin. Infect. Dis.* **32:**643–646.

7. Bhargava, S., A. K. Gupta, and P. N. Tandon. 1982. Tuberculous meningitis—a CT study. *Br. J. Radiol.* **55:**189–196.

8. Bishburg, E., G. Sunderam, L. B. Reichman, and R. Kapila. 1986. Central nervous system tuberculosis with the acquired immunodeficiency syndrome and its related complex. *Ann. Intern. Med.* **105:**210–213.

9. Blazquez, E. P., M. Rodriguez, and M. J. Mendez Ramos. 1994. Tuberculous choroiditis and acquired immune deficiency syndrome. *Ann. Ophthalmol.* **26:**50–54.

10. Bonington, A., J. I. Strang, P. E. Klapper, S. V. Hood, W. Rubombora, M. Penny, R. Willers, and E. G. Wilkins. 1998. Use of Roche AMPLICOR *Mycobacterium tuberculosis* PCR in early diagnosis of tuberculous meningitis. *J. Clin. Microbiol.* **36:**1251–1254.

11. Braun, M. M., R. H. Byers, W. L. Heyward, C. A. Ciesielski, A. B. Bloch, R. L. Berkelman, and D. E. Snider. 1990. Acquired immunodeficiency syndrome and extrapulmonary tuberculosis in the United States. *Arch. Intern. Med.* **150:**1913–1916.

12. British Thoracic Association. 1981. A controlled trial of six months chemotherapy in pulmonary tuberculosis. *Br. J. Dis. Chest* **75:**141–153.

13. Centers for Disease Control and Prevention. 2005. Extrapulmonary tuberculosis cases and percentages by site of disease: reporting areas, 2005. Centers for Disease Control and prevention, Atlanta, GA. http://www.cdc.gov/tb/surv2005/PDF/tabl27.pdf.

14. Centers for Disease Control and Prevention. 2009. Trends in tuberculosis—United States, 2008. *MMWR Morb. Mortal. Wkly. Rep.* **58:**249–253.

15. Centers for Disease Control and Prevention. 2010. *Data Statistics: Tuberculosis (TB) Is One of the World's Deadliest Diseases.* Centers for Disease Control and Prevention, Atlanta, GA. http://www.cdc.gov/tb/surv/statistics/default.htm.

16. Chan, K. H., R. T. Cheung, R. Lee, W. Mak, and S. L. Ho. 2005. Cerebral infarcts complicating tuberculous meningitis. *Cerebrovasc. Dis.* **19:**391–395.

17. Chatterjee, V. K. K., D. R. Buchanan, A. I. Friedmann, and M. Green. 1986. Ocular toxicity following ethambutol in standard dosage. *Br. J. Dis. Chest* **80:**288–290.

18. Dastur, D. K. 1983. Neurosurgically relevant aspects of pathology and pathogenesis of intracranial and intraspinal tuberculosis. *Neurosurg. Rev.* **6:**103–110.

19. Dastur, D. K., D. K. Manghani, and P. M. Udani. 1995. Pathology and pathogenetic mechanisms in neurotuberculosis. *Radiol. Clin. N. Am.* **33:**733–752.

20. Dube, M. P., P. D. Holtom, and R. A. Larsen. 1992. Tuberculous meningitis in patients with and without human immunodeficiency virus infection. *Am. J. Med.* **93:**520–524.

21. Ellard, G. A., M. J. Humphries, and B. W. Allen. 1993. Cerebrospinal fluid drug concentrations and the treatment of tuberculous meningitis. *Am. Rev. Respir. Dis.* **148:**650–655.

22. Farinha, N. J., K. A. Razali, H. Holzel, G. Morgan, and V. M. Novelli. 2000. Tuberculosis of the central nervous system in children: a 20-year survey. *J. Infect.* **41:**61–68.

23. Girgis, N. I., Z. Farid, M. E. Kilpatrick, Y. Sultan, and I. A. Mikhail. 1991. Dexamethasone adjunctive treatment for tuberculous meningitis. *Pediatr. Infect. Dis. J.* **10:**179–183.

24. Goldzieher, J. W., and J. R. Lisa. 1947. Gross cerebral hemorrhage and vascular lesions in acute tuberculous meningitis and meningo-encephalitis. *Am. J. Pathol.* **23:**133–145.

25. Harder, E., M. Z. Al-Kawi, and P. Carney. 1983. Intracranial tuberculoma: conservative management. *Am. J. Med.* **74:**570–576.

26. Hinman, A. R. 1975. Tuberculous meningitis at Cleveland Metropolitan General Hospital, 1959–1963. *Am. Rev. Respir. Dis.* **95:**670–673.

27. Humphries, M. 1992. The management of tuberculous meningitis. *Thorax* **47:**577–581.

28. Kaneko, K., O. Onodera, T. Miyatake, and S. Tsuji. 1990. Rapid diagnosis of tuberculous meningitis by polymerase chain reaction (PCR). *Neurology* **40:**1617–1618.

29. Karandanis, D., and J. A. Shulman. 1976. Recent survey of infectious meningitis in adults: review of laboratory findings in bacterial, tuberculous, and aseptic meningitis. *South. Med. J.* **69:**449–456.

30. Katrak, S. M., P. K. Shembalkar, S. R. Bujwe, and L. D. Bhandarkar. 2000. The clinical, radiological and pathological profile of tuberculous meningitis in patients with and without human immunodeficiency virus infection. *J. Neurol. Sci.* **181:**118–126.

31. Kennedy, D. H., and R. J. Fallon. 1979. Tuberculous meningitis. *JAMA* **241:**264–268.

32. Kent, S. J., S. M. Crowe, A. Yung, C. R. Lucas, and A. M. Mijch. 1993. Tuberculous meningitis: a 30-year review. *Clin. Infect. Dis.* **17:**987–994.

33. Kingsley, D. P., W. A. Hendrickse, B. E. Kendall, M. Swash, and V. Singh. 1987. Tuberculous meningitis: role of CT in management and prognosis. *J. Neurol. Neurosurg. Psychiatry* **50:**30–36.

34. Kocen, R. S., and M. Parsons. 1970. Neurological complications of tuberculosis: some unusual manifestations. *Q. J. Med.* **39:**17–30.

35. Kumar, R., N. Kohli, H. Thavnani, A. Kumar, and B. Sharma. 1996. Value of CT scan in the diagnosis of meningitis. *Indian Pediatr.* **33:**465–468.

36. Lamprecht, D., J. F. Schoeman, P. Donald, and H. Hartzenberg. 2001. Ventriculoperitoneal shunting in childhood tuberculous meningitis. *Br. J. Neurosurg.* **15:**119–125.

37. Mitchison, D. A. 2000. Role of individual drugs in the chemotherapy of tuberculosis. *Int. J. Tuberc. Lung Dis.* **4:**796–806.

38. Noordhoek, G. T., A. H. Kolk, G. Bjune, D. Catty, J. W. Dale, P. E. Fine, P. Godfrey-Faussett, S. N. Cho, T. Shinnick, and S. B. Svenson. 1994. Sensitivity and specificity of PCR for detection of *Mycobacterium tuberculosis*: a blind comparison study among seven laboratories. *J. Clin. Microbiol.* **32:**277–284.

39. Offenbacher, H., F. Fazekas, R. Schmidt, R. Kleinert, F. Payer, G. Kleinert, and H. Lechner. 1991. MRI in tuberculous meningoencephalitis: report of four cases and review of the neuroimaging literature. *J. Neurol.* **238:**340–344.

40. Ozateş, M., S. Kemaloglu, F. Gürkan, U. S. Ozkan, and M. M. Simşek. 2000. CT of the brain in tuberculous meningitis. A review of 289 patients. *Acta Radiol.* **41:**13–17.

41. Pai, M., L. L. Flores, N. Pai, A. Hubbard, L. W. Riley, and J. M. Colford, Jr. 2003. Diagnostic accuracy of nucleic acid amplification tests for tuberculous meningitis: a systematic review and meta-analysis. *Lancet Infect. Dis.* **3:**633–643.

42. Poltera, A. A. 1977. Thrombogenic intracranial vasculitis in tuberculous meningitis. A 20 year "post mortem" survey. *Acta Neurol. Belg.* **77:**12–24.

43. Porkert, M. T., M. Sotir, P. Parrott-Moore, and H. M. Blumberg. 1997. Tuberculous meningitis at a large inner city medical center. *Am. J. Med. Sci.* **313:**325–331.

44. Rahman, N. U. 1980. Atypical forms of spinal tuberculosis. *J. Bone Joint Surg. (Br.)* **62:**162–165.

45. Rich, A. R., and H. A. McCordock. 1933. The pathogenesis of tuberculous meningitis. *Bull. Johns Hopkins Hosp.* **52:**5–37.

46. Rieder, H. L., D. E. Snider, Jr., and G. M. Cauthen. 1990. Extrapulmonary tuberculosis in the United States. *Am. Rev. Respir. Dis.* **141**:347–351.

47. Schoeman, J., P. Donald, L. van Zyl, M. Keet, and J. Wait. 1991. Tuberculous hydrocephalus: comparison of different treatments with regard to ICP, ventricular size and clinical outcome. *Dev. Med. Child Neurol.* **33**:396–405.

48. Schoeman, J., R. Hewlett, and P. Donald. 1988. MR of childhood tuberculous meningitis. *Neuroradiology* **30**:473–477.

49. Schoeman, J. F., L. E. Van Zyl, J. A. Laubscher, and P. R. Donald. 1997. Effect of corticosteroids on intracranial pressure, computed tomographic findings, and clinical outcome in young children with tuberculous meningitis. *Pediatrics* **99**:226–231.

50. Sharma, S. K., A. Mohan, A. Sharma, and D. K. Mitra. 2005. Miliary tuberculosis: new insights into an old disease. *Lancet Infect. Dis.* **5**:415–430.

51. Slavin, R. E., T. J. Walsh, and A. Pollak. 1980. Late generalized tuberculosis: a clinical pathologic analysis and comparison of 100 cases in the pre-antibiotic and antibiotic eras. *Medicine* **59**:352–366.

52. Smith, J., and R. Godwin-Austen. 1980. Hypersecretion of anti-diuretic hormone due to tuberculous meningitis. *Postgrad. Med. J.* **56**:41–44.

53. Tandon, P. N., and S. Bhargava. 1985. Effect of medical treatment on intracranial tuberculoma—a CT study. *Tubercle* **66**:85–97.

54. Teoh, R., M. J. Humphries, and G. O'Mahony. 1987. Symptomatic intracranial tuberculoma developing during treatment of tuberculosis: a report of 10 patients and review of the literature. *Q. J. Med.* **63**:449–460.

55. Thwaites, G. E., T. T. Chau, and J. J. Farrar. 2004. Improving the bacteriological diagnosis of tuberculous meningitis. *J. Clin. Microbiol.* **42**:378–379.

56. Thwaites, G. E., N. T. Lan, N. H. Dung, H. T. Quy, D. T. Oanh, N. T. Thoa, N. Q. Hien, N. T. Thuc, N. N. Hai, N. D. Bang, N. N. Lan, N. H. Duc, V. N. Tuan, C. H. Hiep, T. T. Chau, P. P. Mai, N. T. Dung, K. Stepniewska, N. J. White, T. T. Hien, and J. J. Farrar. 2005. Effect of antituberculosis drug resistance on response to treatment and outcome in adults with tuberculous meningitis. *J. Infect. Dis.* **192**:79–88.

57. Thwaites, G. E., D. B. Nguyen, H. D. Nguyen, T. Q. Hoang, T. T. Do, T. C. Nguyen, Q. H. Nguyen, T. T. Nguyen, N. H. Nguyen, T. N. Nguyen, N. L. Nguyen, H. D. Nguyen, N. T. Vu, H. H. Cao, T. H. Tran, P. M. Pham, T. D. Nguyen, K. Stepniewska, N. J. White, T. H. Tran, and J. J. Farrar. 2004. Dexamethasone for the treatment of tuberculous meningitis in adolescents and adults. *N. Engl. J. Med.* **351**:1741–1751.

58. Traub, M., A. C. Colchester, D. P. Kingsley, and M. Swash. 1984. Tuberculosis of the central nervous system. *Q. J. Med.* **53**:81–100.

59. Udani, P. M., and D. K. Dastur. 1970. Tuberculous encephalopathy with and without meningitis. Clinical features and pathological correlations. *J. Neurol. Sci.* **10**:541–561.

60. van Dyk, A. 1988. CT of intracranial tuberculoma with specific reference to the 'target sign.' *Neuroradiology* **30**:329–336.

61. Verdon, R., S. Chevret, J. P. Laissy, and M. Wolff. 1996. Tuberculous meningitis in adults: review of 48 cases. *Clin. Infect. Dis.* **22**:982–988.

62. Wadia, N. H., and D. K. Dastur. 1969. Spinal meningitides with radiculomyelopathy. Part I—clinical and radiological features. *J. Neurol. Sci.* **8**:239–260.

63. Weisberg, L. A. 1984. Granulomatous diseases of the CNS as demonstrated by computerized tomography. *Comput. Radiol.* **8**:309–317.

64. Whelan, M. A., and J. Stern. 1981. Intracranial tuberculoma. *Radiology* **138**:75–81.

Chapter 19

Tuberculous Lymphadenitis and Parotitis

W. Garrett Hunt

HISTORICAL PERSPECTIVES

What great difficulty we meet with in the cure of the Kings Evill, with the daily experience both of Physicians and Chirurgeons doth shew. . . .When upon trial he shall find the contumaciousness of the disease which frequently diluded his best care and industry, he will find reason of acknowledging the goodness of God; who hath dealth so beautifully with this nation, in giving the Kings of it at least from Edward the Confessor downward (if not for a longer time) an extraordinary power in the miraculous Cure thereof.

Richard Wiseman, 17th-century surgeon (33)

Scrofula, defined as tuberculosis of the lymphatic glands, has afflicted humans for thousands of years. Hippocrates (460 to 377 BCE) mentioned scrofulous tumors in his writing, and Herodotus (484? to 425? BCE) described the exclusion of those afflicted with leprous or scrofulous lesions from the general population. This illness was known as the King's Evil during the Middle Ages in Europe because of the apparent cure of many cases following the king's royal touch. Clovis I of France (466 to 511 CE) is the first recorded king to use the royal touch to cure scrofula after his baptism in 496 CE. The royal touch was practiced by English sovereigns from Edward the Confessor to Queen Anne (35), and historians have recorded vivid accounts of the crushing mobs who gathered to see the royal touch. Charles II of England is reputed to have applied the royal touch 90,798 times. After being touched, patients received a gold piece, which was to protect them from subsequent scrofulous attacks. It was often the job of the parish rector to select needy patients and to ensure that they were more desirous of a cure for their scrofula than of the golden coin about their necks (35).

Not until the 19th century, when pathology emerged as a science, was the tuberculous etiology of scrofula recognized. As late as the first half of the 19th century, the German physician Johan Lucas

Schulman erroneously differentiated scrofula from tuberculosis as a different family of blood-borne diseases (32). A variety of internal and external causes of scrofula were proposed, including hereditary lymphatic temperament, contagion, degeneration of the syphilitic virus, food and drink, dirt, excretions, and atmospheric influence. In 1846 in England, scrofula most frequently afflicted children between ages 2 and 15 years. Of 133,000 children examined, 24% showed obvious scars of scrofula or had enlarged cervical glands (32). Once a scrofulous node erupted through the skin, the illness became a repulsive, long-term disability because the resulting ulcers intermittently exuded a thick, sour-smelling pus. It is little wonder that this potentially disfiguring, chronic disease was regarded by the public and by some physicians as the manifestation of an inherited dysfunction of the constitution or even of degeneracy (32).

EPIDEMIOLOGY

Tuberculosis of the lymph nodes is the most common form of extrapulmonary tuberculosis. Surveys in the United States and Canada have shown lymph node involvement to represent 5 to 9% of all reported cases of tuberculosis (17). Despite declining rates of tuberculosis in the United States during the past decade (11), the incidence of tuberculosis has increased worldwide, resulting in an increased incidence of tuberculous lymphadenitis (18, 19, 34). In contrast, tuberculosis of the parotid glands, first described in 1894 (12), remains a rare occurrence, reported primarily in single or small case studies and identified mostly in parotidectomy specimens (12, 21, 23, 49).

Historically, lymph node tuberculosis has been identified most commonly in children. However, in numerous recent studies from developed countries, the peak age range is between 20 and 40 years of

W. Garrett Hunt • College of Medicine, The Ohio State University, Section of Infectious Diseases, Nationwide Children's Hospital, 700 Children's Drive, ED 162, Columbus, OH 43205.

age (18). This shift in age probably reflects the falling incidence of childhood tuberculosis in developed countries. In contrast, children still compose a high percentage of cases of scrofula in areas of endemic tuberculosis (28) in developing countries or areas where immigration from developing countries has increased (34).

It has long been recognized that primary (childhood) versus secondary (adult) tuberculosis is distinctly different relative to lymph node involvement. In untreated primary tuberculosis of children, almost all patients have enlargement of hilar or paratracheal lymph nodes (or both) apparent on chest roentgenograms (24, 47). Extrapulmonary lymphadenitis develops in 5% of patients within 6 months of tuberculous infection (31). Infected nodes commonly become greatly enlarged and caseous. Lymph node involvement occurs shortly after the onset of primary infection. A total of 50 to 80% of children with cervical lymph node involvement have radiographic evidence of active pulmonary tuberculosis (24, 34, 47). In contrast, adult tuberculous cervical lymphadenitis is accompanied by an abnormal chest radiograph less than 30% of the time (18), and these changes usually represent old, healed tuberculosis, suggesting that node disease results from reactivation of previous infection.

Ethnic origin and gender also seem to have a major bearing on the risk of developing tuberculous lymphadenitis. Within the United States, Canada, Australia, and the United Kingdom, a majority of cases occur in persons born on the Indian and Asian subcontinents. In a national British survey, tuberculous lymphadenitis accounted for about 40% of the cases of tuberculosis in immigrants of Asian origin (37). The influx of Asian immigrants to Canada has been one of the major reasons for the sustained incidence of lymph node tuberculosis in that country despite a decline in pulmonary tuberculosis. In addition to a higher risk of tuberculosis, persons born in Africa or Southeast Asia appear to have a predilection for developing lymphadenitis (20). Within a population of U.S. naval personnel with active tuberculosis, Asians have a disproportionately high rate of lymph node versus pulmonary involvement (10) (Table 1). Although males predominate in cases of pulmonary tuberculosis, most studies of peripheral lymph node tuberculosis describe a greater than 2:1 female/male case ratio (20). In the developed world, then, those at the highest risk for having lymph node tuberculosis are Indian, Asian, or African women between the ages of 20 and 40 years. Persons infected with human immunodeficiency virus (HIV) have a high risk for developing tuberculosis. It has been estimated that among persons with active tuberculosis, HIV type 1-infected patients represent 8% of the worldwide

Table 1. Racial distribution of tuberculous lymphadenitis and pulmonary tuberculosis in U.S. naval personnel[a]

Race	Distribution of tuberculosis (%)	
	Lymph node	Pulmonary
White	7	55
Black	7	10
Asian	79	31
Other	7	4

[a]Adapted from reference 10.

total and 30 to 60% of cases in Africa (1, 19). Extrapulmonary tuberculosis appears to be much more frequent in patients with HIV infection. Isolated extrapulmonary localizations, particularly lymphadenitis, are described for 53 to 63% of tuberculosis cases in HIV type 1-infected patients and more frequently in severely immunocompromised HIV patients (1).

PATHOLOGY

A nearly uniform event following infection by *Mycobacterium tuberculosis* is spread from the primary focus to regional lymph nodes. This often results in a greater volume of diseased tissue in regional lymph nodes than at the original site of infection. From the regional nodes, organisms may continue to spread via the lymphatic system to other nodes or may pass through the nodes and reach the bloodstream in small numbers, from which they may spread to virtually any organ in the body. This form of lymphatic and hematogenous dissemination is usually self-limited. More than 90% of primary infections in humans heal without symptomatic disease. Reactivation tuberculosis may develop as a late recrudescence from dormant organisms in lymph nodes that were invaded during the primary infection. Increased expression of interleukin 10 and transforming growth factor beta may downregulate microbicidal functions, thus favoring the survival and persistence of bacilli in the cellular microenvironment of granulomas (38). Lymphadenitis due to *M. tuberculosis* is associated with a downregulation of memory T cells (CD45RO), reduced macrophage activity, and reduced expression of suppressor of cytokine stimulation 3 (41). These functions may play a role in the long-term bacterial replication and altered immune modulation characteristic of the disease.

Tuberculous infection in the parotid gland usually develops following infection of intraparotid lymph nodes. The intraparotid lymphoid tissue becomes infected following spread through the lymphatics from a focus of mycobacterial infection in a tonsil, gingival sulcus, or break in the oral mucosa (23). As the capsule of the infected lymph tissue breaks down, parotitis may ensue. Direct infection of the parotid gland may also follow hematogenous seeding or occur by communication via the salivary ducts from autoinoculation with infected sputum (21, 49).

Historically, lymph node and parotid tuberculosis was caused mainly by *Mycobacterium bovis*, but nearly all tuberculous lymphadenitis is now due to *M. tuberculosis*. Because infection with *M. tuberculosis* usually begins in the lungs, the regional nodes draining the pulmonary parenchyma are most commonly infected. These nodes include a peribronchial group, filling the hilar regions of both lungs; a subcarinal group, at the angle of the bifurcation of the trachea behind the right pulmonary artery; and a paratracheal group, adjacent to the trachea within the posterior mediastinum. These nodes may all be involved in endobronchial tuberculosis, which occurs most commonly in children but is being described with increasing frequency for adults (18, 24, 47).

Even though mediastinal nodes are the most common primary regional draining sites, they account for only 5% of reported cases of lymph node tuberculosis. Instead, clinically apparent tuberculous lymphadenitis most frequently involves nodes of the head and neck, typically those in the anterior or posterior cervical chains and supraclavicular region (18, 24, 34, 47). Because localized primary infections of the head and neck are unusual, infection in these nodes probably results from the generalized lymphatic spread following a primary pulmonary infection. It has been suggested that paratracheal lymph nodes communicate with deep cervical nodes and abdominal nodes (46). Among 54 patients with primary tuberculosis in the right upper lobe, a location that drains primarily to the right paratracheal lymph node, 14 had involvement of the deep cervical nodes on the same side and 3 had involvement of the abdominal nodes (46).

In the uncommon occurrence of axillary, inguinal, or other noncervical peripheral node tuberculosis, a focus of infection distal to the infected node is often identified. Preauricular adenitis suggests a scalp, eye, or lacrimal duct infection (2, 51). Epitrochlear lymphadenitis may follow infections on the forearm or hand (15). Axillary lymph nodes are involved with lesions of the arms, chest wall, or mammary glands (29, 44). Inguinal lymph nodes may become infected following lesions on the feet or legs or following genital infection (50).

The major pathological events of lymph node tuberculosis include compression of surrounding tissue, caseation and breakdown of nodes, and fibrosis from healing of the eroded nodes. Mortality is uncommon, but morbidity and chronic illness are the rule. Probably the best example of the severe pathological events associated with lymph node tuberculosis

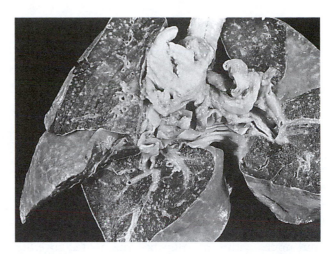

Figure 1. Autopsy specimen of endobronchial tuberculosis. A large caseous lymph node is attached to and compresses the right mainstem and right upper-lobe bronchi.

is found in endobronchial disease of children (24, 30). In the child whose body is unable to contain the progressive multiplication and spread of tubercle bacilli, the onset of delayed hypersensitivity is accompanied by marked hyperemia and swelling of the regional nodes, with external compression of the trachea and bronchi. When the centers of the nodes develop necrosis and caseation, marked perinodal inflammation leads to node adherence to the outer surface of the airways (Fig. 1). As the nodes begin to erode through the bronchial wall, submucosal tubercles, intraluminal polyps, and granulation tissue appear (Fig. 2). Ultimately, nodes may perforate the

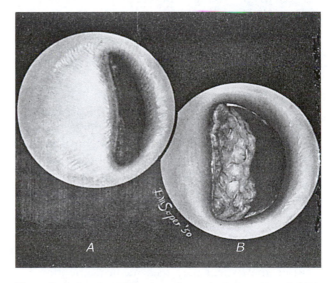

Figure 2. A drawing of the bronchoscopic appearance of childhood endobronchial tuberculosis. (A) Loss of lumen size owing to external compression by a tuberculous peribronchial lymph node; (B) erosion of the lymph node through the bronchial wall with intraluminal granulation tissue. Reprinted from *Tuberculosis in White and Negro Children* (22a) by permission of Harvard University Press.

bronchial wall, causing caseous tissue to extrude into the bronchial lumen, with possible bronchial obstruction or spread of caseous tissue to other areas of the lung. With healing of the involved nodes and bronchus, fibrosis usually leads to permanent bronchial stenosis or bronchiectasis. Lymph node enlargement within the mediastinum may also be accompanied by compression of major blood vessels, impingement on the phrenic or recurrent laryngeal nerves, occlusion of lymphatic drainage, or erosion into the chest wall and sternum.

Involvement of the superficial lymph nodes usually results in enlarging mass lesions. If infected lymph nodes remain untreated, swelling progresses and nodes within a group become matted together and adherent to the overlying skin. Eventually, the overlying skin develops a purplish discoloration, the center of the mass become soft, and caseous material soon ruptures into surrounding tissue or through the skin. This is the classical appearance of scrofula.

CLINICAL ILLNESS

More than 90% of superficial tuberculous lymph nodes are found in the head and neck regions (18). In order of decreasing frequency, these include anterior and posterior cervical, supraclavicular, submandibular, and, occasionally, preauricular or submental nodes (26). Several nodes within a group are usually involved, and bilateral adenitis is common, particularly in young children. Generalized lymphadenopathy and hepatosplenomegaly occur in less than 5% of most series. It should be noted, however, that in children with miliary tuberculosis, generalized lymphadenopathy may be found in 10 to 15% of cases (45).

The symptoms associated with tuberculous lymphadenitis depend largely on the location of involved nodes. In both adults and children, the primary presenting symptom of cervical lymphadenitis is a painless, slowly progressive swelling in the neck (3) (Fig. 3). Several weeks may pass before the nodes are sufficiently enlarged to warrant medical attention. In less than 20% of patients, there are associated symptoms such as weight loss, temperature elevation, anorexia, fatigue, malaise, or pain. If the nodes are allowed to progress through the stages of caseation and erosion, the patient may seek medical attention because of the chronic damage from the resulting ulcer or sinus tract. In a more recent series, this occurred less than 10% of the time (26).

With peribronchial or paratracheal lymph node enlargement, presenting symptoms are somewhat dependent on age. In the adult, enlarging nodes

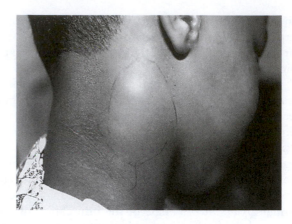

Figure 3. A 9-year-old Somali boy with bilateral posterior cervical tuberculous lymphadenitis (one side shown). Photo courtesy of Dwight Powell, M.D.

rarely impinge on the bronchial lumen to cause respiratory symptoms. Instead, illness is manifested as weight loss, fever, low-grade night sweats, chronic chest pain, malaise, anorexia, or asymptomatic abnormal-looking pulmonary radiographs (18). In children, symptomatic endobronchial tuberculosis is most common in those under 4 years of age and symptoms arise from airway compromise (24, 47). Coughing, often severe and paroxysmal, is the most frequent symptom. With progressive obstruction of the airway lumen, the child may experience wheezing, stridor, dyspnea, and eventually respiratory distress with hypoxia and cyanosis due to pulmonary atelectasis.

Other uncommon presenting symptoms of tuberculous lymphadenitis include chyluria due to obstruction of the thoracic duct, chronic abdominal pain and low-grade fever due to retroperitoneal lymphadenitis, progressive jaundice due to biliary obstruction, chronic chest pain caused by intercostal lymph node involvement, a neck mass with dysphagia caused by a traction diverticulum of the esophagus or retropharyngeal abscess, vocal card paralysis, nasopharyngeal mass, or generalized lymph node enlargement suggesting reticulohistiocytic tumors.

On physical examination, peripheral tuberculous nodes are initially firm or rubbery, discrete, and nontender. The painless quality usually persists despite caseation and erosion through the skin. Occasionally in young children, the nodes may be swollen and tender at the time of presentation owing to secondary bacterial infections (31). The physical appearance of superficial tuberculous lymphadenitis has been classified into five stages by Jones and Campbell (27): stage 1, enlarged, firm, mobile, discrete nodes showing nonspecific reactive hyperplasia; stage 2, larger, rubbery nodes fixed to surrounding tissue owing to periadenitis; stage 3, central softening due to abscess formation; stage 4, collar stud abscess formation; and stage 5, sinus tract formation. The majority of cases fall into stages 2 and 3 at the time of their initial presentation (28).

Tuberculous parotitis rarely presents as acute glandular swelling. More often, chronic parotitis develops as an asymptomatic localized lesion enlarging over months to years (14, 21, 48, 49). These masses are often difficult to distinguish from parotid tumors. In 25 to 50% of cases, chronically draining sinus tracts may develop that mimic a true branchial cleft fistula. Most patients show few signs of systemic or pulmonary tuberculosis. Mild tenderness or spontaneous pain may develop, and late in the course of the swelling, the size of the mass may increase rapidly (57).

DIAGNOSIS

The differential diagnosis of tuberculous lymphadenitis or parotitis is extensive. Consideration must be given to alternative infections (nontuberculous mycobacteria [NTM], viruses, chlamydia, bacteria, fungi, and *Toxoplasma*), neoplasms (lymphoma, sarcoma, adenoma, Warthin's tumor, Hodgkin's disease, and metastatic carcinoma), drug reactions (hydantoin), sarcoidosis, nonspecific reactive hyperplasia, and nonlymphoid neck or parotid swelling (Sjögren's syndrome, sialosis, branchial arch cyst, cystic hygroma, and carotid body tumor). In the differentiation of tuberculous disease from other forms of adenitis, medical or social history and chest radiographs may be helpful, particularly for the young child. More than 80% of children with tuberculous lymphadenitis have a history of exposure to active tuberculosis and chest radiographs showing evidence of recent or active tuberculosis (24, 46). These findings are uncommon in adults: less than 20% have a history of tuberculous contact, and less than 30% have chest radiograph abnormalities (18). Tuberculin skin testing is the most definitive noninvasive diagnostic procedure, yielding positive results in more than 90% of persons with tuberculous lymphadenitis.

Occasionally, lymphadenitis caused by *M. tuberculosis* may be difficult to distinguish from that caused by NTM, a more common problem in children (43). Tuberculous lymphadenitis rarely manifests as unilateral involvement of the superior anterior cervical nodes in the digastric triangle, a finding typical of lymphadenitis caused by NTM. Other helpful clues in this distinction are shown in Table 2. Although differential skin testing with tuberculin and NTM antigens has proven useful, NTM antigens are not currently available for routine use.

Table 2. Comparative features of tuberculous and nontuberculous mycobacterial cervical lymphadenitis

Feature	Tuberculous	Nontuberculous
Age	Any, but peaks at 20–40 yrs	1–6 yrs
Sex	Females predominate	Equal between sexes
Race	Asians and blacks predominate	None
Tuberculosis exposure	Common in children	Uncommon
Systemic symptoms	Uncommon	Uncommon
Node involvement	Anterior and posterior cervical, supraclavicular, bilateral	Jugulodigastric, unilateral
Chest roentgenogram	Abnormal in most children, one-third abnormal in adults	Normal
Tuberculin skin test	Usually positive	Commonly positive

When diagnosis of tuberculous lymphadenitis remains in doubt, biopsy material must be submitted for histology, culture, and potentially PCR. Total excisional biopsy is optimal because an incomplete biopsy nearly always results in ulcerations or sinus tract formation. Ideally, the solid portion of the node should be cultured and processed for histopathology, whereas the frankly caseous portion of the node should be stained with rhodamine-auramine and examined by fluorescent microscopy for mycobacteria. The histology of mycobacterial adenitis may include nonspecific lymphoid infiltrates, small noncaseating granulomas, or typical Langhans giant cells in areas of extensive caseous necrosis. Tuberculous and NTM-infected nodes cannot be differentiated histologically, and distinction from other granulomatous diseases may be difficult. It is, therefore, essential that the biopsy specimen be handled expeditiously in a knowledgeable microbiology laboratory to maximize the possibility of positive culture results.

Fine-needle aspiration of lymph nodes or parotid glands for cytology and culture (6, 22) in conjunction with tuberculin skin test results may be an effective method of diagnosis in geographical areas where tuberculous disease is prevalent. Cytologic findings identify granulomatous changes in 50 to 80% of patients with tuberculous lymphadenitis, but acid-fast bacilli are identified in only 30 to 60% and cultures are positive for only 20 to 80% (6, 39). Thus, other causes of granulomatous lymphadenitis must be excluded in a majority of patients unless the tuberculin skin test is strongly positive. A recent systematic review found that nucleic acid amplification tests for tuberculous lymphadenitis produce highly variable and inconsistent results, precluding the determination of clinically meaningful results (16). However, several methods hold out some promise. The use of PCR dot–enzyme-linked immunosorbent assay versus Ziehl-Neelsen staining or culture of specimens from needle aspiration of tuberculous lymph nodes increased the rate of identification of M. tuberculosis to 70 to 80% (6, 25). In addition, a culture-enhanced assay combining a 15-day broth incubation with the GenoType Mycobacteria Direct test achieved a sensitivity, specificity, positive predictive value, and negative predictive value of 88.6, 100, 100, and 97.9%, respectively, when using a positive diagnosis of tuberculosis as the "gold standard" (42).

When assessing hilar or mediastinal lymph node involvement, sputum and gastric aspirate cultures are usually found to be negative, and diagnosis is best made by excisional biopsy of an involved lymph node with mediastinoscopy or open thoracotomy. If respiratory symptoms or chest radiographs indicate bronchial obstruction, bronchoscopy should be performed to remove any polyps or granulation tissue seen in the bronchial lumen (30) for histology and culture.

TREATMENT

Management of tuberculous lymphadenitis and parotitis involves appropriate use of antituberculous chemotherapy with the judicious use of surgical excision in a minority of patients. When superficial lymphadenitis is detected before extensive caseation, periadenitis, or erosion has occurred, chemotherapy is nearly always curative. During chemotherapy, up to 25% of patients may have the appearance of new nodes or enlargement, fluctuation, or drainage of existing nodes (13). This potential complication usually occurs in the first few weeks or months of therapy, but occasionally it develops later, even after a year. Documented microbiological treatment failure or relapse is rare, however, and these events do not usually require additional chemotherapy, steroids, or surgery (54). The American Thoracic Society, CDC, Infectious Diseases Society of America, and World Health Organization recommend a 6-month regimen of therapy for all patients with tuberculosis lymphadenitis caused by drug-susceptible organisms (7, 54). For adult patients, four basic regimens are recommended, including various combinations of isoniazid (INH), rifampin (RIF), pyrazinamide (PZA), and ethambutol (EMB). These recommendations are based on two prospective controlled studies that have demonstrated successful treatment with combinations of INH, RIF, PZA, and EMB or streptomycin, for 6 months versus 9 months. In 157 adults with cervical, axillary,

or chest wall lymph node tuberculosis monitored for 9 to 30 months after therapy, no differences in outcome were demonstrated between the group treated daily for 6 months versus two groups treated daily for 9 months (9). Similarly, in 91 adults with cervical lymph node tuberculosis monitored for a median of 21 months, no differences in outcome were noted between groups treated thrice weekly for 6 months versus 9 months (56).

For pediatric patients, prospective, controlled trials are limited, but a critical review of evidence for short-course therapy of tuberculous adenitis in children (36) recommends following World Health Organization guidelines (54). These guidelines include 2 months of induction therapy with INH-RIF-PZA and 4 months of maintenance therapy with INH-RIF daily or three times weekly.

Most patients infected with drug-sensitive M. tuberculosis appear to be effectively managed with a 6-month course of combination drug therapy. Data are too few to establish guidelines for treatment of drug-resistant organisms; such cases have generally been excluded from analysis in published studies. For further details of therapy, please refer to other resources (4, 53). There are no published trials of therapy for parotitis, so guidelines for lymphadenitis should be followed.

If not done for diagnostic purposes, surgery should be limited to those individuals who fail to show improvement after an adequate course of chemotherapy or who have discomfort from enlarged or tense, fluctuant nodes (5). Even nodes with sinus tracts and chronic drainage should undergo an attempted trial of chemotherapy prior to surgical removal because initial excision does not seem to affect outcome. If performed, the surgery of choice is always complete excision of the involved nodes and surrounding tissue. Incision plus drainage carries the same risk of ulceration or chronic sinus drainage as partial surgical excision.

Tuberculous lymph nodes in the mediastinum should also be treated the same as pulmonary tuberculosis. Furthermore, mediastinal sonography appears to be a valuable tool to monitor response to treatment in children (8). Endobronchial tuberculosis in children may represent a unique situation in which antituberculous chemotherapy alone may not result in prompt or satisfactory resolution of the illness (30, 40). It is speculated that extensive caseation in the peribronchial lymph nodes makes it difficult for drugs to reach all of the infected tissue. This condition may therefore merit the use of corticosteroids in combination with antituberculous therapy to help control the inflammatory response and resulting bronchial compression. In the only controlled study of its kind,

Table 3. Prednisone therapy for children
with severe endobronchial tuberculosis[a]

Dosage (mg/kg of body wt/day)	Duration (days)
3.0	3
2.0	3
1.0	24
0.5	4
0.25	3
Total	37

[a]To be used only in addition to antituberculous chemotherapy.
Adapted from reference 41.

Nemir and colleagues demonstrated that administering corticosteroids within the first 4 months of illness to children with endobronchial tuberculosis resulted in significantly more rapid resolution of disease (40). Unfortunately, no data are available to determine whether there is a beneficial effect on the long-term outcome in terms of bronchiectasis and bronchial stenosis. The recommended corticosteroid regimen is outlined in Table 3.

Finally, surgery may also have a role in endobronchial tuberculosis in both adults and children. Bronchoscopy in skilled hands may be important for removing intraluminal polyps, granulation tissue, and frank caseous necrotic tissue. For some children, repeated bronchoscopic procedures may be necessary to maintain bronchial patency (30). Rarely, a child or adult with an eroded bronchial wall requires intrathoracic surgery to remove the caseous nodes and patch the bronchial wall erosion (55).

CONCLUSIONS

Tuberculous lymphadenitis, a disease of great historical interest, may now occur more frequently because of the high prevalence of tuberculosis and extrapulmonary tuberculosis in patients with HIV infection. It is most common in young adult Asian or black females and usually presents as painless, slowly evolving lymph node enlargement in the head and neck region but may involve any nodes in the body, particularly those in the mediastinum. Tuberculous parotitis is a rare cause of parotid swelling, usually detected following parotidectomy. Scrofula must be differentiated from a variety of tumors, nontumor masses, and infectious diseases, particularly cervical lymphadenitis caused by NTM. Although history, epidemiology, clinical presentation, chest radiographs, tuberculin skin testing, and gamma interferon release assays may provide a satisfactory diagnosis, fine-needle aspiration or excisional biopsy may be necessary for histology, culture, and possibly PCR. When used, nucleic acid amplification techniques need to be applied in conjunction with conventional methods and interpreted within the context of clinical suspicion. Partial biopsies or incision and drainage should be avoided to prevent ulceration or chronic sinus drainage. Treatment involves the use of combination antituberculous chemotherapy, with occasional need for surgical excision.

REFERENCES

1. **Aaron, L., D. Saadoun, and I. Calatroni.** 2004. Tuberculosis in HIV-infected patients: a comprehensive review. *Clin. Microbiol. Infect.* 10:388–398.
2. **Abrol, R., N. M. Nagarkar, and H. Mohan.** 2002. Primary bilateral tuberculous dacryocystitis with preauricular lymphadenopathy: a diagnostic difficulty of recent times. *Otolaryngol. Head Neck Surg.* 126:201–203.
3. **Al-Serhani, A. M.** 2001. Mycobacterial infection of the head and neck: presentation and diagnosis. *Laryngoscope* 111:2012–2016.
4. **American Thoracic Society, Centers for Disease Control and Prevention, and Infectious Diseases Society of America.** 2003. Treatment of tuberculosis. *Am. J. Respir. Crit. Care Med.* 167:603–662.
5. **Ammari, F. F., A. H. B. Hani, and K. I. Ghariebeh.** 2003. Tuberculosis of the lymph glands of the neck: a limited role for surgery. *Otolaryngol. Head Neck Surg.* 128:576–580.
6. **Bezabih, M., D. W. Mariam, and S. G. Selassie.** 2002. Fine needle aspiration cytology of suspected tuberculous lymphadenitis. *Cytopathology* 13:284–290.
7. **Blumberg, H. M., W. J. Burman, and R. E. Chaisson.** 2004. American Thoracic Society/Centers for Disease Control and Prevention/Infectious Diseases Society of America: treatment of tuberculosis. *Am. J. Respir. Crit. Care Med.* 169:316–317.
8. **Bosch-Marcet, J., X. Serres-Creixams, V. Borras-Perez, M. T. Coll-Sibina, M. Guitet-Julia, and E. Coll-Rosell.** 2007. Value of sonography for follow-up of mediastinal lymphadenopathy in children with tuberculosis. *J. Clin. Ultrasound* 35:118–127.
9. **Campbell, I. A., L. P. Ormerod, and J. A. R. Friend.** 1993. Six months versus nine months chemotherapy for tuberculosis of lymph nodes: final results. *Respir. Med.* 87:621–623.
10. **Cantrell, R. W., J. H. Hensen, and D. Reid.** 1975. Diagnosis and management of tuberculous cervical adenitis. *Arch. Otolaryngol.* 101:53–57.
11. **Centers for Disease Control and Prevention.** 2004. Trends in tuberculosis—United States, 1998–2003. *MMWR Morb. Mortal. Wkly. Rep.* 53:209–214. (Erratum, 53:246.)
12. **Chatterjee, A., V. Meera, and Q. Trent.** 2001. Parotid abscess caused by *Mycobacterium tuberculosis*. *Pediatr. Infect. Dis. J.* 20:912–914.
13. **Cho, O., K. Park, Y. Kim, E. H. Song, E. Y. Jang, E. J. Lee, Y. P. Chong, S. Choi, S. Lee, J. H. Woo, Y. S. Kim, and S. Kim.** 2009. Paradoxical responses in non-HIV-infected patients with peripheral lymph node tuberculosis. *J. Infect.* 59:56–61.
14. **Coen, L. D.** 1987. Tuberculosis of the parotid gland in a child. *J. Pediatr. Surg.* 22:367–368.
15. **Crum, N. F.** 2003. Tuberculosis presenting as epitrochlear lymphadenitis. *Scand. J. Infect. Dis.* 35:888–890.
16. **Daley, P., S. Thomas, and M. Pai.** 2007. Nucleic acid amplification tests for the diagnosis of tuberculous lymphadenitis: a systematic review. *Int. J. Tuberc. Lung Dis.* 11:1166–1176.

17. Farer, L. S., P. M. Lowell, and M. P. Meador. 1979. Extrapulmonary tuberculosis in the United States. *Am. J. Epidemiol.* **109:**205–217.

18. Geldmacher, H., C. Taube, and C. Kroeger. 2002. Assessment of lymph node tuberculosis in northern Germany. *Chest* **121:** 1177–1182.

19. Glynn, J. R., A. C. Crampin, and B. M. Ngwira. 2004. Trends in tuberculosis and the influence of HIV infection in northern Malawi, 1988–2001. *AIDS* **18:**1459–1463.

20. Gonzalez, O. Y., L. D. Teeter, and B. T. Thanh. 2003. Extrathoracic tuberculosis lymphadenitis in adult HIV seronegative patients: a population-based analysis in Houston, Texas, USA. *Int. J. Tuberc. Lung Dis.* **7:**987–993.

21. Hamdan, A. L., U. Hadi, and N. Shabb. 2002. Tuberculous parotitis: a forgotten entity. *Otolaryngol. Head Neck Surg.* **126:**581–582.

22. Handa, U., S. Kumar, and R. S. Punia. 2001. Tuberculous parotitis: a series of five cases diagnosed on fine needle aspiration cytology. *J. Laryngol. Otol.* **115:**235–237.

22a. Hardy, J. B. 1958. *Tuberculosis in White and Negro Children.* Harvard University Press, Cambridge, MA.

23. Hunter, D. C., and J. M. Thomas. 1993. Tuberculosis in the parotid region. *Br. J. Surg.* **80:**1008.

24. Inselman, L. S., and E. L. Kendig. 1998. Disorders of the respiratory tract in children, p. 883. *In* V. Chernick and T. F. Boat (ed.), *Tuberculosis.* W. B. Saunders, Philadelphia, PA.

25. Jain, A., R. K. Verma, and V. Tiwari. 2003. Development of a new antigen detection dot-ELISA for diagnosis of tubercular lymphadenitis in fine needle aspirates. *J. Microbiol. Methods* **53:**107–112.

26. Jha, B. C., A. Dass, and N. M. Nagarkar. 2001. Cervical tuberculous lymphadenopathy: changing clinical pattern and concepts in management. *Postgrad. Med. J.* **77:**185–187.

27. Jones, P. G., and P. E. Campbell. 1962. Tuberculous lymphadenitis in childhood: the significance of anonymous mycobacteria. *Br. J. Surg.* **50:**202.

28. Kabra, S. K., R. Lodha, and V. Seth. 2002. Tuberculosis in children—what has changed in last 20 years? *Indian J. Pediatr.* **69**(Suppl. 1):S5–S10.

29. Khanna, R., G. V. Prasanna, and P. Gupta. 2002. Mammary tuberculosis: report on 52 cases. *Postgrad. Med. J.* **78:**422–424.

30. Lincoln, E. M., L. C. Harris, and S. Bovornkitti. 1958. Endobronchial tuberculosis in children. *Am. Rev. Tuberc.* **77:**271.

31. Lincoln, E. M., and E. M. Sewell. 1963. *Tuberculosis in Children.* McGraw-Hill, New York, NY.

32. Lomax, L. 1977. Hereditary or acquired disease? Early nineteenth century debates on the cause of infantile scrofula and tuberculosis. *J. Hist. Med.* **32:**356–374.

33. Major, R. H. 1945. *Classic Descriptions of Disease,* 3rd ed. Charles C Thomas, Springfield, IL.

34. Maltezou, H. C., P. Spyridis, and D. A. Kafetzis. 2000. Extrapulmonary tuberculosis in children. *Arch. Dis. Child.* **83:**342–346.

35. Maulitz, R. O., and S. R. Maulitz. 1973. The King's Evil in Oxfordshire. *Med. Hist.* **17:**87–89.

36. McMaster, P., and D. Isaacs. 2000. Critical review of evidence for short course therapy for tuberculous adenitis in children. *Pediatr. Infect. Dis. J.* **19:**401–404.

37. Medical Research Council Tuberculosis and Chest Diseases Unit. 1980. National survey of tuberculosis notifications in England and Wales. *Br. Med. J.* **281:**895–898.

38. Mustafa, T., S. J. Mogga, S. G. M. Mfinanga, O. Morkve, and S. Sviland. 2005. Immunohistochemical analysis of cytokines and apoptosis in tuberculous lymphadenitis. *Immunology* **117:**454–462.

39. Nataraj, G., S. Kurup, and A. Pandit. 2002. Correlation of fine needle aspiration cytology, smear and culture in tuberculous lymphadenitis: a prospective study. *J. Postgrad. Med.* **48:**113–116.

40. Nemir, R. L., J. Cardona, and F. Vaziri. 1967. Prednisone as an adjunct in the chemotherapy of lymph node bronchial tuberculosis in childhood: a double-blind study. *Am. Rev. Respir. Dis.* **95:**402.

41. Nicol, A. F., G. J. Nuovo, J. M. Coelho, V. C. Rolla, and C. Horn. 2008. SOCS in situ expression in tuberculous lymphadenitis in an endemic area. *Exp. Mol. Pathol.* **3:**240–244.

42. Noussair, L., F. Bert, and V. Leflon-Guibout. 2009. Early diagnosis of extrapulmonary tuberculosis by a new procedure combining broth culture and PCR. *J. Clin. Microbiol.* **47:** 1452–1457.

43. Powell, D. A. 2004. Nontuberculous mycobacteria, p. 975. *In* R. E. Behrman, R. M. Kliegman, and H. B. Jenson (ed.), *Nelson Textbook of Pediatrics.* W. B. Saunders, Philadelphia, PA.

44. Prasoon, D. 2003. Tuberculosis of the intercostal lymph nodes. *Acta Cytol.* **47:**51–55.

45. Schuit, K. E. 1979. Miliary tuberculosis in children: clinical and laboratory manifestation in 19 patients. *Am. J. Dis. Child.* **133:**583–585.

46. Starke, J. D., and K. C. Smith. 2004. Tuberculous and other mycobacterial infections, p. 1337. *In* R. D. Feigin, J. D. Cherry, G. L. Demmler, and S. L. Kaplan (ed.), *Textbook of Pediatric Infectious Diseases,* 5th ed. W. B. Saunders, Philadelphia, PA.

47. Starke, T. R. 2004. Tuberculosis, p. 731. *In* A. A. Gershon, P. J. Hotez, and S. L. Katz (ed.), *Infectious Diseases in Children.* C. V. Mosby, St. Louis, MO.

48. Suleiman, A. M. 2001. Tuberculous parotitis: report of 3 cases. *Br. J. Oral Maxillofac. Surg.* **39:**320–323.

49. Suoglu, Y., B. Erdamar, and I. Colhan. 1998. Pathology in focus. Tuberculosis of the parotid gland. *J. Laryngol. Otol.* **112:** 588–591.

50. Thami, G. P., S. Kaur, and A. J. Kanwar. 2002. Isolated inguinal tuberculous lymphadenitis. *J. Eur. Acad. Dermatol. Venereol.* **16:**284–301.

51. Whitford, J., and D. Hansman. 1977. Primary tuberculosis of the conjunctiva. *Med. J. Aust.* **1:**486–487.

52. Reference deleted.

53. **World Health Organization.** 2006. *Guidance for National Programmes on the Management of Tuberculosis in Children.* World Health Organization, Geneva, Switzerland.

54. **World Health Organization.** 2003. *Treatment of Tuberculosis: Guidelines for National Programmes,* 3rd ed. WHO/CDS/TB 2003.313. World Health Organization, Geneva, Switzerland.

55. Yurdakul, Y., and A. Aytac. 1979. Surgical repair of the tracheobronchial compression by tuberculous lymph nodes. *Br. J. Dis. Chest* **73:**305–308.

56. Yurn, A. P. W., S. H. W. Wong, and C. M. Tam. 1997. Prospective randomized study of twice weekly six-month and nine-month chemotherapy for cervical tuberculous lymphadenopathy. *Otolaryngol. Head Neck Surg.* **116:**189–192.

57. Zheng, J. W., and Q. H. Zhang. 1995. Tuberculosis of the parotid gland: a report of 12 cases. *J. Oral Maxillofac. Surg.* **53:** 849–851.

Chapter 20

Urogenital Tuberculosis

ANDRÉ A. FIGUEIREDO, ANTÔNIO M. LUCON, AND MIGUEL SROUGI

INTRODUCTION

Tuberculosis has a worldwide distribution, without cyclical or seasonal variations and with greater prevalence in regions of high population densities and poor socioeconomic and sanitary status. It is estimated that 30% of the world's population (1.7 billion people) are carriers of *Mycobacterium tuberculosis* (39). In spite of the availability of pharmacological treatment and of technological breakthroughs, the last three decades have witnessed a recrudescence of the infection, due to the emergence of resistant bacilli, human migration, and the AIDS epidemic. In fact, tuberculosis is still a serious challenge to the world public health, chiefly in developing countries (28).

Starting with a pulmonary focus, 2 to 20% of patients develop urogenital tuberculosis through hematogenous spread to the kidneys, prostate, and epididymis; through the descending collecting system to the ureters, bladder, and urethra; and through the ejaculatory ducts to the genital organs (28, 39). Urogenital tuberculosis occurs at all age ranges, but it is predominant in males in their fourth and fifth decades (17). It is a serious, insidious disease, generally developing symptoms only at a late stage, which leads to a diagnostic delay with consequent urogenital organ destruction; there are reports of patients with renal failure as their initial clinical presentation (17).

Although the condition has been long recognized by nephrologists, urologists, and infectious disease specialists, urogenital tuberculosis is still largely unknown. Even when suggestive findings such as hematuria, sterile pyuria, and recurrent urinary infections are present, we rarely remember this diagnostic possibility. Greater knowledge of the features of urogenital tuberculosis then becomes relevant and should emphasize the importance of an early diagnosis.

EPIDEMIOLOGY

Extrapulmonary tuberculosis occurs in 10% of tuberculosis cases. Urogenital tuberculosis is responsible for 30 to 40% of extrapulmonary tuberculosis cases, being second only to lymph node involvement (7, 28, 54, 55). Urogenital tuberculosis occurs in 2 to 20% of patients with pulmonary tuberculosis (2, 9, 24, 31, 54). While in developed countries the urogenital cases constitute 2 to 10% of cases of pulmonary tuberculosis, the figures are 15 to 20% in developing countries (2, 9, 24, 54).

ETIOPATHOGENESIS

Mycobacterium tuberculosis, an acid-fast aerobic bacillus, is the most virulent mycobacterial pathogen in humans. Its slow replication accounts for the insidious nature of the infection and its resistance to ordinary antibiotics, since the latter work during bacterial division. Although the bacillus can stay dormant in the host, not producing symptoms for a long time, reactivation may follow impairment of immunity (28). Other mycobacteria, such as *Mycobacterium bovis*, important where unpasteurized milk is consumed (7), are less virulent to humans and are only rarely responsible for urogenital lesions.

Once inhaled, the bacilli multiply in the pulmonary alveoli, with primary granuloma formation (28, 39). As few as one to five bacilli in the alveolus may result in infection. Primary pulmonary tuberculosis is usually clinically silent and self-limited. From this pulmonary focus, bacillemia ensues and leads to bacillus implants in other organs. At this point, colonization of the renal and prostate parenchyma may occur. After 6 months, spontaneous cicatrization of primary pulmonary tuberculosis occurs, and the

André A. Figueiredo • Núcleo Interdisciplinar de Pesquisa em Urologia and Department of Morphology, Federal University of Juiz de Fora, Minas Gerais—Brazil, Rua Irineu Marinho 365, apto 801—bloco 3, Bom Pastor—Juiz de Fora, MG 36021, Brazil.
Antônio M. Lucon and Miguel Srougi • Division of Urology, University of São Paulo Medical School, Av Dr. Enéas de Carvalho Aguiar, 255, 7 Andar, sala 710 F., São Paulo, SP 05403-000, Brazil.

patient enters a latent phase, with a 5% likelihood of disease reactivation in the following 2 years and a 5% additional likelihood of reactivation thereafter. In most active cases of both pulmonary and extrapulmonary disease, latent foci are reactivated by malnutrition, diabetes mellitus, steroid and immunosuppressant use, and immunodeficiency (29, 39).

In the pathophysiology of urogenital tuberculosis, there is gradual development of the initial forms, from minimal urogenital damage and few symptoms to severe disease with contracted bladder, bilateral renal injury, and possible end-stage renal failure (17). A clear understanding of this course is paramount to highlight the importance of early diagnosis. After hematogenous spread from the pulmonary focus, there is colonization of the renal parenchyma, with initially bilateral, cortical, glomerular, and pericapillary renal lesions that are concomitant with other hematogenic foci in the prostate and other organs beyond the urogenital system (45, 50). These foci generally cicatrize, and a latent period ensues, unless there is immunodeficiency and systemically symptomatic miliary tuberculosis develops, with constitutional symptoms and multiple renal abscesses, as has been seen in AIDS patients (Fig. 1) (2, 39). In fact, 25 to 62% of patients with miliary tuberculosis have renal lesions with multiple bilateral foci (45, 61). The latent period between pulmonary infection with bacillemia and clinical urogenital tuberculosis is 22 years on average, ranging from 1 to 46 years, according to the moment when immunity falls and the latent renal foci are reactivated (9).

After reactivation of the renal foci, infection progresses from a single focus, affecting one kidney and sparing the other (50). This accounts for the greater frequency of unilateral renal tuberculosis (Fig. 2) (9, 23). Contiguous involvement of the collecting system

leads to bacilluria and descending unilateral spread to the ureter and bladder. In ureteral tuberculosis, multiple stenoses develop throughout the ureter, with ureteral obstruction, ureterohydronephrosis, and consequent risk of renal functional loss. With infection progression, there is bladder damage with progressive fibrosis characterizing a more advanced form known as contracted bladder (Fig. 3 and 4) (16). Progression of bladder tuberculosis reduces bladder capacity and compliance, with distortion of the ureterovesical junctions and development of vesicoureteral reflux; the reflux almost always involves only the initially spared kidney, since ureteral stenosis protects against the radiological manifestation of reflux. Reflux which is secondary to a contracted bladder transforms the collecting system (ureter and pyelocaliceal junction) into an extension of the capacity of the contracted bladder, with ascending transmission of intravesical pressure (16). Unidentified and untreated reflux damages the kidney through infection or transmission of intravesical pressure, leading to end-stage renal failure. In a study of 25 cases of tuberculosis-related contracted bladder (16), the patients with bilateral renal tuberculosis had bilateral ureterohydronephrosis caused by ureteral obstruction on one side (first kidney to be involved) and by high-degree vesicoureteral reflux on the other (second kidney to be involved), pointing to secondary loss of function of one of the kidneys because of vesicoureteral reflux (Fig. 3 and 4). Thus, if diagnosis and treatment do not occur at the initial stages of the infection, urogenital tuberculosis may severely damage the urogenital organs, from unilateral renal loss to contracted bladder-related end-stage renal failure.

AFFECTED ORGANS

Tuberculosis may affect the entire male urinary and genital tracts. Table 1 shows the frequencies of male urinary and genital tract involvement (9, 23, 46).

Urogenital tuberculosis most frequently affects the kidneys, renal infection being slowly progressive, asymptomatic, and highly destructive, with instances of unilateral renal loss of function and renal failure on diagnosis (35). Kidney destruction might be due to progression of a focal lesion, with caseous granuloma formation, fibrosis, and renal cavitation. Yet, obstruction of the collecting system, which may be distal when due to ureteral stenosis or proximal when there are intrarenal stenoses, is the main cause of tuberculosis-related renal dysfunction (3, 44, 55).

Although unilateral renal involvement predominates in tuberculosis (9, 23), bilateral damage may occur, with risk of renal failure. Bilateral renal

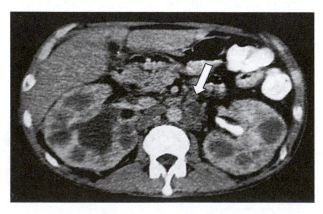

Figure 1. Post-contrast phase of abdominal CT in an AIDS patient, with bilateral renal abscesses and dilatation of the collecting system on the right. Retroperitoneal lymph node enlargement with central necrosis is apparent (arrow). From reference 20, with permission.

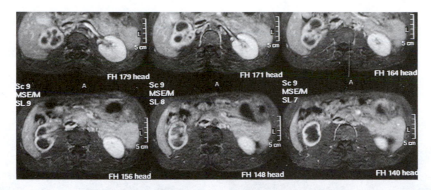

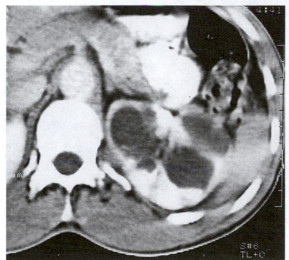
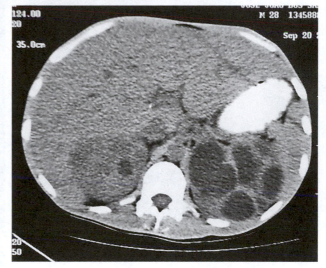

Figure 2. MRI (A) and CT (B and C) of patients with unilateral renal tuberculosis, with dilatation of the collecting system (caliectasis) and thinning of the renal parenchyma. There is no dilatation of the renal pelvis. From reference 20, with permission.

tuberculosis may be due to three mechanisms. (i) The first is exacerbation of the hematogenous spread period, with the formation of multiple predominantly bilateral parenchymatous foci, seen in patients with immunodeficiency and miliary tuberculosis (Fig. 1) (45). (ii) The second is bilateral focus reactivation with progressive descending spread to the collecting system and bilateral ureteral stenoses, without the presence of a contracted bladder. This presentation is extremely rare: Conte et al. (11) describe a patient with postrenal renal failure due to tuberculosis-related bilateral stenosis of the collecting system, which resolved after specific treatment, and Chattopadhyay et al. (8) describe a case of right autonephrectomy due

Table 1. Frequency of affected urogenital organs

Affected organ	Findings in indicated study		
	Christensen, 1974, United States (9)	García-Rodriguez et al., 1994, Spain (23)	Mochalova and Starikov, 1997, Russia (46)
Total (men)	102 (72)	81 (51)	4,298 (2,888)
Kidney (%)	60.8	93.8	100
Bilateral (%)	29	14.5	83.4
Unilateral (%)	71	85.5	16.6
Ureter (%)	18.6	40.7	NR[a]
Bladder (%)	15.7	21	10.6
Prostate[b] (%)	26.4	2	49.5
Epididymis[b] (%)	22.2	11.8	55.5
Seminal vesicles (%)	6.9	0	NR
Urethra (%)	1.4	2	21.4

[a]NR, not reported.
[b]In relation to male patients.

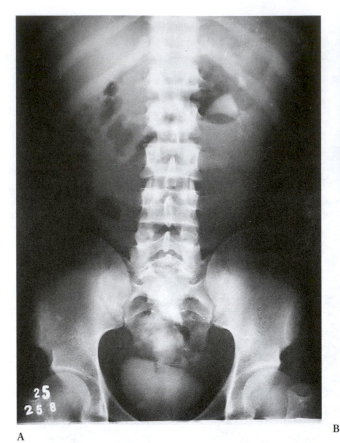

A

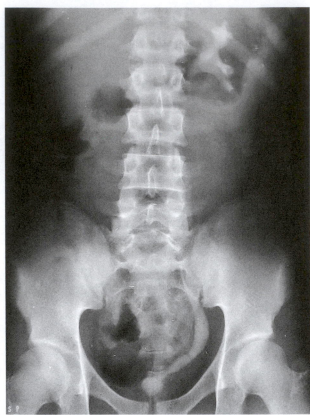

B

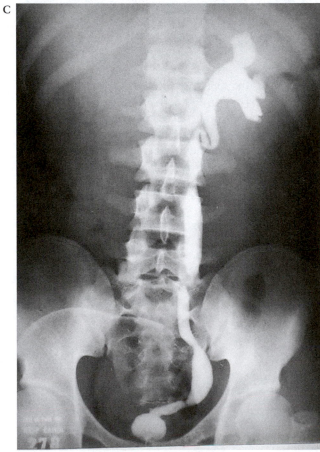

C

Figure 3. Sequential exams of patient with urogenital tuberculosis. (A) Initial intravenous urography (IU) with right kidney dysfunction and normal left kidney and bladder. (B) IU after 10 months, with development of contracted bladder and ureterohydronephrosis on the left. (C) Voiding cystography showing high-grade vesicoureteral reflux on the left as a cause of dilatation of the collecting system. From reference 20, with permission.

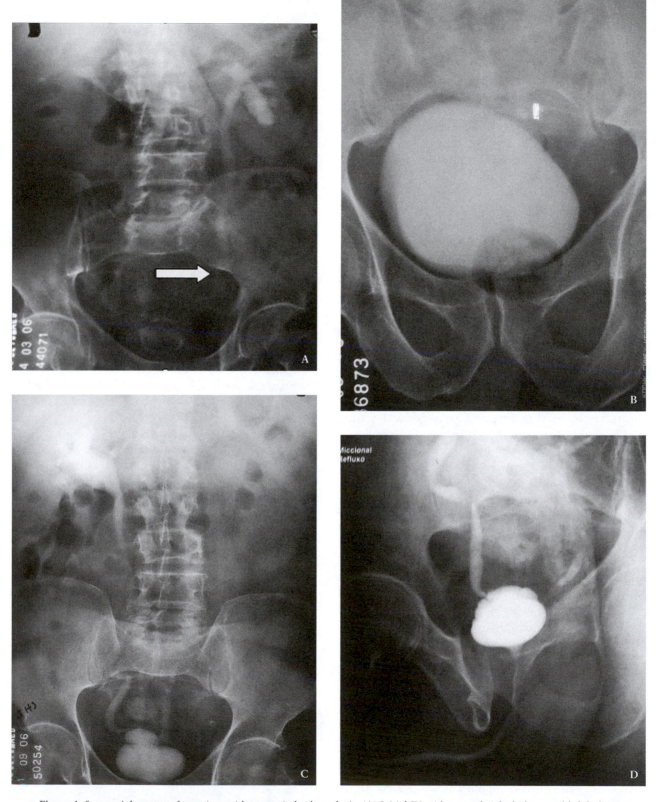

Figure 4. Sequential exams of a patient with urogenital tuberculosis. (A) Initial IU with normal right kidney and left kidney with ureterohydronephrosis due to stenosis of the middle ureter (arrow) and intrarenal stenoses without pelvic dilatation (typical tuberculosis feature). (B) Cystography with normal bladder and no reflux. (C and D) IU and voiding cystography after 6 months without treatment, showing renal dysfunction on the left and ureterohydronephrosis on the right, with contracted bladder and bilateral vesicoureteral reflux (high grade on the right) as a cause of ureterohydronephrosis. From reference 20, with permission.

to obstruction associated with infundibular stenosis of the contralateral kidney. In both cases, there was no bladder tuberculosis. (iii) The third is unilateral renal involvement, with descending spread to the ipsilateral ureter and bladder and then retrograde spread to the contralateral kidney through reflux (16). The last is the main mechanism of bilateral renal damage in tuberculosis. Accordingly, bilateral renal damage in tuberculosis is generally asymmetric, with one of the kidneys more severely damaged (multiple stenoses of the collecting system and asymmetric calyceal dilatation), whereas the other kidney is less involved, with reflux-related ureterohydronephrosis (16). There is a rare subset of patients with bilateral renal tuberculosis who may develop acute or chronic renal failure with histological findings of diffuse interstitial nephritis, with or without granuloma formation but without radiological findings suggestive of tuberculosis, except for renal atrophy in some cases. These cases differ from the classic clinical and radiological presentations of urogenital tuberculosis, since voiding symptoms and radiological alterations are not prominent, and the bacillus can rarely be found in the urine. Diagnosis is generally made on histopathology of a sample obtained through renal biopsy (37, 41).

Ureteral and bladder tuberculosis involvement is secondary to renal disease and consequent descending infection through the collecting or lymphatic systems. Descending lymphatic spread was demonstrated in pigs which received direct renal inoculation of the bacillus and developed ureteral tuberculosis even after total occlusion of the ureter (69). In ureteral tuberculosis, multiple stenoses develop throughout the ureter, with predominance of the anatomical narrowings such as the vesicoureteral junction and, to a lesser extent, the ureterorenal junction and the mid-ureter (7, 35). Ureteral stenosis is the main cause of renal dysfunction in tuberculosis, occurring in up to 93.7% of all cases (7). In bladder tuberculosis, there is an acute inflammatory process with hyperemia, ulceration, and tubercle formation in the vicinity of the ureteral meatus, with subsequent fibrosis of the bladder wall (7, 28).

In spite of constant urethral exposure to the urinary bacilli, urethral tuberculosis occurs in only 1.9 to 4.5% of all cases of urogenital tuberculosis, and never as an isolated entity. Acute urethritis and urethral discharge with associated prostatic tuberculosis, or chronically developing urethral stenosis and fistulae, are the most common clinical presentations (34, 64).

Tuberculosis affects the entire male genital tract, with lesions in the prostate, seminal vesicles, vas deferens, epididymis, Cooper glands, penis, and testicles, the last through contiguity with the epididymis, since the blood-testicle barrier plays a protective role. Genital tuberculosis occurs through hematogenous spread to the prostate and epididymis or through the urinary system to the prostate and spread from the ejaculatory ducts to the seminal vesicles, vas deferens, and epididymis (40, 59). Genital tuberculosis may be accompanied by renal lesions, but it may manifest in isolation (17). The frequency of genital organ involvement varies according to the criteria used. The prostate is histologically involved in 39.5 to 50% of subjects with urogenital tuberculosis, while epididymitis is the most common clinical manifestation, because prostate tuberculosis is usually subclinical (45, 46, 61).

In prostate contamination, hematogenous spread is more frequent than through the urinary system (63). In an experimental and clinical observational study, bacillus injection in the subcapsular and intracortical renal regions of rabbits was observed to lead to tuberculous prostate foci concomitant with foci in other organs, and discrete renal foci without communication with the urinary collecting system. In the clinical cases, the prostate lesion was not accompanied by mucosal or submucosal impairment of the prostatic urethra, being situated instead in the lateral and peripheral regions, while urethral ulcerative lesions with prostate involvement were only seen in more advanced cases with vesical tuberculosis (Fig. 5) (63). In prostatic tuberculosis there is caseous necrosis with calcification and development of fibrosis with gland hardening (36). Prostatic tuberculosis is usually asymptomatic and diagnosed as an incidental prostatectomy finding in patients older than those with urogenital tuberculosis (30, 36, 38). Prostatic abscesses are rare but occur in AIDS patients (65).

The epididymis is affected in 10 to 55% of men with urogenital tuberculosis, and scrotal changes are

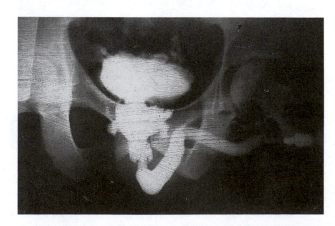

Figure 5. Voiding urethrocystography showing contracted bladder, no vesicoureteral reflux, and prostate tuberculosis, with dilatation and irregularities of the prostatic urethra. From reference 20, with permission.

the main sign on physical examination (9, 23, 29, 46). Epididymal tuberculosis is bilateral in 34% of the cases, presenting as a nodule or scrotal hardening in all patients, scrotal fistula in half the cases, and hydrocele in only 5% (58). The presence of a scrotal fistula is a telltale sign of tuberculosis.

Because of ejaculatory duct obstruction with oligo-azoospermia and low-volume ejaculate due to obstruction of the ejaculatory ducts, infertility may be the first symptom of tuberculosis. Multiple stenoses in the ejaculatory duct system make reconstruction impossible and are an indication for assisted reproduction (7, 40, 53). Leukospermia is a less frequent and earlier mechanism underlying tuberculosis-related infertility (40).

Penile tuberculosis is rare, developing after direct contact or secondary to another urogenital focus, with the appearance of an erythematous papule that may ulcerate. Infiltration of the cavernous bodies may lead to penis deformity and urethral fistulae, a situation that may be confused with penile carcinoma (56, 66).

FEMALE GENITAL TUBERCULOSIS

The incidence of female genital tuberculosis ranges from 0.002 to 0.56% among hospitalized women and from 0.2% to a relevant 21% among those with infertility. The condition affects women of childbearing age, with a predominance in the 20- to 40-year age range (1, 47).

Female genital tuberculosis is secondary to hematogenous spread from a primary focus, generally in the lungs or, less commonly, through lymphatic spread from tuberculosis of abdominal organs. However, primary genital tuberculosis might develop after sexual intercourse with a man with tuberculosis of the penis or epididymis. After initial involvement of the fallopian tube, the infection may involve the endometrium and, more rarely, the myometrium, reaching the ovarian cortex through contiguity. The fallopian tubes are affected in 90 to 100% of the cases, normally in a bilateral fashion, with a predominance of lesions in the ampulla (greater vascular supply), followed by the isthmus. In 50 to 70% of the cases, there is a uterine lesion with a predominance of endometrial lesions, the myometrium being more rarely affected. Ovarian tuberculosis is usually a sequela of tubal tuberculosis, when tubo-ovarian masses develop. Vulvar or vaginal tuberculosis is exceedingly rare (1, 47).

Genital tuberculosis generally presents clinically as infertility (40 to 76%), pelvic or abdominal pain (50 to 55%), and menstrual disorders (20 to 25%).

Infertility is the main manifestation of the disease, resulting from tubal obstruction or the presence of adhesions and synechiae of the uterine cavity. On radiology, hysterosalpingography may show findings suggestive of tuberculosis: obstruction of the fallopian tube, multiple constrictions along the fallopian tube, and adhesion, deformity, and obliteration of the uterine cavity without previous history of curettage. A pelvic mass mimicking an ovarian tumor may develop in genital tuberculosis. Histopathological diagnosis may be made after uterine curettage or biopsy of the fallopian tube. Culture of menstrual fluid is also feasible. Yet, when there is a suspicion of tuberculosis on clinical and radiological grounds alone, treatment may be started, even without histological or bacteriological confirmation (1, 47).

Pharmacotherapy is the mainstay of treatment for female genital tuberculosis, surgery being reserved for voluminous tubo-ovarian abscesses. Pharmacotherapy and tubal surgery do not restore fertility; assisted reproduction, chiefly in vitro fertilization with embryo transfer, is indicated in such cases. Yet, there is anecdotal evidence of parity after treatment of tubal tuberculosis (1, 47).

CLINICAL FEATURES

In a recent review (18) of 9,178 patients described in 39 case series (6 in Latin America, 7 in Africa, 14 in Asia, 4 in the United States, and 8 in Europe), urogenital tuberculosis was seen to affect two males to each female, with a mean age of 40.7 years (range, 5 to 90 years). In only 36.5% of the cases was there clinical history or radiological evidence of previous tuberculosis. Therefore, in most cases, urogenital tuberculosis cannot be suspected on the basis of a history of previous pulmonary disease. Symptoms arise when there is bladder impairment, once, as far as tuberculosis is concerned, the kidneys are mute while the bladder plays the role of the vocal cords (24). Storage symptoms (frequency, nocturia, and urgency) are thus the most common manifestations, followed by hematuria and low back pain, occurring in 50.5, 35.6, and 34.4%, respectively. On physical examination, up to 48.9% of subjects have some scrotal abnormality, with a lump, epididymal hardening, or fistula, which points to the importance of these signs (Table 2).

Autopsy studies revealed that only 50% of the patients with renal tuberculosis were symptomatic, with only 18% having received a clinical diagnosis (45). This diagnostic delay is due to the insidious progression of the disease, paucity and nonspecificity of symptoms, lack of physicians' awareness,

Table 2. Comparison of patients from developed and developing countries[b]

Feature or parameter	Total	Developed	Developing	P[a]
No.	9,178	3,048	1,832	
Men	64.8%	62.9%	60.6%	0.02
Women	35.2%	37.1%	39.4%	0.02
Median age (yrs)	40.7	42.7	39.8	
Range (yrs)	5–90	7–90	5–83	
Previous tuberculosis	36.5%	37.9%	49.1%	<0.01
Symptoms and signs				
Storage symptoms	50.5%	44.3%	55.2%	<0.01
Hematuria	35.6%	24.5%	44.3%	<0.01
Lumbar pain	34.4%	28.7%	42.3%	<0.01
Scrotal mass	48.9%	20.6%	25.0%	0.19
Fever and malaise	21.9%	23.2%	19.9%	0.28
No urinary symptoms	6.4%	8.4%	0%	<0.01
Diagnosis				
Urine	64.2%	79.0%	55.4%	<0.01
Histopathology	21.9%	7.8%	38.3%	<0.01
Clinico-radiographic	10.4%	9.6%	11.3%	0.36
Normal kidneys	15.2%	18.9%	13.2%	<0.01
Unilateral nonfunctioning kidney	26.9%	22.7%	33.3%	<0.01
Renal failure	7.4%	1.9%	13.6%	<0.01
Contracted bladder	8.6%	4.0%	13.6%	<0.01
Surgery	54.9%	56.6%	50.0%	<0.01
Ablative surgery	27.2%	35.0%	43.7%	<0.01

[a]P, significance level through chi square test.
[b]From reference 18, with permission.

poor care-seeking behavior, and difficult bacteriological diagnosis because of sporadic bacilluria with few organisms (31, 55). Therefore, diagnosis is rarely made before severe urogenital lesions develop (17). A total of 7.4% of patients with urogenital tuberculosis develop end-stage chronic renal failure (Table 2).

Comparison of the disease features between developing countries and developed ones (with the exception of Russia, which has intermediate characteristics) shows significant differences. Patients from developing countries are more likely to have specific symptoms and receive late histological diagnoses. In such countries tuberculosis is consequently more severe, with a greater frequency of renal failure, unilateral renal obstruction, ablative surgeries, and contracted bladder and a lower frequency of normal upper collecting systems (Table 2). These data underlie the relationship between the severity of urogenital tuberculosis and the timing of the diagnosis.

Although urogenital tuberculosis affects all age ranges, there are few cases in children, because of the long interval between pulmonary infection and renal tuberculosis (17). Recurrent urinary tract infection or urinary tract infection that does not respond to conventional antibiotics, pyuria with negative urine cultures (sterile pyuria), hematuria, and epididymoorchitis are findings suggestive of urogenital tuberculosis in the pediatric population (8).

IMMUNOSUPPRESSION

Immunosuppression favors the development of tuberculosis, which, in these cases, has a unique course, with greater risk of hematogenous spread and extrapulmonary tuberculosis (32). AIDS is now the main factor leading to tuberculosis development. Besides reactivating latent foci, human immunodeficiency virus (HIV)-related immunosuppression may lead to rapid progression of a new infection or reinfection (32). Between 20 and 50% of HIV-infected patients worldwide have active tuberculosis (42, 67). Urogenital tuberculosis seems to be very important in AIDS patients. In the United States, of 1,282 tuberculosis patients seen between 1991 and 1997 in an inner-city hospital, 46% were coinfected with HIV, and, among the patients with urogenital tuberculosis, two-thirds had AIDS (51). In autopsy studies of 46 AIDS patients in Brazil, 54.3% had tuberculosis, with the disseminated form as the most frequent presentation, whereas an astounding 23.9% of AIDS patients had bilateral renal granulomas (42). In contrast with HIV-negative subjects, HIV-positive patients with tuberculosis are younger, have more constitutional symptoms (fever, bacteremia, and fatigue), show more diffuse pulmonary involvement, develop lymph node enlargement and disseminated tuberculosis more frequently, and have higher mortality rates (32). As for urogenital tuberculosis, HIV-positive patients are younger and more prone to developing kidney and prostate abscesses (51).

From 0.5 to 4.0% of patients with post-renal transplant immunosuppression develop tuberculosis in developed countries, figures that rise to 3.8 to 11.8% in developing countries (13, 14). In transplant patients, pleuropulmonary and disseminated tuberculosis are more common, although urogenital tuberculosis may predominate in developing countries (13, 14). Post-renal transplant patients with urogenital tuberculosis present clinically with fever and without voiding symptoms in two-thirds of cases, and without typical radiological findings in the renal graft. Contrasting with the classic cases of urogenital tuberculosis, only around 20% of these patients have voiding symptoms (13, 14). In a comparison of 72 nonimmunosuppressed patients with urogenital tuberculosis with 8 immunosuppressed patients (4 with AIDS and 4 post-renal transplant), the latter had a predominance of constitutional symptoms, disseminated tuberculosis, and multiple parenchymatous renal foci, with a lower frequency of involvement of the collecting system (Table 3). Therefore, immunosuppressed patients develop a form of urogenital tuberculosis that has distinctive clinical and radiological features, resembling severe bacterial infection, with bacteremia and visceral metastatic foci (19).

LABORATORY AND RADIOLOGICAL WORKUP

For around 10.4% of patients with urogenital tuberculosis, diagnosis is presumptive and based on suggestive clinical, laboratory, and radiological data, without microbiological or histological confirmation (18).

Identification of the tuberculosis bacillus in the urine is achieved through Ziehl-Neelsen's acid-fast staining technique or through urine culture in Lowenstein-Jensen medium (48, 49). The former is quick, with 96.7% specificity but only 42.1 to 52.1% sensitivity (48, 49). Culture is the diagnostic "gold standard" for urogenital tuberculosis. Because bacilluria is sporadic and faint, three to six early morning midstream samples are required. Sensitivity varies widely, from 10.7 to 90%, and the results can take 6 to 8 weeks to be obtained (17, 31).

Some findings in urine examination, such as pyuria, hematuria, acid urine, and negative culture, suggest that urogenital tuberculosis may be present in up to 93% of patients (17). Yet, the suspicion of tuberculosis should not be based on these findings alone, because alterations in the urine have been described in only 22 to 27.6% of cases (15, 48). Usual pathogens are yielded by urine culture for 20 to 40% of urogenital tuberculosis cases and for up to 50% of females (17).

Table 3. Features of immunocompromised and nonimmunocompromised patients with urogenital tuberculosis[a]

Feature	Nonimmunocompromised	Immunocompromised		P
		AIDS	Transplantation	
No.	72	4	4	
Median age (yrs)	35	26	51.5	
Symptoms and Signs				
Storage symptoms	76.4%	37.5%		0.033
Hematuria	58.3%	37.5%		0.288
Lumbar pain	30.6%	25.0%		1.000
Fever	43.1%	87.5%		0.024
Scrotal mass	22.0%	0.0%		0.591
No urological symptoms	5.6%	37.5%		0.019
Duration of symptoms, <6 mo	2.8%	87.5%		<0.001
Previous tuberculosis	26.4%	25.0%		1.00
Disseminated tuberculosis	18.1%	62.5%		0.012
Diagnosis				
Urine	50.0%	50.0%		1.000
Histopathology	33.3%	50.0%		0.441
Clinico-radiographic	16.7%	0.0%		0.599
Cortical kidney lesions	6.2%	87.5%		<0.001
Bilateral	3.1%	37.5%		0.008
Unilateral/grafted	3.1%	50.0%		0.001
Excretory kidney	93.8%	12.5%		<0.001
Lesions	37.5%	12.5%		0.248
Bilateral	56.3%	0.0%		0.005
Unilateral				
Contracted bladder	65.3%	12.5%		0.001
Mortality	4.2%	12.5%		0.350

[a]From reference 19, with permission.

PCR for *Mycobacterium tuberculosis* identification in the urine, a highly sensitive and specific technique in which small bits of genetic material are amplified, has become the ideal diagnostic tool, as it gives results in 24 to 48 h and allows for the diagnosis to be made even when there are few bacilli, features that make it a potentially ideal method for the diagnosis of urogenital tuberculosis (31, 49). Compared to culture, it was 95.6% sensitive and 98.1% specific (49). Compared to bacteriological, histological, or clinico-radiological diagnoses, it was 94.3% sensitive and 85.7% specific (31). Yet, in a systematic review including the analysis of new PCR tests for the diagnosis of urogenital tuberculosis, specificity was high, but sensitivity was variable. In spite of the potential role of PCR in the diagnosis of urogenital tuberculosis, there is no present evidence supporting the diagnosis of the condition without culture confirmation (12).

Intradermal injection of tuberculin, a tuberculosis bacillus-derived purified protein, leads to a late hypersensitivity-like local inflammatory reaction with hard nodular formation after 48 to 72 h. Patients are classified according to the induration diameter as nonreactors (below 5 mm), weak reactors (between 5 and 10 mm), and strong reactors (over 10 mm). The exam is not diagnostic, though, once *M. bovis* BCG-vaccinated subjects are reactors; further, when a nonvaccinated subject reacts, this merely indicates previous contact with the bacillus. Yet, when a previously weak reactor becomes a strong one, it indicates recent infection (28, 39). The tuberculin test may contribute to the diagnosis of urogenital tuberculosis in countries without widespread BCG vaccination, a situation in which the test is positive in 85 to 95% of patients with urogenital tuberculosis (54, 61).

Cystoscopy with biopsy is a low-morbidity procedure that may be performed when there is clinical suspicion of tuberculosis and bacillus-negative urine culture, being more useful in the acute phase. The most frequent findings are local hyperemia, mucosal erosion and ulceration, tubercle formation, and irregularity of the ureteral meatuses. Vesical biopsy is only 18.5 to 52% sensitive, though (31, 60).

Imaging techniques are up to 91.4% sensitive for urogenital tuberculosis diagnosis, with intravenous urography and abdominal computerized tomography being used more (31). Findings suggestive of urogenital tuberculosis are calyceal irregularities; infundibular stenosis; pseudotumor or renal scarring; renal loss of function; renal cavitation; urinary tract calcification (present in 7 to 19% of the cases); collecting system thickening, stenosis, or dilatation; contracted bladder; and lesions in other organs beyond the urinary tract, such as lymph nodes, spleen, liver, and vertebrae (17, 20, 31). The simultaneous finding of kidney and bladder lesions is characteristic of tuberculosis, and the earliest findings are outline irregularity and calyceal dilatation due to infundibular stenosis (31).

Multiple stenoses of the collecting urinary system from the renal pelvis to the ureterovesical junction are the findings most suggestive of urogenital tuberculosis, occurring in 60 to 84% of cases (20). In spite of this variability, urogenital tuberculosis involves the urinary tract in a sequential pattern as described above. After unilateral renal and ureteral involvement, with thickening and stenosis of the collecting system leading to hydronephrosis and renal parenchyma atrophy, there may be bladder damage, with diffuse thickening of the bladder walls and development of vesicoureteral reflux, usually unilaterally to the as-yet-undamaged kidney. High-grade reflux may lead to ureterohydronephrosis, reflux nephropathy, and end-stage renal failure (16). Phases in the urogenital involvement of tuberculosis can then be characterized. Radiological investigation of 20 patients with urogenital tuberculosis showed four types of presentation (20): (i) bilateral renal tuberculosis with predominance of parenchymatous involvement (Fig. 1); (ii) unilateral renal tuberculosis without vesical or contralateral renal involvement (Fig. 2); (iii) unilateral renal tuberculosis and contracted bladder, with a radiologically normal contralateral kidney; and (iv) bilateral renal tuberculosis and contracted bladder, with unilateral renal dysfunction and ureterohydronephrosis of the contralateral kidney due to high-grade reflux. In two of these patients disease progress was radiologically demonstrated (Fig. 3 and 4). Understanding these phases is important for early diagnosis, when such complications and more complex reconstructive surgery may be avoided.

Epididymal tuberculosis presents on ultrasonography as a hypoechoic lesion involving the whole epididymis or just its head, with a heterogeneous texture and concomitant testicular involvement in 38.9% of the cases (10).

PHARMACOLOGICAL TREATMENT

The pharmacological treatment of urogenital tuberculosis should be started after microbiological or histological diagnosis has been made and even before diagnostic confirmation, when clinical, laboratory, and radiological data warrant a presumptive diagnosis (72). Bactericidal (e.g., isoniazid, rifampin, pyrazinamide, and streptomycin) and bacteriostatic (e.g., ethambutol and ethionamide) drugs are used (17, 28, 39). Since there is 80% relapse with a single drug, 25% with two drugs, and 10% with a triple regimen (54), the most conservative approach is to initiate a four-drug regimen, i.e., isoniazid, rifampin, pyrazinamide, and ethambutol or streptomycin. After 2 weeks of treatment, no bacilli can be identified in the urine (28). Although the optimal treatment duration has not been defined, shorter-term treatments have replaced the traditional 18- and 24-month treatments formerly recommended, and infection with susceptible organisms can usually be managed with regimens suitable for pulmonary tuberculosis as discussed in chapter 7. Shorter-term regimens are justified because of the good renal vascularization, high urinary concentration of the drugs used, low bacillary load in the urine, lower cost and toxicity, higher compliance, and efficacy similar to that of longer-duration regimens (51, 68). Four- to six-month treatments with nephrectomy of the excluded kidney have afforded relapse rates lower than 1% (26, 62, 72). Malnutrition and poor social conditions warrant treatment for longer than 9 months, as relapse rates may be as high as 22% after a 6-month regimen and 19% after 1 year (24, 25).

Microbiological relapse of urogenital tuberculosis may occur after initial urine sterilization, even after prolonged treatment and nephrectomy of the excluded kidneys (22, 24, 70). Relapses occur in up to 6.3% of the cases, after a mean of 5.3 years of treatment (range, 11 months to 27 years) with bacilli that are sensitive to the drugs initially used (6, 25). Most authors recommend a 10-year follow-up period after pharmacological treatment, because of the possibility of late relapse and the advantage of early treatment of initial lesions in the asymptomatic phase of relapse (6, 22, 24, 70). The development of antimicrobial resistance, caused by too short a treatment regimen (up to 60% of the patients), is one of the factors responsible for tuberculosis recrudescence (28).

Pharmacological treatment may cure small renal foci and unblock the collecting system (17, 22). Nevertheless, it has been known since the 1970s that pharmacological treatment may aggravate the renal lesions just a few weeks after its start, with fibrosis leading to obstruction of the collecting system and vesical contraction and with worsening of frequency and development of renal dysfunction (35, 54, 70). Therefore, the placement of a double J stent, to prevent worsening obstruction and consequent renal dysfunction, must be considered during the pharmacological treatment of patients with ureteral stenosis.

SURGICAL TREATMENT

Over half (54.9%) the patients with urogenital tuberculosis undergo surgery, a figure that ranges from 8 to 95%, according to the timing of diagnosis (18). In the series where surgery was less frequent, the patients were diagnosed when still asymptomatic, with lower rates of renal lesions (18). On the other hand, when the diagnosis is delayed, the silent progression of the disease leads to organ destruction, with a greater frequency of surgical interventions (18).

Surgery may be ablative, with removal of the tuberculosis-destroyed kidney or epididymis, or reconstructive for unblocking the collecting system or augmenting the contracted bladder (28, 52). The last decades have witnessed a decrease in the number of ablative surgeries and an increase in the number of reconstructive ones (27). The patient should be operated on after at least 4 to 6 weeks of pharmacological treatment (17, 28, 72).

Most authors recommend nephrectomy without ureterectomy in cases of unilateral renal dysfunction to avoid relapse, eliminate irritative voiding symptoms, treat hypertension, and avoid abscess formation (22, 35, 38, 70, 72). Because systemic arterial hypertension is more frequent in patients with urogenital tuberculosis in whom unilateral renal dysfunction develops, nephrectomy can be curative of this condition in up to 64.7% of the cases (22). Relapse is more likely when a nonfunctioning kidney is not removed, because the pharmacological treatment may not sterilize all tuberculous foci, viable bacilli having been identified in kidneys from 8 weeks to 9 months of treatment (21, 55, 70). Conversely, after monitoring 35 patients for up to 22 years, without any complication, some authors recommend kidney preservation if there is no pain, infection, or bleeding (5, 15).

Urinary collecting system obstruction is the main cause of kidney loss of function, the likelihood of renal function recovery in this situation being low (15). In selected cases of severe renal function reduction, however, urinary diversion may preserve these kidneys for later reconstruction (55). The positive prognostic factors for functional recovery of obstructed kidneys are distal ureteral stenosis, cortical thickness greater than 5 mm, and glomerular filtration rate above 15 ml/min, as assessed by the nephrostomy output or renal scintigraphy (55, 70). On the other hand, intrarenal stenoses almost always lead to renal dysfunction (35). In the rare instances in which an early diagnosis is made, percutaneous nephrostomy is 80% successful, and a segment of ileum may be interposed between the bladder and the dilated calices (33, 71).

Ureteral stenosis is treated with dilatation or endoscopic incision, with a 50 to 90% success rate, or with reconstructive surgery (28, 35).

Around 9% of the patients with urogenital tuberculosis have fibrosis of the bladder wall, with capacity reduction and increased frequency of micturition (18). Bladder augmentation is the treatment of choice for contracted bladder due to tuberculosis, with the use of a gastric, ileal, or colonic segment, which is spherically reshaped before anastomosis, to afford greater volume and less reservoir pressure (16).

PERSPECTIVES

After the discovery of specific drugs for tuberculosis treatment in the mid-20th century, there was a profound change in the profile of urogenital tuberculosis, with mortality reduction, cure of initial lesions, reduction of ablative surgeries, and increase in the number of reconstructive surgeries. In recent decades, however, there was no significant change, in spite of technological breakthroughs (57). Since the 1960s, early diagnosis of urogenital tuberculosis has been known to afford greater renal preservation (35). The systematic search for urogenital tuberculosis in patients with pulmonary disease yields 10% culture positivity for the bacillus, with 66.7% of patients asymptomatic and 58% having a normal urine exam and absence of lesions on intravenous urography (4). In two other series, in which cultures were obtained routinely and not as part of any symptom investigation, a greater frequency of asymptomatic patients without lesions on intravenous urography was found (6, 15). Although bacilluria is invariably associated with renal lesion, detection of preclinical bacilluria allows for earlier diagnosis at a time when the initial lesions are amenable to cure and the severe, destructive course of urogenital tuberculosis may be averted (24, 43). A systematic search for the detection of initial cases of urogenital tuberculosis, regardless of symptoms, must be emphasized. A better definition of groups at greater risk (subjects with previous pulmonary tuberculosis or immunosuppression) should be the subject of future studies. We propose that any patient presenting with gross hematuria, persistent microscopic hematuria or pyuria, recurrent urinary tract infection, and persistent irritative micturition symptoms be investigated for urogenital tuberculosis, with six urine samples being collected for culture or PCR. We also propose a periodic urine examination for hematuria or pyuria in patients with previous pulmonary tuberculosis or immunosuppressed subjects (AIDS or posttransplantation).

REFERENCES

1. **Aliyu, M. H., S. H. Aliyu, and H. M. Salihu.** 2004. Female genital tuberculosis: a global review. *Int. J. Fertil.* 49:123–136.

2. **Alvarez, S., and W. R. McCabe.** 1984. Extrapulmonary tuberculosis revisited: a review of experience at Boston City and other hospitals. *Medicine* 63:25–55.

3. **Barrie, H. J., W. K. Kerr, and G. L. Gale.** 1967. The incidence and pathogenesis of tuberculous strictures of the renal pyelus. *J. Urol.* 98:584–589.

4. **Bentz, R. R., D. G. Dimcheff, J. Nemiroff, A. Tsang, and J. G. Weg.** 1975. The incidence of urine cultures positive for *Mycobacterium tuberculosis* in a general tuberculosis patient population. *Am. Rev. Respir. Dis.* 3:647–650.

5. **Bloom, S., H. Wechsler, and J. K. Lattimer.** 1970. Results of long-term study of nonfunctioning tuberculous kidneys. *J. Urol.* 104:654–657.

6. **Butler, M. R., and D. O'Flynn.** 1975. Reactivation of genitourinary tuberculosis. *Eur. Urol.* 1:14–17.

7. **Carl, P., and L. Stark.** 1997. Indications for surgical management of genitourinary tuberculosis. *World J. Surg.* 21:505–510.

8. **Chattopadhyay, A., V. Bhatnagar, S. Agarwala, and D. K. Mitra.** 1997. Genitourinary tuberculosis in pediatric surgical practice. *J. Pediatr. Surg.* 32:1283–1286.

9. **Christensen, W. I.** 1974. Genitourinary tuberculosis. Review of 102 cases. *Medicine* 53:377–390.

10. **Chung, J. J., M. J. Kim, T. Lee, H. S. Yoo, and J. T. Lee.** 1997. Sonographic findings in tuberculous epididymitis and epididynorchitis. *J. Clin. Ultrasound* 25:390–394.

11. **Conte, G., M. Iavarone, D. Santorelli, and L. De Nicola.** 1997. Acute renal failure of unknown origin. Don't forget renal tuberculosis. *Nephrol. Dial. Transplant.* 12:1260–1261.

12. **Dinnes, J., J. Deeks, H. Kunst, A. Gibson, E. Cummins, N. Waugh, F. Drobniewski, and A. Lalvani.** 2007. A systematic review of rapid diagnostic tests for detection of tuberculosis infection. *Health Technol. Assess.* 11:1–196.

13. **Dowdy, L., M. Ramgopal, T. Hoffman, G. Ciancio, G. Burke, D. Roth, C. Mies, B. Jones, and J. Miller.** Genitourinary tuberculosis after renal transplantation: report of 3 cases and review. *Clin. Infect. Dis.* 32:662–666.

14. **El-Agroudy, A. E., A. F. Refaie, O. M. Moussa, and M. A. Ghoneim.** 2003. Tuberculosis in Egyptian kidney transplant recipients: study of clinical course and outcome. *J. Nephrol.* 16:404–411.

15. **Ferrie, B. G., and J. S. H. Rundle.** 1985. Genito-urinary tuberculosis in Glasgow 1970 to 1979: a review of 230 patients. *Scott. Med. J.* 30:30–34.

16. **Figueiredo, A. A., A. M. Lucon, and M. Srougi.** 2006. Bladder augmentation for the treatment of chronic tuberculous cystitis. Clinical and urodynamic evaluation of 25 patients after long term follow-up. *Neurol. Urodyn.* 25:433–440.

17. **Figueiredo, A. A., A. M. Lucon, C. M. Gomes, and M. Srougi.** 2008. Urogenital tuberculosis: patient classification in seven different groups according to clinical and radiological presentation. *Int. Braz. J. Urol.* 34:422–432.

18. **Figueiredo, A. A., A. M. Lucon, R. Falci, Jr., and M. Srougi.** 2008. Epidemiology of urogenital tuberculosis worldwide. *Int. J. Urol.* 15:827–832.

19. **Figueiredo, A. A., A. M. Lucon, R. Falci, Jr., D. S. Ikejiri, W. C. Nahas, and M. Srougi.** 2009. Urogenital tuberculosis in immunocompromised patients. *Int. Urol. Nephrol.* 41:327–333.

20. **Figueiredo, A. A., A. M. Lucon, A. N. Arvellos, C. O. P. Ramos, A. C. T. Toledo, R. Falci, Jr., F. E. Q. Recaverren, J. M. B. Netto, and M. Srougi.** 2010. A better understanding of urogenital tuberculosis pathophysiology based on radiological findings. *Eur. J. Radiol.* 76:246–257.

21. Fischer, M., and J. Flamm. 1990. The value of surgical therapy in the treatment of urogenital tuberculosis. *Urologe A* **29:**261–264.

22. Flechner, S. M., and J. G. Gow. 1980. Role of nephrectomy in the treatment of non-functioning or very poorly functioning unilateral tuberculous kidney. *J. Urol.* **123:**822–825.

23. Garcia-Rodríguez, J. Á., J. E. García Sanchez, and J. L. Muñoz Bellido. 1994. Genitourinary tuberculosis in Spain: review of 81 cases. *Clin. Infect. Dis.* **18:**557–561.

24. Gokalp, A., E. Y. Gultekin, and S. Ozdamar. 1990. Genitourinary tuberculosis: a review of 83 cases. *Br. J. Clin. Pract.* **44:**599–600.

25. Gokce, G., H. Kilicaerslan, S. Ayan, F. Tas, R. Akar, K. Kaya, and E. Y. Gultekin. 2002. Genitourinary tuberculosis: review of 174 cases. *Scand. J. Infect. Dis.* **34:**338–340.

26. Gow, J. G. 1979. Genitourinary tuberculosis: a 7-year review. *Br. J. Urol.* **51:**239–244.

27. Gow, J. G., and S. Barbosa. 1984. Genitourinary tuberculosis. A study of 1117 cases over a period of 34 years. *Br. J. Urol.* **56:**449–455.

28. Gow, J. G. 1998. Genitourinary tuberculosis, p. 807–836. *In* P. C. Walsh, A. B. Retik, E. D. Vaughan, and A. J. Wein (ed.), *Campbell's Urology*, 7th ed. W. B. Saunders Company, Philadelphia, PA.

29. Gueye, S. M., M. Ba, C. Sylla, A. K. Ndoye, P. A. Fall, J. J. Diaw, and A. Mensah. 1998. Epididymal manifestations of urogenital tuberculosis. *Prog. Urol.* **8:**240–243.

30. Hemal, A. K., M. Aron, M. Nair, and S. N. Wadhwa. 1998. Autoprostatectomy: an unusual manifestation in genitourinary tuberculosis. *Br. J. Urol.* **82:**140–141.

31. Hemal, A. K., N. P. Gupta, T. P. Rajeev, R. Kumar, L. Dar, and P. Seth. 2000. Polymerase chain reaction in clinically suspected genitourinary tuberculosis: comparison with intravenous urography, bladder biopsy, and urine acid fast bacilli culture. *Urology* **56:**570–574.

32. Henn, L., F. Nagel, and F. D. Pizzol. 1999. Comparison between human immunodeficiency virus positive and negative patients with tuberculosis in Southern Brazil. *Mem. Inst. Oswaldo Cruz* **94:**377–381.

33. Hwang, T. K., and Y. H. Park. 1994. Endoscopic infundibulotomy in tuberculous renal infundibular stricture. *J. Urol.* **151:**852–854.

34. Indudhara, R., S. Vaidyanathan, and B. D. Radotra. 1992. Urethral tuberculosis. *Urol. Int.* **48:**436–438.

35. Kerr, W. K., G. L. Gale, and K. S. S. Peterson. 1969. Reconstructive surgery for genitourinary tuberculosis. *J. Urol.* **101:**254–266.

36. Kostakopoulos, A., G. Economou, D. Picramenos, C. Macrichoritis, P. Tekerlekis, and N. Kalliakmanis. 1998. Tuberculosis of the prostate. *Int. Urol. Nephrol.* **30:**153–157.

37. Larsen, C. P., R. K. Moreira, R. A. Hennigar, and V. Bijol. 2008. Kidney biopsy findings in a patient with fever, bilateral pulmonary infiltrates, and acute renal failure. *Am. J. Kidney Dis.* **51:**524–529.

38. Lee, Y. H., W. C. Huang, J. S. Huang, J. S. Wang, C. C. Yu, B. P. Jiaan, and J. K. Huang. 2001. Efficacy of chemotherapy for prostatic tuberculosis—a clinical and histologic follow-up study. *Urology* **57:**872–877.

39. Leite, O. H. M. 2001. Tuberculosis. *Problems Gen. Surg.* **18:**69–78.

40. Lubbe, J., C. Ruef, W. Spirig, M. Dubs, and C. Sigg. 1996. Infertility as the first symptom of male genito-urinary tuberculosis. *Urol. Int.* **56:**204–206.

41. Mallinson, W. J. W., R. W. Fuller, D. A. Levison, L. R. I. Baker, and W. R. Cattell. 1980. Diffuse interstitial renal tuberculosis —an unusual cause of renal failure. *Q. J. Med.* **198:**137–148.

42. Marques, L. P. J., L. S. Rioja, C. A. B. Oliveira, and O. R. Santos. 1996. AIDS-associated renal tuberculosis. *Nephron* **74:**701–704.

43. Medlar, E. M., and K. T. Sasano. 1924. Experimental renal tuberculosis, with special reference to excretory bacilluria. *Am. Ver. Tuberc.* **10:**370–377.

44. Medlar, E. M. 1926. Cases of renal infection in pulmonary tuberculosis: evidence of healed tuberculous lesions. *Am. J. Pathol.* **2:**401–411.

45. Medlar, E. M., D. M. Spain, and R. W. Holliday. 1949. Postmortem compared with clinical diagnosis of genito-urinary tuberculosis in adult males. *J. Urol.* **61:**1078–1088.

46. Mochalova, T. P., and I. Y. Starikov. 1997. Reconstructive surgery for treatment of urogenital tuberculosis: 30 years of observation. *World J. Surg.* **21:**511–515.

47. Mondal, S. K., and T. K. Dutta. 2009. A ten year clinicopathological study of female genital tuberculosis and impact on fertility. *J. Nepal Med. Assoc.* **48:**52–57.

48. Mortier, E., J. Pouchot, L. Girard, Y. Boussougant, and P. Vinceneux. 1996. Assessment of urine analysis for the diagnosis of tuberculosis. *Br. Med. J.* **312:**27–28.

49. Moussa, O. M., I. Eraky, M. A. El-Far, H. G. Osman, and M. A. Groneim. 2000. Rapid diagnosis of genitourinary tuberculosis by polymerase chain reaction and non-radioactive DNA hybridization. *J. Urol.* **164:**584–588.

50. Narayana, A. S. 1982. Overview of renal tuberculosis. *Urology* **19:**231–237.

51. Nzerue, C., J. Drayton, R. Oster, and K. Hewan-Lowe. 2000. Genitourinary tuberculosis in patients with HIV infection: clinical features in an inner-city hospital population. *Am. J. Med. Sci.* **320:**299–303.

52. O'Flynn, D. 1970. Surgical treatment of genito-urinary tuberculosis: a report on 762 cases. *Br. J. Urol.* **42:**667–671.

53. Pryor, J. P., and W. F. Hendry. 1991. Ejaculatory duct obstruction in subfertile males: analysis of 87 patients. *Fertil. Steril.* **65:**725–730.

54. Psihramis, K. E., and P. K. Donahoe. 1986. Primary genitourinary tuberculosis: rapid progression and tissue destruction during treatment. *J. Urol.* **135:**1033–1036.

55. Ramanathan, R., A. Kumar, R. Kapoor, and M. Bhandari. 1998. Relief of urinary tract obstruction in tuberculosis to improve renal function. Analysis of predictive factors. *Br. J. Urol.* **81:**199–205.

56. Ramesh, V., and R. Vasanthi. 1989. Tuberculous cavernositis of the penis: case report. *Genitourin. Med.* **65:**58–59.

57. Ross, J. C. 1953. Renal tuberculosis. *Br. J. Urol.* **25:**277–292.

58. Ross, J. C., J. G. Gow, and C. A. St. Hill. 1961. Tuberculous epididymitis. A review of 170 patients. *Br. J. Urol.* **48:**663–666.

59. Schubert, G. E., T. Haltaufderheide, and R. Golz. 1992. Frequency of urogenital tuberculosis in an unselected autopsy series from 1928 to 1949 and 1976 to 1989. *Eur. Urol.* **21:**216–223.

60. Shapiro, A. L., and V. I. Viter. 1989. Cystoscopy and endovesical biopsy in renal tuberculosis. *Urol. Nefrol. (Mosk)* **1:**12–15.

61. Simon, H. B., A. J. Weinstein, M. S. Pasternak, M. N. Swartz, and L. J. Kunz. 1977. Genitourinary tuberculosis. *Am. J. Med.* **63:**410–420.

62. Skutil, V., J. Varsa, and M. Obsitnik. 1985. Six-month chemotherapy for urogenital tuberculosis. *Eur. Urol.* **11:**170–176.

63. Sporer, A., and O. Auerbach. 1978. Tuberculosis of prostate. *Urology* **11:**362–365.

64. Symes, J. M., and J. P. Blandy. 1973. Tuberculosis of the male urethra. *Br. J. Urol.* **45:**432–436.

65. Trauzzi, S. J., C. J. Kay, D. G. Kaufman, and F. C. Lowe. 1994. Management of prostatic abscess in patients with human immunodeficiency syndrome. *Urology* **43:**629–633.

66. **Vasanthi, R., and V. Ramesh.** 1991. Tuberculous infection of the male genitalia. *Australas. J. Dermatol.* **32:**81–83.

67. **Watters, D. A.** 1997. Surgery for tuberculosis before and after human immunodeficiency virus infection: a tropical perspective. *Br. J. Surg.* **84:**8–14.

68. **Weinberg, A. C., and S. D. Boyd.** 1988. Short-course chemotherapy and role of surgery in adult and pediatric genitourinary tuberculosis. *Urology* **31:**95–102.

69. **Winblad, B., and M. Duchek.** 1975. Spread of tuberculosis from obstructed and non-obstructed upper urinary tract. *Acta Pathol. Microbiol. Scand. A* **83:**229–236.

70. **Wong, S. H., and W. Y. Lau.** 1980. The surgical management of non-functioning tuberculous kidneys. *J. Urol.* **124:**187–191.

71. **Wong, S. H., and S. L. Chan.** 1981. Pan-caliceal ileoneocystostomy—a new operation for intrapelvic tuberculotic strictures of the renal pelvis. *J. Urol.* **126:**734–736.

72. **Wong, S. H., W. Y. Lau, G. P. Poon, S. T. Fan, K. K. Ho, T. F. Yiu, and S. L. Chan.** 1984. The treatment of urinary tuberculosis. *J. Urol.* **131:**297–301.

Tuberculosis and Nontuberculous Mycobacterial Infections, 6th ed.
Edited by David Schlossberg
© 2011 ASM Press, Washington, DC

Chapter 21

Musculoskeletal Tuberculosis

MICHAEL K. LEONARD, JR., AND HENRY M. BLUMBERG

INTRODUCTION

Musculoskeletal tuberculosis (TB) accounts for approximately 10% of all extrapulmonary TB cases in the United States and is the third most common site of extrapulmonary TB after pleural and lymphatic disease. Vertebral involvement (tuberculous spondylitis, or Pott's disease) is the most common type of skeletal TB, accounting for about half of all cases of musculoskeletal TB. The presentation of musculoskeletal TB may be insidious over a long period and the diagnosis may be elusive and delayed, as TB may not be the initial consideration in the differential diagnosis. The diagnosis is often confused with malignancy. Concomitant pulmonary involvement may not be present, thus confusing the diagnosis even further.

Ancient skeletal remains dating back several thousand years have preserved the history of skeletal TB. Egyptian mummies are some of the oldest specimens and demonstrate evidence of spinal TB, as well as psoas abscesses (107). PCR has confirmed that these ancient lesions are due to *Mycobacterium tuberculosis* and not *Mycobacterium bovis* as others have suggested (21). There is also evidence of skeletal TB, including vertebral disease, in pre-Columbian, New World remains (55). Molecular diagnostic studies have also confirmed these lesions as *M. tuberculosis* (29, 95). These findings demonstrate that TB was present in the New World prior to the arrival of Europeans, which had been disputed for some time.

Vertebral TB was described by Hippocrates in ancient Greece. Sir Percivall Pott in 1779 was the first to describe the modern presentation of the clinical aspects of vertebral TB when he described a patient that had spinal deformity with paraplegia. He even proposed drainage of adjacent paraspinal abscesses, which frequently are seen in skeletal TB, and reported improvement in symptoms after the procedure (34). It was not until the late 19th century, after the description of the tubercle bacillus in 1882 by Robert Koch, that Pott's disease was linked to illness caused by *M. tuberculosis*.

EPIDEMIOLOGY

The incidence of TB in the United States declined significantly during most of the 20th century and into the 21st century. However, in the mid-1980s through the early 1990s, there was a resurgence of this ancient disease. Between 1985 and 1992 there were an additional 40,000 cases of TB in the United States that were unexpected. This resurgence of TB was due to several factors, including the human immunodeficiency virus (HIV) epidemic and a breakdown in the public health infrastructure in the United States for TB control due to decreases in funding. As cases of pulmonary TB increased, a rise in the number of extrapulmonary disease cases, including musculoskeletal TB, was seen. Enhanced efforts at TB control (including increased funding) were implemented in response to the resurgence and led to a subsequent decline in TB cases and incidence in the United States beginning in 1993. In 2009, a total of 11,540 TB cases were reported in the United States, for a TB rate of 3.8 cases per 100,000 population, which is the lowest ever reported (14). The majority of TB cases in the United States (approximately 60%) now occur among foreign-born persons, reflecting the global TB epidemic (14). The large majority of extrapulmonary TB cases, including musculoskeletal TB, diagnosed in the United States also occur among foreign-born persons.

In 2009, a total of 8,535 TB cases were pulmonary TB, of which 7,133 (83.6%) were culture positive. Of 2,297 extrapulmonary TB cases, 1,630

Michael K. Leonard, Jr., and Henry M. Blumberg • Division of Infectious Diseases, Emory University School of Medicine, Atlanta, GA 30303.

(71.0%) were culture positive. The site of disease or culture status was unknown for 708 cases. From 2008 to 2009, culture-positive pulmonary cases decreased 13.6% (8,257 to 7,133), culture-negative pulmonary TB cases decreased 17.5% (1,700 to 1,402), culture-positive extrapulmonary TB cases decreased 8.3% (1,777 to 1,630), culture-negative extrapulmonary TB cases decreased 3.1% (688 to 667), and cases with unknown site of disease or culture status increased 48.7% (476 to 708) (14). Bone and joint TB cases have accounted for 2 to 3% of all reported TB cases in the United States (Table 1); in some series reported from outside the United States, >6% of TB cases have been due to bone and joint disease (44). Data from the preantibiotic era demonstrated that half of those with musculoskeletal TB had evidence of coexisting pulmonary disease (59). As the number of reported TB cases and incidence of TB disease have decreased in the United States, an increasing racial disparity has been noted, with the majority of cases occurring among minorities and the foreign-born. Foreign-born persons and racial/ethnic minorities have TB disease disproportionate to their respective populations. In 2009, the TB rate in foreign-born persons was nearly 11 times higher than in U.S.-born persons. The rates among Hispanics and blacks were approximately eight times higher than among non-Hispanic whites, and rates among Asians were nearly 26 times higher (14). Reports from the United States and United Kingdom have indicated that about three-fourths of all patients with musculoskeletal TB are foreign-born (98). This is important

for clinicians to remember, as multiple studies have shown that immigrants (i.e., foreign-born persons) have accounted for an increasing percentage of extrapulmonary TB cases and the diagnosis is often delayed (14, 17, 44, 98). Extrapulmonary TB is more common among patients with HIV infection, but musculoskeletal TB is not necessarily increased in HIV-seropositive patients compared to those that are HIV seronegative (61). Tumor necrosis factor alpha inhibitors have been shown to greatly increase the risk of disseminated TB disease among patients with latent TB infection, and recent reports have noted that this includes the development of serious musculoskeletal infections (36).

In countries where TB is endemic, older children and young adults are most commonly affected with musculoskeletal TB, while in developed countries the disease is often seen in older persons (63). Historically, musculoskeletal TB was a disease of children and adolescents, often seen developing within a few years after primary infection. In developing countries this is still often the case, whereas in the developed countries, musculoskeletal TB most commonly results from reactivation. Osteoarticular lesions result from hematogenous spread of a primary infection. Any bone, joint, or bursa can be infected, but the spine, hip, and knee, in order of frequency, are the preferred sites of infection, representing 70 to 80% of infections (22, 63). The diagnosis of musculoskeletal TB is often delayed due to the indolent nature of the disease and low clinical suspicion in areas with a low incidence of TB disease. In a series of 194 patients from India with musculoskeletal TB, 30% of cases occurred during the second decade of life, 22% in the first decade, 18% in the third decade, and 14% in the fourth decade (2). However, in developed countries with a lower prevalence of TB, musculoskeletal TB is seen more frequently in the adult age group, especially among foreign-born persons.

Vertebral or spinal TB is the most common type of musculoskeletal TB, accounting for about 50% of cases in most series. In Los Angeles County, California, a total of 220 cases of musculoskeletal TB were registered between 1990 and 1995; the distribution of sites was as follows: 118 (54%) had vertebral TB, 56 (26%) had joint involvement (29 cases [13%] with knee involvement, 18 [8%] with hip involvement, and 9 [4%] with wrist involvement), and 10 (4%) had soft tissue/muscle involvement (Table 2) (22). A report from India with 194 cases noted of musculoskeletal TB reported the distribution of cases as follows: 49% had vertebral disease, 34 (18%) had involvement of the knee, 32 (16%) had hip involvement, 15 (8%) had ankle/foot involvement, 8 (4%)

Table 1. Number and proportion of musculoskeletal TB cases in the United States, 1993 to 2008[a]

Yr	No. of bone/joint/skeletal TB cases	% of U.S. cases due to bone/joint/skeletal TB	Total TB cases reported (U.S.)
1993	644	2.56	25,108
1994	574	2.37	24,205
1995	547	2.41	22,728
1996	561	2.64	21,211
1997	514	2.60	19,751
1998	498	2.72	18,286
1999	482	2.75	17,501
2000	457	2.80	16,308
2001	439	2.75	15,945
2002	469	3.11	15,057
2003	436	2.93	14,871
2004	405	2.79	14,500
2005	391	2.79	14,067
2006	380	2.23	13,727
2007	344	2.59	13,288
2008	356	2.75	12,904

[a]Source: Centers for Disease Control and Prevention.

Table 2. Anatomic site of musculoskeletal TB reported in Los Angeles County from 1990 to 1995

Group	Site	No.	% of group	% of total
I. Spine ($n = 118$)	Cervical	6	5	3
	Thoracic	45	38	21
	Lumbar	65	55	30
	Sacrum	2	2	1
II. Peripheral joints ($n = 78$)	Hip	18	23	8
	Knee	29	37	13
	Ankle	5	6	2
	Foot	7	9	3
	Shoulder	4	5	2
	Elbow	5	6	2
	Wrist	9	12	4
	Finger	1	1	0.5
III. Other ($n = 24$)	Other bone/soft/tissue/	14	58	6
	muscle	10	42	4

had elbow involvement, 4 (2%) had hand involvement, and 3 (1%) had wrist involvement (2). Other sites in this series with two or fewer cases included the ileum, shoulder, rib, pubis, calcaneus, femur, and sacro-iliac joint. TB can also cause disease of the peripheral joints, skull, and ribs, but these are less common manifestations (32).

PATHOGENESIS

The common lesion in skeletal TB consists of both osteomyelitis and arthritis. Bone involvement usually is the result of hematogenous spread of *M. tuberculosis* (especially occurring following primary infection), but bone and joint involvement can also be due to lymphatic drainage or secondary to a contiguous focus of disease. The growth plates (metaphyses) receive the richest blood supply and are most often the initial site of infection. Tubercle bacilli invade the end arteries, causing an endarteritis and bone destruction through the epiphysis. After crossing the epiphysis, bacilli can drain into the joint space, resulting in tuberculous arthritis, or form a sinus tract after being released from the destroyed bone. *M. tuberculosis* does not produce any cartilage-destroying enzymes as are seen in pyogenic infections. If the infection progresses without treatment, abscesses surrounding the joint or bone may develop. These are often described as being "cold" abscesses. The abscesses may rupture, forming sinus tracts which have long been associated with musculoskeletal TB. Healing of musculoskeletal TB, especially of the joints, involves the formation of fibrous scar tissue. Calcifications are also frequently seen in healed lesions, especially if an abscess, infected bursa, or paraspinous mass was involved. A calcified psoas muscle in someone with healed Pott's

disease (spinal TB) is a classic example of this. The same hematogenous spread of tubercle bacilli can also primarily infect the synovium, bursae, or tendon sheaths, although this occurs much less frequently than bone involvement.

In children, the main route of infection in skeletal TB is through hematogenous spread from a primary source. Children may also experience musculoskeletal TB from reactivation of a quiescent focus after the development of latent TB infection, as occurs not uncommonly among adults. Children historically have been most affected with musculoskeletal TB because of the increased vascularity of their bones during growth, thus making them more susceptible during the period of hematogenous dissemination (e.g., following primary infection). Large weight-bearing bones and joints are the most commonly affected. Muscles are rarely primarily infected in adults or children, but tuberculous myositis may occur secondarily from contiguous bone infection or a draining sinus tract, as is seen with psoas muscle involvement that occurs secondary to Pott's disease (9).

After the dissemination of bacilli to the bone, a granulomatous inflammatory response ensues. Biopsies of bone samples from those with skeletal TB reveal few organisms compared with pulmonary TB. The infected area consists of abscess and granulation tissue, and histology demonstrates giant cells, epithelioid histiocytes, and a mantle of lymphocytes and plasma cells, with an outer layer of proliferating fibroblasts and granulation tissue. As the area of infection enlarges, the center becomes necrotic, resulting in an area of caseating necrosis. This caseation may progress to cause bone expansion and eventually destruction of the cortex. A pathological feature of tuberculous osteomyelitis is that there is no bone regeneration (sclerosis) or periosteal reaction (27).

PATHOPHYSIOLOGY

Tuberculous Spondylitis

Sir Percivall Pott described the classic presentation of vertebral TB in 1779 as destruction of two or more contiguous vertebrae and apposed end plates, commonly associated with a paraspinal mass or abscess (83). In 1936, Compere and Garrison from the University of Chicago provided classic descriptions of vertebral TB, comparing radiologic findings with pathology and autopsy findings (19). They also compared findings at autopsy of patients with tuberculous spondylitis and pyogenic infections. Their descriptions of tuberculous spondylitis noted that the anterior portion of the vertebral body is much more commonly affected than the posterior components of the vertebrae. From this site, TB may spread to adjacent intervertebral disks. More than one vertebra is usually involved because of the contiguous spread along the anterior longitudinal ligaments. Skip lesions can also occur.

Tuberculous spondylitis begins with infection of the subchondral bone that then spreads to the cortex. The cartilage resists destruction by *M. tuberculosis* and despite there being a rich blood supply to the vertebrae, there is no blood supply to the disk (89). The anterior portion of the vertebral body is the most affected, with sparing of the posterior components. Involvement of the posterior components (i.e., laminae, pedicles, transverse processes, and spinous processes) is rare (86). In children, the intervertebral disk is vascularized—therefore, tuberculous diskitis in children may be the result of primary infection. In adults, the disk is avascular and disk disease is due to the contiguous spread of infection from the vertebral body. The narrowing disk space visible in adults on plain radiography is more often due to collapse of the vertebral end plate than to destruction of the disk itself (13). Collapse of the anterior spinal elements results in a kyphotic deformity, giving the hunchback appearance and gibbus deformity associated with Pott's disease. TB of the vertebral skeleton causes lytic destruction without new bone formation (sclerosis). The infection can extend to the soft tissue, forming paraspinal abscesses. The degree of the kyphosis is proportional to the initial loss of vertebral body volume and continues until the vertebral bodies meet anteriorly or until the caseous material and granulation tissue mature into bone (11).

Vertebral TB most commonly involves the thoracic and lumbar regions of the spine. Historically, the thoracic vertebrae have been the most commonly affected area of the spine. Some reports have indicated that the thoracic spine is involved in about 50% of spinal TB cases, whereas the lumbar spine is involved in 25% of cases (103). Cervical and sacral involvement occurs less frequently. However, other more recent reports have suggested that among adults, lumbar involvement may be most common. Of 118 cases of vertebral TB reported from a series in Los Angeles, 65 patients had lumbar tuberculous spondylitis, 45 thoracic, 6 cervical, and 2 sacral. Cervical involvement is frequently associated with retropharyngeal abscess and severe neurologic defects (6).

Spinal deformity and paraplegia/quadriplegia are the most common and serious complications of TB of the spine. Rarely does it result directly from the kyphotic defect unless it is severe enough to cause subluxation of the spine. Paraplegia can be due to compression of the spinal canal by an adjacent abscess, sequestra of the vertebral body or disk, or direct dural invasion. Cervical vertebral TB is highly associated with early and severe neurologic compromise (105).

Paraspinal abscesses are quite common in vertebral TB, occurring in more than 90% of cases. The abscess may extend anteriorly to adjacent ligaments and soft tissues, or it may also extend posteriorly into the epidural space. Because the abscesses can spread beneath the ligament, distant sites may be involved. There are also reports of tuberculous paraspinal abscesses eroding into internal organs or to the body surface (12). Lumbar disease may spread into or beneath the psoas-iliac muscle, causing abscesses in the thigh. Sacral lesions have been reported to extend into the perineum.

Pyogenic abscesses differ from vertebral TB in several ways. Pyogenic abscesses destroy the disk rapidly, resulting in early disk space narrowing. Calcification of a large paraspinous abscess which may be seen with TB is not a prominent feature of a pyogenic abscess. In a study comparing pyogenic, tuberculous, and brucellar vertebral osteomyelitis in Spain, patients with vertebral TB were found to be more likely to have a prolonged clinical course, thoracic segment involvement, absence of fever, presence of spinal deformity, neurologic deficit, and paraspinal or epidural masses (18).

Tuberculous Osteomyelitis and Arthritis

Tuberculous osteomyelitis may extend to a joint or tenosynovium. In adults the lesion may be single and affect any bone, including long bones, the pelvis, ribs, and skull. In children, multiple lesions in long bones dominate, but the bones of the hands and feet may be affected. Tuberculous dactylitis (involvement of the short bones of the hands or feet) is more common among children than adults. Tuberculous osteomyelitis has a predilection for the metaphysis of long bones such as the femur, tibia, and ulna. In children, TB may violate the growth plate and lesions of the epiphysis may extend into the joint space. Destruction of the epiphyseal growth plates in children can also result in shortening of the affected limb. Although uncommon, TB can also involve the ribs and skull. The skull contains little cancellous bone which is usually affected by *M. tuberculosis*. Disease involving the skull occurs more often in children and anecdotally may be associated with head trauma (62). In a review of 223 cases of TB involving the skull, Strauss found that only 15 had associated central nervous system disease (10 with meningitis and 5 with cerebral TB). This is thought to be due to the dura being resistant to infection with *M. tuberculosis* (96). TB of the ribs can occur either by hematogenous seeding of the ribs or in some cases due to contiguous spread in a patient with pulmonary disease. TB of the ribs (Fig. 1) is an uncommon manifestation of the disease but is the second most common cause of nontraumatic rib lesions after malignancy (7). A closed cystic form of skeletal TB can occur, especially in the long bones, and may not have associated sclerosis, osteopenia, or abscess/sinus tract formation as in other forms of skeletal TB. This form of TB is more likely to occur in children and may be misdiagnosed as a malignancy (38, 106).

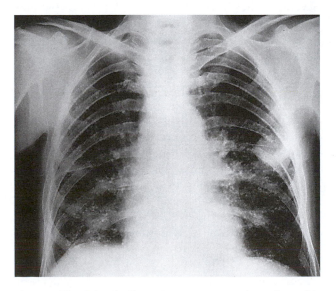

Figure 1. TB of the rib. Shown is a postero-anterior radiographic view of the chest of a man after 3 months of successful antituberculous chemotherapy. Note the mass in the left chest with destruction of a portion of the adjacent rib. A biopsy and culture confirmed TB. The mass resolved with continued therapy.

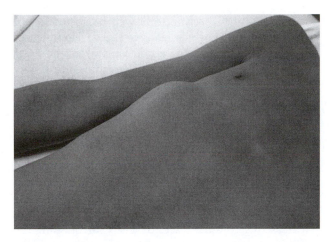

Figure 2. This photograph demonstrates a cold abscess of the chest wall in a patient with TB. Aspiration of this mass yielded material that was AFB smear positive, and the culture yielded *M. tuberculosis.*

Tuberculous osteomyelitis is frequently complicated by tuberculous arthritis (discussed below) as well as by the development of cold abscesses that may form around the adjacent bone process and can rupture creating draining sinus tracts (Fig. 2). Cold abscesses are composed of white blood cells, products of caseating necrosis from the tubercle, bone debris, and tubercle bacilli. Cold abscesses appear to occur commonly among HIV-infected patients.

Several reports have noted an association between mechanical factors such as trauma and the development of skeletal TB. In a Canadian study of 99 patients with skeletal TB, 30 had a history of trauma preceding their presentation and 7 had a recent history of intra-articular steroid injection (30). This may also explain why weight-bearing joints are most frequently involved. Trauma may be associated with skeletal TB because of resulting increased vascularity, decreased resistance, or unmasking of latent infection (22, 62).

Tuberculous Arthritis

Tuberculous arthritis most typically involves large weight-bearing joints such as the hip and the knee, although any other joint may be affected. Invasion of the joint space may be either hematogenous seeding or indirectly from lesions in epiphyseal bone (in adults) or metaphyseal bone (in children) eroding into the joint space. Contiguous spread of TB from other organs to bones may also occur. In long bones, hematogenous spread commonly affects the synovium, causing an erosive deforming arthritis that is monoarticular in about 90% of cases. Initially the synovium develops an inflammatory reaction, followed by formation of granulation tissue, which leads to the development of a pannus. The pannus can erode the margins and surface of the joint. As the effusion develops, fibrin may precipitate, forming "rice bodies" seen in the synovial fluid, bursae, and tendon sheaths. Rice bodies are not unique to TB, as they can also be seen in rheumatoid arthritis. The infection then spreads to the epiphysis and upper metaphysis on either side of the joint through the periarticular vasculature. The granulation tissue erodes and eventually destroys the cartilage, eventually leading to demineralization of the bone and caseating necrosis. In advanced and late disease, para-osseous cold abscesses develop surrounding the joints. Spontaneous drainage of cold abscesses results in sinus tract formation.

Poncet's Disease (Poncet's Arthritis)

Poncet's disease is a reactive polyarthritis usually associated with extrapulmonary TB (e.g., visceral or disseminated TB) in the absence of any evidence of mycobacterial infection of the joints. Poncet's disease was originally described by Charcot in 1864 and Lancereaux in 1871, but Anton Poncet first gave a detailed description of this syndrome when he described polyarthritis occurring in a 15-year-old with suppurative TB of the hip in 1897 (50). Poncet's arthritis is a reactive form of arthritis and is a separate entity from TB directly affecting joint spaces. Usually it occurs during acute TB infection and is a polyarticular process associated with fever. Erythema nodosum may be a hallmark of disease. The pathogenesis of Poncet's disease is unclear. As noted, joint fluid analysis does not reveal the presence of M. tuberculosis disease in the joint space, and clinical symptoms resolve with antituberculous therapy. In a recent review, extrapulmonary TB was present in half of the patients with Poncet's disease and only 6% of the patients presented with erythema nodosum (58).

Tuberculous Myositis

Tuberculous myositis is an uncommon manifestation of the disease and usually the result of contiguous infection, especially seen in Pott's disease (49, 93). Tuberculous myositis can also be "primary" (i.e., a cause of pyomyositis), resulting from hematogenous spread, but this is a less common manifestation of disease and much less likely to occur than myositis due to secondary or contiguous spread (4, 9). The tuberculous lesion of primary myositis may present as a solitary nodule with epithelioid granuloma and caseating necrosis or a cystic formation containing a gelatinous material enclosed by a thick wall (54). The

most common presentation of tuberculous myositis is a psoas abscess due to a complication of and contiguous spread from tuberculous spondylitis; this may extend below the inguinal ligament (49). Tuberculous myositis has been reported more frequently among HIV-infected patients (65).

CLINICAL FEATURES

The onset of musculoskeletal TB is usually an insidious process that often takes months and occasionally years from the first symptoms to the time of diagnosis. Presentation depends upon the stage of the disease, site of the disease, and presence of complications such as neurologic deficits, abscesses, or sinus tracts. Local pain and tenderness are generally the presenting symptoms, followed by impairment of function and swelling of the affected part. Regional muscle wasting and joint deformity are common findings. In some cases, a painless cold abscess (Fig. 2) may be the only presenting clinical feature for an extended period. Systemic symptoms such as fever, night sweats, and weight loss may be seen with early disease but are more likely to occur with advanced cases. About half of the cases of musculoskeletal TB have evidence of active or healed pulmonary TB (2). A single site of involvement is generally seen, but multiple locations are not uncommon. Multiple lesions occur more often in those who are immunocompromised, including persons with HIV infection. Several studies have reported that >90% of patients with musculoskeletal TB were tuberculin skin test positive (30, 66); however, these studies were largely carried out in the pre-HIV era.

Tuberculous Spondylitis

Tuberculous spondylitis remains the most common manifestation of musculoskeletal TB. The progression of disease is usually slow and insidious and the main symptom, back pain, is not specific. This frequently results in delayed diagnosis, resulting in diagnosis from weeks to years after the onset of symptoms. Pertuiset et al. reported a median of 4 months' duration of symptoms prior to diagnosis, with a range of 1 week to 3 years among 103 patients with spinal TB, and noted weight loss in 48%, fever (>38°C) in 31%, and night sweats in 18% (91). As the disease advances, cold abscesses, neurologic deficits, sinus tract formation, and kyphotic deformities can develop. Cold abscesses of the paraspinal tissues or psoas muscle abscesses may be large and protrude under the inguinal ligament when a patient is examined for the first time. Some degree of kyphosis is frequently present. Weakness and paralysis of the lower extremities may occur early during the course of the disease. HIV infection has not been shown to alter the clinical presentation or course of tuberculous spondylitis (61).

On physical examination, there may be focal tenderness over the spinal processes as well as back spasm. Fluctuance, erythema, and focal warmth on exam are unusual findings, as the spinal infection typically involves the anterior column of the spine (68). Range-of-motion testing may produce severe pain, and especially with advanced disease, focal kyphosis can be seen on physician examination. Neurologic symptoms may be subtle at first and progress over time. Initially these include numbness and tingling in the lower extremities or a subjective sense of weakness with activity. With more advanced disease there is evidence of spinal cord compression which can result in paraplegia. Between 10 and 25% of patients in reported case series have had paraplegia (91). Patients with cervical disease are prone to developing neurologic compromise very quickly and may develop retropharyngeal abscesses (6, 37, 87). Cervical TB can also manifest as torticollis, dysphagia, hoarseness, and cranial nerve 12 palsy, depending upon which level of the cervical spine is affected (64). The degree of neurologic damage correlates with prognosis, with those presenting with complete motor loss being unlikely to recover neurologically. Extrinsic cord compression can occur due to vertebral subluxation, collapse of a vertebral body, or an extradural abscess.

Tuberculous Arthritis

Tuberculous arthritis usually occurs as a monoarthritis mostly of weight-bearing joints such as the knee, hip, or ankle. It is slowly progressive and characterized by painful, boggy swelling caused by synovial hypertrophy and effusion (Fig. 3). Eventually ankylosis of the joint may occur. Periarticular abscesses and draining sinus tracts are late findings. Pain is such a prominent symptom that it may lead to immobility of the affected joint. Prolonged immobility may eventually lead to deformity, especially of the knee and hip. Tuberculous arthritis clinically can mimic other processes such as gout or juvenile rheumatoid arthritis, making the diagnosis confusing and delayed (5). Polyarticular tuberculous arthritis has been reported but is rare (101).

Tuberculous Osteomyelitis

Tuberculous osteomyelitis often occurs in conjunction with tuberculous arthritis, but it can occur as a distinct entity without joint involvement. In

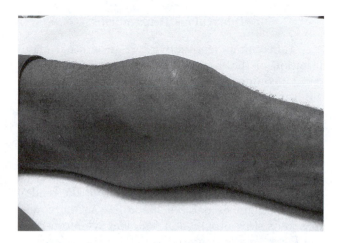

Figure 3. Swollen knee of a patient with tuberculous arthritis. An HIV-infected patient presented with a painful, swollen knee. He had a recent history of trauma to the knee. On examination the knee was warm and an effusion was present. Culture of the synovial fluid following arthrocentesis grew *M. tuberculosis.*

adults, tuberculous osteomyelitis without joint involvement usually presents as a single lesion, usually in the metaphysis of long bones (e.g., femur and humerus), although the ribs, pelvis, skull, mastoid and mandible can be affected. In children, older adults, and immunocompromised persons, including those with HIV infection, the lesions may be multiple (41). In children the lesions may affect the short bones of the hands and feet; tuberculous dactylitis has been reported to occur in adults but is unusual. Patients with widespread lesions may be misdiagnosed as having a malignant process. Bacterial superinfection can also mask the diagnosis and presentation, as there are a number of reports of infection due to coexisting *Staphylococcus aureus* and TB (8, 35).

Tuberculous osteomyelitis usually manifests with pain and swelling adjacent to the bone, with eventual limitation of movement of the affected limb. Symptoms may be present for 6 to 24 months before a diagnosis is made. Fever, weight loss, and night sweats are often present. Abscesses and sinus tracts may occur, often later in the course. Tuberculous involvement of the skull may be associated with headaches and soft tissue masses. TB involving the ribs manifests with chest pain and sometimes with a "cold" chest wall mass (Fig. 2). Infection of bones of the head and neck, especially mastoids and mandible, has been reported to result from tuberculous otitis and disease involving the oral cavity. Facial paralysis can occur secondarily to tuberculous mastoiditis (15). TB of the temporomandibular joint has also been reported as a cause of chronic temporomandibular joint pain (104). TB of the sternum can manifest as anterior chest pain (69).

Tuberculous Tenosynovitis

Tuberculous tenosynovitis is an unusual manifestation of the disease. When it occurs, it may occur in conjunction with another form of skeletal TB, such as TB of the carpal bones in the hand or, rarely, hematogenous spread to the synovium (52). Carpal tunnel syndrome is a common presentation of tuberculous synovitis (53, 94). Carpal tunnel syndrome occurs when the median nerve, going through the flexor compartment of the wrist, is compressed secondarily to thickening and edema of the tendon sheath. Diagnosis is often made late in the course due to its slow progression, indolent symptoms, and the fact that the diagnosis may be delayed because infectious causes are not considered initially (46). Presenting symptoms include swelling, followed by wrist pain, numbness and tingling of the fingers, and decreased range of motion (52). Other causes of carpal tunnel syndrome in the differential diagnosis include trauma, diabetes, amyloidosis, and sarcoidosis. Another presentation of tuberculous tenosynovitis is a ganglion formation along the volar carpal ligament that manifests with soft tissue swelling above the flexor retinaculum (20).

DIAGNOSIS

A high index of suspicion is needed for the diagnosis of musculoskeletal TB, especially given the insidious onset of symptoms and reports of a long duration between onset of symptoms and diagnosis of disease. In countries with a high burden of TB disease, musculoskeletal complaints may be attributed to TB correctly based on clinical and radiologic examination. In the developed world with a lower incidence of TB, the diagnosis may not be initially considered and the diagnosis is frequently delayed. Any bone or joint may be involved, but the spine and weight-bearing joints are the most common sites of infection. Pain is the most common complaint that leads a patient to seek medical care, and TB should be considered in the differential diagnosis of the cause of skeletal pain. Interestingly, local pain, swelling, and limitation of movement may even on occasion precede radiographic findings by up to 8 weeks (100). Cold abscesses can occur and sometimes with draining sinus tracts, but this is usually seen in advanced, untreated disease or among patients with HIV infection. The differential diagnosis of musculoskeletal TB includes other infectious causes of musculoskeletal disease (bacterial, fungal, and other mycobacterial pathogens), as well as malignancy, rheumatologic conditions, and sarcoidosis.

Imaging techniques, which include conventional radiography, computed tomography (CT), and magnetic resonance imaging (MRI), are useful in evaluation of patients with suspected musculoskeletal TB and other skeletal diseases. Use of newer techniques such as CT, MRI, and CT-guided fine-needle aspiration biopsy has revolutionized the diagnostic approach and has resulted in more accurate results and much less invasive procedures than when only plain radiography and open biopsy were available. Previously, conventional radiography had been the mainstay in the diagnosis of tuberculous arthritis and osteomyelitis. However, MRI is now accepted as the imaging modality of choice for diagnosis of tuberculous spondylitis and other types of musculosketal TB and can demonstrate the extent of the disease of tuberculous spondylitis and soft tissue TB (23, 25). MRI may be very helpful in providing diagnostic clues in the evaluation of spondylodiscitis, as it may easily demonstrate anterior corner destruction, the relative preservation of the intervertebral disk, multilevel involvement with or without skip lesions, and a large soft tissue abscess, as these are all arguments in favor of a tuberculous spondylitis (versus a pyogenic infection). Since there are no pathognomonic radiographic findings, the diagnosis is usually made by tissue biopsy and/or culture data (63). Needle aspiration and biopsy can confirm the diagnosis with the findings of caseating granuloma and the presence of acid-fast bacilli (AFB). A positive culture for *M. tuberculosis* provides definitive evidence of tuberculous disease and allows antimicrobial susceptibility testing to be performed, which is essential for helping to prescribe optimal therapy. Fine-needle aspiration biopsy of involved bone (often CT directed) to obtain specimens for culture is useful diagnostically as well as for the draining of abscesses in certain situations (42). In addition to modern culture techniques performed on specimens obtained by biopsy of involved tissues, the use of molecular diagnostics to detect the presence of *M. tuberculosis* has the potential to improve the ability to diagnose skeletal and other types of musculoskeletal TB. While nucleic acid amplification tests have demonstrated high sensitivity and specificity for AFB smear-positive respiratory specimens, there are few data on the utility of these tests for extrapulmonary TB (88). This is especially the case for the use of these molecular diagnostic tests for musculoskeletal TB. The currently commercially available and FDA-approved nucleic acid amplification tests are not approved for use in extrapulmonary TB, including musculoskeletal cases. Further data are needed on the utility of these tests in the aid of diagnosis of musculoskeletal TB.

Tuberculous Spondylitis

Plain radiography is often the first imaging technique employed by clinicians when considering tuberculous spondylitis. At least 50% of the vertebra needs to be destroyed before it can be detected on plain radiography, making this an insensitive diagnostic tool (Fig. 4) (27). Plain radiography may reveal several features indicative of tuberculous spondylitis, such as osteoporotic end plates, involvement of multiple levels, and anterior destruction leading to collapse (Table 3). Sometimes a paravertebral abscess or enlarged psoas muscle may be observed on plain radiography. Plain radiography will show calcifications in abscesses if they are present. Atypical features that may be seen on radiography include involvement of posterior elements, single vertebral involvement, and an "ivory" vertebra, which is the result of diffuse sclerosis (40).

Nuclear medicine imaging is not very useful in diagnosing tuberculous spondylitis because of its

Table 3. Radiographic characteristics of tuberculous spondylitis

Multiple levels involved
Lytic destruction of anterior portion of vertebral body
Disk space narrowing
Vertebral end plate osteoporosis
Increased anterior wedging
Collapse of vertebral bodies
Paravertebral shadow of an abscess sometimes with calcification
Enlarged psoas muscle shadow often with calcifications

low sensitivity and is not recommended as a diagnostic imaging modality in the evaluation of patients with spondylitis. CT scanning is superior to both plain radiography and nuclear medicine imaging. CT has also proved useful in determining the extent of soft tissue infection such as abscesses and draining sinus tracts, as well as soft tissue calcifications (Fig. 5). Irregular lytic lesions, sclerosis, and disk collapse all can be demonstrated on CT. CT is also very helpful in providing guidance for percutaneous drainage and biopsy of vertebra-associated lesions and abscesses (16).

As noted above, MRI is now accepted as the imaging modality of choice for the evaluation of patients with suspected tuberculous spondylitis and may be very useful in the evaluation of soft tissue TB (27). Contrast-enhanced MRI scanning is the optimal test for defining intraspinal extension, focal myelopathy, and spinal cord or nerve root compression (63). Paravertebral abscesses are often seen at multiple levels and show peripheral enhancement with central necrosis on contrast-enhanced images (83). MRI allows the entire spine to be viewed and provides high-contrast resolution. By comparing T1 and T2 weighted images, one can accurately differentiate

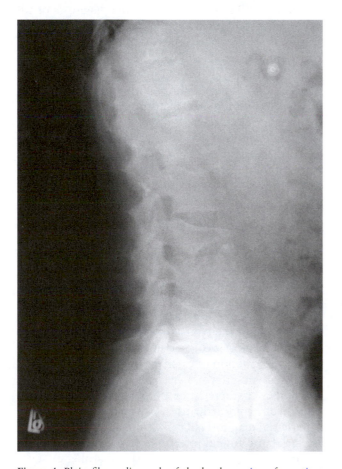

Figure 4. Plain film radiograph of the lumbar spine of a patient with tuberculous spondylitis demonstrating anterior end plate destruction, sclerosis, loss of disk space, and evidence of bony debris. These finding are suggestive of tuberculous spondylitis. A CT-directed biopsy was performed to obtain material for cultures, which yielded *M. tuberculosis*.

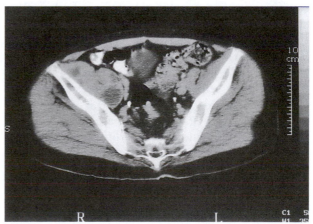

Figure 5. CT evaluation of patients with tuberculous spondylitis. CT demonstrates a large right psoas abscess in an HIV-infected patient with tuberculous spondylitis of the lumbar spine. A percutaneous drain was placed into the psoas abscess, and the fluid culture yielded *M. tuberculosis*.

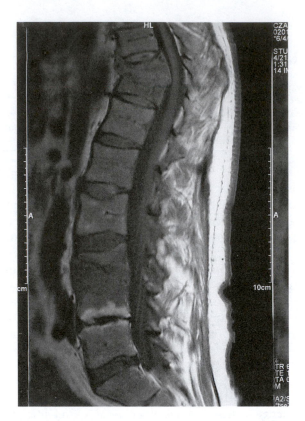

Figure 6. MRI of a patient with multifocal tuberculous spondylitis who has both thoracic and lumbar spine involvement which is not contiguous (i.e., skip lesions). The thoracic lesion reveals anterior collapse of adjacent vertebrae and a gibbus formation leading to kyphosis. There is also evidence of lumbar disease in this patient.

Table 4. Imaging features associated with tuberculous spondylitis[a]

Imaging features suggestive of tuberculous spondylitis versus other infectious etiologies
  More than one vertebra involved
  Multicentric involvement
  Relative sparing of the disk
  Large paravertebral abscess
  Paravertebral osseous debris
  Subligamentous spread
  Heterogenous signal intensity on MRI
  Rim enhancement pattern on MRI

Imaging features suggestive of tuberculous spondylitis versus neoplastic disease
  Paravertebral abscess
  Paravertebral osseous debris
  Subligamentous spread
  Predominant distribution adjacent to end plates or vertebral corners

[a]Table adapted from reference 40.

various diseased tissues, delineate clearly vertebral bodies, and detect marrow infiltration, intervertebral disks, intraspinal contents, posterior vertebral components, meningeal involvement, and paraspinal tissues (Fig. 6). The early inflammatory bone marrow changes that are able to be viewed with MRI also allow for an earlier radiologic diagnosis of tuberculous spondylitis (27). MRI best demonstrates the origin of the pathological tissue causing spinal cord compression (Fig. 6A) by differentiating pus and granulation tissue from the bony, disk, or fibrotic causes of compression, thus helping to avoid unnecessary and aggressive surgical decompression (45).

Newer imaging techniques are helpful in distinguishing tuberculous spondylitis from other infectious etiologies and from neoplastic processes (Table 4). Two distinct patterns of vertebral TB may be seen. The first is the classic finding of spondylodiscitis, characterized by destruction of two or more contiguous vertebrae and opposed end plates, disk infection, and commonly a paraspinal mass or collection. The second pattern, increasing in frequency, is an atypical form of spondylitis without disk involvement (24). The combination of clinical findings, characteristic lesions on plain radiography, CT, and MRI,

and sometimes either with a positive tuberculin skin test or gamma interferon release assay or evidence of pulmonary TB strongly suggests the diagnosis of tuberculous spondylitis. Diagnostic imaging modalities (e.g., CT) as described above can also be helpful by providing means for a directed biopsy to definitively make the diagnosis by obtaining material for pathological examination, culture, and susceptibility testing. It is essential to obtain appropriate specimens for mycobacterial cultures in order to establish a definitive diagnosis. In spinal TB, a CT-guided biopsy often yields the diagnosis. Open spinal biopsy is generally reserved for cases of difficult diagnosis or when surgical therapy is otherwise indicated (63, 103).

Tuberculous Arthritis

The classic triad of juxta-articular osteoporosis, peripheral osseous erosion, and gradual narrowing of the joint space are radiologic characteristics of tuberculous arthritis which were described by Phemister and Hatcher in 1933 (92). The joint space is preserved early in the course of tuberculous arthritis, as opposed to most pyogenic infections, in which there is early destruction of cartilage due to the production of proteolytic enzymes by bacterial pathogens. The radiologic characteristics of pyogenic, tuberculous, and rheumatoid arthritis are shown in Table 5. The differential diagnosis of tuberculous arthritis includes bacterial and fungal infections of the joint as well as noninfectious processes (e.g., rheumatologic). Pyogenic (bacterial) arthritis is usually a monoarticular process as is seen with tuberculous arthritis, but the time course is usually more acute in those with a pyogenic bacterial infection than the more chronic and initially indolent course seen among patients with

Table 5. Radiologic characteristics in the differential diagnosis of tuberculous arthritis

Condition	Radiologic result		
	Osteoporosis	Marginal erosions	Joint space narrowing
TB	+	+	Late, mild
Pyogenic	+/−	+	Early, significant
Rheumatoid arthritis	+	+	Early, significant
Gout	Mild, absent	+	0

tuberculous arthritis. Trauma or bacteremia is frequently associated with pyogenic arthritis. *Nocardia* spp., *Brucella* spp., and *Sporothrix schenckii* can also cause a chronic monoarthritis resembling TB. In addition to pyogenic and other inflammatory processes, pigmented villonodular synovitis, which can cause synovial thickening and joint erosions, needs to be included in the radiographic differential diagnosis of TB arthritis (40).

Radiologic studies may provide some clues to the diagnosis as discussed above (Table 5) but cannot definitively differentiate bacterial from tuberculous arthritis. Because the process begins with synovial thickening and an effusion, joint space swelling is the first radiographic sign. Bone sequestration and dense triangular collections may be found at the edge of the joint. Marginal erosions are especially prominent in the weight-bearing joints (Fig. 7). Sclerosis is usually not seen in tuberculous arthritis except in children, in whom a layered periosteal reaction can be seen (27, 47). Eventually severe joint destruction and fibrous ankylosis occur when the process is left untreated (Fig. 8 and 9).

Martini and Ouahes (66) summarized the radiologic changes of tuberculous arthritis in the following classification, which also reflects the pathogenesis of the infectious process:

- Stage I: no bony lesions, localized osteoporosis
- Stage II: one or more erosions or lytic lesions in the bone; discrete diminution of the joint space
- Stage III: involvement and destruction of the whole joint without gross anatomic disorganization
- Stage IV: gross anatomic disorganization

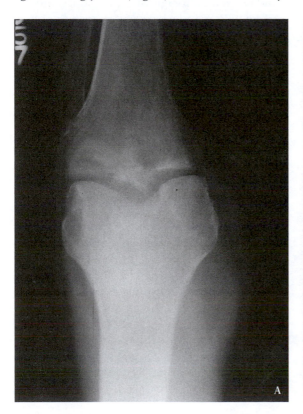
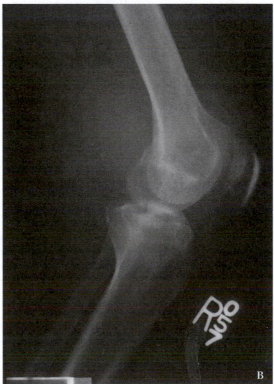

Figure 7. Radiographs of the knee of a patient with tuberculous arthritis. (A) Plain radiograph of the knee shown in Fig. 3. Marginal erosions are visible, along with soft tissue swelling.

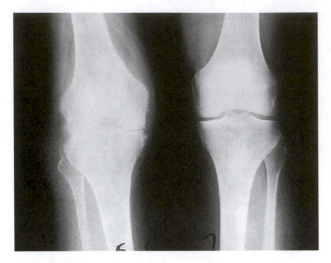

Figure 8. TB of the knee. The radiograph shows findings of TB (left) and the normal knee (right). Note the narrowed joint space, lytic bone destruction in the distal femur and proximal tibia, and soft tissue swelling in the abnormal knee, which had shown clinical evidence of TB for more than 10 years (but the patient had not undergone treatment).

CT imaging of the joint may be useful for evaluating bony destruction and soft tissue swelling or abscess and any evidence of bony sequestration (Fig. 10). MRI can detect earlier changes, especially synovial thickening and periarticular soft tissue changes, and has even been shown to demonstrate rice bodies in the joint space (82). An absence of marrow enhancement on MRI along with bony erosions is suggestive of tuberculous arthritis rather than a pyogenic process (47). MRI may reveal hemosiderin deposits in the synovium and demonstrate the erosions that occur with advanced disease and are often centrally located. As discussed below, a definitive diagnosis should be made. Pursuing arthrocentesis in

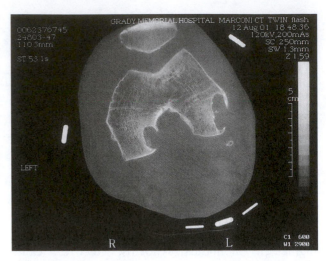

Figure 10. CT of the knee of a patient with tuberculous arthritis. CT imaging of the knee shows extensive marginal destruction as well as erosions.

order to obtain appropriate specimens (e.g., synovial fluid) or performing a synovial biopsy in order to obtain specimens for bacterial, fungal, and mycobacterial culture is crucial in establishing a definitive diagnosis and in order to recover the organism to make a microbiological diagnosis so that susceptibility testing can be performed. In articular TB, the synovial fluid is often nondiagnostic and biopsy and culture of the synovium and periarticular bone are often necessary to make the diagnosis (63).

Tuberculous Osteomyelitis

Radiographically, tuberculous osteomyelitis is often confused with malignancy, especially if the lesions are diffuse and lytic. Plain radiographs may

A

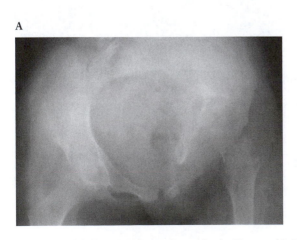

B

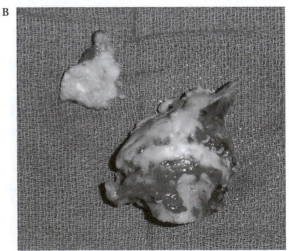

Figure 9. TB of the hip. (A) Plain radiograph of a 12-year-old girl who presented with an abnormal gait for several months. The left femoral head is completely destroyed. (B) Operative specimen of the destroyed femoral head.

Table 6. Differential diagnosis of cystic bone lesions

Cystic TB
Syphilis
Eosinophilic granuloma
Sarcoidosis
Cystic angiomatosis
Multiple myeloma
Neoplasm (metastatic, lymphoma, neuroblastoma)
Fungal infection (blastomycosis and coccidioidomycosis)

show osteoporosis, lytic lesions, sclerosis, and periostitis. Sequestra may appear as spicules of increased radiodensity within the area of destruction. Cystic lesions may be seen, especially in children and young adults. The differential diagnosis of cystic bone lesions is shown in Table 6. The lesions in children are less well defined than in adults, in whom well-defined margins of sclerosis are usually present (38). Multifocal disease is an uncommon presentation and occurs primarily in children and the immunocompromised (84, 99). MRI is useful in detecting osteomyelitis early because of changes in the bone marrow. The normal marrow fat signal on T1 weighted images is replaced by low signal intensity, with corresponding high signal intensities on T2 weighted images and enhancement of T1 weighted images after gadolinium (27). Tuberculous lesions are rarely seen in the hands and feet, but tuberculous dactylitis occurring in children is a well-recognized entity. The typical radiologic appearance is a ballooned-out configuration of "spina ventosa" in which the dissolution of bone causes absorption of trabeculae and expansion of the affected digit (84).

Tuberculous Myositis

Tuberculous myositis is usually discovered secondarily to a known skeletal focus. Primary myositis can occur, especially in the immunocompromised patient, whereas secondary tuberculous myositis, which is much more common, is usually seen in conjunction with vertebral TB. The differential diagnosis of primary myositis or pyomyositis is shown in Table 7. Plain radiography may show calcifications or, in the case of a psoas abscess, an enlarged psoas shadow.

Table 7. Differential diagnosis of primary myositis

TB
Actinomycosis
Sarcoidosis
Malignancy (sarcoma)
Bursa or tendon cyst
Hematoma
Pyogenic myositis
Melioidosis

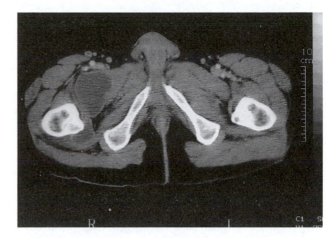

Figure 11. CT imaging of a psoas muscle abscess. The CT shows the lower extremities in a patient with lumbar tuberculous spondylitis who has a psoas abscess that extends into the right thigh.

CT imaging shows a well-marginated tumor-like lesion, either hypodense or isodense compared with normal muscle (Fig. 5 and 11). MRI shows a distinct mass that can be of either lower or higher density than the muscle depending on the T1 or T2 weighted image (1). CT and MRI cannot really differentiate tuberculous myositis from other causes of muscle lesions, but the diagnosis may be highly suspected in the proper clinical setting (e.g., TB at a contiguous or distant site (54). Ultimately, a definitive diagnosis needs to be based on histologic and microbiological studies. Psoas abscesses are often associated with vertebral TB, but other etiologies should be considered as well (Table 8). CT and MRI are both useful in detecting a psoas abscess. A calcified psoas muscle on plain film is pathognomonic of a tuberculous abscess secondary to vertebral disease (39).

Mycobacteriological and Histologic Diagnosis

Radiologic methods may suggest a diagnosis of TB, but bacteriological or histologic confirmation is required to prove the diagnosis. Every attempt should be made to establish a microbiologically confirmed diagnosis (i.e., recovery of *M. tuberculosis* from

Table 8. Etiologies of a psoas muscle abscess

Vertebral TB (Pott's disease)
Diverticulitis
Appendicitis
Crohn's disease
Postpartum infection
Neoplasm of spine or bowel
Renal calculi
Hematoma
Pyogenic infection (especially *Staphylococcus aureus*)
Actinomycosis

culture) so that an isolate is available for susceptibility testing. A presumptive diagnosis can be made by observing caseating granulomas with or without AFB on histologic examination of specimens. However, granulomas in musculoskeletal specimens do not always indicate infection with *M. tuberculosis*. Other diseases producing synovial granulomas include fungal diseases, infection with nontuberculous mycobacteria, sarcoidosis, traumatic fat necrosis, brucellosis, and foreign-body giant cell reactions. In developing countries where TB is highly endemic and resources, including imaging and diagnostic capabilities, are limited, the diagnosis of musculoskeletal TB is often based on the clinical and radiologic (i.e., plain film) findings.

Differentiating pyogenic, tuberculous, or inflammatory arthritis can be difficult radiographically, and ultimately a microbiological diagnosis needs to be made. For tuberculous arthritis, synovial fluid examination is the first procedure performed. As noted above, biopsy of the synovium may be required to establish a diagnosis of tuberculous arthritis. Synovial fluid in early stages of disease appears xanthochromic, and as the disease process advances the fluid becomes yellow-white and thick and gelatinous in nature because of the presence of degenerated cartilage and bony debris (102). An elevated protein over 2.5 g/dl is a uniform finding. The joint fluid glucose level is thought to be low compared to serum levels; the synovial fluid glucose is usually 40 mg/dl less than the blood glucose among patients with tuberculous arthritis. The synovial fluid white blood cell count can vary widely, with the average being in the range of 10,000 to 20,000/ml, but white blood cell counts up to 50,000 to 100,000/ml (in the range of what is often reported for bacterial or "septic" arthritis) have been reported. All of these findings can also be consistent with rheumatoid arthritis as well. For these reasons, a bacteriological and/or histologic diagnosis is imperative.

AFB staining of synovial fluid has a sensitivity that is low but is thought to be higher than that seen in examination of fluid from other serosal membranes (e.g., pleura, pericardium, and peritoneum). Synovial biopsy and culture had a higher yield, with 94% of specimens having a positive histology and yielding a positive culture for *M. tuberculosis*. Open biopsy and fine-needle aspiration biopsy also have a high likelihood of yielding a positive culture (>90%) but are generally not required. Mondal reported a series of 116 fine-needle aspiration biopsies in which TB was diagnosed in 38 patients; metastatic tumor was diagnosed in the remaining 78 patients. Thirty-four of the 38 patients with tuberculous arthritis had cultures positive for *M. tuberculosis* (89%), and 11 (39%)

were smear positive for AFB. The remaining four cases of tuberculous arthritis were confirmed histologically, and the patients demonstrated improvement with antituberculous treatment (81). Masood performed fine-needle aspiration biopsy for diagnosis of bone and soft tissue lesions in 11 patients, and 64% were smear positive for AFB and 84% were culture positive; the author concluded that fine-needle biopsy is as good as open biopsy and less invasive (67). As noted, additional data are needed on the utility of molecular diagnostic techniques (e.g., nucleic acid amplification tests) for the diagnosis of tuberculous arthritis.

Debeaumont showed that the total bacterial population of an infected spine may comprise less than 1 million organisms, whereas an expectorated sputum specimen may produce up to 300,000 bacilli in 1 ml (26). The lower burden of organisms may help explain why it is sometimes difficult to recover tubercle bacilli in paraspinal or psoas abscesses and draining sinus tracts. The yield from culturing material from a sinus tract can be increased if the specimen is collected with a syringe rather than a swab (85). The low bacillary burden also implies that there is a lower chance of developing drug-resistant TB in skeletal disease than in pulmonary TB.

TREATMENT

Early diagnosis and initiation of appropriate antituberculous therapy are important, as early treatment can prevent loss of function and mobility. There is now abundant evidence to show that musculoskeletal TB, detected early, can be cured by chemotherapy without the previously expected, inevitable sequelae of deformity in the spine or ankylosis in the limb joints. Even if minor radiologic changes have occurred, full restoration of function without deformity can be confidently expected if the diagnosis is made early enough. Simple survival of the patient in a moderately disabled condition is no longer acceptable. Early diagnosis may indeed be the greatest contribution that surgery has to make to the modern management of musculoskeletal TB.

The basic principles that underlie the treatment of pulmonary TB also apply to extrapulmonary forms of the disease (10). Regimens that are effective for the treatment of drug-susceptible pulmonary TB are appropriate for the treatment of susceptible musculoskeletal TB. Several studies have examined the treatment of bone and joint TB and have shown that 6- to 9-month (short-course) regimens containing rifampin are at least as effective as 18-month regimens that do not contain rifampin (76, 77, 79).

Because of the difficulties in assessing response, however, some experts tend to favor the 9-month duration (10). Concomitant use of corticosteroids in the treatment of persons with bone and joint disease is not recommended (10). There are few reports of multidrug-resistant skeletal TB, but the same treatment principles should apply.

Tuberculous Spondylitis

Historical perspective

Before the availability of effective antituberculous chemotherapy, Pott's disease was treated with immobilization using prolonged bed rest or a body cast. In Dobson's series of 914 patients, all received prolonged immobilization, with either a brace or a body plaster cast, and 54 underwent a spinal fusion (28). The mortality rate was 20%, and 22% were readmitted for relapses. Antituberculous chemotherapy was gradually introduced into the treatment of osteoarticular TB after the studies of Cannetti and Debeaumont demonstrated the effect of chemotherapy in osteoarticular disease (13a, 26). Hodgson et al. described the first series combining a surgical approach using an anterior approach for decompression and autologous bone grafting for fusion with chemotherapy and reported a high success rate (43). Konstam and Blesovsky were the first to report an ambulatory, medical approach for tuberculous spondylitis (56). They reported treatment of 207 patients with isoniazid and p-aminosalicylic acid (PAS) for at least 12 months (until there was radiographic improvement) and did not include bracing or immobilization as part of the therapy. Surgery was performed only in 27 patients who needed abscesses drained. Eighty-six percent of patients exhibited complete recovery. For the first time it was demonstrated that patients with vertebral TB could be cured with chemotherapy alone and without prolonged immobilization or a complicated surgical procedure.

It was this divergence of opinion and practice that led the British Medical Research Council to set up a series of randomized controlled clinical trials in different centers (70–75, 78, 80). Patients included in these research studies had evidence of active TB of the thoracic or lumbar spine. These studies were carried out in Korea, Zimbabwe (then called Rhodesia), South Africa, and Hong Kong. All patients received chemotherapy (in most studies this consisted of 18 months of isoniazid and PAS supplemented with streptomycin during the first 3 months for some patients). The methods of treatment were determined by the therapy available at that time plus locally available resources and included outpatient

antituberculous therapy; chemotherapy with immobilization by bed rest or body casts; chemotherapy and conservative debridement of infected bone without fusion; and, in Hong Kong and South Africa, chemotherapy with "radical surgery." The radical surgical therapy consisted of anterior resection, debridement of granulation tissue and nonviable bone, and autologous bone strut grafting (70, 77). Nonoperative treatment produced a favorable status in 67% of subjects at 18 months, 85% at 3 years, and 88% at 5 years. The continued improvement that became apparent with the passage of time, from 67% to 85 to 90% at 5 to 10 years, is a valid warning against panic if all does not seem well at the end of the initial period of chemotherapy. No statistically significant difference could be shown at any stage between the results in patients who underwent 6 months of inpatient care, 9 months in plaster jackets, or neither. In addition, no statistically significant advantage could be shown from the addition of streptomycin to PAS and isoniazid. It was therefore concluded that in this series of cases, from the point of view of the preservation of life and health, ambulant outpatient chemotherapy gave excellent results, as judged over a period of 5 years, in patients whose drug taking had been supervised as strictly as possible under the prevailing conditions. Debridement by open operation with or without anterior spinal fusion, in addition to chemotherapy, gave no better ultimate results than did ambulant outpatient treatment. Favorable outcome in these studies was defined as "full physical activity with clinically and radiographically quiescent disease, with no sinuses, abscesses or myelopathy with functional impairment, all without modification of the allocated regimen" (72).

Radical surgery, as performed in Hong Kong, gave similar results in the long term so far as preservation of life and health is concerned. The Hong Kong operation consisted of anterior resection, debridement of infected bone, and autologous bone grafting. At the end of the period of chemotherapy (18 months), 89% of patients had already reached a favorable status; at 3 years, 87% of patients had a favorable status; and at 5 years, 89% were considered to have a favorable status. The Hong Kong operation in conjunction with non-rifampin-based regimens (in the era before the availability of rifampin), however, produced certain distinct advantages: (i) abscesses, including mediastinal abscesses, resolved more rapidly than after conservative treatment and even after debridement; (ii) bony fusion occurred much earlier; and (iii) most importantly, kyphosis did not worsen (70). The "Hong Kong" radical procedure was also performed in South Africa, but unlike in the reports from Hong Kong, did not show advantages over debridement alone. On the basis of the results of these trials, in the era before the availability of rifampin, spinal TB was best treated by a combination of appropriate chemotherapy and the Hong Kong radical operation if, and only if, adequate surgical expertise, anesthesia, and nursing facilities were available. If not, surgery was to be avoided.

Modern therapy for tuberculous spondylitis

Stimulated by the efficacy of short-course chemotherapy for pulmonary TB with isoniazid and rifampin, the British Medical Research Council Working Party started a second series of trials in Hong Kong, Korea, and South India (76, 77, 79). In Hong Kong, all patients underwent the radical operation with either 6 or 9 months of chemotherapy with isoniazid and rifampin supplemented by streptomycin for 6 months. In Korea, only ambulatory chemotherapy with a regimen of 6 or 9 months of isoniazid plus rifampin was compared with a regimen of 9 or 18 months of isoniazid plus PAS or ethambutol. In Madras (now Chennai), South India, ambulatory chemotherapy with a regimen of 6 or 9 months of isoniazid and rifampin was compared with a regimen of 6 or 9 months of isoniazid plus rifampin and the Hong Kong radical operation. After 3 years, all studies showed that >95% had favorable results for regimens containing isoniazid and rifampin (76, 77, 79). These results confirmed the efficacy of a short course of rifampin-based regimens, 6 or 9 months, for spinal TB. The resolution of sinuses and abscesses present on admission was more rapid in patients treated with isoniazid plus rifampin than in patients treated with isoniazid plus PAS or ethambutol. There was no recurrence in patients prescribed rifampin-containing regimens. The resolution of myelopathy was very good in ambulatory regimens, with 83 to 88% of patients making a full recovery. There was no clear evidence that 9 months of treatment with isoniazid plus rifampin had any advantages over 6 months of treatment. Primary resistance to isoniazid and streptomycin was a problem, particularly in the Hong Kong studies.

Thus, on the basis of the results of these more recent randomized trials carried out by the Medical Research Council Working Party on Tuberculosis of the Spine, tuberculous spondylitis of the thoracolumbar spine due to drug-susceptible organisms is best treated by a rifampin-based regimen including isoniazid and rifampin for a period of 6 to 9 months, supplemented by pyrazinamide for 2 months (and ethambutol pending susceptibility results), similar to those regimens used in the treatment of pulmonary TB (see chapter 7). Among patients taking rifampin-based short-course regimens, there was no demonstrated additional benefit of surgical debridement or radical operation (resection of the spinal focus and bone grafting) in combination with chemotherapy compared with chemotherapy alone (79). In addition, myelopathy with or without functional impairment most often responds to chemotherapy. In two studies conducted in Korea, 24 of 30 patients in one study (76) and 74 of 85 patients in an earlier study (90) had complete resolution of myelopathy or complete functional recovery when treated medically. In some circumstances, however, surgery appears to be beneficial and may be indicated. Such situations include failure to respond to chemotherapy with evidence of ongoing infection, the relief of cord compression in patients with persistence or recurrence of neurologic deficits, or instability of the spine (10).

Despite the large number of patients enrolled in the Medical Research Council trials, patients with obvious myelopathy were excluded, so there are no controlled trials evaluating the role of surgery when paresis is present. Paresis is now generally considered a surgical indication (10). Other accepted indications for surgery include failure to respond to chemotherapy with evidence of ongoing infection, the relief of cord compression in patients with neurologic deficits, paraspinal abscesses and psoas abscesses requiring drainage, or the instability of the spine. Late neurologic compromise resulting from kyphosis after the disease is no longer active is also an indication for surgical decompression.

Patients with tuberculous spondylitis of the cervical spine were not included in the Medical Research Council studies, in part because of the low incidence of cervical disease. In two case series which reported on a total of 46 patients with upper and lower cervical TB, all patients received antituberculous chemotherapy and surgery (33, 48). Medical therapy consisted of isoniazid plus rifampin for 12 to 15 months or isoniazid plus PAS for 15 to 21 months. Of the six patients with upper cervical disease, four recovered without sequelae. There were 40 patients with lower cervical disease; all experienced a meaningful clinical and radiologic recovery. Twelve patients with cord compression experienced full neurologic recovery. Treatment recommendations for cervical TB are based on case series (33, 48, 51). Surgical intervention of the cervical spine is often indicated because of the likely association of neurologic deficits, frequent abscesses that can cause respiratory compromise, and the relative instability of the cervical spine, although in some cases, such as those reported by Jain et al. (51), there can be recovery without surgical intervention, as was reported for about two-thirds of the patients in their series. An anterior approach is considered the treatment of choice. A laminectomy should be avoided because it is not as effective in relieving cord compression and can lead to instability of the cervical spine.

Tuberculous Arthritis and Osteomyelitis

There are no controlled trials assessing treatment of musculoskeletal TB, with the exception of tuberculous spondylitis, which is discussed above. Based on experience from treating tuberculous spondylitis and the experience with treating other forms of extrapulmonary disease, it is recommended that treatment of drug-susceptible tuberculous arthritis and osteomyelitis be carried out using rifampin-based short-course regimens similar to those that are used for the treatment of pulmonary disease. Surgery is generally reserved for diagnosis and when necessary to drain an abscess that is not responding to medical therapy or to drain a large abscess to relieve pressure (3). Late treatment or inadequate treatment results in ankylosis of the affected joint by fibrosis or bony fusion. The function of the affected joint is compensated by other joints which in the long term are overused and may become painful because of degenerative arthritis. Recent technical developments have stimulated interest in indications for arthroplasty in joints with old, healed TB (31, 60, 97). Su et al. reported 16 cases of patients with a history of TB of the knee who underwent total knee replacement; eight patients had a preoperative diagnosis of TB and had received at least 2 months of antituberculous medications, and eight were diagnosed at the time of the operation. Five patients, four of whom did not receive antituberculous chemotherapy at the time of the operation, suffered a recurrence of disease after arthroplasty (97). There are no formal recommendations, but some experts have suggested that patients requiring total arthroplasty for quiescent TB receive perioperative chemotherapy for at least 3 weeks before and at least 6 to 9 months after surgery to minimize the risk of reactivation (57).

CONCLUSION

The diagnosis of musculoskeletal TB is often delayed because of failure to consider the diagnosis. Early diagnosis of bone and joint disease is important in order to minimize the risk of deformity and enhance outcome. The introduction of new imaging modalities, including CT and MRI, has enhanced the diagnostic evaluation of patients with musculoskeletal TB and for directed biopsies of affected areas of the musculoskeletal system. Obtaining appropriate specimens for culture is essential in an effort to establish a definitive diagnosis and recover *M. tuberculosis* for susceptibility testing. A total of 6 to 9 months of a rifampin-based regimen, similar to those used for the treatment of pulmonary TB, is recommended for the treatment of musculoskeletal disease. Randomized trials of tuberculous spondylitis have demonstrated that such regimens are efficacious. These data and those from the treatment of pulmonary TB have been extrapolated to form the basis of treatment regimen recommendations for other forms of musculoskeletal TB. Finally, ensuring adherence to chemotherapy is essential for good outcomes; therefore, directly observed therapy is recommended for the treatment of all persons with musculoskeletal TB.

REFERENCES

1. **Abdelwahab, I. F., S. Bianchi, C. Martinoli, M. Klein, and G. Hermann.** 2006. Atypical extraspinal musculoskeletal tuberculosis in immunocompetent patients: part II, tuberculous myositis, tuberculous bursitis, and tuberculous tenosynovites. *Can. Assoc. Radiol. J.* 57:278–286.

2. **Agarwal, R. P., N. Mohan, R. K. Garg, S. K. Bajpai, S. K. Verma, and Y. Mohindra.** 1990. Clinicosocial aspect of osteoarticular tuberculosis. *J. Indian Med. Assoc.* 88:307–309.

3. **Aguirre, M., J. Bago, and N. Martin.** 1989. Tuberculosis of the knee. Surgical or conservative treatment? *Acta Orthop. Belg.* 55:22–25.

4. **Ahmed, J., and J. Homans.** 2002. Tuberculosis pyomyositis of the soleus muscle in a fifteen-year-old boy. *Pediatr. Infect. Dis. J.* 21:1169–1171.

5. **Al-Matar, M. J., D. A. Cabral, and R. E. Petty.** 2001. Isolated tuberculous monoarthritis mimicking oligoarticular juvenile rheumatoid arthritis. *J. Rheumatol.* 28:204–206.

6. **Al Soub, H.** 1996. Retropharyngeal abscess associated with tuberculosis of the cervical spine. *Tuber. Lung Dis.* 77:563–565.

7. **Asnis, D. S., and A. Niegowska.** 1997. Tuberculosis of the rib. *Clin. Infect. Dis.* 24:1018–1019.

8. **Babhulkar, S. S., and S. K. Pande.** 2002. Unusual manifestations of osteoarticular tuberculosis. *Clin. Orthop. Relat. Res.* May:114–120.

9. **Belzunegui, J., I. Plazaola, E. Uriarte, and J. M. Pego.** 1995. Primary tuberculous muscle abscess in a patient with systemic lupus erythematosus. *Br. J. Rheumatol.* 34:1177–1178.

10. **Blumberg, H. M., W. J. Burman, R. E. Chaisson, C. L. Daley, S. C. Etkind, L. N. Friedman, P. Fujiwara, M. Grzemska, P. C. Hopewell, M. D. Iseman, R. M. Jasmer, V. Koppaka, R. I. Menzies, R. J. O'Brien, R. R. Reves, L. B. Reichman, P. M. Simone, J. R. Starke, and A. A. Vernon.** 2003. American Thoracic Society/Centers for Disease Control and Prevention/Infectious Diseases Society of America: treatment of tuberculosis. *Am. J. Respir. Crit. Care Med.* 167:603–662.

11. **Boachie-Adjei, O., and R. G. Squillante.** 1996. Tuberculosis of the spine. *Orthop. Clin. N. Am.* 27:95–103.

12. **Burke, H. E.** 1950. The pathogenesis of certain forms of extrapulmonary tuberculosis; spontaneous cold abscesses of the chest wall and Pott's disease. *Am. Rev. Tuberc.* 62:48–67.

13. **Calderone, R. R., and J. M. Larsen.** 1996. Overview and classification of spinal infections. *Orthop. Clin. N. Am.* 27:1–8.

13a. **Cannetti, G., J. Debeyre, and S. D. Seze.** 1957. Sterilization of lesions in osteo-articular tuberculosis by antibacillary chemotherapy. *Rev. Tuberc.* 21:1337–1344. (In French.)

14. **Centers for Disease Control and Prevention.** 2010. Decrease in reported tuberculosis cases—United States, 2009. *MMWR Morb. Mortal. Wkly. Rep.* 59:289–294.

15. **Chernoff, W. G., and L. S. Parnes.** 1992. Tuberculous mastoiditis. *J. Otolaryngol.* 21:290–292.

16. **Clementsen, P., M. Hansen, C. Conrad, and O. Myhre.** 1988. Percutaneous drainage of tuberculous abscess of the psoas muscle. *Tubercle* 69:63–65.

17. Colmenero, J. D., M. E. Jimenez-Mejias, J. M. Reguera, J. Palomino-Nicas, J. D. Ruiz-Mesa, J. Marquez-Rivas, A. Lozano, and J. Pachon. 2004. Tuberculous vertebral osteomyelitis in the new millennium: still a diagnostic and therapeutic challenge. *Eur. J. Clin. Microbiol. Infect. Dis.* **23:**477–483.

18. Colmenero, J. D., M. E. Jimenez-Mejias, F. J. Sanchez-Lora, J. M. Reguera, J. Palomino-Nicas, F. Martos, J. Garcia de las Heras, and J. Pachon. 1997. Pyogenic, tuberculous, and brucellar vertebral osteomyelitis: a descriptive and comparative study of 219 cases. *Ann. Rheum. Dis.* **56:**709–715.

19. Compere, E. L., and M. Garrison. 1936. Correlation of pathologic and roentgenologic findings in tuberculosis and pyogenic infections of the vertebrae: the fate of the intervertebral disk. *Ann. Surg.* **104:**1038–1067.

20. Cramer, K., J. G. Seiler III, and M. A. Milek. 1991. Tuberculous tenosynovitis of the wrist. Two case reports. *Clin. Orthop. Relat. Res.* **January:**137–140.

21. Crubezy, E., B. Ludes, J. D. Poveda, J. Clayton, B. Crouau-Roy, and D. Montagnon. 1998. Identification of *Mycobacterium* DNA in an Egyptian Pott's disease of 5,400 years old. *C. R. Acad. Sci. III* **321:**941–951.

22. Davidson, P. T., and I. Horowitz. 1970. Skeletal tuberculosis. A review with patient presentations and discussion. *Am. J. Med.* **48:**77–84.

23. De Backer, A. I., K. J. Mortele, F. M. Vanhoenacker, and P. M. Parizel. 2006. Imaging of extraspinal musculoskeletal tuberculosis. *Eur. J. Radiol.* **57:**119–130.

24. De Backer, A. I., K. J. Mortele, I. J. Vanschoubroeck, D. Deeren, F. M. Vanhoenacker, B. L. De Keulenaer, P. Bomans, and M. M. Kockx. 2005. Tuberculosis of the spine: CT and MR imaging features. *JBR-BTR* **88:**92–97.

25. De Backer, A. I., F. M. Vanhoenacker, and D. A. Sanghvi. 2009. Imaging features of extraaxial musculoskeletal tuberculosis. *Indian J. Radiol. Imaging* **19:**176–186.

26. Debeaumont, A. 1966. Bacteriology of osteoarticular tuberculosis under chemotherapy. *Bibl. Tuberc.* **22:**125–188. (In French.)

27. De Vuyst, D., F. Vanhoenacker, J. Gielen, A. Bernaerts, and A. M. De Schepper. 2003. Imaging features of musculoskeletal tuberculosis. *Eur. Radiol.* **13:**1809–1819.

28. Dobson, J. 1951. Tuberculosis of the spine; an analysis of the results of conservative treatment and of the factors influencing the prognosis. *J. Bone Joint Surg. Br.* **33-B:**517–531.

29. Donoghue, H. D., M. Spigelman, C. L. Greenblatt, G. Lev-Maor, G. K. Bar-Gal, C. Matheson, K. Vernon, A. G. Nerlich, and A. R. Zink. 2004. Tuberculosis: from prehistory to Robert Koch, as revealed by ancient DNA. *Lancet Infect. Dis.* **4:**584–592.

30. Reference deleted.

31. Eskola, A., S. Santavirta, Y. T. Konttinen, K. Tallroth, and S. T. Lindholm. 1988. Arthroplasty for old tuberculosis of the knee. *J. Bone Joint Surg. Br.* **70:**767–769.

32. Evanchick, C. C., D. E. Davis, and T. M. Harrington. 1986. Tuberculosis of peripheral joints: an often missed diagnosis. *J. Rheumatol.* **13:**187–189.

33. Fang, D., J. C. Leong, and H. S. Fang. 1983. Tuberculosis of the upper cervical spine. *J. Bone Joint Surg. Br.* **65:**47–50.

34. Fang, H. S., G. B. Ong, and A. R. Hodgson. 1964. Anterior spinal fusion: the operative approaches. *Clin. Orthop. Relat. Res.* **35:**16–33.

35. Franco-Paredes, C., and H. M. Blumberg. 2001. Psoas muscle abscess caused by *Mycobacterium tuberculosis* and *Staphylococcus aureus*: case report and review. *Am. J. Med. Sci.* **321:**415–417.

36. Franco-Paredes, C., A. Diaz-Borjon, M. A. Senger, L. Barragan, and M. Leonard. 2006. The ever-expanding association between rheumatologic diseases and tuberculosis. *Am. J. Med.* **119:**470–477.

37. Garcia, S., A. Combalia, A. Serra, J. M. Segur, and R. Ramon. 1997. Unusual locations of osteoarticular tuberculosis. *Arch. Orthop. Trauma Surg.* **116:**321–323.

38. Gonzalez Herranz, J., D. M. Farrington, J. Angulo Gutierrez, and P. Rodriguez Ferrol. 1997. Peripheral osteoarticular tuberculosis in children: tumor-like bone lesions. *J. Pediatr. Orthop. B* **6:**274–282.

39. Graves, V. B., and M. H. Schreiber. 1973. Tuberculous psoas muscle abscess. *J. Can. Assoc. Radiol.* **24:**268–271.

40. Griffith, J. F., S. M. Kumta, P. C. Leung, J. C. Cheng, L. T. Chow, and C. Metreweli. 2002. Imaging of musculoskeletal tuberculosis: a new look at an old disease. *Clin. Orthop. Relat. Res.* **May:**32–39.

41. Gros, T., V. Soriano, E. Gabarre, J. Tor, and M. Sabria. 1992. Multifocal tubercular osteitis in a female patient infected with the human immunodeficiency virus. *Rev. Clin. Esp.* **191:**35–37. (In Spanish.)

42. Handa, U., S. Garg, H. Mohan, and S. K. Garg. 2010. Role of fine-needle aspiration cytology in tuberculosis of bone. *Diagn. Cytopathol.* **38:**1–4.

43. Hodgson, A. R., F. E. Stock, H. S. Fang, and G. B. Ong. 1960. Anterior spinal fusion. The operative approach and pathological findings in 412 patients with Pott's disease of the spine. *Br. J. Surg.* **48:**172–178.

44. Hodgson, S. P., and L. P. Ormerod. 1990. Ten-year experience of bone and joint tuberculosis in Blackburn 1978–1987. *J. R. Coll. Surg. Edinb.* **35:**259–262.

45. Hoffman, E. B., J. H. Crosier, and B. J. Cremin. 1993. Imaging in children with spinal tuberculosis. A comparison of radiography, computed tomography and magnetic resonance imaging. *J. Bone Joint Surg. Br.* **75:**233–239.

46. Hoffman, K. L., A. G. Bergman, D. K. Hoffman, and D. P. Harris. 1996. Tuberculous tenosynovitis of the flexor tendons of the wrist: MR imaging with pathologic correlation. *Skeletal Radiol.* **25:**186–188.

47. Hong, S. H., S. M. Kim, J. M. Ahn, H. W. Chung, M. J. Shin, and H. S. Kang. 2001. Tuberculous versus pyogenic arthritis: MR imaging evaluation. *Radiology* **218:**848–853.

48. Hsu, L. C., and J. C. Leong. 1984. Tuberculosis of the lower cervical spine (C2 to C7). A report on 40 cases. *J. Bone Joint Surg. Br.* **66:**1–5.

49. Huang, D. Y. 1990. Tuberculous muscle abscess: an unusual presentation of tuberculosis. *Am. J. Med.* **88:**57N–59N.

50. Isaacs, A. J., and R. D. Sturrock. 1974. Poncet's disease—fact or fiction? A re-appraisal of tuberculous rheumatism. *Tubercle* **55:**135–142.

51. Jain, A. K., S. Kumar, and S. M. Tuli. 1999. Tuberculosis of spine (C1 to D4). *Spinal Cord* **37:**362–369.

52. Jaovisidha, S., C. Chen, K. N. Ryu, P. Siriwongpairat, P. Pekanan, D. J. Sartoris, and D. Resnick. 1996. Tuberculous tenosynovitis and bursitis: imaging findings in 21 cases. *Radiology* **201:**507–513.

53. Klofkorn, R. W., and J. C. Steigerwald. 1976. Carpal tunnel syndrome as the initial manifestation of tuberculosis. *Am. J. Med.* **60:**583–586.

54. Kobayashi, H., Y. Kotoura, M. Hosono, T. Tsuboyama, H. Sakahara, and J. Konishi. 1995. Solitary muscular involvement by tuberculosis: CT, MRI, and scintigraphic features. *Comput. Med. Imaging Graph.* **19:**237–240.

55. Konomi, N., E. Lebwohl, K. Mowbray, I. Tattersall, and D. Zhang. 2002. Detection of mycobacterial DNA in Andean mummies. *J. Clin. Microbiol.* **40:**4738–4740.

56. Konstam, P. G., and A. Blesovsky. 1962. The ambulant treatment of spinal tuberculosis. *Br. J. Surg.* **50:**26–38.

57. **Kramer, S. B., S. H. S. Lee, and S. B. Abramson.** 2004. Nonvertebral infections of the musculoskeletal system by *Mycobacterium tuberculosis*, p. 577–586. *In* W. N. Rom and S. M. Garay (ed.), *Tuberculosis*, 2nd ed. Lippincott Williams & Wilkins, Philadelphia, PA.

58. **Kroot, E. J., J. M. Hazes, E. M. Colin, and R. J. Dolhain.** 2007. Poncet's disease: reactive arthritis accompanying tuberculosis. Two case reports and a review of the literature. *Rheumatology* (Oxford) **46:**484–489.

59. **Lafond, E. M.** 1958. An analysis of adult skeletal tuberculosis. *J. Bone Joint Surg. Am.* **40-A:**346–364.

60. **Laforgia, R., J. C. Murphy, and T. R. Redfern.** 1988. Low friction arthroplasty for old quiescent infection of the hip. *J. Bone Joint Surg. Br.* **70:**373–376.

61. **Leibert, E., N. W. Schluger, S. Bonk, and W. N. Rom.** 1996. Spinal tuberculosis in patients with human immunodeficiency virus infection: clinical presentation, therapy and outcome. *Tuber. Lung Dis.* **77:**329–334.

62. **LeRoux, P. D., G. E. Griffin, H. T. Marsh, and H. R. Winn.** 1990. Tuberculosis of the skull—a rare condition: case report and review of the literature. *Neurosurgery* **26:**851–855; discussion, 855–856.

63. **Ludwig, B., and A. A. Lazarus.** 2007. Musculoskeletal tuberculosis. *Dis. Mon.* **53:**39–45.

64. **Lukhele, M.** 1996. Tuberculosis of the cervical spine. *S. Afr. Med. J.* **86:**553–556.

65. **Lupatkin, H., N. Brau, P. Flomenberg, and M. S. Simberkoff.** 1992. Tuberculous abscesses in patients with AIDS. *Clin. Infect. Dis.* **14:**1040–1044.

66. **Martini, M., and M. Ouahes.** 1988. Bone and joint tuberculosis: a review of 652 cases. *Orthopedics* **11:**861–866.

67. **Masood, S.** 1992. Diagnosis of tuberculosis of bone and soft tissue by fine-needle aspiration biopsy. *Diagn. Cytopathol.* **8:**451–455.

68. **McLain, R. F., and C. Isada.** 2004. Spinal tuberculosis deserves a place on the radar screen. *Cleve. Clin. J. Med.* **71:**537–539, 543–549.

69. **McLellan, D. G., K. B. Philips, C. E. Corbett, and M. S. Bronze.** 2000. Sternal osteomyelitis caused by *Mycobacterium tuberculosis*: case report and review of the literature. *Am. J. Med. Sci.* **319:**250–254.

70. **Medical Research Council Working Party on Tuberculosis of the Spine.** 1982. A 10-year assessment of a controlled trial comparing debridement and anterior spinal fusion in the management of tuberculosis of the spine in patients on standard chemotherapy in Hong Kong. Eighth report of the Medical Research Council Working Party on Tuberculosis of the Spine. *J. Bone Joint Surg. Br.* **64:**393–398.

71. **Medical Research Council Working Party on Tuberculosis of the Spine.** 1985. A 10-year assessment of controlled trials of inpatient and outpatient treatment and of plaster-of-Paris jackets for tuberculosis of the spine in children on standard chemotherapy. Studies in Masan and Pusan, Korea. Ninth report of the Medical Research Council Working Party on Tuberculosis of the Spine. *J. Bone Joint Surg. Br.* **67:**103–110.

72. **Medical Research Council Working Party on Tuberculosis of the Spine.** 1973. A controlled trial of ambulant out-patient treatment and in-patient rest in bed in the management of tuberculosis of the spine in young Korean patients on standard chemotherapy: a study in Masan, Korea. First report of the Medical Research Council Working Party on Tuberculosis of the Spine. *J. Bone Joint Surg. Br.* **55:**678–697.

73. **Medical Research Council Working Party on Tuberculosis of the Spine.** 1974. A controlled trial of anterior spinal fusion and debridement in the surgical management of tuberculosis of the spine in patients on standard chemotherapy: a study in Hong Kong. Fourth report of the Medical Research Council Working Party on Tuberculosis of the Spine. *Br. J. Surg.* **61:**853–866.

74. **Medical Research Council Working Party on Tuberculosis of the Spine.** 1978. A controlled trial of anterior spinal fusion and debridement in the surgical management of tuberculosis of the spine in patients on standard chemotherapy: a study in two centres in South Africa. Seventh report of the Medical Research Council Working Party on Tuberculosis of the Spine. *Tubercle* **59:**79–105.

75. **Medical Research Council Working Party on Tuberculosis of the Spine.** 1973. A controlled trial of plaster-of-Paris jackets in the management of ambulant outpatient treatment of tuberculosis of the spine in children on standard chemotherapy. A study in Pusan, Korea. Second report of the Medical Research Council Working Party on Tuberculosis of the Spine. *Tubercle* **54:**261–282.

76. **Medical Research Council Working Party on Tuberculosis of the Spine.** 1993. Controlled trial of short-course regimens of chemotherapy in the ambulatory treatment of spinal tuberculosis. Results at three years of a study in Korea. Twelfth report of the Medical Research Council Working Party on Tuberculosis of the Spine. *J. Bone Joint Surg. Br.* **75:**240–248.

77. **Medical Research Council Working Party on Tuberculosis of the Spine.** 1986. A controlled trial of six-month and nine-month regimens of chemotherapy in patients undergoing radical surgery for tuberculosis of the spine in Hong Kong. Tenth report of the Medical Research Council Working Party on Tuberculosis of the Spine. *Tubercle* **67:**243–259.

78. **Medical Research Council Working Party on Tuberculosis of the Spine.** 1976. A five-year assessment of controlled trials of in-patient and out-patient treatment and of plaster-of-Paris jackets for tuberculosis of the spine in children on standard chemotherapy. Studies in Masan and Pusan, Korea. Fifth report of the Medical Research Council Working Party on tuberculosis of the spine. *J. Bone Joint Surg. Br.* **58-B:**399–411.

79. **Medical Research Council Working Party on Tuberculosis of the Spine.** 1999. Five-year assessment of controlled trials of short-course chemotherapy regimens of 6, 9 or 18 months' duration for spinal tuberculosis in patients ambulatory from the start or undergoing radical surgery. Fourteenth report of the Medical Research Council Working Party on Tuberculosis of the Spine. *Int. Orthop.* **23:**73–81.

80. **Medical Research Council Working Party on Tuberculosis of the Spine.** 1978. Five-year assessments of controlled trials of ambulatory treatment, debridement and anterior spinal fusion in the management of tuberculosis of the spine. Studies in Bulawayo (Rhodesia) and in Hong Kong. Sixth report of the Medical Research Council Working Party on Tuberculosis of the Spine. *J. Bone Joint Surg. Br.* **60-B:**163–177.

81. **Mondal, A.** 1994. Cytological diagnosis of vertebral tuberculosis with fine-needle aspiration biopsy. *J. Bone Joint Surg. Am.* **76:**181–184.

82. **Moore, S. L., and M. Rafii.** 2003. Advanced imaging of tuberculosis arthritis. *Semin. Musculoskeletal Radiol.* **7:**143–153.

83. **Moore, S. L., and M. Rafii.** 2001. Imaging of musculoskeletal and spinal tuberculosis. *Radiol. Clin. N. Am.* **39:**329–342.

84. **Morris, B. S., R. Varma, A. Garg, M. Awasthi, and M. Maheshwari.** 2002. Multifocal musculoskeletal tuberculosis in children: appearances on computed tomography. *Skeletal Radiol.* **31:**1–8.

85. **Mousa, H. A.** 1998. Tuberculosis of bones and joints: diagnostic approaches. *Int. Orthop.* **22:**245–246.

86. Naim-ur-Rahman. 1980. Atypical forms of spinal tuberculosis. *J. Bone Joint Surg. Br.* **62-B:**162–165.

87. Neumann, J. L., and D. P. Schlueter. 1974. Retropharyngeal abscess as the presenting feature of tuberculosis of the cervical spine. *Am. Rev. Respir. Dis.* **110:**508–511.

88. Pai, M., and D. I. Ling. 2008. Rapid diagnosis of extrapulmonary tuberculosis using nucleic acid amplification tests: what is the evidence? *Future Microbiol.* **3:**1–4.

89. Palmer, P. E. S. 2001. *The Imaging of Tuberculosis: With Epidemiological, Pathological, and Clinical Correlation.* Springer-Verlag, New York, NY.

90. Pattison, P. R. M. 1986. Pott's paraplegia: an account of the treatment of 89 consecutive patients. *Paraplegia* **24:**77–91.

91. Pertuiset, E., J. Beaudreuil, F. Liote, A. Horusitzky, F. Kemiche, P. Richette, D. Clerc-Wyel, I. Cerf-Payrastre, H. Dorfmann, J. Glowinski, J. Crouzet, T. Bardin, O. Meyer, A. Dryll, J. M. Ziza, M. F. Kahn, and D. Kuntz. 1999. Spinal tuberculosis in adults. A study of 103 cases in a developed country, 1980–1994. *Medicine* (Baltimore) **78:**309–320.

92. Phemister, D. B., and C. H. Hatcher. 1933. Correlation of the pathological findings in the diagnostic of tuberculous arthritis. *Am. J. Roentgenol. Radium Ther. Nucl. Med.* **29:**736–740.

93. Plummer, W. W., S. Sanes, and W. S. Smith. 1934. Hematogenous tuberculosis of skeletal muscle; report of the case with involvement of gastrocnemius muscle. *J. Bone Joint Surg. Am.* **16:**631–639.

94. Rashid, M., S. U. Sarwar, E. U. Haq, M. Z. Islam, T. A. Rizvi, M. Ahmad, and K. Shah. 2006. Tuberculous tenosynovitis: a cause of carpal tunnel syndrome. *J. Pak. Med. Assoc.* **56:**116–118.

95. Salo, W. L., A. C. Aufderheide, J. Buikstra, and T. A. Holcomb. 1994. Identification of *Mycobacterium tuberculosis* DNA in a pre-Columbian Peruvian mummy. *Proc. Natl. Acad. Sci. USA* **91:**2091–2094.

96. Strauss, D. C. 1933. Tuberculosis of the flat bones of the vault of the skull. *Surg. Gynecol. Obstet.* **57:**384–398.

97. Su, J. Y., T. L. Huang, and S. Y. Lin. 1996. Total knee arthroplasty in tuberculous arthritis. *Clin. Orthop. Relat. Res.* February:181–187.

98. Talbot, J. C., Q. Bismil, D. Saralaya, D. A. Newton, R. M. Frizzel, and D. L. Shaw. 2007. Musculoskeletal tuberculosis in Bradford—a 6-year review. *Ann. R. Coll. Surg. Engl.* **89:**405–409.

99. Tiwari, A., A. Sud, S. Mehta, R. K. Kanojia, and S. K. Kapoor. 2007. Multifocal skeletal tuberculosis presenting as multiple bone cysts. *Ann. Acad. Med. Singapore* **36:**1038–1039.

100. Tuli, S. M. 2002. General principles of osteoarticular tuberculosis. *Clin. Orthop. Relat. Res.* May:11–19.

101. Valdazo, J. P., F. Perez-Ruiz, A. Albarracin, G. Sanchez-Nievas, J. Perez-Benegas, M. Gonzalez-Lanza, and J. Beltran. 1990. Tuberculous arthritis. Report of a case with multiple joint involvement and periarticular tuberculous abscesses. *J. Rheumatol.* **17:**399–401.

102. Wallace, R., and A. S. Cohen. 1976. Tuberculous arthritis: a report of two cases with review of biopsy and synovial fluid findings. *Am. J. Med.* **61:**277–282.

103. Watts, H. G., and R. M. Lifeso. 1996. Tuberculosis of bones and joints. *J. Bone Joint Surg. Am.* **78:**288–298.

104. Wu, H., Q. Z. Wang, and Y. Jin. 1998. Tuberculosis of the temporomandibular joint. *Oral Surg. Oral Med. Oral Pathol. Oral Radiol. Endod.* **85:**243.

105. Wurtz, R., Z. Quader, D. Simon, and B. Langer. 1993. Cervical tuberculous vertebral osteomyelitis: case report and discussion of the literature. *Clin. Infect. Dis.* **16:**806–808.

106. Zahraa, J., D. Johnson, J. E. Lim-Dunham, and B. C. Herold. 1996. Unusual features of osteoarticular tuberculosis in children. *J. Pediatr.* **129:**597–602.

107. Zink, A., C. J. Haas, U. Reischl, U. Szeimies, and A. G. Nerlich. 2001. Molecular analysis of skeletal tuberculosis in an ancient Egyptian population. *J. Med. Microbiol.* **50:**355–366.

Tuberculosis and Nontuberculous Mycobacterial Infections, 6th ed.
Edited by David Schlossberg
© 2011 ASM Press, Washington, DC

Chapter 22

Cardiovascular Tuberculosis

John A. Crocco

Cardiovascular tuberculosis is an uncommon extrapulmonary manifestation of mycobacterial disease. With the advent of AIDS, which has increased the incidence of mycobacterial disease (28, 37, 66, 76, 100, 102, 108), particularly of the extrapulmonary type (3, 8, 25, 33, 35, 39, 71, 95, 101, 107, 121, 122, 134, 136), one can expect an increase in cardiovascular tuberculosis. Nevertheless, cardiovascular tuberculosis is a rare complication of AIDS in the United States (3, 33, 70). Pericardial tuberculosis is the disease present in the greatest percentage of patients with cardiovascular tuberculosis (18, 54, 72, 93, 109). In the United States and other developed countries, most patients with AIDS and pericarditis with effusion have an idiopathic cause. However, in Africa, 86 to 100% of patients with AIDS and pericarditis with effusion have *Mycobacterium tuberculosis* as the etiology (91). Tuberculosis of the aorta (50, 117) and myocardium (110) are reported but extremely unusual forms of cardiovascular tuberculosis.

PERICARDIAL TUBERCULOSIS

Pericardial tuberculosis is defined as pericardial tissue or fluid culture positive for *Mycobacterium tuberculosis*; pericardial biopsy specimens demonstrating acid-fast organisms, caseating granulomata, or both; extrapericardial bacteriological or histologic evidence of active tuberculosis in conjunction with major pericardial effusion or pericardial thickening by echocardiography; or a combination thereof. Tuberculosis of the pericardium arises by contiguous, lymphogenous, or hematogenous spread from areas separate from the pericardium. The acute manifestations are associated with polymorphonuclear followed in about 3 to 5 days by a lymphocytic exudative pericardial effusion. In the subacute stage, there is caseation necrosis with the lying down of a fibrinous exudate. Later in the course of the disease,

organization occurs and constrictive pericarditis with tamponade can occur.

Pericardial tuberculosis is rare, occurring in less than 1% of cases of tuberculosis (18, 72, 93, 109), and may be life threatening. Since the 1960s, great strides have been made in the diagnosis and treatment of tuberculosis; death from tuberculosis in the United States now occurs in less than 3% of all patients with this disease (93). Pericardial tuberculosis is associated with a 14 to 40% mortality rate with most treatment regimens (61, 93, 109, 116, 131). In sub-Saharan Africa, Mayosi and associates (88) found that the overall mortality rate in patients with presumed pericardial tuberculosis was 26%. The major independent predictors of death were an additional proven nontuberculosis final diagnosis, presence of clinical signs of human immunodeficiency virus (HIV) infection, coexistent pulmonary tuberculosis, and older age. A trend toward an increase in death rates occurred in patients who were hemodynamically unstable. This trend was decreased in patients who underwent pericardiocentesis.

There are two major reasons for the high death rate in pericardial tuberculosis. First, there is difficulty in establishing the diagnosis of tuberculous pericarditis. Second, pericardial inflammation often has dire effects on the mechanical efficiency of the heart.

The individual clinical features of tuberculous pericarditis are nonspecific. When they are analyzed together, however, they often suggest the diagnosis. Most patients are middle-aged (72). There appears to be a predilection for black males, as evidence by a 12:1 preponderance of blacks in one series at a large New York City hospital, even after correction for geographic and racial distributions (109).

The most common symptoms are weight loss, cough, dyspnea, orthopnea, chest pain, and ankle swelling (59, 64, 81, 102, 109). The last four symptoms serve as diagnostic clues (59, 64, 73, 81, 102, 109) because they occur more frequently in

John A. Crocco • UMDNJ—Robert Wood Johnson Medical School, New Brunswick, NJ 08854.

tuberculous pericarditis than in pulmonary tuberculosis without pericarditis.

The most prevalent signs are fever, tachycardia, cardiomegaly, and signs of a pleural effusion (6, 64, 81, 102, 109). In a study of 35 patients with pericardial tuberculosis, 25 patients had a pleural effusion and 9 (36%) had tuberculous pleuritis on pleural biopsy or autopsy (109). Percutaneous needle and thoracoscopic biopsies of the pleural space appear to be aids in the diagnosis of pericardial infection. Distant heart sounds, pericardial friction rub, and paradoxical pulse, which are more specific signs of pericarditis and possible tamponade, occurred in a minority of patients (102, 109). They were much more common in patients with tamponade.

In the recent past, the enzyme adenosine deaminase (ADA) has been found to be specifically elevated in pleural (92, 97, 99), peritoneal (84), pericardial (67, 83, 113), and meningeal (98) fluids of tuberculous origin. Martinez-Vazquez and colleagues (83) looked at ADA levels of pericardial fluid of tuberculous origin versus those of idiopathic, neoplastic, or miscellaneous nontuberculous origin. The mean pericardial fluid ADA level in patients with tuberculous pericarditis was 96.8 (standard deviation, 1.54) IU/liter, and the ADA level for pericardial fluid of nontuberculous origin was 2 to 20 IU/liter. Komsuoglu and coworkers (69) performed a similar study and found that those patients with tuberculous pericarditis had a mean pericardial effusion ADA value of 126 ± 16.68 IU/liter, versus 29.5 ± 13.4 IU/liter for patients with other causes of pericarditis. The difference was statistically significant between the groups ($P < 0.0001$), indicating that the ADA value has a 100% sensitivity and 91% specificity. The studies of Koh and coworkers (68) yielded similar results, showing that an ADA value in pericardial fluid of 40 IU/liter or more had a sensitivity of 93% and a specificity of 97% in the diagnosis of tuberculous pericarditis. They also showed that ADA levels could be of great value in the early diagnosis of pericardial tuberculosis, particularly when the results of the clinical and laboratory tests are negative. They also noted significant elevation of pericardial fluid carcinoembryonic antigen values in patients with malignant disease involving the pericardium. Inoue and associates (66) and Isaka and colleagues (67) obtained similar results in their studies. Pericardial effusion ADA levels appear to be helpful in the diagnosis of tuberculous pericarditis.

Other forms of testing have been used in addition to ADA. These include pericardial fluid and tissue lysozyme (LYS), gamma interferon (IFN-γ), and PCR in the diagnosis of pericardial tuberculosis. Aggeli and associates (1) in Greece have used a combination of ADA and LYS levels in pericardial fluid in order to compare their effectiveness in the diagnosis of idiopathic, neoplastic, and tuberculous pericarditis. Seven patients had tuberculous, 4 had neoplastic, and 30 had idiopathic pericarditis. A cutoff value of 72 IU/liter for pericardial fluid ADA was associated with a 100% sensitivity and a 94% specificity in the diagnosis of pericardial tuberculosis. A cutoff value of 6.5 μg/dl for pericardial fluid LYS had a sensitivity of 100% and a specificity of 92% in the diagnosis of this disease. These authors felt that both pericardial ADA and LYS need to be taken into account for an early diagnosis. Burgess (22) in South Africa studied pericardial fluid obtained via pericardiocentesis with echocardiographic direction in 110 patients with large pericardial effusions from various causes. Their diagnoses varied, with 64 with tuberculous pericarditis, 12 with malignant disease, 5 with nontuberculous effusions, 10 with idiopathic effusions, and 19 with effusions from other causes. ADA and IFN-γ levels were significantly higher in effusions from patients with tuberculous pericarditis than in patients with other forms of pericarditis ($P < 0.05$ for ADA and $P > 0.005$ for IFN-γ). A cutoff value of 30 IU/liter for pericardial fluid ADA was associated with a sensitivity of 94%, a specificity of 68%, and a positive predictive value of 80% in the diagnosis of pericardial tuberculosis. A cutoff of 200 pg/liter for pericardial fluid IFN-γ was associated with a sensitivity and specificity of 100% in the diagnosis of pericardial tuberculosis. Burgess concluded that pericardial fluid levels of ADA and IFN-γ were useful in the diagnosis of pericardial tuberculosis. Reuter and associates (104) found similar results in their studies. Biglino and colleagues (17) suggested that an IFN-γ enzyme-linked immunospot assay on pericardial fluid cells might be used as a diagnostic assay in patients suspected of having tuberculous pericarditis. Tuon and coauthors (138) evaluated the utility of ADA activity in pericardial fluid as a diagnostic marker in tuberculous pericarditis via a systematic review with meta-analysis. Of 31 studies reviewed, 5 were selected for further scrutiny. The sensitivity and specificity of this methodology were 88 and 83%, respectively, and the summary receiver operating characteristics curve presented an area with a tendency toward 1 (0.9539). With these data they felt that the clinical value of ADA activity in pericardial fluid was an adjunctive diagnostic marker of tuberculous pericarditis.

Nucleic acid amplification methods such as PCR are now being used to detect tuberculosis in fluids and tissue (1, 2, 24, 74, 142). Cegielski et al. (24) at Duke examined 36 specimens of pericardial fluid and 19 specimens of pericardial tissue from 20 patients, 16 of whom had tuberculous pericarditis and 4 of whom had another diagnosis. Culture studies

(Lowenstein-Jensen and Middlebrook solid media and BACTEC radiometric broth), histologic studies, and PCR studies were performed on these tissues. Tuberculosis was correctly diagnosed in 15 of 16 (93%) by culture, 13 of 16 (81%) by PCR, and 13 of 15 (87%) by histology. PCR was performed on fluid and tissue specimens using the IS*6110*-based primers for *Mycobacterium tuberculosis* complex. There was one false-positive PCR reading for a patient with *Staphylococcus aureus* pericarditis. If individual specimens were considered as the unit of analysis, *Mycobacterium tuberculosis* was found by culture in 30 of 43 (70%) specimens tested and by PCR in 14 of 28 (50%) specimens tested ($P > 0.05$). PCR was significantly higher with tissue specimens (12 of 15, or 80%) than with fluid specimens (2 of 13, or 15%) ($P = 0.02$). The authors concluded that the accuracy of PCR came close to that of culture and histology but was considerably better in tissue specimens than in fluid specimens. They felt that studies of PCR should be pursued and noted the poor sensitivity of PCR in analyzing pericardial fluid. Lee and colleagues (74) in South Korea looked at pericardial fluid PCR and ADA in the diagnosis of pericardial tuberculosis. They studied 67 patients with pericarditis: 12 (18%) with tuberculosis, 20 (30%) with neoplastic disease, and 35 (52%) with idiopathic disease. ADA was significantly higher in pericardial fluid from patients with tuberculous pericarditis than it was in patients without tuberculosis. An ADA cutoff value of 40 IU/liter was associated with an 83% (10 of 12) sensitivity and a 78% (43 of 57) specificity for pericardial tuberculosis. Pericardial PCR was positive for tuberculosis for 9 of 12 patients with pericardial tuberculosis (a 75% sensitivity) and negative for tuberculosis for 55 of 55 patients with nontuberculous pericarditis (a specificity of 100%). These authors point out that PCR is as sensitive as but more specific than ADA in the diagnosis of pericardial tuberculosis. They also point out that ADA levels are higher in rheumatoid arthritis, sarcoidosis, and some empyemas as well as in tuberculous pericarditis. They conclude that PCR testing of pericardial fluid is a rapid, reliable method of identifying pericardial tuberculosis. Zamurian and coauthors (142) studied 30 patients with constrictive pericarditis in an attempt to detect *Mycobacterium tuberculosis* in paraffin-embedded pericardial tissue via a new histopathological examination and PCR amplification of the *Mycobacterium tuberculosis* genome. Five of the 30 patients had tuberculosis, and 4 of the 5 had a positive PCR. The sensitivity of PCR was 80%. They concluded that nuclear amplification techniques such as PCR appear to be promising.

Further evaluation of PCR techniques in the diagnosis of pericardial tuberculosis using IS*6110*

as well as other primers of *Mycobacterium tuberculosis* complex or mycobacterial interspersal repeat unit genotyping (12) to detect DNA specific for *Mycobacterium tuberculosis* is needed. It is known that IS*6110*-based typing requires subculturing of the isolates for several weeks to obtain sufficient DNA. Mycobacterial interspersal repeat unit genotyping has a discriminatory power almost equal to that of IS*6110*-based genotyping. It is technically simpler and can be applied directly to *Mycobacterium tuberculosis* cultures without DNA amplification. It is hoped that in the future PCR techniques will be rapid, more specific, and less expensive than at present.

The chest radiograph is frequently characterized by cardiomegaly, especially in the presence of a pericardial effusion. A "water bottle" configuration to the cardiac silhouette may be visible. Various studies have found cardiomegaly in up to 95% of patients (52, 53, 102, 131).

Pericardial effusion is a common finding in tuberculosis of the pericardium (59, 64, 81, 99, 102, 109). A pericardial effusion is clinically manifested by distant heart sounds, a friction rub that may disappear or become clearly audible, and an apical pulse that ceases to be palpable. If the pericardial effusion is large, percussion may reveal an area of dullness and auscultation may reveal an area of tubular breathing at the angle of the left scapula (Ewart's sign), which are likely caused by compression of the underlying lung.

The most feared complication of pericardial effusion is cardiac tamponade, wherein the accumulated fluid seriously obstructs the flow of blood into the ventricles. The result is a fall in cardiac output and systemic venous congestion that are clinically manifest in falling arterial pressure, a rising venous pressure, distended cervical neck veins on inspiration (Kussmal's sign), and a paradoxical pulse (a fall in systolic arterial pressure on inspiration). Although a paradoxical pulse is a hallmark of cardiac tamponade, it is not pathognomonic, because it can occur in various forms of restrictive cardiomyopathy, chronic obstructive airway disease, and severe bronchial asthma. Various investigators (20, 40, 52, 61, 67, 78, 96, 108, 131) have recorded pericardial tamponade in 10 to 40% of patients with tuberculous pericarditis.

The procedure of significant value in diagnosing and monitoring pericardial effusion is the echocardiogram, which is safe, rapid, and most sensitive in detecting small amounts of fluid (15). An echo-free space may occur, most often posteriorly and frequently anteriorly as well. Larrieu and colleagues (72) showed that echocardiography was 100% accurate in diagnosing pericardial effusion. Chia and associates (31) thought that two-dimensional echocardiography allows better recognition of fluid distribution in the pericardial cavity than the M-mode echocardiogram. Agrawal and coworkers (2) used echocardiography to demonstrate a resolving intrapericardial mass in a tuberculous pericardial effusion. Martin and associates (82) suggested that two-dimensional echocardiograms demonstrate not only anterior and posterior effusions in patients with tuberculosis but also echodense structures lining the visceral and parietal pericardium and protruding into the pericardial space. Komsuoglu and colleagues (69) monitored 20 patients with tuberculous pericarditis with effusion for 12 to 18 months via echocardiography. Pre- and post-therapy studies revealed that only 2 patients still had small effusions. Liu and coworkers (77) studied 53 patients with pericardial effusions, 21 of whom had tuberculous pericarditis and 32 of whom had nontuberculous pericarditis. They found that thickening of the pericardium and the presence of fibrinous strands on the echocardiogram had a high positive predictive value for tuberculous pericarditis compared to nontuberculous pericarditis. An exudative coating was highly sensitive for tuberculous pericarditis, but its specificity was low. These authors felt that an echocardiographic examination was useful in providing information about the nature of a pericardial effusion.

Gallium-67 scans of chest, computer tomography (CT) of the chest, and magnetic resonance imaging (MRI) have also been used to diagnose pericarditis and pericardial effusion (16, 60, 76, 118, 125, 133, 135, 140). In a patient with a pericardial effusion, CT scanning and MRI can provide information additional to the findings on an echocardiogram. These include enlargement (equal to or greater than 10 mm) with mating and hypodense centers and sparing of the hilar lymph nodes on CT examination as well as assessment of the extent of pericardial inflammation and myocardial involvement on MRI. Both of these modalities can better image the pericardium and more accurately measure pericardial thickening.

Angiocardiography is also an effective means of localizing a pericardial effusion, but it is time-consuming, invasive, often uncomfortable, and at times associated with significant morbidity. Radionuclide angiography shows a gated blood pool and a fluid-filled pericardial space when a pericardial effusion is present. MRI can directly image the pericardium and thereby demonstrate abnormal thickening of the pericardium (44, 140).

Hemodynamic findings during cardiac catheterization are often normal in pericardial tuberculosis (20). When constrictive pericarditis is present, however, ventricular filling is not impeded until later in diastole. If cardiac tamponade occurs, ventricular filling is impeded throughout diastole. Central venous and right and left atrial pressure pulses show an M-shaped contour in constrictive pericarditis as well as prominent "x" and "y" descents followed by a rapid rise in pressure during early diastole. In addition to reduced stroke volume, ventricular end-diastolic pressures, and mean atrial, pulmonary vein, and systemic vein pressures are elevated to almost equal amounts. The ventricular pressure pulse shows the characteristic "square-root sign" in diastole. With cardiac tamponade, the most prominent deflection is the "x" trough, whereas there is absence of the "y" descent in the jugular venous pulse and absence of the square-root sign in the ventricular pulse during diastole.

Other significant procedures in diagnosis are electrocardiogram findings, purified protein derivative (PPD) intermediate skin testing, pericardial aspirate culture, and pericardial biopsy (109). Electrocardiographic T-wave inversion consistent with but not diagnostic for pericarditis is a common abnormality (84%) (109). Low-voltage QRS waves may also be visible. PPD of intermediate strength (PPD-intermediate) yields positive results in most patients (80 to 100%) (52, 53, 109, 131). A negative PPD-intermediate test result is common in a patient with pericardial tuberculosis and AIDS because of the increased degree of anergy in patients with AIDS (26).

Pericardial fluid is obtained via pericardiocentesis that is performed to establish an etiology, relieve tamponade, or both. In tuberculous pericarditis, the effusion is usually a lymphocytic exudate that may be bloody or blood-tinged (52, 109, 131). It usually has a high protein content and a low sugar level. Culture of pericardial fluid was positive for up to 50% of patients in three studies (109, 113, 131). This percentage could not be duplicated in other studies.

Pericardial biopsy has also been advocated in the diagnosis of pericarditis (40, 93, 102, 113, 131). Between 1950 and 1970, many investigators thought that examination of the entire pericardium at pericardiectomy or autopsy was required to definitively diagnose tuberculosis (29, 41, 118). Fredriksen and associates (55) reviewed the cases of 20 patients with pericardial effusion who underwent pericardiocentesis and percutaneous open pericardial window with pericardial biopsy. Biopsy provided a specific etiological diagnosis in 2 (10%), and 13 (65%) had at least one serious complication postoperatively. Pericardiocentesis was uncomplicated and yielded a specific diagnosis in four patients (20%).

Reuter and coauthors (105) performed open pericardial biopsies in 36 patients with large pericardial effusions via pericardiocentesis, which was followed by daily intermittent catheter drainage. Tuberculous pericarditis was found in 25 of these patients, 5 of whom were also HIV positive. Thirteen of the 20 HIV-negative patients with tuberculous pericardial effusions (65%) demonstrated granulomatous lesions, compared with 2 of the 5 HIV-positive patients (40%). Those authors concluded that coinfection with HIV affects the histopathology of pericardial tuberculosis and leads to a decrease in the sensitivity of the test.

In view of the significant morbidity and poor diagnostic yield from pericardial windows, Fredriksen and associates (55) proposed specific recommendations for pericardiocentesis and percutaneous open pericardial window with biopsy. These included relief of tamponade and establishment of the causative factor of pericardial effusion as the main indications for pericardiocentesis. Percutaneous pericardial window with biopsy was indicated for drainage of a purulent pericardial effusion, for recurrent tamponade after pericardiocentesis, and for chronic effusion after unproductive pericardiocentesis. More recent studies have attempted to shed more light on the usefulness of pericardial biopsy. In 1988, Strang and colleagues (131) found that 33 (70%) of 47 pericardial biopsy samples from patients with pericardial tuberculosis had histologic evidence of tuberculosis (e.g., caseating granulomata). Sagrista-Sauleda and co-authors (113), also in 1988, found evidence of tuberculosis in all three pericardial biopsies performed on patients with tuberculous pericarditis and the six pericardiectomies performed in this series. All showed the presence of tuberculosis on histologic examination.

Endrys and associates (48) have presented a new technique for multiple pericardial biopsies. In the cardiac catheterization laboratory the pericardium is punctured, air is allowed to enter the pericardial space, and a bioptome is inserted to obtain multiple biopsy specimens (an average of eight) of the parietal pericardium. This is all performed under fluoroscopy. The air is aspirated from the pericardial space at the end of the procedure, and a sheath is left in place until daily fluid drainage is less than 30 ml. Eighteen biopsies were performed, with six revealing tuberculosis, two cancer, and one mesothelioma. The other nine biopsies were noncontributory but excluded malignancy. None of the nine patients exhibited malignancy during follow-up.

The introduction of pericardioscopy and its use in creating a pericardial window for diagnosis and treatment of pericardial effusions as well as obtaining multiple pericardial biopsies (e.g., 18 to 20) has opened a new era in the management of all forms of pericarditis, including the tuberculous form. It has improved the results obtained from pericardial biopsies because pericardioscopy allows for multiple biopsy samples to be taken from the parietal and even visceral pericardium under direct vision (119).

Seferovic and colleagues (119) compared the use of pericardial biopsy under fluoroscopic control with a standard number (3 to 6 per patient) of pericardial samples (group 1), the use of pericardioscopic guidance with standard sampling (4 to 6 per patient) (group 2), and pericardioscopic guidance with extensive sampling (18 to 20 per patient) (group 3). Pericardial biopsies were of the parietal pericardium. The 49 patients studied suffered from malignant disease as well as tuberculosis. There were 12 patients in group 1, 22 in group 2, and 15 in group 3. For group 1 patients a new diagnosis and etiology of pericarditis were determined in 8.3% of patients, a clinical diagnosis confirmed in 33.3% of patients, and a false-negative result (no useful information) in 58.3%. For group 2 patients a new diagnosis was established in 26.3% of patients, etiology was revealed in 40.9%, a clinical diagnosis was confirmed in 36.4%, and a pericardial biopsy false negative in 36.4%. For group 3 patients a new diagnosis was established in 40%, etiology was uncovered in 53%, a clinical diagnosis was confirmed in 53.3%, and no useful information was found in 6.3%. There were no major complications. There were minor complications of nonsustained ventricular tachycardia in 4.7%, pain during the placement of the pericardioscopy sheath in 56.7%, and transient fever in 35.1%. This study demonstrates that periocardioscopically directed pericardial biopsies with extensive sampling (18 to 20 per patient) provided a significantly improved diagnostic capability. Further evaluation of this methodological advance in tuberculous pericarditis is indicated.

Mayosi and associates (86, 135) have proposed a protocol for an integrated etiological approach to be used in patients with a suspected tuberculous pericardial effusion in tuberculosis-endemic and -nonendemic areas.

The first step is an initial evaluation which includes a chest roentgenogram, echocardiogram, CT scan, and/or MRI of the chest, a right scalene node biopsy (if pericardial fluid is not accessible and lymphadenopathy is present), and culture of sputum, gastric aspirate, and/or urine (in all patients), as well as HIV testing, white blood cell count, and globulin testing. A tuberculin test is not helpful regardless of the background prevalence of tuberculosis.

The second step is a therapeutic pericardiocentesis, especially in the presence of tamponade, a diagnostic pericardiocentesis with culture of fluid for acid-fast bacilli, biochemical tests to distinguish a transudate from an exudates (fluid and serum protein and lactate dehydrogenase), white blood cell count and cytology of pericardial fluid, and indirect tests for tuberculosis (ADA, IFN-γ, or LYS assay).

The third step is a pericardial biopsy. A therapeutic biopsy should be performed as part of the surgical drainage with severe tamponade relapsing after pericardiocentesis or requiring open drainage of pericardial fluid for whatever reason. A diagnostic biopsy is not required in areas where tuberculosis is endemic, and empirical therapy can be started right away. A diagnostic biopsy is needed in patients with greater than 3 weeks of illness and without an etiologic diagnosis being reached by other tests.

The fourth step is empirical antituberculosis chemotherapy. This is recommended in areas where tuberculosis is endemic for exudative pericardial effusions, after excluding uremia, malignancy, and trauma. It is also recommended in an area where tuberculosis is endemic and pericardiocentesis is not available for a patient with a tuberculous pericarditis index of more than 6 points (weight loss = 1 point, night sweats = 1 point, fever = 2 points, white blood cell count of less than 10×10^9/liter = 3 points, serum globulin of more than 40 g/liter = 3 points). In non-tuberculosis-endemic areas, empirical antituberculosis chemotherapy is not recommended when systemic investigation fails to reveal a diagnosis of tuberculous pericarditis.

THERAPY

The American Thoracic Society, the Centers for Disease Control and Prevention, and the Infectious Diseases Society of America (5) recommend that patients with pericardial tuberculosis receive a 6-month regimen (2 months of isoniazid [INH], rifampin [RIF], pyrazinamide [PZA], and ethambutol followed by 4 months of INH and RIF) as initial therapy unless the organisms are known or strongly suspected of being resistant to first-line drugs. They also recommended as adjunctive therapy for tuberculous pericarditis corticosteroid therapy for the first 11 weeks of antituberculosis treatment. The dosage of corticosteroids used was prednisone at 60 mg/day (or equivalent dose of prednisolone) for 4 weeks, followed by 30 mg/day for 4 weeks, 15 mg/day for 2 weeks, and 5 mg/day for the final week.

Because current antituberculosis treatment is most effective in eradicating mycobacteria, prompt diagnosis and institution of therapy are imperative. Difficulty in the diagnosis of pericardial tuberculosis often results in the late institution of therapy and therefore is, in part, responsible for the high mortality rate of this disease. Another major cause of the high mortality rate is that the pericardial inflammation interferes with the mechanical efficiency of the heart, particularly when pericardial tamponade occurs.

Mycobacteria grow slowly, and therefore, there is a lag time between institution of antituberculosis medication and elimination of the organisms. Abortion of the inflammatory response is not immediate. This interval or lag time is critical in terms of mortality. The pericardial inflammation that occurs is a potential risk because the rapid accumulation of fluid with tamponade and induction of arrhythmias may compromise cardiac performance.

In order to suppress a pericardial reaction and minimize its sequelae, corticosteroids have been introduced. These drugs have been found to be efficacious in the treatment and control of pericardial effusions in many different varieties of pericarditides (7, 43, 56, 75, 109, 131, 137, 139). In pulmonary and pleural tuberculosis, the addition or corticosteroids together with antituberculosis drugs results in a more rapid resolution of disease (9, 11, 21, 56, 85, 94, 109). Experimental evidence has shown that cortisone reduced the host reaction to mycobacterial infections and minimized exudation, fibrin deposition, and proliferation of granulation tissue (9, 11, 21, 34, 36, 45, 94, 103, 109, 127, 131).

In tuberculous pericarditis, corticosteroids nonspecifically suppress the inflammation, thereby lessening the hemodynamic sequelae as the antituberculosis drugs eliminate the organisms. The exudation of fluid abates and reabsorption of fluid commences. A noticeable decrease in heart size often occurs within 2 to 3 days, and the size may return to normal within 2 weeks. Defervescence is rapid and arrhythmias are controlled within 2 to 3 days. The corticosteroids may be withdrawn over the next 11 weeks without recrudescence of symptoms of tuberculous pericarditis. At the same time, the mycobacteria, which evoke the inflammatory reaction in this disease, are eradicated by the concomitant use of antituberculosis drugs. Upon withdrawal of corticosteroids, occasionally pulmonary tuberculosis may be aggravated transiently, which abates quickly with continuous antituberculosis therapy.

A number of authors have had success with corticosteroid therapy in addition to antituberculosis treatment in the management of tuberculous pericarditis (7, 42, 43, 109, 122, 131, 137, 139). In a study of 28 patients who received chemotherapy for tuberculous pericarditis, 10 patients were treated with a three-drug regimen alone and 18 were treated with three antituberculosis drugs and prednisone (109). In the first group 4 patients died, 2 of whom were in a group of 4 requiring pericardiectomy. There were no deaths in the prednisone-treated group, 14 improved without surgery, and 4 required pericardiectomy.

In 1959, Schrire (122) in Cape Town, South Africa, studied 28 patients with pericardial effusion from suspected tuberculous pericarditis who were treated with antituberculosis medications and were also alternately, but not blindly, given adjunctive corticosteroids or no corticosteroids. At first the group receiving the corticosteroids received a loading dose of 300 mg of cortisone per day and then a maintenance dose of 100 mg per day for several weeks. At a later date the regimen was changed. Prednisone was given at first at a dosage of 60 mg per day, and then a maintenance dosage of 30 mg per day was used. Four patients in the corticosteroid group needed a pericardiectomy due to constrictive pericarditis. The author did not provide information regarding the characteristics of the patients, the basis for the diagnosis of tuberculous pericarditis, or the length of follow-up.

In 1987 Strang and colleagues (132) studied 143 patients with active constrictive tuberculous pericarditis without significant pericardial effusion. This was a double-blind study comparing the use of corticosteroids or placebo as a supplement to 6 months of antituberculosis medication in the treatment of active constrictive tuberculous pericarditis and the need for pericardiectomy. The antituberculosis drug regimen included INH, streptomycin, RIF, and PZA for the initial 14 weeks and INH and RIF for the remainder of the 6 months. Twenty-nine of the 143 patients were excluded for multiple reasons. One hundred fourteen were monitored and their status was reassessed at up to 24 months. Fifty-three received adjunctive corticosteroids, and 61 received placebo. The outcome of these studies included more rapid improvement with prednisolone characterized by the rate of fall in the mean pulse rate, the rate at which jugular venous pressure fell to normal, and the rate at which the level of physical activity became normal. At follow-up, which occurred at up to 24 months, death from pericarditis occurred in 2 (4%) patients on prednisolone and 7 (11%) on placebo. Pericardiectomy was required in 11 (21%) patients in the prednisolone group and 18 (30%) in the placebo group. A favorable status was present at 24 months in 50 (94%) patients on prednisolone and 52 (82%) patients on placebo. The authors (101) recommended that in the absence of any contraindications, antituberculosis medications should be supplemented with adjunctive corticosteroids.

In 1988, Strang and colleagues (131) studied 240 patients with active tuberculous pericarditis with pericardial effusion. The regimen used was the same as the antituberculosis medication, prednisolone, and placebo regimen used in the 1987 study by Strang and associates (132). In this study 42 patients were excluded for various reasons. Those patients who were willing were then either allocated to open pericardial biopsy and complete drainage of pericardial fluid on admission or percutaneous pericardiocentesis, which was required for substantial cardiac embarrassment with restricted physical activity or tamponade. Complete open drainage on admission abolished the need for pericardiocentesis but did not influence the need for subsequent pericardiectomy for constriction and did not influence the risk of death. The patients who did not have open drainage on admission had the following outcomes. Over the 24 months that these patients were monitored, death from pericarditis occurred in 2 (3%) patients taking adjunctive prednisolone and 10 (14%) patients taking placebo ($P < 0.05$). Six (18%) patients on adjunctive prednisolone required a pericardiectomy, versus 9 (12%) patients on placebo ($P < 0.05$). Seven (9%) patients on prednisolone required repeat pericardiocentesis, versus 17 (23%) patients on placebo ($P < 0.05$).

Strang and colleagues (130) analyzed their data regarding 363 patients, 143 of whom had constrictive tuberculous pericarditis without a pericardial effusion (132) and 240 of whom had tuberculous pericarditis with a pericardial effusion (131) 10 years after the original double-blind, placebo-controlled, randomized study to determine whether early benefits were maintained and to study any further differences emerging after the first 2 years of follow-up. The 10-year follow-up rate was 96%. In the patients with constriction but no pericardial effusion, the adverse-outcome rates were 19/70 (27%) in the prednisolone group and 28/73 (38%) in the placebo group ($P = 0.15$), and the mortality rates were 2/70 (3%) in the prednisolone group and 8/73 (11%) in the placebo group ($P = 0.098$). In patients with pericardial effusion, patients with open pericardial drainage and prednisolone had adverse effects 19% of the time (4/29), patients with no open pericardial drainage and placebo had adverse effects 52% of the time (14/27), patients with open pericardial drainage and placebo had adverse effects 11% of the time (4/35), and patients with no open pericardial drainage and prednisolone had adverse effects 19% of the time (6/31). Open pericardial drainage eliminated the need for repeat pericardiocentesis. In the 176 patients with pericardial effusions, an adverse outcome occurred in those without drainage who were receiving prednisolone 19% of the time (17/88) and in those without drainage who were receiving placebo 40% of the time (35/88) ($P = 0.003$). In 9 (10%) patients on prednisolone that had a repeat pericardiocentesis, there was an adverse outcome. Twenty (23%) patients placed on placebo had adverse reactions ($P = 0.025$). These authors (130) concluded after multivariate survival analysis of patients stratified by type of pericarditis that prednisolone reduced the overall death rate after adjusting for age and sex ($P = 0.044$). Also, at 10 years the great majority of surviving patients in all treatment groups were either fully active or out and about, even if activity was restricted. The authors again favored use of adjunctive corticosteroids in addition to antituberculosis chemotherapy in patients with tuberculous pericarditis, provided there was no contraindication. They did state that a limitation to their study was the accuracy of the diagnosis, since in the constrictive group (132) 84% had evidence of definitive tuberculosis (histologic in 40%) and in the effusion group (130) 73% had definitive evidence of tuberculosis (bacteriological in 57%).

In 2000, Hakim et al. (62) in Zimbabwe studied 58 patients with effusive tuberculous pericarditis who were infected with HIV. All received antituberculosis therapy, but one-half received prednisolone for 6 weeks and one-half received placebo in a double-blind randomized placebo-controlled trial. Prednisolone was given in a dosage of 60 mg/day for the first week and tapered by 10 mg/day each week thereafter. In this study 5 patients in the prednisolone group and 10 patients in the placebo group died over an 18-month period ($P = 0.07$). The prednisolone group had a significantly more rapid resolution of hepatomegaly and elevated jugular venous pressure and more rapid improvement in physical activity. The authors concluded that treatment of effusive tuberculous pericarditis in HIV-infected patients should include not only standard antituberculosis therapy but also prednisolone.

In 1999, Chen and colleagues (30) in Taiwan studied 22 patients with tuberculous pericarditis. These patients were evaluated by echocardiography; 17 showed a pericardial effusion ("shaggy" in 8 and "non-shaggy" in 9), whereas 5 showed constrictive pericarditis. Patients with a shaggy tuberculous pericardial effusion had a medium duration between onset of symptoms and diagnosis compared to those with a nonshaggy effusion. Antituberculosis treatment and 20 to 30 mg/day of prednisolone were used in 11 patients, 2 of whom developed constrictive pericarditis. Treatment with antituberculosis medicine but without prednisolone resulted in constrictive pericarditis in 5 of 6 patients. The authors concluded that antituberculosis medication with prednisolone resulted in a significant decrease in constrictive pericarditis, particularly in patients with a shaggy tuberculous pericardial effusion compared with those who did not receive prednisolone. However, they also showed that patients with a nonshaggy tuberculous pericardial effusion did not exhibit the same benefit.

In 2002 Mayosi (87) reviewed four randomized or quasirandomized trials (62, 122, 131, 132) using meta-analysis to compare the effectiveness of corticosteroids versus placebo therapy in the treatment of tuberculous pericarditis. Of 469 patients studied, the corticosteroid recipients had a statistically higher chance of being alive with no functional impairment at 2 years after treatment than did those receiving placebo. However, in a sensitivity analysis including patients lost to follow-up, the effect of treatment was not sustained. Furthermore, the benefits of corticosteroid treatments on reaccumulation of pericardial effusion and its progression to constrictive pericarditis did not reach statistical significance. The author felt that corticosteroids might have a beneficial effect on mortality and morbidity in tuberculous pericarditis but that these trials were not large enough to be conclusive. Mayosi felt that a large placebo-controlled trial was needed to conclusively prove that corticosteroid therapy results in a statistically significant improvement in the treatment of pericardial tuberculosis.

In 2003 Ntsekhe and colleagues (90), in their systemic review of the use of corticosteroids in patients with tuberculous pericarditis, which mirrored the analysis of Mayosi (87), noted that the use of corticosteroids in addition to antituberculosis chemotherapy in tuberculous pericarditis decreased the death rate, decreased the need for repeat pericardiocentesis, and decreased the need for pericardiectomy compared to these rates in patients receiving placebo and antituberculosis chemotherapy. They commented that these data or point estimates suggested that there was a large benefit (about 50%) in terms of morbidity and mortality when corticosteroids were added to antituberculosis chemotherapy in patients with tuberculous pericarditis. However, Ntsekhe and associates (90) felt that these findings were statistically inconclusive because of the small number of patients studied. Other problems arose from the limitation of bacteriological and histopathological confirmation of the diagnosis of active tuberculosis in 30 to 60% of patients in the four trials reviewed (62, 122, 129, 131, 132).

Corticosteroids are successful in suppressing ongoing inflammation, but they cannot reverse damage that has occurred prior to treatment. Repair by fibrosis can still take place, and blood, fibrin, and other exudative substances that are already present can result in continuous deleterious influences. In such circumstances, surgical intervention in the form of pericardiectomy is the best method for controlling mechanical compression. There are many excellent descriptions of the surgical technique, but it must be emphasized that the earlier the pericardiectomy is performed in patients that do not respond to medical therapy, the better the overall results (4, 13, 19, 23, 40, 65, 72, 78, 88, 93, 96, 102, 109, 113–115, 126, 131).

Whether or not corticosteroids will diminish the likelihood of late constrictive pericarditis is not known because resolution of this problem requires a large number of untreated patients as well as a large number of antituberculosis drug-treated patients, equal numbers of whom do and do not receive corticosteroids. Death among untreated patients with tuberculous pericarditis is common. Therefore, little information is available to gauge what percentage of patients that heal spontaneously later develop pericardial constriction. The report of Hageman and colleagues (61) suggests that antituberculosis drug-treated patients infrequently developed constriction. This conclusion is not secure without a minimum follow-up of 5 years and preferably 20 years to assess the true incidence of this complication. If residual fibrosis resulting from tuberculosis can be used as an index for predicting the likelihood of late constriction, the use of corticosteroids in pleural and pulmonary tuberculosis would suggest that these drugs do not significantly alter these residues and therefore probably will not prevent constriction to any greater degree than antituberculosis drugs alone.

Any patient who experiences signs and symptoms of pericarditis, whose tuberculin skin test result is positive, and whose chest radiograph is characterized by a pulmonary infiltrate, a pleural effusion, or both should be empirically regarded as having tuberculous pericarditis until proven otherwise. Prompt treatment with antituberculosis drugs should be initiated. Prednisone, 60 mg/day or its equivalent, is administered concomitantly. This dose is maintained for 4 weeks and is progressively reduced to discontinuation in 11 weeks. It has to be recognized that corticosteroid treatment is not a panacea in the management of tuberculous pericarditis and does not always eliminate the necessity for pericardiocentesis, ancillary agents to control heart failure, or even pericardiectomy. The need for the latter is dictated by close evaluation of the clinical response to treatment.

The need for pericardiectomy is not universal in tuberculous pericarditis. In the majority of studies that address the need for pericardiectomy in this disease, this surgical procedure was performed in 10 to 50% (23, 40, 61, 78, 102, 109, 126, 131). The indication for the procedure was constrictive pericarditis, cardiac tamponade, or both.

In the recent past investigators have looked at idiopathic chronic pericardial effusions (111), acute cardiac tamponade (128), and effusive-constrictive pericarditis (112). In reviewing large idiopathic pericardial effusions, Sagrista-Sauleda et al. (111) looked at the natural history and treatment of this problem. They defined this malady as a collection of pericardial fluid that persists more than 3 months and does

not have an apparent cause. They concluded that this condition can be well treated for long periods in many patients but that severe tamponade can occur at any time. They noted that large pericardial effusions can resolve with pericardiocentesis alone, but that recurrence is common and that when a large pericardial effusion occurs after pericardiocentesis, pericardiectomy should be considered. Spodick (128), in reviewing pericardial tamponade, considered this medical problem as a slow or rapid compression of the heart due to pericardial accumulation of fluid, pus, blood, clots, or gas as a result of effusion, trauma, or rupture of the heart. He felt that the causes of this situation are diverse, with traumatic tamponade likely to occur after cardiac surgery and tuberculous tamponade more common in Africa but rare in the United States. His recommendation for treatment included drainage of the pericardial contents, preferably by needle pericardiocentesis under the guidance of echocardiographic, fluoroscopic, or CT imaging. If the heart cannot be reached by needle or catheter, surgical drainage is required. Surgical drainage is also needed for intrapericardial bleeding, clotted hemopericardium, and recurrences of tamponade. Sagrista-Sauleda et al. (112) discuss the problem of effusive-constrictive pericarditis, an uncommon syndrome characterized by a concomitant tamponade caused by a tense pericardial effusion and constriction caused by the visceral pericardium. The hallmark of this abnormality is persistent elevation of diastolic pressures after the removal of pericardial fluid has returned the intrapericardial pressures to normal. They felt that evolution to persistent constriction was frequent and that the idiopathic form may resolve spontaneously, but that extensive pericardiectomy with particular attention to the extent of involvement of the visceral pericardium was the best treatment in patients requiring surgery. In the surgical patient, special attention should be paid to the extent of visceral pericardial involvement and the need for extensive epicardiectomy.

In order to determine the need for pericardiectomy in tuberculous pericarditis, the following course of action has been promulgated (109). The patient's heart size is monitored by radiography at least every 2 weeks, usually more frequently, and this reading is correlated with determination of right-sided heart pressures. If there is a persistently large heart and decreased cardiac performance supervenes, pericardiectomy is performed. If no change in heart size is observed by the 12th week of therapy, pericardiectomy is recommended. Similarly, if the heart size regresses but the venous pressure rises, the operation is performed. In this situation, extensive epicardiectomy may be needed, with particular attention to the visceral pericardium as described by Sagrista-Sauleda et al. (112).

In patients whose heart size is decreased but in whom elevated venous pressure is stable, careful frequent observation is continued until the venous pressure returns to normal. If heart failure supervenes and/or venous pressure is not normal by the 12th week of therapy, pericardiectomy is performed. Patients whose heart size has decreased but has not reached normal are maintained on antituberculosis chemotherapy and monitored carefully as long as their venous pressure remains normal and they are asymptomatic.

The problem of AIDS has arisen in recent years and has had a great effect on tuberculosis (26, 27, 47, 80). AIDS has been associated with a significant worldwide increase in tuberculosis, especially of the extrapulmonary type (26, 27). Tuberculous pericarditis has not escaped this problem (8, 25, 33, 38, 51, 101, 107, 120). Treatment of *Mycobacterium tuberculosis* in patients with AIDS has appeared to some investigators to be just as effective as in tuberculosis patients without AIDS (6, 28, 47, 79, 100, 124). However, more recent data (58, 91, 106, 141) have challenged that opinion. Gandhi and his associates (58) feel that the most recent reports of HIV infection and drug-resistant tuberculosis in low-income areas of South Africa demonstrate that the epidemic of HIV infection in this area when combined with the severe problem of multidrug-resistant tuberculosis (MDR TB) and extensively drug-resistant tuberculosis has resulted in a severe crisis. They found that the KwaZulu-Natal locale in South Africa was characterized by a high prevalence of HIV infection and a high prevalence of drug-resistant tuberculosis. The mortality rates in patients coinfected with HIV as well as multidrug-resistant tuberculosis (265 patients) or extensively drug-resistant tuberculosis (374 patients) were 71 and 83%, respectively. Many of the deaths in these drug-resistant groups occurred within 30 days of sputum collection. However, it takes 6 to 8 weeks to diagnose drug-resistant tuberculosis by conventional culture and to obtain drug susceptibility testing results. As a result, many of these drug-resistant patients die before a diagnosis of tuberculosis is made, and if they survive, they often merely receive first-line drugs, as the drug susceptibility tests have not yet returned to show which medications will be effective. These authors suggest that there is a great need for a low-cost, rapid point-of-care test that is sensitive in HIV-infected patients and that this test must be able to be used in peripheral health care centers. Other things needed are new rapid tuberculosis assays for drug resistance as well as tests that are sensitive in tubercle bacillus smear-negative settings.

Also important are atypical mycobacteria, particularly of the *Mycobacterium avium-intracellulare* type, which are often poorly responsive to chemotherapy. Of 11 patients reported on by Anderson and Virmanani (6), 2 had *M. avium-intracellulare* as the causative organism.

In recent presentations of tuberculous pericarditis in 185 patients with HIV infections, a number of investigators (91, 106, 141) have questioned the effectiveness of the addition of corticosteroid treatment in the treatment of patients who have tuberculous pericarditis and who are already receiving antituberculosis medication. These patients were from 15 referral hospitals in sub-Saharan Africa (Cameroon, Nigeria, and South Africa). They were enrolled in the Investigation of the Management of Pericarditis in Africa (IMPI Africa) registry. Their diagnosis of HIV infection and tuberculous pericarditis and the treatment of such were at the discretion of the physician who cared for the patient (observational study). Eleven of the 185 (6%) patients were lost to follow-up. The remaining 174 (94%) had complete survival data. Ninety-six (52%) were serologically tested for an HIV infection. Fifty-three (55%) were positive and 43 were negative. Ten (19%) of the 53 received antiretroviral therapy. One hundred two (59%) received corticosteroids together with antituberculosis chemotherapy. The other 43 (41%) received antituberculosis chemotherapy without corticosteroids. The mortality rate in the group who did not receive corticosteroids was 40%, and the mortality rate in the group that did receive corticosteroids was 17%. However, the results of this study when analyzed statistically showed that the use of adjunctive corticosteroids did not have a significant independent effect on survival. The problems with this study are in some ways similar to those of previous studies (62, 122, 129, 131). This study lacks random allocation of patients, whereas others (62, 122, 129) were properly randomized. This study was not adequately powered to assess the effects of corticosteroids in tuberculous pericarditis. Other problems included absence of confirmation of pericardial tuberculosis and a paucity of data to support a diagnosis of tuberculosis and/or HIV infection. This was explained as a lack of funds for HIV serological testing and microbiological testing for tuberculosis in a large number of participants in sub-Saharan Africa as well as in many other poorly industrialized or nonindustrialized nations. The authors stated that there are real-life experiences in many African countries where there are frequent shortages of medication, medical equipment, and often basic medical care. This is unfortunate and should be corrected by economic assistance from affluent nations. However, this does not change the data, which lack scientific rigor.

If one looks closely at the method of treatment of pericardial tuberculosis, it is readily apparent that the majority of investigations in this area lack statistical power to define whether the use of corticosteroids in addition to antituberculosis chemotherapy in pericardial tuberculosis has been definitively proven. It is obvious that further studies are needed particularly with regard to the addition of adjunctive corticosteroids to the management of tuberculous pericarditis. Another form of investigation, namely, pericardioscopy with direct visualization of the area of the pericardium to be biopsied, requires further study in tuberculous pericarditis. Finally, the relationships among tuberculous pericarditis, HIV infection, use of antituberculosis medication, and adjuvant corticosteroids also need further study. The effects of RIF on HIV patients who are receiving highly active antiretroviral therapy are well known and can result in both inadequate antituberculosis drug dosage and toxicity from overdosage or vice versa. Use of corticosteroids in patients receiving inadequate antituberculosis medications could be disastrous. Proper use of pericardiocentesis, use of pericardial windows, need for early pericardiectomy, and use of pericardioscopy with biopsy need to be addressed in a clear succinct manner.

At present, many investigators favor the use of adjunctive corticosteroids in the treatment of tuberculous pericarditis because of the trends that show a decrease in morbidity and mortality with this type of management. They accept the lack of statistical confirmation and controversy with regard to corticosteroid usage but point to the trends in this area which favor adjunctive corticosteroid therapy. Other investigators have a less favorable opinion and are concerned with the effects of adjunctive corticosteroids in patients with HIV because in their area of practice HIV infections are extremely common in patients with tuberculous pericarditis. A major note of caution is important for patients with tuberculous pericarditis on antiretroviral therapy because of the problem with RIF and some antiretroviral drugs. Physicians must be aware that when antiretroviral drugs are used, RIF may be contraindicated in some antituberculosis regimens and that if this is true, another antituberculosis drug(s) should be used as a replacement for RIF or an antiretroviral regimen should be used that does not adversely interact with RIF. If this limitation is realized and steps are taken to avoid it, the addition of corticosteroids to the antituberculosis regimen should be acceptable.

Finally, it is important that future studies in the use of antituberculosis drugs and adjunctive corticosteroids in patients with tuberculous pericarditis be of sufficient size, randomized, well controlled, and double blind. They should include a definitive diagnosis which microbiologically and/or histopathologically demonstrates tuberculosis and that demonstrates HIV infection serologically; also, the evidence

for pericarditis should be clearly defined so that there is no question that the analysis performed is accurate and statistically significant. This is a tall task, but in view of the problem of tuberculous pericarditis, it is a necessary one.

TUBERCULOSIS OF THE AORTA AND MYOCARDIUM

More than 100 patients with tuberculosis of the aorta have been reported (32, 46, 49, 123). About half of these patients experience aneurysmal dilation of the thoracic or abdominal aorta. Most of these patients are diagnosed on postmortem examination. Those with aneurysm formation usually die from rupture and exsanguination.

The mechanism of development of aortic tuberculosis is believed to be via contiguous spread from tuberculous lymph nodes, pulmonary tuberculosis, vertebral tuberculosis, pericardial tuberculosis, pleural tuberculosis, or a combination thereof. Hematogenous spread to the aortic intima or vasa vasorum is thought to be uncommon. The rarity of aortic tuberculosis in patients with miliary tuberculosis seems to support this contention. Tuberculosis usually spreads from a contiguous focus into the aorta, usually creating a false aneurysm. The most frequent complication of these aneurysms is rupture, especially into the gastrointestinal tract.

Whenever signs and symptoms of an aortic aneurysm are present in a patient with active tuberculosis elsewhere in the body, particularly in the thorax, tuberculous aortitis must be considered. Aortography must be performed immediately for an early definitive diagnosis because the arterial wall can necrose rapidly.

Treatment should include antituberculosis drugs. With the diagnosis of an aortic aneurysm, management also involves resection of the aneurysm to prevent rupture.

In an Indian study, a pericardial abscess was reported for 13 patients with pericardial tuberculosis (57). Eleven patients had histologic confirmation, and 4 others had extrapulmonary tuberculosis present in the form of mediastinal or retroperitoneal lymphadenopathy with central necrosis. In the 13 patients there were 15 abscesses. Nine were in the right atrioventricular groove, and 5 were in the left atrioventricular groove. The lesions were demonstrated in these areas by CT scan and/or by MRI. Eight of the 13 responded well to antituberculosis chemotherapy, and 5 needed adjunctive surgery. One patient who presented in New York Heart Association class IV with cardiac failure died on the second postoperative day. A pericardial abscess can occur when the unevenness of the adhesions between the visceral and parietal layers of the pericardium results in loculation of pericardial fluid. If this area contains pus and debris, it is referred to as an abscess. The treatment of these patients includes a partial or complete pericardiectomy with debridement and drainage of the abscess contents.

Another form of cardiovascular tuberculosis that has been reported recently is tuberculosis of the myocardium (10, 14, 63, 110). It has usually been diagnosed postmortem, although with the advent of endomyocardial biopsy, antemortem diagnoses have been made (10). Treatment of myocardial tuberculosis is via antituberculosis chemotherapy.

Unless there is vigilance in seeking out these patients who have tuberculosis and cardiovascular disease, the mortality rate will remain high. Proper management and prevention of complications require early diagnosis as well as early treatment.

REFERENCES

1. **Aggeli, C., C. Pisavos, S. Bril, D. Hasapis, A. Frogpidalo, C. Stenfanodis, and P. Toulouzas.** 2000. Relevance of adenosine deaminase and lysozyme measurements in the diagnosis of tuberculous pericarditis. *Cardiology* **94**:81–85.

2. **Agrawal, S., A. Radhakrishnan, and N. Sinha.** 1990. Echocardiographic demonstration of resolving intrapericardial mass in tuberculous pericarditis. *Int. J. Cardiol.* **26**:240–241.

3. **Alvarez, S., and W. R. McCabe.** 1984. Extrapulmonary tuberculosis revisited. A review of experience of Boston and other hospitals. *Medicine* (Baltimore) **63**:25–55.

4. **Alzeer, A. M., and A. M. Fitzgerald.** 1993. Corticosteroids and tuberculosis: risks and use as adjunct therapy. *Tuber. Lung Dis.* **74**:6–11.

5. **American Thoracic Society/Centers for Disease Control/Infectious Diseases Society of America.** 2003. Treatment of tuberculosis. *Am. J. Respir. Crit. Care Med.* **167**:603–662.

6. **Anderson, D. W., and R. Virmani.** 1990. Progress in pathology: emerging patterns of heart disease in patients with acquired immunodeficiency syndrome. *Hum. Pathol.* **21**:253–259.

7. **Angel, J. H., L. S. Chu, and H. A. Lyons.** 1961. Corticotropin in the treatment of tuberculosis: a controlled study. *Arch. Intern. Med.* **180**:353–369.

8. **Antony, S. J., and D. W. Haas.** 1995. Tuberculous pericarditis in an HIV infected patient. *Scand. J. Infect. Dis.* **27**:411–413.

9. **Aspin, J., and H. O'Hara.** 1958. Steroid-treated tuberculous effusion. *Br. J. Tuberc.* **52**:81–83.

10. **Bali, H. K., S. Wahi, and B. K. Sharma.** 1990. Myocardial tuberculosis presenting as restrictive cardiomyopathy. *Am. Heart J.* **120**:703–706.

11. **Ballabio, C. H., and G. Sala.** 1954. Le indicazione al trattamento locale della pleurite e pericarditiessudatie con idracortisone acetato. *Minerva Med.* **45**:1839–1846.

12. **Barnes, P. F., and M. D. Cave.** 2003. Molecular epidemiology of tuberculosis. *N. Engl. J. Med.* **349**:1149–1156.

13. **Bauer, H., R. Sachs, and M. M. Cummings.** 1956. *Tuberculous Pericarditis among Veterans: Veteran's Administration Transactions of the Fifteenth Conference on Chemotherapy of Tuberculosis*, vol. 15, p. 138. Veteran's Administration, Washington, DC.

14. **Bennett, J. M., D. F. Nande, and A. DeVilliers.** 1989. Recurrence of two myocardial aneurysms infected with tuberculosis after a previous aneurysmectomy. *Clin. Cardiol.* **12**:605–606.

15. **Berger, M., I. Bobak, M. Jelveh, and E. Goldberg.** 1978. Pericardial effusion diagnosed by echocardiography. *Chest* **72**:1744–1779.

16. **Bertolaccini, T., M. Chimenti, and S. Bianchi.** 1993. Gallium-67 scintigraphy in an AIDS patient presenting with tuberculous pericarditis. *J. Nucl. Biol.* **37**:245–248.

17. **Biglino, A., P. Crivelli, E. Concialdi, C. Bolla, and C. Montrucchio.** 2008. Clinical usefulness of ELISPOT assay on pericardial fluid in a case of suspected tuberculous pericarditis. *Infection* **36**:601–604.

18. **Blake, S., S. Bonor, H. O'Neill, P. Hanley, I Drury, M. Flanagan, and J. Garrett.** 1983. Aetiology of chronic constrictive pericarditis. *Br. Heart J.* **50**:273–276.

19. **Blakemore, W. S., M. F. Zinsser, C. K. Kirby, W. B. Whitaker, and J. Johnson.** 1978. Pericardiectomy for relapsing pericarditis and chronic constrictive pericarditis. *J. Thorac. Cardiovasc. Surg.* **39**:26–34.

20. **Braunwald, E.** 2008. Pericardial disease, p. 1489–1495. *In* A. S. Fauci, E. Braunwald, D. J. Kasper, S. L. Hauser, D. L. Longo, J. L. Jameson, and J. Loscalzo (ed.), *Harrison's Principles of Internal Medicine*, 17th ed. McGraw-Hill, New York, NY.

21. **British Tuberculosis Association, Research Committee.** 1963. Trial of corticotropin and prednisone with chemotherapy in pulmonary tuberculosis: a two year radiographic follow-up. *Tubercle* **44**:484–486.

22. **Burgess, L.** 2000. The use of adenosine deaminase and interferon-gamma as diagnostic tools for tuberculous pericarditis. *Chest* **122**:900–905.

23. **Carson, T. J., G. F. Murray, and S. B. Wilcox.** 1974. The role of surgery in tuberculous pericarditis. *Ann. Thorac. Surg.* **17**:163–167.

24. **Cegielski, J. P., B. Devlin, A. J. Morris, J. N. Kitinya, U. P. Pulipaka, L. E. Lema, and L. B. Reller.** 1997. Comparison of PCR, culture, and histology for diagnosis of tuberculous pericarditis. *J. Clin. Microbiol.* **35**:3254–3257.

25. **Cegielski, J. P., J. Lwakatara, C. S. Dukes, L. E. Lema, G. J. Lallinger, J. N. Kitinya, L. B. Reller, and F. Sheriff.** 1994. Tuberculous pericardial effusion associated with and without HIV infection. *Tuber. Lung Dis.* **75**:429–434.

26. **Centers for Disease Control.** 1989. Tuberculosis and human immunodeficiency virus infection: recommendations of the Advisory Committee for the Elimination of Tuberculosis (ACET). *MMWR Morb. Mortal. Wkly. Rep.* **38**:236–238.

27. **Centers for Disease Control.** 1987. Tuberculosis and acquired immunodeficiency syndrome—New York City. *MMWR Morb. Mortal. Wkly. Rep.* **36**:785–795.

28. **Chaisson, R. E., G. F. Schecter, A. Theuer, G. Echenberg, and P. C. Hopewell.** 1987. Tuberculosis in patients with acquired immunodeficiency syndrome: clinical features, response to therapy and survival. *Am. Rev. Respir. Dis.* **136**:570–574.

29. **Cheitlin, M. D., L. J. Serfos, S. S. Sbar, and S. P. Glasser.** 1968. Tuberculous pericarditis: is limited pericardial biopsy sufficient for diagnosis? *Am. Rev. Respir. Dis.* **98**:287–290.

30. **Chen, L. Y., Y. S. Liaw, and H. L. Kao.** 1999. Constrictive pericarditis in patients with tuberculous pericarditis. *J. Formos. Med. Assoc.* **98**:599–605.

31. **Chia, B. I., M. Chod, H. Tan, and B. Ee.** 1984. Echocardiographic abnormalities in tuberculous pericardial effusion. *Am. Heart J.* **107**:1034–1035.

32. **Choudhary, S. K., A. Bhan, S. Talwar, M. Goyal, S. Sharma, and P. Venugopal.** 2001. Tubercular pseudoaneurysm of the aorta. *Ann. Thorac. Surg.* **72**:1239–1244.

33. Coulter, J. B., K. Walsh, S. J. King, and P. Shears. 1996. Tuberculous pericarditis in a child. *J. Infect.* **32:**157–160.

34. Cummings, M. M., P. C. Hudgkins, M. C. Whorton, and W. H. Sheldon. 1952. The influence of cortisone and streptomycin on experimental tuberculosis in the albino rat. *Am. Rev. Tuberc.* **65:**596–602.

35. Dalli, E., A. Quesada, and G. Juan. 1987. Tuberculous pericarditis as the first manifestation of the acquired immunodeficiency syndrome. *Am. Heart J.* **114:**905–906.

36. D'Arcy Hart, P., and R. J. W. Rees. 1950. Enhancing effect of cortisone on tuberculosis in the mouse. *Lancet* **ii:**391–395.

37. Davidson, P. T. 1990. Treating tuberculosis: what drugs, for how long? *Ann. Intern. Med.* **112:**393–395.

38. D'Cruz, I. A., E. E. Sengupta, C. Abrahams, H. K. Reddy, and P. V. Turlipati. 1988. Cardiac involvement including tuberculous pericardial effusion, complicating acquired immunodeficiency syndrome. *Am. Heart J.* **112:**1100–1102.

39. deMiguel, J., J. D. Pedriera, V. Campos, A Perez-Gomez, and J. A. Lorenzo-Porto. 1990. Tuberculous pericarditis and AIDS. *Chest* **97:**1273.

40. Desai, H. N. 1979. Tuberculous pericarditis: a review of 100 cases. *S. Afr. Med. J.* **55:**877–880.

41. Deterling, R. A., Jr., and G. H. Humphreys. 1955. Factors in the etiology of constrictive pericarditis. *Circulation* **12:**30–33.

42. Dooley, D. P., J. L. Carpenter, and S. Rademacher. 1997. Adjunctive corticosteroid therapy for tuberculosis: a critical appraisal of the literature. *Clin. Infect. Dis.* **25:**872–887.

43. Dressler, W. 1959. The post-myocardial infarction syndrome. *Arch. Intern. Med.* **103:**28–42.

44. D'Silva, S. A., Z. M. Nalladaru, D. B. Dalvi, P. A. Ksle, and A. G. Tendolkar. 1992. MRI as a guide to surgical approach in tuberculous pericardial abscess. *Scand. J. Thorac. Cardiovasc. Surg.* **26:**229–231.

45. Ebert, R. H. 1952. In vivo observation of the effect of cortisone in experimental tuberculosis, using the rabbit ear chamber technique. *Am. Rev. Tuberc.* **65:**64–74.

46. Efredmidis, S. C., S. Lakshmanan, and J. T. Hsu. 1979. Tuberculous aortitis: a rare cause of mycotic aneurysm of the aorta. *Am. J. Roentgenol.* **127:**859–861.

47. Ellner, J. J. 1990. Tuberculosis in the time of AIDS: the facts and the message. *Chest* **98:**1051–1052.

48. Endrys, J., M. Simo, M. Z. Shafie, B. Uthaman, Y Kiwan, T. Chugh, S. M. Ali, K. Spacek, A. M. Yousef, and G. Cheridin. 1988. New non-surgical technique for multiple pericardial biopsies. *Cath. Cardiovasc. Dig.* **12:**92–94.

49. Estrera, A. S., M. R. Platt, and L. J. Mills. 1979. Tuberculous aneurysms of the descending aorta. *Chest* **75:**386–388.

50. Felson, B., T. Akers, G. Hall, J. T. Schreiber, R. E. Greene, and C. S. Pedrosa. 1977. Mycotic tuberculous aneursym of the thoracic aorta. *JAMA* **237:**1104–1108.

51. Flora, G. S., T. Modilevsky, A. Antoniskis, and P. F. Barnes. 1990. Undiagnosed tuberculosis in patients with human immunodeficiency virus infection. *Chest* **98:**1056–1059.

52. Fowler, N. O., and G. T. Manitsas. 1973. Infectious pericarditis. *Prog. Cardiovasc. Dis.* **16:**323–336.

53. Fowler, N. O. 1985. *The Pericardium in Health and Disease.* Futura, Mount Kisco, NY.

54. Fowler, N. O. 1991. Tuberculous pericarditis. *JAMA* **266:**99–103.

55. Fredriksen, R. T., L. S. Cohen, and C. B. Mullins. 1971. Pericardial windows or pericardiocentesis for pericardial effusions. *Am. Heart J.* **82:**158–162.

56. Freedberg, C. K. 1966. Pericardial disease, p. 956. *In* C. K. Freedberg (ed.), *Diseases of the Heart*, 3rd ed. W. B. Saunders, Philadelphia, PA.

57. Galati, G., and S. Sharma. 2004. Pericardial abscess occurring after tuberculous pericarditis: image morphology on computed tomography and magnetic resonance imaging. *Clin. Radiol.* **59:**514–519.

58. Gandhi, N. R., N. S. Shah, J. R. Andrews, V. Vella, A. P. Moll, M. Scott, D. Weissman, C. Marra, U. G. Laloo, and G. H. Freidland on behalf of the Tugela Ferry Care and Research (FT CARES) Collaboration. 2010. HIV coinfection in multidrug- and extensively drug-resistant tuberculosis results in high mortality. *Am. J. Respir. Crit. Care Med.* **181:**80–86.

59. Girling, D. J., J. H. Darbyshire, M. J. Humphries, Sr., and J. Mahoney. 1988. Extrapulmonary tuberculosis. *Br. Med. Bull.* **44:**738–756.

60. Haase, D., T. J. Marrie, R. Martin, and O. Hayne. 1981. Gallium scanning in tuberculous pericarditis. *Clin. Nucl. Med.* **6:**275.

61. Hageman, J. H., N. H. D'Esopo, and W. W. Glenn. 1964. Tuberculosis of the pericardium: a long-term analysis of forty-four proved cases. *N. Engl. J. Med.* **270:**327–332.

62. Hakim, J. G., J. Ternouth, E. Mushangi, S. Siziya, V. Robertson, and A. Malin. 2000. Double blind randomized placebo-controlled trial of adjunctive prednisolone in treatment of effusive tuberculous pericarditis in HIV seropositive persons. *Heart* **84:**183–188.

63. Halim, M. A., E. M. Mercer, and G. A. Guinn. 1985. Myocardial tuberculoma with rupture and pseudoaneurysm formation—successful surgical treatment. *Br. Heart J.* **54:**603–604.

64. Harris, L. F. 1987. Tuberculous pericarditis, a unique experience. *Ala. Med.* **57:**16–23.

65. Hatcher, C. R., Jr., R. B. Logue, W. D. Logan, P. N. Symbas, K. A. Masour, and O. A. Abbott. 1971. Pericardiectomy for recurrent pericarditis. *J. Thorac. Cardiovasc. Surg.* **62:**371–378.

66. Inoue, T., K. Iga, K. Hori, T. Matsumara, H. Gen, Y. Kohri, and T. Iwata. 1993. Tuberculous pericarditis: importance of adenosine deaminase activity in pericardial fluid. *Intern. Med.* **32:**675–677.

67. Isaka, N., R. Tanaka, M. Nakamura M, M. Sugausa, T. Konishi, and T. Nakano. 1990. A case of tuberculous pericarditis—use of adenosine deaminase activity (ADA) in early diagnosis. *Heart Vessels* **5:**247–248.

68. Koh, K. K., E. J. Kim, C. H. Cho, H. Chul, M. J. Choi, S. K. Cho, S. S. Kim, C. J. Lee, S. H. Jin, J. M. Kim, H. S. Nam, and Y. H. Lee. 1994. Adenosine deaminase and carcinoembryonic antigen in pericardial effusion diagnosis, especially in tuberculous pericarditis. *Circulation* **89:**2728–2735.

69. Komsuoglu, B., O. Goldeli, K. K. Kulan, and S. S. Komsuoglu. 1995. The diagnostic and prognostic value of adenosine deaminase in tuberculous pericarditis. *Eur. Heart J.* **16:**1126–1130.

70. Kramer, F., T. Modilevsky, A. R. Waliany, J. M. Leedman, and P. F. Barnes. 1990. Delayed diagnosis of tuberculosis in patient with human immunodeficiency virus. *Am. J. Med.* **89:**451–456.

71. Kwan, T., M. M. Karve, and O. Emerole. 1993. Cardiac tamponade in patients infected with HIV. *Chest* **104:**1059–1062.

72. Larrieu, A. J., G. F. Tyers, E. H. Williams, and J. R. Derrick. 1980. Recent experience with tuberculous pericarditis. *Ann. Thorac. Surg.* **29:**464–468.

73. Lazarus, A., and B. Thiagar. 2007. Tuberculosis of pericardium, larynx, and other uncommon sites. *Dis. Mon.* **53:**46–54.

74. Lee, J. H., C. W. Lee, S. G. Lee, H. S. Yang, M. K. Hong, J. J. Kim, S. W. Park, and H. S. Chi, and S. J. Park. 2002. Comparison of polymerase chain reaction with adenosine deaminase activity in pericardial fluid for the diagnosis of tuberculous pericarditis. *Am. J. Med.* **113:**519–521.

75. Legrand, R., M. Linquette, and J. Desruelles. 1954. A propos de deux cas de pericardite tuberculeuse traités par la cortisone. *France Med.* **17:**37–38.

76. Lin, D. S., and R. E. Tipton. 1983. Ga-67 cardiac uptake. *Clin. Nucl. Med.* 8:603–604.

77. Liu, P., Y. Li, W. Tsai, Tsai, T. Chao, Y. Yung, and J. Chen. 2001. Usefulness of echocardiographic intrapericardial abnormalities in the diagnosis of tuberculous pericardial effusion. *Am. J. Cardiol.* 87:1133–1135.

78. Long, R., M. Younes, N. Patton, and E. Hershfield. 1989. Tuberculous pericarditis: long-term outcome in patients who received medical therapy alone. *Am. Heart J.* 117:1133–1139.

79. Louie, E., L. B. Rich, and R. S. Holzman. 1987. Tuberculosis in non-Haitian patients with acquired immunodeficiency syndrome in a New York City Hospital. *Chest* 91:176–180.

80. Mann, J., D. E. Snider, A. Francis, T. C. Quinn, R. L. Colebunders, P. Piot, J. W. Curren, N. Nzilambi, N. Basenga, and M. Malonga. 1986. Association between HTLV-III/LAV infection and tuberculosis in Zaire. *JAMA* 256:346.

81. Martin, R. P., R. Bowden, K. Filly, and R. L. Popp. 1980. Intrapericardial abnormalities in patients with pericardial effusion: findings by two-dimensional echocardiography. *Circulation* 61:568–572.

82. Martin, R. P., H. Rakowski, J. French, and R. L. Popp. 1978. Localization of pericardial effusion with wide-angle phase array echocardiography. *Am. J. Cardiol.* 42:904–905.

83. Martinez-Vazquez, J. M., E. Ribera, I. Ocana, R. M. Segura, R. Serrat, and J. Sagrista. 1986. Adenosine deaminase activity in tuberculous pericarditis. *Thorax* 41:888–889.

84. Martinez-Vazquez, J. M., I. Ocana, and E. Ribera. 1984. Diagnostico temprano de la tuberculosis pleuroperitoneal mediante to determinacion de adenosina desaminasa. *Med. Clin.* (Barcelona) 83:578–580.

85. Mathur, K. S., R. Prasad, and J. S. Mathur. 1960. Intrapleural cortisone in tuberculous pleural effusion. *Tubercle* 41:358–362.

86. Mayosi, B., L. Burgess, and A. Doubell. 2005. Tuberculous pericarditis. *Circulation* 112:3608–3616.

87. Mayosi, B. M. 2002. Interventions for treating tuberculous pericarditis. *Cochrane Database Syst. Rev.* 4:CD000526.

88. Mayosi, B. M., C. S. Wiysonge, M. Ntsekhe, F. Gumedze, J. A. Volmink, G. A. Maartens, A. Aje, B. M. Thomas, K. M. Thomas, A. A. Awotedu, B. Thembela, P. Mntla, F. Maritz, K. N. Blackett, D. C. Knowonlack, V. C. Burch, K. Rebe, A. Parrish, K. Sliwa, B. Z. Vezi, N. Alam, B. G. Brown, T. Gould, T. Visser, N. P. Magula, and J. Patrick. 2008. Mortality in patients treated for tuberculous pericarditis in sub-Saharan Africa. *S. Afr. J. Med.* 98:36–40.

89. Miller, J. I., K. A. Mansour, and C. R. Hatcher, Jr. 1982. Pericardiectomy: current indications, concepts and results in a university setting. *Ann. Thorac. Surg.* 34:140–145.

90. Ntsekhe, M., C. Wiysonge, J. A. Volmink, P. J. Commerford, and B. M. Mayosi. 2003. Adjuvant corticosteroids for tuberculous pericarditis. *Q. J. Med.* 96:593–599.

91. Ntsekhe, M., and J. Hakim. 2005. Impact of human immunodeficiency virus infection on cardiovascular disease in Africa. *Circulation* 105:3602–3607.

92. Ocana, I., J. M. Martinez-Vazquez, R. M. Segura, T. Fernandez-Dasilla, and J. A. Capdevila. 1983. Adenosine deaminase in pleural fluids: test for diagnosis of tuberculous pleural effusion. *Chest* 84:51–53.

93. Ortbals, D. W., and L. V. Avioli. 1979. Tuberculous pericarditis. *Arch. Intern. Med.* 139:231–234.

94. Paley, S. S., J. P. Mihaly, E. L. Mais, S. A. Gittens, and B. Lupini. 1959. Prednisone in the treatment of tuberculous effusions. *Am. Rev. Tuberc.* 79:307–314.

95. Pedro-Botet, J., T. Auguet, J. Coll, J. S. Poris, and J. Rabies-Prat. 1993. Tuberculous pericarditis as the first manifestation of AIDS. *Infection* 21:334–335.

96. Permanyer, G., J. Sagrista-Sauleda, and J. Soler-Soler. 1985. Primary acute pericardial disease: a prospective study of 231 consecutive patients. *Am. J. Cardiol.* 56:623–630.

97. Petersson, T., K. Ojala, and T. H. Weber. 1984. Adenosine deaminase in the diagnosis of pleural effusion. *Acta Med. Scand.* 215:299–304.

98. Piras, M. A., and C. Gakis. 1973. Cerebrospinal fluid adenosine deaminase activity in tuberculous meningitis. *Enzyme* 14:314–317.

99. Piras, M. A., C. Gakis, A. Budroni, and G. Andreoni. 1978. Adenosine deaminase activity in pleural effusions: an aid to differential diagnosis. *Br. Med. J.* 2:1751–1752.

100. Pitchenik, A. E., J. Burr, M. Suarez, D. Fertel, G. Gonzalaz, and C. Moas. 1987. Human lymphotrophic T-cell virus-III (HTLV-III) seropositivity and related disease among 71 consecutive patients in whom tuberculosis was diagnosed. A prospective study. *Am. Rev. Respir. Dis.* 135:875–879.

101. Posniak, A. L., J. Weinberg, M. Mahari, P. Niell, B. Houston, and A. Latif. 1994. Tuberculous pericardial effusion associated with HIV infection: a sign of disseminated disease. *Tuber. Lung Dis.* 75:297–300.

102. Quale, J. M., G. Y. Lipschik, and A. E. Heurich. 1987. Management of tuberculous pericarditis. *Ann. Thorac. Surg.* 43:653–655.

103. Ragan, C., E. L. Howes, and C. M. Plotz. 1949. Effect of cortisone on production of granulation tissue in the rabbit. *Proc. Soc. Exp. Biol. Med.* 72:718–721.

104. Reuter, H., L. Burgess, W. van Wuuren, and A. Doubell. 2006. Diagnosing tuberculous pericarditis. *Q. J. Med.* 99:827–839.

105. Reuter, H., L. Burgess, V. Schneider, W. van Vuuren, and A. Doubell. 2006. The role of histopathology in establishing the diagnosis of tuberculous pericardial effusions in the presence of HIV. *Histopathology* 48:295–302.

106. Reuter, H. 2008. Tuberculous pericarditis and HIV infection in Africa. *S. Afr. J. Med.* 98:29–30.

107. Richter, C., B. Nodosi, A. S. Mwammy, and R. K. Mbwambo. 1991. Extrapulmonary tuberculosis—a simple diagnosis? A retrospective study at Dar es Salaam, Tanzania. *Trop. Geogr. Med.* 43:375–378.

108. Rieder, H. L., G. M. Cauthen, A. B. Block, C. H. Cole, D. Holtzman, D. E. Snider, W. J. Bigler, and J. J. Wittle. 1989. Tuberculosis and acquired immunodeficiency syndrome—Florida. *Arch. Intern. Med.* 149:1268–1273.

109. Rooney, J. J., J. A. Crocco, and H. A. Lyons. 1970. Tuberculous pericarditis. *Ann. Intern. Med.* 72:73–78.

110. Rose, A. G. 1987. Cardiac tuberculosis: a study of 19 patients. *Arch. Pathol. Lab. Med.* 111:422–426.

111. Sagrista-Sauleda, J., J. Angel, G. Permanyer-Miralda, and J. Soler-Soler. 1999. Long-term follow-up of idiopathic pericardial effusion. *N. Engl. J. Med.* 341:2054–2059.

112. Sagrista-Sauleda, J., J. Angel, A. Sanchez, and G. Permanyer-Miralda. 2004. Effusive constrictive pericarditis. *N. Engl. J. Med.* 350:469–475.

113. Sagrista-Sauleda, J., G. Permanyer-Mirald, and J. Soler-Soler. 1988. Tuberculous pericarditis: ten year experience with a prospective protocol for diagnosis and treatment. *J. Am. Coll. Cardiol.* 11:724–728.

114. Scannell, J. G. 1959. Surgical treatment of tuberculous pericarditis, p. 7–59. *In* A. A. Luisada (ed.), *Cardiology, an Encyclopedia of the Cardiovascular System*, vol. 3. McGraw-Hill, New York, NY.

115. Scannell, J. G., G. S. Meyers, and A. L. Friedlich. 1952. Significance of pulmonary hypertension in constrictive pericarditis. *Surgery* 32:184–194.

116. Schepers, G. H. W. 1962. Tuberculous pericarditis. *Am. J. Cardiol.* 9:248–276.

117. Schlossberg, D., and T. Aaron. 1991. Aortitis caused by *Mycobacterium fortuitum*. *Arch. Intern. Med.* 151:1010–1011.

118. Schwartz, M. J., H. R. May, and H. F. Fitzpatrick. 1963. Pericardial biopsy. *Arch. Intern. Med.* 112:917–923.

119. Seferovic, P., A. Ristic, A. Maksimovic, V. Tatu, M. Ostojic, and V. Kanjuth. 2003. Diagnostic value of pericardial biopsy: improvement with extensive sampling enabled by pericardioscopy. *Circulation* 107:978–983.

120. Serrano-Heranz, R., A. Camino, I. Vilacosta, A. Lopez-Castelanos, and V. Roca. 1995. Tuberculous tamponade and AIDS. *Eur. Heart J.* 16:430–432.

121. Shafer, R. W., D. S. Kim, J. P. Weiss, and J. Quale. 1991. Extrapulmonary tuberculosis in patients with human immunodeficiency virus infection. *Medicine* (Baltimore) 70:384–397.

122. Shrire, V. 1959. Experimental pericarditis at Groote Schuur Hospital, Cape Town: an analysis of 160 cases over a 6 year period. *S. Afr. J. Med.* 33:810–817.

123. Silbergleit, A., A. Arbulu, B. A. Defever, and E. G. Nedwicki. 1975. Tuberculous aortitis: surgical resection of an abdominal false aneurysm. *JAMA* 193:331–333.

124. Snider, D. E., P. C. Hopewell, and J. Mills. 1987. Mycobacterioses and the acquired immunodeficiency syndrome: a joint position paper of the American Thoracic Society and the Centers for Disease Control. *Am. Rev. Respir. Dis.* 136:492–496.

125. Solomon, A., J. Weiss, D. Stern, and E. Barmier. 1983. Computerized tomography in pericardial disease. *Heart Lung* 12:513–515.

126. Sonnenberg, F. A., and S. G. Parker. 1986. Elective pericardiectomy for tuberculous pericarditis: should the snappers be snipped? *Med. Decis. Making* 6:110–123.

127. Spain, D. M., and N. Molomut. 1950. Effects of cortisone on the development of tuberculous lesions in guinea pigs and on their modification by streptomycin therapy. *Am. Rev. Tuberc.* 62:337–344.

128. Spodick, D. H. 2003. Acute cardiac tamponade. *N. Engl. J. Med.* 349:684–690.

129. Strang, J. I. G. 1994. Rapid resolution of tuberculous pericardial effusion with high dose prednisone and anti-tuberculosis chemotherapy. *J. Infect.* 28:251–254.

130. Strang, J. I. G., A. J. Nunn, D. A. Johnson, A. Casbard, D. G. Gibson, and D. J. Girling. 2004. Management of tuberculous constrictive pericarditis and tuberculous pericardial effusion in Transkei: results of 10 years follow-up. *Q. J. Med.* 97:525–535.

131. Strang, J. I. G., H. H. S. Kakaza, D. G. Gibson, B. W. Allen, D. A. Mitchison, D. J. Evans, D. J. Girling, A. J. Nunn, and W. Fox. 1988. Controlled clinical trial of complete open surgical drainage and of prednisone in treatment of tuberculous pericardial effusion in Transkei. *Lancet* ii:759–764.

132. Strang, J. I. G., H. H. H. Kakaza, D. G. Gibson, D. J. Girling, A. J. Nunn, and W. Fox. 1987. Controlled trial of prednisolone as adjunct in treatment of tuberculous pericarditis in Transkei. *Lancet* ii:1418–1422.

133. Suchet, I. B., and T. A. Horowitz. 1992. CT in tuberculous constrictive pericarditis. *J. Comput. Assist. Tomogr.* 16:391–400.

134. Supervia, A., I. Campodarve, M. Shaath, L. Mellibovsky, M. Caldelass, and J. Bruguera. 1993. Tuberculous pericarditis as the first manifestation of AIDS: the indication for diagnostic pericardiocentesis. *Rev. Clin. Esp.* 192:150–151.

135. Syed, F., and B. Mayosi. 2007. A modern approach to tuberculous pericarditis. *Prog. Cardiovasc. Dis.* 50:218–236.

136. Taelman, H., A. Kagame, J. Batungwanayo, A. Nyaribareja, M. Abdel-Aziz, P. Blanche, J. Bogaerts, and P. van de Perve. 1990. Pericardial effusion in HIV infection. *Lancet* 335:924.

137. Tourniaire, A., J. Blum, and G. Gros. 1958. Pericardite tuberculeuse en voie d'organisation symphysaire guerie par l'association medicamenteuse streptomycin-deltacortisone. *Lyon Med.* 90:5–10.

138. Tuon, F., M. Litvoc, and M. Lopes. 2006. Adenosine deaminase and tuberculous pericarditis—a systematic review with meta-analysis. *Acta Trop.* 99:67–74.

139. Voegtlin, R., M. Simler, and R. Hauswald. 1955. Pericardite tuberculeuse aigue: effet de la cortisone. *Strasbourg Med.* 6:242–246.

140. Winkler, M., and C. B. Higgins. 1987. Suspected intracardiac masses: evaluation by MR imaging. *Radiology* 165:117–121.

141. Wiysonge, C., M. Nteshke, F. Gumedze, K. Sliwa, K. Blackett, P. Cummerford, and J. Volmink. 2006. Contemporary use of adjunctive corticosteroids in tuberculous pericarditis. *Int. J. Cardiol.* 124:388–390.

142. Zamurian, M., M. Moktarian, H. Motazedian, A. Monabati, and G. Rezaian. 2007. Constrictive pericarditis: detection of *Mycobacterium tuberculosis* in paraffin-embedded pericardial tissue by polymerase chain reaction. *Clin. Biochem.* 40:355–358.

Tuberculosis and Nontuberculous Mycobacterial Infections, 6th ed.
Edited by David Schlossberg
© 2011 ASM Press, Washington, DC

Chapter 23

Gastrointestinal Tuberculosis

Eric H. Choi and Walter J. Coyle

INTRODUCTION

Intestinal involvement by tuberculosis (TB) remains a prevalent and clinically relevant disease entity in certain areas of the world and in specific at-risk patient populations. Although the most common forms of extrapulmonary TB (EPTB) include lymph node, pleural, disseminated, pericardial, and meningeal TB, gastrointestinal TB is believed to be the next most frequent form (62, 201, 222). Although there is much variability in the prevalence of intestinal TB by geographic location and by the population's risk profile, the true prevalence of the disease is difficult to ascertain because many patients with pulmonary TB may be asymptomatic from their intestinal involvement (8, 103). This requires a very high index of suspicion, as a delay in diagnosis can have detrimental results. When patients do become symptomatic, their presentation may lack any specific signs or symptoms to direct the clinician to intestinal TB; furthermore, as TB can involve any part of the gastrointestinal tract, the manifestations are protean (199).

PATHOGENESIS

Mycobacterial infections of the gastrointestinal tract occur in one of several ways: (i) swallowing of infected sputum in a patient with active pulmonary disease, (ii) hematogenous or lymphatic spread from a distant focus, (iii) direct extension from a contiguous site, or (iv) ingestion of milk products infected with *Mycobacterium bovis* (82). The latter mechanism is rare in the United States and other developed nations due to the pasteurization of milk and tuberculin testing of the herd population, although a United Kingdom study demonstrated that *M. bovis* was responsible for 0.5 to 1.5% of cases of culture-confirmed TB cases from 1990 to 2003 (59). Milk products remain a viable means of mycobacterial infection in some countries, particularly in those cultures in which raw milk is consumed as part of local tradition (8). Ethiopian cattle owners that consumed the raw milk of their cattle were found to be at a >3-fold-greater risk of TB infection than those who consumed boiled milk (69).

Some authors have described two types of enteric TB: a primary form, usually from ingestion of the bovine bacillus, and a secondary form due to spread of the human bacillus from active pulmonary disease (7). As mentioned, the primary form is extremely rare in the United States and, when it does occur, likely represents a reinfection from a previous and no longer apparent focus of TB or from an unrecognized pulmonary infection (82). Only 16 to 30% of patients with intestinal TB have evidence of concurrent active pulmonary disease (70, 76, 82, 186, 191, 199), but this is highly variable and may reflect the rigidity of the criteria used in the studies to make the diagnosis (150, 178). Some studies have suggested that 31 to 50% of patients with smear-positive cavitating pulmonary TB also have tuberculous enteritis with a statistically significant correlation between the severity of lung disease and the likelihood of intestinal involvement (105, 159, 205). The proportion of patients with concurrent pulmonary and intestinal TB may be under-recognized as a result of the asymptomatic nature of intestinal TB, which may proceed unnoticed and resolve with the appropriate treatment of the pulmonary disease (105, 186).

The entire gastrointestinal tract from the esophagus to anus can be involved (44, 126, 174, 212). The ileocecal region is the most common location, affected in 44 to 93% of cases (7, 125, 150). The colon and small bowel alone are the next most frequent sites of infection, and the esophagus and stomach are rarely involved (7, 76). The mycobacteria have a fatty capsule, which resists digestion and interferes with release early in the gastrointestinal tract, explaining the rarity of proximal gastrointestinal lesions (199). The narrow lumen and relative stasis of the ileocecal region allow digestion of the capsule and efficient

Eric H. Choi and Walter J. Coyle • Scripps Clinic Torrey Pines, 10666 N. Torrey Pines Rd., N203, LaJolla, CA 92037.

absorption of the organism. Abundant lymphatic tissue for which the organism has an affinity further enhances infections at this site (96). Once in the submucosa, the bacillus colonizes the Peyer's patches and initiates an inflammatory response, forming granulomas. The tubercles undergo caseous necrosis and release organisms into the lymphatics, allowing migration to regional nodes where further granulomata form. As the tubercles enlarge, the bowel wall becomes markedly thickened and small papillary elevations form in the mucosa. Combined with an associated endarteritis and lymphangitis, the superficial mucosa becomes edematous and circumferentially ulcerated. As the ulcers heal, deposition and contraction of collagen in the submucosa can lead to stricture formation (96, 127, 199). Thus, tuberculous enteritis can be classified grossly as ulcerative, hypertrophic, mixed ulcerohypertrophic, and fibrotic (76, 125). The ulcerative form is more likely to be found in the small intestine and the hypertrophic form in the cecum (32, 199).

EPIDEMIOLOGY AND RISK FACTORS FOR GASTROINTESTINAL TUBERCULOSIS

A recognized clinical entity for centuries, the impact of TB on global health was significantly truncated by specific measures targeting improved living conditions, the increased pasteurization of milk and the widespread distribution of anti-TB medications in the latter part of the 20th century. Although TB was deemed a "rare" disease in United States in the 1960s and 1970s (82), the world has witnessed a recent resurgence of TB, directly related to the rise in human immunodeficiency virus (HIV) prevalence (220). It has been estimated that TB is the leading cause of death in AIDS patients at 11% (54), and in Africa, one-third of HIV patient deaths are attributed to disseminated TB (19, 119, 166). The incidence of EPTB, including gastrointestinal TB, has paralleled this increase in pulmonary TB incidence. Gastrointestinal TB appears to present more frequently and in a more severe form in the HIV-infected population secondary to a deficiency in the host immune response (62).

The prevalence of gastrointestinal TB appears to vary significantly by geography. In North America, gastrointestinal involvement by TB appears to be one of the least prevalent types of extrapulmonary infection (65, 222), whereas it remains a more significant problem in parts of the Middle East, Africa, and Asia. In Saudi Arabia, gastrointestinal TB represented the most common location of EPTB with 15.8% of cases affecting the alimentary tract (8). In a group of Indian AIDS patients, autopsies demonstrated a 14%

prevalence of intestinal TB (110). In more industrialized nations, the prevalence appears to be considerably lower. A retrospective autopsy study in Japan demonstrated a 1.6% prevalence of gastrointestinal TB among patients with a history of active or remote TB infection (198); while in Canada, intestinal TB represented only 4.2% of the cases of extrapulmonary disease (5).

The variability in the prevalence of gastrointestinal TB may, in part, be due to the variable prevalence of TB, lower socioeconomic status, and immunocompromised states in these countries (1, 120). The immunocompromised state includes HIV/AIDS but is also increasingly inclusive of patients under treatment with anti-tumor necrosis factor agents (53, 95, 194) and solid organ transplant patients, such as renal (93, 192, 226), cardiac (227), and liver transplants (80, 118, 148). Because the immunosuppressant agents used in the posttransplant patient target cell-mediated immunity, the response to mycobacterial infections is blunted (80, 148). Studies demonstrate the overall incidence of TB in organ transplant recipients to be 0.35 to 2.3%, with a mortality rate ranging from 0 to 40% (48, 51, 80, 148, 228). Several transplant database studies suggest that renal transplant patients appear to be at a particular risk for pulmonary TB and EPTB, although the absolute numbers of intestinal TB cases were low. A review of 2,333 renal transplantations in southern China revealed 41 cases of TB and 21 cases of EPTB; only one of the 21 cases of EPTB had gastrointestinal involvement (48). A similar Korean study over a 22-year time period demonstrated 78 TB cases of which 24 were EPTB; only 2 of the EPTB cases were intestinal TB cases (153).

Within industrialized nations, an additional risk factor is immigration from a region of high prevalence (105, 125, 127). In the United Kingdom, where there is a low incidence of EPTB, South Asians represented 91% of all the cases of intestinal TB (164). In the United States in 2008, 59% of all new cases of TB were in foreign-born patients and 48.8% of those patients were from Mexico, the Philippines, Vietnam, and India, areas with high endemicity for TB (223). Despite reports of increased cases of abdominal and intestinal TB in the early 1990s (82), current CDC data suggest a continuous downward trend in the incidence of all forms of the disease, both pulmonary and extrapulmonary. Interestingly, although the absolute number of TB and EPTB cases has decreased, the proportion of extrapulmonary cases amongst all cases of TB slightly increased from 16% to 20% between 1993 and 2008 (223).

Several reports indicate that female gender may be an additional risk factor for intestinal TB (58, 135,

216, 225). In Nepal, where 45% of the total population is estimated to be infected with TB, being female was identified as an independent risk factor for EPTB in a retrospective analysis of a single, high-volume referral center (195). This finding is consistent with a French study, which also noted a female predominance for EPTB (43). Interestingly, these results belie the findings of other studies, which demonstrate an equal to slightly greater number of males affected (7, 32, 76, 117, 124, 178, 186, 195, 205, 208). A putative explanation for these differences may exist in cultural differences and varying social norms of certain regions and time periods, which may increase the exposure of one sex to possible tuberculous infections over the other (70).

Age may also play a factor in one's risk for gastrointestinal TB. In Western Nepal, over a 3-year period, more than 40% of the cases of EPTB were found in the population of patients less than 25 years old, while the older than 50 years old cohort represented only 21.7% of the cases of EPTB (195). In these patients, gastrointestinal TB was noted to be the second most common site of TB involvement with 14.8% of cases (195). A U.S. study demonstrated that being under the age of 18 alone was associated with a twofold-increased risk for EPTB (78).

CLINICAL MANIFESTATIONS

Diagnosing gastrointestinal TB is a challenge, as it frequently presents with vague, nonspecific symptoms, and there are no pathognomonic signs for enteric TB (96). It has often been described as presenting in "protean" manifestations (8, 23, 199), and it is very difficult to differentiate from other inflammatory conditions that affect the gastrointestinal tract. Compound the nonspecific presentation of the disease with the relative rarity of intestinal TB, and TB is often not even considered in the differential diagnosis (211, 213). The presentation of gastrointestinal TB often resembles that of other disease entities; case reports of intestinal TB presenting as a mimic of esophageal cancer (114), esophageal ulcers (172), submucosal tumors (94, 133), ulcerated gastric masses (100), linitis plastica (200), colorectal cancer (52, 67, 92), Crohn's disease (109, 113, 187, 219, 229), sarcomas (82), and appendicitis (108, 115, 125) abound in the literature.

Studies have shown that physicians entertained the diagnosis in less than 40% of patients on initial presentation, which resulted in a delay in treatment (31, 178). As a result, the majority of patients present chronically with symptoms present for several weeks to months (134). The longest reported period of symptoms prior to presentation was 15 years (178). Acute and acute-on-chronic presentations are also observed, and in a large case series by Bhansali (32), these were seen 19 and 28% of the time, respectively. A delay in diagnosis and the subsequently delay in treatment can result in significant morbidity and mortality (125). In-hospital mortality alone can be 14%, and overall mortality is 19 to 38% in patients with ileocecal TB, the most common form of intestinal TB (9, 115).

The complications of intestinal TB are diverse and frequently encountered with ample case reports of bleeding (30, 90, 132, 192), luminal obstruction (156, 158), intussusception (141), perforation (25, 52, 74, 180), stricturing disease (3, 4, 11, 57), and fistulae (17, 27, 130, 138). Even a case of chronic inflammatory demyelinating polyneuropathy associated with intestinal tuberculosis has been reported (50).

Patients with gastrointestinal TB can also present asymptomatically. One study from Japan reported a case series of 11 consecutive patients over a 15-year period that were diagnosed with intestinal TB by colonoscopy; only one patient had clinical symptoms of anorexia and weight loss, while the other 10 patients were asymptomatic (176). Similarly, one case report describes a patient with a cavitary lung mass on computed tomography (CT) who underwent a positron emission tomography (PET) scan to rule out lung cancer and was found to have an incidental finding of increased 18F-fluorodeoxyglucose (FDG) activity in the ileocecal area, which on subsequent surgical resection was found to be ileocecal TB (97). Another case series reported that 53% of enteric TB cases were detected unexpectedly during surgery for an unrelated diagnosis (186).

Because TB can affect any part of the gastrointestinal tract, the presenting symptoms will often vary depending on the affected anatomic location of the disease. However, in one Indian study, regardless of the gastrointestinal location of TB involvement, patients most commonly presented with abdominal pain, fever, and weight loss, in order of decreasing frequency (205). These results parallel numerous studies that note abdominal pain as the most common symptom, seen in 70 to 100% patients (7, 32, 61, 70, 76, 124, 134, 150). The pain is usually colicky and intermittent in nature and may represent subacute intestinal obstruction. It is frequently located in the right lower quadrant or periumbilical regions, although it may be retrosternal or epigastric in the rare cases of esophageal or gastric involvement, respectively (61, 70, 94, 100, 200). Anorexia and weight loss are seen in a majority of patients, while symptoms of nausea, vomiting, and fevers are seen in about 40% of patients

Table 1. Symptoms of gastrointestinal tuberculosis

Parameter	Value for study by (reference):									
	Fräki and Peltokallio (71)	Findlay et al. (70)	Al-Bahrani and Al-Saleem (7)	Gilinsky et al. (76)	Palmer et al. (150)	Patel et al. (156)	Zhou and Luo (229)	Leung et al. (115)	Tripathi and Amarapurkar (205)	Weighted avg
No. of subjects	33	52	50	46	42	250	30	22	110	
Abdominal pain (%)	91	81	96	80	100	79	30	82	83	81
Weight loss (%)	55	40	96	83	52	58	93	55	54	62
Fever (%)	39	16	16	50	60	64	37	45	58	51
Nausea and vomiting (%)	36	19	72	50	45			18		42
Diarrhea (%)	42			48		22	30	55	29	29
Constipation (%)	27			20				18		22

(Table 1). A change in bowel habits is encountered in 42 to 76% of affected patients, with diarrhea more common than constipation (7, 61, 76, 115, 134, 156).

On physical exam, an abdominal mass may be palpable; the frequency of this sign encompasses a broad range in the literature, varying from 1.8 to 72% (115, 150, 205, 209). The higher range of abdominal mass frequency may in part be related to the heterogeneity of the literature in separating cases of luminal TB from cases of peritoneal TB involvement, which can often present as an abdominal mass on account of the inflammatory and reactive fibrotic changes within the peritoneum (see chapter 24). A case series involving 173 confirmed cases of luminal TB (excluding cases of peritoneal TB) in India noted that an abdominal mass was noted in only 12% of cases (156). Abdominal distension is also frequently seen in the peritoneal form of disease; however, cases of intestinal TB can present with distension secondary to intestinal obstruction or ileus (141, 156, 158). The presentation of a "doughy" abdomen is a classic presentation, although it is a rare and unreliable physical finding, suggesting intraperitoneal inflammation (8, 117, 134, 168).

The results of laboratory testing frequently reflect a chronic inflammatory process, although examinations of the erythrocyte sedimentation rate and C-reactive protein levels in these patients are usually too nonspecific to be clinically helpful (9, 70). The finding of an elevated erythrocyte sedimentation rate can vary from 19 to 92% (7, 70, 124, 125, 208). Leukocytosis is rare and may signify a complication, such as a perforation (61, 178). Stool testing for occult blood is positive in 28 to 75% of those investigated (76, 178), and anemia can be a common finding, with hemoglobin values ranging from 10 to 11 mg/dl with microcytic indices. Numerous studies report the rate of anemia as ranging from 31 to 70% (32, 70, 76, 208). Hypoalbuminemia occurs in the majority of cases and reflects a combination of malnutrition due

to poor oral intake, malabsorption, and lymphatic disease (70, 76, 117, 134). Alkaline phosphatase levels have been reported to be elevated in some series (55, 132), but it is unclear whether the source of enzyme elevation was liver, intestine, or bone, as fractionation was not performed. In a minority of patients, all laboratory examinations can be normal; one Turkish study noted that 12.8% of their patients with documented gastrointestinal TB had completely normal laboratory test values (208).

The results of skin testing with purified protein derivative (PPD) vary widely with the population studied. For example, only 23% of patients were PPD positive in a series from Saudi Arabia (134), while 72% of patients from the University of Michigan were PPD positive (150). In a case series of 26 pediatric patients with gastrointestinal TB, 88% of the patients had positive PPD skin testing. In addition to the uncertain sensitivity of PPD testing for enteric TB, the specificity is also frequently compromised by a history of previous disease or prior vaccination with *M. bovis* bacillus Calmette-Guérin (BCG).

ESOPHAGUS

The first primary case of esophageal TB was described in 1837 on an autopsy by Denonvilliers (79). Primary TB of the esophagus is a rare occurrence, with most cases in the literature reporting cases of secondary esophageal TB as a result of direct extension of mediastinal or pulmonary TB into the esophagus (66, 125, 170). The rarity of esophageal TB is believed to be secondary to the peristaltic effects of the esophagus to clear contents through into the stomach, the coating of the esophagus with a layer of saliva and mucus as well as the esophagus' protective squamous epithelium (79, 175). In one case series, esophageal TB only constituted one of the cases (0.34%) among the 297 cases of gastrointestinal TB (125).

There are no specific symptoms that suggest esophageal TB. The most commonly reported symptoms are dysphagia, weight loss, anorexia, retrosternal pain, and fever (68, 131, 157, 210), while odynophagia was an infrequent complaint (114). Symptoms of a cough, particularly with eating, may signal the presence of a tracheoesophageal fistula. The most common complications associated with esophageal TB include fistulae (aortoesophageal, tracheoesophageal, and esophagomediastinal), strictures, ulcerations, and perforation (131, 163). Half of the patients with esophageal TB reported by Devarbhavi et al. were found to have an associated esophagotracheal fistula or an esophagomediastinal sinus (61). Massive hematemesis from erosion into the thoracic aorta or from aortoesophageal fistulae has been reported with esophageal hemorrhaging occurring both spontaneously and following the initiation of antituberculous therapy (45, 46, 86, 146).

The endoscopic appearance of esophageal TB is most commonly a mucosal ulceration, although mucosal infiltration by *Mycobacteria* with or without stricture formation is also seen (21, 41, 114, 210). The middle one-third of the esophagus is the most common location for tuberculous involvement (18, 131, 182). In a minority of cases, the focus of TB involvement, presenting as an ulcerative or hypertrophied lesion, is mistakenly identified as a submucosal mass (94) or malignant lesion (114, 131). Intramural pseudodiverticulosis has also been reported in association with primary esophageal TB (207). A recent report of mediastinal-esophageal fistulae formation after endoscopic ultrasound (EUS)–fine-needle aspiration (FNA) of TB of the mediastinum suggests another possible complication after endoscopy in patients with TB (215). When performing an endoscopy on any patient with a suspected case of TB, it is important to protect endoscopic personnel from possible infection by aerosolized *Mycobacteria* by using appropriate respiratory protection.

Radiographic tests can reveal displacement of the esophagus by mediastinal lymph nodes, sinus tracts, and fistulae into the mediastinum or bronchial tree. The mucosal architecture can be evaluated by barium studies, although these findings can be very subtle. The most common finding on barium swallow is extrinsic compression of the esophagus, but traction diverticula, strictures, sinus/fistulous tracts and pseudotumoral mass lesions have been reported (137). CT provides details of esophageal wall thickening and nodal enlargement as well as mediastinal and pulmonary involvement (218). In a case series of 32 patients, chest CT demonstrated mediastinal lymphadenopathy involving 2 or more groups of lymph nodes in 14 patients (137).

The diagnosis and various medical therapies for esophageal TB are discussed in later sections. Medical therapy is generally considered the mainstay of treatment, and surgical therapy is reserved for those individuals with large or nonhealing fistulae, recurrent or massive hemorrhage, or obstruction (28, 88, 112). The first case of successful nonsurgical therapy with anti-TB medications alone as treatment for a tracheoesophageal fistula was in 1976 (217). When fistulae are very large or not responsive to medical therapy, the usual approach is a right thorocotomy with primary resection and closure (112); one series noted a 90% success rate of esophageal fistula closures with medical therapy alone (61). There is limited literature on the use of esophageal or bronchial stents in the setting of esophageal TB (171). Successful placement of an esophageal endoprosthesis was recently reported in a patient who refused surgery (165), although complications of stent migration and resultant esophageal perforation need to be considered (171).

STOMACH

The stomach is a rare site for mycobacterial infections. Earlier literature suggested an incidence of 0.004 to 0.1% in resected specimens and 0.03 to 0.5% in autopsy cases (81, 149, 196); however, more recent literature reports a greater incidence, especially in patients with immunosuppression (40, 82, 150). Gastric lesions are usually associated with concomitant pulmonary or disseminated disease (105), although several reports of sporadic gastric TB exist (12, 100, 101, 116). The relative resistance of the stomach to tuberculous involvement has been attributed to multiple factors, including the low pH, the absence of lymphatic follicles, the integrity of the gastric mucosa, and the rapid emptying process of the stomach (81, 105, 200).

The symptoms of patients are often nonspecific, with reports of primary gastric TB presenting with bleeding (81), fever of unknown origin (173), gastric cancer (101, 147), linitis plastica (200), symptoms of peptic ulcer disease (100), perforation (75, 185), and gastric outlet obstruction (12, 224). Gastric outlet obstruction is believed to be secondary to mycobacterial infiltration, secondary fibrosis, and localized edema in the region of the pyloric outlet (81, 196). As a result, obstruction tends to occur most frequently in the hypertrophic form of gastric TB (2, 167, 200). In one case series from India, 61% of all patients with gastric TB presented with gastric outlet obstruction and another 26% presented with gastrointestinal bleeding (167).

The lesser curvature of the antrum and the pylorus (particularly the posterior wall) are the most frequent locations of tuberculous infection, with fundic involvement being very rare (75, 100). Gastric manifestations of TB include most commonly the ulcerative and hypertrophic subtypes of gastric TB (2). Ulcerations can be single or multiple (100) and are usually superficial, rarely extending beyond the submucosa or muscle layer (200); consequently, perforation is a rare, but reported, sequela of gastric TB (75, 81).

The diagnosis is either suspected or confirmed by histopathologic examination of endoscopic mucosal biopsy specimens, brush cytology, and culture of biopsy specimens (116, 168, 184), although submucosal foci of TB can be difficult to reach with endoscopic biopsy forceps (173). A patient who had a 5-mm prepyloric nodule with negative Ehrlich Ziehl-Neelsen staining and cultures of the biopsy specimens was ultimately diagnosed on the basis of a PCR for *Mycobacterium tuberculosis* complex DNA (29). PCR analysis of gastric aspirates has also been used to confirm the diagnosis with an overall specificity of approximately 85% (202). Antimicrobial treatment is discussed in a later section, but surgery remains an important adjunct to medical therapy. Surgery is usually required for gastric outlet obstruction, and the most common procedures described are gastrojejunostomy or antrectomy with Billroth II reconstruction (2, 149). There is one reported case of successful treatment of outlet obstruction with medical and endoscopic therapy without surgical intervention (81) as well as a report of a subcardiac TB nodule which completely resolved with 12 months of anti-TB medications (116).

SMALL INTESTINE

The small bowel is a frequent site of involvement with gastrointestinal TB. The likelihood of infection increases as one moves distally, with the likelihood of TB involvement in the ileum being three times higher than in the jejunum (32, 105). In India, it has been noted that among 173 cases of confirmed gastrointestinal TB, only 2% of cases involved the duodenum, whereas the ileocecal region was involved 49% of the time (156). A study from New York City in the early 1990s demonstrated duodenal involvement by TB to be 0.3%, whereas jejunoileal and ileocecal involvement were 35 and 42%, respectively (82). A rare case of isolated TB of the ampulla of Vater masquerading as a periampullary carcinoma has been reported (204). Although the ileum is usually involved in conjunction with the cecum, isolated ileal involvement is

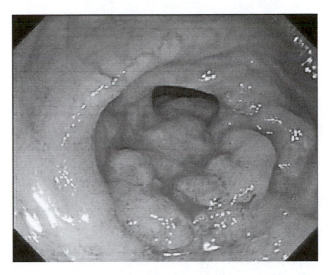

Figure 1. Endoscopic image of tuberculous involvement of the ileocecal valve and proximal colon. (Courtesy of Si Young Song, Kyung Joo Lee, and Moon Jae Chung.)

observed in up to one-third of cases of small intestinal TB (61, 76, 156).

The presentation of tuberculous enteritis is usually insidious, and when apparent, the clinical symptoms are most likely due to a specific complication (156). Obstruction is the most frequent complication and, in one surgical series, has been described in up to 44% of cases (6). The obstructive process is gradual, and the bowel may adapt to the progressive luminal narrowing (61). When obstruction occurs, it is most frequently in the ileocecal valve (Fig. 1), and on endoscopic view, the ileocecal valve has a patulous appearance with a classic, fish mouth deformity (Fig. 2) (4). Pathologically, tuberculous enteritis typically presents

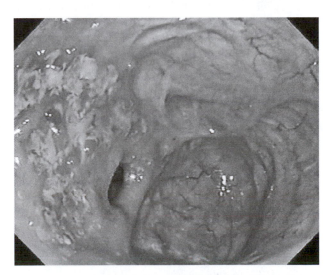

Figure 2. Endoscopic image of a patulous ileocecal valve with a classic, fish mouth deformity and an ascending colon with mucosal erythema and nodularity secondary to TB. (Courtesy of Si Young Song, Kyung Joo Lee, and Moon Jae Chung.)

as either an ulcerative (in the jejunum or ileum) or a hypertrophic (ileocecal) phenotype. Both pathologic morphologies can result in obstructive symptoms. This is attributed not only to circumferential stricturing from secondary fibrotic changes but also due to focal nodular mucosal inflammation and extrinsic compression from adenopathy (38, 62, 168, 179). Strictures can be multiple, with three or more strictures present in 28% of cases (32). Enterolith formation is rare, occurring proximal to a stricture due to intestinal stasis, and suggests a chronic process. The symptoms of obstruction from TB are similar to other causes of intestinal obstruction and include nausea, vomiting, and abdominal pain (38, 158). On physical examination, abdominal distension and signs of hyperperistalsis are universally present, although guarding is usually absent. The finding of abdominal tenderness can be highly variable (32).

Perforation in small intestinal TB is the second most common complication after obstruction. The clinical presentation may be surprisingly nonspecific and variable; however, most reports suggest abdominal pain as the primary symptom in 85 to 100% of cases (32, 64). Although one report of 300 patients demonstrated an incidence of perforation to be 7.6% (32), other reports have noted intestinal perforation secondary to TB involvement to be as high as 25 to 32.7% (77, 205), with mortality after perforation approaching 30% (127). Multiple sites of perforation are not uncommon, occurring in 25 to 40% of the cases; the mortality in this setting appears to be higher, attributable to either an increased burden of intraperitoneal soilage or a more aggressive infection due to a higher degree of host immune deficiency (72, 160, 161). There are multiple reports of perforation in the context of ongoing antituberculous therapy, and the putative mechanism is a dramatic reduction in the intestinal wall inflammation before a sufficient fibrous response, resulting in a compromise in intestinal wall integrity (199).

The clinical scenario of a patient with pulmonary TB, presenting with an acute abdomen or signs of peritonitis, should raise strong concern for a perforated tuberculous ulcer (181). The absence of radiographic evidence of pulmonary disease or pneumoperitoneum does not rule out the diagnosis and should not deter the clinician from further investigation. In fact, in one series of 8 patients with documented perforation from intestinal TB, only 2 patients presented with the classic finding of subdiaphragmatic free air (77). The lack of reliability in this radiographic finding in assessing for perforation in intestinal TB may be due to the fibrotic and adhesive changes associated with the chronic inflammation of intestinal TB, which limits the spread of intraluminal

contents and intraperitoneal air (161). Accordingly, in a series of 28 patients with enteric TB and perforation, it was noted that 23 of the perforations were contained with only 5 demonstrating free leakage into the peritoneum (138).

Life-threatening upper and lower gastrointestinal bleeding from ulceration of the small intestine has been reported but remains an uncommon complication (144, 151, 192). Mucosal ulcerations resulting from inflammatory changes from tuberculous involvement are accompanied by an obliterative endarteritis, which makes hemorrhaging a less likely outcome. However, in areas where TB is endemic, such as India, it appears that despite the rarity of overt gastrointestinal hemorrhaging in developed countries, intestinal TB can be a common etiology for either obscure or overt gastrointestinal bleeding. In one case series from a tertiary hospital in eastern India, among 40 patients presenting for evaluation for obscure gastrointestinal bleeding, 10% of patients had intestinal TB (169). In another case series from India, involving 91 patients with massive gastrointestinal hemorrhaging, 8 patients were found to have ileal TB (14). Fistulae from the small intestine to vascular structures, such as the aorta and mesenteric arteries, are the etiologies of cases of massive gastrointestinal hemorrhage, typically associated with a high mortality (91, 106, 206). Although a case of hemorrhaging from isolated gastric varices secondary to jejunal TB-related splenic vein thrombosis has been documented, it remains a rare presentation (188).

Fistulae are rare occurrences. In two Indian studies, involving 173 and 110 cases of confirmed intestinal TB, there was only one documented case of fistula formation (156, 205). Enterocutaneous fistulae are the most common, followed by enteroenteric and enterocolonic fistulae (138). Fistulae from the duodenum to the biliary tree (10, 47, 130) and from the duodenum to the kidneys (33, 140) have been described. Since fistulae are also seen as a complication of Crohn's disease, their presence in tuberculous enteritis further adds to the complexity in differentiating these two diseases.

Malabsorption is suspected to occur in approximately 20% of cases (1, 31) but is more difficult to diagnose than the aforementioned complications due to a lack of definitive radiologic or surgical findings. Intestinal TB is the second most common cause for malabsorption in South Africa and India (25), and the pathogenesis most likely involves a combination of bacterial overgrowth from stricturing, decreased absorptive surface area secondary to diffuse mucosal ulceration and inflammation, lymphatic congestion, and bypassing of intestinal segments via fistulous tracts (32, 122). Tandon et al. demonstrated that greater rates of malabsorption in intestinal TB occurred in those patients with high-grade intestinal obstruction compared to low-grade or no obstruction (203). Furthermore, when these patients underwent surgical correction of their obstruction, the malabsorption was also corrected. The authors suggest that the concurrence of intestinal obstruction, malabsorption, and bacterial overgrowth point to a "stagnant loop syndrome" in which the luminal obstruction leads to stagnation of luminal contents, causing bacterial overgrowth and subsequently malabsorption (203). Besides causing diarrhea, malabsorption leads to a hypoproteinemic state with a consequently higher rate of postsurgical mortality and subtherapeutic serum levels of antituberculous drugs. One author even recommends using the lack of an expected urine color change with the use of rifampin as a screen for malabsorption in patients with intestinal TB (31).

ILEAL TB VERSUS CROHN'S DISEASE

The clinical dilemma of differentiating ileal TB from Crohn's disease has been a notoriously difficult one. Both disease processes can involve a chronic process of bowel wall inflammation, intermittent luminal obstruction, and fibrostenotic disease. Furthermore, the radiographic, clinical, and pathologic presentation may be identical. The importance in distinguishing the two disease processes is further highlighted because the treatment is vastly different (16, 20). In fact, the immunosuppressant medications used in the treatment of Crohn's disease are potentially toxic medications and may exacerbate intestinal TB (53, 95). Although an empiric trial of anti-TB medications may be initiated before a definitive diagnosis of ileal Crohn's disease is made (154, 190), this strategy inherently results in a delay in treatment in patients who are ultimately diagnosed with Crohn's disease. Although intestinal TB was uncommon in industrialized countries in the past and a similar infrequency in Crohn's disease was seen in developing nations, this has dramatically changed with the emergence of the AIDS epidemic and the rapid trends toward globalization as a result of population shifts from immigration (221). These factors have resulted in a significant overlap in the epidemiology of these two disease entities that was previously not observed, resulting in an increased importance of physicians' abilities to differentiate between ileal Crohn's and TB.

A number of studies have investigated whether the colonoscopic appearance of the intestinal mucosa could differentiate between the two disease processes. On colonoscopy and ileoscopy, intestinal TB and Crohn's colitis can both present with mucosal ulcerations, nodularity, mucosal edema, ileocecal valve and cecal deformity, fibrous bands, strictures, and pseudopolyps in the ileocecal area (11, 128, 187). Studies have investigated whether the disease processes demonstrated any features typical or characteristic of these usual endoscopic findings, which would allow adequate differentiation (123). Studies have described ulcerations in intestinal TB to be more likely to extend in a transverse or circumferential manner, while Crohn's ulcerations were longitudinal in appearance (35, 113, 136, 190). One prospective study, which investigated the colonoscopic findings in patients with nonspecific ulcers in the ileocecum, found the only endoscopic feature with statistical significance in patients to differentiate Crohn's disease from intestinal TB was an aphthous-appearing ulcer, which more likely represented Crohn's disease than intestinal TB in 66.7% versus 22.2% of patients, respectively (154). A Korean study of 88 patients who were diagnosed with either Crohn's or intestinal TB demonstrated that having fewer than 4 segments involved and transverse ulcerations were most suggestive of intestinal TB, while demonstration of anorectal lesions, aphthous ulcers, and longitudinal ulcers were the most statistically significant in predicting a diagnosis of Crohn's disease (113).

COLON

Colonic TB can involve any portion of the large bowel; however, the ileocecal region is the most common site of intestinal involvement, followed by the ascending colon. The sigmoid colon and rectum are less commonly involved (82, 92). Various studies have noted overall colonic involvement to occur in 20 to 33% of cases of intestinal TB (82, 156), and two-thirds of cases are observed in the context of pulmonary disease (49, 176).

Colonic TB can be asymptomatic (176) or present with nonspecific symptoms of acute or chronic abdominal pain, fever, weight loss, diarrhea, nausea, vomiting, and rarely, hematochezia. Endoscopy can assist in the diagnosis by providing not only a pathologic specimen but also characteristic images consistent with colonic TB. Classically on colonoscopy, the appearance of colonic TB is circumferential, white- to yellowish-based ulcers with surrounding inflammation, nodules, and edema (136, 183, 214). Tuberculous colitis has also been described as having multiple small pink nodules with moderate erythema, friability of the surrounding mucosa, pseudopolyposis, and stenoses (Fig. 3) (49, 190, 214). Segmental colitis has been reported in 19 to 26% of patients with colonic TB (35, 39), involving every location throughout the

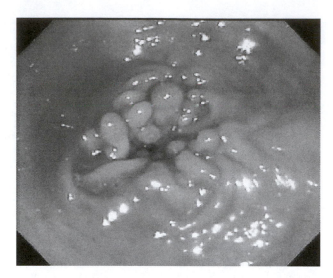

Figure 3. Colonoscopic image of pseudopolyposis and stenosis from TB involvement of the transverse colon. (Courtesy of Si Young Song, Kyung Joo Lee, and Moon Jae Chung.)

colon, including the appendix (3, 108). In the majority of patients with segmental tuberculous colitis, the affected colonic segment was usually solitary and measured 4 to 8 cm (35, 39). A marked hypertrophy of the mucosa along with stenosis due to chronic colonic TB can be easily misdiagnosed as malignancy (52, 67, 181, 190). An even more rare circumstance of coexistent colonic TB and colon carcinoma has been reported (98).

Complications of colonic TB include obstruction, hemorrhage, fistula formation, and perforation (52, 74, 90, 92, 132, 138). Obstruction is the most common complication reported in 15 to 60% of series and has a predilection to occur in short segmental areas with tight stenoses (11, 105, 117, 190, 214). Hemorrhage is unusual and massive bleeding even rarer (14, 143, 162); the low rate of bleeding is believed to be secondary to the obliterative endarteritis caused by the chronic mycobacterial infection. Colonic TB often requires surgical intervention for its complications. In a large surgical series, 58% of colonic TB subjects required either a hemicolectomy or a segmental resection. A fistulotomy was required in 10%, and in an additional 12% of subjects, the surgical procedure played a critical diagnostic role (49).

DIAGNOSIS

The diagnosis of intestinal TB should be considered in anyone with abdominal symptoms from an area where TB is endemic. Patients with a prior exposure or known infection should increase one's clinical suspicion of extrapulmonary disease and be further evaluated if clinical clues point to mucosal

disease. With the increased use of immunosuppressant medications and diseases of immunodeficiency, reactivation of latent TB infection is always a concern and real possibility. Endoscopic evaluation is best facilitated by multiple biopsies, the specimens of which should be sent for histology, acid-fast bacillus (AFB) stain/culture, and PCR (24, 35, 79, 136, 181, 183). Under ideal circumstances, the mucosal biopsy specimens taken during endoscopy would demonstrate AFB or caseous necrosis to enable the diagnosis of intestinal TB; however, the sensitivity of these findings is very low (104, 159). The classic histology of caseating granulomas may not be seen if the endoscopic biopsies are superficial, as the granulomas of intestinal TB may be located in the submucosa, which highlights the importance of multiple deep biopsies to increase diagnostic yield. The concurrent use of AFB staining and histologic findings of caseous necrosis from endoscopic biopsies for diagnosis only marginally increases the sensitivity for intestinal TB. In one retrospective series from Korea, the sensitivity of the findings of caseous necrosis and AFB positivity were only 11.1% and 17.3%, respectively (113). Among 225 patients who were ultimately diagnosed with intestinal TB, only 23.1% of patients had either of the findings (caseous necrosis or AFB positivity) to enable the diagnosis of intestinal TB, and the addition of *Mycobacterium* culture only increased the sensitivity to 38.7%. Despite the low sensitivity of AFB staining, it remains a useful adjunct in clinical practice because of its high specificity, and it should remain an important component of testing with endoscopic biopsy specimens (8).

PCR analyses of mucosal biopsy specimens from endoscopy have been shown to be a valuable tool in improving diagnostic yield with a high specificity of 95% (13). PCR has also been found to be more sensitive than acid-fast stains and culture in diagnosing intestinal TB (15, 29, 73). Some studies have proposed the use of a serologic enzyme-linked immunospot assay, which detects with a specificity of >90% the gamma interferon made in response to exposure to specific mycobacterial tuberculosis antigens, increasing the diagnostic yield in cases when the diagnosis of intestinal TB versus Crohn's disease is uncertain (34, 109, 189).

Radiographic imaging studies usually provide corollary information to prompt further investigation but rarely establish the diagnosis because of the nonspecific signs of intestinal TB. Radiologic findings are rarely pathognomonic for TB but can be suggestive of intestinal TB in the appropriate clinic context and when the clinical suspicion is high. For example, multiple radiographic tests, including barium enema, CT, and magnetic resonance imaging of the abdomen, have been shown to be helpful in aiding in the diagnosis of colonic TB (26, 122). Although many of the findings observed in these tests will be nonspecific for intestinal TB, there are some frequently encountered signs which may suggest intestinal TB, such as ulcerations, nodularity, tumor-like lesions, deformity to the ileocecal region, strictures, and fistulae (8, 142, 156). Barium studies can demonstrate findings of spasm and hypermobility with ileocecal valve deformity and edema, while double-contrast studies frequently reveal ulcerations with elevated margins and linear ulcers arranged perpendicularly to the longitudinal axis of the colon (42, 142). Foci of luminal narrowing can often be appreciated with areas of proximal dilation.

CT scans are now more commonly being used than barium studies (Fig. 4). One study commented that, by using CT, one can increase the yield of differentiating intestinal TB from ileal Crohn's disease: CT provided the correct diagnosis in 81% of cases with a previous indeterminate finding on barium study (121). The most common CT finding was abdominal lymphadenopathy, and several studies noted the finding of abdominal lymphadenopathy in 60 to 88% of patients with documented intestinal TB, most frequently in the parapancreatic, mesenteric, and paracaval lymph nodes (39, 107, 111). The enlarged lymph nodes also frequently presented with findings consistent with caseous necrosis, which on CT manifested as central hypoattenuation. Intestinal TB can also manifest with an asymmetric thickening pattern to the bowel wall on CT scan, which has been suggested as a sign of more severe tuberculous involvement (27, 58). In 2009, one group reported the first case of ileocecal and proximal colonic tuberculosis as examined by CT colonography (virtual colonoscopy) and described circumferential bowel wall thickening with mild enhancement of the intestinal wall, mucosal

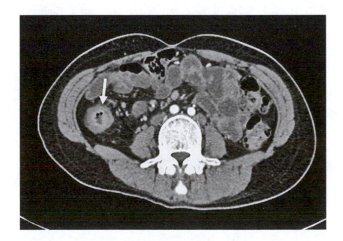

Figure 4. CT scan demonstrating segmental and circumferential wall thickening of the proximal colon due to TB involvement. (Courtesy of Si Young Song, Kyung Joo Lee, and Moon Jae Chung.)

nodularity, edema, and incompetence of the ileocecal valve, as well as an area of circumferential superficial ulceration (102). CT enteroclysis is a particularly useful tool given the propensity of TB to localize in the small intestine. One large study of 265 cases of proven small intestinal TB demonstrated that the most common findings on CT enteroclysis were strictures, adhesions, and ulcers at 62.7, 21.8, and 9.1%, respectively (139). These findings were better defined by CT enteroclysis than barium studies as enteroclysis was found to have the ability to test the distensibility of the small bowel in areas of prestenotic dilatation, where minimal strictures can often be present—a finding not as easily demonstrated by conventional barium follow-through examinations (37, 139).

Magnetic resonance images can also demonstrate caseating granulomas, which on T2-weighted images appear as a hyperdense center surrounded by a hypodense rim (58, 62). PET scans have also been useful in localizing EPTB (145), particularly when there is no pulmonary disease and the clinical suspicion of intestinal TB is low (85). In a case report of an elderly woman, a PET scan was performed for a lung mass and incidentally uncovered an abnormal accumulation of FDG within the ileocecal region, which facilitated the decision to pursue colonoscopic biopsies to confirm the diagnosis of intestinal TB (97).

Endoscopic ultrasound is a modality that has been in practice for over 30 years, which continues to witness an increase in its application. The addition of an ultrasound probe at the distal tip of the endoscope provides it the ability to observe anatomical structures outside the confines of the gastrointestinal tract. Although EUS has been found to be useful in the diagnosis of granulomatous diseases, such as histoplasmosis (177), less is known about its role in intestinal TB. EUS is limited to the upper gastrointestinal tract and the distal colon because the endoscope is a side-viewing device and thus, the passage of the endoscope is not under direct visualization. Upper gastrointestinal tract and rectal TB are significantly rarer than small intestinal TB, and thereby, the rarity of these conditions has limited the description of EUS characteristics and the diagnostic capability of EUS in intestinal TB. One Turkish group described two cases of esophageal TB in which they noted the EUS features of esophageal wall thickening with the concomitant presence of multiple large mediastinal lymph nodes (22). Another key feature was the loss of an ultrasonographic border between the lymph nodes and the adjacent esophageal wall (22, 83). The mediastinal lymph nodes can be round or oval shaped, heterogeneous or homogenously hypoechoic but typically have regular borders with some fine central calcifications (22).

EUS also allows for the acquisition of cytology specimens by FNA, a proven modality for the diagnosis of intestinal TB (84). EUS-FNA holds the theoretical advantage of a higher diagnostic yield than endoscopic brush biopsies because it can access the submucosa and extraintestinal locations of TB, although no studies directly comparing the two modalities have been performed. Other studies have demonstrated the utility of percutaneous FNA, and although this represents a valuable diagnostic tool, EUS-FNA is a less-invasive alternative (56, 87, 89, 129).

TREATMENT

Antituberculous medical therapy is extensively covered elsewhere (see chapter 7). Most experts recommend therapy similar to that used for active pulmonary TB; however, the data on duration of therapy remain controversial. Although some retrospective data have suggested that short-course chemotherapy (6 months duration of antituberculous medications) is sufficient (60), much of the data is gathered from other sites of extrapulmonary involvement and not directly from studies involving cases of intestinal TB (155, 193, 197). As a result, there remains a disinclination among some clinicians to treat gastrointestinal TB with short-course chemotherapy because the clinical response to therapy is often ill-defined (63). One recent prospective trial randomized 90 patients with intestinal TB to either 6 or 9 months of therapy with isoniazid, rifampin, and ethambutol with pyrazinamide during the first 2 months (152). The intention-to-treat analysis revealed that the 6-month therapy was as effective as 9-month therapy in patients with intestinal TB, with the additional benefits of reduced treatment cost and increased compliance.

Surgery is used as an adjunct for significant bleeding, obstruction, abscess formation, and fistulae that are large or refractory to antimicrobial drugs. Although endoscopic balloon dilatation therapy, applied to strictures of the ileocecal valve and the colon from TB involvement, has been reported, there remains a paucity of data on prospective endoscopic therapy in terms of safety and feasibility (4, 36). Both surgery and endoscopic intervention need to be tailored to the specific site of infection and the type of lesion involved.

SUMMARY

Gastrointestinal TB is a fascinating disease which can be observed in both the clinical context of active pulmonary disease and as a primary infection with no pulmonary involvement. It represents a significant clinical challenge because of the recent resurgence of tuberculosis as well as the diagnostic challenges it poses. A high clinical suspicion remains the most powerful tool in an era of medicine when reliance on technology increases. Antimicrobial therapy is the mainstay of therapy, but surgical and endoscopic intervention are frequently required for intestinal TB. Gastrointestinal TB is truly the "great mimic" and continues to require the astute clinical acumen of skillful clinicians to diagnose and treat it.

REFERENCES

1. Abdul-Ghaffar, N. U., T. T. Ramadan, and A. A. Marafie. 1998. Abdominal tuberculosis in Ahmadi, Kuwait: a clinico-pathological review. *Trop. Doct.* **28:**137–139.
2. Agrawal, S., S. V. Shetty, and G. Bakshi. 1999. Primary hypertrophic tuberculosis of the pyloroduodenal area: report of 2 cases. *J. Postgrad. Med.* **45:**10–12.
3. Ahn, S. B., D. S. Han, C. S. Eun, S. Y. Bang, Y. C. Lee, K. N. Rim, Y. G. Lee, and T. Y. Kim. 2007. A case of acute appendicitis due to intestinal stricture after intestinal tuberculosis treatment. *Korean J. Gastroenterol.* **50:**277–279.
4. Akarsu, M., and H. Akpinar. 2007. Endoscopic balloon dilatation applied for the treatment of ileocecal valve stricture caused by tuberculosis. *Dig. Liver Dis.* **39:**597–598.
5. Akgun, Y. 2005. Intestinal and peritoneal tuberculosis: changing trends over 10 years and a review of 80 patients. *Can. J. Surg.* **48:**131–136.
6. Akinoğlu, A., and I. Bilgin. 1988. Tuberculous enteritis and peritonitis. *Can. J. Surg.* **31:**55–58.
7. Al-Bahrani, Z. R., and T. Al-Saleem. 1982. Intestinal tuberculosis in Iraq: a study of 50 cases. *Int. Surg.* **67**(Suppl. 4): 483–485.
8. al Karawi, M. A., A. E. Mohamed, M. I. Yasawy, D. Y. Graham, S. Shariq, A. M. Ahmed, A. al Jumah, and Z. Ghandour. 1995. Protean manifestation of gastrointestinal tuberculosis: report on 130 patients. *J. Clin. Gastroenterol.* **20:**225–232.
9. Almadi, M. A., S. Ghosh, and A. M. Aljebreen. 2009. Differentiating intestinal tuberculosis from Crohn's disease: a diagnostic challenge. *Am. J. Gastroenterol.* **104:**1003–1012.
10. Al Nakib, B., G. S. Jacob, H. Al Liddawi, and J. Commen. 1982. Choledochoduodenal fistula due to tuberculosis. *Endoscopy* **14:**64–65.
11. Alvares, J. F., H. Devarbhavi, P. Makhija, S. Rao, and R. Kottoor. 2005. Clinical, colonoscopic, and histological profile of colonic tuberculosis in a tertiary hospital. *Endoscopy* **37:**351–356.
12. Amarapurkar, D. N., N. D. Patel, and A. D. Amarapurkar. 2003. Primary gastric tuberculosis—report of 5 cases. *BMC Gastroenterol.* **3:**6.
13. Amarapurkar, D. N., N. D. Patel, A. D. Amarapurkar, S. Agal, R. Baigal, and P. Gupte. 2004. Tissue polymerase chain reaction in diagnosis of intestinal tuberculosis and Crohn's disease. *J. Assoc. Physicians India* **52:**863–867.
14. Anand, A. C., P. K. Patnaik, V. P. Bhalla, R. Chaudhary, A. Saha, and V. S. Rana. 2001. Massive lower intestinal bleeding—a decade of experience. *Trop. Gastroenterol.* **22:**131–134.
15. Anand, B. S., F. E. Schneider, F. A. El-Zaatari, R. M. Shawar, J. E. Clarridge, and D. Y. Graham. 1994. Diagnosis of intestinal tuberculosis by polymerase chain reaction on endoscopic biopsy specimens. *Am. J. Gastroenterol.* **89:**2248–2249.

16. **Anand, S. S., and I. C. Pathak.** 1961. Surgical treatment of abdominal tuberculosis with special reference to ileocaecal tuberculosis. A record of one hundred cases treated surgically. *J. Indian Med. Assoc.* **37:**423–429.

17. **Angamuthu, N., and S. A. Olakkengil.** 2003. Coloduodenal fistula: an uncommon sequel of colonic tuberculosis. *Indian J. Gastroenterol.* **22:**231–232.

18. **Annamalai, A., and S. Shreekumar.** 1972. Tuberculosis of the esophagus. *Am. J. Gastroenterol.* **57:**166–168.

19. **Ansari, N. A., A. H. Kombe, T. A. Kenyon, N. M. Hone, J. W. Tappero, S. T. Nyirenda, N. J. Binkin, and S. B. Lucas.** 2002. Pathology and causes of death in a group of 128 predominantly HIV-positive patients in Botswana, 1997-1998. *Int. J. Tuberc. Lung Dis.* **6:**55–63.

20. **API Consensus Expert Committee.** 2006. API TB consensus guidelines 2006: management of pulmonary tuberculosis, extra-pulmonary tuberculosis and tuberculosis in special situations. *J. Assoc. Physicians India* **54:**219–234.

21. **Audouin, J., and J. Poulain.** 1950. Stenosing tuberculosis of the esophagus, apparently primary, cured by esophagectomy. *Arch. Mal. Appar. Dig. Mal. Nutr.* **39:**231–236.

22. **Aydin, A., F. Tekin, O. Ozutemiz, and A. Musoglu.** 2006. Value of endoscopic ultrasonography for diagnosis of esophageal tuberculosis: report of two cases. *Dig. Dis. Sci.* **51:**1673–1676.

23. **Badaoui, E., T. Berney, L. Kaiser, G. Mentha, and P. Morel.** 2000. Surgical presentation of abdominal tuberculosis: a protean disease. *Hepatogastroenterology* **47:**751–755.

24. **Balamurugan, R., S. Venkataraman, K. R. John, and B. S. Ramakrishna.** 2006. PCR amplification of the IS*6110* insertion element of *Mycobacterium tuberculosis* in fecal samples from patients with intestinal tuberculosis. *J. Clin. Microbiol.* **44:**1884–1886.

25. **Bani-Hani, M. G., A. Al-Nowfal, and S. Gould.** 2009. High jejunal perforation complicating tuberculous abdominal cocoon: a rare presentation in immune-competent male patient. *J. Gastrointest. Surg.* **13:**1373–1375.

26. **Bargalló, N., C. Nicolau, P. Luburich, C. Ayuso, C. Cardenal, and F. Gimeno.** 1992. Intestinal tuberculosis in AIDS. *Gastrointest. Radiol.* **17:**115–118.

27. **Barreiros, A. P., B. Braden, C. Schieferstein-Knauer, A. Ignee, and C. F. Dietrich.** 2008. Characteristics of intestinal tuberculosis in ultrasonographic techniques. *Scand. J. Gastroenterol.* **43:**1224–1231.

28. **Bashi, S. A., M. B. Laajam, I. A. Joharjy, and A. K. Abdullah.** 1985. Tuberculous oesophagopulmonary communication: effectiveness of antituberculous chemotherapy. A case report and review of literature. *Digestion* **32:**145–148.

29. **Baylan, O., G. Kilciler, A. Albay, A. Tuzun, O. Kisa, and K. Dagalp.** 2009. Polymerase chain reaction based diagnosis of primary gastric tuberculosis in an 80-year-old woman: a case report and review of the literature. *New Microbiol.* **32:**217–221.

30. **Beppu, K., T. Osada, K. Matsumoto, T. Shibuya, N. Sakamoto, M. Kawabe, A. Nagahara, M. Otaka, T. Ogihara, and S. Watanabe.** 2009. Gastrointestinal tuberculosis as a cause of massive bleeding. *Med. Sci. Monit.* **15:**CS151–CS154.

31. **Bernhard, J. S., G. Bhatia, and C. M. Knauer.** 2000. Gastrointestinal tuberculosis: an eighteen-patient experience and review. *J. Clin. Gastroenterol.* **30:**397–402.

32. **Bhansali, S. K.** 1977. Abdominal tuberculosis. Experiences with 300 cases. *Am. J. Gastroenterol.* **67:**324–337.

33. **Bhargava, B. N., F. S. Mehta, and P. C. Gupta.** 1982. Pyeloduodenal fistula secondary to renal tuberculosis. *J. R. Coll. Surg. Edinb.* **27:**242–243.

34. **Bhargava, D. K., S. Dasarathy, M. D. Shriniwas, A. K. Kushwaha, H. Duphare, and B. M. Kapur.** 1992. Evaluation of enzyme-linked immunosorbent assay using mycobacterial saline-extracted antigen for the serodiagnosis of abdominal tuberculosis. *Am. J. Gastroenterol.* **87:**105–108.

35. **Bhargava, D. K., A. K. Kushwaha, S. Dasarathy, Shriniwas, and P. Chopra.** 1992. Endoscopic diagnosis of segmental colonic tuberculosis. *Gastrointest. Endosc.* **38:**571–574.

36. **Bhasin, D. K., B. C. Sharma, S. Dhavan, A. Sethi, S. K. Sinha, and K. Singh.** 1998. Endoscopic balloon dilation of ileal stricture due to tuberculosis. *Endoscopy* **30:**S44.

37. **Boudiaf, M., A. Jaff, P. Soyer, Y. Bouhnik, L. Hamzi, and R. Rymer.** 2004. Small-bowel diseases: prospective evaluation of multi-detector row helical CT enteroclysis in 107 consecutive patients. *Radiology* **233:**338–344.

38. **Brandt, M. M., P. N. Bogner, and G. A. Franklin.** 2002. Intestinal tuberculosis presenting as a bowel obstruction. *Am. J. Surg.* **183:**290–291.

39. **Breiter, J. R., and J. J. Hajjar.** 1981. Segmental tuberculosis of the colon diagnosed by colonoscopy. *Am. J. Gastroenterol.* **76:**369–373.

40. **Brody, J. M., D. K. Miller, R. K. Zeman, R. S. Klappenbach, M. H. Jaffe, L. R. Clark, S. B. Benjamin, and P. L. Choyke.** 1986. Gastric tuberculosis: a manifestation of acquired immunodeficiency syndrome. *Radiology* **159:**347–348.

41. **Brullet, E., B. Font, M. Rey, A. Ferrer, and A. Nogueras.** 1993. Esophageal tuberculosis: early diagnosis by endoscopy. *Endoscopy* **25:**485.

42. **Burrill, J., C. J. Williams, G. Bain, G. Conder, A. L. Hine, and R. R. Misra.** 2007. Tuberculosis: a radiologic review. *Radiographics* **27:**1255–1273.

43. **Cailhol, J., B. Decludt, and D. Che.** 2005. Sociodemographic factors that contribute to the development of extrapulmonary tuberculosis were identified. *J. Clin. Epidemiol.* **58:**1066–1071.

44. **Candela, F., P. Serrano, J. M. Arriero, A. Teruel, D. Reyes, and R. Calpena.** 1999. Perianal disease of tuberculous origin: report of a case and review of the literature. *Dis. Colon Rectum* **42:**110–112.

45. **Catinella, F. P., and C. F. Kittle.** 1988. Tuberculous esophagitis with aortic aneurysm fistula. *Ann. Thorac. Surg.* **45:**87–88.

46. **Chase, R. A., M. H. Haber, J. C. Pottage, Jr., J. A. Schaffner, C. Miller, and S. Levin.** 1986. Tuberculous esophagitis with erosion into aortic aneurysm. *Arch. Pathol. Lab. Med.* **110:**965–966.

47. **Chaudhary, A., A. Bhan, N. Malik, J. B. Dilawari, and S. K. Khanna.** 1989. Choledocho-duodenal fistula due to tuberculosis. *Indian J. Gastroenterol.* **8:**293–294.

48. **Chen, S. Y., C. X. Wang, L. Z. Chen, J. G. Fei, S. X. Deng, J. Qiu, J. Li, G. O. Chen, H. M. Fu, and C. M. Xie.** 2008. Tuberculosis in southern Chinese renal-transplant recipients. *Clin. Transplant.* **22:**780–784.

49. **Chen, W. S., S. Y. Leu, H. Hsu, J. K. Lin, and T. C. Lin.** 1992. Trend of large bowel tuberculosis and the relation with pulmonary tuberculosis. *Dis. Colon Rectum* **35:**189–192.

50. **Chong, V. H., T. P. Joseph, P. U. Telisinghe, and A. Jalihal.** 2007. Chronic inflammatory demyelinating polyneuropathy associated with intestinal tuberculosis. *J. Microbiol. Immunol. Infect.* **40:**377–380.

51. **Clemente, W. T., L. C. Faria, S. S. Lima, E. G. Vilela, A. S. Lima, L. F. Velloso, M. D. Sanches, and O. L. Cançado.** 2009. Tuberculosis in liver transplant recipients: a single Brazilian center experience. *Transplantation* **87:**397–401.

52. **Cömert, F. B., M. Cömert, C. Külah, O. Taşcilar, G. Numanoğlu, and S. Aydemir.** 2006. Colonic tuberculosis mimicking tumor perforation: a case report and review of the literature. *Dig. Dis. Sci.* **51:**1039–1042.

53. **Cooper, J., B. Flückiger, B. Traichl, P. A. Diener, P. Otto, and J. von Kempis.** 2009. Abdominal pain in a patient with an-

kylosing spondylitis under treatment with infliximab. *J. Clin. Rheumatol.* **15:**244–246.

54. Corbett, E. L., C. J. Watt, N. Walker, D. Maher, B. G. Williams, M. C. Raviglione, and C. Dye. 2003. The growing burden of tuberculosis: global trends and interactions with the HIV epidemic. *Arch. Intern. Med.* **163:**1009–1021.

55. Croker, J., C. O. Record, and J. T. Wright. 1978. Ileo-caecal tuberculosis in immigrants. *Postgrad. Med. J.* **54:**410–412.

56. Das, D. K., C. S. Pant, B. Rath, S. Parkash, T. James, and P. Sodhani. 1993. Fine-needle aspiration diagnosis of intra-thoracic and intra-abdominal lesions: review of experience in the pediatric age group. *Diagn. Cytopathol.* **9:**383–393.

57. Das, K., S. Puri, and A. S. Puri. 2006. Gastrointestinal: multiple colonic strictures caused by tuberculosis. *J. Gastroenterol. Hepatol.* **21:**476.

58. De Backer, A. I., K. J. Mortelé, B. L. De Keulenaer, L. Henckaerts, and L. Verhaert. 2006. CT and MR imaging of gastrointestinal tuberculosis. *JBR-BTR* **89:**190–194.

59. de la Rua-Domenech, R. 2006. Human Mycobacterium bovis infection in the United Kingdom: incidence, risks, control measures and review of the zoonotic aspects of bovine tuberculosis. *Tuberculosis* (Edinburgh) **86:**77–109.

60. Demir, K., A. Okten, S. Kaymakoglu, D. Dincer, F. Besisik, U. Cevikbas, S. Ozdil, G. Bostas, Z. Mungan, and Y. Cakaloglu. 2001. Tuberculous peritonitis - reports of 26 cases, detailing diagnostic and therapeutic problems. *Eur. J. Gastroenterol. Hepatol.* **13:**581–585.

61. Devarbhavi, H. C., J. F. Alvares, and M. Radhikadevi. 2003. Esophageal tuberculosis associated with esophagotracheal or esophagomediastinal fistula: report of 10 cases. *Gastrointest. Endosc.* **57:**588–592.

62. Donoghue, H. D., and J. Holton. 2009. Intestinal tuberculosis. *Curr. Opin. Infect. Dis.* **22:**490–496.

63. Dutt, A. K., D. Moers, and W. W. Stead. 1986. Short-course chemotherapy for pleural tuberculosis. Nine years' experience in routine treatment service. *Chest* **90:**112–116.

64. Eggleston, F. C., M. C. Deodhar, and A. Kumar. 1983. Tuberculous perforation of the bowel - results in 21 cases. *Trop. Gastroenterol.* **4:**164–167.

65. Enarson, D. A., M. J. Ashley, S. Grzybowski, E. Ostapkowicz, and E. Dorken. 1980. Non-respiratory tuberculosis in Canada. Epidemiologic and bacteriologic features. *Am. J. Epidemiol.* **112:**341–351.

66. Eng, J., and S. Sabanathan. 1991. Tuberculosis of the esophagus. *Dig. Dis. Sci.* **36:**536–540.

67. Ergun, M., M. Cindoruk, H. Alagozlu, S. Unal, T. Karakan, and A. Dursun. 2008. Hypertrophic colonic tuberculosis mimicking tumourous mass. *Colorectal Dis.* **10:**735–736.

68. Eroğlu, A., C. Kürkçüoğlu, N. Karaoğlanoğlu, O. Yilmaz, and N. Gürsan. 2002. Esophageal tuberculosis abscess: an unusual cause of dysphagia. *Dis. Esophagus* **15:**93–95.

69. Fetene, T., N. Kebede, and G. Alem. 13 November 2009. Tuberculosis infection in animal and human populations in three districts of western Gojam, Ethiopia. *Zoonoses Public Health.* doi:10.1111/j.1863-2378.2009.01265.x. [Epub ahead of print.]

70. Findlay, J. M., N. V. Addison, D. K. Stevenson, and Z. A. Mirza. 1979. Tuberculosis of the gastrointestinal tract in Bradford, 1967-77. *J. R. Soc. Med.* **72:**587–590.

71. Fräki, O., and P. Peltokallio. 1975. Intestinal and peritoneal tuberculosis: report of two cases. *Dis. Colon Rectum.* **18:**685–693.

72. Friedenberg, K. A., J. O. Draguesku, M. Kiyabu, and J. E. Valenzuela. 1993. Intestinal perforation due to Mycobacterium tuberculosis in HIV-infected individuals: report of two cases. *Am. J. Gastroenterol.* **88:**604–607.

73. Gan, H. T., Y. Q. Chen, Q. Ouyang, H. Bu, and X. Y. Yang. 2002. Differentiation between intestinal tuberculosis and Crohn's disease in endoscopic biopsy specimens by polymerase chain reaction. *Am. J. Gastroenterol.* **97:**1446–1451.

74. García-Díaz, R. A., J. L. Ruiz-Gómez, J. C. Rodríguez-Sanjuan, D. García-Palomo, and M. Gómez-Fleitas. 2006. Perforation of the colon caused by intestinal tuberculosis. *Dis. Colon Rectum.* **49:**927.

75. Geo, S. K., R. Harikumar, T. Varghese, P. Rajan, and K. P. Aravindan. 2005. Isolated tuberculosis of gastric cardia presenting as perforation peritonitis. *Indian J. Gastroenterol.* **24:**227–228.

76. Gilinsky, N. H., I. N. Marks, R. E. Kottler, and S. K. Price. 1983. Abdominal tuberculosis. A 10-year review. *S. Afr. Med. J.* **64:**849–857.

77. Gilinsky, N. H., M. D. Voigt, D. H. Bass, and I. N. Marks. 1986. Tuberculous perforation of the bowel. A report of 8 cases. *S. Afr. Med. J.* **70:**44–46.

78. Gonzalez, O. Y., G. Adams, L. D. Teeter, T. T. Bui, J. M. Musser, and E. A. Graviss. 2003. Extra-pulmonary manifestations in a large metropolitan area with a low incidence of tuberculosis. *Int. J. Tuberc. Lung Dis.* **7:**1178–1185.

79. Gordon, A. H., and J. B. Marshall. 1990. Esophageal tuberculosis: definitive diagnosis by endoscopy. *Am. J. Gastroenterol.* **85:**174–177.

80. Grauhan, O., R. Lohmann, P. Lemmens, N. Schattenfroh, S. Jonas, H. Keck, R. Raakow, J. Langrehr, W. Bechstein, and G. Blumhardt. 1995. Mycobacterial infection after liver transplantation. *Langenbecks Arch. Chir.* **380:**171–175.

81. Gupta, B., S. Mathew, and S. Bhalla. 1990. Pyloric obstruction due to gastric tuberculosis—an endoscopic diagnosis. *Postgrad. Med. J.* **66:**63–65.

82. Horvath, K. D., R. L. Whelan, S. Weinstein, A. L. Basner, S. M. Staugaitis, and E. Greenebaum. 1995. Isolated sigmoid tuberculosis. Report of a case. *Dis. Colon Rectum.* **38:**1327–1330.

83. Huang, S. P., Y. J. Zhao, S. H. Lu, J. L. Cheng, and Y. L. Feng. 2009. Pulmonary miliary tuberculosis and intestinal tuberculosis co-infected with AIDS. *J. Dig. Dis.* **10:**225–227.

84. Hussain, T., A. Salamat, M. A. Farooq, F. Hassan, and M. Hafeez. 2009. Indications for endoscopic ultrasound and diagnosis on fine-needle aspiration and cytology. *J. Coll. Physicians Surg. Pak.* **19:**223–227.

85. Ichikawa, T., H. Takagi, and M. Mori. 2009. Abdominal tuberculosis in the absence of pulmonary involvement shown by 2-[fluorine 18] fluoro-2-deoxy-D-glucose positron emission tomography. *Clin. Gastroenterol. Hepatol.* **7:**A20.

86. Iwamoto, I., Y. Tomita, M. Takasaki, K. Mine, Y. Koga, K. Nabeshima, and Y. Takechi. 1995. Esophagoaortic fistula caused by esophageal tuberculosis: report of a case. *Surg. Today* **25:**381–384.

87. Jain, S., N. Kumar, D. K. Das, and S. K. Jain. 1999. Esophageal tuberculosis. Endoscopic cytology as a diagnostic tool. *Acta Cytol.* **43:**1085–1090.

88. Jain, S. K., S. Jain, M. Jain, and A. Yaduvanshi. 2002. Esophageal tuberculosis: is it so rare? Report of 12 cases and review of the literature. *Am. J. Gastroenterol.* **97:**287–291.

89. Javid, G., G. M. Gulzar, B. Khan, A. Shah, and M. A. Khan. 1999. Percutaneous sonography-guided fine needle aspiration biopsy of colonoscopic biopsy-negative colonic lesions. *Indian J. Gastroenterol.* **18:**146–148.

90. Joshi, M. A., D. Balsarkar, A. Abhyankar, D. G. Pereira, N. Avasare, C. Pradhan, P. Subramanyan, T. T. Changlani, H. L. Deshmukh, R. G. Shirahatti, and B. Biswas. 1998. Massive rectal bleeding due to jejunal and colonic tuberculosis. *Trop. Gastroenterol.* **19:**168–170.

91. Kahn, S. A., and B. S. Kirschner. 2006. Massive intestinal bleeding in a child with superior mesenteric artery aneurysm and gastrointestinal tuberculosis. *J. Pediatr. Gastroenterol. Nutr.* **43:**256–259.

92. Kamani, L., A. Ahmed, M. Shah, S. Hasan, and W. Jafri. 2007. Rectal tuberculosis: the great mimic. *Endoscopy* **39**(Suppl. 1):E227–E228.

93. Kandutsch, S., A. Feix, M. Haas, M. Häfner, G. Sunder-Plassmann, and A. Soleiman. 2004. A rare cause of anemia due to intestinal tuberculosis in a renal transplant recipient. *Clin. Nephrol.* **62:**158–161.

94. Kang, M. J., and S. Y. Yi. 2008. Esophageal tuberculosis presenting as a submucosal tumor. *Clin. Gastroenterol. Hepatol.* **6:**A26.

95. Karagiannis, S., D. Papaioannou, S. Goulas, D. Psilopoulos, and C. Mavrogiannis. 2008. Intestinal tuberculosis in a patient on infliximab treatment. *Gastrointest. Endosc.* **67:**1178–1179.

96. Kasulke, R. J., W. J. Anderson, S. K. Gupta, and M. L. Gliedman. 1981. Primary tuberculous enterocolitis. Report of three cases and review of the literature. *Arch. Surg.* **116:**110–113.

97. Katagiri, Y., S. Hachinohe, and K. Nakajima. 2006. A case of lung tuberculosis which also incidentally found intestinal tuberculosis by 18F-fluorodeoxyglucose-positron emission tomography. *Nippon Shokakibyo Gakkai Zasshi* **103:**420–425.

98. Kaushik, R., R. Sharma, and A. K. Attri. 2003. Coexisting tuberculosis and carcinoma of the colon: a report of two cases and a review of the literature. *Trop. Gastroenterol.* **24:**137–139.

99. Reference deleted.

100. Khan, F. Y., A. AlAni, A. Al-Rikabi, A. Mizrakhshi, M. El-Mudathir Osman. 2008. Primary gastric fundus tuberculosis in immunocompetent patient: a case report and literature review. *Braz. J. Infect. Dis.* **12:**453–455.

101. Kim, S. E., K. N. Shim, S. J. Yoon, S. A. Jung, T. H. Kim, K. Yoo, and H. Moon. 2006. A case of gastric tuberculosis mimicking advanced gastric cancer. *Korean J. Intern. Med.* **21:**62–67.

102. Kim, T. H., J. K. Kim, and J. H. Lee. 2009. Education and imaging. Gastrointestinal: CT colonography in ileocecal tuberculosis. *J. Gastroenterol. Hepatol.* **24:**699.

103. Kim, Y. S., Y. H. Kim, K. M. Lee, J. S. Kim, Y. S. Park, and IBD Study Group of the Korean Association of the Study of Intestinal Diseases. 2009. Diagnostic guideline of intestinal tuberculosis. *Korean J. Gastroenterol.* **53:**177–186.

104. Kirsch, R., M. Pentecost, P. D. M. Hall, D. P. Epstein, G. Watermeyer, and P. W. Friederich. 2006. Role of colonoscopic biopsy in distinguishing between Crohn's disease and intestinal tuberculosis. *J. Clin. Pathol.* **59:**840–844

105. Klimach, O. E., and L. P. Ormerod. 1985. Gastrointestinal tuberculosis: a retrospective review of 109 cases in a district general hospital. *Q. J. Med.* **56:**569–578.

106. Kodaira, Y., T. Shibuya, K. Matsumoto, K. Uchiyama, T. Tenjin, N. Yamada, and S. Tanaka. 1997. Primary aortoduodenal fistula caused by duodenal tuberculosis without an abdominal aortic aneurysm: report of a case. *Surg. Today* **27:**745–748.

107. Koh, D. M., P. R. Burn, G. Mathews, M. Nelson, and J. C. Healy. 2003. Abdominal computed tomographic findings of Mycobacterium tuberculosis and Mycobacterium avium intracellulare infection in HIV seropositive patients. *Can. Assoc. Radiol. J.* **54:**45–50.

108. Kuntanapreeda, K. 2008. Tuberculous appendicitis presenting with lower gastrointestinal hemorrhage—a case report and review of the literature. *J. Med. Assoc. Thai.* **91:**937–942.

109. Lai, C. C., T. C. Lee, C. H. Hsiao, C. H. Liao, C. H. Chou, C. K. Tan, H. P. Wang, and P. R. Hsueh. 2009. Differential diagnosis of Crohn's disease and intestinal tuberculous by enzyme-linked immunospot assay for interferon-gamma. *Am. J. Gastroenterol.* **104:**2121–2122.

110. Lanjewar, D. N., B. S. Anand, R. Genta, M. B. Maheshwari, M. A. Ansari, S. K. Hira, and H. L. DuPont. 1996. Major differences in the spectrum of gastrointestinal infections associated with AIDS in India versus the west: an autopsy study. *Clin. Infect. Dis.* **23:**482–485.

111. Leder, R. A., and V. H. Low. 1995. Tuberculosis of the abdomen. *Radiol. Clin. North Am.* **33:**691–705.

112. Lee, J. H., D. H. Shin, K. W. Kang, S. S. Park, and D. H. Lee. 1992. The medical treatment of a tuberculous tracheo-oesophageal fistula. *Tuber. Lung Dis.* **73:**177–179.

113. Lee, Y. J., S. K. Yang, S. J. Myung, J. S. Byeon, I. G. Park, J. S. Kim, G. H. Lee, H. Y. Jung, W. S. Hong, J. H. Kim, and Y. I. Min. 2004. The usefulness of colonoscopic biopsy in the diagnosis of intestinal tuberculosis and pattern of concomitant extra-intestinal tuberculosis. *Korean J. Gastroenterol.* **44:**153–159.

114. Leung, V. K., W. H. Chan, T. L. Chow, I. S. Luk, T. N. Chau, and T. K. Loke. 2006. Oesophageal tuberculosis mimicking oesophageal carcinoma. *Hong Kong Med. J.* **12:**473–476.

115. Leung, V. K., S. T. Law, C. W. Lam, I. S. Luk, T. N. Chau, T. K. Loke, W. H. Chan, and S. H. Lam. 2006. Intestinal tuberculosis in a regional hospital in Hong Kong: a 10-year experience. *Hong Kong Med. J.* **12:**264–271.

116. Lin, O. S., S. S. Wu, K. T. Yeh, and M. S. Soon. 1999. Isolated gastric tuberculosis of the cardia. *J. Gastroenterol. Hepatol.* **14:**258–261.

117. Lingenfelser, T., J. Zak, I. N. Marks, E. Steyn, J. Halkett, and S. K. Price. 1993. Abdominal tuberculosis: still a potentially lethal disease. *Am. J. Gastroenterol.* **88:**744–750.

118. Lu, W., C. T. Wai, M. Da Costa, P. A. Tambyah, K. Prabhakaran, and K. H. Lee. 2005. Tuberculosis post-liver transplantation: a rare but complicated disease. *Ann. Acad. Med. Singapore* **34:**213–215.

119. Lucas, S. B., A. Hounnou, C. Peacock, A. Beaumel, G. Djomand, J. M. N'Gbichi, K. Yeboue, M. Hondé, M. Diomande, C. Giordano, et al. 1993. The mortality and pathology of HIV infection in a west African city. *AIDS* **7:**1569–1579.

120. Machado, N., C. S. Grant, and E. Scrimgeour. 2001. Abdominal tuberculosis—experience of a University hospital in Oman. *Acta Trop.* **80:**187–190.

121. Makanjuola, D. 1998. Is it Crohn's disease or intestinal tuberculosis? CT analysis. *Eur. J. Radiol.* **28:**55–61.

122. Makanjuola, D., I. al Orainy, R. al Rashid, and K. Murshid. 2004. Radiological evaluation of colonic strictures: impact of dilation on diagnosis. *Endoscopy* **36:**1099–1103.

123. Makharia, G. K., S. Srivastava, P. Das, P. Goswami, U. Singh, M. Tripathi, V. Deo, A. Aggarwal, R. P. Tiwari, V. Sreenivas, and S. D. Gupta. 2010. Clinical, endoscopic, and histological differentiations between Crohn's disease and intestinal tuberculosis. *Am. J. Gastroenterol.* **105:**642–651.

124. Mandal, B. K., and P. F. Schofield. 1977. Abdominal tuberculosis in Britain. *Br. Med. J.* **2:**319.

125. Marshall, J. B. 1993. Tuberculosis of the gastrointestinal tract and peritoneum. *Am. J. Gastroenterol.* **88:**989–999.

126. Mathew, S. 2008. Anal tuberculosis: report of a case and review of literature. *Int. J. Surg.* **6:**e36–e39.

127. McGee, G. S., L. F. Williams, J. Potts, S. Barnwell, and J. L. Sawyers. 1989. Gastrointestinal tuberculosis: resurgence of an old pathogen. *Am. Surg.* **55:**16–20.

128. Misra, S. P., V. Misra, M. Dwivedi, and S. C. Gupta. 1999. Colonic tuberculosis: clinical features, endoscopic appearance and management. *J. Gastroenterol. Hepatol.* **14**:723–729.

129. Misra, S. P., V. Misra, M. Dwivedi, and M. Singh. 1998. Fine-needle aspiration biopsy of colonic masses. *Diagn. Cytopathol.* **19**:330–332.

130. Miyamoto, S., J. Furuse, Y. Maru, H. Tajiri, M. Muto, M. Yoshino. 2001. Duodenal tuberculosis with a choledocho-duodenal fistula. *J. Gastroenterol. Hepatol.* **16**:235–238.

131. Mokoena, T., D. M. Shama, H. Ngakane, and J. V. Bryer. 1992. Oesophageal tuberculosis: a review of eleven cases. *Postgrad. Med. J.* **68**:110–115.

132. Monkemuller, K. E., and J. B. Lewis, Jr. 1996. Massive rectal bleeding from colonic tuberculosis. *Am. J. Gastroenterol.* **91**:1439–1441.

133. Moore, A. R., F. M. Rogers, D. Dietrick, and S. Smith. 2008. Extrapulmonary tuberculosis in pregnancy masquerading as a degenerating leiomyoma. *Obstet. Gynecol.* **111**:550–552.

134. Muneef, M. A., Z. Memish, S. A. Mahmoud, S. A. Sadoon, R. Bannatyne, and Y. Khan. 2001. Tuberculosis in the belly: a review of forty-six cases involving the gastrointestinal tract and peritoneum. *Scand. J. Gastroenterol.* **36**:528–532.

135. Musellim, B., S. Erturan, E. Sonmez Duman, and G. Ongen. 2005. Comparison of extra-pulmonary and pulmonary tuberculosis cases: factors influencing the site of reactivation. *Int. J. Tuberc. Lung Dis.* **9**:1220–1223.

136. Naga, M. I., H. H. Okasha, Z. Ismail, M. El-Fatatry, S. Hassan, and B. E. Monir. 2001. Endoscopic diagnosis of colonic tuberculosis. *Gastrointest. Endosc.* **53**:789–793.

137. Nagi, B., A. Lal, R. Kochhar, D. K. Bhasin, M. Gulati, S. Suri, and K. Singh. 2003. Imaging of esophageal tuberculosis: a review of 23 cases. *Acta Radiol.* **44**:329–333.

138. Nagi, B., A. Lal, R. Kochhar, D. K. Bhasin, B. R. Thapa, and K. Singh. 2002. Perforations and fistulae in gastrointestinal tuberculosis. *Acta Radiol.* **43**:501–506.

139. Nagi, B., K. S. Sodhi, R. Kochhar, D. K. Bhasin, and K. Singh. 2004. Small bowel tuberculosis: enteroclysis findings. *Abdom. Imaging* **29**:335–340.

140. Nair, K. V., C. G. Pai, K. P. Rajagopal, V. N. Bhat, and M. Thomas. 1991. Unusual presentations of duodenal tuberculosis. *Am. J. Gastroenterol.* **86**:756–760.

141. Nakamura, S., K. Yanagihara, K. Izumikawa, M. Seki, H. Kakeya, Y. Yamamoto, Y. Miyazaki, N. Suyama, and S. Kohno. 2008. Severe pulmonary tuberculosis complicating ileocecal intussusception due to intestinal tuberculosis: a case report. *Ann. Clin. Microbiol. Antimicrob.* **7**:16.

142. Nakano, H., E. Jaramillo, M. Watanabe, I. Miyachi, K. Takahama, and M. Itoh. 1992. Intestinal tuberculosis: findings on double-contrast barium enema. *Gastrointest. Radiol.* **17**:108–114.

143. Namisaki, T., H. Yoshiji, M. Fujimoto, H. Kojima, K. Yanase, M. Kitade, Y. Ikenaka, M. Toyohara, J. Yamao, T. Tsujimoto, T. Tsuruzono, H. Kitano, K. Matsumura, Y. Matsumura, and H. Fukui. 2004. Two cases of colonic tuberculosis presenting with massive melena. *Int. J. Clin. Pract.* **58**:1162–1164.

144. Narayani, R. I., and C. Brady III. 2002. GI bleeding from ileocecal Mycobacterium tuberculosis. *Gastrointest. Endosc.* **55**:83.

145. Netherland, N. A., and S. Peter. 2009. Education and imaging. Gastrointestinal: positron emission tomography (PET) in intestinal tuberculosis: masquerading hot spots. *J. Gastroenterol. Hepatol.* **24**:1798–1799.

146. Newman, R. M., P. R. Fleshner, F. E. Lajam, and U. Kim. 1991. Esophageal tuberculosis: a rare presentation with hematemesis. *Am. J. Gastroenterol.* **86**:751–755.

147. Okoro, E. O., and O. F. Komolafe. 1999. Gastric tuberculosis: unusual presentations in two patients. *Clin. Radiol.* **54**:257–259.

148. Ozbülbül, N. I., M. Ozdemir, and N. Turhan. 2008. CT findings in fatal primary intestinal tuberculosis in a liver transplant recipient. *Diagn. Interv. Radiol.* **14**:221–224.

149. Palmer, E. D. 1950. Tuberculosis of the stomach and the stomach in tuberculosis; a review with particular reference to gross pathology and gastroscopic diagnosis. *Am. Rev. Tuberc.* **61**:116–130.

150. Palmer, K. R., D. H. Patil, G. S. Basran, J. F. Riordan, and D. B. Silk. 1985. Abdominal tuberculosis in urban Britain—a common disease. *Gut* **26**:1296–1305.

151. Park, J. K., S. H. Lee, S. G. Kim, H. Y. Kim, J. H. Lee, J. H. Shim, J. S. Kim, H. C. Jung, and I. S. Song. 2005. A case of intestinal tuberculosis presenting massive hematochezia controlled by endoscopic coagulation therapy. *Korean J. Gastroenterol.* **45**:60–63.

152. Park, S. H., S. K. Yang, D. H. Yang, K. J. Kim, S. M. Yoon, J. W. Choe, B. D. Ye, J. S. Byeon, S. J. Myung, and J. H. Kim. 2009. Prospective randomized trial of six-month versus nine-month therapy for intestinal tuberculosis. *Antimicrob. Agents Chemother.* **53**:4167–4171.

153. Park, Y. S., J. Y. Choi, C. H. Cho, K. H. Chang, Y. G. Song, Y. S. Kim, and J. M. Kim. 2004. Clinical outcomes of tuberculosis in renal transplant recipients. *Yonsei Med. J.* **45**:865–872.

154. Park, Y. S., D. W. Jun, S. H. Kim, H. H. Lee, Y. J. Jo, M. H. Song, N. I. Kim, and J. S. Lee. 2008. Colonoscopy evaluation after short-term anti-tuberculosis treatment in nonspecific ulcers on the ileocecal area. *World J. Gastroenterol.* **14**:5051–5058.

155. Parthasarathy, R., K. Sriram, T. Santha, R. Prabhakar, P. R. Somasundaram, and S. Sivasubramanian. 1999. Short-course chemotherapy for tuberculosis of the spine. A comparison between ambulant treatment and radical surgery—ten-year report. *J. Bone Joint Surg. Br.* **81**:464–471.

156. Patel, N., D. Amarapurkar, S. Agal, R. Baijal, P. Kulshrestha, S. Pramanik, and P. Gupte. 2004. Gastrointestinal luminal tuberculosis: establishing the diagnosis. *J. Gastroenterol. Hepatol.* **19**:1240–1246.

157. Peixoto, P. C., P. S. Ministro, A. D. Sadio, E. M. Cancela, R. N. Araújo, J. L. Machado, A. H. Castanheira, A. T. Silva, R. D. Nunes, M. T. Carvalho, and A. F. Caldas. 2009. Esophageal tuberculosis: an unusual cause of dysphagia. *Gastrointest. Endosc.* **69**:1173–1176.

158. Petrosyan, M., and R. J. Mason. 2006. Tuberculous enteritis presenting as small-bowel obstruction. *Clin. Gastroenterol. Hepatol.* **4**:xxiii.

159. Pettengell, K. E., C. Larsen, M. Garb, F. G. Mayet, A. E. Simjee, and D. Pirie. 1990. Gastrointestinal tuberculosis in patients with pulmonary tuberculosis. *Q. J. Med.* **74**:303–308.

160. Porter, J. M., R. J. Snowe, and D. Silver. 1972. Tuberculous enteritis with perforation and abscess formation in childhood. *Surgery* **71**:254–257.

161. Porter, K. A., J. Henson, and F. K. Chong. 1990. Perforated gastrointestinal tuberculosis. *Dig. Dis. Sci.* **35**:1046–1048.

162. Rabkin, D. G., J. M. Caiati, J. A. Allendorf, and M. Treat. 2003. Intractable hematochezia: an unusual presentation of intestinal tuberculosis. *Surgery* **133**:592–593.

163. Ramakantan, R., and P. Shah. 1990. Tuberculous fistulas of the pharynx and esophagus. *Gastrointest. Radiol.* **15**:145–147.

164. Ramesh, J., G. S. Banait, and L. P. Ormerod. 2008. Abdominal tuberculosis in a district general hospital: a retrospective review of 86 cases. *QJM* **101**:189–195.

165. Rämö, O. J., J. A. Salo, J. Isolauri, M. Luostarinen, and S. P. Mattila. 1996. Tuberculous fistula of the esophagus. *Ann. Thorac. Surg.* **62:**1030–1032.

166. Rana, F. S., M. P. Hawken, C. Mwachari, S. M. Bhatt, F. Abdullah, L. W. Ng'ang'a, C. Power, W. A. Githui, J. D. Porter, and S. B. Lucas. 2000. Autopsy study of HIV-1-positive and HIV-1-negative adult medical patients in Nairobi, Kenya. *J. Acquir. Immune Defic. Syndr.* **24:**23–29.

167. Rao, Y. G., G. K. Pande, P. Sahni, and T. K. Chattopadhyay. 2004. Gastroduodenal tuberculosis management guidelines, based on a large experience and a review of the literature. *Can. J. Surg.* **47:**364–368.

168. Rasheed, S., R. Zinicola, D. Watson, A. Bajwa, and P. J. McDonald. 2007. Intra-abdominal and gastrointestinal tuberculosis. *Colorectal Dis.* **9:**773–783.

169. Ray, G., P. K. Banerjee, U. C. Ghoshal, K. Dhar, B. B. Pal, A. D. Biswas, U. Das, M. L. Saha, A. N. Acharya, and S. Majumdar. 2001. Etiology and management of obscure gastrointestinal bleed—an appraisal from eastern India. *Indian J. Gastroenterol.* **20:**90–93.

170. Rosario, M. T., C. L. Raso, and G. M. Comer. 1989. Esophageal tuberculosis. *Dig. Dis. Sci.* **34:**1281–1284.

171. Rosario, P., J. Song, W. Wittenborn, and F. Christian. 1996. Tracheoesophageal fistula in AIDS: stent versus primary repair. *AIDS Patient Care STDS* **10:**334–335.

172. Rövekamp, B. T., K. van der Linde, J. Dees, S. E. Overbeek, M. van Blankenstein, and E. J. Kuipers. 2005. A solitary tuberculous ulcer in the oesophagus. *Eur. J. Gastroenterol. Hepatol.* **17:**435–439.

173. Salpeter, S. R., R. M. Shapiro, and J. D. Gasman. 1991. Gastric tuberculosis presenting as fever of unknown origin. *West. J. Med.* **155:**412–413.

174. Samarasekera, D. N., and P. R. Nanayakkara. 2008. Rectal tuberculosis: a rare cause of recurrent rectal suppuration. *Colorectal Dis.* **10:**846–847.

175. Sathiyasekaran, M., and S. Shivbalan. 2004. Esophageal tuberculosis. *Indian J. Pediatr.* **71:**457–458.

176. Sato, S., K. Yao, T. Yao, R. J. Schlemper, T. Matsui, T. Sakurai, and A. Iwashita. 2004. Colonoscopy in the diagnosis of intestinal tuberculosis in asymptomatic patients. *Gastrointest. Endosc.* **59:**362–368.

177. Savides, T. J., F. G. Gress, L. J. Wheat, S. Ikenberry, and R. H. Hawes. 1995. Dysphagia due to mediastinal granulomas: diagnosis with endoscopic ultrasonography. *Gastroenterology* **109:**366–373.

178. Schulze, K., H. A. Warner, and D. Murray. 1977. Intestinal tuberculosis: experience at a Canadian teaching institution. *Am. J. Med.* **63:**735–745.

179. Schwartz, D. C., and P. R. Pfau. 2003. Multifocal intestinal tuberculosis. *Gastrointest. Endosc.* **58:**100.

180. Sefr, R., P. Rotterová, and J. Konecný. 2001. Perforation peritonitis in primary intestinal tuberculosis. *Dig. Surg.* **18:**475–479.

181. Segal, I., L. O. Tim, J. Mirwis, D. G. Hamilton, and A. Mannell. 1981. Pitfalls in the diagnosis of gastrointestinal tuberculosis. *Am. J. Gastroenterol.* **75:**30–35.

182. Seivewright, N., J. Feehally, and A. C. Wicks. 1984. Primary tuberculosis of the esophagus. *Am. J. Gastroenterol.* **79:**842–843.

183. Shah, S., V. Thomas, M. Mathan, A. Chacko, G. Chandy, B. S. Ramakrishna, and D. D. Rolston. 1992. Colonoscopic study of 50 patients with colonic tuberculosis. *Gut* **33:**347–351.

184. Sharma, B. L., H. Prasad, D. K. Bhasin, and K. Singh. 2000. Gastroduodenal tuberculosis presenting with massive hematemesis in a pregnant woman. *J. Clin. Gastroenterol.* **30:**336.

185. Sharma, D., A. Gupta, B. K. Jain, V. Agrawal, P. Dargan, L. Upreti, and V. Arora. Tuberculous gastric perforation: report of a case. *Surg. Today* **34:**537–541.

186. Sherman, S., J. J. Rohwedder, K. P. Ravikrishnan, and J. G. Weg. 1980. Tuberculous enteritis and peritonitis. Report of 36 general hospital cases. *Arch. Intern. Med.* **140:**506–508.

187. Sibartie, V., W. O. Kirwan, S. O'Mahony, W. Stack, and F. Shanahan. 2007. Intestinal tuberculosis mimicking Crohn's disease: lessons relearned in a new era. *Eur. J. Gastroenterol. Hepatol.* **19:**347–349.

188. Singh, K., S. A. Zargar, D. Bhasin, A. K. Malik, B. Nagi, and S. M. Bose. 1990. Isolated splenic vein thrombosis with natural shunt caused by jejunal tuberculosis. *Trop. Gastroenterol.* **11:**39–43.

189. Singh, V., A. K. Jain, R. K. Lal, V. K. Srivastava, S. Khanna, S. Gupta, and J. P. Gupta. 1990. Serodiagnosis of gut tuberculosis. *J. Assoc. Physicians India* **38:**267–269.

190. Singh, V., P. Kumar, J. Kamal, V. Prakash, K. Vaiphei, and K. Singh. 1996. Clinicocolonoscopic profile of colonic tuberculosis. *Am. J. Gastroenterol.* **91:**565–568.

191. Sircar, S., V. A. Taneja, and U. Kansra. 1996. Epidemiology and clinical presentation of abdominal tuberculosis—a retrospective study. *J. Indian Med. Assoc.* **94:**342–344.

192. Siu, Y. P., M. K. Tong, Y. L. Kwok, K. T. Leung, T. H. Kwan, C. S. Lam, and T. C. Au. 2008. An unusual case of both upper and lower gastrointestinal bleeding in a kidney transplant recipient. *Transpl. Infect. Dis.* **10:**276–279.

193. Skutil, V., J. Varsa, and M. Obsitník. 1985. Six-month chemotherapy for urogenital tuberculosis. *Eur. Urol.* **11:**170–176.

194. Sorrentino, D., C. Avellini, and E. Zearo. 2004. Colonic sarcoidosis, infliximab, and tuberculosis: a cautionary tale. *Inflamm. Bowel Dis.* **10:**438–440.

195. Sreeramareddy, C. T., K. V. Panduru, S. C. Verma, H. S. Joshi, and M. N. Bates. 2008. Comparison of pulmonary and extrapulmonary tuberculosis in Nepal- a hospital-based retrospective study. *BMC Infect. Dis.* **8:**8.

196. Subei, I., B. Attar, G. Schmitt, and H. Levendoglu. 1987. Primary gastric tuberculosis: a case report and literature review. *Am. J. Gastroenterol.* **82:**769–772.

197. Sunakorn, P., S. Pongparit, and S. Wongrung. 1980. Short course chemotherapy in tuberculous meningitis: a pilot trial. *J. Med. Assoc. Thai.* **63:**340–345.

198. Suzuki, H., K. Nagao, and M. Miyazaki. 2002. The current status and problems of the intestinal tuberculosis through a review of the Annual of the Pathological Autopsy Cases in Japan. *Kekkaku* **77:**355–360.

199. Tabrisky, J., R. R. Lindstrom, R. Peters, and R. S. Lachman. 1975. Tuberculous enteritis. Review of a protean disease. *Am. J. Gastroenterol.* **63:**49–57.

200. Talukdar, R., S. Khanna, N. Saikia, and J. C. Vij. 2006. Gastric tuberculosis presenting as linitis plastica: a case report and review of the literature. *Eur. J. Gastroenterol. Hepatol.* **18:**299–303.

201. Tam, C. M., C. C. Leung, K. Noertjojo, S. L. Chan, and M. Chan-Yeung. 2003. Tuberculosis in Hong Kong—patient characteristics and treatment outcome. *Hong Kong Med. J.* **9:**90.

202. Tan, M. F., W. C. Ng, S. H. Chan, and W. C. Tan. 1997. Comparative usefulness of PCR in the detection of Mycobacterium tuberculosis in different clinical specimens. *J. Med. Microbiol.* **46:**164–169.

203. Tandon, R. K., R. Bansal, B. M. Kapur, and Shriniwas. 1980. A study of malabsorption in intestinal tuberculosis: stagnant loop syndrome. *Am. J. Clin. Nutr.* **33:**244–250.

204. Tewari, M., R. R. Mishra, V. Kumar, A. G. Kar, and H. S. Shukla. 2009. Isolated tuberculosis of the ampulla of vater masquerading as periampullary carcinoma: a case report. *JOP* **10**:184–186.

205. Tripathi, P. B., and A. D. Amarapurkar. 2009. Morphological spectrum of gastrointestinal tuberculosis. *Trop. Gastroenterol.* **30**:35–39.

206. Tsai, T. J., H. C. Yu, K. H. Lai, G. H. Lo, P. I. Hsu, and T. Y. Fu. 2008. Primary aortoduodenal fistula caused by tuberculous aortitis presenting as recurrent massive gastrointestinal bleeding. *J. Formos. Med. Assoc.* **107**:77–83.

207. Upadhyay, A. P., R. S. Bhatia, A. Anbarasu, P. Sawant, P. Rathi, and S. A. Nanivadekar. 1996. Esophageal tuberculosis with intramural pseudodiverticulosis. *J. Clin. Gastroenterol.* **22**:38–40.

208. Uygur-Bayramicli, O., G. Dabak, and R. Dabak. 2003. A clinical dilemma: abdominal tuberculosis. *World J. Gastroenterol.* **9**:1098–1101.

209. Uzunkoy, A., M. Harma, and M. Harma. 2004. Diagnosis of abdominal tuberculosis: experience from 11 cases and review of the literature. *World J. Gastroenterol.* **10**:3647–3649.

210. Vahid, B., N. Huda, and A. Esmaili. 2007. An unusual case of dysphagia and chest pain in a non-HIV patient: esophageal tuberculosis. *Am. J. Med.* **120**:e1–e2.

211. Vanderpool, D. M., and J. P. O'Leary. 1988. Primary tuberculous enteritis. *Surg. Gynecol. Obstet.* **167**:167–173.

212. Vanhoenacker, F. M., A. I. De Backer, B. Op de Beeck, M. Maes, R. Van Altena, D. Van Beckevoort, P. Kersemans, and A. M. De Schepper. 2004. Imaging of gastrointestinal and abdominal tuberculosis. *Eur. Radiol.* **14**(Suppl. 3):E103–E115.

213. Veeragandham, R. S., F. P. Lynch, T. G. Canty, D. L. Collins, and W. M. Danker. 1996. Abdominal tuberculosis in children: review of 26 cases. *J. Pediatr. Surg.* **31**:170–175.

214. Villanueva Sáenz, E., P. Martínez Hernández Magro, J. Fernando Alvarez-Tostado Fernández, and M. Valdés Ovalle. 2002. Colonic tuberculosis. *Dig. Dis. Sci.* **47**:2045–2048.

215. von Bartheld, M. B., K. W. van Kralingen, R. A. Veenendaal, L. N. Willems, K. F. Rabe, and J. T. Annema. 2010. Mediastinal-esophageal fistulae after EUS-FNA of tuberculosis of the mediastinum. *Gastrointest. Endosc.* **71**:210–212.

216. Wig, K. L., N. L. Chitkara, S. P. Gupta, K. Kishore, and R. L. Manchanda. 1961. Ileocecal tuberculosis with particular reference to isolation of Mycobacterium tuberculosis. With a note on its relation to regional ileitis (Crohn's disease). *Am. Rev. Respir. Dis.* **84**:169–178.

217. Wigley, F. M., H. W. Murray, R. B. Mann, G. P. Saba, H. Kashima, and J. J. Mann. 1976. Unusual manifestation of tuberculosis: TE fistula. *Am. J. Med.* **60**:310–314.

218. Williford, M. E., W. M. Thompson, J. D. Hamilton, and R. W. Postlethwait. 1983. Esophageal tuberculosis: findings on barium swallow and computed tomography. *Gastrointest. Radiol.* **8**:119–122.

219. Wong, W. M., K. C. Lai, W. C. Yiu, B. C. Wong, F. L. Chan, and C. L. Lai. 2007. Intestinal tuberculosis mimicking fistulizing Crohn's disease. *J. Gastroenterol. Hepatol.* **22**:137–139.

220. World Health Organization. 2009. *2009 Update Tuberculosis Facts.* World Health Organization, Geneva, Switzerland. http://www.who.int/tb/publications/2009/tbfactsheet_2009update_one_page.pdf. Accessed 27 January 2010.

221. World Health Organization. 2009. *Global Tuberculosis Control: a Short Update to the 2009 Report.* World Health Organization, Geneva, Switzerland. http://www.who.int/tb/publications/global_report/2009/update/tbu_9.pdf. Accessed 27 January 2010.

222. World Health Organization. 2007. *Improving the Diagnosis and Treatment of Smear-Negative Pulmonary and Extrapulmonary Tuberculosis among Adults and Adolescents.* World Health Organization, Geneva, Switzerland. http://whqlibdoc.who.int/hq/2007/WHO_HTM_TB_2007.379_eng.pdf. Accessed 27 January 2010.

223. World Health Organization. 2009. *Morbidity Trend Tables United States.* World Health Organization, Geneva, Switzerland. http://www.cdc.gov/tb/statistics/reports/2008/pdf/4_MorbTrend.pdf. Accessed 2 February 2010.

224. Woudstra, M., A. J. van Tilburg, and J. S. Tjen. 1997. Two young Somalians with gastric outlet obstruction as a first manifestation of gastroduodenal tuberculosis. *Eur. J. Gastroenterol. Hepatol.* **9**:393–396.

225. Yang, Z., Y. Kong, F. Wilson, B. Foxman, A. H. Fowler, C. F. Marrs, M. D. Cave, and J. H. Bates. 2004. Identification of risk factors for extrapulmonary tuberculosis. *Clin. Infect. Dis.* **38**:199–205.

226. Yilmaz, E., A. Balci, S. Sal, and H. Cakmakci. 2003. Tuberculous ileitis in a renal transplant recipient with familial Mediterranean fever: gray-scale and power doppler sonographic findings. *J. Clin. Ultrasound* **31**:51–54.

227. Zedtwitz-Liebenstein, K., B. Podesser, M. Peck-Radosavljevic, and W. Graninger. 1999. Intestinal tuberculosis presenting as fever of unknown origin in a heart transplant patient. *Infection* **27**:289–290.

228. Zhang, X. F., Y. Lv, W. J. Xue, B. Wang, C. Liu, P. X. Tian, L. Yu, X. Y. Chen, and X. M. Liu. 2008. Mycobacterium tuberculosis infection in solid organ transplant recipients: experience from a single center in China. *Transplant. Proc.* **40**:1382–1385.

229. Zhou, Z. Y., and H. S. Luo. 2006. Differential diagnosis between Crohn's disease and intestinal tuberculosis in China. *Int. J. Clin. Pract.* **60**:212–214.

Tuberculosis and Nontuberculous Mycobacterial Infections, 6th ed.
Edited by David Schlossberg
© 2011 ASM Press, Washington, DC

Chapter 24

Tuberculous Peritonitis

Urvashi Vaid and Gregory C. Kane

INTRODUCTION

Abdominal tuberculosis (TB), more common in the developing world (10, 24, 53), is not entirely uncommon in United States and Europe. Patients with AIDS, immigrants from areas of endemicity, Native Americans on reservations, the urban poor, and the elderly are at particular risk (36, 42). TB rates have decreased from 52.6 cases per 100,000 population in 1953 to 4.2 per 100,000 population in 2008 (CDC 2009) despite a temporary resurgence in the late 80s and early 90s. Interestingly, the proportion of extrapulmonary TB has increased (from 16% in 1993 to 20% in 2008). Peritoneal TB accounts for 6.1% of all extrapulmonary TB (CDC 2009). Symptoms and signs of peritoneal TB are nonspecific, and a high index of suspicion needs to be maintained to make the diagnosis in a timely manner. In this chapter, we review the epidemiology, pathogenesis, clinical features, available diagnostic techniques, and therapy of tuberculous peritonitis.

EPIDEMIOLOGY

Of all sites affected by extrapulmonary TB, the abdomen is the sixth most common after lymphatic, genitourinary, bone and joint, miliary, and meningeal involvement (36). TB was on the decline until it made a resurgence as a result of the AIDS epidemic between 1985 and 1992 (CDC 2009). One hundred thirty-two cases of peritoneal TB were reported between 1963 and 1986, which represented 3.3% of all extrapulmonary TB cases (42). Since then, the numbers have been rising in developed (26) and developing (24) countries. More recently, peritoneal TB was found to represent 6.1% of all extrapulmonary TB in the United States from data collected between 1993 and 2008 (CDC 2009). Tuberculous peritonitis is predominantly a disease affecting young adults in the third and fourth decades of life but can occur at any age (13, 30, 46, 57). Several case series of peritoneal TB in children report a low incidence in children. One retrospective study found 26 cases between 1980 and 1993 in three teaching hospitals in San Diego, CA (58). Interestingly, 80% of mycobacterial isolates from this study were identified as *Mycobacterium bovis* and the rest were *Mycobacterium tuberculosis*. In four large case series from the developing world, women were affected more frequently than men, accounting for 57% to 67% of reported cases (10, 24, 47, 53). More recently in developed countries, this trend has reversed, with men accounting for as many or more cases than women (13, 15, 57).

The development of peritoneal TB has been associated with several comorbidities. Fifty percent of patients with human immunodeficiency virus (HIV)/AIDS have extrapulmonary manifestations of TB. In comparison, only 10 to 15% of non-HIV-infected patients develop extrapulmonary disease (11). Tuberculous peritonitis as the initial manifestation of HIV infection was reported first in 1992 (54). Alcoholic liver disease has been shown to be associated with peritoneal TB, though not causally, by Shakil et al. (51). In this study, 62% of patients had underlying alcoholic liver disease. Nearly three-quarters of Native Americans were believed to be heavy alcohol consumers in one series (35). Another high-risk group is patients with end-stage renal disease on continuous ambulatory peritoneal dialysis (CAPD) (56). In one series, 14 of 790 patients on CAPD were diagnosed with peritoneal TB between 1994 and 2000 (33). Other risk factors include diabetes mellitus, underlying malignancy, and the use of corticosteroids and/or other immunosuppressants (1, 11, 42, 50).

Urvashi Vaid and Gregory C. Kane • Department of Pulmonary and Critical Care Medicine, Thomas Jefferson University, Philadelphia, PA 19107.

PATHOGENESIS

Peritoneal TB is thought to be the result of reactivation of latent foci established in the peritoneum via hematogenous spread to the mesenteric lymph nodes from previous pulmonary infection. Ingestion of bacilli, with subsequent passage through Peyer's patches in intestinal mucosa to mesenteric lymph nodes, is another possible route of infection, as is contiguous spread from infected lymph nodes or ileocecal TB (27, 42, 49). Less frequently, direct spread from genitourinary sites (fallopian tubes) or hematogenous spread from active pulmonary disease or miliary TB can occur (41, 46); 15 to 20% of patients with abdominal TB have active pulmonary disease (4, 34). The organism is principally *Mycobacterium tuberculosis*, but *Mycobacterium bovis* has been reported to cause abdominal TB via ingestion of unpasteurized milk (55, 58).

CLINICAL FEATURES

Peritoneal TB is an insidious disease with a subacute presentation. The average duration of symptoms prior to diagnosis extends from weeks to months (24). Several case series report the two most common symptoms to be abdominal pain (31% to 94%) and fever (45% to 100%) (13, 15, 17, 46, 57). Other systemic symptoms of weight loss, fatigue, malaise, and anorexia are more prominent with peritoneal TB than with other forms of abdominal TB (27). Diarrhea is unusual but may be present in one-fifth of patients (46). A minority have symptoms of coexistent pulmonary TB, including cough and hemoptysis.

Physical examination often reveals ascites (73%) and abdominal tenderness (47.7%) (17, 46). The classic "doughy" abdomen is rare (5 to 13%). Peritoneal TB has been classified as the more common "wet type," which is characterized by ascites, and the less common "plastic or fibroadhesive type," which manifests as abdominal masses comprised of adherent bowel loops (41). The absence of signs of chronic liver disease, including palmar erythema, spider angiomata, and dilated abdominal wall veins, should increase clinical suspicion for TB peritonitis.

The tuberculin skin test may be positive in about 50% of patients (1, 15, 32, 34, 51). Mild to moderate normocytic, normochromic anemia is common, and the erythrocyte sedimentation rate (ESR) is universally elevated (46). Chest roentgenograms (CXR) may be abnormal in anywhere from 19% to 83% of patients. Chow et al. reported CXR findings of active or healed TB in a third of patients (15).

Table 1. Clinical and laboratory features of tuberculous peritonitis[a]

Feature type	Feature	Frequency or sensitivity (%)[b]
Clinical		
	Systemic symptoms	
	Fever	59
	Weight loss	61
	Abdominal symptoms	
	Abdominal pain	64.5
	Diarrhea	Up to 21
	Signs	
	Abdominal tenderness	47.7
	Ascites	73
	Abdominal mass	6–40
Laboratory		
	Positive purified protein derivative skin test	38
	Abnormal chest radiograph	19–83
	Ascitic fluid	
	Protein, >3 g%	84–100
	Lymphocyte predominance	68
	ADA	Up to 100
	AFB smear	3
	Culture	35
	Gamma interferon assay	93

[a]Data are from references 1, 4, 6, 10, 16, 19, 32, 34, 43, 46, 48, 51, and 53.
[b]Data for clinical features are frequencies; data for laboratory features are sensitivities.

Ascitic fluid typically is a straw-colored lymphocytic exudate with a serum-ascitic albumin gradient (SAAG) of less than 1.1 and a protein level of >2.5 to 3 g/dl (41, 46). Cell counts range from 500 to 1,500 cells/mm^3 and are predominantly lymphocytes (40 to 92%) (15, 46), except in patients with renal failure, where neutrophils predominate (14, 33). Ascitic fluid that is bloody, chylous, or purulent and with leukocyte counts as low as 10 cells has also been reported (6, 26). Table 1 summarizes the classical clinical and laboratory features of TB peritonitis.

DIAGNOSIS

The diagnosis of peritoneal TB entails maintaining a high index of clinical suspicion. Microbiological or pathological confirmation is usually required to make a definitive diagnosis. The gold standard remains laparoscopy and peritoneal biopsy (16, 46, 47).

Ultrasonographic appearances of peritoneal TB include ascites (either free or loculated, seen in 30 to 100%) (3, 23), echogenic debris with multiple fine strands of fibrin (40), and/or peritoneal thickening (8). Computed tomography (CT) is more sensitive in the detection of bowel thickening and abdominal lymphadenopathy (18, 52). Both imaging modalities can be used to guide fine-needle aspiration of ascitic fluid or peritoneal biopsy specimens. Features on CT when used in combination (mesenteric macronodules, smooth peritoneal thickening, lymph nodal masses with hypodense centers, splenic lesions, and calcifications) may help distinguish peritoneal TB from peritoneal carcinomatosis (22, 45).

Aspiration of ascitic fluid with subsequent microbiological examination with staining for acid-fast bacilli (AFB) and cultures is frequently a step in the diagnosis of peritoneal TB. AFB stains and cultures are notoriously insensitive in identifying the organism, with reported sensitivities of 3% for stains (1, 46) and 35% for cultures (46). The yield may increase when larger volumes of ascitic fluid are cultured. Singh et al. reported an 83% positivity rate by culturing 1 liter of peritoneal fluid (53). The diagnosis may be delayed further because *M. tuberculosis* requires 4 to 8 weeks to grow on traditional media. Fortunately, the use of the BACTEC radiometric system has reduced this time to 2 weeks.

Laparoscopy allows peritoneal inspection as well as the option of pathological and microbiological confirmation of the diagnosis. Laparoscopic examination and biopsy confirm tuberculous peritonitis in 85 to 90% of cases (9, 34, 47, 59). The laparoscopic appearances have been classified into three types: thickened peritoneum with scattered whitish miliary nodules and ascites (66%), thickened peritoneum with ascites and adhesions (21%), and the fibro-adhesive type where the peritoneum is markedly thickened with yellowish nodules and cheesy material with extensive adhesions (13%) (9). Sanai and Bzeizi reported a 93% sensitivity and 98% specificity of laparoscopic examination in making the diagnosis of peritoneal TB from data accumulated from 402 patients in 11 studies (46). Complications of laparoscopy include bowel perforation, bleeding, infection, and death but are rare, seen in <3% of cases. Complications may be more common in the fibro-adhesive type (37, 46). Laparoscopic biopsy should be performed whenever possible for histological and/or microbiological confirmation. Sensitivities for peritoneal biopsy are similar to laparoscopic inspection (41).

More recently, noninvasive tests to detect peritoneal TB have become available. A meta-analysis by Riquelme et al. reported the sensitivity and specificity of adenosine deaminase (ADA) levels in ascitic fluid to be 100% and 97%, respectively, when cut-off values of 36 to 40 IU/liter were used (43). Similarly, high levels of gamma interferon in ascitic fluid have been shown to be of similar value (31, 48).

The differential diagnosis of tuberculous peritonitis includes the differential diagnosis of ascites as well as the differential diagnosis of granulomatous peritonitis. On initial clinical presentation, malignancy, for example, carcinomatosis peritonei or ovarian cancer, may be the first concern. Interestingly, increased serum CA-125 levels have been reported in patients with peritoneal TB (12, 38). Also, malignant ascites is frequently a bloody exudate. Another important differential is end-stage liver disease with ascites and spontaneous bacterial peritonitis (SBP). The presentation of SBP is more acute and can be diagnosed by examination of the ascitic fluid (>250 neutrophils or a positive Gram stain or culture).

Granulomatous peritonitis on histopathology may not always be secondary to *M. tuberculosis*. The differential includes starch peritonitis from surgical gloves, peritoneal sarcoid, and nontuberculous mycobacterial peritonitis in patients undergoing CAPD (7, 21, 25, 29, 39, 44, 60). In these cases, microbiological confirmation becomes imperative.

TREATMENT

The treatment of peritoneal TB is primarily medical. Antituberculous regimens used are identical to those for pulmonary TB (5; see chapter 7). The role of corticosteroids is controversial, and empiric data are lacking (20). Singh et al. reported no fibrotic complications in the 23 patients randomized to receive steroids compared to 4 fibrotic complications in patients not on steroids (53). A delay in the initiation of medical therapy can result in significant morbidity and even mortality (2). More than 80% of patients deteriorated clinically while being evaluated in one series, and the overall mortality was reported to be 35% (15). Surgical intervention is reserved for complications arising from adhesions and inflammation, including bowel perforation, intestinal obstruction, fistulae, abscesses, and hemorrhage (28, 41).

CONCLUSION

Tuberculous peritonitis, though rare in the United States, continues to be reported in certain high-risk populations which include patients with AIDS or cirrhosis, patients on CAPD, recent immigrants, and those on immunosuppression. The diagnosis of this disease requires a high index of suspicion and should be considered in the differential of ascites with a lymphocyte predominance and a SAAG of <1.1 mg/dl. Microbiological or pathological confirmation remains the gold standard for diagnosis. Ascitic fluid cultures have low yield, but peritoneoscopy with biopsy or cultures frequently confirms the diagnosis. Newer techniques with future application include ADA and gamma interferon levels in ascitic fluid. Ultrasound and CT are frequently used to guide fluid aspiration and biopsies. Six months of treatment with antituberculous therapy is adequate except in cases of drug-resistant TB. The role of steroids remains controversial. Surgical approaches may be required to deal with complications, including bowel perforation, intestinal obstruction from adhesions, fistula formation, or bleeding.

REFERENCES

1. Aguado, J. M., F. Pons, F. Casafont, G. San Miguel, and R. Valle. 1990. Tuberculous peritonitis: a study comparing cirrhotic and noncirrhotic patients. *J. Clin. Gastroenterol.* 12: 550–554.

2. Ahmad, M., and A. Ahmed. 1999. Tuberculous peritonitis: fatality associated with delayed diagnosis. *South. Med. J.* 92: 406–408.

3. Akhan, O., F. B. Demirkazik, A. Demirkazik, N. Gulekon, M. Eryilmaz, M. Unsal, and A. Besim. 1990. Tuberculous peritonitis: ultrasonic diagnosis. *J. Clin. Ultrasound* 18:711–714.

4. al Karawi, M. A., A. E. Mohamed, M. I. Yasawy, D. Y. Graham, S. Shariq, A. M. Ahmed, A. al Jumah, and Z. Ghandour. 1995. Protean manifestation of gastrointestinal tuberculosis: report on 130 patients. *J. Clin. Gastroenterol.* 20:225–232.

5. American Review of Respiratory Disease. 1986. American Thoracic Society. Treatment of tuberculosis and tuberculosis infection in adults and children. *Am. Rev. Respir. Dis.* 134: 355–363.

6. Bastani, B., M. R. Shariatzadeh, and F. Dehdashti. 1985. Tuberculous peritonitis--report of 30 cases and review of the literature. *Q. J. Med.* 56:549–557.

7. Bates, B. 1965. Granulomatous peritonitis secondary to corn starch. *Ann. Intern. Med.* 62:335–347.

8. Batra, A., M. S. Gulati, D. Sarma, and S. B. Paul. 2000. Sonographic appearances in abdominal tuberculosis. *J. Clin. Ultrasound* 28:233–245.

9. Bhargava, D. K., Shriniwas, P. Chopra, S. Nijhawan, S. Dasarathy, and A. K. Kushwaha. 1992. Peritoneal tuberculosis: laparoscopic patterns and its diagnostic accuracy. *Am. J. Gastroenterol.* 87:109–112.

10. Borhanmanesh, F., K. Hekmat, K. Vaezzadeh, and H. R. Rezai. 1972. Tuberculous peritonitis. Prospective study of 32 cases in Iran. *Ann. Intern. Med.* 76:567–572.

11. Braun, M. M., R. H. Byers, W. L. Heyward, C. A. Ciesielski, A. B. Bloch, R. L. Berkelman, and D. E. Snider. 1990. Acquired immunodeficiency syndrome and extrapulmonary tuberculosis in the United States. *Arch. Intern. Med.* 150:1913–1916.

12. Candocia, S. A., and G. Y. Locker. 1993. Elevated serum CA 125 secondary to tuberculous peritonitis. *Cancer* 72:2016–2018.

13. Chen, H. L., M. S. Wu, W. H. Chang, S. C. Shih, H. Chi, and M. J. Bair. 2009. Abdominal tuberculosis in southeastern Taiwan: 20 years of experience. *J. Formos. Med. Assoc.* 108:195–201.

14. Cheng, I. K., P. C. Chan, and M. K. Chan. 1989. Tuberculous peritonitis complicating long-term peritoneal dialysis. Report of 5 cases and review of the literature. *Am. J. Nephrol.* 9:155–161.

15. Chow, K. M., V. C. Chow, L. C. Hung, S. M. Wong, and C. C. Szeto. 2002. Tuberculous peritonitis-associated mortality is high among patients waiting for the results of mycobacterial cultures of ascitic fluid samples. *Clin. Infect. Dis.* 35:409–413.

16. Chow, K. M., V. C. Chow, and C. C. Szeto. 2003. Indication for peritoneal biopsy in tuberculous peritonitis. *Am. J. Surg.* 185:567–573.

17. Demir, K., A. Okten, S. Kaymakoglu, D. Dincer, F. Besisik, U. Cevikbas, S. Ozdil, G. Bostas, Z. Mungan, and Y. Cakaloglu. 2001. Tuberculous peritonitis--reports of 26 cases, detailing diagnostic and therapeutic problems. *Eur. J. Gastroenterol. Hepatol.* 13:581–585.

18. Denton, T., and J. Hossain. 1993. A radiological study of abdominal tuberculosis in a Saudi population with special reference to ultrasound and computed tomography. *Clin. Radiol.* 47:409–414.

19. Dineen, P., W. P. Homan, and W. R. Grafe. 1976. Tuberculous peritonitis: 43 years' experience in diagnosis and treatment. *Ann. Surg.* 184:717–722.

20. Dooley, D. P., J. L. Carpenter, and S. Rademacher. 1997. Adjunctive corticosteroid therapy for tuberculosis: a critical reappraisal of the literature. *Clin. Infect. Dis.* 25:872–887.

21. Falcone, E. L., A. Alam, and N. Tangri. 2008. Mycobacterium avium complex-associated peritonitis in a patient on continuous ambulatory peritoneal dialysis. *Clin. Nephrol.* 69:387–390.

22. Ha, H. K., J. I. Jung, M. S. Lee, B. G. Choi, M. G. Lee, Y. H. Kim, P. N. Kim, and Y. H. Auh. 1996. CT differentiation of tuberculous peritonitis and peritoneal carcinomatosis. *AJR Am. J. Roentgenol.* 167:743–748.

23. Hulnick, D. H., A. J. Megibow, D. P. Naidich, S. Hilton, K. C. Cho, and E. J. Balthazar. 1985. Abdominal tuberculosis: CT evaluation. *Radiology* 157:199–204.

24. Ihekwaba, F. N. 1993. Abdominal tuberculosis: a study of 881 cases. *J. R. Coll. Surg. Edinb.* 38:293–295.

25. Iyer, S., K. Afshar, and O. P. Sharma. 2008. Peritoneal and pleural sarcoidosis: an unusual association - review and clinical report. *Curr. Opin. Pulm. Med.* 14:481–487.

26. Jayanthi, V., C. S. Probert, K. S. Sher, A. C. Wicks, and J. F. Mayberry. 1993. The renaissance of abdominal tuberculosis. *Dig. Dis.* 11:36–44.

27. Kapoor, V. K. 1998. Abdominal tuberculosis. *Postgrad. Med. J.* 74:459–467.

28. Khan, A. R., L. M. Morris, S. G. Keswani, I. R. Khan, L. Le, W. C. Lee, and J. P. Hunt. 2009. Tuberculous peritonitis: a surgical dilemma. *South. Med. J.* 102:94–95.

29. Klink, B., and C. J. Boynton. 1990. Starch peritonitis. A case report and clinicopathologic review. *Am. Surg.* 56:672–674.

30. Lazarus, A. A., and B. Thilagar. 2007. Abdominal tuberculosis. *Dis. Mon.* 53:32–38.

31. Liao, C. H., C. H. Chou, C. C. Lai, Y. T. Huang, C. K. Tan, H. L. Hsu, and P. R. Hsueh. 2009. Diagnostic performance of an enzyme-linked immunospot assay for interferon-gamma in extrapulmonary tuberculosis varies between different sites of disease. *J. Infect.* 59:402–408.

32. Lisehora, G. B., C. C. Peters, Y. T. Lee, and P. J. Barcia. 1996. Tuberculous peritonitis--do not miss it. *Dis. Colon Rectum* 39: 394–399.

33. Lui, S. L., S. Tang, F. K. Li, B. Y. Choy, T. M. Chan, W. K. Lo, and K. N. Lai. 2001. Tuberculosis infection in Chinese patients undergoing continuous ambulatory peritoneal dialysis. *Am. J. Kidney Dis.* 38:1055–1060.

34. Manohar, A., A. E. Simjee, A. A. Haffejee, and K. E. Pettengell. 1990. Symptoms and investigative findings in 145 patients

with tuberculous peritonitis diagnosed by peritoneoscopy and biopsy over a five year period. *Gut* **31**:1130–1132.

35. Marrie, T. J., and E. S. Hershfield. 1978. Tuberculous peritonitis in Manitoba. *Can. J. Surg.* **21**:533–536.

36. Mehta, J. B., A. Dutt, L. Harvill, and K. M. Mathews. 1991. Epidemiology of extrapulmonary tuberculosis. A comparative analysis with pre-AIDS era. *Chest* **99**:1134–1138.

37. Mimica, M. 1992. Usefulness and limitations of laparoscopy in the diagnosis of tuberculous peritonitis. *Endoscopy* **24**:588–591.

38. O'Riordan, D. K., A. Deery, A. Dorman, and O. E. Epstein. 1995. Increased CA 125 in a patient with tuberculous peritonitis: case report and review of published works. *Gut* **36**:303–305.

39. Perazella, M., T. Eisen, and E. Brown. 1993. Peritonitis associated with disseminated *Mycobacterium avium* complex in an acquired immunodeficiency syndrome patient on chronic ambulatory peritoneal dialysis. *Am. J. Kidney Dis.* **21**:319–321.

40. Pereira, J. M., A. J. Madureira, A. Vieira, and I. Ramos. 2005. Abdominal tuberculosis: imaging features. *Eur. J. Radiol.* **55**:173–180.

41. Rasheed, S., R. Zinicola, D. Watson, A. Bajwa, and P. J. McDonald. 2007. Intra-abdominal and gastrointestinal tuberculosis. *Colorectal Dis.* **9**:773–783.

42. Rieder, H. L., G. M. Cauthen, G. D. Kelly, A. B. Bloch, and D. E. Snider, Jr. 1989. Tuberculosis in the United States. *JAMA* **262**:385–389.

43. Riquelme, A., M. Calvo, F. Salech, S. Valderrama, A. Pattillo, M. Arellano, M. Arrese, A. Soza, P. Viviani, and L. M. Letelier. 2006. Value of adenosine deaminase (ADA) in ascitic fluid for the diagnosis of tuberculous peritonitis: a meta-analysis. *J. Clin. Gastroenterol.* **40**:705–710.

44. Robinson, E. K., and R. W. Ernst. 1954. Boeck's sarcoid of the peritoneal cavity; a case report. *Surgery* **36**:986–991.

45. Rodriguez, E., and F. Pombo. 1996. Peritoneal tuberculosis versus peritoneal carcinomatosis: distinction based on CT findings. *J. Comput. Assist. Tomogr.* **20**:269–272.

46. Sanai, F. M., and K. I. Bzeizi. 2005. Systematic review: tuberculous peritonitis--presenting features, diagnostic strategies and treatment. *Aliment. Pharmacol. Ther.* **22**:685–700.

47. Sandikci, M. U., S. Colakoglu, Y. Ergun, S. Unal, H. Akkiz, S. Sandikci, and S. Zorludemir. 1992. Presentation and role of peritoneoscopy in the diagnosis of tuberculous peritonitis. *J. Gastroenterol. Hepatol.* **7**:298–301.

48. Sathar, M. A., A. E. Simjee, Y. M. Coovadia, P. N. Soni, S. A. Moola, B. Insam, and F. Makumbi. 1995. Ascitic fluid gamma interferon concentrations and adenosine deaminase activity in tuberculous peritonitis. *Gut* **36**:419–421.

49. Scully, R. E., E. J. Mark, W. F. McNeely, S. H. Ebeling, and L. D. Phillips. 1998. Case records of the Massachusetts General Hospital. Weekly clinicopathological exercises. Case 3-1998. A 31-year-old woman with a pleural effusion, ascites, and persistent fever spikes. *N. Engl. J. Med.* **338**:248–254.

50. Senn, L., T, Kovacsovics, P. E. Tarr, and P. Meylan. 2009. Peritoneal tuberculosis after imatinib therapy. *Arch. Intern. Med.* **169**:312–313.

51. Shakil, A. O., J. Korula, G. C. Kanel, N. G. Murray, and T. B. Reynolds. 1996. Diagnostic features of tuberculous peritonitis in the absence and presence of chronic liver disease: a case control study. *Am. J. Med.* **100**:179–185.

52. Sheikh, M., F. Abu-Zidan, M. al-Hilaly, and A. Behbehani. 1995. Abdominal tuberculosis: comparison of sonography and computed tomography. *J. Clin. Ultrasound* **23**:413–417.

53. Singh, M. M., A. N. Bhargava, and K. P. Jain. 1969. Tuberculous peritonitis. An evaluation of pathogenetic mechanisms, diagnostic procedures and therapeutic measures. *N. Engl. J. Med.* **281**:1091–1094.

54. Soubani, A. O., and A. E. Glatt. 1992. Tuberculous peritonitis as an initial manifestation of HIV infection. *N. Y. State J. Med.* **92**:269–270.

55. Stout, J. E., C. W. Woods, A. A. Alvarez, A. Berchuck, and C. Dukes Hamilton. 2001. Mycobacterium bovis peritonitis mimicking ovarian cancer in a young woman. *Clin. Infect. Dis.* **33**:E14–E16.

56. Talwani, R., and J. A. Horvath. 2000. Tuberculous peritonitis in patients undergoing continuous ambulatory peritoneal dialysis: case report and review. *Clin. Infect. Dis.* **31**:70–75.

57. Tan, K. K., K. Chen, and R. Sim. 2009. The spectrum of abdominal tuberculosis in a developed country: a single institution's experience over 7 years. *J. Gastrointest. Surg.* **13**:142–147.

58. Veeragandham, R. S., F. P. Lynch, T. G. Canty, D. L. Collins, and W. M. Danker. 1996. Abdominal tuberculosis in children: review of 26 cases. *J. Pediatr. Surg.* **31**:170–175.

59. Wolfe, J. H., A. R. Behn, and B. T. Jackson. 1979. Tuberculous peritonitis and role of diagnostic laparoscopy. *Lancet* **i**:852–853.

60. Wong, M., and S. W. Rosen. 1962. Ascites in sarcoidosis due to peritoneal involvement. *Ann. Intern. Med.* **57**:277–280.

Tuberculosis and Nontuberculous Mycobacterial Infections, 6th ed.
Edited by David Schlossberg
© 2011 ASM Press, Washington, DC

Chapter 25

Tuberculosis of the Liver, Biliary Tract, and Pancreas

THOMAS H. TAYLOR, DALIA IBRAHIM, AND JAMES H. LEWIS

HISTORY OF HEPATOBILIARY TUBERCULOSIS

Involvement of the liver in patients with *Mycobacterium tuberculosis* has been described for more than 100 years. One of the earliest descriptions was published in Guy's Hospital Reports by Thomas Addison in 1836 (292). Autopsy studies during the latter half of the 19th and early 20th century, an era of great interest in morbid anatomy, demonstrated granulomas and a variety of other lesions in the livers of patients dying with tuberculosis (226, 236, 288, 292). The reports by Gillman and Gillman (96) and subsequently by many others (83, 141) on the use of needle biopsy of the liver to demonstrate tuberculous lesions have made the procedure a valuable tool for diagnosis of the disease, especially in cases of cryptic miliary tuberculosis without recognized pulmonary involvement (166). Although isolated hepatobiliary tuberculosis was described infrequently in years past (99, 108), a number of detailed reviews attest to its continued importance in the clinical spectrum of the disease (8, 30, 77, 165, 199).

With the advent of the AIDS epidemic, the increase in homelessness, and increasing immigration of persons from developing countries, the rate of new cases of tuberculosis that had been declining began to increase between 1984 and 1994 (270). As many as two-thirds of patients with AIDS and tuberculosis have extrapulmonary involvement (42, 266). The rate of new cases of tuberculosis, as described by Gordon Snider, is enormous, with nearly 8 million new cases estimated to have occurred by the end of the 20th century, many of which were associated with human immunodeficiency virus (HIV) infection. Atypical mycobacteria, especially *Mycobacterium avium* complex, continue to play an important role in the course of AIDS, especially with respect to liver involvement (119, 130).

This chapter reviews the clinical, biochemical, and histopathologic spectrum of tuberculosis and atypical mycobacteria involving the liver and pancreaticobiliary tract, as well as the hepatotoxicity caused by antituberculosis therapy. Classic *M. tuberculosis* infection in persons not infected with HIV precedes the discussion of the disease in patients with HIV and AIDS and other immunocompromised persons, such as liver transplant recipients.

SPECTRUM OF HEPATOBILIARY AND PANCREATIC TUBERCULOSIS

The liver can be involved in all forms of tuberculosis (i.e., pulmonary, extrapulmonary, and miliary). In addition, infection confined predominantly to the liver or biliary tract has been recognized with some regularity, especially in areas where tuberculosis remains endemic. A variety of hepatic lesions have been recorded (Table 1). These include the lesions long known to be regularly associated with tuberculosis (i.e., granulomas, Kupffer cell hyperplasia, sinusoidal infiltration, caseous necrosis, and steatosis), as well as the less common ones, peliosis hepatis, and amyloidosis. Additional lesions associated with tuberculosis that have come into focus are those caused by adverse effects of drugs used for treatment. With the advent of effective therapy for tuberculosis after World War II, the pattern and prognosis of tuberculosis have undergone striking changes (133, 187), as will be discussed.

EVIDENCE OF HEPATIC INVOLVEMENT

Granulomas

Prevalence

The reported prevalence of hepatic granulomas (tubercles) in biopsy material from patients with tuberculosis has ranged from 0% to 100% of studied

Thomas H. Taylor • Division of Gastroenterology, Georgetown University Hospital, Washington, DC 20007. **Dalia Ibrahim** • Department of Internal Medicine, Georgetown University Hospital, Washington, DC 20007. **James H. Lewis** • Division of Hepatology, Department of Medicine, Georgetown University Hospital, Washington, DC 20007.

Table 1. Histopathologic spectrum of hepatobiliary tuberculosis

Granulomas
Granulomatous hepatitis
Tuberculomas
Caseous necrosis
Tuberculous abscess
Cholangitis
Cholecystitis
Pancreatitis
Fulminant hepatic failure
Nonspecific changes
    Fatty change
    Focal necrosis
    Kupffer cell hyperplasia
    Sinusoidal inflammation
    Free acidophilic bodies
    Portal fibrosis
    Giant hepatocytes
    Amyloidosis
    Glycogenated nuclei
    Peliosis hepatis
Coincidental lesions
    Alcoholic liver disease and cirrhosis
    Viral hepatitis
    Nodular regenerative hyperplasia
    Hemosiderosis
Hepatotoxicity secondary to antituberculous therapy
    Bacillus Calmette-Guérin-induced granulomatous hepatitis
    Drug-induced hepatitis (isoniazid, *para*-aminosalicyclic acid,
        rifampin, pyrazinamide
    Drug-induced fibrosis (streptomycin)

cases (Tables 2 and 3). Pulmonary tuberculosis involves the liver less frequently than does miliary tuberculosis, with an average of approximately 20% for pulmonary tuberculosis and 68% for extrapulmonary or miliary disease. It has been suggested that hepatic invasion in patients with pulmonary tuberculosis occurs only terminally, a view based on the observations of Torrey (288) and Mather and colleagues (171) that no granulomas could be demonstrated in autopsy material from patients with active

pulmonary tuberculosis dying of unrelated causes. Indeed, in most series employing liver biopsy, staining (see Fig. 4) or culture is positive far less frequently in patients with pulmonary tuberculosis than among those with the miliary form of the disease. Identification of the organism in patients with pulmonary tuberculosis has ranged from 0% in several large series to a high of almost 20% in others (Table 4). The figures for demonstrating the organism among patients with miliary tuberculosis range from 20% to 50% (Tables 4 and 5). The ability to demonstrate mycobacteria by staining is usually associated with the presence of caseous necrosis (77, 144). Caseation is thought to occur as a result of overwhelming acute dissemination of mycobacterial organisms; hence, it is present more often in cases with miliary involvement.

The relative rarity of caseation in hepatic granulomas in nonmiliary tuberculosis is presumably the reason for the difficulty in demonstrating the acid-fast bacilli (AFB). Nevertheless, Alexander and Galambos (6) were able to identify acid-fast organisms in the liver of 2 of 11 patients with pulmonary tuberculosis (18%) with and without hepatic granulomas. They have also reported the greatest success in demonstrating the organisms by stain and culture in miliary cases, doing so in 53 of 67 cases with hepatic granulomas. In their series, liver biopsy afforded the first morphologic evidence of tuberculosis in 82.5% of cases and provided the first bacteriologic proof of tuberculosis in 52.5% of miliary cases. In 45% of their patients, a positive liver biopsy provided the only laboratory evidence for systemic granulomatous disease. Granulomas have been demonstrated in an appreciable proportion of patients surviving their disease. The wide variation in reported prevalence has been attributed to the relative diligence with which granulomas had been sought. For example, the 93%

Table 2. Biopsy incidence of hepatic granulomas in pulmonary tuberculosis

Author(s) (reference)	Yr	No. of patients	% with granulomas
Van Buchem (295)	1949	9	0
Klatskin and Yesner (141)	1950	8	25
Seife et al. (247)	1951	70	13
Finkh et al. (83)	1953	25[a]	8
Ban (21)	1955	59	20
Haex and Van Beek (110)	1955	45	93
Mather et al. (171)	1955	34	3
Von Oldershausen et al. (298)	1955	248	19
Arora et al. (14)	1956	50[b]	12
Buckingham et al. (38)	1956	13	15
Salib et al. (232)	1961	39	0
Bowry et al. (35)	1970	32	25
Abdel-Dayem et al. (2)	1997	29	45

[a]Received antituberculous therapy.
[b]Included both pulmonary and extrapulmonary tuberculosis.

Table 3. Biopsy incidence of hepatic granulomas in extrapulmonary, localized hepatic, and miliary tuberculosis

Author(s) (reference)	Yr	No. of patients	% with granulomas	Type of tuberculosis
Haex and Van Beek (110)	1955	189	93	Extrapulmonary
Arora et al. (14)	1956	50	12	Extrapulmonary
Buckingham et al. (38)	1956	22	40	Extrapulmonary
Korn et al. (144)	1959	30	80	Extrapulmonary
Bowry et al. (35)	1970	5	80	Extrapulmonary
Klatskin and Yesner (141)	1950	4	100	Miliary
Mather et al. (171)	1955	22	68	Miliary and meningeal
Von Oldershausen et al. (298)	1955	93	25.3	Miliary
Biehl (33)	1958	7	100	Miliary
Munt (187)	1971	9	67	Miliary
Gelb et al. (94)	1973	38	81.6	Miliary
Alvarez and Carpio (8)	1983	130	100	Localized hepatobiliary
Essop et al. (77)	1984	96	96	Localized hepatobiliary
Palmer et al. (203)	1985	90	9	Abdominal-peritoneal
Maharaj et al. (165)	1987	41	88	Localized hepatic
al-Karawi et al. (7)	1995	130	14.6	Localized abdominal
Lundstedt et al. (164)	1996	112	10	Localized abdominal
Sinha et al. (263)	2003	143	102	Extrapulmonary

Table 4. Demonstration of hepatic AFB in pulmonary tuberculosis

Author(s) (reference)	Yr	% with granulomas with caseation	% with positive Ziehl-Neelsen stain	% with positive culture
Seife et al. (247)	1951	13 (9 of 70)	0	
Buckingham et al. (38)	1956	23 (29 of 128)		
Guckian and Perry (106)	1966	29 (9 of 31)	13 (4 of 31)	
Bowry et al. (35)	1970	0 (0 of 32)		
Gelb et al. (94)	1970	37 (14 of 38)		
Munt (187)	1971	50 (3 of 6)		
Alexander and Galambos (6)	1973	Majority of 20	18 (2 of 11)	0 (0 of 10)

Table 5. Caseating granulomas in hepatic biopsy material in localized hepatic and miliary tuberculosis

Author(s) (reference)	Yr	No. of patients with granulomas	No. with caseating granulomas (%)	No. or % with positive AFB stain or culture
Korn et al. (144)	1959	6	6 (100)	2 of 9
Klatskin and Yesner (141)	1950	4	3 (75)	1 of 3
Munt (187)	1971	9	3 (33)	3 of 3
Gelb et al. (94)	1973	38	14 (37)	1 of 1
Biehl (33)	1958	7	7 (100)	None
Hersch (114)	1964	200	86 of 114 (75) at autopsy	5 of 6 at autopsy, 6 of 29 at autopsy
Guckian and Perry (106)	1966	33 of 34	30 of 34 (88)	1 positive tuberculosis culture
Alexander and Galambos (6)	1973	39	Most of 39	61%
Alvarez and Carpio (8a)	1983	130	97 (75)	2 of 30
Essop et al. (76)	1984	92	77 (83)	9%
Palmer et al. (203)	1985	8	0	1 of 8
Maharaj et al. (165)	1987	36	(52)	59%
Huang et al. (123)	2003	5	4	1

prevalence reported by Haex and Van Beek (110) seems attributable to their having examined more than 100 sections from each biopsy specimen as well as having included "epithelioid cell subtubercles" as granulomas. An increased yield of hepatic granulomas also has been reported with a fluorescent staining technique as described by Yamaguchi and Braunstein

(307). The inclusion of patients, in some series, who had undergone previous antituberculous chemotherapy (83), on the other hand, could lead to a falsely low estimate of the prevalence of granulomas because complete resolution of diffuse granulomatosis following successful therapy may occur within a few months (77, 198, 265, 314).

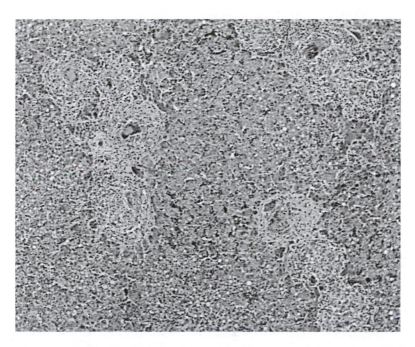

Figure 1. Low-power photomicrograph of the liver of an infant with miliary tuberculosis showing multiple granulomas. Moderate steatosis attributable to severe malnutrition is also present. (Courtesy of K. G. Ishak.)

Character of granulomas

Tuberculous granulomas are composed of mononuclear (epithelioid) cells, surrounded by lymphocytes with or without Langerhans' multinucleated giant cells (Fig. 1 and 2). They range in size from 0.05-mm microgranulomas (104) to 12-cm tuberculomas (314) but are generally 1 to 2 mm in diameter.

Central necrosis of the tubercle sometimes develops. It is characteristically granular and cheesy, hence, the term "caseous." Caseous necrosis (Fig. 3 and 4) occurs with more regularity in miliary tuberculosis (Table 5) than in other forms of the disease (156). The notion that tuberculous granulomas form in a similar fashion to foreign body granulomas—serving to encircle and "wall off" material that cannot be destroyed—is

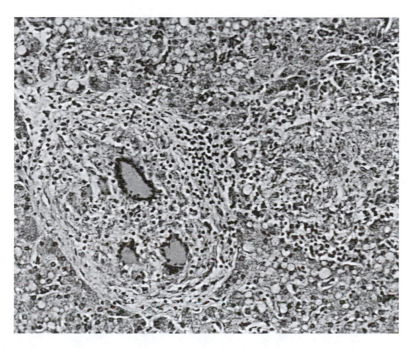

Figure 2. Section from the liver in Fig. 1 showing two noncaseating hepatic granulomas, one with Langerhans' giant cells. (Courtesy of K. G. Ishak.)

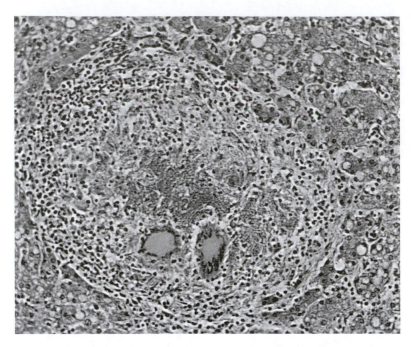

Figure 3. Higher magnification of a granuloma from Fig. 1 showing central caseous necrosis. (Courtesy of K. G. Ishak.)

a view that is undergoing significant change (60). The dynamics of tuberculosis (TB) granuloma formation and function have been brought to light by recent studies by Egen et al. (73), who have produced live images of a mycobacterial infection in a murine host. These investigations using the in vivo liver have demonstrated that blood-borne *Mycobacterium bovis* BCG is rapidly phagocytized by Kupffer cells, which in turn recruit other macrophages to the area and also attract T lymphocytes to form aggregates of the originally-infected Kupffer cells, other macrophages, and motile T cells that appear to wander through the granuloma. The clinical significance of these innate and adaptive immune responses in the context of mycobacterial containment and escape is the subject of ongoing investigation (60).

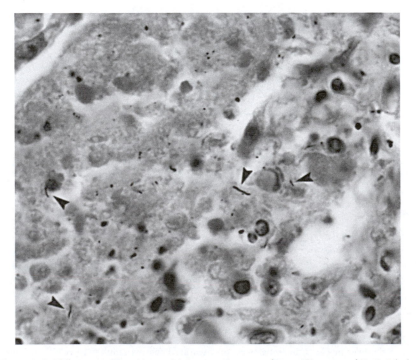

Figure 4. Acid-fast organisms (arrows) in a caseating granuloma. (Courtesy of K. G. Ishak.)

Nonspecific Hepatic Lesions

A high incidence of histologic abnormalities other than hepatic granulomas is often observed in pulmonary, extrapulmonary, and miliary tuberculosis (Table 6). Nearly 75% of patients with pulmonary involvement can be shown to have one or more nonspecific lesions, such as Kupffer cell hyperplasia, sinusoidal inflammation or dilatation, fatty metamorphosis, focal necrosis, periportal fibrosis, acidophilic bodies or amyloidosis (35), and even peliosis hepatis (77). In miliary tuberculosis, such changes receive less attention, although Buckingham and associates (38) found "nonspecific reactive hepatitis" (i.e., focal and diffuse degenerative changes, Kupffer cell hypertrophy, and portal and periportal cellular infiltrates) in 45% of 32 patients with miliary tuberculosis.

Kupffer cell hyperplasia with stellate radiation into adjacent sinusoids has been variously called "retothelial" or "histiocytic" nodules. These cells in a rounded configuration have been regarded as an early lesion in the formation of microgranulomas (144). Although not pathognomonic of tuberculosis, their presence has been reported in 80% to 91% of patients with pulmonary disease (231, 238).

Infiltration of the sinusoids with lymphocytes occurred in 44% of patients studied by Bowry and coworkers (35). Such sinusoidal inflammation has been called "nonspecific reactive hepatitis" by Buckingham and colleagues (38). It is usually observed only with moderate or severe pulmonary disease but may occur with miliary involvement. *Sinusoidal dilatation* is a nonspecific abnormality that also has been associated with neoplastic hepatic processes and hepatic congestion.

The incidence of *fatty metamorphosis* in pulmonary tuberculosis has ranged from 14% to 44%. It has generally been focal and mild. Alcoholism and malnutrition in patients with tuberculosis, rather than the tuberculosis per se, are probably responsible for the steatosis. The rarity of fatty metamorphosis in modern biopsy series, despite its frequency in the former necropsy-based data, supports this view.

Focal necrosis of hepatocytes is common. It may be acute (poorly circumscribed foci of necrotic cells with polymorphonuclear infiltration) or subacute (more discrete foci with lymphocyte predominance).

Periportal fibrosis has been described in patients with pulmonary tuberculosis (231) and with predominantly hepatic involvement (77). *Cirrhosis* may be present but probably precedes the tuberculosis lesions. Indeed, it had been previously suggested that cirrhosis might predispose patients toward the development of tuberculosis. There is, however, no convincing evidence that tuberculosis can lead to cirrhosis. Nevertheless, the possibility remains that fibrosis and architectural distortion secondary to hepatic involvement may result in a histologic picture similar to that of severe granulomatous involvement by sarcoidosis (141, 230) or that attributed to the hepatic involvement of brucellosis (173). In addition, radiocolloid scans of the liver in patients with hepatic tuberculosis may closely mimic the changes visible with cirrhosis (78). Little attention, however, is given today to the earlier concept of "tuberculosis cirrhosis" (135).

Free acidophilic bodies were seen in 2 of 32 patients in the report of Bowry and colleagues (35) and in the studies of Korn and associates (144). These rounded, deeply eosinophilic staining bodies are the remains of degenerating liver cells and are commonly visible in viral and drug-induced hepatitis.

A rare change occurring in miliary tuberculosis is the presence of giant hepatocytes, reported by Pintos and coauthors (212). Such giant hepatocytes are more often characteristic of neonatal hepatitis (256).

Glycogenated nuclei were seen in 3% of patients in one series (247). This change is also nonspecific and is more common in diabetic patients and in some patients receiving corticosteroids.

Amyloidosis was seen in 10% of one autopsy series (292) and in smaller numbers of patients with chronic untreated pulmonary tuberculosis in the reports by Ban (21) and Buckingham and coworkers (38). Essop and colleagues (77) recorded a 1% prevalence among patients with predominantly localized hepatic tuberculosis. Detectable by various special stains, amyloidosis most likely represents a response to the chronic infection.

Peliosis hepatis, the presence of blood-filled lakes in the liver, is today a lesion seen predominantly in patients who have been taking anabolic or contraceptive steroids. Older reports have drawn attention to the association of peliosis with the terminal state of diseases characterized by "wasting," namely, tuberculosis and carcinomatosis (275). In one series, the prevalence was recorded as 2% (77).

Granulomatous hepatitis is a term that has been applied to the presence of multiple granulomas in the liver (131, 294). We think that a more exact use of the term would restrict it to granulomatous involvement accompanied by sinusoidal and other parenchymal cellular infiltrates and by parenchymal injury, including acidophilic bodies. Such lesions occur in miliary tuberculosis, brucellosis, histoplasmosis, Q fever, and other infections (166). In sarcoidosis (141), however, and in many of the patients with pulmonary tuberculosis, granulomas may be the only hepatic lesions present, in which case the histologic description would be better given as simply hepatic granulomas.

Table 6. Nonspecific hepatic lesions in pulmonary tuberculosis

Author(s) (reference)	Yr	Kupffer cell hyperplasia	Sinusoidal dilation	Fatty change	Focal necrosis	Periportal fibrosis	Acidophilic bodies	Glycogen nuclei	Amyloid	Peliosis	Siderosis
Ullom (292)	1909			35%					10%		
Torrey (288)	1916										
Saphir (236)	1929	80%		34%		67%					
Jones and Peck (135)	1944			42%							
Seife et al. (247)	1951			14%	62%	14%		3%			
Schaffner et al. (242)	1953	91%			70%			13%			
Ban (untreated) (21)	1955	0/34		35%	12	36					
Arora et al. (14)	1956			36%							
Buckingham et al. (38)	1956								6%		
Hersch (114)	1964										28% at biopsy; 47% at autopsy
Bowry et al. (35)	1970	16%	44%	44%	16%	12%	6%				
Essop et al. (77)	1984			42%		20%			1%	2%	

Table 7. Tuberculosis as a cause of hepatic granulomas

Author(s) (reference)	Yr	Country	No. of cases	Proportion (%) TB
Harrington et al. (111)	1982	Multiple	1,129	20
Cunningham et al. (56)	1982	Scotland	77	10
Anderson et al. (11)	1988	Australia	59	7
Satti et al. (240)	1990	Saudi Arabia	59	32
Sartin and Walker (238)	1991	United States	88	3
McCluggage and Sloan (172)	1994	Ireland	163	0.1
Guglielmi et al. (107)	1994	Italy	15	6.7
Sabharwal et al. (231)	1995	India	51	55
Mert et al. (177)	2001	Turkey	56	36
Gaya et al. (93)	2003	United Kingdom	63	8
Dourakis et al. (68)	2006	Greece	66	1.5
Drebber et al. (69)	2008	Germany	442	0.7
Sanai et al. (235)	2008	Saudi Arabia	66	43
Martin-Blondel et al. (168)	2010	France	21	4.8

Although tuberculosis is a major cause of hepatic granulomas in most series, its frequency is highly variable and depends on the population studied. Sartin and Walker (238) reported only a 3% incidence of tuberculosis in a series of 88 patients with granulomas at the Mayo Clinic. Other series reported frequencies ranging from 0.7% to 55% of patients (Table 7). In a review of granulomatous hepatitis by Drebber and colleagues (69) in 2008, tuberculosis accounted for 0.7% of 442 cases in Germany. In another review of granulomatous hepatitis by Harrington et al. (111) in 1982, tuberculosis accounted for approximately 20% of hepatic granulomas in 8 series totaling 1,129 patients. The largest percentage was found in a series from India (231), where a tubercular cause of hepatic granulomas was found in 55% of 51 patients.

Biochemical Abnormalities in Tuberculosis

Biochemical evidence of hepatic dysfunction in tuberculosis has been observed in a large number of cases (Table 8), although in general the biochemical values themselves correlate poorly with the specific type of hepatobiliary tuberculosis and are considered of limited diagnostic value (165). Nevertheless, it remains useful to review the liver-related tests that have traditionally been used as potential markers of tuberculous involvement. The bromosulfophthalein (BSP) retention test was a popular one in years past and was the most common hepatic functional abnormality seen (275). In contrast with extrapulmonary tuberculosis, in which impaired BSP excretion has been noted to be characteristic, pulmonary tuberculosis, even with the presence of hepatic granulomas, usually has not been accompanied by impaired liver function. Also, there has been no correlation between serum alkaline phosphatase levels and hepatic granulomas in pulmonary or localized hepatic tuberculosis (165).

However, in immunocompromised patients with hepatic tuberculosis, the serum alkaline phosphatase level was significantly higher than that in immunocompetent patients (297).

Abnormal serum protein levels are characteristic of tuberculosis. Hyperglobulinemia is frequent, occurring in up to 50% of patients with pulmonary tuberculosis and in up to 80% of patients with extrapulmonary and, especially, miliary disease. The elevation reflects the elevated gamma globulin fraction, a regular marker of chronic infection. Indeed, tuberculosis is one of the recognized causes of extreme hyperglobulinemia, and Schaffner and colleagues (242) have drawn attention to the usefulness of serum globulin level as a measure of intensity of nonspecific host reaction to the infection.

Serum cholesterol levels are variably affected. They are elevated in 10% to 20% and decreased in 21% to 40% of cases, as reported by Seife and associates (247) and Schaffner and coworkers (242).

Hyperbilirubinemia in pulmonary tuberculosis is uncommon and is generally mild. Mild hyperbilirubinemia (less than 3 mg/dl) was found in 13% of 123 miliary patients reported by Hersch (114) and in 5% of 63 patients with both miliary and pulmonary tuberculosis reported by Guckian and Perry (106). Nearly one-fourth of a group of patients with miliary tuberculosis reported by Munt (187) had elevations of serum bilirubin, all slight. Jaundice mimicking extrahepatic obstruction is an infrequent clinical presentation of localized tuberculous hepatitis, usually resulting from common bile duct obstruction due to compression by tuberculomas or enlarged lymph nodes at the porta (8, 16, 77, 211). Jaundice of this type, however, is rare outside areas of endemicity.

Serum aminotransferases (serum glutamic-oxaloacetic transaminase [SGOT], serum glutamic-pyruvic transaminase [SGPT]) are usually normal in

Table 8. Hepatic function tests and biochemical abnormalities in tuberculosis

Author(s) (reference)	Yr	No. of patients	Abnormal BSP retention	Elevated alkaline phosphatase	Bilirubin <3 mg	Bilirubin >3 mg	Elevated SGOT/SGPT	Increased globulin	Cholesterol High	Cholesterol Low	Tuberculosis type
Hurst et al. (127)	1947	17	23%	55%	100%						Pulmonary
Klatskin and Yesner (141)	1950	4	75%	67%				67%			Miliary
Galen et al. (91)	1950	53	19%								Pulmonary
Seife et al. (247)	1951	70	14.30%	14.30%				50%	21.40%	10%	Pulmonary (treated)
Schaffner et al. (242)	1953	23						74%	40%	20%	Pulmonary (treated)
Ban (21)	1955	35	71%	0							Pulmonary (treated)
Ban (21)	1955	25	60%	0							Pulmonary (treated)
Korn et al. (144)	1959	50	85.70%	40.90%	26.7%			75%			Extrapulmonary
Hersch (114)	1964	123	100%	72% (18 of 25)		13%		50%	40%	20%	Miliary
Hersch (114)	1964	20	100%	87.5% (7 of 8)	14%	6%		43% (3 of 7)			Localized
Guckian and Perry (106)	1966	63		56%	50%		50% (slight)	60%			Hepatic
Bowry et al. (35)	1970	32	49%	16%	0	0	0	45%			Granulomatous hepatitis
Munt (187)	1971	69	54.50%	34%	23%	0	93%				Pulmonary
Irani and Dobbins (130a)	1979	9	12.50%	44%			12.50%	62.50%			Miliary
Essop et al. (77)	1984	96		Most (6- to 10-fold)							Combined
Alvarez and Carpio (8)	1983	130	55%	75%	65%	65%	35%/35%	81%			Localized
Maharaj et al. (165)	1987	41		87% (20% > 3×)	15%			78%			Localized

patients with pulmonary tuberculosis in the absence of alcoholic liver disease or other drug toxicity. In acute miliary disease, transaminase levels are slightly increased. As a general rule, however, there is no correlation between the degree or incidence of biochemical abnormalities and the extent of histologic injury in pulmonary, localized hepatic, or miliary tuberculosis (35, 77, 144).

Clinical Symptoms and Signs

No specific symptoms can be related to the hepatic abnormalities in pulmonary tuberculosis, although, of course, the constitutional symptoms associated with the underlying tuberculosis (fever, chills, fatigue, abdominal pain, and weight loss) are common (106). Hepatomegaly occurs in approximately 50% of patients, and the spleen is enlarged in 25% to 40%. Physical manifestations of chronic alcoholism and malnutrition may be present. Patients with hepatic involvement due to granulomatous hepatitis may have fever of unknown origin (259). In localized hepatic tuberculosis, as previously mentioned, the clinical presentation may simulate alcoholic or viral hepatitis (77), amebic (280) or pyogenic liver abscess (79, 220), metastatic disease or primary hepatocellular carcinoma (62, 78, 80, 124, 125, 143, 307), extrahepatic obstructive jaundice (8, 16, 77, 209), and rarely, an "acute abdomen" (217). Sanai et al. (235) evaluated signs and symptoms associated with hepatic granulomas in 66 patients. Fever, weight loss, and fatigue were significantly more common in hepatic granulomas caused by TB than those by viral causes (77% versus 9%, $P = 0.0002$; 69% versus 9%, $P = 0.001$; and 69% versus 18%, $P = 0.01$, respectively). In addition, fever and weight loss were significantly more common in tuberculous hepatic granulomas than hepatic granulomas that were deemed idiopathic, though fatigue was statistically the same in each group (77% versus 33%, $P = 0.04$; 69% versus 22%, $P = 0.02$; and 69% versus 33%, $P > 0.05$, respectively).

THE LIVER IN RELATION TO THE SITE OF TUBERCULOSIS

Pulmonary Tuberculosis

Tuberculosis confined to the lungs involves the liver less often than does miliary tuberculosis. Hepatic granulomas are found at biopsy in about 20% of patients, but tubercle bacilli are rarely demonstrable by strain or culture (Table 5). A characteristic but nonspecific histologic manifestation of pulmonary tuberculosis is the presence of localized areas of Kupffer cell hyperplasia, yielding lesions called retothelial or histiocytic nodules. Biochemical abnormalities in patients with pulmonary tuberculosis may include elevated levels of alkaline phosphatase and hyperglobulinemia. Jaundice is rare as a manifestation of hepatic involvement due to pulmonary tuberculosis alone.

Localized Extrapulmonary Tuberculosis

Korn and colleagues (144) described three patterns of hepatic dysfunction in 50 patients with extrapulmonary tuberculosis: (i) elevated alkaline phosphatase and BSP retention associated with space-occupying granulomas, (ii) abnormal flocculation test results and hyperglobulinemia associated with chronic localized tuberculous infections such as osteomyelitis, and (iii) a combination of the two, simulating intrinsic liver disease without overt jaundice. Hepatic granulomas were present in 80% of patients, and most (87.5%) had impaired BSP excretion. Large caseating granulomas were more frequent in patients with the greatest degree of hepatic dysfunction. They found granulomas in 14 of 15 patients with raised alkaline phosphatase levels. However, the biochemical abnormality was an insensitive measure of hepatic granulomas because 10 of 15 patients without elevated alkaline phosphatase levels also had granulomas. Nonspecific abnormalities such as Kupffer cell hyperplasia and diffuse sinusoidal inflammation were common.

Abnormalities in one or more liver function or serum protein tests were present in all patients studied by Korn and colleagues (144). Serum bilirubin was elevated in 26.7% (highest value, 5.0 mg/dl), and slight jaundice was detected in three patients. Values for aminotransferases were only slightly elevated in most patients with extrapulmonary tuberculosis.

Palmer and associates (203) described 90 patients admitted to a London hospital with abdominal tuberculosis, most of whom were Asian immigrants. Liver biopsy often provided histologic confirmation in cases wherein the diagnosis was in doubt. Eight patients presented with fever and elevated alkaline phosphatase and had a histologic picture consistent with granulomatous hepatitis. The granulomas were noncaseating; tubercle bacilli were identified in biopsy tissue in only one patient.

Localized Hepatobiliary Tuberculosis

A subset of patients with extrapulmonary tuberculosis has the infection confined solely or predominantly to the liver or biliary tract. Terry and Gunnar (283) reported a dozen cases in 1957. They referred to this form of infection as *primary miliary tuber-culosis* of the liver and defined it as "a condition in which there is hematogenous dissemination of tuber-culosis of the liver with minimal involvement of other organs." Although inapparent sites of infection usually remained clinically silent, 4 of their 12 patients died with tuberculous spread to other organs. "Atypical tuberculosis of the liver" was the term proposed by Cleve and coworkers (52) to "designate exclusive or principal involvement of the liver by tuberculous infection leading to clinical manifestations of hepatic disease." Cinque and colleagues (51) suggested that tubercle bacilli reach the liver via the portal vein or hepatic artery. Indeed, in autopsy cases in which tuberculosis has been confined clinically to the liver, abdominal and mediastinal lymph node involvement may be found and may result in miliary spread.

Although rare in the United States (30), this form of localized hepatic tuberculosis is not infrequently encountered in areas with high rates of infection. For example, the prevalence of localized hepatic involvement in tuberculosis was 2.3% in 820 patients seen over an 8-year period in Saudi Arabia, with the diagnosis confirmed by endoscopic or laparoscopic biopsy in most cases (7). Liver involvement was present in 14.6% of these persons overall with abdominal tuberculosis. Among 112 patients with abdominal symptoms due to tuberculosis, 10% had macronodular focal hepatic lesions, often associated with hepatomegaly as seen on abdominal imaging studies (164). The report by Alvarez and Carpio (8) from the Philippines describes the clinical and histologic features of 130 patients with localized hepatobiliary tuberculosis seen over a 20-year period at the Santo Thomas University Hospital in Manila. In 82% of cases, the diagnosis was clinically suspected prior to histologic confirmation. The two major forms of presentation included (i) a hard nodular liver with fever and weight loss simulating cancer in 65% of patients and (ii) chronic recurrent jaundice mimicking extrahepatic obstruction in 35%. A 2:1 male predominance was observed, and the majority of patients were in the 11- to 30-year age range. Symptoms were generally present for 1 to 2 years prior to the diagnosis.

Percutaneous liver biopsy was performed in 71 persons and confirmed the diagnosis in 48 (67%). Laparoscopy yielded the correct diagnosis in 49 of 53 patients (92%), with the hepatic lesions appearing as cheesy, white, irregular nodules. In a few patients, however, what grossly appeared to be a tuberculoma was actually metastatic cancer on biopsy. Interestingly, a positive AFB stain was recorded in only 2 of 30 cases, although the mere presence of caseating granulomata was considered diagnostic by the authors.

Hepatic calcifications were efficient in 49% of patients. They appeared as rounded calcific densities with ill-defined margins scattered throughout the liver. Radiocolloid liver scan revealed filling defects in 52%. In three persons in whom hepatic arteriography was performed to exclude cancer, an avascular mass was seen, in contrast with the neovascularity usually expected with malignancy.

Hepatic enzyme abnormalities were seemingly dependent on whether or not jaundice was present; jaundice usually resulted from enlarged lymph nodes obstructing the common bile duct near the hepatoduodenal ligament or porta hepatis. Serum aminotransferase values were elevated in more than 90%, and alkaline phosphatase was raised in 100% of patients with jaundice. In contrast, only 5% of nonjaundiced patients had abnormal aminotransferase levels, and alkaline phosphatase values were elevated in only 60%. The presence or absence of jaundice also influenced the response to treatment. Seventy-five percent of nonjaundiced patients responded to conventional drug therapy, compared with only 25% with jaundice. Six of 45 jaundiced patients required surgical intervention for biliary decompression.

Overall, 12% of patients died, most owing to respiratory failure, a few secondary to tuberculous peritonitis, and approximately one-third due to portal hypertension and variceal hemorrhage. All of these last patients had cirrhosis. Although fatal variceal hemorrhage has been linked to tuberculous hepatic involvement by others (211), no causal relationship between tuberculosis and cirrhosis has been demonstrated (225).

Essop and his colleagues in South Africa (77) reviewed the clinical features of 96 patients with what they called "tuberculous hepatitis," that is, a predominantly hepatic presentation during acute miliary tuberculosis or chronic hepatic presentation during acute miliary tuberculosis or chronic hepatic tuberculosis secondary to reactivation of the disease. This form of tuberculosis represented 1.2% of all cases seen over a 6-year period. Physical signs and symptoms included tender hepatomegaly and fever in most patients. Splenomegaly was present in 45%. Right hypochondrial pain was common and led to exploratory laparotomy in two patients who presented with obstructive jaundice and an acute abdomen, respectively. Fourteen percent of the group had abdominal symptoms exclusively, 22% had respiratory symptoms, and 12% had only fever, sweats, malaise, and weight loss. Most patients had a combination of these three symptom complexes.

Granulomas were present on biopsy or at laparotomy or autopsy in 96% of patients, provided the first evidence of systemic granulomatous disease in

16 cases, and helped diagnose pulmonary disease in another 13 patients. This high incidence of granulomas was largely due to the exclusion of cases with primary pulmonary or extra-abdominal tuberculosis with incidental hepatic involvement. Caseation was present in 83% of patients, but tubercle bacilli were demonstrable by stain in only 9% of cases (those with the greatest number of granulomas and highest degree of caseation).

Other histologic findings included fatty change in 42% and portal fibrosis in 20%. Peliosis hepatis and amyloidosis were rare. Coexisting liver disease included cirrhosis in eight patients, alcoholic hepatitis in six, and hepatoma in one.

Serum alkaline phosphatase was moderately elevated (6-fold to 10-fold) in the majority of patients, and hyperbilirubinemia was present in about 25%. Hyponatremia was a common presenting laboratory abnormality.

The cumulative mortality rate was 42% for the patients in this series; mortality was highest in those with acute miliary tuberculosis; age below 20 years; a predisposing factor such as steroid therapy, chronic renal failure, or diabetes mellitus; and the presence of coagulopathy. Hepatic enzymes were not useful in predicting patient survival.

Huang et al. (123) described 5 patients with a local nodular form of hepatic tuberculosis from Taiwan over a 4-year period. All 5 patients underwent surgery and had a preoperative diagnosis of malignant hepatic neoplasm and a postoperative histological diagnosis of chronic granulomatous inflammation suggestive of tuberculosis. None of them had a known previous history of tuberculosis. All were positive for *M. tuberculosis* by PCR analysis of the liver tissue. This report as well as others (143) highlights the difficulty in correctly diagnosing hepatic tuberculosis. It is often confused with primary or metastatic carcinoma of the liver. A high index of suspicion is required for diagnosis, which can be made by histology and bacterial studies as well as by PCR techniques.

Tuberculomas

Tuberculomas may occur as solitary or multiple nodules in patients with primary miliary tuberculosis of the liver or secondary to reactivation of hepatic foci of infection. As mentioned previously, lesions may have a diameter of up to 12 cm (314) and may undergo central caseation leading to abscess formation (79, 113, 150, 219, 272). Symptoms of fever, malaise, and weight loss are common. Less often, abdominal pain and diarrhea occur. Hepatomegaly is frequent. Uncommon presenting signs have included portal hypertension, jaundice, and a palpable abdominal mass.

Jaundice, when present, has been attributed to tuberculomas at the porta hepatis, causing obstruction to bile flow (77). Rarely, these lesions bleed, leading to a clinical presentation of an acute abdomen with progressive anemia (217). Outside areas of endemicity, the diagnosis is often not suspected and is usually confirmed serendipitously with the finding of tuberculomas at laparotomy or at autopsy.

Biochemical parameters of hepatic injury are not prominently abnormal. Alkaline phosphatase levels are generally only slightly increased or normal, a pattern characteristic of space-occupying lesions of the liver. Filling defects on liver scan or angiography may suggest primary or metastatic carcinoma. Indeed, there are several reports of tuberculous pseudotumors (62, 78, 300, 301), including at least one instance wherein hepatic tuberculomas resembled malignant disease arteriographically (72). More commonly, tuberculomas are confused with an amebic or pyogenic liver abscess (79, 220, 280). Blind percutaneous liver biopsy has generally not been helpful in confirming the diagnosis (32, 70). Bhargava and colleagues (31), among others, reported the use of aspiration cytology at the time of laparoscopy to make the diagnosis in areas where the infection is common. Bacteriologic confirmation is difficult, and there are only a few reported instances of positive acid-fast stains or cultures (220). Zipser and coworkers (314) suggest that because of the condition's resemblance to metastatic disease, culture is often not attempted. However, they note that with successful antituberculous therapy, complete resolution of tuberculomas can be expected within 6 to 9 months. In addition, percutaneous drainage of tubercular abscess has been shown as an effective alternative to surgery (220). It should be pointed out that in regions where tuberculosis is endemic, the finding of caseating hepatic granulomata is generally sufficient to confirm the diagnosis, regardless of the results of AFB staining or cultures (77).

Treska and colleagues (290) report an asymptomatic isolated liver tuberculoma that initially responded to antituberculous therapy (ATT) but subsequently relapsed, and a second focus was found at this time adjacent to the middle hepatic vein. The patient was subsequently treated successfully with partial hepatic resection. The patient continued ATT postoperatively, and postoperative imaging at 2 months showed resolution of the 2-cm focus, confirmed again at 5 months postoperatively, at which time they stopped ATT. At last follow-up, 10 months out, the patient had normal post-op findings of the liver with no evidence of disease.

Several reports describe the sonographic, computed tomographic (CT), and magnetic resonance imaging (MRI) appearance of macroscopic tuberculosis of the liver (36, 164, 185, 191). Ultrasonographic features that suggest a diagnosis of tuberculoma include a mass with irregular calcifications, the presence of ascites, splenomegaly with enlarged lymph nodes, and resolution of the lesion or lesions following antituberculous therapy (36). CT findings include low-density, solid, heterogeneous, and sometimes partially calcified lesions with a thickened wall and either no or minimal enhancement by contrast. Irregular calcifications are also characteristic. High-density ascites relating to high ascitic protein content is also a useful clue (36). In children, single or multiple low-attenuation intrahepatic lesions, hepatomegaly, ascites, and a positive tuberculin skin test result suggest the diagnosis of tuberculosis rather than disseminated malignancy (152, 185).

Murata and colleagues (188) described the MRI findings in one patient with surgically proven tuberculomas who had hypoechoic lesions in the lesion seen initially, as described by Kawamori and colleagues (139). The lesions were hyperintense on weighted T2 images, indicating the tuberculomas can be of either increased or decreased signal intensity on MRI.

The role of endoscopic retrograde cholangiopancreatography (ERCP) has been emphasized in patients with suspected tuberculous strictures of the common bile duct who present with obstructive jaundice (17) (see "Tuberculosis of the bile ducts," below).

Miliary Tuberculosis

Hepatic involvement in disseminated tuberculosis is very common (30, 142, 218, 253). Granulomas have been demonstrated in 75% to 100% of patients with miliary disease (Table 5). Characteristically, miliary lesions are small (1 to 2 mm), epithelioid granulomas. The proportion of patients with caseous necrosis has varied from 33% to 100%, depending on the series. Nonspecific hepatic lesions such as Kupffer cell hyperplasia and fatty metamorphosis also are common.

As with pulmonary and localized extrapulmonary disease, impaired BSP excretion is the most frequent biochemical abnormality in miliary tuberculosis. Alkaline phosphatase elevations occur in approximately 50% of cases. There is a poor correlation between hepatic function tests and liver histology in cases with miliary involvement. The clinical features of acute miliary infection localized predominantly to the liver have been reviewed by Essop and colleagues (77) and Alvarez and Carpio (8) (see "Localized Hepatobiliary Tuberculosis," above). Rarely has disseminated tuberculosis presented as hepatic failure. A case report described a Japanese patient who presented with jaundice, deteriorated rapidly, and died just 3 days after admission (17).

Miliary tuberculosis presenting as fulminant hepatitis

Fulminant hepatic failure caused by tuberculosis was described by Curry and Alcott (57) in 1955. Although deaths due to miliary tuberculosis are not infrequent, deaths specifically attributable to acute hepatic failure are unusual (17, 98, 128). Hussain and colleagues (128) describe a 54-year-old woman who presented with a 5-day history of right-upper-quadrant pain, vomiting, and mild jaundice. Two months earlier, her hepatic enzyme levels had been normal. Twenty years earlier, she had been treated for active pulmonary tuberculosis with a 2-year drug regimen. On presentation, her bilirubin was elevated threefold, alkaline phosphatase twice normal, and aspartate aminotransferase (AST) five times normal, along with hypoalbuminemia, hyponatremia, and hypoprothrombinemia. Acetaminophen levels were "negative," and all hepatitis viral serology was "negative." Her chest radiograph appeared normal, and an ultrasound scan showed an enlarged liver. She deteriorated clinically over the next 8 days, with her AST peaking at 1,790 IU/liter and her serum sodium falling to a low of 114 mEq/liter. A transjugular biopsy showed caseating granulomas, but AFB cultures remained negative. She was treated aggressively for tuberculosis but continued to deteriorate and experienced renal failure along with stage IV coma, and she died 13 days after presentation. Autopsy revealed the presence of AFB in multiple organs, with the liver showing coagulative necrosis with more than 50% of the parenchyma destroyed by caseating necrosis. Culture of the liver grew *M. tuberculosis*.

Congenital Tuberculosis

Reports of congenital and neonatal tuberculosis are scant (63, 285) but continue to appear (12, 29, 47, 50, 301). Debre and colleagues (63) reported an infant who died with disseminated tuberculosis of the liver, spleen, lung, and hilar lymph nodes 7 weeks after being born to a mother with long-standing pulmonary tuberculosis. Although the child was separated from the mother immediately after delivery, jaundice was observed during the first week of the infant's life, and it was concluded that there had been transplacental transmission of tubercle bacilli. When prompt treatment is initiated, the prognosis is good, as has been illustrated by 2 cases (12, 50). Recently, Berk and Sylvester (29) reported a neonate with congenital tuberculosis who presented with fulminant hepatic failure without respiratory compromise and was successfully treated with antitubercular therapy despite profound hepatic compromise.

Histologically, neonatal tuberculosis of the liver is characterized by diffuse, large, caseating granulomas containing numerous tubercle bacilli accompanied by fatty metamorphosis (209). Hepatomegaly, jaundice, and failure to thrive in an infant born to a mother with active tuberculosis should alert the clinician to the diagnosis.

Atypical Mycobacterial Infection

Rarely is a mycobacterial organism other than *M. tuberculosis* isolated from the liver. McNutt and Fudenberg (176) have drawn attention to the fact that atypical mycobacteria most commonly cause localized pulmonary infection and generally do not result in disseminated disease. Stewart and Jackson (278) reported hepatic and splenic tuberculosis due to *Mycobacterium kansasii* diagnosed at autopsy in a patient with a myeloproliferative disease. In general, however, *M. kansasii* does not produce hepatic disease, even in HIV-infected persons (42, 152). Although *M. kansasii* can be cultured from the necrotic tuberculous lesions, no other gross pathologic or clinical features distinguish the infection from that due to *M. tuberculosis* (152, 267).

M. avium is the most common organism associated with nontuberculous mycobacterial infection. Although rarely reported between 1940 and 1980, with only a few dozen cases in the literature, the advent of AIDS has brought a plethora of new cases to light (119, 130) (see "Hepatic Mycobacterial Infection in AIDS").

The portal of entry is thought to be the gastrointestinal tract and possibly the respiratory tree. Hematogenous dissemination is common, with fever, weight loss, local pain, cough, and night sweats being frequent presenting symptoms. Hepatosplenomegaly has been recorded in 35% to 45% of patients, and jaundice was noted in 8% of patients in the series reviewed by Horsburgh (119). The diagnosis can be achieved by several methods, but liver biopsy may be the most rapid and efficient, as illustrated by case reports in references 121 and 252. Caseation was infrequent in all tissues examined, and AFB were rarely visible. Culture was positive in only about 25% of cases.

In contrast with *M. avium* infection in association with AIDS, more than two-thirds of patients without AIDS have responded to therapy (most having received cycloserine as part of the treatment regimen), although patients with large numbers of organisms were more likely to experience therapy failure (119). Other atypical mycobacteria that may involve the liver include *Mycobacterium scrofulaceum* (208), *Mycobacterium gordonae* (148), *Mycobacterium xenopi*, *Mycobacterium fortuitum* (180), and *Mycobacterium chelonae* (152).

Granulomatous Hepatitis Induced by Bacillus Calmette-Guérin

Granulomatous involvement of the liver has been reported in 12% to 28% of patients receiving bacillus Calmette-Guérin (BCG) as immunotherapy for neoplastic disease (34, 85, 93, 102, 126, 201). Flippin and colleagues (85) reported that asymptomatic granulomatous hepatitis usually occurs within several months after the last BCG inoculation. The clinical appearance of constitutional symptoms, hepatomegaly, mildly elevated serum transaminase and bilirubin values, and moderately elevated alkaline phosphatase levels, focal defects, or nonhomogeneous uptake on technetium liver scan plus the presence of granulomas, hepatocellular necrosis, lymphohistiocytic aggregates, and Kupffer cell hyperplasia represent the clinicopathologic spectrum of granulomatous hepatitis due to BCG.

The exact mechanism for the development of granulomatous disease following BCG therapy is not known. A role for both viable BCG bacilli and hypersensitivity reaction has been proposed. O'Brien and Hyslop (197) note that an intense inflammatory reaction occurs at the site of vaccination, and BCG organisms often remain viable for weeks to months and may disseminate to various organs. The role that associated immunosuppressive chemotherapy plays in predisposition to systemic BCG infection is unclear. Rarely have acid-fast BCG bacilli been demonstrated in hepatic or lymph node tissue (85). Hunt and associates (126) proposed that BCG preparations are antigenic and that granulomas develop as a result of the hypersensitivity response to these antigens.

Patients with symptomatic granulomatous hepatitis have a high rate of morbidity, and several fatalities have been reported (85, 175). O'Brien and Hyslop (197) warn that an early sign of BCG "overdose" may be the development of anergy to tuberculin purified protein derivative (PPD). Isoniazid (INH) and methanol extraction residue (MER) given concurrently during BCG inoculation have each been shown to protect against the development of granulomatous hepatitis (146, 271).

Severe and life-threatening disseminated BCG infection with granulomatous hepatitis has been reported with local immunotherapy using BCG for urinary bladder cancer therapy (102). This patient was successfully treated with empirical antitubercular therapy in combination with a short course of steroids.

Tuberculosis of the Hepatobiliary Pancreatic Tract

Tuberculosis of the bile ducts

Prior to 1900, biliary tuberculosis was commonly found at autopsy. Since the turn of the 20th century, however, the reported incidence has been low. Stemmerman (277) found only 45 instances in 1,500 autopsies of patients with tuberculosis, yielding an incidence of approximately 3%. In that series, the incidence of bile duct tuberculosis rose 7% in cases with miliary involvement. The distribution of periportal tubercles in those cases with bile duct involvement was not significantly different from cases having no bile duct involvement (47% versus 43%), and there was no consistent relationship between the weight of the liver and either the size or the number of biliary abscesses.

The typical pathologic picture of bile duct (tubular) tuberculosis as reported by Stemmerman (277) is one of multiple small cavities (1 to 20 mm) containing greenish necrotic material. Rarely do these biliary abscesses reach a large size (up to 12 cm), and rarely can a bile ductule be traced directly to the cavity. Microscopically, caseation and bile pigment are usually present within the cavity. Bile ductule and capillary remnants may be visible within the caseous process. The abscess capsule varies in thickness, being widest when bile duct proliferation and collagen bundles are present. AFB, when found, are usually demonstrated at the junction of the outer capsule and the caseous inner wall.

Signs and symptoms attributable to bile duct tuberculosis are uncommon. Only three of the 45 patients reported by Stemmerman had clinical jaundice (6.7%), and only one-third had hepatomegaly. However, tuberculosis of other organs drained by the portal circulation was present in 41 of 45 cases, including caseous tuberculosis of mesenteric lymph nodes in 89%, tuberculous ulcerations of the intestinal tract in 73%, and tuberculous peritonitis in 27%.

The pathogenesis of bile duct tuberculosis has been linked to two possible mechanisms. Rosenkranz and Howard (227) showed that periportal tubercles could rupture into the walls of contiguous bile ductules, thereby giving rise to an abscess cavity. They thought that the excretion of AFB into the bile was always due to microscopic ruptures of this kind. Other workers postulated that the bile ducts may be infected primarily. Stemmerman (277) favored the theory that bile abscesses arise from tubercle bacilli, having gained entry into small bile ductules from the blood stream or lymphatics.

Jaundice due to hepatobiliary tuberculosis

Jaundice is rare in tuberculosis (35, 55, 89, 144). Nevertheless, it has become axiomatic that visible jaundice, when present, may imply ductal obstruction in the absence of other hepatic or drug-induced injury. Patients with elevated bilirubin levels usually have cholestasis associated with the parenchymal damage due to tuberculous infection. Curry and Alcott (57) suggested that the intrahepatic type of jaundice was usually associated with acute, fulminating miliary disease, as illustrated by a case presenting as fulminant hepatitis (17). The jaundice that has been occasionally noted in instances of chronic pulmonary tuberculosis generally has been attributed to the generalized dissemination of tubercle bacilli that occurs preterminally.

Jaundice due to intrahepatic cholestasis is usually mild (serum bilirubin levels being <5 to 6 mg/dl), and it is often clinically inapparent. In contrast, deep jaundice may occur when the larger biliary ducts are involved or when enlarged lymph nodes obstruct the porta hepatis (77). There are several reports of tuberculous lymphadenitis involving the porta hepatis causing obstructive jaundice with bilirubin levels greater than 20 mg/dl (1, 8, 52, 142, 189, 190, 207, 273, 309). Pineda and Dalmacio-Cruz (211) and Alvarez and Carpio (8) emphasized the potential complication of portal hypertension with ascites, splenomegaly, and ruptured esophageal varices that occurred in several of their patients with tuberculous involvement of the porta hepatis leading to biliary cirrhosis. Portal lymph nodes may be involved by direct contiguous spread from the gallbladder or by hematogenous or lymphatic spread from organs drained by these nodes.

Occasionally, jaundice has been reported secondary to a bile duct stricture in patients with known tuberculosis. Bearer and colleagues (24) described the ERCP findings in a Filipino immigrant with obstructive jaundice who was found to have a common bile duct stricture in the presence of granulomatous hepatitis. A diagnosis of tuberculosis was confirmed by aspirate and culture from the bile. The stricture persisted despite antituberculous therapy, and biliary cirrhosis developed, as was seen on follow-up liver biopsy. As a result, a biliary stent was inserted, which normalized the hepatic enzymes within a period of 2 months. Stanley and colleagues (273) have also reported the treatment of a tuberculous bile duct stricture using an endoprosthesis. Colovic and colleagues (54) report a case of obstructive jaundice with severe narrowing of the distal common bile duct (CBD) seen on ERCP. During open surgery, the stricture was found to be secondary to TB lymphadenitis causing compression and inflammation of the lymph nodes and the CBD complicated by caseation of the lymph nodes causing fistulation into the CBD. The narrowed distal CBD was resected, the distal end oversewn, and the proximal end anastomosed with a Roux-en-Y jejunal limb followed by ATT with good results through 2.5 years of follow-up.

Multiple intrahepatic biliary strictures, areas of dilation, beading, and ectasia resembling sclerosing cholangitis or cholangiocarcinoma are also described (8, 30, 115). Biliary strictures may occur in the hilar region or distal common bile duct with dilation of the intrahepatic ducts. Arora and colleagues (15) report a 23-year-old male who presented with anorexia, icterus, brown urine, clay-colored stool, and weight loss. Chest X ray was negative, and he had no history of TB infection. Total bilirubin was 12.1 mg% with a direct fraction of 9 mg%, alkaline phosphatase was 2,122 IU/liter, AST was 166 IU/liter, and alanine aminotransferase (ALT) was 95 IU/liter. Imaging showed dilated intrahepatics with a block at the porta hepatis, right portal vein thrombosis, and collapsed distal common bile duct. Clinicoradiologic diagnosis of a cholangiocarcinoma Klatskin's tumor was made, and the patient was sent to diagnostic and exploratory laparoscopy with resection. The pathology, however, showed no tumor to be present, and PCR for TB was positive, allowing a diagnosis of a tubercular lesion at the porta hepatis to be made. Tubercular cholangitis is extremely rare (257). It is thought to occur as a result of rupture of a caseating granuloma from the portal tract into the bile duct. Clinical features resemble bacterial cholangitis, with right upper quadrant pain, fever, and jaundice.

Tuberculosis of the gallbladder

The gallbladder is an uncommon site of tuberculous infection. Leader (150), in reviewing the literature in 1951, noted that fewer than 40 cases have been reported. The majority of cases were women over 30 years of age. Gallstones were present in more than one-half of cases, and the most commonly reported symptoms and signs included epigastric pain made worse by eating and right upper quadrant tenderness. Saluja et al. (233) report 3 cases of TB of the gallbladder with a clinical presentation that included abdominal pain (2), fever (1), anorexia (1), weight loss (1), melena (1), hepatomegaly (1), and a gallbladder mass (1).

Rarely has tuberculosis been isolated to the gallbladder. Most cases occur in association with other organ involvement, including tuberculous peritonitis. Cholecystitis is the most frequent preoperative diagnosis, and cholangitis has also been reported. Miliary tuberculosis presenting as acute cholecystitis was reported by Garber and colleagues (92).

Treatment usually requires cholecystectomy in combination with antituberculous therapy. Complications such as tuberculous abscess of the gallbladder require prompt surgical attention.

Cryptic miliary tuberculosis clinically mimicking a case of cholecystitis with sepsis has been reported (258). Pulmonary tuberculosis with gallbladder involvement presenting as acute cholecystitis and cholelithiasis was reported in a 14-year-old girl by Rozmanic et al. (229). A rare case of hepatobiliary tuberculosis presenting as a gallbladder tumor has also been described (27).

Tuberculosis of the pancreas

Tuberculosis of the pancreas or of the peripancreatic lymph nodes is infrequent compared to the liver. We were able to identify 130 cases reported in the literature from 1966 to 2009 (Table 9). One explanation for the lower prevalence is that pancreatic enzymes destroy mycobacteria (304). Pancreatic involvement can be isolated to the gland, a part of miliary tuberculosis, or a site of reactivated disease. The most likely mechanism of spread is lymphohematogenous dissemination from an occult focus in the lungs (64, 88, 223, 291). Men and women are affected equally (149, 245), with a mean age of around 40 years. Reported cases of pancreatic tuberculosis are predominantly seen from northeast Asia or immigrants to Europe and the United States from countries where tuberculosis is endemic (149). Patients with HIV infection have a greater incidence of atypical and extrapulmonary tuberculosis. Tubercular pancreatic abscess as an initial AIDS-defining disorder in patients infected with HIV has been reported (132).

The clinical manifestations of pancreatic tuberculosis depend on the type of involvement, acute or chronic pancreatitis, and focal mass lesion mimicking carcinoma portal hypertension. Symptoms may include acute or chronic abdominal pain, weight loss, recurrent vomiting, obstructive jaundice, and occasionally fever of unknown origin. Most cases have a high sedimentation rate and tuberculin skin tests are positive in over 70% of cases (149, 245). The most frequent clinical presentation is a pancreatic mass mimicking carcinoma (64, 88, 223, 291). Less often, acute or chronic pancreatitis is described (88, 223, 245). Portal hypertension secondary to portal vein compression or thrombosis is rare (304). A majority of cases involve the head and/or body of the pancreas; isolated involvement of the tail of the pancreas is uncommon.

Radiologic findings are often nonspecific. Focal pancreatic lesions in pancreatic tuberculosis are usually demonstrated by ultrasound or CT closely mimicking pancreatic carcinoma or mucinous tumors of the pancreas (304). Occasionally, the pancreatic mass is diagnosed on imaging as a pancreatic abscess (213, 245). Pombo et al. (213) retrospectively reviewed the CT findings of 6 patients with pancreatic tuberculosis, 3 of whom had AIDS. Findings included focal mass lesions, multiple small low-attenuation pancreatic

Table 9. Pancreatic tuberculosis as reported in the literature

Author(s) (reference[s])	Yr	No. of cases	Clinical presentation	Type of involvement			Pancreatic pathology		Outcome	
				Imaging focal mass	Isolated	Disseminated	Caseating granulomas	Positive AFB smear or *M. tuberculosis* culture	Treated successfully with ATT for 6–12 mo	Mortality
Ladas et al. (149)	1966–97	41	Abdominal pain (60%), fever (40%), weight loss (37%), jaundice (23%)	91%	100%		100%	38%		7%
Ladas et al. (149)	1997	2	Abdominal pain (1), fever (1), weight loss (2), anemia (1)	2	2		2	2	2	
Rezeig (223)	1998	4	Abdominal pain (4), fever (1), weight loss (2), jaundice (1)	4	4		4	3	4	
Woodfield et al. (304)	2004	3	Abdominal pain (3), fever (1), weight loss (2), jaundice (2)	3	3		3	2	3	
Pombo et al. (213)	1998	6	Abdominal pain (4), fever (3), weight loss (3), jaundice (4), diarrhea (1), HIV+ (3)	4	2	4	6	6	5	1
Demir et al. (64)	2001	2	Abdominal pain (2), fever (2), weight loss (2)	2	2		2		2	
Schneider et al. (245)	2002	2	Portal hypertension (1)	2	2		2	1	1	
El Mansari et al. (75)	2003	2	Abdominal pain (1), weight loss (1), jaundice (1)	2	2		2		1	1
Kumar et al. (147)	2003	2	Abdominal pain (1), fever (2), weight loss (2), jaundice (1), HIV+ (1)	2	2		2	1	1	1
Pramesh et al. (215)	2002	2								
Franco-Pardes et al. (88)	2002	2		2					2	
Xia et al. (306)	2002	16	Abdominal pain (75%), fever (50%), weight loss (69%), jaundice (31%), back pain (38%)	100%	100%	Liver, spleen, bile duct involvement in 42%	75%	30%	100%	
Chaudhary et al. (45)	2002	9	Mimicking pancreatic carcinoma (5), acute pseudocyst (1), pancreatic abscess (1)		9				8	1
Lo et al. (162)	1998	2	GIB[a] (1)	2					2	
Saluja et al. (233)	2007	7	Abdominal pain (5), jaundice (3), fever (2), anorexia (2), weight loss (3), enlarged supraclavicular lymph nodes (2), hepatomegaly (3), palpable gallbladder (2), abdominal mass (1)	3					4	
Others[b] (18, 22, 25, 37, 46, 48, 53, 58, 61, 65, 86, 118, 134, 138, 145, 161, 202, 205, 206, 221, 224, 234, 248, 254, 260, 261, 264, 282, 291, 311)	1998–2009	29	Abdominal pain (15), fever (9), weight loss (9), jaundice (8), HIV+ (2), dyspepsia and sour eructations (1), dysphagia (1), anorexia (1), back pain (1), bilious vomiting (1), history of pulmonary TB 30 yr prior with negative chest X ray (1), duodenal stenosis with pancreatico-duodenal fistula (1), acute pancreatitis (2), recurrent pancreatitis (1), post-liver transplant (1), periampullary mass (1)	24	21	Significant portal and retroperitoneal adenopathy and multiple cystic lesions in the spleen and liver (1), peripancreatic and porta hepatis multicystic lesions (1), peripancreatic and para-aortic lymphadenopathy (1)	17	14, PCR+ (7)	22	

[a]GIB, gastrointestinal bleeding.
[b]Single case reports.

nodules, or diffuse enlargement of glands in AIDS patients, whereas a nonspecific focal mass lesion was seen in HIV-seronegative patients. Low-attenuation peripancreatic or periportal adenopathy with peripheral rim enhancement in conjunction with signs of disseminated tuberculosis were ancillary features that supported a diagnosis of pancreatic tuberculosis.

A definitive diagnosis of pancreatic tuberculosis is only achieved with histologic confirmation (304). However, the success rate of image-guided fine-needle aspiration cytology in diagnosing pancreatic tuberculosis is only approximately 50% (134, 245). In cases of pancreatic abscesses, clinical correlation and aspiration are necessary to differentiate between a pyogenic and tuberculous abscess. If tuberculosis is not confirmed by aspiration cytology or core biopsy, then laparoscopy may prove to be helpful. However, even with the use of appropriate preoperative and intraoperative investigations, the diagnosis is often only made at the time of pancreatic resection (64, 291).

Hemobilia secondary to tuberculosis

Hemobilia (biliary tract hemorrhage) has been associated with various inflammatory and vascular lesions of the biliary tree, but only two cases of tuberculosis-related hemobilia have been described. Agrawal and associates (3) reported hemobilia following a percutaneous needle biopsy of the liver in a patient with disseminated tuberculosis. They argued that diffuse involvement of the liver was the primary cause of the hemobilia, postulating that one or more necrotic foci might have spontaneously eroded into a portal blood vessel and bile duct simultaneously. However, percutaneous liver biopsy by itself has been associated with hemobilia (74, 153, 154), and there seems little reason to relate this extraordinarily rare event to the tuberculosis. Das et al. (59) reported hemobilia in a patient with disseminated tuberculosis presenting initially with nonlocalizable massive upper gastrointestinal bleeding but subsequently found to have pancreatitis, pleural effusion, and hemobilia, which were treated successfully. Hepatic artery mycotic aneurysm of tubercular etiology is also reported (26).

Hepatic Mycobacterial Infection in AIDS

Histologic material obtained via liver biopsy or at autopsy in patients with AIDS has revealed hepatic pathology in the majority (66, 97, 105, 151, 158, 200, 222, 246). Although most lesions are nonspecific, the findings of hepatic granulomata have been relatively commonplace, and the diagnosis of M. *tuberculosis* and M. *avium* infection is now being made with regularity (13, 42, 130, 234, 249, 266, 279).

Mycobacterium tuberculosis in HIV and AIDS

Persons infected with HIV are susceptible to infection with tuberculosis, both from reactivation of a latent disease and from newly acquired infections that can progress rapidly (42). Infection rates up to 1,000-fold higher have been reported in HIV-positive persons than in those not infected with HIV (167). Selwyn and colleagues (249) found that 15% of HIV-positive intravenous drug users with a positive tuberculin test result developed active tuberculosis over a 2-year period, compared with none of the similar group of HIV-seronegative persons. Similarly, in a study of 1,130 HIV-seropositive persons without AIDS monitored for a median of 53 months, Markowitz and colleagues (167) found that patients with CD4 counts of less than 200 cells/mm^3 and PPD-positive patients were at high risk for tuberculosis.

Although M. *tuberculosis* in an HIV-infected patient is primarily a pulmonary infection, extrapulmonary sites of disease are common. Between 25% and 70% of HIV-associated M. *tuberculosis* cases have extrapulmonary disease, a finding that fulfills current Centers for Disease Control and Prevention (CDC) surveillance criteria for the diagnosis of AIDS (42, 147, 214). Hepatosplenomegaly is frequently present in HIV-positive patients and thus is relatively nonspecific for the diagnosis of a mycobacterial infection. The most common extrapulmonary sites of involvement in patients with AIDS are lymph nodes, blood, bone marrow, the urinary tract, the liver, and the central nervous system. Extrapulmonary involvement is associated with poorer prognosis than in pulmonary tuberculosis alone in these patients because extrapulmonary disease is associated with a greater degree of immune deficiency (42). Clinically and pathologically, generalized tuberculosis in the setting of AIDS is characterized by unusual features or the lack of typical features described for disseminated tuberculosis in patients who do not have AIDS. As a result, many cases remain undiagnosed until postmortem examinations (268).

A retrospective analysis of all patients with AIDS and tuberculosis in San Francisco between 1981 and 1988 by Small and coworkers (266) found a prevalence of M. *tuberculosis* at 2.2% (132 of 6,103 AIDS cases). Patients with M. *tuberculosis* infection were more likely to be African American or Hispanic and to have intravenous drug abuse as a risk factor. Eighty percent were born in the United States. Fifty-nine percent of these patients developed tuberculosis prior to any other AIDS-defining disease, and nearly 30% of this group had extrapulmonary involvement. Approximately one-third had pulmonary tuberculosis, and the remaining one-third had both pulmonary and extrapulmonary disease. Nearly 50% of patients who experienced *M. tuberculosis* infection prior to any other infection had a positive tuberculin test result. Of those with extrapulmonary involvement, liver biopsy was diagnostic in a number of patients. Although site specifics were not given in this review, the percentage of acid-fast stains from extrapulmonary sites that were positive was only 16% compared with 75% positivity for culture. In an autopsy series consisting of 29 patients with AIDS and a confirmed diagnosis of tuberculosis, hepatic involvement was seen in 45% (2). African-American ethnicity is an independent risk factor for extrapulmonary tuberculosis. Mortality at 6 months correlates in part with dissemination of *M. tuberculosis* and the severity of underlying comorbidities (100).

Vilaichone et al. (297) compared the clinical spectrum of hepatic tuberculosis between immunocompetent and immunocompromised patients. Fever, weight loss, hepatomegaly, disproportionate elevation of alkaline phosphatase, and reverse albumin-globulin ratios were common in hepatic tuberculosis. Noncaseating granulomas without detection of AFB was a common finding in both groups; however, disproportionate elevation of alkaline phosphatase was significantly higher in the immunocompromised hosts. PCR techniques showed a sensitivity of 86% and a specificity of 100% in the diagnosis of hepatic tuberculosis.

Several atypical features of *M. tuberculosis* infection in HIV-positive persons were noted in the series by Small and colleagues (266). The first was that the 30% with extrapulmonary involvement was a substantially higher figure than the 13% reported in patients without AIDS from the San Francisco area. The other major difference was that although HIV-positive persons did not appear to respond any differently to antituberculous medication, they experienced a much higher incidence of adverse drug reactions (18%) than that reported for patients not infected with HIV (3.7%). Skin rashes accounted for 56% of adverse reactions, but hepatitis developed in 26%. Rifampin (RIF) was the most common drug associated with an adverse reaction, requiring its discontinuation. INH was withdrawn in 4% and ethambutol in 1%. Sixty percent of all adverse reactions occurred within the first month of treatment, and 95% were evident by the end of the second month. Of the 125 patients who received antituberculous therapy, eight (6.4%) died of tuberculosis-related causes (with six of eight deaths occurring in the first month of treatment). Overall, treatment failure occurred in just 1% and relapse in 5%, which was not different from patients without the AIDS

Liberato et al. (159) compared characteristics of pulmonary tuberculosis in HIV-seropositive and -seronegative patients in a northeastern region of Brazil. Patients with pulmonary tuberculosis and HIV infection were mostly male, showed higher frequency of weight loss (>10 kg), and had a higher rate of nonreactive result to the tuberculin skin test, a higher frequency of negative sputum smear examination for AFB, and negative sputum culture for *M. tuberculosis*. Treatment failure was more common in those who were HIV positive. The association between extrapulmonary and pulmonary tuberculosis was more frequent in those who were seropositive for HIV than in those without HIV infection (30% versus 1.6%).

The higher incidence of adverse reactions to antituberculous medications in patients with AIDS has also been noted with other antimicrobials, such as trimethoprim-sulfamethoxazole and pentamidine, among others (239) (see below). As noted by Small and colleagues (266), HIV-infected persons with AIDS appear to be at increased risk of hepatotoxicity from antituberculous therapy. Ozick and colleagues (202) observed that the combination of INH and RIF produced hepatocellular injury (defined as an ALT level of >200 IU/liter) in 11% of patients in New York City, several of whom were under the age of 35. Amarapurkar and colleagues (9) described a tuberculous abscess of the liver associated with HIV infection that had features similar to tuberculous abscesses that have developed in the non-HIV-infected population.

Obstructive jaundice due to tuberculosis is usually seen in immunocompetent patients due to tubercular hilar adenopathy or biliary stricture. Recently, Probst et al. (216) reported a patient with obstructive jaundice in AIDS who was diagnosed by ERCP and endoscopic aspiration of bile. AFB were detected in direct smears and identified as *M. tuberculosis* by PCR and by traditional culture. The patient was treated with antituberculous therapy with resolution of jaundice; however, she died after 4 weeks from suspected tuberculous sepsis.

Mycobacterium avium complex in AIDS

Disseminated infection with *M. avium* complex (MAC) is the most common systemic bacterial infection complicating AIDS in the United States (130). The annual incidence of MAC is up to 20% after an AIDS-defining illness has occurred (120). Since the seminal report by Greene and colleagues (104) in 1982 first brought MAC to light as an opportunistic infection, numerous reports have followed. Although MAC is rarely reported as the initial opportunistic infection in AIDS, disseminated MAC has been present in up to 50% of patients with AIDS coming to autopsy, with the antemortem diagnosis being confirmed in 30% to 40% (43) (Table 10). According

Table 10. Hepatic *Mycobacterium avium* in AIDS

Author(s) (reference)	Total no. studied	No. with *M. avium* infection	No. with granulomas	No. with positive AFB stain	No. with positive culture	
					With granuloma	Without granuloma
Greene et al. (104)	5	4	3	3	3	1
Glasgow et al. (97)	42	8	9	6		3 of 6
Reichert et al. (222)	9	3	0	3	2	
Lebovics et al. (151)	25	4	3	3	3	1
Lewis et al. (158)	9	2	1	2	1	1
Hawkins et al. (112)	366	67	NSR[a]	NSR	6 of 6 (biopsy), 32 of 42 (autopsy)	
Orenstein et al. (200)	10	6	6	6	5	
Guarda et al. (105)	13	1	NSR	1 (bone marrow)	1 (bone marrow)	
Schneiderman et al. (246)	85	8 (biopsy), 6 (autopsy)	7 (biopsy), 1 (autopsy)	NSR		NSR
Chang et al. (44)	28	8	11	2		
Tarantino et al. (281)	12	5		12		

[a]NSR, not specifically reported.

to Horsburgh (119), this increased incidence is not only due to improved diagnostic methods but also reflects improved treatment regimens that may have influenced the decision to pursue the diagnosis. In addition, the introduction of antiretroviral therapies has increased survival among HIV-infected patients because *M. avium* typically occurs late in the course of AIDS. Such therapy also has permitted the diagnosis in increasing numbers of patients with *M. avium* disease

In contrast with *M. tuberculosis* in AIDS, which results largely from reactivation of a previous focus of infection, disseminated *M. avium* infection is usually the result of primary infection. The organism is ubiquitous in nature and is acquired by exposure to environmental sources such as food, water, soil, and house dust. The portal of entry is considered to be the gastrointestinal tract because local gastrointestinal infections are common. The organism disseminates hematogenously and has a predilection for parasitizing macrophages. As a result, reticuloendothelial system involvement is a hallmark of infection. Microscopically, the liver (and other organs) is filled with large numbers of distended histiocytes teeming with AFB as seen on Ziehl-Neelsen staining (Fig. 5). Tissue loads are estimated to be as high as 10^9 to 10^{10}

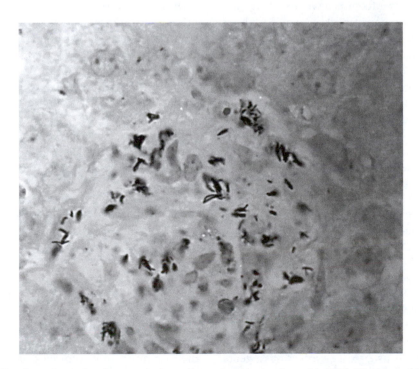

Figure 5. *Mycobacterium avium* in a poorly formed granuloma in a patient with AIDS. (Courtesy of I. K. Ishak.)

colony-forming units per gram, with little evidence of granuloma formation or surrounding inflammatory response. Although phagocytosis of the organism appears to be normal, macrophage-mediated killing is apparently severely impaired. Histologically, the large numbers of organisms are present amid a minimal inflammatory response resembling that of lepromatous leprosy (12, 108). Caseation necrosis is rarely observed in the liver, being described more commonly in pulmonary *M. avium* infections (119).

The most common clinical presentation of *M. avium* is persistent fever with or without night sweats and weight loss. The likelihood of disseminated disease is greater than 70% in febrile patients with AIDS in whom *Pneumocystis carinii*, cytomegalovirus, and other pathogens are excluded. Chronic diarrhea and abdominal pain suggest gastrointestinal involvement. Extrahepatic obstruction may produce a cholangitis or an acalculous cholecystitis picture. Severe anemia is another hallmark of *M. avium* infection, and frequent transfusions may be required. The diagnosis is confirmed by culture of peripheral blood, which has a sensitivity ranging from 86% to 96%. Bone marrow smear and culture are the best indicators for early dissemination. The liver as well as the bone marrow and lymph nodes remain important potential diagnostic biopsy sites. Tarantino et al. (281) evaluated fine-needle aspiration biopsy in disseminated mycobacterial infection in patients with HIV infection. Spleen and/or lymph node aspiration biopsy indicated the specific diagnosis in 100% of patients. Patients with disseminated *M. avium* infection have a significantly shortened survival compared with patients without AIDS and *M. avium* infection. At autopsy, however, death is seldom seen to be a direct result of the organism because causes of death are similar to those in patients with AIDS who do not have the infection. The shortened survival is presumably the result of severe malnutrition and weight loss associated with the organism (119).

Jaundice due to hepatic involvement by *M. avium* is rare. Bilirubin values were normal in all cases of *M. avium* infection reported by Glasgow and colleagues (97) despite a florid granulomatous reaction involving about 40% of the hepatic parenchyma in one patient. Lewis and coworkers (158) described jaundice in one patient with disseminated *M. avium* infection involving the liver, but a concomitant cytomegalovirus infection was also present. Serum alkaline phosphatase values have been elevated in nearly all cases of hepatic *M. avium* (97), although the enzyme levels are not specific for *M. avium*, having been recorded in response to a hypersensitivity reaction to sulfonamide therapy as well as to other infectious agents such as histoplasmosis (151).

One of the important differences between *M. tuberculosis* and *M. avium* infection in AIDS is the relative lack of response of *M. avium* to conventional antituberculous therapy. Most early reports observed either a poor or absent response for most patients (13, 104, 112, 140, 180, 196, 302). This lack of clinical responsiveness may have been a reflection of the severe immune dysfunction of these patients because *M. avium* typically occurs late in the course of AIDS when cell counts are at their lowest. CD4$^+$ cell counts of less than 60/mm^3 are typical of patients with disseminated *M. avium* infection, and the infection is rare in patients having more than 200 CD4$^+$ cells. This explains why *M. avium* usually occurs *after* rather than concurrently *with* Kaposi's sarcoma or *P. carinii* pneumonia, which typically occurs in patients with greater than 100 CD4$^+$ cells. With improvements in patient survival due to antiretroviral therapy, an improved response to multidrug regimens has been observed with *M. avium* infection (119, 251). In addition, alkaline phosphatase (reflective of hepatic involvement) may normalize following treatment (119).

Other mycobacteria

Although *M. avium* is the predominant nontuberculous mycobacterial infection in AIDS, a number of other atypical mycobacteria, including *M. fortuitum*, *M. gordonae*, *M. xenopi*, and *M. chelonae*, have also caused disseminated disease in AIDS. *M. kansasii*, however, rarely if ever leads to liver disease or other extrapulmonary involvement. For example, in a study of 17 patients with pulmonary infection due to *M. kansasii*, none had laboratory evidence of hepatic dysfunction (152). As with *M. avium*, a majority of patients infected with *M. kansasii* had lymphocyte counts of less than 200/mm^3, indicating advanced immunosuppression.

Tuberculosis Occurring in Liver Transplant Patients (See Also Chapter 33)

The overall incidence of tuberculosis developing in solid organ transplant recipients around the world is estimated to be 1% to 4%, although the incidence of tuberculosis affecting the transplanted liver ranges from 0.9 to 2.3% (4, 262). A recent systematic review by Holty et al. (117) that included 81 reports of posttransplant infection found that approximately 1% of liver transplant patients develop active MTB infection. Both adult and pediatric liver transplant recipients appear to be at risk for tuberculosis because of their immunocompromised state (173, 176). In a case series of 550 liver transplant patients monitored for a 5-year period in New York City, Meyers and colleagues (179) diagnosed the new onset of tuberculosis in four persons for a prevalence of 0.7%. One person had evidence of miliary tuberculosis in the peritoneum at the time of transplantation. The transplantation was performed, and the patient was treated successfully. In the other three patients, tuberculosis developed between 2 months and 57 months after transplantation, and one of these patients experienced a tuberculous liver abscess. The rate of infection with tuberculosis was similar to the 1.2% (5 of 462 cases) reported by Grauhan and colleagues (103) in Germany. Among 42 patients in San Francisco who underwent liver biopsy following liver transplantation and who were found to have granulomas, one patient had tuberculosis, for a prevalence of 2.4% (82). The majority of epithelioid granulomas or microgranulomas in the parenchyma (an overall prevalence of 50%) were associated with hepatocyte necrosis but without a specific infection being identified.

Recent data suggest that the incidence of tuberculosis in transplant recipients is 3- to 100-fold higher than in the general population (28, 122, 262). The majority of cases occur within the first 12 months after transplantation; although in a retrospective review of 760 transplant cases, in which 15 developed active *M. tuberculosis* infection, the median duration from transplant to diagnosis was 31 months (122). Nonrenal transplantation, rejection within 6 months before the onset of tuberculosis, and type of primary immunosuppressive regimen are predictors of posttransplant tuberculosis (262). Disseminated tuberculosis is common in the posttransplant setting. Holty et al. (117) found that more than 60% of liver transplant recipients with active *M. tuberculosis* infection have extrapulmonary involvement. Receipt of OKT3 or anti-T-cell antibodies is a significant predisposing factor (262).

The most likely cause of tuberculosis in organ transplant recipients is reactivation of old quiescent disease (262). Ironically, fewer than one-third of all liver transplant recipients have a known tuberculin skin testing (TST) result (117). Other causes may include nosocomial exposure and transmission by cadaveric or living donors with tuberculosis (262).

Of greater concern than active tuberculosis developing posttransplant is the risk of hepatotoxicity associated with INH prophylaxis, which is discussed later. Hepatic enzyme abnormalities associated with drug therapy can be confused with transplant rejection. The rationale for INH prophylaxis in liver transplant recipients is the fact that a majority of patients are anergic and on immunosuppressive therapy, which places them at high risk for acquiring tuberculosis. The policy at many institutions is to treat

active tuberculosis or patients who have evidence of old tuberculosis on chest radiograph as well as those who have a positive PPD result in the pretransplant period. Meyers and colleagues (179) also suggest that recipients of livers from donors with active tuberculosis should undergo treatment after transplantation. Because of the risk of INH hepatotoxicity in immunocompromised patients (244), some institutions recommend that surveillance mycobacterial cultures and smears be obtained following liver transplantation as an alternative to the prophylactic use of INH. In a study conducted by Torre-Cisneros et al. (286) of 100 liver transplant patients over the first 180 days after a transplant, only a single patient was identified by sputum or urine AFB smears and cultures as having active tuberculosis and was promptly treated. No patient who remained culture negative experienced an active tuberculosis infection according to this approach.

Routine preoperative screening for tuberculosis via TST and prophylactic treatment of patients with positive results are controversial because TST is an imperfect identifier of patients at risk of tuberculosis (28, 287). Holty et al. (117) report that of liver transplant patients with active *M. tuberculosis* infection and known TST, only 37% have a positive test. Another controversial aspect of preoperative TST and prophylactic treatment of positive tests is the increased risk of INH hepatitis in liver transplant recipients. However, a case control study demonstrated the safety and efficacy of INH chemoprophylaxis administered during liver transplant candidacy (262). Aggressive management is required to prevent tuberculosis in transplant candidates. Based on retrospective data (287), patients who inadvertently undergo transplantation can be effectively treated when diagnosed early.

Clinically significant hepatotoxicity requiring discontinuation of INH was seen in 41% to 83.3% in post-liver transplant patients (178, 262), but 8 of 15 liver biopsies in the series reported by Singh et al. (262) demonstrated acute or chronic rejection plus granulomas or only granulomas in patients receiving INH-containing regimens. In the series by Meyers and colleagues (178) from New York City, liver biopsy revealed drug-induced hepatitis in 5 of 6 (88%) patients and rejection in 3 of 6 (50%) patients. Therefore, these data suggest that a presumptive diagnosis of INH hepatotoxicity may not be accurate for liver transplant recipients and liver biopsy should be considered for the evaluation of elevated liver enzymes levels, since multiple etiologies could account for the occurrence of abnormal liver enzyme levels in these patients. Bolstering this approach, Holty et al. (117) found that in patients treated for latent

M. tuberculosis with INH, severe hepatotoxicity occurred in only 1%.

While managing patients with active tuberculosis in the posttransplant setting, reduction of immunosuppression appears to be critical (284). In addition, experience from a large transplant center in the United States reveals that liver transplant patients have poor tolerance for conventional therapy due to inherent toxicity of these agents and their concomitant bouts of organ rejection. Nonconventional therapy consisting mainly of ethambutol and ofloxacin for a mean length of 9 months yielded remarkably good results in 6 patients who developed drug-induced hepatotoxicity with conventional agents (178). In their systematic review, Holty et al. found that approximately 35% of liver transplant patients with active *M. tuberculosis* infection will have their ATT regimens altered or stopped because of hepatotoxicity; however, the long-term sequelae of antibiotic-related hepatotoxicity are rare.

Active tuberculosis in the posttransplant setting is associated with high mortality. Singh et al. (262) reported a mortality rate of 29% on the basis of compilation of published reports in the literature. Meyers et al. (178) and Verma et al. (296) also reported similar mortality rates from post-liver transplant tuberculosis in adults and pediatric transplant recipients in the United States. Holty et al. (117) found that the short-term mortality rate for liver transplant recipients with active tuberculosis is 31%. Disseminated infection, prior rejection, and receipt of OKT3 or anti-T-cell antibodies are significant predictors of mortality in patients with tuberculosis (262). Survivors were more likely to have received multidrug tuberculosis induction regimens or to have been diagnosed within 1 month of symptom onset (117).

ASSOCIATED AND COINCIDENTAL HEPATIC LESIONS IN TUBERCULOSIS

Alcoholic Hepatitis and Cirrhosis

Rolleston and McNee (225) found that nearly 30% of patients dying of cirrhosis had demonstrable tuberculosis infections, most commonly pulmonary and peritoneal. It was their contention that the cirrhosis was present prior to the tuberculosis and that the cirrhosis served to predispose patients to the infectious process. They supported their view by citing the lack of firm evidence that tuberculosis leads to cirrhosis in humans. To date, such evidence continues to be lacking, despite the earlier acceptance of the term "tuberculous cirrhosis" (137).

Alcoholism commonly has been associated with tuberculosis, having been recorded in up to 54% of

patients with the infection (95, 114, 187, 247). Accordingly, the coexistence of histologic features of alcoholic liver disease (including steatosis and cirrhosis with hepatic granulomas) is to be expected. Indeed, Korn and colleagues (144) suggested that the fatty changes in the livers of patients with tuberculosis may be the result of concomitant alcohol ingestion. Alcohol also increases the risk of hepatotoxicity from INH and other antituberculous therapy, as is discussed later.

Viral Hepatitis

Tuberculosis does not appear to predispose patients to viral hepatitis, but outbreaks may occur in tuberculosis hospitals. Fitzgerald and associates (84) described an outbreak of hepatitis B involving 37 of 64 hospitalized tuberculosis patients that spread to both hospital staff members and close contacts of infected persons. Several patients experienced a carrier state for longer than 6 months. A high incidence of chronic hepatitis B surface antigen (HbsAg) carriage in tuberculosis patients has been noted by Petera and colleagues (209) and McGlynn and coworkers (174), especially among persons from high-risk groups. There is little likelihood that coincidental chronic viral hepatitis might result in biochemical and clinical features that might be mistaken for tuberculous involvement of the liver, and histologic differences would, of course, clarify the situation. Hepatic steatosis due to concomitant non-A, non-B hepatitis may be an important cause of the macrovesicular fat in some patients with tuberculosis (151). Chronic asymptomatic HbsAg carriers receiving INH therapy, although at one time considered to be at increased risk of hepatic injury, were not found to have higher SGOT levels than those not receiving INH in one study (174).

Severe hepatotoxicity, however, was reported from the combination of INH and RIF in HbsAg-positive patients from Taiwan who were being treated for active tuberculosis (305). The number of fatal cases led the authors to speculate that improved cellular immunity following successful antituberculous therapy may, in some patients, have precipitated a severe reactivation of hepatitis B with death due to viral injury rather than to drug toxicity.

Pan and colleagues (204) looked at 47 TB patients with hepatitis B virus (HBV) infection and 170 TB patients without HBV infection and divided them into two different treatment groups: HPBES (INH, RIF, pyrazinamide, ethambutol, streptomycin) and HLAMKO (INH, rifabutin, ofloxacin, levofloxacin). The rate of hepatotoxicity was 59% in the patients with HBV and TB and only 24% in the TB patients without HBV. The incidence of liver dysfunction was

46.1% in the HBPES group and only 12.7% in the HLAMKO group, which the authors claim supports the use of HLAMKO as the regimen of choice for TB treatment in patients with chronic HBV.

Cirrhosis

Patients with cirrhosis may be more susceptible to TB related to immune system dysfunction. Cho et al. (49) found that extrapulmonary TB was more common in patients with cirrhosis than those without liver disease (31% versus 12%; $P = 0.02$). However, the clinical and radiographic manifestations and response to treatment did not differ between the groups. The frequency of hepatotoxicity was higher in cirrhotics treated with regimens that contained RIF and isoniazid, but the difference was not statistically significant.

Cirrhosis has also been described as a possible risk factor for the development of drug-resistant tuberculosis (192). In addition, patients with cirrhosis have been treated with ofloxacin for tuberculosis, which may be safer than traditional antituberculous therapy in patients with underlying liver disease (20, 21).

Other Hepatic Lesions

Amyloidosis has been described in the livers of up to 10% of patients with hepatic tuberculosis (292). In some patients, the amyloid infiltration has been extensive, producing marked hepatomegaly. Most cases have occurred in patients with long-standing advanced disease, often involving the intestinal tract (135). Currently available treatment for tuberculosis would make amyloidosis a rare complication today.

Nodular regenerative hyperplasia of the liver is an uncommon lesion characterized by diffuse nodularity of the parenchyma with portal fibrosis. Hepatocyte atrophy may be present in some lobules and regenerative nodules in others. Although the pathogenesis is unknown, nodular regenerative hyperplasia has been described in a variety of disorders, including tuberculosis (228, 276, 299). Whether or not the relationship to tuberculosis is fortuitous is not clear.

Hemosiderosis of the liver has been described in as many as 47% of autopsy cases and 28% of needle biopsy specimens in African patients with hepatic tuberculosis. It should be noted, however, that this high incidence occurred in a population containing a large proportion of Bantus, who are known to have a high incidence of hemosiderosis (114). Tuberculosis by itself probably does not lead to hepatic iron deposition. An interesting report by Gordeuk and colleagues (101) reanalyzed an iron overload study

originally conducted in 714 black South Africans in the 1920s to determine whether or not tuberculosis was related to the hepatic and splenic iron associated with hepatocellular carcinoma in these patients. They concluded that iron overload in these patients was probably a risk factor for death from hepatocellular carcinoma as well as from tuberculosis.

HEPATIC INJURY DUE TO ANTITUBERCULOUS THERAPY

Hepatic injury due to antituberculosis drugs has a bearing on liver disease associated with TB because it extends its spectrum. A common definition of antituberculosis drug-induced hepatotoxicity is a treatment-emergent increase in serum alanine aminotransferase greater than three or five times the upper limit of normal, with or without symptoms of hepatitis, respectively (289).

The reported incidence of antituberculosis drug-induced hepatotoxicity varies between 2% and 28% (289). The incidence is higher in developing countries, with rates ranging from 8% to 39%, compared to developed countries at 3% to 4%, despite similar regimens used (170). Risk factors for hepatotoxicity from these drugs are advanced age, female sex, malnutrition, HIV, and preexistent liver disease (19, 289). Other risk factors include that of alcoholism, HBV, and HCV, extensive pulmonary parenchymal disease, and hypoalbuminemia (19). It is still difficult nonetheless to predict what patient will develop hepatotoxicity during tuberculosis treatment (289).

The incidence of acute hepatitis in patients receiving antituberculosis treatment varies widely depending on the grade of aminotransferase elevations. Moreover, what is perceived as anti-TB drug-induced hepatotoxicity may not be drug induced all the time. Acute viral hepatitis is an important confounding illness which clinically, biochemically, and histologically mimics drug-induced hepatotoxicity (237).

Sharma and colleagues (255) have reported on this safe use of reintroducing treatment for tuberculosis among patients with hepatotoxicity. In their study from India of 175 patients who developed drug-induced liver injury (DILI) from TB drugs, they utilized three different regimens including isoniazid, RIF, and pyrazinamide at full dose, as well as the regimens recommended by the American Thoracic Society and the British Thoracic Society. The American Thoracic Society recommends sequential reintroduction with RIF at maximum dosage from day 1, isoniazid at maximum dosage from day 8, and pyrazinamide at maximum dosage from day 15. The British Thoracic Society recommends isoniazid at 100 mg/day from day 1 and maximum dosage from day 4, RIF at 150 mg/day from day 8 and maximum dosage from day 11, and pyrazinamide at 500 mg/day from day 15 and maximum dosage from day 18. These investigators found that 11% of retreated patients had recurrent DILI, but there was no difference between the regimens. Pretreatment albumin was the only predictor of future recurrent DILI in this series. They concluded that even though DILI may have initially occurred with the full-dose regimen, therapy can be reintroduced in patients who are in need of active treatment.

Active TB is usually treated with multiple drugs, which therefore limits the data on toxicity rates of antituberculosis drugs individually, except for that of isoniazid, which has been widely used as a prophylactic monotherapy for latent TB infections. Nevertheless, a reasonably clear picture has emerged for several drugs (313).

Para-aminosalicylic acid can lead to a syndrome of acute hepatocellular injury with jaundice accompanied by clinical manifestations that have led to the syndrome being dubbed "pseudomononucleosis," with fever, rash, lymphadenopathy, eosinophilia, and lymphocytosis with "atypical" lymphocytes. The incidence has been estimated to approach 1%, and the mechanism can reasonably be deduced to be hypersensitivity (312). In contrast with the case of INH, no age relationship was apparent. The relative abandonment of this drug makes the hepatic injury of more historic and pathophysiologic interest than of clinical importance.

Isoniazid

INH causes acute hepatocellular jaundice in about 1% of all recipients, and at least 10% experience more trivial, anicteric hepatic injury. Clinical features are virtually indistinguishable from acute viral hepatitis, with malaise, anorexia, and nausea with or without vomiting developing prior to the onset of jaundice. Fever and hepatomegaly are much less common. Biochemically, the condition also resembles acute viral hepatitis, with jaundice being a presenting feature in approximately 10% of patients. Case fatality rates of approximately 10% occur in persons who experience jaundice with massive hepatic necrosis, leading to a fatal outcome (183).

Susceptibility to INH hepatotoxicity seems importantly age related, with children and adolescents under the age of 20 being far less susceptible than older persons. Young adults, aged 20 to 35 years, have shown an incidence of overt icteric liver damage of approximately 0.5%, whereas adults over the age of 35 show at least twice that incidence and those over 50 have an incidence that approaches 3%. Reports

highlight the fact that young persons are indeed susceptible to INH injury, however, including the development of fatal hepatotoxicity. Snider and Caras (269) reviewed the medical literature from 1965 to 1989 that dealt with INH hepatotoxicity. In addition, they searched Food and Drug Administration files and a number of other databases and discovered a total of 177 deaths attributed to INH during this period. Of the 153 patients whose age was known, 9.2% were under the age of 20, 12.4% were aged 20 to 34, 17.6% were aged 35 to 49, 37.9% were aged 50 to 64, and 23% were over the age of 65. Women constituted nearly 70% of all the fatal cases. The racial mix was 40% non-Hispanic Caucasian, 38% African American, 15% Hispanic, 4% Native American, and only 1% Asian. Among women aged 15 to 44 years in this series, 38% were within 1 year of having given birth. Others have also found an increased risk in postpartum females and in women in general (90). This series suggested that deaths from untreated tuberculosis were 25 times more likely than the risk of dying from INH hepatotoxicity based on the assumption that 5% of untreated infected persons experienced clinical tuberculosis. Chronic hepatitis C and B and HIV independently have been shown to increase the risk of INH-induced hepatotoxicity (81, 90, 293, 303, 308). Female sex and birthplace in Asia are additional risk factors for first-line antitubercular agent-induced hepatotoxicity (308).

Antituberculosis agents are among the most common causes of non-acetaminophen-related acute liver failure leading to emergency liver transplantation. In a recent review of the United Network for Organ Sharing database, INH led the list (181). According to the most recent CDC report, during 2004 to 2008, a total of 17 serious liver injuries were reported in patients receiving INH therapy; five patients underwent liver transplantation, and five died, including one liver transplant recipient (40).

Barcena and colleagues report the outcome of seven cases of fulminant hepatic failure secondary to tuberculosis prophylaxis or treatment. Five of them were transplanted, and only one died due to reasons not related to tuberculosis. The other four cases were alive at the end of follow-up (mean, 455 days; range, 162 to 797 days) (23).

The management of tuberculosis in liver-transplanted patients differs from that of the general population due to an immunocompromised status and a higher potential hepatotoxicity. The classical public health approach of short-course therapy with very effective drugs (isoniazid and rifampin) could be considered for those patients who present with tuberculosis some years after transplantation. Liver function must be closely monitored due to increased hepatotoxicity. In patients who present with tuberculosis in the following weeks or months after transplantation, the toxicity of antituberculous drugs could be confounded with other allograft dysfunctions, but a very effective therapy should be employed initially. A gentle sustained approach of longer therapies with second-line drugs should be reserved for patients transplanted due to toxicity of antituberculous drugs (23).

The question of considering active tuberculosis as a contraindication to liver transplantation is a matter of debate. Based on the scarce information in the literature, universal recommendations are not available on this issue. Therefore, each case should be individualized (23).

The mechanism of hepatic injury due to INH appears to be metabolic idiosyncrasy rather than hypersensitivity (157). Although it was previously thought that susceptibility was increased among rapid acetylators (184), more recent studies have failed to substantiate any relationship between hepatic toxicity and acetylator phenotype in children or adults (67, 109, 169, 250). Nevertheless, occasional dissenting reports continue to appear (136, 184). Alcoholics appear to be at increased risk of INH toxicity, most likely by inducing its metabolism. Similarly, INH has potentiated the toxicity of acetaminophen, probably through the induction of the P450 2E1 cytochrome pathway that is responsible for the toxic acetaminophen metabolite (189, 195). Cytochrome P450 2E1 genetic polymorphism may be associated with susceptibility to INH-induced hepatitis (124). The risk of hepatitis from INH is also seen in patients also taking other antituberculous drugs, especially RIF and pyrazinamide (PZA). Ozick and colleagues (202) found that the combination of INH and RIF in patients with AIDS led to an 11% incidence of hepatocellular injury, defined as ALT greater than 200 IU/liter. Similarly, children receiving combination therapy appear to be at increased risk of hepatic injury from INH and RIF. In India, Parthasarathy and colleagues (207) found that the incidence of hepatic injury from daily regimens of INH and RIF was up to 39% in children being treated for tuberculous meningitis, 10% with spinal tuberculosis, and up to 8% of those being treated for pulmonary tuberculosis. The risk of hepatic injury was highest among those receiving daily therapy compared with twice-weekly regimens. In their series, there was no indication that PZA added to the hepatotoxic potential as it appears to do in adults (see below).

A report by Moulding and colleagues (186) from California that chronicles 20 deaths from INH over a 14-year period continues to highlight the need for careful monitoring in patients receiving chemoprophylaxis with INH. In this series of fatal cases, females outnumbered males by more than two to one, with the individual patients ranging in age from 15 to 55 years. Four deaths occurred in postpartum females who had started INH prophylaxis during pregnancy and continued it following delivery. Eight of the 20 deaths (40%) occurred in patients under the age of 35, which was considerably higher than expected. The authors made the important observation that in many of these patients, vomiting and abdominal pain were not considered specific symptoms of hepatitis, and this may have added to a delay in the diagnosis. In addition, management errors, such as not seeing patients on a monthly basis and providing several months' worth of medication at a single visit for convenience, may also have contributed to a delay in diagnosing serious hepatic injury. When therapy is properly monitored, however, it is thought that the risk of INH injury is significantly reduced (186).

Rifampin

Treatment of latent tuberculosis infection (LTBI) with rifampin for 4 months is an alternative to the standard 9-month regimen of INH. Several studies have demonstrated the efficacy of the 4-month rifampin regimen and have also shown that it is less hepatotoxic than INH. Previous studies of rifampin treatment of LTBI suggest a very low incidence of hepatotoxicity, including a lower incidence than INH. The incidence of increases in transaminases associated with rifampin treatment of LTBI has ranged from 0% to 0.4%. Hepatotoxicity associated with rifampin may range from hyperbilirubinemia without hepatocellular damage to moderate elevations in transaminases or, rarely, clinically significant hepatitis (87).

RIF is frequently used in combination with INH as well as other agents. Although RIF is thought to increase the likelihood that INH will lead to hepatic injury (5, 274), probably through induction of the cytochrome system that enhances conversion of INH to its toxic metabolite, RIF has also produced occasional instances of idiosyncratic, acute hepatocellular injury (243). The clinical manifestations are those of acute viral hepatitis similar to the symptoms occurring with INH. However, these signs and symptoms generally occur within a month of initiating treatment with RIF, whereas INH injury usually does not occur until the second month (85% of cases). In addition to its ability to produce hepatocellular damage, RIF can also interfere with bilirubin uptake and excretion as a benign effect (243, 312), although marked hyperbilirubinemia can lead to anxiety on the part of both patient and physician.

Pyrazinamide

PZA may cause severe hepatitis when used as a single agent but, importantly, appears to increase the risk of fatal hepatotoxicity when used in combination with INH and RIF (32, 77). Durand and colleagues (71) reported 18 cases of fulminant or subfulminant hepatic failure secondary to antituberculous therapy. Nine patients received INH and RIF, and nine received the combination of INH plus RIF and PZA. Only two of the nine who received PZA survived, whereas eight of nine receiving only INH and RIF survived. These authors concluded that PZA potentiated the toxicity of INH and RIF. Survival in these cases was inversely related to the time to onset of jaundice, with survivors becoming jaundiced within the first 15 days of therapy. They recommend avoiding PZA in patients with abnormal hepatic or renal status and suggest that biochemical monitoring be performed on a weekly basis during the first 2 months of treatment. PZA should be discontinued if the ALT rises above threefold the upper limits of normal in these patients. Mitchell and colleagues (182) from Kings College Hospital described four additional patients with acute liver failure from the combination of INH, RIF, and PZA, two of whom died. Rechallenge was performed in three of the patients and was noted to be positive. Based on the unacceptably high rate of severe hepatotoxicity, including fatal liver failure from the combination of rifampin and pyrazinamide, the CDC recommends that pyrazinamide not be used to treat latent TB (39, 129).

It is unknown what enzyme systems are involved in pyrazinamide-induced liver toxicity and whether the hepatotoxicity is caused by pyrazinamide or its metabolites. In a rat study, pyrazinamide inhibited the activity of several cytochrome P450 isoenzymes (2B, 2C, 2E1, 3A), but a study with human liver microsomes showed that pyrazinamide has no inhibitory effect on the cytochrome P450 isoenzymes (289).

Second-Line Agents

Clarithromycin is currently being used to prevent and treat *M. avium* infections (210, 251). It has been described as causing a cholestatic illness in a patient being treated for *M. chelonae*. That patient was inadvertently rechallenged with clarithromycin and experienced a recurrence of cholestasis (310). Macrolide antibiotics in general have long been known to cause cholestatic injury (157, 312).

Fluoroquinolones are frequently used to replace agents in first-line anti-TB regimens in patients with TB who have drug-induced hepatic dysfunction. Fluoroquinolones are not recommended as first-line therapies and are reserved for treatment of drug-resistant TB or as a substitute drug for patients who are intolerant to first-line drugs. Levofloxacin and moxifloxacin are newer fluoroquinolones with high bactericidal activity against *Mycobacterium tuberculosis*. The safety profile of fluoroquinolones, when used as short-course treatment for bacterial infection, has been well established. However, the safety profile of long-term use (duration, 12 weeks) of these agents has not been well studied. Although fluoroquinolones may induce mild elevation of liver function test values in previous studies, they have not been shown to impose an additional risk of hepatotoxicity in patients with TB. But the safety of levofloxacin and moxifloxacin in patients with TB and DILI associated with first-line anti-TB treatment is not known (116).

Reversible aminotransferase elevations among the fluoroquinolones may occur in up to 2 to 3% of cases. Severe hepatocellular injury and cholestasis have been reported to occur in less than 1% of all fluoroquinolone recipients, excluding trovafloxacin, which was withdrawn due to its hepatotoxicity. Clinically significant hepatotoxicity has been reported with ciprofloxacin, trovafloxacin, norfloxacin, ofloxacin, enoxacin, levofloxacin, and gatifloxacin, with large population denominators. The mechanism of fluoroquinolone hepatotoxicity is believed to be a hypersensitivity reaction, often manifested by eosinophilia (241).

Monitoring for Isoniazid and Combination Antituberculous Chemotherapy

With proper clinical and biochemical monitoring, it is thought that the risk of INH and combination chemotherapy-induced hepatic injury can be significantly reduced (186). Data indicate that the incidence of clinical hepatitis is lower than was previously thought. Hepatitis occurred in only 0.1 to 0.15% of 11,141 persons receiving INH alone as treatment for latent tuberculosis infection in an urban tuberculosis control program (194). The most recent guidelines of the American Thoracic Society, CDC, and Infectious Diseases Society of America (10) do not recommend routine monitoring for INH, RIF, or PZA, unless the patient has baseline elevation of liver enzymes, clinical symptoms, or is felt to be at higher risk due to chronic hepatitis B or C. The American Thoracic Society has independently refined their recommendations (241) to encourage baseline and follow-up monitoring for those with a history of chronic liver disease (hepatitis B and C, alcoholic hepatitis, and cirrhosis), chronic use of alcohol, HIV infection with highly active antiretroviral therapy, pregnant women, and those who are up to 3 months postpartum and baseline testing on an individual basis in patients receiving other medications and for those with chronic medical conditions, and they acknowledge that some experts monitor healthy patients older than 35 at baseline and monthly or on a 1-, 3-, and 6-month basis.

As a practical matter, we agree with the recommendations that if acute hepatitis occurs, INH, RIF, and/or PZA should be discontinued immediately, serologic tests for hepatitis A, B, and C should be performed, with hepatitis E. Sarda and colleagues (237) reviewed 2,906 patients with normal liver-associated tests treated for TB; 102 (3.5%) patients developed acute hepatitis while on ATT. Of the 102 patients with acute hepatitis, 15 (14.7%) had viral hepatitis present, interestingly hepatitis A (1), B (2), C (3), and E (8). In addition, the patient should be questioned carefully regarding symptoms of biliary tract disease, exposure to other potential hepatotoxins, especially alcohol and hepatotoxic medications. Alternative antitubercular regimens should be used until the cause of the hepatitis is identified. Once AST/ALT levels decrease to <2 times the upper limit of normal and symptoms have significantly improved, the first-line medications should be restarted in sequential fashion at weekly intervals beginning with RIF and ending with PZA. However, if symptoms recur or ALT increases to >2 times the upper limit of normal or a significant increase in bilirubin/alkaline phosphatase levels occurs, the last drug added should be discontinued. If RIF and INH are tolerated, and the hepatitis was severe, PZA should be assumed to be responsible and should be discontinued (155).

Support for these recommendations, however, is based on a number of reports of persons who, despite not being in the traditional high-risk groups (especially patients under the age of 35), have developed severe and even fatal hepatic injury. For example, many of the patients reported by the CDC from New York City were young and did not drink alcohol (41). Similarly, several of the fatal cases reported by Moulding and colleagues (186) were under the age of 35. Mitchell and colleagues (182) noted that even monthly monitoring would not have prevented two of their four fatalities, nor would it have prevented 11 of the 18 fatal cases described by Durand and colleagues (71) using these guidelines. These and other authors (193) have called for more-frequent biochemical monitoring. In France, it has been recommended since 1993 that biochemical testing be performed weekly rather than monthly for the first month in patients receiving INH and for the first 2 months if PZA is used in combination (71). If the ALT values rise above threefold or if serum bilirubin increases,

then INH and PZA should be stopped. PZA should not be used for more than 2 months' duration in any case (155). Mitchell and coworkers (182) called for African American and Hispanic females, postpartum females, and women on estrogen therapy to be monitored more closely because hepatic enzyme abnormalities are thought to occur well ahead of symptoms and therefore offer a window of opportunity to discontinue the antituberculous medications prior to the development of fulminant hepatic failure.

Prophylaxis of Hepatotoxicity Due to Antituberculosis Therapy

Finding a medication to prevent the hepatotoxicity of antituberculosis therapy has proven elusive. There has been much focus in the alternative medicine arena with multiple compounds proposed as hepatoprotective. Liu and colleagues (160) systematically reviewed ingredients and evaluation studies; 85 articles met criteria for inclusion and evaluated 30 distinct preparations including silymarin (extract of milk thistle). Their evaluation shows that the majority of these studies are small and poorly conducted. They conclude that there is no reliable evidence to support taking liver protection drugs with TB treatment and that some of these drugs may do harm. We do not recommend taking liver protection drugs. However, we recognize that patients may seek to take these medications with or without the knowledge of their provider. If a patient is insistent, a discussion of the lack of proven efficacy and potential unknown harm is warranted. Clearly, use of any "prophylactic" agent in the setting of antituberculosis treatment does not preclude recommended monitoring.

REFERENCES

1. Abascal, I., F. Martin, L. Abreu, F. Pereira, J. Herrera, T. Ratia, and J. Menendez. 1988. Atypical hepatic tuberculosis presenting as obstructive jaundice. *Am. J. Gastroenterol.* 83:1183–1186.
2. Abdel-Dayem, H. M., S. Naddaf, M. Aziz, B. Mina, T. Turoglu, M. F. Akisik, W. S. Omar, L. DiFabrizio, V. LaBombardi, and J. S. Kempf. 1997. Sites of tuberculous involvement in patients with AIDS: autopsy findings and evaluation of gallium imaging. *Clin. Nucl. Med.* 22:310–314.
3. Agrawal, H. S., J. W. Benson, and J. J. Major. 1967. An unusual case of hemobilia: hepatic tuberculosis with hemorrhage. *Arch. Surg.* 95:202–206.
4. Aguada, J. M., J. A. Herrero, J. Gavalda, J. Torre-Cisneros, M. Blanes, G. Rufí, A. Moreno, M. Gurguí, M. Hayek, C. Lumbreras, and C. Cantarell. 1997. Clinical presentation and outcome of tuberculosis in kidney, liver and heart transplant recipients in Spain. *Transplantation* 63:1278.
5. Akaard, D. S., T. Wilcke, and M. Dossing. 1995. Hepatotoxicity caused by the combined action of isoniazid and rifampicin. *Thorax* 50:213–214.

6. Alexander, I. F., and I. T. Galambos. 1973. Granuloma-tous hepatitis: the usefulness of liver biopsy in the diagnosis of tuberculosis and sarcoidosis. *Am. J. Gastroenterol.* **59:** 23–30.

7. al Karawi, M. A., A. B. Mohamed, M. I. Yasawy, D. Y. Graham, S. Shariq, A. M. Ahmed, A. al Jumah, and Z. Ghandour. 1995. Protean manifestation of gastrointestinal tuberculosis: report on 130 patients. *J. Clin. Gastroenterol.* **20:**225–232.

8. Alvarez, S. Z., and R. Carpio. 1983. Hepatobiliary tuberculosis. *Dig. Dis. Sci.* **28:**193–200.

9. Amarapurkar, D. N., K. B. Chopra, A. Y. Phadke, S. Sahni, S. R. Prabhu, and R. H. Kalro. 1995. Tuberculous abscess of the liver associated with HIV infection. *Indian J. Gastroenterol.* **14:**21–22.

10. American Thoracic Society, CDC, and Infectious Diseases Society of America. 2003. Treatment of tuberculosis. *Am. J. Respir. Crit. Care Med.* **167:**603–662.

11. Anderson, C. S., J. Nicholls, R. Rowland, and J. T. LaBrooy. 1988. Hepatic granulomas: a 15-year experience in the Royal Adelaide Hospital. *Med. J. Aust.* **148:**71–74.

12. Ariede, K. I. 1990. Congenital miliary tuberculosis. *Ann. Trop. Paediatr.* **10:**363–368.

13. Armstrong, D., J. W. N. Gold, J. Dryjanski, E. Whimbey, B. Polsky, C. Hawkins, A. E. Brown, E. Bernard, and T. E. Kiehn. 1985. Treatment of infections in patients with the acquired immunodeficiency syndrome. *Ann. Intern. Med.* **103:**738–745.

14. Arora, M. M., A. Ali, A. J. D'Souza, and K. N. Pawar. 1956. Clinical, functional and needle biopsy studies of the liver in tuberculosis. *J. Indian Med. Assoc.* **26:**341–344.

15. Arora, R., A. Sharma, P. Bhowate, V. K. Bansal, S. Guleria, and A. K. Dinda. 2008. Hepatic tuberculosis mimicking Klatskin tumor: a diagnostic dilemma. *Indian J. Pathol. Microbiol.* **51:** 382–385.

16. Arrese, M., F. Lopez, R. Rossi, E. Traipe, and F. Cruz. 1997. Extrahepatic cholestasis attributable to tuberculous adenitis. *Am. J. Gastroenterol.* **92:**912–913.

17. Assada, Y., T. Hayashi, A. Sumiyoshi, M. Aburaya, and E. Shishime. 1991. Miliary tuberculosis presenting as fever and jaundice with hepatic failure. *Hum. Pathol.* **22:**92–94.

18. Babu, R. K., and V. John. 2001. Pancreatic tuberculosis: case report and review of the literature. *Trop. Gastroenterol.* **22:** 213–214.

19. Baghaei, P., P. Tabarsi, E. Chitsaz, M. Saleh, M. Marjani, S. Shemirani, M. V. Pooramiri, M. Kazempour, P. Farnia, F. Fahimi, D. Mansouri, and M. Masjedi. 2010. Incidence, clinical and epidemiological risk factors, and outcome of drug-induced hepatitis due to antituberculous agents in new tuberculosis cases. *Am. J. Ther.* **17:**17–22.

20. Bagnato, G. F., E. DiCesare, S. Gulli, and D. Cucinotta. 1995. Long-term treatment of pulmonary tuberculosis with ofloxacin in a subject with liver cirrhosis. *Monaldi Arch. Chest Dis.* **50:**279–281.

21. Ban, B. 1955. Hepatic damage in chronic pulmonary tuberculosis. *Am. Rev. Tuberc.* **72:**71–90.

22. Baraboutis, I., and A. Skoutelis. 2004. Isolated tuberculosis of the pancreas. *JOP* **5:**155–158.

23. Barcena, R., E. Oton, M. Angeles Moreno, J. Fortún, M. Garcia-Gonzalez, A. Moreno, and E. de Vicente. 2005. Is liver transplantation advisable for isoniazid fulminant hepatitis in active extrapulmonary tuberculosis? *Am. J. Transplant.* **5:** 2796–2798.

24. Bearer, E. D., T. J. Savides, and J. A. McCutchan. 1996. Endoscopic diagnosis and management of hepatobiliary tuberculosis. *Am. J. Gastroenterol.* **91:**2602–2604.

25. Beaulieu, S., E. Chouillard, B. Petit-Jean, R. L. Vitte, and C. Eugene. 2004. Pancreatic tuberculosis: a rare cause of pseudo-neoplastic obstructive jaundice. *Gastroenterol. Clin. Biol.* **28:** 295–298.

26. Beeresha, L. H. Ghotekar, T. K. Dutta, S. K. Verma, and S. Elangovan. 2000. Hepatic artery aneurysm of tubercular etiology. *J. Assoc. Physicians India* **48:**247–248.

27. Ben, R. J., T. Young, and H. S. Lee. 1995. Hepatobiliary tuberculosis presenting as a gall bladder tumor. *Scand. J. Infect. Dis.* **27:**415–417.

28. Benito, N., O. Sued, A. Moreno, J. P. Horcajada, J. González, M. Navasa, and A. Rimola. 2002. Diagnosis and treatment of latent tuberculosis infection in liver transplant recipients in an endemic area. *Transplantation* **74:**1381–1386.

29. Berk, D. R., and K. G. Sylvester. 2004. Congenital tuberculosis presenting as progressive liver dysfunction. *Pediatr. Infect. Dis. J.* **23:**78–80.

30. Bernhard, J. S., G. Bhatia, and M. C. Knauer. 2000. Gastrointestinal tuberculosis: an eighteen patient experience and review. *J. Clin. Gastroenterol.* **30:**397–402.

31. Bhargava, D. K., K. Venna, and A. N. Malaviya. 1983. Solitary tuberculoma of liver: laparoscopic, histologic, and cytologic diagnosis. *Gastrointest. Endosc.* **29:**329–330.

32. Bhargava, S. P., and M. L. Sharma. 1962. Multiple tuberculoma of liver: a case report. *J. Indian Med. Assoc.* **38:**54–55.

33. Biehl, J. P. 1958. Miliary tuberculosis: a review of sixty-eight adult patients admitted to a municipal general hospital. *Am. Rev. Tuberc.* **77:**605–624.

34. Bodurtha, A., Y. H. Kin, I. F. Laucius, R. A. Donato, and M. J. Mastrangelo. 1974. Hepatic granulomas and other hepatic lesions associated with BCG immunotherapy for cancer. *Am. J. Clin. Pathol.* **6:**727–752.

35. Bowry, S., C. H. Chan, H. Weiss, S. Katz, and H. J. Zimmerman. 1970. Hepatic involvement in pulmonary tuberculosis: histologic and functional characteristics. *Am. Rev. Respir. Dis.* **101:**941–948.

36. Brauner, M., M. D. Buffard, V. Jeantils, I. Legrand, and C. Gotheil. 1989. Sonography and computed tomography of macroscopic tuberculosis of the liver. *J. Clin. Ultrasound* **17:** 563–568.

37. Brugge, W. R., P. R. Mueller, and J. Misdraji. 2004. Case 8-2004: a 28-year-old man with abdominal pain, fever, and mass in the region of pancreas. *N. Engl. J. Med.* **350:**1131–1138.

38. Buckingham, W. B., G. C. Turner, W. B. Knapp, Q. D. Young, and F. Schaffner. 1956. Liver biopsy in a tuberculosis hospital. *Dis. Chest* **29:**675–683.

39. Centers for Disease Control and Prevention. 2003. CDC update: adverse event data and revised American Thoracic Society/CDC recommendations against the use of rifampicin and pyrazinamide for treatment of latent tuberculosis infection–United States, 2003. *MMWR Morb. Mortal. Wkly. Rep.* **52:** 735–739.

40. Centers for Disease Control and Prevention. 2010. Severe isoniazid-associated liver injuries among persons being treated for latent tuberculosis infection - United States, 2004—2008. *MMWR Morb. Mortal. Wkly. Rep.* **59:**224–229.

41. Centers for Disease Control and Prevention. 1993. Severe isoniazid-associated hepatitis: New York, 1991-1993. *MMWR Morb. Mortal. Wkly. Rep.* **42:**545–547.

42. Chaisson, R. E., and G. Slutkin. 1989. Tuberculosis and human immunodeficiency virus infection. *J. Infect. Dis.* **159:**96–100.

43. Chaisson, R. E., R. D. Moore, D. D. Richman, J. Keruly, and T. Creagh. 1992. Incidence and natural history of Mycobacte-

rium avium-complex infections in patients with advanced human immunodeficiency virus disease treated with zidovudine. *Am. Rev. Respir. Dis.* **146:**285–289.

44. Chang, Y. G., P. J. Chen, C. C. Hung, M. Y. Chen, M. Y. Lai, and D. S. Chen. 1999. Opportunistic hepatic infections in AIDS patients with fever of unknown origin. *J. Formos. Med. Assoc.* **98:**5–10.

45. Chaudhary, A., S. S. Negi, A. K. Sachdev, and R. Gondal. 2002. Pancreatic tuberculosis: still a histopathological diagnosis. *Dig. Surg.* **19:**389–392.

46. Chen, C. H., C. C. Yang, Y. H. Yeh, J. C. Yang, and D. A. Chou. 1999. Pancreatic tuberculosis with obstructive jaundice—a case report. *Am. J. Gastroenterol.* **94:**2534–2536.

47. Chen, H. J., N. C. Chiu, H. A. Kao, and T. Y. Wang. 2004. Perinatal tuberculosis in a three-month-old infant. *J. Formos. Med. Assoc.* **103:**144–147.

48. Cheng, J., K. Tadi, M. Halpern, M. Feurdean, J. McNelis, and J. Brensilver. 2008. Pancreatic tuberculosis in a human immunodeficiency virus positive patient: a case report. *World J. Gastroenterol.* **14:**939–940.

49. Cho, Y. J., S. M. Lee, C. G. Yoo, Y. W. Kim, S. K. Han, Y. S. Shim, and J. J. Yim. 2007. Clinical characteristics of tuberculosis in patients with liver cirrhosis. *Respirology* **12:**401–405.

50. Chou, Y. H. 2002. Congenital tuberculosis proven by percutaneous liver biopsy: report of a case. *J. Perinat. Med.* **30:**423–425.

51. Cinque, T. J., N. E. Gary, and V. S. Palladino. 1964. "Primary" miliary tuberculosis of the liver. *Am. J. Gastroenterol.* **42:**611–619.

52. Cleve, E. A., J. R. Gibson, and W. M. Webb. 1954. Atypical tuberculosis of the liver with jaundice. *Ann. Intern. Med.* **41:**251–260.

53. Coelho, J. C., J. C. Wiederkehr, M. B. Parolin, E. Balbi, and A. E. Nassif. 1999. Isolated tuberculosis of the pancreas after orthotopic liver transplantation. *Liver Transpl. Surg.* **5:**153–155.

54. Colovic, R., N. Grubor, R. Jesic, M. Micev, T. Jovanovic, N. Colovic, and H. D. Atkinson. 2008. Tuberculous lymphadenitis as a cause of obstructive jaundice: a case report and literature review. *World J. Gastroenterol.* **14:**3098–3100.

55. Cruice, J. M. 1914. Jaundice in tuberculosis. *Am. J. Med. Sci.* **147:**720–726.

56. Cunnigham, D., P. R. Mills, E. M. Quigley, R. S. Patrick, G. Watkinson, J. F. MacKenzie, and R. I. Russell. 1982. Hepatic granulomas: experience over a 10-year period in the West of Scotland. *Q. J. Med.* **51:**162–170.

57. Curry, F. J., and D. Alcott. 1955. Tuberculosis hepatitis with jaundice: report of 2 cases. *Gastroenterology* **28:**1037–1042.

58. Dang, S., M. Atiq, M. Saccente, K. W. Olden, and F. Aduli. 2009. Isolated tuberculosis of the pancreas: a case report. *JOP* **10:**64–66.

59. Das, D., S. K. Mandal, D. Majumdar, and B. K. De. 2003. Disseminated tuberculosis presenting as hemobilia, successfully treated with arterial embolization. *J. Assoc. Physicians India* **51:**229–231.

60. Davis, J. M., and L. Ramakrishnan. 2008. "The very pulse of the machine": the tuberculous granuloma in motion. *Immunity* **28:**146–148.

61. D'Cruz, S., A. Sachdev, L. Kaur, U. Handa, A. Bhalla, and S. S. Lehl. 2003. Fine needle aspiration diagnosis of isolated pancreatic tuberculosis: a case report and review of the literature. *JOP* **4:**158–162.

62. DeBray, J., M. Krulik, and J. F. Bernard. 1972. La tuberculose pseudo tumorale du foie: a propos d'une observation personnelle. *Semin. Hop. Paris* **48:**3165–3167.

63. Debre, R., M. Furiet-Laforet, and P. Royer. 1948. Congenital transplacental tuberculosis of icteric form. *Arch. Fr. Pediatr.* **5:**225–231.

64. Demir, K., S. Kaymakoglu, F. Besisik, Z. Durakoglu, S. Ozdil, Y. Kaplan, G. Boztas, Y. Cakaloglu, and A. Okten. 2001. Solitary pancreatic tuberculosis in immunocompetent patients mimicking pancreatic carcinoma. *J. Gastroenterol. Hepatol.* **16:**1071–1074.

65. Desai, C. S., M. Lala, A. Joshi, P. Abraham, D. Desai, R. B. Deshpande, and S. R. Shah. 2004. Co-existence of periampullary carcinoma with peripancreatic tuberculous lymphadenopathy. *JOP* **5:**145–147.

66. Devars du Mayne, J. F., C. Marche, C. Penalba, D. Vittecoq, G. Saimot, and M. Cerf. 1985. Liver disease in acquired immune deficiency syndrome: study of 20 cases. *Presse Med.* **14:**1177–1180.

67. Dickinson, D. S., W. C. Bailey, and B. I. Hirschowitz. 1981. Risk factors for isoniazid (INH)-induced liver dysfunction. *J. Clin. Gastroenterol.* **3:**271–279.

68. Dourakis, S. P., R. Saramadou, A. Alexopoulou, G. Kafiri, M. Deutsch, J. Koskinas, and A. J. Archimandritis. 2007. Hepatic granulomas: a 6-year experience in a single center in Greece. *Eur. J. Gastroenterol. Hepatol.* **19:**101–104.

69. Drebber, U., H. U. Kasper, J. Ratering, I. Wedemeyer, P. Schirmacher, H. P. Dienes, and M. Odenthal. 2008. Hepatic granulomas: histological and molecular pathological approach to differential diagnosis: a study of 442 cases. *Liver Int.* **28:**828–834.

70. Duckworth, W. C. 1964. Tuberculosis of the liver. *S. Afr. Med. J.* **38:**945.

71. Durand, F., J. Bernuau, D. Passayre, D. Samuel, J. Belaiche, C. Degott, H. Bismuth, J. Belghiti, B. Erlinger, B. Rueff, and J. P. Benhamou. 1995. Deleterious influence of pyrazinamide on the outcome of patients with fulminant or sub-fulminant liver failure during anti-tuberculous treatment including isoniazid. *Hepatology* **21:**929–932.

72. Dwek, J. H., L. S. Schechter, and M. E. Grinberg. 1981. Hepatic angiography in a patient with tuberculosis of the liver. *Am. J. Gastroenterol.* **75:**307–308.

73. Egen, J. G., A. G. Rothfuchs, C. G. Feng, N. Winter, A. Sher, and R. N. Germain. 2008. Macrophage and T cell dynamics during development and disintegration of mycobacterial granulomas. *Immunity* **28:**271–284.

74. Elfe, P. M., W. G. van Aken, D. M. Agenant, and G. N. Tijtgat. 1980. Hemobilia after liver biopsy: early detection in a patient with mild hemophilia A. *Arch. Intern. Med.* **140:**839–840.

75. El Mansari, O., M. T. Tajdine, I. Mikou, and M. I. Janati. 2003. Pancreatic tuberculosis: report of two cases. *Gastroenterol. Clin. Biol.* **27:**548–550.

76. Essop, A. R., J. Hodkinson, J. Posen, I. Segal, and P. Macerollo. 1983. Simultaneous hepatic tuberculosis, cirrhosis and hepatoma: a case report. *S. Afr. Med. J.* **64:**1102–1104.

77. Essop, A. R., J. A. Posen, J. H. Hodkinson, and I. Segal. 1984. Tuberculosis hepatitis: a clinical review of 96 cases. *Q. J. Med.* **53:**465–477.

78. Essop, A. R., J. A. Posen, I. Savitch, J. Levin, and M. C. Kew. 1984. Radiocolloid liver imaging in tuberculous hepatitis. *Clin. Nucl. Med.* **9:**81–84.

79. Essop, A. R., I. Segal, J. Posen, and N. Noormohamed. 1983. Tuberculous abscess of the liver: a case report. *S. Afr. Med. J.* **63:**825–826.

80. Fernandes, J. D., R. A. Nebesar, S. G. Wall, and P. T. Minihan. 1984. Report of tuberculous hepatitis presenting as metastatic disease. *Clin. Nucl. Med.* **9:**345–357.

81. Fernandez-Villar, A., B. Sopena, R. Vazquez, F. Ulloa, E. Fluiters, M. Mosteiro, C. Martínez-Vázquez, and L. Piñeiro. 2003. Isoniazid hepatotoxicity among drug users: the role of hepatitis C virus. *Clin. Infect. Dis.* 36:293–298.

82. Ferrell, L. D., R. Lee, C. Brixko, N. M. Bass, J. R. Lake, J. P. Roberts, N. Ascher, and J. Rabkin. 1995. Hepatic granulomas following liver transplantation: clinical-pathologic features in 42 patients. *Transplantation* 60:926–933.

83. Finkh, E. S., S. J. Baker, and M. M. P. Ryan. 1953. The value of liver biopsy in the diagnosis of tuberculosis and sarcoidosis. *Med. J. Aust.* 2:369–374.

84. Fitzgerald, G. R., H. Grimes, M. Reynolds, H. Hitchcock, and C. F. McCarthy. 1975. Hepatitis-associated-antigen-positive hepatitis in a tuberculosis unit. *Gut* 16:421–428.

85. Flippin, T., B. Mukherji, and Y. Dayal. 1980. Granulomatous hepatitis as a late complication of BCG immunotherapy. *Cancer* 46:1759–1762.

86. Foo, F. J., C. S. Verbeke, J. A. Guthrie, A. Ala, and K. V. Menon. 2007. Pancreatic and peripancreatic tuberculosis mimicking malignancy. *JOP* 8:201–205.

87. Fountain, F. F., E. A. Tolley, A. R. Jacobs, and T. H. Self. 2009. Rifampin hepatotoxicity associated with treatment of latent tuberculosis infection. *Am. J. Med. Sci.* 337:317–320.

88. Franco-Pardes, C., M. Leonardo, R. Jurado, H. M. Blumberg, and R. M. Smith. 2002. Tuberculosis of the pancreas: report of 2 cases and review of the literature. *Am. J. Med. Sci.* 323:54–58.

89. Frank, B. B., and E. C. Raffensperger. 1965. Hepatic granulomata: report of a case with jaundice improving on antituberculosis therapy and review of the literature. *Arch. Intern. Med.* 115:223–234.

90. Franks, A. L., N. J. Binkin, D. E. Snider, Jr., W. M. Rokaw, and S. Becker. 1989. Isoniazid hepatitis among pregnant and postpartum Hispanic patients. *Public Health Rep.* 104:151–155.

91. Galen, R. S., D. Weimer, and S. A. Hartmap. 1950. Functional hepatic impairment in pulmonary tuberculosis. *Dis. Chest* 17:524–531.

92. Garber, H. I., G. R. Mason, and W. H. Bouchelle. 1981. "Primary" miliary tuberculosis of the liver presenting as acute cholecystitis. *Maryland State Med. J.* 3:73–74.

93. Gaya, D. R., D. Thorburn, K. A. Oien, A. J. Morris, and A. J. Stanley. 2003. Hepatic granulomas: a 10 year single center experience. *J. Clin. Pathol.* 56:850–853.

94. Gelb, A. F., C. Leffler, A. Brewin, V. Mascatello, and H. A. Lyons. 1973. Miliary tuberculosis. *Am. Rev. Respir. Dis.* 108:1327–1333.

95. Gelb, A. M., N. Brazenas, H. Sussman, and R. Wallach. 1970. Acute granulomatous disease of the liver. *Am. J. Dig. Dis.* 15:842–847.

96. Gillman, T., and J. Gillman. 1945. Modified liver aspiration biopsy apparatus and technique, with special reference to its clinical applications as assessed by 500 biopsies. *S. Afr. J. Med. Sci.* 10:53–66.

97. Glasgow, B. J., K. Anders, L. F. Layfleld, K. D. Steinsapir, G. L. Gitnick, and K. J. Lewin. 1985. Clinical and pathologic findings of the liver in the acquired immune deficiency syndrome (AIDS). *Am. J. Clin. Pathol.* 83:582–588.

98. Godwin, J. E., A. A. Coleman, and S. A. Sahn. 1991. Miliary tuberculosis presenting as hepatic and renal failure. *Chest* 99:752–754.

99. Gold, J., A. Widgerson, E. Lehman, and I. R. Schwartz. 1957. Tuberculosis hepatitis: report of a case and review of the literature. *Gastroenterology* 33:113–120.

100. Gonzalez, O. Y., G. Adams, L. D. Teeter, T. T. Bui, J. M. Musser, and E. A. Graviss. 2003. Extra-pulmonary manifestations in a large metropolitan area with a low incidence of tuberculosis. *Int. J. Tuberc. Lung Dis.* 7:1178–1185.

101. Gordeuk, V. R., C. E. McLaren, A. P. MacPhail, G. Deichsel, and T. H. Bothwell. 1996. Associations of iron overload in Africa with hepatocellular carcinoma and tuberculosis: Strachan's 1929 thesis revisited. *Blood* 87:3470–3476.

102. Gottke, M. U., P. Wong, C. Muhn, M. Jabbari, and S. Morin. 2000. Hepatitis in disseminated bacillus Calmette-Guerin infection. *Can. J. Gastroenterol.* 14:333–336.

103. Grauhan, O., R. Lohmann, T. Lemmens, N. Schattenfroh, S. Jonas, H. Keck, R. Raakow, J. Langrehr, W. Bechstein, and G. Blumhardt. 1995. Mycobacterial infection after liver transplantation. *Langenbecks Arch. Chir.* 380:171–175.

104. Greene, J. B., G. S. Sidh, S. Lewin, J. F. Levine, H. Masur, M. S. Simberkoff, P. Nicholas, R. C. Good, S. B. Zolla-Pazner, A. A. Pollock, M. L. Tapper, and R. S. Holzman. 1982. Mycobacterium avium intracellulare: a cause of disseminated life threatening infection in homosexuals and drug abusers. *Ann. Intern. Med.* 97:539–546.

105. Guarda, L. A., M. A. Luna, J. L. Smith, P. W. Mansell, F. Gyorkey, and A. N. Roca. 1984. Acquired immune deficiency syndrome: postmortem findings. *Am. J. Clin. Pathol.* 81:549–557.

106. Guckian, J. C., and J. E. Perry. 1966. Granulomatous hepatitis: an analysis of 63 cases and review of the literature. *Ann. Intern. Med.* 65:1081–1100.

107. Guglielmi, V., O. G. Manghisi, M. Pirrelli, and M. L. Caruso. 1994. Granulomatous hepatitis in a hospital population in southern Italy. *Pathologica* 86:271–278.

108. Gulati, P. D., and P. B. Vyas. 1965. Tuberculosis of the liver. *J. Indian Med. Assoc.* 43:144–145.

109. Gurumurthy, P., M. S. Kirshnamurthy, O. Nazareth, R. Parthasarathy, G. R. Sarma, P. R. Somasundaram, S. P. Tripathy, and G. A. Ellard. 1984. Lack of relationship between hepatic toxicity and acetylator phenotype in three thousand South Indian patients during treatment with isoniazid for tuberculosis. *Am. Rev. Respir. Dis.* 129:58–61.

110. Haex, A. J. C., and C. Van Beek. 1955. *Tuberculosis and Aspiration Liver Biopsy.* Bohn, Haarlem, The Netherlands.

111. Harrington, P. T., J. J. Gutierrez, C. H. Ramirez-Ronda, R. Quiñones-Soto, R. H. Bermúdez, and J. Chaffey. 1982. Granulomatous hepatitis. *Rev. Infect. Dis.* 4:638–655.

112. Hawkins, C. C., J. W. M. Gold, E. Whimbey, T. E. Kiehn, P. Brannon, R. Cammarata, A. E. Brown, and D. Armstrong. 1986. Mycobacterium avium complex infections in patients with the acquired immunodeficiency syndrome. *Ann. Intern. Med.* 105:184–188.

113. Hennan, P., V. Pugliese, R. Laurino Neto, M. C. Machado, and H. W. Pinotti. 1995. Nodular form of local hepatic tuberculosis: case report. *J. Trop. Med. Hyg.* 98:141–142.

114. Hersch, C. 1964. Tuberculosis of the liver: a study of 200 cases. *S. Afr. Med. J.* 38:857–863.

115. Hickey, N., J. G. McNulty, H. Osborne, and J. Finucane. 1999. Acute hepatobiliary tuberculosis: a report of two cases and review of the literature. *Eur. Radiol.* 9:886–889.

116. Ho, C. C., Y. C. Chen, F. C. Hu, C. J. Yu, P. C. Yang, and K. T. Luh. 2009. Safety of fluoroquinolone use in patients with hepatotoxicity induced by anti-tuberculosis regimens. *Clin. Infect. Dis.* 48:1526–1533.

117. Holty, J. E., M. K. Gould, L. Meinke, E. B. Keeffe, and S. J. Ruoss. 2009. Tuberculosis in liver transplant recipients: a systematic review and meta-analysis of individual patient data. *Liver Transplant.* 15:894–906.

118. Hong, S. G., J. S. Kim, M. K. Joo, K. G. Lee, K. H. Kim, C. R. Oh, J. J. Park, and Y. T. Bak. 2009. Pancreatic tuberculosis

masquerading as pancreatic serous cystadenoma. *World J. Gastroenterol.* **15**:1010–1013.

119. Horsburgh, C. R., Jr. 1991. Mycobacterium avium complex infection in the acquired immunodeficiency syndrome. **324:** 1332–1338.

120. Horsburgh, C. R., Jr., B. Metchock, S. M. Gordon, J. A. Havlik, Jr., J. E. McGowan, Jr., and S. E. Thompson III. 1994. Predictors of survival in patients with AIDS and disseminated Mycobacterium avium complex disease. *J. Infect. Dis.* **170:** 573–577.

121. Hsieh, S. M., C. C. Hung, M. Y. Chen, P. R. Hsueh, S. C. Chang, and K. T. Luh. 1999. The role of tissue studies in facilitating early initiation of antimycobacterial treatment in AIDS patients with disseminated tuberculosis disease. *Int. J. Tuberc. Lung Dis.* **3**:521–527.

122. Hsu, M. S., J. L. Wang, W. J. Ko, P. H. Lee, N. K. Chou, S. S. Wang, S. H. Chu, and S. C. Chang. 2007. Clinical features and outcome of tuberculosis in solid organ transplant recipients. *Am. J. Med. Sci.* **334**:106–110.

123. Huang, W. T., C. C. Wang, W. J. Chen, Y. F. Cheng, and H. L. Eng. 2003. The nodular form of hepatic tuberculosis: a review with five additional new cases. *J. Clin. Pathol.* **56**:835–839.

124. Huang, Y. S., H. D. Chern, W. J. Su, J. C. Wu, S. C. Chang, C. H. Chiang, F. Y. Chang, and S. D. Lee. 2003. Cytochrome P450 2E1 genotype and the susceptibility to antituberculosis drug-induced hepatitis. *Hepatology* **37**:924–930.

125. Hulnick, D. H., A. J. Megibow, D. P. Naidich, S. Hilton, K. C. Cho, and E. J. Balthazar. 1985. Abdominal tuberculosis: CT evaluation. *Radiology* **157**:199–204.

126. Hunt, J. S., M. J. Silverstein, F. C. Sparks, C. M. Haskell, Y. H. Pilch, and D. L. Morton. 1973. Granulomatous hepatitis: a complication of BCG immunotherapy. *Lancet* **ii**:820–821.

127. Hurst, A., H. M. Maier, and S. A. Lough. 1947. Studies of hepatic function in pulmonary tuberculosis. *Am. J. Med. Sci.* **214**:431–435.

128. Hussain, W., D. Mutimer, R. Harrison, S. Hubscher, and J. Neuberger. 1995. Fulminant hepatic failure caused by tuberculosis. *Gut* **36**:792–794.

129. Ijaz, K., J. A. Jereb, L. A. Lambert, W. A. Bower, P. R. Spradling, P. D. McElroy, M. F. Iademarco, T. R. Navin, and K. G. Castro. 2006. Severe or fatal liver injury in 50 patients in the United States taking rifampicin and pyrazinamide for latent tuberculosis infection. *Clin. Infect. Dis.* **42**:346–355.

130. Inderlied, C. B., C. A. Kemper, and L. E. M. Bennudez. 1993. The Mycobacterium avium complex. *Clin. Microbiol. Rev.* **6**: 266–310.

130a.Irani, S. K., and W. O. Dobbins III. 1979. Hepatic granulomas: a review of 73 patients from one hospital and survey of the literature. *J. Clin. Gastroenterol.* **1**:131–143.

131. Ishak, K. G., and H. J. Zimmerman. 1988. Drug-induced and toxic granulomatous hepatitis. *Baillieres Clin. Gastroenterol.* **2**:463–480.

132. Jaber, B., and R. Gleckman. 1995. Tuberculous pancreatic abscess as an initial AIDS-defining disorder in a patient infected with the human immunodeficiency virus: a case report and review. *Clin. Infect. Dis.* **20**:890–894.

133. Jacques, J., and J. M. Slan. 1970. The changing pattern of miliary tuberculosis. *Thorax* **25**:237–240.

134. Jenney, A. W., R. W. Pickles, M. E. Hellard, D. W. Spelman, A. J. Fuller, and W. J. Spicer. 1998. Tuberculous pancreatic abscess in an HIV antibody-negative patient: case report and review. *Scand. J. Infect. Dis.* **30**:99–104.

135. Jones, K., and W. M. Peck. 1944. Incidence of fatty liver in tuberculosis with special reference to tuberculosis enteritis. *Arch. Intern. Med.* **74**:371–374.

136. Karnamoto, T., T. Suou, and C. Hirayama. 1986. Elevated serum aminotransferase induced by isoniazid in relation to isoniazid acetalator phenotype. *Hepatology* **6**:295–298.

137. Karsner, H. T. 1943. Morphology and pathogenesis of hepatic cirrhosis. *Am. J. Clin. Pathol.* **13**:569–606.

138. Kaushik, N., K. Schoedel, and K. McGrath. 2006. Isolated pancreatic tuberculosis diagnosed by endoscopic ultrasound-guided fine needle aspiration: a case report. *JOP* **7**:205–210.

139. Kawamori, Y., O. Matsui, K. Kitagawa, M. Kadoya, T. Takashima, and T. Yamahana. 1992. Macronodular tuberculoma of the liver: CT and MR findings. *AJR Am. J. Roentgenol.* **158**:311–313.

140. Kiehn, T. E., F. F. Edwards, P. Brannon, A. Y. Tsang, M. Maio, J. W. Gold, E. Whimbey, B. Wong, J. K. McClatchy, and D. Armstrong. 1985. Infections caused by Mycobacterium avium complex in immunocompromised patients: diagnosis by blood culture and fecal examination, antimicrobial susceptibility test, and morphological and seroagglutination characteristics. *J. Clin. Microbiol.* **21**:168–173.

141. Klatskin, G., and R. Yesner. 1950. Hepatic manifestations of sarcoidosis and other granulomatous diseases: a study based on histologist examination of tissue obtained by needle biopsy of the liver. *Yale J. Biol. Med.* **23**:207–248.

142. Kohen, M. D., and K. A. Altrnan. 1973. Jaundice due to a rare case: tuberculous lymphadenitis. *Am. J. Gastroenterol.* **59**:48–53.

143. Kok, K. Y., and S. K. Yapp. 1999. Isolated hepatic tuberculosis: report of 5 cases and review of literature. *J. Hepatobiliary Pancreat. Surg.* **6**:195–198.

144. Korn, R. J., W. F. Kellow, P. Heller, B. Chomet, and H. J. Zimmerman. 1959. Hepatic involvement in extrapulmonary tuberculosis: histologic and functional characteristics. *Am. J. Med.* **27**:60–71.

145. Kouraklis, G., A. Glinavou, A. Karayiannakis, and G. Karatzas. 2001. Primary tuberculosis of the pancreas mimicking a pancreatic tumor. *Int. J. Pancreatol.* **29**:151–153.

146. Krown, S. E., E. Y. Hilal, and C. M. Pinsky. 1978. Intralesional injection of methanol extraction residue of bacille Calmette-Guerin (MER) into cutaneous metastasis of malignant melanoma. *Cancer* **42**:2648–2660.

147. Kumar, R., D. Kapoor, J. Singh, and N. Kumar. 2003. Isolated tuberculosis of the pancreas: a report of two cases and review of the literature. *Trop. Gastroenterol.* **24**:76–78.

148. Kurnik, P. B., U. Padmanabh, C. Bonatsos, C. Bonatsos, and M. H. Cynamon. 1983. Mycobacterium gordonae as a human hepatoperitoneal pathogen, with a review of the literature. *Am. J. Med. Sci.* **285**:45–48.

149. Ladas, S. D., E. Vaidakis, C. Lariou, K. Anastasiou, G. Chalevelakis, D. Kintzonidis, and S. A. Raptis. 1998. Pancreatic tuberculosis in non-immunocompromised patients: report of two cases and a literature review. *Eur. J. Gastroenterol. Hepatol.* **10**:973–976.

150. Leader, S. A. 1951. Tuberculosis of the liver and gallbladder with abscess formation: a review and case report. *Ann. Intern. Med.* **37**:594–605.

151. Lebovics, E., S. N. Thung, F. Schafner, and P. W. Radensky. 1985. The liver in the acquired immunodeficiency syndrome: a clinical and histologic study. *Hepatology* **5**:293–298.

152. Levine, V., and R. E. Chaisson. 1991. Mycobacterium kansasii: a cause of treatable pulmonary disease associated with advanced human immunodeficiency virus (HIV) infection. *Ann. Intern. Med.* **114**:861–868.

153. Levinson, J. D., G. Olsen, J. W. Terman, C. R. Cleaveland, C. P. Graham, Jr., and K. J. Breen. 1972. Hemobilia secondary to percutaneous liver biopsy. *Arch. Intern. Med.* **120**: 396–400.

154. Lewis, J., V. Varma, H. Tice, W. Steinberg, and R. Reba. 1982. Hepatobiliary scanning in hemobilia-induced acute cholecystitis. *Gastrointest. Radiol.* 7:168–171.

155. Lewis, J. H. 2002. The rational use of potentially hepatotoxic medications in patients with underlying liver disease. *Exper. Opin. Drug Saf.* 1:159–172.

156. Lewis, J. H. 2007. Hepatic granulomas, p. 1425–1448. *In* E. R. Schiff, M. F. Sorrell, and W. C. Maddrey (ed.), *Schiff's Diseases of the Liver*, 10th ed. Lippincott, Williams and Wilkins, Baltimore, MD.

157. Lewis, J. H., and H. J. Zimmerman. 1989. Drug-induced liver disease. *Med. Clin. North Am.* 73:775–792.

158. Lewis, J. H., B. J. Winston, M. A. Garone, and A. Farhood. 1985. The liver in AIDS: a clinicopathologic correlation. *Gastroenterology* 88:1675.

159. Liberato, I. R., M. F. de Albuquerque, A. R. Campelo, and H. R. de Melo. 2004. Characteristics of pulmonary tuberculosis in HIV seropositive and seronegative patients in a Northeastern region of Brazil. *Rev. Soc. Bras. Med. Trop.* 37: 46–50.

160. Liu, Q., P. Garner, Y. Wang, B. Huang, and H. Smith. 2008. Drugs and herbs given to prevent hepatotoxicity of tuberculosis therapy: systematic review of ingredients and evaluation studies. *BMC Public Health* 8:365.

161. Liu, Q., H. Zhenping, and B. Ping. 2003. Solitary pancreatic tuberculous abscess mimicking pancreatic cystadenocarcinoma: a case report. *BMC Gastroenterol.* 3:16.

162. Lo, S. F., A. K. Ahchong, C. N. Tang, and A. W. Yip. 1998. Pancreatic tuberculosis: case reports and review of the literature. *J. R. Coll. Surg. Edinb.* 43:65–68.

163. Reference deleted.

164. Lundstedt, C., R. Nyman, J. Brismar, C. Hugosson, and I. Kagevi. 1996. Imaging of tuberculosis. II. Abdominal manifestations in 112 patients. *Acta Radiol.* 37:489–495.

165. Maharaj, B., O. P. Leary, and D. J. Pudifin. 1987. A prospective study of hepatic tuberculosis in 41 African-American patients. *Q. J. Med.* 63:517–522.

166. Mansuy, M. M., and W. J. Seiferth. 1950. Miliary tuberculosis of the liver: liver biopsy as an adjunct to diagnosis. *Am. J. Med. Sci.* 220:293–297.

167. Markowitz, N., N. I. Hansen, P. C. Hopewell, J. Glassroth, P. A. Kvale, B. T. Mangura, T. C. Wilcosky, J. M. Wallace, M. J. Rosen, and L. B. Reichman. 1997. Incidence of tuberculosis in the United States among HIV-infected persons. *Ann. Intern. Med.* 126:123–132.

168. Martin-Blondel, G., B. Camara, J. Selves, M. A. Robic, S. Thebault, D. Bonnet, and L. Alric. 2010. Etiology and outcome of liver granulomatosis: a retrospective study of 21 cases. *Rev. Med. Interne* 31:97–106.

169. Martinez-Roig, A., J. Carni, J. Llorens-Terol, R. de la Torre, and F. Perich. 1986. Acetylation phenotype and hepatotoxicity in the treatment of tuberculosis in children. *Pediatrics* 77: 912–915.

170. Marzuki, O. A., A. R. Fauzi, S. Ayoub, and M. Kamarul Imran. 2008. Prevalence and risk factors of anti-tuberculosis drug-induced hepatitis in Malaysia. *Singapore Med. J.* 49: 688–693.

171. Mather, G., J. Dawson, and C. Hoyle. 1955. Liver biopsy in sarcoidosis. *Q. J. Med.* 24:331–350.

172. McCluggage, W. G., and J. M. Sloan. 1994. Hepatic granulomas in Northern Ireland: a thirteen year review. *Histopathology* 25:219–228.

173. McCullough, N. B., and C. W. Eisele. 1951. Brucella leading to cirrhosis of the liver. *Arch. Intern. Med.* 88:793–802.

174. McGlynn, K. A., E. D. Lustbader, and W. T. London. 1985. Immune responses to hepatitis B virus and tuberculosis infections in Southeast Asian refugees. *Am. J. Epidemiol.* 122: 1032–1036.

175. McKhann, C. F., C. G. Hendrickson, L. E. Spitler, A. Gunnarsson, D. Banerjee, and W. R. Nelson. 1975. Immunotherapy of melanoma with BCG: two fatalities following intralesional injection. *Cancer* 35:514–520.

176. McNutt, D. R., and H. H. Fudenberg. 1971. Disseminated scotochromogen infection and unusual myeloproliferative disorder. *Ann. Intern. Med.* 75:737–744.

177. Mert, A., R. Ozaras, M. Bilir, V. Tahan, A. Cetinkaya, S. Yirmibescik, G. Ozbay, and H. Senturk. 2001. The etiology of hepatic granulomas. *J. Clin. Gastroenterol.* 32:275–276.

178. Meyer, B. R., G. A. Papanicolau, P. Sheiner, S. Emre, and C. Miller. 2000. Tuberculosis in orthotopic liver transplantation patients: increased toxicity of recommended agents; cure of disseminated infection with nonconventional regimens. *Transplantation* 69:64–69.

179. Meyers, B. R., M. Halpern, P. Sheiner, M. H. Mendelson, E. Neibart, and C. Miller. 1994. Tuberculosis in liver transplant patients. *Transplantation* 58:301–306.

180. Minamoto, G., and D. Armstrong. 1986. Combating infections in patients with AIDS: update on the evolving epidemiology, issues in screening, and therapy. *J. Crit. Illness* 1:37–48.

181. Mindikoglu, A. L., L. S. Magder, and A. Regev. 2009. Outcome of liver transplantation for drug-induced acute liver failure in the United States: analysis of the United Network for Organ Sharing database. *Liver Transplant.* 15:719–729.

182. Mitchell, I., J. Wendon, S. Fitt, and R. Williams. 1995. Antituberculous therapy and acute liver failure. *Lancet* 345:555–556.

183. Mitchell, J. R., K. G. Ishak, and W. R. Snodgrass. 1976. Isoniazid liver injury: clinical spectrum, pathology and probable pathogenesis. *Ann. Intern. Med.* 84:181–192.

184. Mitchell, J. R., U. P. Thorgeirsson, M. Black, J. A. Timbrell, W. R. Snodgrass, W. Z. Potter, H. R. Jollow, and H. R. Keiser. 1975. Increased incidence of isoniazid hepatitis in rapid acetylators: possible relation to hydrazine metabolites. *Clin. Pharmacol. Ther.* 18:70–79.

185. Moskovic, E. 1990. Macronodular hepatic tuberculosis in a child: computed tomographic appearances. *Br. J. Radiol.* 63: 656–658.

186. Moulding, T. S., A. G. Redeker, and G. C. Kanel. 1989. Twenty isoniazid-associated deaths in one state. *Am. Rev. Respir. Dis.* 140:700–705.

187. Munt, P. W. 1971. Miliary tuberculosis in the chemotherapy era: with a clinical review in 69 American adults. *Medicine* 51:139–155.

188. Murata, Y., I. Yamada, Y. Sumiya, Y. Shichijo, and Y. Suzuki. 1996. Abdominal macronodular tuberculomas: MR findings. *J. Comput. Assist. Tomogr.* 20:643–646.

189. Murphy, R., R. Swartz, and P. B. Watkins. 1990. Severe acetaminophen toxicity in a patient receiving isoniazid. *Ann. Intern. Med.* 113:799–800.

190. Murphy, T. F., and G. F. Gray. 1980. Biliary tract obstruction due to tuberculous adenitis *Am. J. Med.* 68:452–454.

191. Nagai, H., S. Shimizu, H. Kawamoto, M. Yamanoue, T. Tsuchiya, and M. Yamamoto. 1989. A case of solitary tuberculosis of the liver. *Jpn. J. Med.* 28:251–255.

192. Nishioka, S. A. 1996. Cirrhosis as a risk factor to drug-resistant tuberculosis. *Eur. Respir. J.* 9:2188–2189.

193. Noble, A. 1995. Antituberculous therapy and acute liver failure. *Lancet* 345:867.

194. Nolan, C. M., S. V. Goldberg, and S. E. Buskin. 1999. Hepatotoxicity associated with isoniazid preventive therapy: a 7-year survey from a public health tuberculosis clinic. *JAMA* 281:1014–1018.

195. Nolan, C. M., R. E. Sandblom, K. E. Thummel, J. T. Slattery, and S. D. Nelson. 1994. Hepatotoxicity associated with acetaminophen usage in patients receiving multiple drug therapy for tuberculosis. *Chest* 105:408–411.

196. O'Brien, R. J., M. A. Lyle, M. W. Johnson, and D. E. Snider. 1985. Ansamycin LM427 therapy in AIDS patients with Mycobacterium avium (MAI) complex infection: a preliminary report, p. 47. *Abstr. Int. Conf. Acquir. Immunodefic. Syndr.*, American College of Physicians, Philadelphia, PA.

197. O'Brien, T. F., and N. E. Hyslop, Jr. 1975. Case records of the Massachusetts General Hospital, case 34-1975. *N. Engl. J. Med.* 293:443–448.

198. Okuda, K., K. Kimura, K. Takara, M. Ohto, M. Omata, and L. Lesmana. 1986. Resolution of diffuse granulomatous fibrosis of the liver with antituberculous chemotherapy. *Gastroenterology* 91:456–460.

199. Oliva, A., B. Durate, O. Jonasson, and V. Nadimpalli. 1990. The nodular form of local hepatic tuberculosis: a review. *J. Clin. Gastroenterol.* 12:166–173.

200. Orenstein, M. S., A. Tavitian, B. Yonk, H. P. Dincsoy, J. Zerega, S. K. Iyer, and E. W. Straus. 1985. Granulomatous involvement of the liver in patients with AIDS. *Gut* 26:1220–1225.

201. Ozbakkaloglu, B., O. Tunger, S. Surucuoglu, M. Lekili, and A. R. Kandiloglu. 1999. Granulomatous hepatitis following bacillus Calmette-Guerin therapy. *Int. Urol. Nephrol.* 31:49–53.

202. Ozick, L. A., L. Jacob, G. M. Comer, T. P. Lee, J. Ben-Zvi, S. S. Donelson, and C. P. Felton. 1995. Hepatotoxicity from isoniazid and rifampin in inner-city AIDS patients. *Am. J. Gastroenterol.* 90:1978–1980.

203. Palmer, K. R., D. H. Patil, A. S. Basran, J. F. Riordan, and D. B. Silk. 1985. Abdominal tuberculosis in urban Britain-a common disease. *Gut* 26:1296–1305.

204. Pan, L., Z. S. Jia, L. Chen, E. Q. Fu, and G. Y. Li. 2005. Effect of anti-tuberculosis therapy on liver function of pulmonary tuberculosis patients infected with hepatitis B virus. *World J. Gastroenterol.* 11:2518–2521.

205. Pandita, K. K., Sarla, and S. Dogra. 2009. Isolated pancreatic tuberculosis. *Indian J. Med. Microbiol.* 27:259–260.

206. Panzuto, F., A. D'Amato, A. Laghi, G. Cadau, G. D'Ambra, D. Aguzzi, R. Iannaccone, R. Montesani, R. Caprilli, and G. Delle Fave. 2003. Abdominal tuberculosis with pancreatic involvement: case report. *Dig. Liver Dis.* 35:283–287.

207. Parthasarathy, R., G. R. Sarma, B. Janardhanam, P. Ramachandran, T. Santha, S. Sivasubramanian, P. R. Somasundaram, and S. P. Tripathy. 1986. Hepatic toxicity in South Indian patients during treatment of tuberculosis with short course regimens containing isoniazid, rifampicin and pyrazinamide. *Tubercle* 67:99–108.

208. Patel, K. M. 1981. Granulomatous hepatitis due to Mycobacterium scrofulaceum: report of a case. *Gastroenterology* 81:156–158.

209. Petera, V., V. Vesely, V. Kulich, and J. Dura. 1972. The clinical and morphological correlations in the Au/SH antigen carriers. *Digestion* 5:227–228.

210. Pierce, M., S. Crampton, D. Henry, L. Heifets, A. LaMarca, M. Montecalvo, G. P. Wormser, H. Jablonowski, J. Jemsek, M. Cynamon, B. G. Yangco, G. Notario, and J. C. Craft. 1996. A randomized trial of clarithromycin as prophylaxis against disseminated Mycobacterium avium complex infection in patients with advanced acquired immunodeficiency syndrome. *N. Engl. J. Med.* 335:384–391.

211. Pineda, F. M., and A. Dalmacio-Cruz. 1966. Tuberculosis of the liver and the porta hepatis: report of 9 cases. *Acta Med. Philipp.* 2:128–139.

212. Pintos, J. F., L. C. Rey, and J. S. Boo. 1972. Tuberculosis miliar hepatica combinada con una proliferacion de hepatocitos gigantes. *Rev. Esp. Enferm. Apar. Dig.* 38:847–854.

213. Pombo, F., M. J. Diaz Candamio, E. Rodriguez, and S. Pombo. 1998. Pancreatic tuberculosis: CT findings. *Abdom. Imaging* 23:394–397.

214. Poprawski, D., P. Pitisuttitum, and S. Transuphasawadikul. 2000. Clinical presentation and outcomes of tuberculosis among HIV-positive patients. *Southeast Asian J. Trop. Med. Public Health* 31(Suppl. 1):140–142.

215. Pramesh, C. S., A. A. Heroor, P. J. Shukla, P. M. Jagannath, and L. J. De Souza. 2002. Pancreatic tuberculosis. *Trop. Gastroenterol.* 23:142–143.

216. Probst, A., W. Schmidbaur, G. Jechart, A. Hammond, J. Zentner, E. Niculescu, and H. Messmann. 2004. Obstructive jaundice in AIDS: diagnosis of biliary tuberculosis by ERCP. *Gastrointest. Endosc.* 60:145–148.

217. Prochazka, M., F. Vyhnanek, V. Vorreith, and M. Jirásek. 1986. Bleeding into solitary hepatic tuberculoma: report of a case treated by resection. *Acta Chir. Scand.* 152:73–75.

218. Proudfoot, A. T., A. J. Akhtar, A. C. Douglas, and N. W. Horne. 1969. Miliary tuberculosis in adults. *Br. Med. J.* 2:273–276.

219. Rab, S. M., and M. Zakaullah Beg. 1977. Tuberculosis liver abscess. *Br. J. Clin. Pract.* 31:157–158.

220. Rahmatulla, R. H., I. A. al-Mofleh, R. S. al-Rashed, M. A. al-Hedaithy, and I. Y. Mayet. 2001. Tuberculous liver abscess: a case report and review of literature. *Gastroenterol. Hepatol.* 13:437–440.

221. Redha, S., R. L. Suresh, J. Subramaniam, and I. Merican. 2001. Pancreatic tuberculosis presenting as recurrent acute pancreatitis. *Med. J. Malaysia* 56:95–97.

222. Reichert, C. M., T. J. O'Leary, D. L. Levens, C. R. Simrell, and A. M. Macher. 1983. Autopsy pathology in the acquired immune deficiency syndrome. *Am. J. Pathol.* 112:357–382.

223. Rezeig, M. A. 1998. Pancreatic tuberculosis mimicking pancreatic carcinoma: four case reports and review of the literature. *Dig. Dis. Sci.* 43:329–331.

224. Riaz, A. A., P. Singh, P. Robshaw, and A. M. Isla. 2002. Tuberculosis of the pancreas diagnosed with needle aspiration. *Scand. J. Infect. Dis.* 34:303–304.

225. Rolleston, H., and J. W. McNee. 1929. *Diseases of the Liver, Gallbladder and Bile Ducts*. Macmillan, London, United Kingdom.

226. Rolleston, H. D. 1905. Tuberculosis of the liver and bile ducts, p. 336–346. *Disease of the Liver, Gallbladder and Bile Ducts*. WB Saunders, Philadelphia, PA.

227. Rosenkranz, K., and L. D. Howard. 1936. Tubular tuberculosis of the liver. *Arch. Pathol.* 22:743–754.

228. Rougier, P., C. Degott, B. Rueff, and J. P. Benhamou. 1978. Nodular regenerative hyperplasia of the liver: report of six cases and review of the literature. *Gastroenterology* 75:169–172.

229. Rozmanic, V., S. Kilvain, V. Ahel, S. Banac, and M. Gazdik. 2001. Pulmonary tuberculosis with gall bladder involvement: a review and case report. *Pediatr. Int.* 43:511–513.

230. Rudzki, C., I. G. Ishak, and H. J. Zimmerman. 1975. Chronic intrahepatic cholestasis of sarcoidosis. *Am. J. Med.* 59:373–387.

231. Sabharwal, B. D., N. Malhotra, R. Garg, and V. Malhotra. 1995. Granulomatous hepatitis: a retrospective study. *Indian J. Pathol. Microbiol.* 38:413–416.

232. Salib, M., P. C. Le Golvan, H. G. Arm, M. Sabour, and E. E. Shehata. 1961. Clinical, histopathological and bacteriological study of the liver in chronic fibrocaseous pulmonary tuberculosis. *J. Egypt. Med. Assoc.* 44:226–232.

233. Saluja, S. S., S. Ray, S. Pal, M. Kukeraja, D. N. Srivastava, P. Sahni, and T. K. Chattopadhyay. 2007. Hepatobiliary and pancreatic tuberculosis: a two-decade experience. *BMC Surg.* 7:10.

234. Sanabe, N., Y. Ikematsu, Y. Nishiwaki, H. Kida, G. Murohisa, T. Ozawa, S. Hasegawa, T. Okawada, T. Toritsuka, and S. Waki. 2002. Pancreatic tuberculosis. *J. Hepatobiliary Pancreat. Surg.* 9:515–518.

235. Sanai, F. M., S. Ashrafi, A. A. Abdo, M. B. Satti, F. Batwa, H. Al-Husseini, A. M. Saleh, and K. I. Bzeizi. 2008. Hepatic granuloma: decreasing trend in a high-incidence area. *Liver Int.* 28:1402–1407.

236. Saphir, O. 1929. Changes in the liver and pancreas in chronic tuberculosis. *Arch. Pathol.* 7:1025–1039.

237. Sarda, P., S. K. Sharma, A. Mohan, G. Makharia, A. Jayaswal, R. M. Pandey, and S. Singh. 2009. Role of acute viral hepatitis as a confounding factor in ATT induced hepatotoxicity. *Indian J. Med. Res.* 129:64–67.

238. Sartin, J. S., and R. C. Walker. 1991. Granulomatous hepatitis: a retrospective review of 88 cases at the Mayo Clinic. *Mayo Clin. Proc.* 66:914–918.

239. Satter, F. R., R. Cowan, D. M. Nielsen, and J. Ruskin. 1988. Trimethoprim-sulfamethoxazole compared with pentamidine for treatment of Pneumocystis carinii pneumonia in the acquired immunodeficiency syndrome: a prospective, noncrossover study. *Ann. Intern. Med.* 109:280–287.

240. Satti, M. B., H. al-Freihi, E. M. Ibrahim, A. Abu-Melha, G. al-Ghassab, H. Y. al-Idrissi, and M. O. al-Sohaibani. 1990. Hepatic granuloma in Saudi Arabia: a clinicopathological study of 59 cases. *Am. J. Gastroenterol.* 85:669–674.

241. Saukkonen, J. J., D. L. Cohn, R. M. Jasmer, S. Schenker, J. A. Jereb, C. M. Nolan, C. A. Peloquin, F. M. Gordin, D. Nunes, D. B. Strader, J. Bernardo, R. Venkataramanan, and T. R. Sterling. 2006. An official ATS statement: hepatotoxicity of antituberculosis therapy. *Am. J. Respir. Crit. Care Med.* 174: 935–952.

242. Schaffner, P., G. C. Turner, D. E. Eshbaugh, W. B. Buckingham, and H. Popper. 1953. Hypergammaglobulinemia in pulmonary tuberculosis. *Arch. Intern. Med.* 92:490–493.

243. Scheuer, P., J. A. Surnmerfield, S. Lal, and S. Sherlock. 1974. Rifampicin hepatitis: a clinical histological study. *Lancet* i: 421–425.

244. Schluger, L. K., P. A. Sheiner, M. Jonas, J. V. Guarrera, I. M. Fiel, B. Meyers, and P. D. Berk. 1996. Isoniazid hepatotoxicity after orthotopic liver transplantation. *Mt. Sinai J. Med.* 63:364–369.

245. Schneider, A., C. von Birgelen, U. Duhrsen, G. Gerken, and M. Rünzi. 2002. Two cases of pancreatic tuberculosis in nonimmunocompromised patients: a diagnostic challenge and a rare cause of portal hypertension. *Pancreatology* 2:69–73.

246. Schneiderman, D. J., D. M. Arenson, and J. P. Cello. 1986. Hepatic disease in patients with the acquired immune deficiency syndrome. *Gastroenterology* 90:1620.

247. Seife, M., B. J. Messier, J. Hoffman, and J. R. Lisa. 1951. A clinical, functional, and needle biopsy study of the liver in pulmonary tuberculosis. *Am. Rev. Tuberc.* 63:202–209.

248. Sekikawa, A., M. Inada, K. Tsuyuoka, M. Nakamura, C. Kurusu, S. Takeshi, O. Yasuhide, Y. Okimoto, and T. Yoshimura. 2001. A case of pancreatic tuberculosis resembling pancreatic serous cystadenoma. *Jpn. J. Gastroenterol.* 98:1298–1303.

249. Selwyn, P. A., V. A. Lewis, and E. E. Schoenbaum. 1988. HIV infection and tuberculosis in intravenous drug users in a methadone program, abstr. 7549. *Proc. IVth Int. Conf. AIDS*, Stockholm, Sweden.

250. Seth, V., and A. Beotra. 1989. Hepatic function in relation to acetylator phenotype in children treated with antitubercular drugs. *Indian J. Med. Res.* 89:306–309.

251. Shafran, S. D., J. Singer, D. P. Zarowny, P. Phillips, I. Salit, S. L. Walmsley, I. W. Fong, M. J. Gill, A. R. Rachlis, R. G. Lalonde, M. M. Fanning, and C. M. Tsoukas. 1996. A comparison of two regimens for the treatment of Mycobacterium avium complex bacteremia in AIDS: rifabutin, ethambutol, and clarithromycin versus rifampin, ethambutol, clofazimine, and ciprofloxacin. *N. Engl. J. Med.* 335:377–383.

252. Shah, S. R., D. A. Rastegar, and T. L. Nicol. 2000. Case report: diagnosis of disseminated Mycobacterium avium complex infection by liver biopsy. *AIDS Reader* 10:669–672.

253. Shan, S. A., and T. A. Neff. 1974. Miliary tuberculosis. *Am. J. Med.* 56:495–505.

254. Shan, Y.-S., E. D. Sy, and P. W. Lin. 2000. Surgical resection of isolated pancreatic tuberculosis presenting as obstructive jaundice. *Pancreas* 21:100–101.

255. Sharma, S. K., R. Singla, P. Sarda, A. Mohan, G. Makharia, A. Jayaswal, V. Sreenivas, and S. Singh. 2010. Safety of 3 different reintroduction regimens of antituberculosis drugs after development of antituberculosis treatment-induced hepatotoxicity. *Clin. Infect. Dis.* 50:833–839.

256. Sherlock, S. (ed.). 1981. *Diseases of the Liver and Biliary System*, 6th ed., p. 395. Blackwell Scientific, Oxford, United Kingdom.

257. Sherlock, S. 1985. The liver in infections, p. 460–461. *In* S. Sherlock (ed.), *Diseases of the Liver and Biliary System*, 7th ed. Blackwell Science, Oxford, United Kingdom.

258. Siemann, M., G. Rabenhorst, A. Bramann, and C. Renk. 1999. A case of cryptic miliary tuberculosis mimicking cholecystitis with sepsis. *Infection* 27:44–45.

259. Simon, H. B., and S. M. Wolff. 1973. Granulomatous hepatitis and prolonged fever of unknown origin: a study of 13 patients. *Medicine* 52:1–21.

260. Singh, B., J. Moodley, S. Batitiang, and R. Chetty. 2002. Isolated pancreatic tuberculosis and obstructive jaundice. *S. Afr. Med. J.* 92:357–359.

261. Singh, D. K., A. Haider, M. Tatke, P. Kumar, and P. K. Mishra. 2009. Primary pancreatic tuberculosis masquerading as a pancreatic tumor leading to Whipple's pancreaticoduodenectomy: a case report and review of the literature. *JOP* 10: 451–456.

262. Singh, N., M. M. Wagener, and T. Gayowski. 2002. Safety and efficacy of isoniazid chemoprophylaxis administered during liver transplant candidacy for the prevention of posttransplant tuberculosis. *Transplantation* 74:892–895.

263. Sinha, S. K., M. Chatterjee, S. Bhattacharya, S. K. Pathak, R. B. Mitra, K. Karak, and M. Mukherjee. 2003. Diagnostic evaluation of extrapulmonary tuberculosis by fine needle aspiration (FNA) supplemented with AFB smear and culture. *J. Indian Med. Assoc.* 101:588, 590–591.

264. Small, G., and D. Wilks. 2001. Pancreatic mass caused by Mycobacterium tuberculosis with reduced drug sensitivity. *J. Infect.* 42:201–202.

265. Small, M. S. 1974. Tuberculosis of liver: scan appearance before and after successful treatment. *J. Nucl. Med.* 15:135–138.

266. Small, P. M., G. F. Schecter, P. C. Goodman, M. A. Sande, R. E. Chaisson, and P. C. Hopewell. 1991. Treatment of tuberculosis in patients with advanced human immunodeficiency virus infection. *N. Engl. J. Med.* 324:289–294.

267. Smith, E. R., and H. A. Penman. 1971. Histological diagnosis of *M. kansasii* lung infection. *Pathology* 3:93.

268. Smith, M. B., M. C. Boyars, S. Veasey, and G. L. Woods. 2000. Generalized tuberculosis in the acquired immunodeficiency syndrome. *Arch. Pathol. Lab. Med.* **124:**1267–1274.

269. Snider, D. E., and G. J. Caras. 1992. Isoniazid associated hepatitis: a review of available information. *Am. Rev. Respir. Dis.* **145:**494–497.

270. Snider, G. L. 1997. Tuberculosis then and now: a personal perspective on the last 50 years. *Ann. Intern. Med.* **126:**237–243.

271. Sparks, F. C., N. E. Albert, and J. H. Breeding. 1977. Effect on isonicotinic acid hydrazide on the intraturnor injection of BCG. *J. Natl. Cancer Inst.* **58:**367–368.

272. Spegel, C. T., and C. U. Tuazon. 1984. Tuberculous liver abscess. *Tubercle* **65:**127–131.

273. Stanley, H. J., P. L. Yantis, and W. H. Marsh. 1984. Periportal tuberculous adenitis: a rare cause of obstructive jaundice. *Gastrointest. Radiol.* **9:**227–229.

274. Steele, M. A., R. F. Burk, and R. M. DesPrez. 1991. Toxic hepatitis with isoniazid and rifampin: a meta-analysis. *Chest* **99:**465–471.

275. Steidl, J., and F. J. Heise. 1933. Studies of liver function in advanced pulmonary tuberculosis. *Am. J. Med. Sci.* **186:**631–640.

276. Steiner, P. E. 1959. Nodular regenerative hyperplasia of the liver. *Am. J. Pathol.* **35:**943–953.

277. Stemmerman, M. 1941. Bile duct tuberculosis. *Q. Bull. Sea View Hosp.* **6:**316–324.

278. Stewart, C., and L. Jackson. 1976. Spleno-hepatic tuberculosis due to *Mycobacterium kansasii*. *Med. J. Aust.* **2:**99–101.

279. Sunderam, G., R. J. McDonald, T. Maniatis, J. Oleske, R. Kapila, and L. B. Reichman. 1986. Tuberculosis as a manifestation of the acquired immunodeficiency syndrome (AIDS). *JAMA* **256:**362–366.

280. Tahiliani, R. R., J. A. Parikh, A. V. Hedge, S. J. Bhatia, K. P. Deodhar, N. M. Kapadia, R. C. Khokhani, and V. B. Damle. 1983. Hepatic tuberculosis simulating hepatic amoebiasis. *J. Assoc. Physicians India* **31:**697–680.

281. Tarantino, L., A. Giorgio, G. de Dtefano, N. Farella, A. Perrotta, and F. Esposito. 2003. Disseminated mycobacterial infection in AIDS patients: abdominal US features and value of fine-needle aspiration biopsy of lymph nodes and spleen. *Abdom. Imaging* **28:**602–608.

282. Teo, L. L., S. K. Venkatesh, and K. Y. Ho. 2007. Clinics in diagnostic imaging (117). *Singapore Med. J.* **48:**687–692.

283. Terry, R. B., and R. M. Gunnar. 1957. Primary miliary tuberculosis of the liver. *JAMA* **164:**150–157.

284. Thora, S., M. Chansoria, and K. K. Kaul. 1985. Congenital tuberculosis: a case with unusual features. *Indian J. Pediatr.* **52:**425–427.

285. Tobias, H., and A. Sherman. 2002. Hepatobiliary tuberculosis, p. 537–547. *In* W. N. Rom and S. M. Garay (ed.), *Tuberculosis*, 2nd ed. Lippincott Williams & Wilkins, Phildelphia, PA.

286. Torre-Cisneros, J., J. J. Caston, J. Moreno, A. Rivero, E. Vidal, R. Jurado, and J. M. Kindelán. 2004. Tuberculosis in the transplant candidate: importance of early diagnosis and treatment. *Transplantation* **77:**1376–1380.

287. Torre-Cisneros, J., M. de la Mata, S. Rufian, J. L. Villanueva Marcos, J. Gutierrez Aroca, M. Casal, G. Miño, and C. Pera. 1995. Importance of surveillance of mycobacterial cultures after liver transplantation. *Transplantation* **60:**1054–1055.

288. Torrey, R. G. 1916. The occurrence of miliary tuberculosis of the liver in the course of pulmonary tuberculosis. *Am. J. Med. Sci.* **151:**549–556.

289. Tostmann, A., M. J. Boeree, R. E. Aarnoutse, W. C. de Lange, A. J. van der Ven, and R. Dekhuijzen. 2008. Antituberculosis drug-induced hepatotoxicity: concise up to date review. *J. Gastroenterol. Hepatol.* **23:**192–202.

290. Treska, V., O. Hes, and J. Nemcova. 2009. Liver tuberculoma. *Bratisl. Lek. Listy* **110:**363–365.

291. Turan, M., M. Sen, A. Koyuncu, C. Aydin, N. Elaldi, and S. Arici. 2002. Pancreatic pseudotumor due to peripancreatic tuberculous lymphadenitis. *Pancreatology* **2:**561–564.

292. Ullom, J. T. 1909. The liver in tuberculosis. *Am. J. Med. Sci.* **137:**694–699.

293. Ungo, J. R., D. Jones, D. Ashkin, E. S. Hollender, D. Bernstein, A. P. Albanese, and A. E. Pitchenik. 1998. Antituberculosis drug-induced hepatotoxicity: the role of hepatitis C virus and the human immunodeficiency virus. *Am. J. Respir. Crit. Care Med.* **157:**1871–1876.

294. Valdez, V. A., and N. E. Herrera. 1978. Granulomatous hepatitis: spectrum of scintigraphic manifestations. *Clin. Nucl. Med.* **3:**392–396.

295. Van Buchem, F. S. P. 1946. On morbid conditions of liver and diagnosis of disease of Besnier-Boeck-Shauman. *Acta Med. Scand.* **124:**168.

296. Verma, A., A. Dhawan, J. J. Wade, W. H. Lim, G. Ruiz, J. F. Price, N. Hadzic, A. J. Baker, M. Rela, N. D. Heaton, and G. Mieli-Vergani. 2000. Mycobacterium tuberculosis infection in pediatric liver transplant recipients. *Pediatr. Infect. Dis.* **19:**625–630.

297. Vilaichone, R. K., W. Vilaichone, S. Tumwasorn, P. Suwanagool, H. Wilde, and V. Mahachai. 2003. Clinical spectrum of hepatic tuberculosis: comparison between immunocompromised and immunocompetent hosts. *J. Med. Assoc. Thai.* **86**(Suppl. 2)**:**S432–S438.

298. Von Oldershausen, H. G., R. von Oldershausen, and A. Tellesz. 1955. Zur Klinik und pathogenetischen Bedeutung der sogenannten "granulomatosen Hepatopathie" bei der Tuberculose. *Klin. Wochenschr.* **33:**104.

299. Wanless, I. R., L. C. Solt, P. Kortan, J. H. Deck, G. W. Gardiner, and E. J. Prokipchuk. 1981. Nodular regenerative hyperplasia of the liver associated with macroglobulinemia. *Am. J. Med.* **70:**1203–1209.

300. Wee, A., B. Nilsson, T. L. Wang, I. Yap, and P. Y. Siew. 1995. Tuberculous pseudotumor causing biliary obstruction: report of a case with diagnosis by fine needle aspiration biopsy and bile cytology. *Acta Cytol.* **39:**559–562.

301. Wissmer, B. 1976. Tuberculosis of the liver, p. 511–514. *In* H. L. Bockus (ed.), *Gastroenterology*, vol. 3. WB Saunders, Philadelphia, PA.

302. Wong, B., F. F. Edwards, T. E. Kiehn, E. Whimbey, H. Donnelly, E. M. Bernard, J. W. Gold, and D. Armstrong. 1985. Continuous high-grade Mycobacterium avium-intracellulare bacteremia in patients with the acquired immune deficiency syndrome. *Am. J. Med.* **78:**35–40.

303. Wong, W. M., P. C. Wu, M. F. Yuen, C. C. Cheng, W. W. Yew, P. C. Wong, C. M. Tam, C. C. Leung, and C. L. Lai. 2000. Antituberculosis drug-related liver dysfunction in chronic hepatitis B infection. *Hepatology* **31:**201–206.

304. Woodfield, J. C., J. A. Windsor, C. C. Godfrey, D. A. Orr, and N. M. Officer. 2004. Diagnosis and management of isolated pancreatic tuberculosis. *Aust. N. Z. J. Surg.* **74:**368–371.

305. Wu, J.-C., S.-D. Lee, P.-F. Yeh, C. Y. Chan, Y. J. Wang, Y. S. Huang, Y. T. Tsai, P. Y. Lee, L. P. Ting, and K. J. Lo. 1990. Isoniazid-rifampin-induced hepatitis in hepatitis B carriers. *Gastroenterology* **98:**502–504.

306. Xia, F., R. T. Poon, S. G. Wang, P. Bie, X. Q. Huang, and J. H. Dong. 2003. Tuberculosis of pancreas and peripancreatic lymph nodes in immunocompetent patients: experience from China. *World J. Gastroenterol.* **9:**1361–1364.

307. Yamaguchi, B. T., and H. Braunstein. 1965. Fluorescent stain for tubercle bacilli in histological sections. II. Diagnostic efficiency in granulomatous lesions of the liver. *Am. J. Clin. Pathol.* **43:**184–187.

308. Yee, D., C. Valiquette, M. Pelletier, I. Parisien, I. Rocher, and D. Menzies. 2003. Incidence of serious side effects from first line antituberculosis drugs among patients treated for active tuberculosis. *Am. J. Respir. Crit. Care Med.* **167:**1472–1477.

309. Yeh, T. S., N. H. Chen, Y. Y. Jan, T. L. Hwang, L. B. Jeng, and M. F. Chen. 1999. Obstructive jaundice caused by biliary tuberculosis: spectrum of the diagnosis and management. *Gastrointest. Endosc.* **50:**105–108.

310. Yew, W. W., C. H. Chau, J. Lee, and C. W. Leung. 1995. Cholestatic hepatitis in a patient who received clarithromycin therapy for a Mycobacterium chelonae lung infection. *Clin. Infect. Dis.* **20:**1073–1074.

311. Yokoyama, T., S. Miyagawa, T. Noike, R. Shimada, and S. Kawasaki. 1999. Isolated pancreatic tuberculosis. *Hepatogastroenterology* **46:**2011–2014.

312. Zimmerman, H. J. 1978. *Hepatotoxicity: the Adverse Effects of Drugs and Other Chemicals on the Liver*, p. 485–495. Appleton-Century-Crofts, New York, NY.

313. Zimmerman, H. J., and J. H. Lewis. 1984. Hepatic toxicity of antimicrobial agents, p. 153–201. *In* R. K. Root and M. A. Sande (ed.), *New Dimensions in Antimicrobial Therapy*. Churchill Livingstone, New York, NY.

314. Zipser, R. D., L. E. Rau, R. R. Ricketts, and L. C. Bevans. 1976. Tuberculous pseudotumors of the liver. *Am. J. Med.* **61:**946–951.

Tuberculosis and Nontuberculous Mycobacterial Infections, 6th ed.
Edited by David Schlossberg
© 2011 ASM Press, Washington, DC

Chapter 26

Cutaneous Tuberculosis

Michael K. Hill and Charles V. Sanders

Cutaneous tuberculosis (TB) is not a well-defined entity but comprises a wide spectrum of clinical manifestations. In the past, much of the confusion regarding cutaneous TB has resulted from misleading, redundant nomenclature and cumbersome, non-clinically oriented classifications of cutaneous disease. These classifications have been based on various criteria, including chronic versus labile disease, localizing versus hematogenous disease, histologic forms of disease, immunologic status of the patient, primary disease versus reinfection, and listing of the various types of cutaneous mycobacteriosis (3, 6, 35). A more clinically relevant classification has been developed that uses three criteria: pathogenesis, clinical presentation, and histologic evaluation (Table 1).

Skin involvement may occur as a result of exogenous inoculation (in non-previously sensitized hosts, regional adenopathy occurs) by contagious spread from a focus underlying the skin, particularly from osteomyelitis, epididymitis, or lymphadenitis, and by hematogenous spread from a distant focus or as a part of a generalized hematogenous dissemination (15, 63). Although it is rare in the United States and accounts for less than 1% of cases in European dermatologic clinics, there has been an increase in the incidence of cutaneous TB (61, 63). Contrary to earlier claims that cutaneous TB is uncommon in the tropics, reports from India, Southeast Asia, and Africa prove otherwise (66).

INOCULATION CUTANEOUS TB FROM AN EXOGENOUS SOURCE

Primary inoculation TB results from the entry of mycobacteria into the skin or, less frequently, the mucosa of a person who has not previously been infected or who has no natural or artificial immunity to *Mycobacterium tuberculosis*. Because the acid-fast bacilli (AFB) cannot penetrate the normal intact skin

barrier, some form of injury is required to initiate the infection. The entry point for AFB is usually through minor skin abrasions, hangnail wounds, impetigo, or furuncles.

Although inoculation can occur in a variety of ways, most reports have involved persons working in medically related professions (Fig. 1). Laennec described his own "prosector's wart" in 1826. TB lesions have followed mouth-to-mouth resuscitation, inoculation, inoculation of laboratory guinea pigs, injection with poorly sterilized needles, ear piercing, intramuscular injections given by a nurse with active TB, tattooing, insect bites, sexual intercourse leading to venereal inoculation TB, and venipuncture in an infant (1, 7, 19, 23, 26–29, 33, 44, 45, 51, 52, 56, 57, 68). Historically, ritualistic circumcision performed by a practitioner with active pulmonary TB has resulted in miliary disease in the infant (28).

Mucocutaneous involvement may account for one-third of the total primary cutaneous TB cases and includes infection of the conjunctiva or of the oral cavity after tooth extraction or after drinking nonpasteurized milk infected with *Mycobacterium bovis* (15, 63, 66, 75).

The pathogenesis of cutaneous TB from an exogenous source is similar to that of other primary diseases. Over 2 to 4 weeks, as the organism multiplies in the skin, a tuberculous chancre slowly develops, initially appearing as a nodule that evolves into an indolent, firm, nontender, sharply delineated ulcer. It also may develop into impetigenous or ichthyotic forms. Lymphatic extension occurs, and lymphadenopathy occurs 3 to 8 weeks after skin inoculation. The purified protein derivative (PPD) skin test result becomes positive, and enlarged lymph nodes may become fluctuant and drain spontaneously. The complex of the tuberculous chancre and regional adenopathy is the cutaneous analog of the primary tubercular infection of the lung, the Gohn complex. Within 2 to 3 years, calcification can be found in draining nodes.

Michael K. Hill • *56 Starbrush Circle, Covington, LA 70433.* **Charles V. Sanders** • Department of Medicine, Louisiana State University School of Medicine, 1542 Tulane Avenue, Suite 421, Box T4M-2, New Orleans, LA 70112.

Table 1. Classification of cutaneous TB and synonymous terms used previously[a]

Classification of cutaneous TB	Clinical appearance	Histology	Associated finding	Terms previously used in literature
Cutaneous TB from exogenous source				
Primary inoculation	Ulcer, nodule, local disease, lymphatic extension	Chronic inflammation, granulomatous inflammation	History of trauma	Primary inoculation TB chancre TB primary complex
Post-primary inoculation	Hyperkeratoic papule, "wart"	Hyperkeratosis	History of trauma	TB verrucosa cutis Warty TB Verruca necrogenica Prosector's wart TB cutis verrucosa
Cutaneous TB from endogenous source				
Contiguous spread	Sinus tract, abscess	Granulomatous inflammation, sinus tract	Underlying infected source	Scrofuloderma TB colliquativa cutis
Autoinoculation	Ulcer at body orifice	Ulceration, granulomatous inflammation	Widespread TB	Orificial TB TB cutis orificialis TB ulcerosa cutis et mucosae
Cutaneous TB from hematogenous spread				
Lupus vulgaris	Multiple nodules and plaques on face, neck	Granulomatous inflammation	May develop carcinoma	Lupus vulgaris TB luposa cutis
Acute hematogenous dissemination	Multiple papules and pustules	Nonspecific inflammation	Acute presentation	Acute miliary TB of the skin TB cutis miliaris disseminate TB cutis acuta generalisata
Nodules or abscesses	Multiple soft tissue abscesses	Granulomatous inflammation	May arise at site of trauma	TB gumma Metastatic tuberculous abscess

[a]Adapted from the work of Beyt et al. (6).

The early histologic picture is an acute neutrophilic reaction with embedded areas of necrosis associated with numerous AFB. Three to six weeks later, the infiltrate becomes granulomatous and caseation necrosis becomes evident. In some instances, the dermal infiltrate is nonspecific. AFB may or may not be present (63).

In patients with preexisting immunity to TB, postprimary cutaneous inoculation usually results, heralded by development of a hyperkeratotic papule—the prosector's wart—which eventually becomes verrucous. The lesion progresses centrifugally in an annular or a serpiginous fashion. Spontaneous resolution is common in the center of the lesion. Unlike in the primary lesion, in the postprimary lesion no associated adenopathy occurs. The postprimary lesion also rarely ulcerates, and spontaneous involution may occur over months to years (45, 63).

CUTANEOUS TB FROM AN ENDOGENOUS SOURCE

Cutaneous infection with TB may result from contiguous involvement of the skin overlying a subcutaneous focus (most commonly tuberculous lymphadenitis) or TB of the bones and joints, or secondary

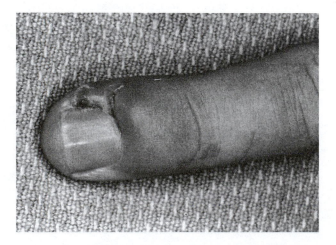

Figure 1. Paronychia in a pathology resident after performing an autopsy on a patient with unsuspected TB. Reprinted with permission from *Archives of Dermatology* (22).

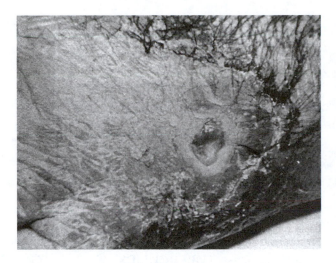

Figure 2. Draining ulcerative lesion over dorsum of the left hand associated with tuberculous osteomyelitis of the fourth and fifth metacarpals. Reprinted with permission from *Medicine* (6).

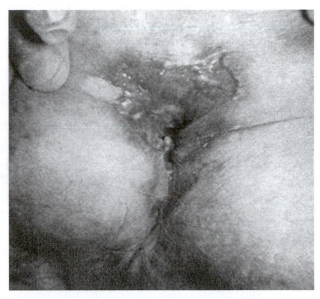

Figure 3. Shallow (10-cm) draining ulcer extending from the ano-rectal line in a patient with external pulmonary TB. Reprinted with permission from *Medicine* (6).

to TB epididymitis (Fig. 2). In the past, the term scrofuloderma was used to describe this condition. Cervical lymph nodes are affected most often, and children are afflicted more frequently than adults (43).

The initial lesion is typically a firm subcutaneous swelling or nodule that, although initially mobile, soon firmly attaches to the overlying skin. It then suppurates, and eventually an indolent chronic draining sinus tract or cutaneous abscess develops. Multiple ulcers may form; these are arranged linearly. Watery, purulent, or caseous discharge may occur from the sinus. Spontaneous healing, if it does occur, may take years to complete.

Histopathologically, caseation necrosis and granuloma formation occur; AFB are demonstrated on special stains. As the lesion ages, granuloma formation may be replaced by a nonspecific chronic inflammatory infiltrate and AFB may become scarce (45, 63). The PPD test result is usually positive, and concurrent pulmonary TB occurs frequently.

Occasionally, cutaneous TB results from the autoinoculation of the mucous membrane and adjoining of the orifices that occurs when viable organisms are either expectorated or passed in patients without significant immunity (41, 66) (Fig. 3). The organisms invade tissue that is normally resistant to infection. In the past, the term orifacial TB was used to describe this condition. The typical patient with this condition is older, lacks PPD reactivity, and has far-advanced pulmonary, intestinal, or genitourinary TB (41, 63). AFB shed from these primary foci are inoculated into the mucocutaneous areas of the orifices at previously traumatized sites. Lesions occur in the oral cavity or perineal/perirectal skin (17, 49, 66); they are ulcerative and painful and do not heal spontaneously.

Nonspecific ulceration and lymphedema occur superficially (45, 66). In most cases, granuloma formation and caseation necrosis are found deep in the dermis. AFB are usually present.

CUTANEOUS TB FROM A HEMATOGENOUS SOURCE

Lupus vulgaris is a particular type of chronic cutaneous TB in a previously sensitized person with a high degree of TB sensitivity. Hematogenous or lymphatic seeding accounts for the majority of cases. Occasionally, lupus vulgaris appears over a primary inoculation site, in a scar of scrofulderma, or after recurrent bacillus Calmette-Guérin vaccinations (9, 30, 34, 38). These lesions are usually solitary plaques or nodules with some ulceration and scarring; they typically appear as "apple jelly" nodules on diascopy and are most commonly located on the face or neck (Fig. 4).

Several diverse presentations of lupus vulgaris have been reported and include psoriasiform lesions, nasal ulcerations, and eventual destruction of the cartilaginous part of the nasal septum, as well as widespread systemic dissemination (4, 18, 20, 74). Because of the broad range of clinical presentations, many cases are misdiagnosed for years (16, 40, 60, 67). The tuberculin skin test result is frequently positive. Malignancy develops in up to 8% of patients with long-standing lupus vulgaris. Squamous cell carcinoma and sarcoma occur occasionally (21, 25, 50). An instance of Hodgkin's disease complicating lupus vulgaris also

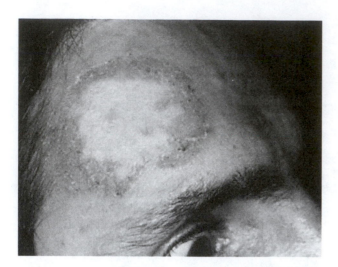

Figure 4. Typical lesion of lupus vulgaris on a patient whose skin biopsy specimen grew *Mycobacterium tuberculosis*.

has been described (59). The histopathological picture of lupus vulgaris is diverse and not always diagnostic. When caseation necrosis is present, it is minimal, and AFB are difficult to demonstrate (62).

An uncommon fulminant form of cutaneous TB, previously known as TB cutis miliaris disseminate, occurs in infants or children after acute hematogenous dissemination of *M. tuberculosis* (15, 53, 77). The initial focus of infection is either pulmonary or meningeal, and it may be preceded by an exanthematous disease such as measles (71). Lesions occur most commonly on the trunk, thigh, buttocks, and genitalia, beginning as papules capped by minute vesicles that eventually rupture and crust (42, 53, 63).

Histologic examination of these lesions reveals a nonspecific inflammatory cellular infiltrate with focal areas of necrotizing vasculitis, and vascular thrombi containing numerous bacilli have been reported (37, 63, 77). The disease is usually fatal, although a few cases of improvement after antituberculous chemotherapy have occurred (31, 63).

Cutaneous hematogenous dissemination of *M. tuberculosis* may present subacutely as soft tissue abscesses or nodules (31, 47, 55, 65, 73). Occasionally the abscess develops at the site of previous trauma, suggesting localization of blood-borne organisms in the injured tissue. Multiple cold abscesses and chronic recurrent perirectal abscesses have been reported to occur in patients with AIDS, and multiple skin nodules from disseminated TB have also occurred in these patients (12, 24, 69, 70). The multiple skin nodules can be nondescript in the patient with AIDS, necessitating a high degree of suspicion on the clinician's part, especially in patients with CD4 counts under 200/ml. In some cases these isolates develop multidrug resistance and become rapidly fatal (2, 11, 36).

TUBERCULOUS MASTITIS

TB of the breast—tuberculosis mastitis—is difficult to recognize and frequently misdiagnosed as breast cancer. It occurs most often in women 20 to 50 years of age who present with a hard, nontender nodule or mass in the breast along with axillary adenopathy (10, 46, 58, 74). The inflammatory lesion may suppurate and drain. Breast involvement is a result of retrograde lymphatic extensions from underlying mediastinal, parasternal, axillary, or cervical lymph nodes. Histologically, granulomatous inflammation and caseation may be found.

TUBERCULIDS

Tuberculids are a group of cutaneous conditions occurring in the presence of TB but containing no stainable or culturable AFB; based on histopathology, then, they were previously regarded as an allergic reaction to the infection. These conditions have included erythema induratum, papulonecrotic tuberculids, and lichen scrofulosorum. Many of these lesions are now thought to be secondary to nontuberculous processes. A possible exception to this is erythema nodosum, which has been attributed to primary TB.

DIAGNOSIS

Because of the varied clinical spectrum and rarity of cutaneous TB, a high index of suspicion is needed to identify skin lesions that may be tubercular in origin and will therefore require biopsy for histopathology purposes as well as AFB stain and culture. In some cases, histopathology shows nonspecific inflammation without granuloma formation. Fluorescent staining with auramine or rhodamine may be useful (32, 76). Enzyme-linked immunosorbent assay for antibodies to PPD and to *M. tuberculosis* antigen 5 also may be helpful (5, 13, 48). Monoclonal antibody assays and the PCR technique have become increasingly useful clinically (64, 72). Recently, for example, PCR amplification has proven to be a rapid and accurate means of identifying *M. tuberculosis* from patients with cutaneous TB (3, 39, 54).

THERAPY

The mainstay of therapy is chemotherapy. Treatment of lupus vulgaris with isoniazid alone has resulted in high cure rates (8, 22). Combination chemotherapy is recommended for patients with extracutaneous disease and multiple skin lesions and for those with profound immunosuppression. The reader is referred to chapter 7 for a detailed discussion. Surgery, which can include excisional biopsy and debridement, also may play a minor adjuvant role in treatment. With the exception of TB cutis miliaris disseminate (discussed above), most forms of cutaneous TB respond to chemotherapy and carry a good prognosis.

A paradoxical skin reaction sometimes occurs in patients undergoing antituberculous therapy, particularly in anergic patients treated for miliary TB: weeks or months into therapy, fluctuant swellings appear that on aspiration yield pus. Smear and culture for *M. tuberculosis* are often positive, and the isolate usually retains its susceptibility to the patient's treatment regimen. This paradoxical response is thought to represent an immunologic phenomenon—not resistance—and typically responds to continued chemotherapy.

REFERENCES

1. Angus, B. J., Y. Yates, C. Conlon, and I. Byren. 2001. Cutaneous tuberculosis of the penis and sexual transmission of tuberculosis confirmed by molecular typing. *Clin. Infect. Dis.* 33: 132–134.

2. Antonori, S., L. Galimberti, G. L. Tudini, A. L. Ridolfo, C. Parravicini, R. Esposoto, and M. Morini. 1995. *Mycobacterium tuberculosis* in AIDS patients. *Eur. J. Clin. Microbiol. Infect. Dis.* 14:911–914.

3. Baselga, E., M. A. Bernadas, N. Margall, and J. M. deMorgas. 1996. Detection of *M. tuberculosis* complex DNA in a lesion resembling sarcoidosis. *Clin. Exp. Dermatol.* 21:235–238.

4. Bateman, D. E., W. Makepeace, and M. Lensa. 1980. Miliary tuberculosis in association with chronic cutaneous tuberculosis. *Br. J. Dermatol.* 103:557–561.

5. Benjamin, R. G., and T. M. Daniel. 1982. Serodiagnosis of tuberculosis using the enzyme-linked immunoabsorbent assay (ELISA) of antibody to *Mycobacterium tuberculosis* antigen-5. *Am. Rev. Respir. Dis.* 126:1013–1016.

6. Beyt, B. E., Jr., D. W. Ortbals, D. J. Santa Cruz, G. S. Kobayashi, A. Z. Eisen, and G. Medoff. 1981. Cutaneous mycobacteriosis: analysis of 34 cases with a new classification of the disease. *Medicine* 60:95–109.

7. Bjornstad, R. 1947. Tubercular primary infection of genitalia: two case reports of venereal genital tuberculosis. *Acta Dermatol. Venereol.* 27:106.

8. Bruck, C., and A. W. Carlson. 1964. Treatment of lupus vulgaris with INH exclusively. *Acta Dermatol. Venereol.* 44:223–225.

9. Caplan, S. E., and C. L. Kauffman. 1996. Primary inoculation tuberculosis after immunotherapy for malignant melanoma with BCG vaccine. *J. Am. Acad. Dermatol.* 35:783–785.

10. Cohen, C. 1977. Tuberculosis mastitis. A review of 34 cases. *S. Afr. Med. J.* 52:12–14.

11. Corbett, E. L., I. Crossley, K. M. DeCock, and R. F. Miller. 1995. Disseminated cutaneous *Mycobacterium tuberculosis* infection in a patient with AIDS. *Genitourin. Med.* 71:308–310.

12. Daikos, G. L., R. B. Uttamchandani, C. Tuda, M. A. Fischl, N. Miller, T. Cleary, and M. J. Saldana. 1998. Disseminated miliary tuberculosis of the skin in patients with AIDS: report of four cases. *Clin. Infect. Dis.* 27:205–208.

13. Daniel, T. M., R. G. Benjamin, S. M. Debanne, Y. Ma, and E. A. Balestrino. 1985. ELISA of IgG antibody to *M. tuberculosis* antigen 5 for serodiagnosis of tuberculosis. *Indian J. Pediatr.* 52:349–355.

14. Deluca, M. 1951. Skin tuberculosis. Etiology, pathogenesis, histology, classification. *Rass. Int. Clin. Ter.* 31:335–340.

15. Dinning, W. J., and S. Marston. 1985. Cutaneous and ocular tuberculosis: a review. *J. R. Soc. Med.* 78:576–581.

16. Duncan, W. C. 1968. Cutaneous mycobacterial infections. *Tex. Med.* 64:66–70.

17. Engleman, W. R., and F. J. Putney. 1972. Tuberculosis of the tongue. *Trans. Am. Acad. Ophthalmol. Otolaryngol.* 76:1384–1386.

18. Fine, R. M., and H. D. Meltzer. 1970. Psoriasiform lupus vulgaris : a case report. *Int. J. Dermatol.* 9:273–277.

19. Fisher, I., and M. Orkin. 1966. Primary tuberculosis of the skin. *JAMA* 195:314–316.

20. Fisher, J. R. 1977. Miliary tuberculosis with unusual cutaneous manifestations. *JAMA* 238:241–242.

21. Forstrom, L. 1969. Carcinomatous changes in lupus vulgaris. *Ann. Clin. Res.* 1:213–219.

22. Forstrom, L. 1969. Isoniazid treatment of lupus vulgaris. A long-term follow-up study. *Ann. Clin. Res.* 1:36–39.

23. Goette, D. K., K. W. Jacobson, and D. R. Doty. 1978. Primary cutaneous inoculation tuberculosis of the skin. *Arch. Dermatol.* 114:567–569.

24. Handwerger, S., D. Mildvan, R. Senie, and F. W. McKinley. 1987. Tuberculosis and the acquired immunodeficiency syndrome at a New York City Hospital: 1978–1985. *Chest* 91:176–180.

25. Harrison, P. V., and J. M. Marks. 2006. Lupus vulgaris and cutaneous lymphoma. *Clin. Exp. Dermatol.* 5:73–76.

26. Heilmaa, K. M., and C. Muschenheim. 1978. Primary cutaneous tuberculosis of the skin. *Arch. Dermatol.* 273:1035–1036.

27. Heycock, J. B., and T. C. Noble. 1961. Four cases of syringe-transmitted tuberculosis. *Tubercle* 42:25–27.

28. Hole, L. E. 1913. Tuberculosis acquired through ritual circumcision. *JAMA* 61:99–102.

29. Hoyt, E. M. 1981. Primary inoculation tuberculosis. *JAMA* 245:1556–1557.

30. Izumi, A. K., and J. Matsunaga. 1982. BCG vaccine-induced lupus vulgaris. *Arch. Dermatol.* 118:171–172.

31. Kennedy, C., and G. K. Knowles. 1975. Miliary tuberculosis presenting with skin lesions. *Br. Med. J.* 3:356.

32. Koch, M. L., and R. H. Cote. 1965. Comparison of fluorescence microscopy with Ziehl-Neelsen stain for demonstration of acid-fast bacilli in smear preparations and tissue sections. *Am. Rev. Respir. Dis.* 91:283–284.

33. Kramer, F., S. Sasse, J. Simms, and J. M. Leedom. 1993. Primary cutaneous tuberculosis after a needlestick injury from a patient with AIDS and undiagnosed tuberculosis. *Ann. Intern. Med.* 119:594–595.

34. Lee, S. M., S. K. Hann, S. Chun, and Y. K. Park. 1994. An unusual form of skin tuberculosis following B.C.G. vaccination. *J. Dermatol.* 21:106–110.

35. Lenzini, L., P. Rottoli, and L. Rottoli. 1977. The spectrum of human tuberculosis. *Clin. Exp. Immunol.* 27:230–237.

36. Libraty, D. H., and T. F. Byrd. 1996. Cutaneous miliary tuberculosis in the AIDS era: case report and review. *Clin. Infect. Dis.* 23:706–710.

37. Lipper, S., D. L. Watkins, and L. B. Kahn. 1980. Nongranulomatous septic vasculitis due to miliary tuberculosis: a pitfall in diagnosis for the pathologist. *Am. J. Dermatopathol.* 2:71–74.

38. Maguire, A. 1968. Lupus marinus: the discovery, diagnosis and treatment of seventeen cases of lupus marinus. *Br. J. Dermatol.* **80**:213–219.

39. Margall, N., E. Baselga, P. Coll, M. A. Barnadas, J. M. de-Moragas, and G. Prats. 1996. Detection of *Mycobacterium tuberculosis* complex DNA by the polymerase chain reaction for rapid diagnosis of cutaneous tuberculosis. *Br. J. Dermatol.* **135**:231–236.

40. Martin, A. R., and E. J. Mark. 1972. Case 43-1972—granulomatous disease in a man from Honduras. *N. Engl. J. Med.* **287**:872–878.

41. McAndrew, P. G., E. O. Adekeye, and A. B. Ajdukiewicz. 1976. Miliary tuberculosis presenting with multifocal oral lesions. *Br. Med. J.* **1**:1320.

42. McCray, M. K., and N. B. Esterly. 1981. Cutaneous eruption in congenital tuberculosis. *Arch. Dermatol.* **117**:460–464.

43. Michelson, H. E. 1924. Scrofuloderma gummosa (tuberculosis colliquativa). *Arch. Dermatol.* **10**:565–578.

44. Minkowitz, S., I. J. Brandt, Y. Rapp, and C. B. Radlauer. 1969. "Prosector's Wart" (cutaneous tuberculosis) in a medical student. *Am. J. Clin. Pathol.* **51**:260–263.

45. Montgomery, H. 1937. Histopathology of various types of cutaneous tuberculosis. *Arch. Dermatol. Syph.* **35**:698–715.

46. Mukerjee, P., R. V. Cohen, and A. H. Niden. 1971. Tuberculosis of the breast. *Am. Rev. Respir. Dis.* **104**:661–667.

47. Munt, P. W. 1972. Miliary tuberculosis in the chemotherapy era: with a clinical review of 69 American adults. *Medicine* **51**:139–155.

48. Nassau, E., E. R. Parsons, and G. D. Johnson. 1976. The detection of antibodies to *Mycobacterium tuberculosis* by microplate enzyme-linked immunosorbent assay (ELISA). *Tubercle* **57**:67–70.

49. Nepomuceno, O. R., J. F. O'Grady, S. W. Eisenberg, and H. E. Bacon. 1971. Tuberculosis of the anal canal: report of a case. *Dis. Colon Rectum* **14**:313–316.

50. Nyfors, A. 1968. Lupus vulgaris, isoniazid and cancer. *Scand. J. Respir. Dis.* **49**:264–269.

51. O'Donnell, T. F., P. F. Jurgenson, and N. H. Weyerich. 1971. An occupational hazard—tuberculosis paronychia. *Arch. Surg.* **103**:757–758.

52. Pereira, C. A., B. Webber, and J. M. Orson. 1976. Primary tuberculosis complex of the skin. *JAMA* **235**:942.

53. Platou, R. V., and R. A. Lennox. 1956. Tuberculosis cutaneous complexes in children. *Am. Rev. Tuberc.* **74**(2 Pt. 2):160–169; discussion, 169–172.

54. Quiros, E., M. C. Maroto, A. Bettinardi, I. Gonzalez, and G. Piedrola. 1996. Diagnosis of cutaneous tuberculosis in biopsy specimens by PCR and southern blotting. *J. Clin. Pathol.* **49**:889–891.

55. Reitbrock, R. C., R. P. M. Dahlmans, F. Smedts, P. J. Frantzen, R. J. Koopman, and J. W. VanderMeer. 1991. Tuberculosis cutis miliaris dissemination as a manifestation of miliary tuberculosis. A literature review and report of a case of recurrent skin lesions. *Rev. Infect. Dis.* **12**:265–269.

56. Rytel, M. W., E. S. Davis, and K. J. Prebil. 1970. Primary cutaneous inoculation tuberculosis. *Am. Rev. Respir. Dis.* **102**:264–267.

57. Sahn, S. A., and D. J. Pierson. 1974. Primary cutaneous inoculation drug-resistant tuberculosis. *Am. J. Med.* **57**:676–678.

58. Schaefer, G. 1955. Tuberculosis of the breast, a review with the additional presentation of ten cases. *Am. Rev. Tuberc.* **72**:810–824.

59. Schein, P. S., and H. R. Vickers. 1972. Lupus vulgaris and Hodgkins disease. *Arch. Dermatol.* **105**:244–246.

60. Schmidt, C. L., M. Ho, and J. R. Pomeranz. 1976. Lupus vulgaris: recovery of living tubercle bacilli 35 years after onset. *Cutis* **18**:221–223.

61. Sehgal, V. N., M. K. Jani, and G. Srivastavia. 1989. Changing patterns of cutaneous tuberculosis. *Int. J. Dermatol.* **28**:231–236.

62. Sehgal, V. N., G. Srivastavia, V. K. Khurana, E. Bhalla, and P. C. Beohar. 1987. An appraisal of epidermologic, clinical, bacteriologic, histopathologic, and immunologic parameters in cutaneous tuberculosis. *Int. J. Dermatol.* **26**:521–526.

63. Sehgal, V. N., and S. A. Wagh. 1990. Cutaneous tuberculosis: current concept. *Int. J. Dermatol.* **29**:237–252.

64. Senturk, N., S. Sahin, and T. Kocagoz. 2002. Polymerase chain reaction in certain tuberculosis: is it a reliable diagnostic method in paraffin-embedded tissue? *Int. J. Dermatol.* **41**:863–867.

65. Shaw, N. M., and A. K. Basu. 1970. Unusual cold abscesses. *Br. J. Surg.* **57**:418–422.

66. Shengold, M. A., and H. Sheingold. 1951. Oral tuberculosis. *Oral Surg.* **4**:239–250.

67. Stevens, C. S., and D. E. V. Ploeg. 1981. Lupus vulgaris: a case that escaped diagnosis for twenty-eight years. *Cutis* **27**:510–511, 514–515, 525.

68. Strand, S. 1946. Tubercular primary lesion on penis—cancer, penis venereal tuberculosis. *Acta Dermatol. Venereol.* **26**:461.

69. Sunderam, G., B. T. Mongura, J. M. Lombardo, and L. B. Reichman. 1987. Failure of four-drug short course tuberculosis chemotherapy in a compliant patient with human immunodeficiency syndrome (AIDS). *Am. Rev. Respir. Dis.* **136**:1475–1478.

70. Sunderam, G., R. J. McDonald, T. Maniatis, J. Oleske, R. Kapila, and L. B. Reichman. 1986. Tuberculosis as a manifestation of the acquired immunodeficiency syndrome (AIDS). *JAMA* **256**:362–366.

71. Sundt, A. 1925. A case of lupus dissematus (post exanthematic miliary tuberculosis cutis). *Br. J. Dermatol.* **37**:316–324.

72. Tan, S. H., B. H. Tan, C. L. Goh, S. H. Tan, K. C. Tan, M. F. Tan, W. C. Ng, and W. C. Tan. 1999. Detection of *Mycobacterium tuberculosis* DNA using polymerase chain reaction in cutaneous tuberculosis. *Int. J. Dermatol.* **38**:122–127.

73. Ward, A. S. 1971. Superficial abscesses formation: an unusual presenting feature of tuberculosis. *Br. J. Surg.* **58**:540–543.

74. Warin, A. P., and E. W. Jones. 1977. Cutaneous tuberculosis of the nose with unusual clinical and histologic features leading to a delay in diagnosis. *Clin. Exp. Dermatol.* **2**:235–242.

75. Weaver, R. A. 1987. Tuberculosis of the tongue. *JAMA* **235**:2418.

76. Wilner, G., S. A. Nassar, A. Siket, and H. A. Azar. 1969. Fluorescent staining for mycobacteria in sarcoid and tubercular granulomas. *Am. J. Clin. Pathol.* **51**:585–590.

77. Yamauchi, T., J. D. Klein, and W. F. Fanell. 1973. Tuberculosis of the skin. *Am. J. Dis. Child.* **125**:855–856.

Chapter 27

Miliary Tuberculosis

SURENDRA K. SHARMA AND ALLADI MOHAN

INTRODUCTION

Miliary tuberculosis (TB) is a lethal form of disseminated TB that results from a massive lymphohematogenous dissemination from a *Mycobacterium tuberculosis*-laden focus (93, 111). The term miliary TB (derived from the Latin word *miliarius*, meaning related to millet seed) was coined by John Jacob Manget (66) in republishing the work of Bonetus (18) in 1700 to describe the resemblance of gross pathological findings to that of innumerable millet seeds in size and appearance (Fig. 1). Traditionally, the miliary pattern on a chest radiograph has been defined as "a collection of tiny discrete pulmonary opacities that are generally uniform in size and widespread in distribution, each of which measures two mm or less in diameter" (130). In 10% of the cases, the nodules may be greater than 3 mm in diameter (57).

Previously, miliary TB was considered to be a disease of infants and children; however, during the last three decades, it has been increasingly recognized in adults as well. Several factors, such as the emergence of human immunodeficiency virus (HIV) infection, the AIDS pandemic, increasing use of immunosuppressive drugs, the effect of bacillus Calmette-Guérin (BCG) vaccination (resulting in a substantial reduction in miliary TB among young vaccinees), increased awareness and use of computed tomography (CT), and wider application of invasive diagnostic methods have been responsible for this change in the epidemiology of miliary TB (111).

Diagnosis of miliary TB requires the presence of a diffuse miliary infiltrate on a chest radiograph or high-resolution CT (HRCT) or histopathological evidence of miliary tubercles in tissue specimens obtained from multiple organs. The myriad clinical manifestations and atypical radiographic findings often delay the diagnosis of miliary TB. Not surprisingly, the rate of mortality from miliary TB has remained high despite effective therapy being available.

EPIDEMIOLOGY

Community-based data on the prevalence of miliary TB are lacking. Data derived from clinical series are hampered by factors such as lack of a "gold standard" for the diagnosis and variation in the nature of invasive methods used for securing tissue to confirm the diagnosis. Autopsy studies contain few data regarding miliary TB in children and frequently include patients with advanced disease or a missed diagnosis. These issues make meaningful comparison of data difficult and should be kept in mind while interpreting epidemiological data. Among immunocompetent adults, miliary TB accounts for less than 2% of all cases of TB and up to 20% of all extrapulmonary TB cases in various clinical studies (6, 39, 43, 54, 62, 78, 121, 132). Among HIV-seropositive and immunosuppressed persons, extrapulmonary TB becomes increasingly common as immunosuppression progresses, and in late HIV infection, extrapulmonary TB accounts for more than 50% of all cases of TB (Fig. 2) (109, 110). Autopsy studies reveal a higher proportion of miliary TB among adult TB cases (10, 24, 46, 47, 61, 120, 134) (Table 1). According to Centers for Disease Control and Prevention (CDC) data (22), the prevalence of miliary TB was 350 cases/year among reported cases of TB during the period from 1975 to 1990; during the period from 1969 to 2002, miliary TB accounted for 1.3 to 2.1% of all reported cases of TB and 7.4 to 10.7% of all reported cases of extrapulmonary TB. During the period from 2000 to 2008, the proportion of miliary TB cases remained constant among all reported cases of TB (1.6 to 2%) and extrapulmonary TB (8.1 to 9.3%) (Fig. 3) (22).

Age

In the preantibiotic era, miliary TB was predominantly a disease of infants and children (9, 20).

Surendra K. Sharma • Department of Medicine, All India Institute of Medical Sciences, New Delhi 110 029, India.
Alladi Mohan • Department of Medicine, Sri Venkateswara Institute of Medical Sciences, Tirupati 517 507, India.

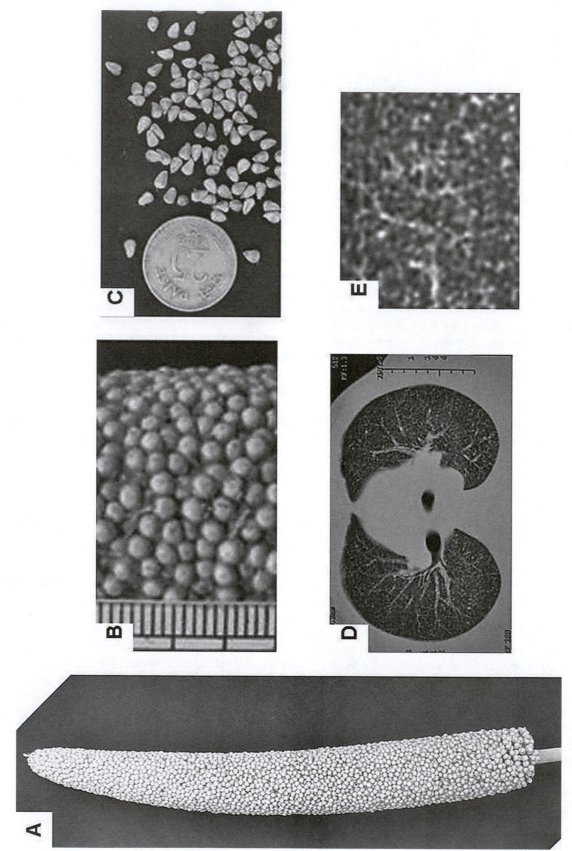

Figure 1. Pearl millet (*Pennisetum typhoides*) seeds are small grains that have an average diameter of <2 mm (A to C). These grains (D and E) correspond to the approximate size of lesions observed in miliary TB on HRCT of the chest.

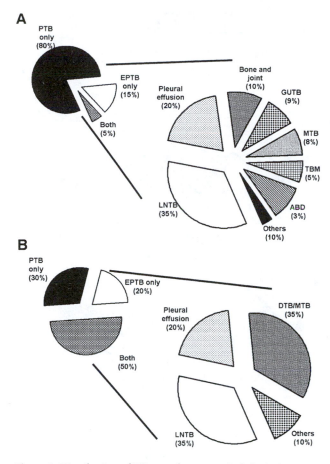

Figure 2. Distribution of TB cases by anatomical site in immunocompetent (A) and immunosuppressed (B) adults. PTB, pulmonary TB; EPTB, extrapulmonary TB; GUTB, genitourinary TB; DTB, disseminated TB; MTB, miliary TB; ABD, abdominal TB; LNTB, lymph node TB. Reproduced with permission from *Indian Journal of Medical Research* (109).

Table 1. Epidemiology of miliary TB

Frequency of miliary TB (%)	Adults		Children (clinical studies[c])
	Autopsy studies[a]	Clinical studies[b]	
Overall	0.3–13.3	1.3–2.0	0.7–41.3
Among TB cases	11.9–40.5	0.64–6.0	1.3–3.2
Among EPTB[d] cases		2.9–20	

[a]Data from references 10, 24, 46, 47, 61, 120, and 134.
[b]Data from references 6, 43, 62, and 78.
[c]Data from references 39, 43, 54, 121, and 132.
[d]EPTB, extrapulmonary TB.

Currently, two peaks are evident–one involving adolescents and young adults and another later in life among elderly persons (1, 5, 6, 16, 21, 34, 37, 39, 41, 43, 51, 54, 62, 63, 72, 76, 78, 79, 87, 89, 102, 111, 121, 124, 126, 132).

Gender

Males seem to be more frequently affected by miliary TB in pediatric as well as adult series (1, 5, 6, 16, 21, 34, 37, 39, 41, 43, 51, 54, 62, 63, 72, 76, 78, 79, 87, 89, 102, 111, 121, 124, 126, 132). A few recent adult series on miliary TB (41, 62, 72, 134) describe a female preponderance, probably reflecting increased awareness and use of health services by women.

Ethnicity

In the United States, a higher incidence of miliary TB has been described for black Americans in some

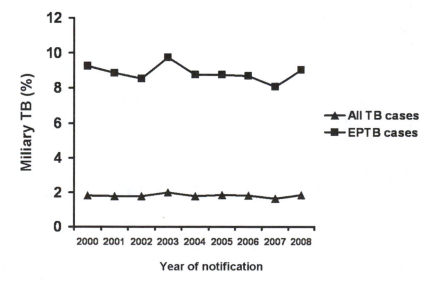

Figure 3. Proportion of miliary TB cases among all reported TB cases and extrapulmonary TB (EPTB) cases. Reprinted with permission from the CDC (22).

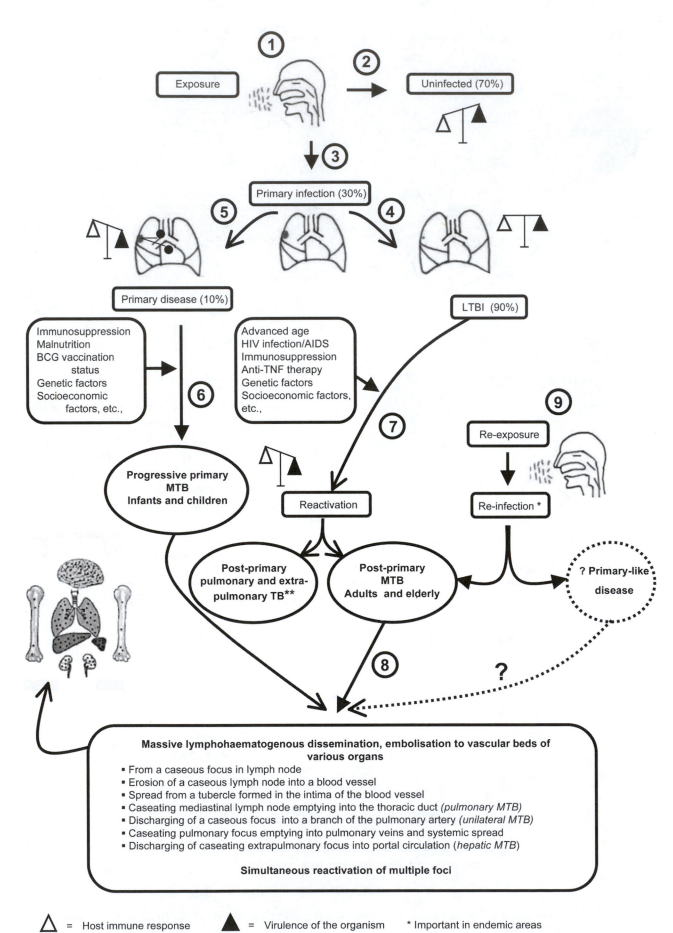

Exposure

① ②
Uninfected (70%)

③
Primary infection (30%)

⑤ ④

Primary disease (10%)

LTBI (90%)

Immunosuppression
Malnutrition
BCG vaccination
   status
Genetic factors
Socioeconomic
   factors, etc.,

Advanced age
HIV infection/AIDS
Immunosuppression
Anti-TNF therapy
Genetic factors
Socioeconomic factors,
etc.,

⑥

⑦

⑨

Re-exposure

Reactivation

Re-infection *

**Progressive primary
MTB
Infants and children**

**Post-primary
pulmonary and extra-
pulmonary TB****

**Post-primary
MTB
Adults and elderly**

**? Primary-like
disease**

⑧

?

**Massive lymphohaematogenous dissemination, embolisation to vascular beds of
various organs**
- From a caseous focus in lymph node
- Erosion of a caseous lymph node into a blood vessel
- Spread from a tubercle formed in the intima of the blood vessel
- Caseating mediastinal lymph node emptying into the thoracic duct *(pulmonary MTB)*
- Discharging of a caseous focus into a branch of the pulmonary artery *(unilateral MTB)*
- Caseating pulmonary focus emptying into pulmonary veins and systemic spread
- Discharging of caseating extrapulmonary focus into portal circulation *(hepatic MTB)*

Simultaneous reactivation of multiple foci

△ = Host immune response   ▲ = Virulence of the organism   * Important in endemic areas
** Organ-restricted TB with adequate host immunity

418

of the earlier publications, though such a trend is not evident from recent data (16, 76, 111). Whether this is due to ethnic variation alone or is the consequence of host genetic factors or other factors such as socio-economic and nutritional status or comorbid illnesses needs further study.

PATHOGENESIS

Miliary TB can develop either at the time of primary infection or later during reactivation of a dormant focus. In areas of endemicity with increased transmission of *Mycobacterium tuberculosis*, reinfection also has an important role in the development of miliary TB. A massive lymphohematogenous dissemination of *Mycobacterium tuberculosis* from a pulmonary or extrapulmonary focus and embolization to the vascular beds of various organ systems result in miliary TB. Rarely, simultaneous reactivation of multiple foci in various organs can also result in miliary TB (Fig. 4) (111). When miliary TB develops during the course of primary disease (early generalization), the disease has an acute onset and is rapidly progressive. During postprimary TB, late generalization can be rapidly progressive (acute miliary TB), episodic, or protracted (chronic miliary TB).

Occasionally, discharge of caseous material from an extrapulmonary site can result in miliary TB. If the caseous material is discharged into the portal circulation, hepatic involvement occurs initially, with the classical pulmonary involvement becoming evident late (111). In neonates, hematogenous spread from infected placenta through the umbilical vein or aspiration of amniotic fluid in utero can cause congenital TB; miliary TB is a common manifestation of congenital TB. Miliary TB may also develop in neonates as a result of acquisition of infection during the perinatal period through aspiration and ingestion of infected maternal genital tissues and fluid and subsequent hematogenous dissemination.

Table 2. Conditions predisposing to or associated with miliary TB

Childhood infections
Malnutrition
HIV/AIDS
Alcoholism
Tobacco smoking
Diabetes mellitus
Chronic renal failure, dialysis
Postsurgery (e.g., gastrectomy[a])
Organ transplantation
Connective tissue disorders
Pregnancy, postpartum
Underlying malignancy
Silicosis

[a]Predisposes to TB in general.

Predisposing Conditions

Several predisposing or associated conditions that have been described for patients with miliary TB are detailed in Table 2 (111).

Iatrogenic Dissemination

The use of certain drugs (29, 64, 128, 133) and several procedures and interventions (11, 43, 74, 88, 118) have been implicated in facilitating hematogenous dissemination and the causation of iatrogenic miliary TB (Table 3). Corticosteroids and immunosuppressive and cytotoxic drugs are increasingly being used at the present time for the treatment of connective tissue disorders and in organ transplant recipients. Miliary TB can develop as a consequence of their use (111). Fatal TB, including miliary TB, has been described to occur in patients with rheumatoid arthritis who were treated with immunomodulator drugs, such as the anti-tumor necrosis factor agents infliximab (133), etanercept (128), and adalimumab (64). A report from the British Society for Rheumatology Biologics Register national prospective observational study (29) among rheumatoid arthritis patients indicates that the rate of development of TB was higher for adalimumab (144 events/100 000

Figure 4. Development of miliary TB. Small droplet nuclei (1 to 5 μm) containing *Mycobacterium tuberculosis* get deposited in the alveoli (1), where host-pathogen interactions occur. Seventy percent of individuals exposed do not get infected (2), whereas 30% develop infection (3). Infection is contained in 90% of those infected (latent TB infection) (4). The remaining 10% develop progressive primary TB (5). During this phase, extensive lymphohematogenous dissemination (6) to various organs can result in miliary TB. People with latent TB infection have a 10% lifetime risk of reactivation of the infection, resulting in postprimary TB (7). Fifty percent of reactivations occur during the first 2 years of primary infection. By contrast, in HIV-infected individuals with latent TB infection, the risk of reactivation is enormously high (approximately 10%/year). Massive lymphohematogenous dissemination during reactivation (8) can also result in miliary TB (progressive postprimary miliary TB). In areas with high transmission rates, reinfection with a new strain of *Mycobacterium tuberculosis* (9) can occur and the cycle is repeated. MTB, miliary TB; TNF, tumor necrosis factor. Reproduced with permission from *Lancet Infectious Diseases* (111).

Table 3. Iatrogenic causes of miliary TB[a]

Drugs
  Corticosteroids
  Immunosuppressive and cytotoxic drugs
  Immunomodulator drugs (e.g., infliximab, etanercept, and
    adalimumab)

Procedures and interventions
  Ureteral catheterization[b]
  Extracorporeal shockwave lithotripsy[c]
  Laser lithotripsy[c]
  Cardiac valve homograft replacement[d]
  Intravesical BCG therapy for urinary bladder carcinoma

[a]Data from references 11, 29, 64, 74, 88, 118, 128, 133, and 143.
[b]Predisposes to TB in general.
[c]Patient had undiagnosed genitourinary TB.
[d]Contamination of homografts probably occurred at the time of harvest
  from cadavers.

person-years) and infliximab (136/100,000 person-years) than etanercept (39/100,000 person-years). The median time to development of TB was lowest for infliximab (5.5 months), followed by etanercept (13.4 months) and adalimumab (18.5 months). Extrapulmonary TB constituted 25 of the 40 (62%) cases; 11 cases (27.5% of all TB cases and 44% of extrapulmonary TB) were disseminated and miliary TB.

Immunopathogenesis

The inadequacy of effector T-cell (Teff cell) response in containment of *Mycobacterium tuberculosis* is thought to be responsible for the development of miliary TB (25, 92, 99, 106). Although both Th1 and Th2 responses are inflammatory reactions, Th1 reactions characterize protective immunity and Th2 reactions seem to have a counterregulatory effect. Miliary TB probably represents the Th2 end of the spectrum. The abundance of Th1 and Th2 polarized Teff cells in the peripheral blood and local disease site(s) among patients with miliary TB has been described previously (99, 106). Interleukin 4, with its ability to downregulate inducible nitric oxide synthase, Toll-like receptor 2, and macrophage activation, may play an important role in the events that determine whether the infection becomes latent or progressive (25, 92, 111). Inadequate T-cell response, particularly at the pathological site(s), is believed to depend on the host immunoregulatory mechanisms. Thus, *Mycobacterium tuberculosis* either can fail to evoke the protective response or can drive the protective mechanisms and then deliberately "sabotage" them, leading to progressive disease (25, 92, 99, 106, 111).

Regulatory T cells (Treg cells) are thought to play a critical role in the immunopathogenesis of miliary TB by suppression of the effector immune response against *Mycobacterium tuberculosis* at the pathological site(s). Increases in frequency of Treg cells ($CD4^+$ $CD25^+$ $FoxP3^+$) and FoxP3 mRNA levels have been described at the local disease site in miliary TB (106). Furthermore, $FoxP3^+$ Treg cells in bronchoalveolar lavage (BAL) fluid from patients with miliary TB predominantly produced interleukin-10 and suppressed the autologous T-cell proliferation in response to *Mycobacterium tuberculosis* antigen (99).

In miliary TB, the attempt by the host to selectively recruit the Teff cells at the pathological site, however, fails to provide an adequate level of effector immunity at the disease site due to efficient and comparable homing of Treg cells ($FoxP3^+$), which inhibit the function of the Teff cells that have infiltrated at the pathological disease site. This probably leads to a state of local immunosuppression and dissemination of disease (99, 106, 111).

Molecular Basis of Dissemination

Several molecular mechanisms have been implicated in the development of miliary TB. These include impaired expansion of γ/δ T cells (15); failure to generate adequate cell-mediated immunity (30); presence of HLA-Bw15 (4), HLA-DRB1*15/16, DRB1*13, and DQB1*0602 (14); absence of HLA-Cw6, HLA-DRB1*10, and DQB1*0501 (14); impaired major histocompatibility complex class II-restricted target cell lysis; and overexuberant lysis of target cell macrophages (56) and LTA+368 G/A polymorphisms (125).

PATHOLOGY

The frequency of organ involvement at autopsy is shown in Table 4 (1, 21, 24, 34, 37, 87, 120). Organs with a high blood flow, such as the spleen, liver, lungs, bone marrow, kidneys, and adrenals, are frequently affected. On gross examination, small, punctate, gray to reddish brown, rounded lesions of more or less uniform size may be seen in the lungs and various organs. The "tubercle" constitutes the histopathological hallmark of miliary TB. When miliary TB is the result of acute massive hematogenous dissemination, the lesions in all viscera appear similar ("soft" or "exudative" tubercles) (13, 90, 111); an obvious caseous focus invading the blood vessel is usually demonstrable, and the lesions often reveal acid-fast bacilli (AFB). When the dissemination is due to the discharge of bacilli into microscopic blood vessels within the caseous lesions, which in turn seed large vessels, the acute soft lesions are found to be admixed with "hard" tubercles. The AFB are seldom

Table 4. Organ system involvement in miliary TB[a]

Variable	Chapman and Whorton (24)[b]	Gelb et al. (34)[b,c]	Campbell (21)[b,c]	Grieco and Chmel (37)[b,c]	Aderele (1)[b,c]	Prout and Benatar (87)[b,c]	Slavin et al. (120)[b]
Yr of publication	1946	1973	1973	1974	1978	1980	1980
No. of autopsies	63	21[d]	23[e]	10[f]	11[g]	34[h]	100
Organ system involvement (%)							
Spleen	100	86	70	80	82	79	100
Liver	100	91	61	60	55	85	97
Lungs	63	100	100	100	100	77	86
Lymph nodes	33	38[i]	39	80	73	79	ND
Bone marrow	84	24	ND	ND	ND	47	77
Kidneys	53	62	43	30	55	56	64
Adrenals	42	14	22	30	ND	29	53
Ocular choroid	ND	ND	ND	ND	ND	ND	50[j]
Thyroid	ND	19	ND	ND	ND	6	14
Breast	ND	ND	ND	ND	ND	ND	13
Pancreas	20	14	ND	ND	ND	ND	12
Heart	10	ND	ND	ND	36	6	10
Prostate	ND	ND	ND	ND	ND	ND	7
Testis	41	ND	ND	ND	ND	ND	5
Pituitary	ND	ND	ND	ND	ND	ND	4
Central nervous system	41	ND	22	ND	36	26	ND

[a]All values expressed as percentages corrected to the nearest round figure. ND, not described.
[b]Autopsy data.
[c]Clinical data.
[d]Autopsy was performed on 21 of the 30 patients who died.
[e]Autopsy was performed on 23 of the 25 patients who died.
[f]Autopsy was performed on 10 patients.
[g]Pediatric series. Autopsy was performed on 11 of the 44 children.
[h]Autopsy was performed on 34 of the 40 patients who died.
[i]Mediastinal lymph nodes.
[j]Fourteen eyes were available for histological examination.

demonstrable in these hard lesions (93, 111). When acute respiratory distress syndrome (ARDS) develops due to miliary TB, hyaline membranes are present in addition to the cellular infiltrate. Occasionally, vasculitic lesions can be discerned in miliary TB patients with TB meningitis (TBM). Choroidal tubercles, when present, are pathognomonic of miliary TB (see below). They are multiple in number and are usually evident in both eyes, mostly in the posterior pole. As the acute infection resolves, the center of the choroidal tubercles may become white or yellow with a surrounding peripheral rim of pigmentation; the margins become sharply delineated and distinct. Subsequently an atrophic scar may develop. Rarely, infective endocarditis, pericarditis, intracardiac mass, or mycotic aneurysm may also be evident at autopsy.

When patients with advanced HIV infection develop miliary TB, the salient pathological features include poor granuloma formation with minimal cellular reaction, severe necrosis, and presence of abundant AFB. Foci of acute TB pneumonia involving air spaces rather than the interstitium are also common in HIV-coinfected patients with miliary TB (109, 110).

CLINICAL MANIFESTATIONS

Adults

The clinical manifestations of miliary TB in adults are protean and nonspecific and can be obscure till late in the disease (Table 5).

Constitutional symptoms

Patients with miliary TB classically present with fever of several weeks' duration, anorexia, weight loss, weakness, and cough (93, 111). Recently, occurrence of daily morning temperature spikes (26) was reported to be characteristic of miliary TB. Occasionally, fever may be absent and the patients may present with progressive wasting strongly mimicking a metastatic carcinoma. Proudfoot et al. (86) suggested "cryptic miliary TB" for this presentation in the pre-CT era. Since its initial description, cryptic miliary TB is increasingly being reported to occur in the elderly (9, 20). Previously, cryptic miliary TB could be diagnosed only at autopsy. However, with the availability of HRCT, these patients can now be diagnosed during their lifetime (102, 111).

Table 5. Presenting symptoms and signs in miliary TB[a]

Variable	Adult series (%)[b]	Pediatric series (%)[c]
Symptoms		
Fever	35–100	61–98
Chills	15–28	ND
Anorexia	24–100	4–81
Weight loss	20–100	4–60
Night sweats	8–100	8–75
Weakness/fatigue	25–100	14–54
Cough/sputum	27–82	17–90
Chest pain	3–49	1–03
Dyspnea	8–100	7–25
Hemoptysis	3–15	1
Headache	2–18	2–8
Altered sensorium	5–26	2–8
Seizures	ND	7–30
Nausea	1–19	ND
Abdominal pain	5–19	3–15
Diarrhea	2–3	ND
Urinary symptoms	2–6	ND
Signs		
Fever	35–100	39–75
Pallor	36–59	31
Cyanosis	1–2	ND
Icterus	5–9	3
Lymphadenopathy	2–30	5
Chest signs	29–84	34–72
Hepatomegaly	14–62	39–82
Splenomegaly	2–32	24–54
Ascites	4–38	6–09
Choroidal tubercles	2–12	2–05
Neurological signs	3–26	19–35

[a]All values are expressed as percentages corrected to the nearest round figure. ND, not described.
[b]Data from references 16, 21, 34, 37, 51, 63, 72, 76, 79, and 87.
[c]Data from references 1, 39, 43, 54, and 89.

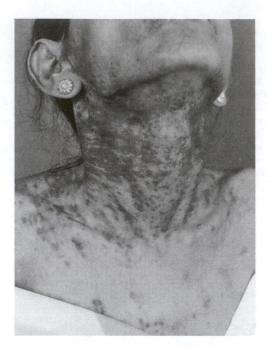

Figure 5. Papulonodular skin lesions in a patient with miliary TB. Skin biopsy confirmed the diagnosis.

Chills and rigors, usually seen in patients with malaria, or sepsis and bacteremia have often been described to occur in adult patients with miliary TB (93, 111). A recent publication (32) documents the utility of a damp shadow sign (where sweat engraved the patient's silhouette on the bed, closely resembling a body's shadow) in raising the suspicion of miliary TB.

Systemic involvement

Since miliary TB can involve many organs, patients present with symptoms and signs referable to various organ systems (Table 5). Dry cough and dyspnea are often present. Sometimes, cutaneous lesions are the only discernible clues to miliary TB (Fig. 5). These include eythematous macules and papules (TB miliaria cutis) (111). Choroidal tubercles, when present, offer a valuable clue to miliary TB as the diagnosis (93, 102, 111). TBM has been described for 10 to 30% of adult patients with miliary TB (1, 5, 16, 21, 34, 37, 41, 51, 62, 63, 72, 76, 79, 87, 89, 102, 120, 124, 126); about one-third of patients presenting with TBM have underlying miliary TB (127). In a recently published study from India (33), the spectrum of neurological involvement in adult patients with miliary TB (n = 60) included TBM with (45%) and without (35%) tuberculoma, and thoracic transverse myelopathy (15%). These observations warrant a careful clinical examination and appropriate investigations to ascertain neurological involvement.

Clinically evident cardiac or renal involvement is uncommon in patients with miliary TB. Overt adrenal insufficiency manifesting as Addison's disease at initial presentation or during anti-TB treatment has also been described to occur in miliary TB (19, 144).

Children

Comparatively fewer published series on childhood miliary TB are available (1, 39, 43, 54, 89) compared to adults (1, 5, 16, 21, 34, 37, 41, 51, 62, 63, 72, 76, 79, 87, 89, 102, 120, 124, 126). Clinical presentation of miliary TB in children (Table 5) is similar to that observed in adults, with some important differences. Miliary TB develops less often in children who have received the BCG vaccination (111). Chills and night sweats, hemoptysis, and productive cough are less common and peripheral lymphadenopathy and hepatosplenomegaly are more common in children with miliary TB than in adults (Table 5). A larger proportion of children with miliary TB (20 to 40%) suffer from TBM (1, 39, 43, 54, 89) than do adults (15 to 30%) (1, 5, 16, 21, 34, 37, 41, 51, 62, 63, 72, 76, 79, 87, 89, 102, 120, 124, 126).

Miliary TB in Immunosuppressed Individuals

The prevalence of miliary TB in persons with early HIV infection (CD4$^+$ cell counts of >200 cells/mm^3) is similar to that observed in immunocompetent individuals. With progression of immunosuppression, in late, advanced stages of HIV infection (CD4$^+$ cell counts of <200 cells/mm^3), miliary TB is seen more often (109–111). Cutaneous involvement, a rare clinical manifestation in HIV-seronegative patients with miliary TB, is more commonly seen in HIV-infected patients with CD4$^+$ cell counts below 100 cells/mm^3 (58, 104, 107, 109–111), in whom these lesions appear as tiny papules or vesiculopapules, described as TB cutis miliaris disseminata, TB cutis acuta generalisita, and disseminated TB of the skin (Fig. 5). Sometimes macular, pustular, or purpuric lesions, indurated ulcerating plaques, and subcutaneous abscesses have been reported (27). In miliary TB patients coinfected with HIV, especially in those with profound immunosuppression, intrathoracic lymphadenopathy and tuberculin anergy are more common; sputum smears are seldom positive and blood culture may grow *Mycobacterium tuberculosis* (58, 104, 107, 109–111). These observations seem to be applicable to other causes of immunosuppression as well. In a study from China (98), miliary TB was present in 31% of immunocompromised patients (*n* = 39), compared to 2.6% of immunocompetent persons (*n* = 79).

ATYPICAL CLINICAL MANIFESTATIONS

Several atypical clinical manifestations have been observed in adult and pediatric patients with miliary TB (Table 6). Atypical clinical presentations often result in a delay in the diagnosis, and miliary TB is often a "missed diagnosis."

Acute Respiratory Distress Syndrome

Miliary TB is a rare but an important treatable cause of ARDS. Although ARDS may develop at any time during the course of miliary TB, it is usually seen at the time of initial presentation (35, 52, 73, 81, 114). Sometimes, ARDS may develop as a component of multiorgan dysfunction syndrome (MODS) due to TB or as a manifestation of immune reconstitution inflammatory syndrome (IRIS) (35, 52, 73, 81, 114).

Table 6. Atypical clinical manifestations and complications in miliary TB[a]

Cryptic miliary TB
Presentation as pyrexia of unknown origin
Incidental diagnosis
ARDS
Air leak syndrome (pneumothorax, pneumomediastinum)
Myelophthisic anemia, myelofibrosis, pancytopenia, immune hemolytic anemia
Acute empyema
Septic shock, MODS
Thyrotoxicosis
Renal failure
Immune complex glomerulonephritis
Sudden cardiac death
Mycotic aneurysm of aorta
Native valve and prosthetic valve endocarditis
Myocarditis, congestive heart failure, intracardiac masses
Cholestatic jaundice
Presentation as focal extrapulmonary TB (e.g., hepatic miliary TB)
Syndrome of inappropriate antidiuretic hormone secretion
Deep vein thrombosis

[a]Data from references 12, 35, 38, 42, 49, 52, 59, 65, 73, 81, 93, 94, 109, 111, and 114.

In a study from two large teaching hospitals at New Delhi and Tirupati in India (114), among patients with TB, prolonged illness, miliary TB, absolute lymphocytopenia, and elevated alanine aminotransferase were found to be independently associated with the development of ARDS. In another study (50) from Korea, higher C-reactive protein levels and an increasing nutritional risk score were found to be independent risk factors for the development of ARDS in patients with miliary TB.

Air Leak Syndromes

Pneumothorax, which may sometimes be bilateral, may be the presenting feature or may sometimes develop while the patient is receiving treatment (38, 59, 93, 111). Typical miliary shadows may not be evident initially and may become apparent once the lung expands. Intrapulmonary rupture of alveoli and consequent air leak that traverses into the mediastinum after spreading along the vascular sheath can result in pneumomediastinum with subcutaneous emphysema which may be fatal (55).

Renal Failure

In patients with miliary TB, apart from being a part of MODS, renal failure may occur due to direct renal parenchymal involvement (65, 111). Renal failure can also develop as a manifestation of IRIS in HIV-infected patients (94). Rarely, renal failure can develop as a consequence of obstructive uropathy caused by the disease process (109).

Hepatic and Gastrointestinal Complications

An asymptomatic rise in hepatic transaminases is common in patients with miliary TB, and anti-TB treatment should not be withheld on this evidence alone. In this scenario, liver functions should be periodically monitored. Fulminant hepatic failure due to widespread liver cell necrosis may, rarely, be the presenting manifestation in miliary TB (12, 42). In some of these patients the characteristic pulmonary lesions that constitute the hallmark of miliary TB are absent, resulting in a delay in diagnosis (12, 42). This could probably be the result of an extrapulmonary focus discharging the tubercle bacilli into the portal circulation, resulting in hepatic miliary TB. Anti-TB drug-induced hepatotoxicity is also common; standard guidelines (95) should be followed in its management. Small intestinal perforations at the site of granulomatous involvement have been described to occur in some patients while on treatment (96).

Cardiovascular Complications

In patients with miliary TB, life-threatening complications such as myocarditis, congestive heart failure, infective endocarditis, pericarditis, intracardiac mass, mycotic aneurysm, and sudden cardiac death have been described to occur (111).

Immune Reconstitution Inflammatory Syndrome

IRIS, occasionally described to occur in HIV-negative individuals with TB, has been reported to occur in 32 to 36% of patients coinfected with HIV and TB within days to weeks of the initiation of highly active antiretroviral therapy (71). Manifestations range from isolated instances of fever to increased or initial appearance of lymphadenopathy, new or worsening pulmonary infiltrates, serositis, cutaneous lesions, and new or expanding central nervous system mass lesions (71, 110). IRIS can be brief or prolonged with multiple recurrences. Acute renal failure (49, 94) or ARDS (35) can develop during the course of IRIS.

APPROACH TO DIAGNOSIS

Even in an area of endemicity, the diagnosis of miliary TB can be difficult, as the clinical symptoms have been nonspecific, the chest radiographs do not always reveal the classical miliary changes and atypical presentations such as ARDS, and shadows larger than miliary on chest radiograph commonly occur. Therefore, a high index of clinical suspicion and a focused diagnostic testing to establish the diagnosis of miliary TB can facilitate early institution of anti-TB treatment, which can be lifesaving.

The following criteria have been suggested for the diagnosis of miliary TB: (i) clinical presentation consistent with a diagnosis of TB, such as pyrexia with evening rise of temperature, weight loss, anorexia, tachycardia, and night sweats of more than 6 weeks' duration responding to anti-TB treatment; (ii) classical miliary pattern on chest radiograph; (iii) bilateral diffuse reticulonodular lung lesions on a background of miliary shadows demonstrable on either plain chest radiograph or HRCT; and (iv) microbiological and/or histopathological evidence of TB (102).

Fundus Examination

Choroidal tubercles are bilateral, pale, grayish white, and oblong patches that are pathognomonic of miliary TB. Though rare (Table 5), their presence is diagnostic of miliary TB (93, 102, 111). Thus, systematic ophthalmoscopic examination after mydriatic administration must be done in every suspected patient with miliary TB to look for this valuable clue to the diagnosis (93, 102, 111).

Sputum, Body Fluid, and Tissue Examination

In patients with suspected miliary TB, attempts must be made to confirm histopathological or microbiological diagnosis. Sputum, other body fluids (such as pleural fluid, pericardial fluid, ascitic fluid, cerebrospinal fluid, joint fluid, pus from cold abscess, and endometrial aspirate), urine, bronchoscopic secretions, blood, and tissue biopsy specimens have all been employed to confirm the diagnosis of disseminated and miliary TB, with various results. In patients with miliary TB, relative diagnostic yields with the conventional microbiological methods from various body fluids and tissues that are commonly tested are listed in Table 7 (1, 2, 5, 6, 16, 21, 34, 37, 39, 41, 43, 51, 54, 62, 63, 72, 76, 78, 79, 87, 89, 102, 111, 117, 121, 124, 126, 132). Rapid culture methods, such as Mycobacteria Growth Indicator Tube (MGIT), may be employed for rapid drug susceptibility testing (DST) (111).

Laboratory Abnormalities

A number of hematological and biochemical abnormalities are known to occur in miliary TB (Table 8) (1, 5, 6, 16, 21, 34, 37, 39, 41, 43, 51, 54, 62, 63, 72, 76, 78, 79, 87, 89, 102, 111, 117, 121, 124, 126, 132), but their significance is controversial. Disseminated intravascular coagulation (73, 114) has been described to occur in patients with miliary TB in the setting of ARDS and MODS and is associated

Table 7. Method of confirmation of diagnosis in adults with miliary TB[a]

Variable	Cumulative yield (%)
Sputum[b]	41.4
Bronchoscopy[b,c]	46.8
Gastric lavage[b]	61.1
Cerebrospinal fluid[b]	21.2
Urine[b]	32.7
Bone marrow[b,d]	66.7
Liver biopsy	88.9
Lymph node biopsy	90.9

[a]Data from references 1, 2, 5, 6, 16, 21, 34, 37, 39, 41, 43, 51, 54, 62, 63, 72, 76, 78, 79, 87, 89, 102, 111, 117, 121, 124, 126, and 132. Criteria for subjecting the patients to these tests were not clearly defined in any of the studies. Often, more than one test was performed for confirming the diagnosis. For histopathological diagnosis, presence of granulomas and caseation, and demonstration of AFB have been variously used to define a positive test.
[b]Yield from smear and culture.
[c]Includes yield from bronchoscopic aspirate, washings, brushings, BAL, and transbronchial lung biopsy.
[d]Yield from aspiration and/or trephine biopsy.

with a high mortality rate. Miliary TB has also been implicated as a cause of pancytopenia and hypoplastic anemia (119). Immune mechanisms have been implicated to cause bone marrow suppression in patients with miliary TB (111). Hypercalcemia has been documented in miliary TB but is uncommon (23).

Hyponatremia in patients with miliary TB may indicate the presence of TBM (76) and may also be a predictor of mortality (102). Hyponatremia in miliary TB has been thought to be due to an acquired disturbance of neurohypophyseal function resulting in unregulated antidiuretic hormone release due to an antidiuretic principle in the lung tissue affected by TB that may either produce antidiuretic hormone or absorb an inappropriately released hormone from the posterior pituitary (97, 135, 138). Recently, rifampin-induced adrenal crisis in a patient with miliary TB and Addison's disease who developed generalized malaise and hyponatremia while she was initiated on anti-TB treatment has also been described (144).

Table 8. Laboratory abnormalities in miliary TB

Hematological abnormality	Biochemical abnormality
Anemia	Hyponatremia
Leukocytosis	Hypoalbuminemia
Neutrophilia	Hyperbilirubinemia
Lymphocytosis	Elevated transaminases
Monocytosis	Elevated serum alkaline
Thrombocytosis	phosphatase
Leukopenia	Hypercalcemia
Lymphopenia	Hypophosphatemia
Thrombocytopenia	Elevated serum ferritin levels
Leukemoid reaction	
Hemophagocytosis	
Elevated ESR and CRP levels[a]	

[a]ESR, erythrocyte sedimentation rate; CRP, C-reactive protein.

Tuberculin Skin Test

Tuberculin anergy is more common in miliary TB than in pulmonary TB and extrapulmonary TB; tuberculin skin test (TST) conversion may occur following successful treatment. In various published pediatric series, tuberculin anergy has ranged from 35 to 74% (1, 39, 43, 54, 89); in published adult series, the corresponding figures have been 20 to 70% (16, 21, 34, 37, 51, 63, 72, 76, 79, 87, 117). However, a positive TST only indicates infection with *Mycobacterium tuberculosis* and does not always indicate active disease.

Gamma Interferon Release Assays

Newer in vitro T-cell-based gamma interferon release assays (IGRAs) appear to be promising in detecting TB infection and appear to have several advantages over the TST. These tests, available in the enzyme-linked immunosorbent assay and enzyme-linked immunospot assay formats, may be useful for patients with miliary TB, especially children, BCG-vaccinated individuals, and persons living with HIV infection and AIDS (28, 75). A positive IGRA test result, however, does not distinguish between latent TB infection and active disease, but a negative IGRA result may be helpful in ruling out a diagnosis of TB (80).

Pulmonary Function and Gas Exchange Abnormalities

Miliary TB is associated with abnormalities of pulmonary function typical of interstitial lung disease, and these may be of a greater magnitude than might be anticipated from the chest radiograph (69, 101, 137). Impairment of diffusion is the most common abnormality and may sometimes be severe (3, 137). Other abnormalities include a mild reduction in flow rates suggestive of peripheral airway involvement (3). During the acute stage, arterial hypoxemia due to widening of the alveolar-arterial oxygen gradient and hypocapnia due to tachypnea are also observed (115).

Cardiopulmonary Exercise Testing

Patients with miliary TB have abnormal cardiopulmonary exercise performance, with lower maximum oxygen consumption, maximal work rate, anaerobic threshold, peak minute ventilation, and breathing reserve and low maximal heart rate (111, 115–117). Other abnormalities include higher respiratory frequency and peak minute ventilation at

Table 9. Chest radiographic abnormalities in miliary TB[a]

Common	Uncommon	Rare
Classical miliary pattern (50%)	Nonmiliary patterns (10–30%)	Other associated findings (<5%)
	Asymmetrical nodular pattern	Intrathoracic lymphadenopathy
	Coalescence of nodules	Pleural effusion
	Mottled appearance	Empyema
	"Snow storm" appearance	Pulmonary parenchymal lesions and cavitation
	Air space consolidation	Segmental consolidation
		Thickening of interlobular septae
		Pneumothroax
		Pneumomediastinum
		Pericardial effusion

[a]Data from references 1, 5, 6, 16, 21, 34, 37, 39, 41, 43, 51, 54, 62, 63, 72, 76, 78, 79, 87, 89, 102, 111, 117, 121, 124, 126, and 132.

submaximal work and high physiological dead space/tidal volume. A demonstrable fall in oxygen saturation (to 4% or more) with exercise has been observed. Following successful anti-TB treatment, these abnormalities had reversed in most of the patients, though they did persist in some of them (115, 116).

Immunological Abnormalities and BAL

A few reports on the cellular characteristics of BAL fluid in patients with miliary TB have been published, and the results presented have conflicted (3, 100, 109). The proportion and absolute number of lymphocytes are substantially increased in BAL fluid. Although a raised CD4$^+$/CD8$^+$ T-lymphocyte ratio and B lymphocytes were reported for BAL fluid in one study (101), a decrease in the CD4$^+$/CD8$^+$ T-lymphocyte ratio was reported in another (3). The small number of patients studied could partly be the reason for these differences. Polyclonal hypergammaglobulinemia with increases in immunoglobulin G (IgG), IgA, and IgM was observed in peripheral blood

and BAL fluid in one study (101). These findings probably result from increased local synthesis by activated B lymphocytes. Increased BAL fluid fibronectin and serum C3 levels as an acute-phase response to ongoing inflammation were observed (84, 101). Lymphocytic alveolitis and increased IgG and IgA levels persisted following anti-TB treatment (101).

Imaging Studies

A miliary pattern on the chest radiograph is often the first clue suggestive of miliary TB. Several other imaging modalities, such as ultrasonography, CT, and magnetic resonance imaging (MRI) help to discern the extent of organ involvement and are also useful in evaluation of response to treatment.

Chest radiograph

A miliary pattern on chest radiograph (93, 111, 130) is the classical feature of miliary TB and is observed for a majority of patients. Subtle miliary

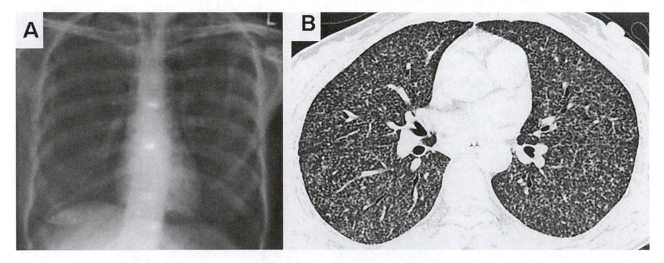

Figure 6. (A) Chest radiograph (postero-anterior view) of a 30-year old woman who presented with a 3-month history of fever with no other localizing clue; (B) HRCT of the same patient showing the classical miliary pattern. Bone marrow biopsy confirmed the diagnosis of miliary TB; *Mycobacterium tuberculosis* was grown on bronchoscopic aspirate culture.

lesions are best delineated in slightly underpenetrated films, especially when the diamond-shaped areas of the lung in between the ribs are carefully scrutinized using bright light (57, 122). The chest radiographic abnormalities in miliary TB are listed in Table 9 (111, 117). Some patients may have normal chest radiographs initially and the classical miliary pattern may evolve over the course of disease (Fig. 6), emphasizing the importance of periodic repeat chest radiographic examination in patients with pyrexia of unknown origin (102, 111).

When patients with miliary TB develop ARDS (Fig. 7), the chest radiograph findings may be identical to those seen in ARDS due to other causes (73, 114). The majority of the patients (88%) in a study reported by Sharma et al. (102) had chest radiographs consistent with miliary TB; in some, these classical radiographic changes evolved over the course of the disease. The diagnosis of miliary TB is easier when the patient presents with classical miliary shadowing on chest radiograph in an appropriate setting. However, the diagnosis may be difficult in those situations where the chest radiograph does not show classical miliary shadows.

In the pre-CT scan era, for up to 50% of the patients, the classical miliary pattern would not be discernible on the chest radiograph, being evident only at the time of autopsy (16, 24, 60, 61, 76, 120). Steiner (122) reasoned that when caseous material, collagen, or both were present in the tubercles, they

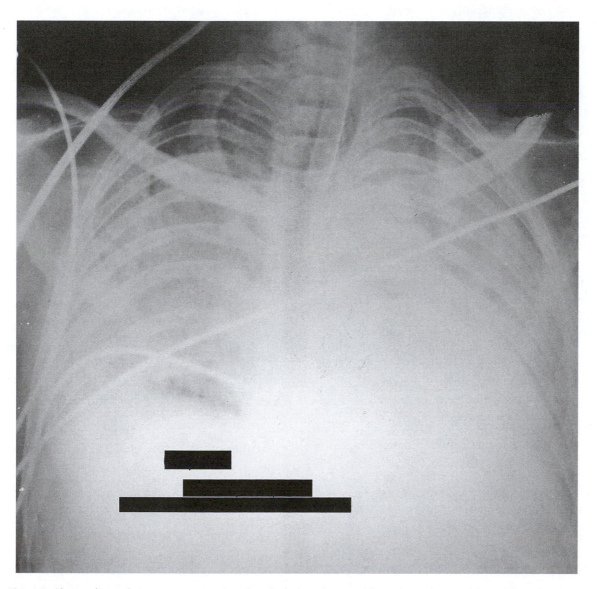

Figure 7. Chest radiograph (antero-posterior view, done bedside with a portable machine) showing bilateral frontal opacities and air space consolidation suggestive of ARDS in an HIV-seropositive patient with miliary TB. Tracheal aspirate smear for AFB and bone marrow biopsy confirmed the diagnosis.

became visible on the chest radiograph. The classical miliary pattern on the chest radiograph represents summation of densities of the tubercles that are perfectly aligned, and imperfectly aligned tubercles result in curvilinear densities and a reticulonodular pattern (48). Rarely, lymphatic obstruction or infiltration can result in a ground glass appearance (85).

Ultrasonography

Ultrasonography helps in detecting associated lesions, such as ascites and pleural effusion which may sometimes be loculated, focal hepatic and splenic lesions, and cold abscess. Ultrasonography guidance also facilitates diagnostic thoracic or abdominal paracentesis to procure pleural or peritoneal fluid for diagnostic testing, especially if the fluid is loculated.

CT and MRI

HRCT and thin-section multidetector row CT have considerably improved the antemortem diagnosis of miliary pattern. HRCT reveals a mixture of both sharply and poorly defined nodules of less than 2 mm that are widely disseminated throughout the lungs, associated with diffuse reticulation (70, 103). The HRCT may reveal a classical miliary pattern even when the chest radiograph looks normal (102, 111) and also facilitates identification of intrathoracic lymphadenopathy, calcification, and pleural lesions. Air trapping has been described on HRCT both at presentation and during follow-up (103) and occurs due to endobronchial involvement of peripheral airways. The interlobular septal thickening or intralobular fine networks that are evident on HRCT in miliary TB seem to be caused by the caseation necrosis in the alveolar walls and interlobular septa. Sometimes in subjects with active postprimary disease, centrilobular nodules and branching linear structures giving a "tree-in-bud" appearance may be evident (70, 103).

Pipavath et al. (82) recently reported the following changes on HRCT in patients with miliary TB (total of 16 patients): miliary pattern ($n = 16$), intrathoracic lymphadenopathy ($n = 8$), alveolar lesions such as ground glass attenuation and/or consolidation ($n = 5$), pleural and pericardial effusions (2 patients each), and peribronchovascular interstitial thickening and emphysema (1 patient each). In this study (82), nodules were randomly distributed in both lung fields in miliary TB, whereas in sarcoidosis, the findings included peribronchovascular interstitial thickening and perilymphatic distribution of the nodules. In another recent study (53), a higher prevalence of interlobular septal thickening, necrotic lymph

nodes, and extrathoracic involvement was observed in HIV-seropositive patients with miliary TB.

MRI and CT have been useful in identifying miliary lesions at extrapulmonary sites. Abdominal CT has been useful in identifying lesions in the liver and spleen, lymphadenopathy, and cold abscesses (111). Unlike in CT of the chest, where the classical nodular lesions of less than 2 mm are evident, miliary lesions in the liver and spleen may appear as discrete hypodense lesions, a few of which may be confluent, sometimes with irregular peripheral rim enhancement (145). MRI of the brain and spine is very useful in the initial evaluation and follow-up of miliary TB patients with TBM or spinal TB and also protects from radiation exposure (111). Image-guided radiological procedures such as fine-needle aspiration for cytological examination and biopsy under CT or MRI guidance are useful for procuring tissue or body fluids for diagnostic testing.

Echocardiography

Two-dimensional transthoracic echocardiography helps to diagnose associated pericardial effusion.

Bronchoscopy

Fiber-optic bronchoscopy, BAL, bronchoscopic aspirate, brushings, and transbronchial lung biopsy are useful in confirming the diagnosis of miliary TB. The cumulative diagnostic yield for various bronchoscopic specimens by smear and culture methods in published studies has been found to be 46.8% (Table 7) (5, 51, 63, 87, 102, 136).

Laparoscopy

When associated abdominal involvement is present, laparoscopy provides an opportunity to visualize the lesions with the naked eye and facilitates biopsy from the liver, peritoneum, omentum, and mesenteric lymph nodes for diagnostic confirmation (44).

Serodiagnostic, Molecular, and Other Methods

Detection of mycobacterial antigens, antibodies, and immune complexes in the blood and body fluids by enzyme-linked immunosorbent assay has been used for diagnosis of miliary TB (111). PCR of cerebrospinal fluid, tissue biopsy specimens, and blood (especially for HIV-infected patients) may be useful for confirmation of diagnosis (109). PCR has been found to be most useful when applied to clean specimens such as cerebrospinal fluid, with which its sensitivity and specificity have been reported to be 0.5 to

0.9 and 1.0, respectively (109). Adenosine deaminase and gamma interferon level estimation in ascitic fluid and pleural fluid can be helpful in the diagnosis of miliary TB (91, 105, 108, 112, 113).

Positron Emission Tomography

Positron emission tomography CT using the radiopharmaceutical ^{18}F-labeled 2-deoxy-D-glucose has been found to be useful to assess the activity of various infectious lesions, including pulmonary TB (36, 45). The utility of positron emission tomography in assessing the activity of lesions that might persist following anti-TB treatment in miliary TB needs to be studied further.

TREATMENT

Miliary TB is uniformly fatal if not treated (93, 111). Standard anti-TB treatment is the cornerstone of management. There is no consensus regarding the optimum duration of treatment. Additionally, there are no published randomized controlled trials assessing the efficacy of the standard World Health Organization (WHO) treatment regimens that are widely used in national tuberculosis control programs worldwide (141, 142). Even less is known regarding the efficacy of standard treatment regimens in the treatment of HIV and miliary TB coinfection.

The American Thoracic Society, the CDC, and the Infectious Diseases Society of America (17) and National Institute for Health and Clinical Excellence (77) guidelines from the United Kingdom recommend 6 months of treatment (2-month intensive phase with isoniazid, rifampin, pyrazinamide, and ethambutol or streptomycin, followed by a 4-month continuation phase with isoniazid and rifampin), whereas the American Academy of Pediatrics (7) advocates 9 months of treatment for newly diagnosed cases of miliary TB without meningeal involvement. When TBM is present, it is suggested that the treatment be extended for 12 months (7, 17, 77). In several parts of the world, patients with miliary TB get treated under national TB control programs, with DOTS using intermittent chemotherapy (141, 142).

In the recently published WHO guidelines for the treatment of TB (140), the use of diagnostic categories I to IV has been done away with and patients are categorized as "new patients" or "previously treated patients." In these guidelines (140), miliary TB is classified as pulmonary TB because there are lesions in the lungs. New patients with miliary TB receive 6 months of daily or intermittent treatment as described above. The guidelines suggested that HIV-coinfected patients

with TB and all TB patients in HIV-prevalent settings should receive daily treatment at least during the intensive phase. However, further evidence is required before endorsing this as a guideline. The guidelines mention that some experts recommend 9 to 12 months of treatment when TBM is present, given the serious risk of disability and mortality, and 9 months of treatment when bone and joint TB is also present. For previously treated patients, the guidelines advocate that specimens for culture and DST should be obtained from all previously treated TB patients at or before the start of treatment. DST should be performed for at least isoniazid and rifampin, and in settings where rapid molecular DST results are available, the results should guide the choice of regimen. Although this duration of treatment may be sufficient for many, each patient needs to be assessed individually, and wherever indicated, treatment duration may have to be extended.

Corticosteroids

No study has specifically evaluated the role of adjunct corticosteroid treatment in patients with miliary TB; only limited evidence is available, including conflicting results. A beneficial response was observed in some studies (123), although such benefit could not be documented in others (68). While associated adrenal insufficiency is an absolute indication for their administration, adjunctive corticosteroid treatment may be beneficial in miliary TB with TBM, large pericardial or pleural effusion, dyspnea and/or disabling chest pain, IRIS, ARDS, immune complex nephritis, and histiocytic phagocytosis syndrome (35, 67, 111).

Antiretroviral Drugs

Coadministration of rifampin may result in dangerously low levels of antiretroviral agents by inducing the hepatic cytochrome P450 pathway. There has been a change in the WHO revised recommendations based on the Grading of Recommendations Assessment, Development and Evaluation (GRADE) system (40) regarding the timing of starting of antiretroviral drugs, the choice of drugs, and the timing of initiation in relation to institution of anti-TB treatment. These new recommendations (139) and the British HIV Association guidelines (83) are shown in Fig. 8.

Mechanical Ventilation

Assisted mechanical ventilation and other interventions may be required for the management of patients with miliary TB who develop ARDS (73, 114).

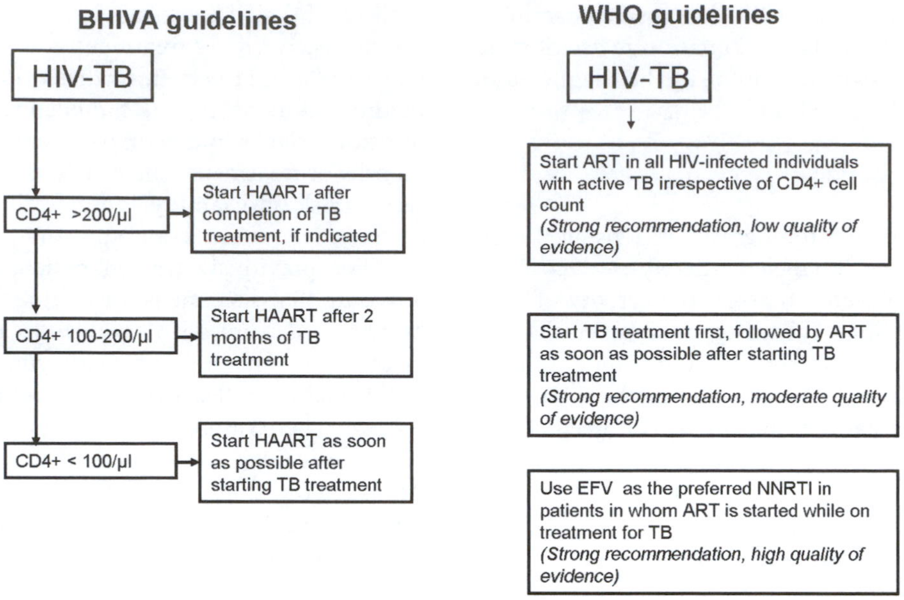

BHIVA guidelines

HIV-TB

CD4+ >200/μl → Start HAART after completion of TB treatment, if indicated

CD4+ 100-200/μl → Start HAART after 2 months of TB treatment

CD4+ < 100/μl → Start HAART as soon as possible after starting TB treatment

WHO guidelines

HIV-TB

Start ART in all HIV-infected individuals with active TB irrespective of CD4+ cell count
(*Strong recommendation, low quality of evidence*)

Start TB treatment first, followed by ART as soon as possible after starting TB treatment
(*Strong recommendation, moderate quality of evidence*)

Use EFV as the preferred NNRTI in patients in whom ART is started while on treatment for TB
(*Strong recommendation, high quality of evidence*)

Figure 8. Guidelines on timing of antiretroviral treatment in patients with HIV-TB coinfection. ART, antiretroviral treatment; BHIVA, British HIV Association; EFV, efavirenz; HAART, highly active antiretroviral treatment. NNRTI, nonnucleoside reverse transcriptase inhibitor. Guidelines are based on references 83 and 139.

Surgery

Surgery is often required to procure specimens for diagnostic testing and to ameliorate complications, such as small bowel perforation, in which it may be lifesaving.

Mortality

The rate of mortality related to miliary TB is about 15 to 20% in children (1, 39, 43, 54, 89) and is slightly higher in adults (25 to 30%) (16, 21, 34, 37, 51, 63, 72, 76, 79, 87). Delay in diagnosis and initiation of specific anti-TB treatment appears to be responsible for a higher mortality rate in miliary TB.

Prognostic Factors

Several factors have been identified as predictors of poor outcome in patients with miliary TB (Table 10). For patients with ARDS due to miliary TB (114), an acute physiological and chronic health evaluation (APACHE II) score greater than 18, an APACHE II score less than or equal to 18 in the

Table 10. Predictors of poor outcome in patients with disseminated or miliary TB

Study (yr) (reference)	Predictor(s) of poor outcome
Gelb et al. (1973) (34)[a]	Stupor, meningismus, increasing age, cirrhosis of liver, leukopenia, leukocytosis
Grieco and Chmel (1974) (37)	Increasing age, presence of underlying disease, history of cough, night sweats
Kim et al. (1990) (51)	Female gender, altered mental status
Maartens et al. (1990) (63)	Age greater than 60 yrs, lymphopenia, thrombocytopenia, hypoalbuminemia, elevated transaminase levels, treatment delay
Sharma et al. (1995) (102)	Dyspnea, chills, temp of >39.3°C, icterus, hepatomegaly, hypoalbuminemia, hyponatremia, elevated serum alkaline phosphatase
Long et al. (1997) (62)	Presence of one or more predisposing conditions[b]
Mert et al. (2001) (72)	Male sex, presence of atypical chest radiographic pattern, delay in instituting anti-TB treatment
Hussain et al. (2004) (41)	Presence of altered mental status, lung crackles, leukocytosis, thrombocytopenia, and need for ventilation
Kim et al. (2008) (50)	High nutritional risk score[c]

[a]No statistical analysis was performed.
[b]Listed in Tables 2 and 3.
[c]A four-point nutritional risk score was defined according to the presence of four nutritional factors: low body mass index (<18.5 kg/m^2), hypoalbuminemia (serum albumin, <30 g/liter), hypocholesterolemia (serum cholesterol, <2.33 mmol/liter), and severe lymphocytopenia (<7 × 10^5 cells/liter). Each risk factor was assigned a value of 1 if present or 0 if absent. Patients with three or four points were classified as having a high nutritional risk score.

presence of hyponatremia, and a PaO$_2$/FIO$_2$ ratio less than or equal to 108.5 have been identified to be predictors of death. Identification of these factors can alert the clinicians managing patients with miliary TB.

PREVENTION

BCG vaccination is effective in reducing the incidence of miliary TB, especially in children (129). However, it is not effective in individuals who have latent TB infection and should not be administered to immunosuppressed hosts. Targeted tuberculin testing is practiced in countries with a low prevalence of TB, such as the United States (8, 17), but anti-TB drug-induced hepatotoxicity is a potential risk with the treatment of latent TB infection. Ongoing research (31, 131) has yet to provide a more effective vaccine than BCG.

REFERENCES

1. Aderele, W. I. 1978. Miliary tuberculosis in Nigerian children. *East Afr. Med. J.* 55:166–171.
2. Ahluwalia, G., S. K. Sharma, S. Dattagupta, and J. N. Pande. 1999. Role of transbronchial lung biopsy in diffuse pulmonary disease: a review of 25 cases during one year. *Indian J. Chest Dis. Allied Sci.* 41:213–217.
3. Ainslie, G. M., J. A. Solomon, and E. D. Bateman. 1992. Lymphocyte and lymphocyte subset numbers in blood and in bronchoalveolar lavage and pleural fluid in various forms of pulmonary tuberculosis at presentation and during recovery. *Thorax* 47:513–518.
4. Al-Arif, L. I., R. A. Goldstein, L. F. Affronti, and B. W. Janicki. 1979. HLA-Bw15 and tuberculosis in a North American black population. *Am. Rev. Respir. Dis.* 120:1275–1278.
5. Al-Jahdali, H., K. Al-Zahrani, P. Amene, Z. Memish, A. Al-Shimemeri, M. Moamary, and A. Alduhaim. 2000. Clinical aspects of miliary tuberculosis in Saudi adults. *Int. J. Tuberc. Lung Dis.* 4:252–255.
6. Alvarez, S., and W. R. McCabe. 1984. Extrapulmonary tuberculosis revisited: a review of experience at Boston City and other hospitals. *Medicine* (Baltimore) 63:25–55.
7. American Academy of Pediatrics Committee on Infectious Diseases. 1992. Chemotherapy for tuberculosis in infants and children. *Pediatrics* 89:161–165.
8. American Thoracic Society. 2000. Targeted tuberculin testing and treatment of latent tuberculosis infection. *MMWR Recommend. Rep.* 49(RR-6):1–51.
9. Anonymous. 1970. Miliary tuberculosis: a changing pattern. *Lancet* i:985–986.
10. Ansari, N. A., A. H. Kombe, T. A. Kenyon, N. M. Hone, J. W. Tappero, S. T. Nyirenda, N. J. Binkin, and S. B. Lucas. 2002. Pathology and causes of death in a group of 128 predominantly HIV-positive patients in Botswana, 1997–1998. *Int. J. Tuberc. Lung Dis.* 6:55–63.
11. Anyanwu, C. H., E. Nassau, and M. Yacoub. 1976. Miliary tuberculosis following homograft valve replacement. *Thorax* 31:101–106.
12. Asada, Y., T. Hayashi, A. Sumiyoshi, M. Aburaya, and E. Shishime. 1991. Miliary tuberculosis presenting as fever and jaundice with hepatic failure. *Hum. Pathol.* 22:92–94.
13. Auerbach, O. 1944. Acute generalized miliary tuberculosis. *Am. J. Pathol.* 20:121–136.
14. Balamurugan, A. 2002. HLA-DR restriction of Th1/Th2 cytokine profile in tuberculosis: impact of genetic diversity. Ph.D. thesis. All India Institute of Medical Sciences, New Delhi, India.
15. Barnes, P. F., C. L. Grisso, J. S. Abrams, H. Band, T. H. Rea, and R. L. Modlin. 1992. Gamma delta T lymphocytes in human tuberculosis. *J. Infect. Dis.* 165:506–512.
16. Biehl, J. P. 1958. Miliary tuberculosis; a review of sixty-eight adult patients admitted to a municipal general hospital. *Am. Rev. Tuberc.* 77:605–622.
17. Blumberg, H. M., W. J. Burman, R. E. Chaisson, C. L. Daley, S. C. Etkind, L. N. Friedman, P. Fujiwara, M. Grzemska, P. C. Hopewell, M. D. Iseman, R. M. Jasmer, V. Koppaka, R. I. Menzies, R. J. O'Brien, R. R. Reves, L. B. Reichman, P. M. Simone, J. R. Starke, and A. A. Vernon for the American Thoracic Society/Centers for Disease Control and Prevention/Infectious Diseases Society of America. 2003. Treatment of tuberculosis. *Am. J. Respir. Crit. Care Med.* 167:603–662.
18. Bonetus, T. 1679. *Sepulchretum sive anatomica practica*, vol. 1. Observatio XLVI. Sumptibus Leonardi Chouët, Genevae.
19. Braidy, J., C. Pothel, and S. Amra. 1981. Miliary tuberculosis presenting as adrenal failure. *J. Can. Med. Assoc.* 82:254–256.
20. Braun, M. M., T. R. Cote, and C. S. Rabkin. 1993. Trends in death with tuberculosis during the AIDS era. *JAMA* 269:2865–2868.
21. Campbell, I. G. 1973. Miliary tuberculosis in British Columbia. *Can. Med. Assoc. J.* 108:1517–1519.
22. Centers for Disease Control and Prevention. 20 March 2010, posting date. *Reported Tuberculosis in the United States.* Centers for Disease Control and Prevention, Atlanta, GA. http://www.cdc.gov/TB/statistics/archived.htm.
23. Chan, C. H., T. Y. Chan, A. C. Shek, T. W. Mak, S. F. Lui, and K. N. Lai. 1994. Severe hypercalcaemia associated with miliary tuberculosis. *J. Trop. Med. Hyg.* 97:180–182.
24. Chapman, C. B., and C. M. Whorton. 1946. Acute generalised miliary tuberculosis in adults. A clinicopathological study based on sixty three cases diagnosed at autopsy. *N. Engl. J. Med.* 235:239–248.
25. Collins, H. L., and S. H. Kaufmann. 2001. The many faces of host responses to tuberculosis. *Immunology* 103:1–9.
26. Cunha, B. A., J. Krakakis, and B. P. McDermott. 2009. Fever of unknown origin (FUO) caused by miliary tuberculosis: diagnostic significance of morning temperature spikes. *Heart Lung* 38:77–82. [Epub ahead of print.]
27. del Giudice, P., E. Bernard, C. Perrin, G. Bernardin, R. Fouché, C. Boissy, J. Durant, and P. Dellamonica. 2000. Unusual cutaneous manifestations of miliary tuberculosis. *Clin. Infect. Dis.* 30:201–204.
28. Dheda, K., R. Z. Smit, M. Badri, and M. Pai. 2009. T-cell interferon-gamma release assays for the rapid immunodiagnosis of tuberculosis: clinical utility in high-burden vs. low-burden settings. *Curr. Opin. Pulm. Med.* 15:188–200.
29. Dixon, W. G., K. L. Hyrich, K. D. Watson, M. Lunt, J. Galloway, A. Ustianowski, and D. P. M. Symmons. 2010. Drug-specific risk of tuberculosis in patients with rheumatoid arthritis treated with anti-TNF therapy: results from the British Society for Rheumatology Biologics Register (BSRBR). *Ann. Rheum. Dis.* 69:522–528. [Epub ahead of print.]
30. Ellner, J. J. 1997. The immune response in human tuberculosis—implications for tuberculosis control. *J. Infect. Dis.* 176:1351–1359.

31. Fletcher, H. A., T. Hawkridge, and H. McShane. 2009. A new vaccine for tuberculosis: the challenges of development and deployment. *J. Bioeth. Inq.* **6**:219–228. [Epub ahead of print.]

32. Flores-Franco, R. A., and L. A. Ríos-Ortiz. 2010. The "damp shadow" sign: another clinical indicator of miliary tuberculosis. *Heart Lung* **39**:87–88. [Epub ahead of print.]

33. Garg, R. K., R. Sharma, A. M. Kar, R. A. Kushwaha, M. K. Singh, R. Shukla, A. Agarwal, and R. Verma. 2010. Neurological complications of miliary tuberculosis. *Clin. Neurol. Neurosurg.* **12**:188–192. [Epub ahead of print.]

34. Gelb, A. F., C. Leffler, A. Brewin, V. Mascatello, and H. A. Lyons. 1973. Miliary tuberculosis. *Am. Rev. Respir. Dis.* **108**:1327–1333.

35. Goldsack, N. R., S. Allen, and M. C. Lipman. 2003. Adult respiratory distress syndrome as a severe immune reconstitution disease following the commencement of highly active antiretroviral therapy. *Sex. Transm. Infect.* **79**:337–338.

36. Goo, J. M., J. G. Im, K. H. Do, J. S. Yeo, J. B. Seo, H. Y. Kim, and J. K. Chung. 2000. Pulmonary tuberculoma evaluated by means of FDG PET: findings in 10 cases. *Radiology* **216**:117–121.

37. Grieco, M. H., and H. Chmel. 1974. Acute disseminated tuberculosis as a diagnostic problem. A clinical study based on twenty-eight cases. *Am. Rev. Respir. Dis.* **109**:554–560.

38. Gupta, P. P., D. Mehta, D. Agarwal, and T. Chand. 2007. Recurrent pneumothorax developing during chemotherapy in a patient with miliary tuberculosis. *Ann. Thorac. Med.* **2**:173–175.

39. Gurkan, F., M. Bosnak, B. Dikici, V. Bosnak, A. Yaramis, M. Ali Tas, and K. Haspolat. 1998. Miliary tuberculosis in children: a clinical review. *Scand. J. Infect. Dis.* **30**:359–362.

40. Guyatt, G. H., A. D. Oxman, G. E. Vist, R. Kunz, Y. Falck-Ytter, P. Alonso-Coello, and H. J. Schünemann for the GRADE Working Group. 2008. GRADE: an emerging consensus on rating quality of evidence and strength of recommendations. *BMJ* **336**:924–926.

41. Hussain, S. F., M. Irfan, M. Abbasi, S. S. Anwer, S. Davidson, R. Haqqee, J. A. Khan, and M. Islam. 2004. Clinical characteristics of 110 miliary tuberculosis patients from a low HIV prevalence country. *Int. J. Tuberc. Lung Dis.* **8**:493–499.

42. Hussain, W., D. Mutimer, R. Harrison, S. Hubscher, and J. Neuberger. 1995. Fulminant hepatic failure caused by tuberculosis. *Gut* **36**:792–794.

43. Hussey, G., T. Chisholm, and M. Kibel. 1991. Miliary tuberculosis in children: a review of 94 cases. *Pediatr. Infect. Dis. J.* **10**:832–836.

44. Ibrarullah, M., A. Mohan, A. Sarkari, M. Srinivas, A. Mishra, and T. S. Sundar. 2002. Abdominal tuberculosis: diagnosis by laparoscopy and colonoscopy. *Trop. Gastroenterol.* **23**:150–153.

45. Ichiya, Y., Y. Kuwabara, M. Sasaki, T. Yoshida, Y. Akashi, S. Murayama, K. Nakamura, T. Fukumura, and K. Masuda. 1996. FDG-PET in infectious lesions: the detection and assessment of lesion activity. *Ann. Nucl. Med.* **10**:185–191.

46. Jacques, J., and T. M. Sloan. 1970. The changing pattern of miliary tuberculosis. *Thorax* **25**:237–240.

47. Jagirdar, J., and D. Zagzag. 2004. Pathology and insights into pathogenesis of tuberculosis, p. 323–344. *In* W. N. Rom and S. M. Garay (ed.), *Tuberculosis*. Lippincott Williams & Wilkins, Philadelphia, PA.

48. Jamieson, D. H., and B. J. Cremin. 1993. High resolution CT of the lungs in acute disseminated tuberculosis and a pediatric radiology perspective of the term "miliary." *Pediatr. Radiol.* **23**:380–383.

49. Jehle, A. W., N. Khanna, J. P. Sigle, K. Glatz-Krieger, M. Battegay, J. Steiger, M. Dickenmann, and H. H. Hirsch. 2004. Acute renal failure on immune reconstitution in an HIV-positive patient with miliary tuberculosis. *Clin. Infect. Dis.* **38**:e32–e35. [Epub ahead of print.]

50. Kim, D. K., H. J. Kim, S. Y. Kwon, H. I. Yoon, C. T. Lee, Y. W. Kim, H. S. Chung, S. K. Han, Y. S. Shim, and J. H. Lee. 2008. Nutritional deficit as a negative prognostic factor in patients with miliary tuberculosis. *Eur. Respir. J.* **32**:1031–1036. [Epub ahead of print.]

51. Kim, J. H., A. A. Langston, and H. A. Gallis. 1990. Miliary tuberculosis: epidemiology, clinical manifestations, diagnosis, and outcome. *Rev. Infect. Dis.* **12**:583–590.

52. Kim, J. Y., Y. B. Park, Y. S. Kim, S. B. Kang, J. W. Shin, I. W. Park, and B. W. Choi. 2003. Miliary tuberculosis and acute respiratory distress syndrome. *Int. J. Tuberc. Lung Dis.* **7**:359–364.

53. Kim, J. Y., Y. J. Jeong, K. I. Kim, I. S. Lee, H. K. Park, Y. D. Kim, and I. H. Seok. 2010. Miliary tuberculosis: a comparison of CT findings in HIV-seropositive and HIV-seronegative patients. *Br. J. Radiol.* **83**:206–211.

54. Kim, P. K., J. S. Lee, and D. J. Yun. 1969. Clinical review of miliary tuberculosis in Korean children: 84 cases and review of the literature. *Yonsei Med. J.* **10**:146–152.

55. Krishnaswami, K. V. 1977. Mediastinal emphysema in miliary tuberculosis. *JAMA* **69**:227–229.

56. Kumararatne, D. S., A. S. Pithie, P. Drysdale, J. S. Gaston, R. Kiessling, P. B. Iles, C. J. Ellis, J. Innes, and R. Wise. 1990. Specific lysis of mycobacterial antigen-bearing macrophages by class II MHC-restricted polyclonal T cell lines in healthy donors or patients with tuberculosis. *Clin. Exp. Immunol.* **80**:314–323.

57. Kwong, J. S., S. Carignan, E. Y. Kang, N. L. Muller, and J. M. Fitzgerald. 1996. Miliary tuberculosis. Diagnostic accuracy of chest radiography. *Chest* **110**:339–342.

58. Lado Lado, F. L., E. Barrio Gomez, E. Carballo Arceo, and A. Cabarcos Ortiz de Barron. 1999. Clinical presentation of tuberculosis and the degree of immunodeficiency in patients with HIV infection. *Scand. J. Infect. Dis.* **31**:387–391.

59. Lakin, B. D., F. A. Riordan, and C. M. John. 2009. Air leak in miliary tuberculosis. *Am. J. Trop. Med. Hyg.* **80**:325.

60. Lee, K. S., T. S. Kim, J. Han, J. H. Hwang, J. H. Yoon, Y. Kim, and S. Y. Yoo. 1999. Diffuse micronodular lung disease: HRCT and pathologic findings. *J. Comput. Assist. Tomogr.* **23**:99–106.

61. Lewison, M., E. B. Frelich, and O. B. Ragins. 1931. Correlation of clinical diagnosis and pathological diagnosis with special reference to tuberculosis: analysis of autopsy findings in 893 cases. *Am. Rev. Tuberc.* **24**:152–171.

62. Long, R., R. O'Connor, M. Palayew, E. Hershfield, and J. Manfreda. 1997. Disseminated tuberculosis with and without a miliary pattern on chest radiograph: a clinical-pathologic-radiologic correlation. *Int. J. Tuberc. Lung Dis.* **1**:52–58.

63. Maartens, G., P. A. Willcox, and S. R. Benatar. 1990. Miliary tuberculosis: rapid diagnosis, hematologic abnormalities, and outcome in 109 treated adults. *Am. J. Med.* **89**:291–296.

64. Malipeddi, A. S., R. Rajendran, and G. Kallarackal. 2007. Disseminated tuberculosis after anti-TNF alpha treatment. *Lancet* **369**:162.

65. Mallinson, W. J., R. W. Fuller, D. A. Levison, L. R. Baker, and W. R. Cattell. 1981. Diffuse interstitial renal tuberculosis—an unusual cause of renal failure. *Q. J. Med.* **50**:137–148.

66. Manget, J. J. 1700. *Sepulchretum sive anatomica practica*, vol. 1. Observatio XLVII. Cramer and Perachon, London, England.

67. Marais, S., R. J. Wilkinson, D. J. Pepper, and G. Meintjes. 2009. Management of patients with the immune reconstitution inflammatory syndrome. *Curr. HIV/AIDS Rep.* **6**:162–171.

68. Massaro, D., S. Katz, and M. Sachs. 1964. Choroidal tubercles. A clue to hematogenous tuberculosis. *Ann. Intern. Med.* 60:231–241.

69. McClement, J. H., A. D. Renzetti, Jr., D. Carroll, A. Himmelstein, and A. Cournand. 1951. Cardiopulmonary function in hematogenous pulmonary tuberculosis in patients with streptomycin therapy. *Am. Rev. Tuberc.* 64:588–601.

70. McGuinness, G., D. P. Naidich, J. Jagirdar, B. Leitman, and D. I. McCauley. 1992. High resolution CT findings in miliary lung disease. *J. Comput. Assist. Tomogr.* 16:384–390.

71. Meintjes, G., S. D. Lawn, F. Scano, G. Maartens, M. A. French, W. Worodria, J. H. Elliott, D. Murdoch, R. J. Wilkinson, C. Seyler, L. John, M. S. van der Loeff, P. Reiss, L. Lynen, E. N. Janoff, C. Gilks, and R. Colebunders for the International Network for the Study of HIV-Associated IRIS. 2008. Tuberculosis-associated immune reconstitution inflammatory syndrome: case definitions for use in resource-limited settings. *Lancet Infect. Dis.* 8:516–523.

72. Mert, A., M. Bilir, F. Tabak, R. Ozaras, R. Ozturk, H. Senturk, H. Aki, N. Seyhan, T. Karayel, and Y. Aktuglu. 2001. Miliary tuberculosis: clinical manifestations, diagnosis and outcome in 38 adults. *Respirology* 6:217–224.

73. Mohan, A., S. K. Sharma, and J. N. Pande. 1996. Acute respiratory distress syndrome in miliary tuberculosis: a 12-year experience. *Indian J. Chest Dis. Allied Sci.* 38:147–152.

74. Morano Amado, L. E., L. Amador Barciela, A. Rodriguez Fernandez, I. Martinez-Sapina Llamas, O. Vazquez Alvarez, and J. Fernandez Martin. 1993. Extracorporeal shock wave lithotripsy complicated with miliary tuberculosis. *J. Urol.* 149:1532–1534.

75. Mori, T. 2009. Usefulness of interferon-gamma release assays for diagnosing TB infection and problems with these assays. *J. Infect. Chemother.* 15:143–155. [Epub ahead of print.]

76. Munt, P. W. 1972. Miliary tuberculosis in the chemotherapy era: with a clinical review in 69 American adults. *Medicine* (Baltimore) 51:139–155.

77. National Institute for Health and Clinical Excellence, National Collaborating Centre for Chronic Conditions. 2006. *Tuberculosis: Clinical Diagnosis and Management of Tuberculosis, and Measures for Its Prevention and Control*, p. 64–76. Royal College of Physicians, London, England.

78. Noertjojo, K., C. M. Tam, S. L. Chan, and M. M. Chan-Yeung. 2002. Extrapulmonary and pulmonary tuberculosis in Hong Kong. *Int. J. Tuberc. Lung Dis.* 6:879–886.

79. Onadeko, B. O., R. Dickinson, and E. O. Sofowora. 1975. Miliary tuberculosis of the lung in Nigerian adults. *East Afr. Med. J.* 52:390–395.

80. Pai, M., R. Joshi, and S. P. Kalantri. 2009. Diagnosis of latent tuberculosis infection: recent advances and future directions, p. 186–199. *In* S. K. Sharma and A. Mohan (ed.), *Tuberculosis*, 2nd ed. Jaypee Brothers Medical Publishers, New Delhi, India.

81. Penner, C., D. Roberts, D. Kunimoto, J. Manfreda, and R. Long. 1995. Tuberculosis as a primary cause of respiratory failure requiring mechanical ventilation. *Am. J. Respir. Crit. Care Med.* 151:867–872.

82. Pipavath, S. N., S. K. Sharma, S. Sinha, S. Mukhopadhyay, and M. S. Gulati. 2007. High resolution CT (HRCT) in miliary tuberculosis (MTB) of the lung: correlation with pulmonary function tests & gas exchange parameters in north Indian patients. *Indian J. Med. Res.* 126:193–198.

83. Pozniak, A. L., R. L. Miller, M. C. I. Lipman, A. R. Freedman, L. P. Ormerod, M. A. Johnson, S. Collins, and S. B. Lucas, on behalf of the BHIVA Guidelines Writing Committee. 2005. BHIVA treatment guidelines for tuberculosis (TB)/HIV infection 2005. *HIV Med.* 6(Suppl. 2):62–83.

84. Prabhakaran, D., S. K. Sharma, K. Verma, and J. N. Pande. 1990. Estimation of fibronectin in bronchoalveolar lavage fluid in various diffuse interstitial lung diseases. *Am. Rev. Respir. Dis.* 141:A51.

85. Price, M. 1968. Lymphangitis reticularis tuberculosa. *Tubercle* 49:377–384.

86. Proudfoot, A. T., A. J. Akhtar, A. C. Douglas, and N. W. Horne. 1969. Miliary tuberculosis in adults. *BMJ* 2:273–276.

87. Prout, S., and S. R. Benatar. 1980. Disseminated tuberculosis. A study of 62 cases. *S. Afr. Med. J.* 58:835–842.

88. Rabe, J., K. W. Neff, K. J. Lehmann, U. Mechtersheimer, and M. Georgi. 1999. Miliary tuberculosis after intravesical bacille Calmette-Guerin immunotherapy for carcinoma of the bladder. *Am. J. Roentgenol.* 172:748–750.

89. Rahajoe, N. N. 1990. Miliary tuberculosis in children. A clinical review. *Paediatr. Indones.* 30:233–240.

90. Rich, A. R. 1951. *The Pathogenesis of Tuberculosis*. Charles C Thomas, Springfield, IL.

91. Riquelme, A., M. Calvo, F. Salech, S. Valderrama, A. Pattillo, M. Arellano, M. Arrese, A. Soza, P. Viviani, and L. M. Letelier. 2006. Value of adenosine deaminase (ADA) in ascetic fluid for the diagnosis of tuberculous peritonitis: a meta-analysis. *J. Clin. Gastroenterol.* 40:705–710.

92. Rook, G. A., R. Hernandez-Pando, K. Dheda, and G. Teng Seah. 2004. IL-4 in tuberculosis: implications for vaccine design. *Trends Immunol.* 25:483–488.

93. Sahn, S. A., and T. A. Neff. 1974. Miliary tuberculosis. *Am. J. Med.* 56:494–505.

94. Salliot, C., I. Guichard, E. Daugas, M. Lagrange, J. Verine, and J. M. Molina. 2008. Acute kidney disease due to immune reconstitution inflammatory syndrome in an HIV-infected patient with tuberculosis. *J. Int. Assoc. Physicians AIDS Care* 7:178–181. [Epub ahead of print.]

95. Saukkonen, J. J., D. L. Cohn, R. M. Jasmer, S. Schenker, J. A. Jereb, C. M. Nolan, C. A. Peloquin, F. M. Gordin, D. Nunes, D. B. Strader, J. Bernardo, R. Venkataramanan, and T. R. Sterling on behalf of the ATS Hepatotoxicity of Antituberculosis Therapy Subcommittee. 2006. An official ATS statement: hepatotoxicity of antituberculosis therapy. *Am. J. Respir. Crit. Care Med.* 174:935–952.

96. Seabra, J., H. Coelho, H. Barros, J. O. Alves, V. Goncalves, and A. Rocha-Marques. 1993. Acute tuberculous perforation of the small bowel during antituberculosis therapy. *J. Clin. Gastroenterol.* 16:320–322.

97. Shalhoub, R. J., and L. D. Antoniou. 1969. The mechanism of hyponatremia in pulmonary tuberculosis. *Ann. Intern. Med.* 70:943–962.

98. Shao, C., J. Qu, and L. He. 2003. A comparative study of clinical manifestations caused by tuberculosis in immunocompromised and non-immunocompromised patients. *Chin. Med. J. (Engl.)* 116:1717–1722.

99. Sharma, P. K., P. K. Saha, A. Singh, S. K. Sharma, B. Ghosh, and D. K. Mitra. 2009. FoxP3+ regulatory T cells suppress effector T-cell function at pathologic site in miliary tuberculosis. *Am. J. Respir. Crit. Care Med.* 179:1061–1070. [Epub ahead of print.]

100. Sharma, S. K., J. N. Pande, and K. Verma. 1988. Bronchoalveolar lavage (BAL) in miliary tuberculosis. *Tubercle* 69:175–178.

101. Sharma, S. K., J. N. Pande, Y. N. Singh, K. Verma, S. S. Kathait, S. D. Khare, and A. N. Malaviya. 1992. Pulmonary function and immunologic abnormalities in miliary tuberculosis. *Am. Rev. Respir. Dis.* 145:1167–1171.

102. Sharma, S. K., A. Mohan, J. N. Pande, K. L. Prasad, A. K. Gupta, and G. C. Khilnani. 1995. Clinical profile, laboratory

characteristics and outcome in miliary tuberculosis. *Q. J. Med.* **88**:29–37.

103. Sharma, S. K., S. Mukhopadhyay, R. Arora, K. Verma, J. N. Pande, and G. C. Khilnani. 1996. Computed tomography in miliary tuberculosis: comparison with plain films, bronchoalveolar lavage, pulmonary functions and gas exchange. *Australas. Radiol.* **40**:113–118.

104. Sharma, S. K., A. Mohan, R. Gupta, A. Kumar, A. K. Gupta, V. K. Singhal, and J. N. Pande. 1997. Clinical presentation of tuberculosis in patients with AIDS: an Indian experience. *Indian J. Chest Dis. Allied Sci.* **39**:213–220.

105. Sharma, S. K., V. Suresh, A. Mohan, P. Kaur, P. Saha, A. Kumar, and J. N. Pande. 2001. A prospective study of sensitivity and specificity of adenosine deaminase estimation in the diagnosis of tuberculosis pleural effusion. *Indian J. Chest Dis. Allied Sci.* **43**:149–155.

106. Sharma, S. K., D. K. Mitra, A. Balamurugan, R. M. Pandey, and N. K. Mehra. 2002. Cytokine polarization in miliary and pleural tuberculosis. *J. Clin. Immunol.* **22**:345–352.

107. Sharma, S. K., and A. Mohan. 2004. Co-infection of human immunodeficiency virus (HIV) and tuberculosis: Indian perspective. *Indian J. Tuberc.* **51**:5–16.

108. Sharma, S. K., and A. Banga. 2004. Diagnostic utility of pleural fluid IFN gamma in tuberculosis pleural effusion. *J. Interferon Cytokine Res.* **24**:213–217.

109. Sharma, S. K., and A. Mohan. 2004. Extrapulmonary tuberculosis. *Indian J. Med. Res.* **120**:316–353.

110. Sharma, S. K., A. Mohan, and T. Kadhiravan. 2005. HIV-TB co-infection: epidemiology, diagnosis and management. *Indian J. Med. Res.* **121**:550–567.

111. Sharma, S. K., A. Mohan, A. Sharma, and D. K. Mitra. 2005. Miliary tuberculosis: new insights into an old disease. *Lancet Infect. Dis.* **5**:415–430.

112. Sharma, S. K., and A. Banga. 2005. Pleural fluid interferon-gamma and adenosine deaminase levels in tuberculosis pleural effusion: a cost-effectiveness analysis. *J. Clin. Lab. Anal.* **19**:40–46.

113. Sharma, S. K., M. Tahir, A. Mohan, D. Smith-Rohrberg, H. K. Mishra, and R. M. Pandey. 2006. Diagnostic accuracy of ascitic fluid IFN-gamma and adenosine deaminase assays in the diagnosis of tuberculous ascites. *J. Interferon Cytokine Res.* **26**:484–488.

114. Sharma, S. K., A. Mohan, A. Banga, P. K. Saha, and K. K. Guntupalli. 2006. Predictors of development and outcome in patients with acute respiratory distress syndrome due to tuberculosis. *Int. J. Tuberc. Lung Dis.* **10**:429–435.

115. Sharma, S. K., and G. Ahluwalia. 2006. Effect of antituberculosis treatment on cardiopulmonary responses to exercise in miliary tuberculosis. *Indian J. Med. Res.* **124**:411–418.

116. Sharma, S. K., and G. Ahluwalia. 2007. Exercise testing in miliary tuberculosis–some facts. *Indian J. Med. Res.* **125**:182–183.

117. Sharma, S. K., and A. Mohan. 2009. Disseminated and miliary tuberculosis, p. 493–518. *In* S. K. Sharma and A. Mohan (ed.), *Tuberculosis*, 2nd ed. Jaypee Brothers Medical Publishers, New Delhi, India.

118. Silverblatt, A., J. A. DeSimone, and T. J. Babinchak. 2002. Acute miliary tuberculosis following laser lithotripsy. *Infect. Med.* **19**:80–82.

119. Singh, K. J., G. Ahluwalia, S. K. Sharma, R. Saxena, V. P. Chaudhary, and M. Anant. 2001. Significance of haematological manifestations in patients with tuberculosis. *J. Assoc. Physicians India* **49**:790–794.

120. Slavin, R. E., T. J. Walsh, and A. D. Pollack. 1980. Late generalized tuberculosis: a clinical pathologic analysis and comparison of 100 cases in the preantibiotic and antibiotic eras. *Medicine* (Baltimore) **59**:352–366.

121. Somu, N., D. Vijayasekaran, T. Ravikumar, A. Balachandran, L. Subramanyam, and A. Chandrabhushanam. 1994. Tuberculous disease in a pediatric referral centre: 16 years experience. *Indian Pediatr.* **31**:1245–1249.

122. Steiner, P. E. 1937. The histopathological basis for the X-ray diagnosability of pulmonary miliary tuberculosis. *Am. Rev. Tuberc.* **36**:692–705.

123. Sun, T. N., J. Y. Yang, L. Y. Zheng, W. W. Deng, and Z. Y. Sui. 1981. Chemotherapy and its combination with corticosteroids in acute miliary tuberculosis in adolescents and adults: analysis of 55 cases. *Chin. Med. J. (Engl.)* **94**:309–314.

124. Swaminathan, S., C. Padmapriyadarsini, C. Ponnuraja, C. H. Sumathi, S. Rajasekaran, V. A. Amerandran, M. V. K. Reddy, and C. N. Deivanayagam. 2007. Miliary tuberculosis in human immunodeficiency virus infected patients not on antiretroviral therapy: clinical profile and response to short course chemotherapy. *J. Postgrad. Med.* **53**:228–231.

125. Taype, C. A., S. Shamsuzzaman, R. A. Accinelli, J. R. Espinoza, and M. A. Shaw. 2010. Genetic susceptibility to different clinical forms of tuberculosis in the Peruvian population. *Infect. Genet. Evol.* **10**:495–504. [Epub ahead of print.]

126. Teklu, B., J. Butler, and J. H. Ostrow. 1977. Miliary tuberculosis. A review of 83 cases treated between 1950 and 1968. *Ethiop. Med. J.* **15**:39–48.

127. Thwaites, G. E., D. B. Nguyen, H. D. Nguyen, T. Q. Hoang, T. T. Do, T. C. Nguyen, Q. H. Nguyen, T. T. Nguyen, N. H. Nguyen, T. N. Nguyen, N. L. Nguyen, H. D. Nguyen, N. T. Vu, H. H. Cao, T. H. Tran, P. M. Pham, T. D. Nguyen, K. Stepniewska, N. J. White, T. H. Tran, and J. J. Farrar. 2004. Dexamethasone for the treatment of tuberculous meningitis in adolescents and adults. *N. Engl. J. Med.* **351**:1741–1751.

128. Toussirot, E., G. Streit, and D. Wendling. 2007. Infectious complications with anti-TNF alpha therapy in rheumatic diseases: a review. *Recent Pat. Inflamm. Allergy Drug Discov.* **1**:39–47.

129. Trunz, B. B., P. Fine, and C. Dye. 2006. Effect of BCG vaccination on childhood tuberculous meningitis and miliary tuberculosis worldwide: a meta-analysis and assessment of cost-effectiveness. *Lancet* **367**:1173–1180.

130. Tuddenham, W. J. 1984. Glossary of terms for thoracic radiology: recommendations of the Nomenclature Committee of the Fleischner Society. *Am. J. Roentgenol.* **143**:509–517.

131. Tyagi, A., B. Dey, and R. Jain. 2009. Tuberculosis vaccine development: current status and future expectations. p. 918–946. *In* S. K. Sharma and A. Mohan (ed.), *Tuberculosis*, 2nd ed. Jaypee Brothers Medical Publishers; New Delhi, India.

132. Udani, P. M., U. S. Bhat, S. K. Bhave, S. G. Ezuthachan, and V. V. Shetty. 1976. Problem of tuberculosis in children in India: epidemiology, morbidity, mortality and control programme. *Indian Pediatr.* **13**:881–890.

133. Uthman, I., N. Kanj, J. El-Sayad, and A. R. Bizri. 2004. Miliary tuberculosis after infliximab therapy in Lebanon. *Clin. Rheumatol.* **23**:279–280.

134. Vasankari, T., K. Liippo, and E. Tala. 2003. Overt and cryptic miliary tuberculosis misdiagnosed until autopsy. *Scand. J. Infect. Dis.* **35**:794–796.

135. Vorherr, H., S. G. Massry, R. Fallet, L. Kaplan, and C. R. Kleeman. 1970. Antidiuretic principle in tuberculous lung tissue of a patient with pulmonary tuberculosis and hyponatremia. *Ann. Intern. Med.* **72**:383–387.

136. Willcox, P. A., P. D. Potgieter, E. D. Bateman, and S. R. Benatar. 1986. Rapid diagnosis of sputum negative miliary tuberculosis using the flexible fibreoptic bronchoscope. *Thorax* **41**:681–684.

137. **Williams, N. H., Jr., C. Kane, and O. H. Yoo.** 1973. Pulmonary function in miliary tuberculosis. *Am. Rev. Respir. Dis.* **107:**858–860.

138. **Winkler, A. W., and D. F. Crankshaw.** 1938. Chloride depletion in conditions other than Addison's disease. *J. Clin. Investig.* **17:**1–6.

139. **World Health Organization.** 2009. *Rapid Advice. Antiretroviral Therapy for HIV Infection in Adults and Adolescents.* World Health Organization, Geneva, Switzerland.

140. **World Health Organization.** 2009. *Treatment of Tuberculosis Guidelines*, 4th ed. WHO/HTM/TB/2009.420. World Health Organization, Geneva, Switzerland.

141. **World Health Organization.** 2003. 20 March 2010, posting date. *Revised Guidelines for National Programmes*, 3rd ed. WHO/CDS/TB/2003.313. Revision approved by STAG, June 2004. World Health Organization, Geneva, Switzerland.

http://www.who.int/docstore/gtb/publications/ttgnp/PDF/tb_2003_313chap4_rev.pdf.

142. **World Health Organization.** 2003. *Treatment of Tuberculosis: Guidelines for National Programmes*, 3rd ed. WHO/CDS/TB/2003.313. World Health Organization, Geneva, Switzerland.

143. **Yekanath, H., P. A. Gross, and J. H. Vitenson.** 1980. Miliary tuberculosis following ureteral catheterization. *Urology* **16:**197–198.

144. **Yokoyama, T., R. Toda, Y. Kimura, M. Mikagi, and H. Aizawa.** 2009. Addison's disease induced by miliary tuberculosis and the administration of rifampicin. *Intern. Med.* **48:**1297–1300. [Epub ahead of print.]

145. **Yu, R. S., S. Z. Zhang, J. J. Wu, and R. F. Li.** 2004. Imaging diagnosis of 12 patients with hepatic tuberculosis. *World J. Gastroenterol.* **10:**1639–1642.

Tuberculosis and Nontuberculous Mycobacterial Infections, 6th ed.
Edited by David Schlossberg
© 2011 ASM Press, Washington, DC

Chapter 28

Endocrine and Metabolic Aspects of Tuberculosis

Christopher Vinnard and Emily A. Blumberg

OVERVIEW

Endocrine and metabolic derangements are infrequent in patients with tuberculosis, but they are important when they occur. The basis for these abnormalities is complex. While *Mycobacterium tuberculosis* has been described to infect virtually every endocrine gland, the incidence of gland involvement is low, especially in the era of effective antituberculous therapy. Furthermore, endocrine and metabolic abnormalities do not always reflect direct infection of the gland but may result from physiological response or as a consequence of therapy. Metabolic disease may also predispose patients to the development of active tuberculosis, particularly in the case of diabetes mellitus. While hormonal therapy may be necessary in some instances, frequently these endocrine complications do not require specific interventions other than antituberculous therapy itself.

ADRENAL GLAND MANIFESTATIONS

Tuberculosis may lead to adrenal insufficiency by direct glandular involvement, by extra-adrenal infection, or as a by-product of antituberculous therapy. When primary adrenal insufficiency is a product of direct glandular involvement, signs and symptoms may not appear until more than 90% of the gland has been destroyed (142). Bilateral adrenal cortex destruction leads to a deficiency in the production of glucocorticoids, mineralcorticoids, and androgens.

In Addison's original description of 11 patients with the constellation of findings that characterizes primary adrenal insufficiency, 6 patients had adrenal tuberculosis. In a review of the adrenal pathology of 566 cases of Addison's disease in 1930, tuberculous adrenalitis was observed in 70% of cases (62). In areas where the incidence of tuberculosis has declined,

the role of tuberculosis as a cause of Addison's disease has likewise decreased.

Several patterns of direct adrenal gland involvement have been described. Primary adrenal insufficiency usually results from chronic infection of the adrenal gland with *M. tuberculosis*, with clinical manifestations becoming apparent years after the initial presentation. Less commonly, adrenal insufficiency may occur as an isolated manifestation of early adrenal involvement (62, 128, 154).

There are four classic histopathological patterns of adrenal tuberculosis: caseating or noncaseating granulomas, glandular enlargement with adrenal destruction by inflammatory granulomas, mass lesions secondary to the development of cold abscesses, and adrenal atrophy from fibrosis related to chronic infection (77). Epithelioid granulomas occur less frequently in the adrenals than in extra-adrenal foci, possibly reflecting the local production of anti-inflammatory steroids (89). Calcification of the gland is a common but not specific finding. Although descriptions of adrenal tuberculosis often focus on cortical involvement, it is important to note that the medulla may also be involved.

Adrenal tuberculosis results from early hematogenous spread; consequently, it is often associated with extra-adrenal infection. In a large autopsy series from Hong Kong, 6% of patients with active tuberculosis had evidence of adrenal infection, and in one-fourth of these patients infection was isolated to the adrenal glands (91). Other case series have found isolated adrenal tuberculosis in 3% of all patients with tuberculosis (3, 62). When infection is not isolated to the adrenals, the most common extra-adrenal manifestations are pulmonary and genitourinary tuberculosis (77). While both adrenal glands are usually involved, they may not be equally affected (14, 77, 81).

Adrenal insufficiency should be verified by demonstrating depressed morning plasma cortisol levels

Emily A. Blumberg and Christopher Vinnard • Division of Infectious Diseases, Department of Medicine, University of Pennsylvania School of Medicine, Philadelphia, PA 19104.

with a diminished response to synthetic adrenocorticotropin (ACTH) (38). Differences in the methods of assessment of adrenal insufficiency have led to a wide range in the reported incidence of pretreatment adrenal insufficiency. When adrenal function is measured appropriately in patients with tuberculosis prior to treatment, primary adrenal insufficiency is uncommonly found (13, 78, 117, 151). An impaired ACTH response has also been observed in the setting of an elevated basal cortisol level, but the clinical significance of this finding is uncertain (119, 161).

The possibility of adrenal tuberculosis should be considered when patients with a history of tuberculosis, either active disease or a positive tuberculin skin test, present with the classic manifestations of adrenal insufficiency: malaise, anorexia, orthostatic hypotension, and hyperpigmentation. The index of suspicion for adrenal insufficiency should be greater in patients with concurrent autoimmune disease, metastatic malignancy, sarcoidosis, amyloidosis, or treatment with potential adrenal suppressants. While human immunodeficiency virus (HIV) is also a cause of adrenal insufficiency, HIV infection did not confer additional risk of adrenal insufficiency among tuberculosis patients in Kenya (65). Laboratory abnormalities may include anemia, hyponatremia, and hyperkalemia. Rarely, patients may present with the acute onset of life-threatening adrenal insufficiency (113, 156).

Computed tomography (CT) is a useful noninvasive adjunct to diagnosis. During the first 2 years of illness, the most common CT findings include noncalcified, enlarged adrenal glands with areas of lucency secondary to necrosis (28, 46, 152). With chronic infection, the typical CT appearance is of shrunken adrenal glands, often with associated calcifications. The incidence of calcifications increases with the duration of illness, and their presence on CT imaging increases the likelihood of a diagnosis of tuberculosis (61). Findings on magnetic resonance imaging (MRI) are less well studied. In a single study of Chinese patients with proven adrenal tuberculosis, 83% of glands demonstrated peripheral enhancement on contrast MRI (162).

The differential diagnosis for adrenal enlargement includes malignancy, hemorrhage, fungal infection, amyloidosis, sarcoidosis, adenomas, hemangiomas, and hyperplasia. Whenever possible, tissue specimens should be obtained for microbiological and pathological analysis, especially in cases in which adrenal involvement is the only evidence of tuberculosis. CT-guided needle aspiration of the adrenal gland has been used successfully to obtain adequate tissue specimens for diagnosis (14, 28).

Treatment recommendations for adrenal tuberculosis are similar to those outlined for pulmonary tuberculosis in all cases, except for children with miliary tuberculosis, for whom treatment in excess of the standard 6-month regimen is recommended (5). Rifampin induces the hepatic enzymes responsible for the metabolism of steroids, thereby potentially increasing the metabolism of glucocorticoids; aldosterone is less likely to be affected (47, 82, 88, 130). Rarely, adrenal crisis has been precipitated by the administration of rifampin (159).

There are several reports of adrenal recovery when patients receive antituberculous therapy early in the course of disease, prior to the destruction of the adrenal gland (8, 36, 109, 156). Similarly, patients with extra-adrenal infection and blunted adrenal responses to ACTH have experienced improvement in adrenal function in response to antituberculous therapy (119). With chronic disease, adrenal gland destruction is usually substantial and treatment is unlikely to result in recovery of adrenal function (19).

THYROID GLAND TUBERCULOSIS

Tuberculosis uncommonly involves the thyroid gland. In a series of selected patients with late generalized tuberculosis occurring in the pre- and post-antibiotic eras, 14% of patients had evidence of thyroid seeding (139). Tuberculosis was seen in 0.1 to 1% of patients with thyroid tissue sampled for any indication (41, 99, 121). In a review of 2,426 Moroccan patients with thyroid tissue sampled, only 8 had evidence of tuberculosis; 5 patients had goiter and 3 patients had an isolated thyroid nodule (49).

Tuberculosis of the thyroid can result from hematogenous dissemination or by direct extension from an active laryngeal or lymph node focus. Five distinct presentations have been described: solitary cold abscess, diffuse goiter (often with caseation), acute abscess, multiple lesions from miliary spread, and chronic fibrosing tuberculosis (83). Miliary disease is the most common presentation, with multiple cold abscesses that mimic the presentation of thyroid carcinoma. Pathologically, tuberculosis causes the formation of epithelioid granulomas, usually with central caseation, Langerhans giant cells, and peripheral lymphocyte cuffing. Acid-fast stains are often positive (11, 74, 79).

Tuberculous thyroiditis and bacterial nontuberculous thyroiditis have important differences in their presenting signs and symptoms (17). Patients with tuberculous thyroiditis are less likely to note pain, thyroid tenderness, and fever than are patients with nontuberculous bacterial thyroiditis. Consequently, the duration of symptoms tends to be greater in patients with tuberculosis. In one comparative series, the mean duration of symptoms prior to diagnosis was 105 days for patients with tuberculosis, compared with 18 days for patients with acute nontuberculous bacterial thyroiditis (79). Patients with tuberculosis report a history of prior thyroid disease less frequently and are more likely to have normal leukocyte counts at the time of diagnosis. Both groups of patients may develop dysphagia, dysphonia, or even recurrent laryngeal nerve palsy related to compression of adjacent structures or fibrosis. These local extrathyroidal findings may be more common in patients with nontuberculous infections (17, 50).

Thyroid function tests are usually normal for patients with tuberculous thyroiditis, but thyrotoxicosis due to rapid release of stored thyroid hormone from the thyroid gland and myxedema caused by thyroid gland destruction have both been reported (11, 79, 99, 107). A review of 76 cases of thyroid tuberculosis previously reported in the literature found that only 4 cases showed evidence of abnormal thyroid function testing (27). The ultrasonographic appearance of tuberculous thyroiditis ranges from solid and heterogenous masses to cystic or hypoechoic lesions (41). Radionuclide thyroid scans typically reveal diminished uptake in the affected tissue (99). Consequently, tuberculous thyroiditis should be considered in patients with solitary cold thyroid nodules after other causes have been excluded, especially in tuberculin-positive patients with normal thyroid function studies.

Fine-needle aspiration for cytology and microbiology is the preferred diagnostic tool for the differentiation of tuberculous thyroiditis from carcinoma and other granulomatous entities, including sarcoidosis, syphilis, and Hashimoto's thyroiditis (41, 99). The definitive diagnosis of tuberculosis depends upon the demonstration of consistent cytopathological changes with either a positive acid-fast stain or culture for *M. tuberculosis*. In countries with a high incidence of tuberculosis, the diagnosis should be suspected and treatment started if epithelioid granulomas with caseation are found, even in the absence of confirmatory acid-fast studies (41). Although early definitions of thyroid tuberculosis required the demonstration of an extrathyroidal focus of infection, this requirement has been suspended in view of the more recent recognition of isolated involvement of the thyroid gland.

Many cases of thyroid tuberculosis have been treated with a combination of surgical and antimicrobial therapy. In most cases, surgery has been performed because the prevailing preoperative diagnosis was malignancy. In cases in which thyroidal tuberculosis was treated solely with standard antituberculous therapy, the response has been favorable, often with resolution of any abnormal results of thyroid

function studies (17, 107). Treatment regimens are identical to those outlined for adrenal tuberculosis.

Thyroid abnormalities may be noted in patients with active tuberculosis who do not have associated infection of the thyroid gland. Pulmonary tuberculosis is not typically associated with significant alterations in thyroid function, although elevations of free triiodothyronine (T_3) and total T_3 have been reported in response to therapy (69). In patients who are hospitalized with tuberculosis, the incidence of euthyroid sick syndrome has been substantial, ranging from 63 to 92% (34, 117). The presence of the euthyroid sick syndrome may serve as an indicator of severity of illness, given a significant association between mortality and diminished T_3 levels at the time of presentation (34). In that study, results of all thyroid studies were normal for survivors after 1 month of therapy.

Antituberculous therapy may also have some effect on thyroid appearance and function. Munkner reported an association between the administration of *p*-aminosalicylic acid and the development of goiter (103). In addition, induction of hepatic microsomal enzymes by rifampin may enhance the extrathyroidal metabolism of thyroid hormones, leading to decreased levels of serum free thyroxine and possibly reverse T_3 (110). Practically, these fluctuations are unlikely to significantly affect the patient's clinical course, and there are no reports of thyroid hormone supplementation being required for patients receiving rifampin.

PITUITARY GLAND TUBERCULOSIS

Pituitary gland tuberculosis is rarely seen. In an 11-year pre-antibiotic era autopsy series involving 14,160 specimens from Cook County Hospital, including 652 cases of pulmonary tuberculosis and 368 cases of tuberculous meningitis, only 2 specimens yielded evidence of anterior pituitary involvement (85). In the selected group of patients with late generalized tuberculosis, Slavin et al. noted a 4% incidence of pituitary involvement (139). It is important to note that in many cases tuberculous involvement of the pituitary is diagnosed purely on pathological grounds, often in the absence of confirmatory microbiology or even of positive acid-fast stains. In a literature review of infections involving the sella turcica, only nine cases included adequate evidence to diagnose tuberculosis definitively (16).

It has been postulated that pituitary tuberculosis can arise from hematogenous seeding, either in the presence or absence of miliary disease, or from direct extension from the sphenoid sinus, brain, or meninges (85). Depending on the pathogenesis, infection can involve the pituitary gland alone or be associated with tuberculosis in an adjacent or distant site.

The clinical presentation of pituitary tuberculosis can vary significantly. Compared with acute nontuberculous bacterial infection, the presentation is typically more indolent (16). Fever is often present. Patients may experience symptoms related to pituitary enlargement, including headache and visual complaints, with or without selective hypopituitarism (16, 120, 122). Sometimes, selective hypopituitarism occurs in the absence of other symptoms (44). Patients may be relatively asymptomatic, and the endocrine abnormalities may be subtle and noted only on detailed investigation. Any portion of the pituitary (including anterior, posterior, and the stalk) or the hypothalamus can be involved; consequently, presentations can vary and include growth retardation, hypogonadism, galactorrhea-amenorrhea related to excess prolactin secretion, diabetes insipidus, and even panhypopituitarism (26, 44, 85, 120, 122). Because of the small numbers of cases reported and the incomplete documentation of many of the reported cases, there is not a pathognomonic presentation associated with pituitary gland tuberculosis.

Although hypopituitarism may result from direct involvement of the pituitary gland, it may also occur in association with tuberculous meningitis (64, 90, 136). According to MRI performed on a small number of patients with a history of tuberculous meningitis and abnormal pituitary function, the pituitary often appeared normal. In some cases, third ventricle dilatation, pituitary atrophy, or enhancement of a portion of the gland or hypothalamus was noted (90).

Pituitary manifestations associated with tuberculous meningitis are variable and unpredictable and may not become apparent until years after recovery. Consequently, the true incidence of pituitary dysfunction following tuberculous meningitis is unknown. In the only detailed assessment of this phenomenon, Lam et al. studied all available patients who experienced tuberculous meningitis prior to the age of 21 years at a single hospital in Hong Kong (90). The investigators were only able to locate 49 of 246 eligible patients, and 10 of 49 patients had evidence of abnormal pituitary function, with growth hormone deficiency being the most common finding.

Infection of the pituitary itself should be suspected when patients with tuberculosis elsewhere present with any signs or symptoms of hypopituitarism. In addition to an assessment of endocrine function, radiologic studies are a useful adjunct to diagnosis. Skull films may demonstrate calcifications in the region of the sella turcica (90, 136). Appearance on CT or MRI suggests intrasellar tumor, and angiography results are normal (16, 55, 120). In some cases, thickening of the pituitary stalk, with or without pituitary extension into the sphenoid sinus, may be noted on CT or MRI (133, 141).

Definitive diagnosis rests on the pathological demonstration of caseating granulomas with documentation of the organism. Acid-fast stains are often negative; consequently, the diagnosis must also be considered if the patient has a positive tuberculin skin test result or evidence of tuberculosis in another location. Whenever possible, confirmatory cultures should be obtained. The differential diagnosis includes other granulomatous diseases of the pituitary, notably sarcoidosis, histiocytosis X, lymphocytic adenohypophysitis, syphilis, and giant cell granuloma (16).

There are no specific treatment recommendations for pituitary tuberculosis. Because of the association with tuberculous meningitis, lumbar puncture should be performed in patients with clinical signs or symptoms suggestive of meningeal involvement. While there are no specific treatment guidelines for pituitary tuberculosis, given the anatomic location it seems advisable to follow the guidelines for the treatment of tuberculous meningitis. In case reports where the diagnosis was made premortem, treatment with standard therapy led to resolution of compressive symptoms, with a return to normal pituitary function (55, 120).

HYPONATREMIA AND SYNDROME OF INAPPROPRIATE ANTIDIURETIC HORMONE

Disorders of sodium have long been associated with tuberculosis. Infrequently, hypernatremia secondary to diabetes insipidus has been recognized in patients with either pituitary tuberculosis or tuberculous meningitis (64, 122). Hyponatremia is more frequently seen in patients with active tuberculosis, with reported incidences of 10.7 and 43% in two large case series (35, 101).

The potential causes of tuberculosis-associated hyponatremia include adrenal insufficiency, the syndrome of inappropriate antidiuretic hormone (SIADH), and cerebral salt wasting. Hyponatremia from adrenal insufficiency is accompanied by hyperkalemia and increased urine potassium excretion, and adrenal function can be assessed by an adrenal stimulation test. When adrenal function is normal, hyponatremia is almost always a consequence of free water intake and retention (inappropriate antidiuresis). SIADH results from ongoing secretion of arginine vasopressin (antidiuretic hormone), from either the pituitary gland or an ectopic site, despite the presence of hyponatremia and extracellular volume expansion (48). Cerebral salt wasting is an alternate explanation for the development of hyponatremia in patients with tuberculous meningitis.

Weiss and Katz first noted the association of pulmonary tuberculosis with SIADH (155). They observed excessive urinary sodium excretion in four patients with active pulmonary tuberculosis and hyponatremia. With marked fluid restriction, the patients experienced an increase in the serum sodium and decrease in urinary sodium excretion, and all surviving patients experienced normalization of their serum sodium levels during antituberculous therapy.

Subsequently, several mechanisms have been proposed for the development of SIADH in patients with pulmonary tuberculosis. First, hypoxemia associated with pulmonary tuberculosis may stimulate baroreceptors, leading to arginine vasopressin release from the posterior pituitary gland (6). This relationship would also explain the development of SIADH in other pulmonary diseases characterized by hypoxemia (including acute respiratory failure and chronic obstructive pulmonary disease) (157). A second possibility is a shift in osmoregulation during active tuberculosis (the "reset osmostat"). Hill et al. measured levels of arginine vasopressin in patients with pulmonary tuberculosis (66). Levels of arginine vasopressin were elevated despite the presence of hyponatremia and subsequently declined after the administration of free water. This response to a hyposmolal stimulus suggests that osmoregulation was functioning, but at a lower set point for serum osmolality. Finally, ectopic production of arginine vasopressin has been proposed as a third mechanism for SIADH in pulmonary tuberculosis, suggested by a case report of SIADH developing in a pulmonary tuberculosis patient with long-standing diabetes insipidus (94).

As with other infections of the central nervous system, hyponatremia is also seen in a significant proportion of patients with tuberculous meningitis. In a pediatric population with tuberculous meningitis, SIADH was noted in 71% of patients and appeared to be a predictor of increased mortality rate (39). A study of adult patients with tuberculous meningitis reported SIADH in 45% of patients (123). An association was observed between SIADH and increased intracranial pressure in children with tuberculous meningitis (40).

The degree of hyponatremia is variable in patients with tuberculosis, and most patients are asymptomatic. In the vast majority of patients, hyponatremia resolves concurrently with response to antituberculosis therapy (66). After ruling out volume depletion as the cause of hyponatremia, water restriction should be considered only in those patients with severe or symptomatic hyponatremia. Additional pharmacological interventions are generally not required. When correction of hyponatremia is indicated for clinical reasons, accepted practice guidelines for the rate of serum sodium correction should be followed (48).

Finally, cerebral salt wasting has been proposed as an alternate, but controversial, explanation for the onset of hyponatremia in patients with central nervous system injury, including tuberculous meningitis (137). Both SIADH and cerebral salt wasting are characterized by hyponatremia, elevated urine osmolality, and elevated urine sodium excretion. However, urine sodium excretion is the putative cause of hyponatremia in cerebral salt wasting, leading to a decrease in extracellular fluid volume (114). This distinction between SIADH and cerebral salt wasting syndrome is difficult to establish given the uncertainty in assessing a patient's extracellular volume status (42, 149). Several investigators have reported the successful treatment of suspected cerebral salt wasting in tuberculous meningitis patients with the administration of hypertonic saline and fludrocortisone (30, 32, 104).

HYPERCALCEMIA

Tuberculosis is a well-described cause of hypercalcemia. In one large series of patients from Hong Kong, 6% of patients with confirmed hypercalcemia had tuberculosis (135). The actual prevalence of hypercalcemia in patients with tuberculosis is difficult to estimate, as concurrent serum albumin levels are not always reported. Moreover, the reported rates vary considerably according to geography. Surveys from India, Hong Kong, the United States, Malaysia, and Greece report prevalence rates between 11 and 48%, with the highest rates occurring in the sunniest climates and in patients receiving supplemental calcium and/or vitamin D (1, 86, 95, 125, 134). In contrast, surveys from Great Britain, Belgium, and Turkey reported a much lower prevalence of hypercalcemia (24, 56, 80).

The majority of the reports of hypercalcemia are for patients with pulmonary tuberculosis, perhaps reflecting the preponderance of pulmonary infection over infection at other sites. Patients with hypercalcemia often demonstrate more extensive pulmonary involvement, but the association with disease severity is inconsistent (86, 131, 135). Hypercalcemia has been less frequently noted in conjunction with extrapulmonary disease, including miliary infection, peritonitis, and osteomyelitis (23, 96, 158). Frequently, hypercalcemia is not noted at the time of diagnosis but occurs early in the course of treatment (131, 135). Initial assessments may not account for disease-related hypoalbuminemia, and hypercalcemia may only appear as the serum albumin increases during treatment, reflecting an improvement in nutritional status (105). Hypercalcemia has also developed following the initiation of antiretroviral therapy in patients coinfected with HIV and tuberculosis (53, 92).

The mechanism of tuberculosis-associated hypercalcemia remains uncertain. Multiple studies have excluded the common causes of hypercalcemia in these patients, including coexisting hyperparathyroidism, malignancy, adrenal insufficiency, milk-alkali syndrome, and hyperthyroidism (1). According to one possible explanation, hypercalcemia develops as a consequence of increased levels of 1,25-dihydroxyvitamin D in patients with pulmonary tuberculosis. In support of this mechanism, several investigators have reported elevated 1,25-dihydroxyvitamin D levels and low to normal 25-hydroxyvitamin D levels in tuberculosis patients with hypercalcemia (52, 58, 70, 115, 127). Hypercalcemia was also more common in tuberculosis patients receiving vitamin D supplementation (1).

In healthy individuals, conversion of 25-hydroxyvitamin D to 1,25-hydroxyvitamin D by the enzyme 1-alpha-hydroxylase takes place in the renal tubules. However, hypercalcemia is frequently reported to occur in tuberculosis patients with chronic kidney disease, including patients receiving peritoneal dialysis or hemodialysis (67, 93, 160). Tuberculosis-associated hypercalcemia has even been observed in anephric patients (52, 58, 115). These findings suggest an extrarenal site of production of 1,25-dihydroxyvitamin D in patients with tuberculosis.

Given that hypercalcemia is also seen in other granulomatous diseases, the granuloma itself may be the site of extrarenal production of 1,25-dihydroxyvitamin D. Macrophages can express the enzyme 1-alpha-hydroxylase, and alveolar macrophages recovered from a patient with active pulmonary tuberculosis were able to synthesize 1,25-dihydroxyvitamin D in vitro (29, 100). A study of peripheral blood mononuclear cells taken from patients with active tuberculosis found an increased rate of conversion of 1,25-dihydroxyvitamin D compared to that in peripheral blood mononuclear cells taken from healthy controls (33).

The physiological role for macrophage production of 1,25-dihydroxyvitamin D is uncertain. According to one proposed mechanism, 1,25-dihydroxyvitamin D enhances the antimycobacterial activity of the monocyte, either as a direct effect or by enhancing cellular responses to gamma interferon (124). Alternatively, more recent work has found that macrophage 1,25-dihydroxyvitamin D production led to an inhibition of nitric oxide (NO) release, and the investigators suggest that NO inhibition provides protection from oxidative injury (33). According to either mechanism, increased intestinal absorption of calcium is a by-product of macrophage 1,25-dihydroxyvitamin D production, leading to the observed association between active tuberculosis and hypercalcemia.

It should also be noted that other studies have refuted the importance of vitamin D in the pathogenesis of tuberculosis-associated hypercalcemia. In clinical trials of patients with active tuberculosis from the United States, Africa, and Belgium, there was no correlation between 1,25-dihydroxyvitamin D levels and serum calcium measurements (43, 56, 145).

Finally, antituberculous therapy influences calcium homeostasis. In healthy individuals, both isoniazid and rifampin reduce circulating levels of 25-hydroxyvitamin D and 1,25-dihydroxyvitamin D (25, 43). Although long-term administration of both drugs to tuberculosis patients affected 25-hydroxyvitamin D levels, the effect of the combination was less than anticipated. Furthermore, levels of 1,25-dihydroxyvitamin D were not affected with long-term administration, and as a result the overall clinical impact was insignificant.

With marked hypercalcemia, patients may develop any of the symptoms characteristically associated with hypercalcemia, including lethargy and even metastatic calcifications (158). In most cases, however, hypercalcemia associated with tuberculosis is mild, and patients typically experience complete resolution within 1 to 7 months of antituberculous therapy without additional intervention (134).

DIABETES MELLITUS

Hyperglycemia is a common occurrence in patients with tuberculosis, and individuals who have no history of diabetes may demonstrate impaired glucose tolerance at the time of diagnosis of tuberculosis. In one study of 506 consecutive patients with active pulmonary tuberculosis, 2% had a history of diabetes mellitus, 5% were found to be newly diabetic, and 16% had impaired glucose tolerance (102). Additional studies have supported the association between active pulmonary infection and glucose intolerance, noting that impaired glucose tolerance resolved with effective antituberculous treatment (60, 112).

Patients with an established diagnosis of diabetes mellitus appear to be at increased risk for the development of tuberculosis. This observation was initially noted in studies from the pretreatment era, including a 1946 survey from Philadelphia, Pennsylvania, in which the incidence of tuberculosis was nearly twofold higher in patients with diabetes (20).

A recent meta-analysis of 13 separate observational studies found that the risk of developing active tuberculosis was three times greater in patients with diabetes (72). While the risk of developing tuberculosis does not appear to be associated with the duration of diabetes, several investigators have observed an association with the severity of diabetes, as measured by daily insulin requirements (20, 51, 111, 146).

Diabetes may lead to increased susceptibility to tuberculosis through several mechanisms. Diabetic patients demonstrate impaired granulocyte chemotaxis, phagocytosis, bactericidal activity, and superoxide production. Furthermore, monocyte/macrophage function may also be impaired. Reduced numbers of circulating peripheral monocytes, decreased phagocytosis, and alterations in surface receptors may all contribute to increased susceptibility to infections with intracellular pathogens (57, 59). Impaired in vitro lymphocyte responses have also been reported for patients with poorly controlled diabetes (31).

Commonly, the presentation of tuberculosis in diabetic patients resembles that in nondiabetic patients. However, some differences have been noted with regard to radiographic findings. Both early and later reports suggested that diabetics were more likely to have involvement of lower lobes, unusual segments of the middle and upper lobes, and multilobar disease (9, 15, 21, 63, 116, 140). Ikezoe et al. compared the CT appearances of pulmonary tuberculosis in diabetic and nondiabetic patients with and without other types of immunocompromise (68). They found that diabetic patients were more likely to have nonsegmental distribution of lesions and multiple cavities within any single lesion. Other investigators have also found an increase in cavity formation in diabetic patients with tuberculosis (148, 153).

The Advisory Committee for Elimination of Tuberculosis includes diabetes mellitus among the clinical conditions that warrant targeted tuberculin testing, with 10 mm of induration as the criterion for a positive tuberculin skin test (4). Patients with well-controlled diabetes appear to respond to standard intradermal testing (118).

While drug regimens for active tuberculosis are identical for diabetic and nondiabetic patients, treatment outcomes may differ. A single study has reported a higher incidence of relapse in diabetics treated with a 9-month regimen (76). In a study from Indonesia comparing tuberculosis patients with and without diabetes, diabetic patients were more likely to remain sputum smear positive after 2 months of therapy and sputum culture positive after 6 months of therapy (2). In contrast, diabetic and nondiabetic patients in the United States had similar rates of 2-month culture conversion (45).

There is also concern that diabetes may lead to differences in pharmacokinetics of the antituberculous drugs. Diabetic patients in Indonesia had lower exposure to rifampin in the continuation phase of treatment than did nondiabetic patients, which may have been a consequence of differences in body weight (18, 108). In the same population, diabetes did not influence the pharmacokinetics of antituberculous drugs during the intensive phase of treatment (126). Two studies have noted an increased incidence of multidrug-resistant tuberculosis among diabetic patients (12, 54). However, other investigators have not found an association between diabetes and multidrug resistance (138, 143, 144, 147).

Finally, diabetes presents additional treatment considerations during antituberculous therapy. Diabetic patients may have increased risk of neuropathy associated with isoniazid, even with concurrent use of pyridoxine (87). Glycemic control may also worsen during antituberculous therapy, as rifampin induces the metabolism of certain oral hypoglycemic agents (71, 106). Diabetic patients should be monitored closely for these developments during treatment for tuberculosis.

CORTICOSTEROIDS AND TUBERCULOSIS

The exact impact of corticosteroid administration on the development and diagnosis of tuberculosis remains somewhat controversial, and the critical dose and duration of corticosteroid exposure associated with tuberculosis reactivation are unknown. In a retrospective study of patients in the United Kingdom receiving corticosteroid treatment for any indication, corticosteroid use within the preceding 6 months was associated with increased odds of developing tuberculosis (73).

Other studies have examined disease-specific risk of tuberculosis duration treatment with corticosteroids. Low-risk patients receiving chronic low dose corticosteroid therapy for treatment of systemic rheumatologic diseases did not have increased reactivation of tuberculosis (7). Higher corticosteroid doses have been associated with reactivation in patients with rheumatic diseases, but the critical dose threshold is unknown (84). Corticosteroid-dependent asthmatics with a history of positive tuberculin skin tests were not at increased risk for the development of active tuberculosis, and use of high-dose inhaled corticosteroids was not associated with reactivation in tuberculin-positive pediatric patients with prior *Mycobacterium bovis* BCG vaccination (10, 129, 132). Finally, there does not appear to be any increased risk for patients with AIDS who are receiving corticosteroids as adjunctive therapy for *Pneumocystis carinii* pneumonia (75, 98).

Corticosteroid administration can decrease the reliability of tuberculin skin testing. Healthy adult volunteers who were known to be tuberculin positive were treated with 40 mg of prednisone per day for 1 month, and inhibition of the response to tuberculin skin testing began at a mean of 14 days and ended 6 days after suspension of steroid therapy (22). Smaller corticosteroid doses affect skin test responses unpredictably (129, 150). Patients who receive alternate-day corticosteroid therapy generally have preserved responses to tuberculin skin testing (97, 129). Of note, patients who are given corticosteroids to treat underlying immunologic disorders may actually experience augmented responses to tuberculin skin testing (150).

The American Thoracic Society recommends targeted tuberculin testing for all patients who receive more than 15 mg of prednisone daily (or its equivalent) for greater than 1 month's duration, with 5 mm of induration as the criterion for a positive test (4). In patients with positive tuberculin skin testing, there is no contraindication to continuing corticosteroid treatment as required for concurrent illnesses, provided that antituberculous therapy is also administered (37).

SUMMARY

The endocrine and metabolic manifestations of tuberculosis are protean. Direct involvement of endocrine glands is only one way in which tuberculosis can affect hormonal and metabolic function. Indirect effects of infection and the impact of treatment on hormonal function must also be considered. Ultimately, treatment plans should be tailored which take into account both the direct and indirect impact of *M. tuberculosis* infection.

REFERENCES

1. Abbasi, A. A., J. K. Chemplavil, S. Farah, B. F. Muller, and A. R. Arnstein. 1979. Hypercalcemia in active pulmonary tuberculosis. *Ann. Intern. Med.* **90:**324–328.
2. Alisjahbana, B., E. Sahiratmadja, E. J. Nelwan, A. M. Purwa, Y. Ahmad, T. H. Ottenhoff, R. H. Nelwan, I. Parwati, J. W. van der Meer, and R. van Crevel. 2007. The effect of type 2 diabetes mellitus on the presentation and treatment response of pulmonary tuberculosis. *Clin. Infect. Dis.* **45:**428–435.
3. Alvarez, S., and W. R. McCabe. 1984. Extrapulmonary tuberculosis revisited: a review of experience at Boston City and other hospitals. *Medicine* (Baltimore) **63:**25–55.
4. American Thoracic Society. 2000. Targeted tuberculin testing and treatment of latent tuberculosis infection. *Am. J. Respir. Crit. Care Med.* **161:**S221–S247.
5. American Thoracic Society/Centers for Disease Control and Prevention/Infectious Disease Society of America. 2003. Treatment of tuberculosis. *Am. J. Respir. Crit. Care Med.* **167:**603–662.
6. Anderson, R. J., R. G. Pluss, A. S. Berns, J. T. Jackson, P. E. Arnold, R. W. Schrier, and K. E. McDonald. 1978. Mechanism of effect of hypoxia on renal water excretion. *J. Clin. Investig.* **62:**769–777.
7. Andonopoulos, A. P., C. Safridi, D. Karokis, and A. Bounas. 1998. Is a purified protein derivative skin and subsequent antituberculous chemoprophylaxis really necessary in systemic rheumatic disease patients receiving corticosteroids? *Clin. Rheumatol.* **17:**181–185.
8. Annear, T. D., and G. P. Baker. 1961. Tuberculous Addison's disease. A case apparently cured by chemotherapy. *Lancet* **ii:** 577–578.
9. Bacakoglu, F., O. K. Basoglu, G. Cok, A. Sayiner, and M. Ates. 2001. Pulmonary tuberculosis in patients with diabetes mellitus. *Respiration* **68:**595–600.
10. Bahceciler, N. N., Y. Nuhoglu, M. A. Nursoy, N. Kodalli, I. B. Barlan, and M. M. Basaran. 2000. Inhaled corticosteroid therapy is safe in tuberculin-positive asthmatic children. *Pediatr. Infect. Dis. J.* **19:**215–218.
11. Barnes, P., and R. Weatherstone. 1979. Tuberculosis of the thyroid: two case reports. *Br. J. Dis. Chest* **73:**187–191.
12. Bashar, M., P. Alcabes, W. N. Rom, and R. Condos. 2001. Increased incidence of multidrug-resistant tuberculosis in diabetic patients on the Bellevue Chest Service, 1987 to 1997. *Chest* **120:**1514–1519.
13. Beadsworth, M. B., J. J. van Oosterhout, M. J. Diver, E. B. Faragher, A. Shenkin, H. C. Mwandumba, S. Khoo, T. O'Dempsey, S. B. Squire, and E. E. Zijlstra. 2008. Hypoadrenalism is not associated with early mortality during tuberculosis treatment in Malawi. *Int. J. Tuberc. Lung Dis.* **12:**314–318.
14. Benini, F., T. Savarin, G. E. Senna, S. Durigato, and L. Vettore. 1990. Diagnostic and therapeutic problems in a case of adrenal tuberculosis and acute Addison's disease. *J. Endocrinol. Investig.* **13:**597–600.
15. Berger, H. W., and M. G. Granada. 1974. Lower lung field tuberculosis. *Chest* **65:**522–526.
16. Berger, S. A., S. C. Edberg, and G. David. 1986. Infectious disease in the sella turcica. *Rev. Infect. Dis.* **8:**747–755.
17. Berger, S. A., J. Zonszein, P. Villamena, and N. Mittman. 1983. Infectious diseases of the thyroid gland. *Rev. Infect. Dis.* **5:** 108–122.
18. Beth Gadkowski, L., and J. E. Stout. 2007. Pharmacokinetics of rifampicin. *Clin. Infect. Dis.* **44:**618–619. (Author's reply, **44:**619.)
19. Bhatia, E., S. K. Jain, R. K. Gupta, and R. Pandey. 1998. Tuberculous Addison's disease: lack of normalization of adrenocortical function after anti-tuberculous chemotherapy. *Clin. Endocrinol.* (Oxford) **48:**355–359.
20. Boucot, K., P. Cooper, and E. Dillon. 1952. Tuberculosis among diabetics. The Philadelphia survey. *Am. Rev. Tuberc.* **65:**1.
21. Boucot, K. R. 1957. Diabetes mellitus and pulmonary tuberculosis. *J. Chronic Dis.* **6:**256–279.
22. Bovornkitti, S., P. Kangsadal, P. Sathirapat, and P. Oonsombatti. 1960. Reversion and reconversion rate of tuberculin skin reactions in correction with the use of prednisone. *Dis. Chest* **38:**51–55.
23. Braman, S. S., A. L. Goldman, and M. I. Schwarz. 1973. Steroid-responsive hypercalcemia in disseminated bone tuberculosis. *Arch. Intern. Med.* **132:**269–271.
24. British Thoracic Association. 1981. A controlled trial of six months of chemotherapy in pulmonary tuberculosis. *Br. J. Dis. Chest* **75:**141–153.

25. Brodie, M. J., A. R. Boobis, C. J. Hillyard, G. Abeyasekera, J. C. Stevenson, I. MacIntyre, and B. K. Park. 1982. Effect of rifampicin and isoniazid on vitamin D metabolism. *Clin. Pharmacol. Ther.* **32:**525–530.

26. Brooks, M. H., J. S. Dumlao, D. Bronsky, and S. S. Waldstein. 1973. Hypophysial tuberculoma with hypopituitarism. *Am. J. Med.* **54:**777–781.

27. Bulbuloglu, E., H. Ciralik, E. Okur, G. Ozdemir, F. Ezberci, and A. Cetinkaya. 2006. Tuberculosis of the thyroid gland: review of the literature. *World J. Surg.* **30:**149–155.

28. Buxi, T. B., R. B. Vohra, Sujatha, S. P. Byotra, S. Mukherji, and M. Daniel. 1992. CT in adrenal enlargement due to tuberculosis: a review of literature with five new cases. *Clin. Imaging* **16:**102–108.

29. Cadranel, J., A. J. Hance, B. Milleron, F. Paillard, G. M. Akoun, and M. Garabedian. 1988. Vitamin D metabolism in tuberculosis. Production of 1,25(OH)2D3 by cells recovered by bronchoalveolar lavage and the role of this metabolite in calcium homeostasis. *Am. Rev. Respir. Dis.* **138:**984–989.

30. Camous, L., N. Valin, J. L. Zaragoza, E. Bourry, E. Caumes, G. Deray, and H. Izzedine. 2008. Hyponatraemic syndrome in a patient with tuberculosis—always the adrenals? *Nephrol. Dial. Transplant.* **23:**393–395.

31. Casey, J. I., B. J. Heeter, and K. A. Klyshevich. 1977. Impaired response of lymphocytes of diabetic subjects to antigen of *Staphylococcus aureus. J. Infect. Dis.* **136:**495–501.

32. Celik, U. S., D. Alabaz, D. Yildizdas, E. Alhan, E. Kocabas, and S. Ulutan. 2005. Cerebral salt wasting in tuberculous meningitis: treatment with fludrocortisone. *Ann. Trop. Paediatr.* **25:**297–302.

33. Chang, J. M., M. C. Kuo, H. T. Kuo, S. J. Hwang, J. C. Tsai, H. C. Chen, and Y. H. Lai. 2004. 1-α,25-Dihydroxyvitamin D3 regulates inducible nitric oxide synthase messenger RNA expression and nitric oxide release in macrophage-like RAW 264.7 cells. *J. Lab. Clin. Med.* **143:**14–22.

34. Chow, C. C., T. W. Mak, C. H. Chan, and C. S. Cockram. 1995. Euthyroid sick syndrome in pulmonary tuberculosis before and after treatment. *Ann. Clin. Biochem.* **32**(Pt. 4):385–391.

35. Chung, D. K., and W. W. Hubbard. 1969. Hyponatremia in untreated active pulmonary tuberculosis. *Am. Rev. Respir. Dis.* **99:**595–597.

36. Coleman, E. N., and G. C. Arneil. 1962. Acute tuberculous adrenocortical failure with clinical recovery. *Lancet* **i:**886–888.

37. The Committee on Therapy. 1968. Adrenal corticosteroids and tuberculosis. *Am. Rev. Respir. Dis.* **97:**484–485.

38. Cooper, M. S., and P. M. Stewart. 2003. Corticosteroid insufficiency in acutely ill patients. *N. Engl. J. Med.* **348:**727–734.

39. Cotton, M. F., P. R. Donald, J. F. Schoeman, C. Aalbers, L. E. Van Zyl, and C. Lombard. 1991. Plasma arginine vasopressin and the syndrome of inappropriate antidiuretic hormone secretion in tuberculous meningitis. *Pediatr. Infect. Dis. J.* **10:**837–842.

40. Cotton, M. F., P. R. Donald, J. F. Schoeman, L. E. Van Zyl, C. Aalbers, and C. J. Lombard. 1993. Raised intracranial pressure, the syndrome of inappropriate antidiuretic hormone secretion, and arginine vasopressin in tuberculous meningitis. *Childs Nerv. Syst.* **9:**10–15; discussion, 15–16.

41. Das, D. K., C. S. Pant, K. L. Chachra, and A. K. Gupta. 1992. Fine needle aspiration cytology diagnosis of tuberculous thyroiditis. A report of eight cases. *Acta Cytol.* **36:**517–522.

42. Dass, R., R. Nagaraj, J. Murlidharan, and S. Singhi. 2003. Hyponatraemia and hypovolemic shock with tuberculous meningitis. *Indian J. Pediatr.* **70:**995–997.

43. Davies, P. D., H. A. Church, R. C. Brown, and J. S. Woodhead. 1987. Raised serum calcium in tuberculosis patients in Africa. *Eur. J. Respir. Dis.* **71:**341–344.

44. Delsedime, M., M. Aguggia, R. Cantello, I. Chiado Cutin, G. Nicola, R. Torta, and M. Gilli. 1988. Isolated hypophyseal tuberculoma: case report. *Clin. Neuropathol.* **7:**311–313.

45. Dooley, K. E., T. Tang, J. E. Golub, S. E. Dorman, and W. Cronin. 2009. Impact of diabetes mellitus on treatment outcomes of patients with active tuberculosis. *Am. J. Trop. Med. Hyg.* **80:**634–639.

46. Doppman, J. L., J. R. Gill, Jr., A. W. Nienhuis, J. M. Earll, and J. A. Long, Jr. 1982. CT findings in Addison's disease. *J. Comput. Assist. Tomogr.* **6:**757–761.

47. Edwards, O. M., R. J. Courtenay-Evans, J. M. Galley, J. Hunter, and A. D. Tait. 1974. Changes in cortisol metabolism following rifampicin therapy. *Lancet* **ii:**548–551.

48. Ellison, D. H., and T. Berl. 2007. Clinical practice. The syndrome of inappropriate antidiuresis. *N. Engl. J. Med.* **356:**2064–2072.

49. El Malki, H. O., R. Mohsine, K. Benkhraba, M. Amahzoune, A. Benkabbou, M. El Absi, L. Ifrine, A. Belkouchi, and S. Balafrej. 2006. Thyroid tuberculosis: diagnosis and treatment. *Chemotherapy* **52:**46–49.

50. Emery, P. 1980. Tuberculous abscess of the thyroid with recurrent laryngeal nerve palsy: case report and review of the literature. *J. Laryngol. Otol.* **94:**553–558.

51. Ezung, T., N. T. Devi, N. T. Singh, and T. B. Singh. 2002. Pulmonary tuberculosis and diabetes mellitus—a study. *J. Indian Med. Assoc.* **100:**376, 378–379.

52. Felsenfeld, A. J., M. K. Drezner, and F. Llach. 1986. Hypercalcemia and elevated calcitriol in a maintenance dialysis patient with tuberculosis. *Arch. Intern. Med.* **146:**1941–1945.

53. Ferrand, R. A., A. Elgalib, W. Newsholme, A. Childerhouse, S. G. Edwards, and R. F. Miller. 2006. Hypercalcaemia complicating immune reconstitution in an HIV-infected patient with disseminated tuberculosis. *Int. J. STD AIDS* **17:**349–350.

54. Fisher-Hoch, S. P., E. Whitney, J. B. McCormick, G. Crespo, B. Smith, M. H. Rahbar, and B. I. Restrepo. 2008. Type 2 diabetes and multidrug-resistant tuberculosis. *Scand. J. Infect. Dis.* **40:**888–893.

55. Flannery, M. T., S. Pattani, P. M. Wallach, and E. Warner. 1993. Case report: hypothalamic tuberculoma associated with secondary panhypopituitarism. *Am. J. Med. Sci.* **306:**101–103.

56. Fuss, M., R. Karmali, T. Pepersack, A. Bergans, P. Dierckx, T. Prigogine, P. Bergmann, and J. Corvilain. 1988. Are tuberculous patients at a great risk from hypercalcemia? *Q. J. Med.* **69:**869–878.

57. Geisler, C., T. Almdal, J. Bennedsen, J. M. Rhodes, and K. Kolendorf. 1982. Monocyte functions in diabetes mellitus. *Acta Pathol. Microbiol. Immunol. Scand. C* **90:**33–37.

58. Gkonos, P. J., R. London, and E. D. Hendler. 1984. Hypercalcemia and elevated 1,25-dihydroxyvitamin D levels in a patient with end-stage renal disease and active tuberculosis. *N. Engl. J. Med.* **311:**1683–1685.

59. Glass, E. J., J. Stewart, D. M. Matthews, A. Collier, B. F. Clarke, and D. M. Weir. 1987. Impairment of monocyte "lectin-like" receptor activity in type 1 (insulin-dependent) diabetic patients. *Diabetologia* **30:**228–231.

60. Gulbas, Z., Y. Erdogan, and S. Balci. 1987. Impaired glucose tolerance in pulmonary tuberculosis. *Eur. J. Respir. Dis.* **71:**345–347.

61. Guo, Y. K., Z. G. Yang, Y. Li, E. S. Ma, Y. P. Deng, P. Q. Min, L. L. Yin, J. Hu, X. C. Zhang, and T. W. Chen. 2007. Addison's disease due to adrenal tuberculosis: contrast-enhanced CT features and clinical duration correlation. *Eur. J. Radiol.* **62:**126–131.

62. Guttman, P. 1930. Addison's disease: a statistical analysis of 566 cases and a study of pathology. *Arch. Pathol.* **10:**742–745.

63. Hadlock, F. P., S. K. Park, R. J. Awe, and M. Rivera. 1980. Unusual radiographic findings in adult pulmonary tuberculosis. *Am. J. Roentgenol.* 134:1015–1018.

64. Haslam, R. H., W. W. Winternitz, and J. Howieson. 1969. Selective hypopituitarism following tuberculous meningitis. *Am. J. Dis. Child.* 118:903–908.

65. Hawken, M. P., J. C. Ojoo, J. S. Morris, E. W. Kariuki, W. A. Githui, E. S. Juma, S. N. Gathua, J. N. Kimari, L. N. Thiong'o, J. G. Raynes, P. Broadbent, C. F. Gilks, L. S. Otieno, and K. P. McAdam. 1996. No increased prevalence of adrenocortical insufficiency in human immunodeficiency virus-associated tuberculosis. *Tuber. Lung Dis.* 77:444–448.

66. Hill, A. R., J. Uribarri, J. Mann, and T. Berl. 1990. Altered water metabolism in tuberculosis: role of vasopressin. *Am. J. Med.* 88:357–364.

67. Hung, Y. M., H. H. Chan, and H. M. Chung. 2004. Tuberculous peritonitis in different dialysis patients in Southern Taiwan. *Am. J. Trop. Med. Hyg.* 70:532–535.

68. Ikezoe, J., N. Takeuchi, T. Johkoh, N. Kohno, N. Tomiyama, T. Kozuka, K. Noma, and E. Ueda. 1992. CT appearance of pulmonary tuberculosis in diabetic and immunocompromised patients: comparison with patients who had no underlying disease. *Am. J. Roentgenol.* 159:1175–1179.

69. Ilias, I., A. Tselebis, A. Boufas, G. Panoutsopoulos, N. Filippou, and J. Christakopoulou. 1998. Pulmonary tuberculosis and its therapy do not significantly affect thyroid function tests. *Int. J. Clin. Pract.* 52:227–228.

70. Isaacs, R. D., G. I. Nicholson, and I. M. Holdaway. 1987. Miliary tuberculosis with hypercalcaemia and raised vitamin D concentrations. *Thorax* 42:555–556.

71. Jaakkola, T., J. T. Backman, M. Neuvonen, J. Laitila, and P. J. Neuvonen. 2006. Effect of rifampicin on the pharmacokinetics of pioglitazone. *Br. J. Clin. Pharmacol.* 61:70–78.

72. Jeon, C. Y., and M. B. Murray. 2008. Diabetes mellitus increases the risk of active tuberculosis: a systematic review of 13 observational studies. *PLoS Med.* 5:e152.

73. Jick, S. S., E. S. Lieberman, M. U. Rahman, and H. K. Choi. 2006. Glucocorticoid use, other associated factors, and the risk of tuberculosis. *Arthritis Rheum.* 55:19–26.

74. Johnson, A. G., M. E. Phillips, and R. J. Thomas. 1973. Acute tuberculous abscess of the thyroid gland. *Br. J. Surg.* 60:668–669.

75. Jones, B. E., E. K. Taikwel, A. L. Mercado, S. U. Sian, and P. F. Barnes. 1994. Tuberculosis in patients with HIV infection who receive corticosteroids for presumed *Pneumocystis carinii* pneumonia. *Am. J. Respir. Crit. Care Med.* 149:1686–1688.

76. Kameda, K., S. Kawabata, and N. Masuda. 1990. Follow-up study of short-course chemotherapy of pulmonary tuberculosis complicated with diabetes mellitus. *Kekkaku* 65:791–803.

77. Kannan, C. 1988. *The Adrenal Gland*, vol. 2. Plenum Medical Book Company, New York, NY.

78. Kaplan, F. J. L., N. S. Levitt, and S. G. Soule. 2000. Primary hypoadrenalism assessed by the 1 microgram ACTH test in hospitalized patients with active pulmonary tuberculosis. *Q. J. Med.* 93:603–609.

79. Kapoor, V. K., K. Subramani, S. K. Das, A. K. Mukhopadhyay, and T. K. Chattopadhyay. 1985. Tuberculosis of the thyroid gland associated with thyrotoxicosis. *Postgrad. Med. J.* 61:339–340.

80. Kelestimur, F., M. Guven, M. Ozesmi, and H. Pasaoglu. 1996. Does tuberculosis really cause hypercalcemia? *J. Endocrinol. Investig.* 19:678–681.

81. Kelestimur, F., O. Ozbakir, A. Saglam, F. Ozturk, and M. Yucesoy. 1993. Acute adrenocortical failure due to tuberculosis. *J. Endocrinol. Investig.* 16:281–284.

82. Keven, K., A. R. Uysal, and G. Erdogan. 1998. Adrenal function during tuberculous infection and effects of antituberculosis treatment on endogenous and exogenous steroids. *Int. J. Tuberc. Lung Dis.* 2:419–424.

83. Khan, E. M., I. Haque, R. Pandey, S. K. Mishra, and A. K. Sharma. 1993. Tuberculosis of the thyroid gland: a clinicopathological profile of four cases and review of the literature. *Aust. N. Z. J. Surg.* 63:807–810.

84. Kim, H. A., C. D. Yoo, H. J. Baek, E. B. Lee, C. Ahn, J. S. Han, S. Kim, J. S. Lee, K. W. Choe, and Y. W. Song. 1998. *Mycobacterium tuberculosis* infection in a corticosteroid-treated rheumatic disease patient population. *Clin. Exp. Rheumatol.* 16:9–13.

85. Kirshbaum, J. D., and H. A. Levy. 1941. Tuberculoma of hypophysis with insufficiency of anterior lobe: a clinical and pathological study of two cases. *Arch. Intern. Med.* 68:1095–1104.

86. Kitrou, M. P., A. Phytou-Pallikari, S. E. Tzannes, K. Virvidakis, and T. D. Mountokalakis. 1982. Hypercalcemia in active pulmonary tuberculosis. *Ann. Intern. Med.* 96:255.

87. Koziel, H., and M. J. Koziel. 1995. Pulmonary complications of diabetes mellitus. Pneumonia. *Infect. Dis. Clin. N. Am.* 9:65–96.

88. Kyriazopoulou, V., O. Parparousi, and A. G. Vagenakis. 1984. Rifampicin-induced adrenal crisis in addisonian patients receiving corticosteroid replacement therapy. *J. Clin. Endocrinol. Metab.* 59:1204–1206.

89. Lack, E. E., and H. P. W. Kozakewich. 1990. Embryology, developmental anatomy, and selected aspects of nonneoplastic pathology, In E. E. Lack (ed.), *Pathology of the Adrenal Glands. Contemporary Issues in Surgical Pathology*, vol. 14. Churchill Livingstone, New York, NY.

90. Lam, K. S., M. M. Sham, S. C. Tam, M. M. Ng, and H. T. Ma. 1993. Hypopituitarism after tuberculous meningitis in childhood. *Ann. Intern. Med.* 118:701–706.

91. Lam, K. Y., and C. Y. Lo. 2001. A critical examination of adrenal tuberculosis and a 28-year autopsy experience of active tuberculosis. *Clin. Endocrinol.* (Oxford) 54:633–639.

92. Lawn, S. D., and D. C. Macallan. 2004. Hypercalcemia: a manifestation of immune reconstitution complicating tuberculosis in an HIV-infected person. *Clin. Infect. Dis.* 38:154–155.

93. Lee, C. T., K. H. Hung, C. H. Lee, H. L. Eng, and J. B. Chen. 2002. Chronic hypercalcemia as the presenting feature of tuberculous peritonitis in a hemodialysis patient. *Am. J. Nephrol.* 22:555–559.

94. Lee, P., and K. K. Ho. 2010. Hyponatremia in pulmonary TB: evidence of ectopic antidiuretic hormone production. *Chest* 137:207–208.

95. Liam, C. K., K. H. Lim, P. Srinivas, and P. J. Poi. 1998. Hypercalcaemia in patients with newly diagnosed tuberculosis in Malaysia. *Int. J. Tuberc. Lung Dis.* 2:818–823.

96. Lin, S. M., S. L. Tsai, and C. S. Chan. 1994. Hypercalcemia in tuberculous peritonitis without active pulmonary tuberculosis. *Am. J. Gastroenterol.* 89:2249–2250.

97. MacGregor, R. R., J. N. Sheagren, M. B. Lipsett, and S. M. Wolff. 1969. Alternate-day prednisone therapy. Evaluation of delayed hypersensitivity responses, control of disease and steroid side effects. *N. Engl. J. Med.* 280:1427–1431.

98. Martos, A., D. Podzamczer, J. Martinez-Lacasa, G. Rufi, M. Santin, and F. Gudiol. 1995. Steroids do not enhance the risk of developing tuberculosis or other AIDS-related diseases in HIV-infected patients treated for *Pneumocystis carinii* pneumonia. *AIDS* 9:1037–1041.

99. Mondal, A., and D. K. Patra. 1995. Efficacy of fine needle aspiration cytology in the diagnosis of tuberculosis of the thyroid gland: a study of 18 cases. *J. Laryngol. Otol.* 109:36–38.

100. Monkawa, T., T. Yoshida, M. Hayashi, and T. Saruta. 2000. Identification of 25-hydroxyvitamin D3 1α-hydroxylase gene expression in macrophages. *Kidney Int.* **58**:559–568.

101. Morris, C. D., A. R. Bird, and H. Nell. 1989. The haematological and biochemical changes in severe pulmonary tuberculosis. *Q. J. Med.* **73**:1151–1159.

102. Mugusi, F., A. B. Swai, K. G. Alberti, and D. G. McLarty. 1990. Increased prevalence of diabetes mellitus in patients with pulmonary tuberculosis in Tanzania. *Tubercle* **71**:271–276.

103. Munkner, T. 1969. Studies on goitre due to para-aminosalicylic acid. *Scand. J. Respir. Dis.* **50**:212–226.

104. Nagotkar, L., P. Shanbag, and N. Dasarwar. 2008. Cerebral salt wasting syndrome following neurosurgical intervention in tuberculous meningitis. *Indian Pediatr.* **45**:598–601.

105. Need, A. G., and P. J. Phillips. 1979. Pulmonary tuberculosis and hypercalcaemia. *Ann. Intern. Med.* **91**:652–653.

106. Niemi, M., J. T. Backman, M. Neuvonen, P. J. Neuvonen, and K. T. Kivisto. 2001. Effects of rifampin on the pharmacokinetics and pharmacodynamics of glyburide and glipizide. *Clin. Pharmacol. Ther.* **69**:400–406.

107. Nieuwland, Y., K. Y. Tan, and J. W. Elte. 1992. Miliary tuberculosis presenting with thyrotoxicosis. *Postgrad. Med. J.* **68**:677–679.

108. Nijland, H. M., R. Ruslami, J. E. Stalenhoef, E. J. Nelwan, B. Alisjahbana, R. H. Nelwan, A. J. van der Ven, H. Danusantoso, R. E. Aarnoutse, and R. van Crevel. 2006. Exposure to rifampicin is strongly reduced in patients with tuberculosis and type 2 diabetes. *Clin. Infect. Dis.* **43**:848–854.

109. Nordin, B. E. 1955. Addison's disease with partial recovery. *Proc. R. Soc. Med.* **48**:1024–1026.

110. Ohnhaus, E. E., and H. Studer. 1983. A link between liver microsomal enzyme activity and thyroid hormone metabolism in man. *Br. J. Clin. Pharm.* **15**:71–76.

111. Olmos, P., J. Donoso, N. Rojas, P. Landeros, R. Schurmann, G. Retamal, M. Meza, and C. Martinez. 1989. Tuberculosis and diabetes mellitus: a longitudinal-retrospective study in a teaching hospital. *Rev. Med. Chil.* **117**:979–983. (In Spanish.)

112. Oluboyo, P. O., and R. T. Erasmus. 1990. The significance of glucose intolerance in pulmonary tuberculosis. *Tubercle* **71**:135–138.

113. Osborne, T. M., and M. J. Sage. 1988. Disseminated tuberculosis causing acute adrenal failure, C.T. findings with post mortem correlation. *Australas. Radiol.* **32**:394–397.

114. Palmer, B. F. 2003. Hyponatremia in patients with central nervous system disease: SIADH versus CSW. *Trends Endocrinol. Metab.* **14**:182–187.

115. Peces, R., and J. Alvarez. 1987. Hypercalcemia and elevated 1,25(OH)2D3 levels in a dialysis patient with disseminated tuberculosis. *Nephron* **46**:377–379.

116. Perez-Guzman, C., A. Torres-Cruz, H. Villarreal-Velarde, and M. H. Vargas. 2000. Progressive age-related changes in pulmonary tuberculosis images and the effect of diabetes. *Am. J. Respir. Crit. Care Med.* **162**:1738–1740.

117. Post, F. A., S. G. Soule, P. A. Willcox, and N. S. Levitt. 1994. The spectrum of endocrine dysfunction in active pulmonary tuberculosis. *Clin. Endocrinol.* (Oxford) **40**:367–371.

118. Pozilli, P., S. Pagani, and P. Aruduini. 1987. In vivo determination of cell mediated immune response in diabetic patients using a multiple intradermal antigen dispenser. *Diabetes Res.* **6**:5–8.

119. Prasad, G. A., S. K. Sharma, A. Mohan, N. Gupta, S. Bajaj, P. K. Saha, N. K. Misra, N. P. Kochupillai, and J. N. Pande. 2000. Adrenocortical reserve and morphology in tuberculosis. *Indian J. Chest Dis. Allied Sci.* **42**:83–93.

120. Ranjan, A., and M. J. Chandy. 1994. Intrasellar tuberculoma. *Br. J. Neurosurg.* **8**:179–185.

121. Rankin, F. W., and A. S. Graham. 1932. Tuberculosis of the thyroid gland. *Ann. Surg.* **96**:625–648.

122. Rickards, A. G., and P. W. Harvey. 1954. Giant-cell granuloma and the other pituitary granulomata. *Q. J. Med.* **23**:425–439.

123. Roca, B., N. Tornador, and E. Tornador. 2008. Presentation and outcome of tuberculous meningitis in adults in the province of Castellon, Spain: a retrospective study. *Epidemiol. Infect.* **136**:1455–1462.

124. Rook, G. A., J. Steele, L. Fraher, S. Barker, R. Karmali, J. O'Riordan, and J. Stanford. 1986. Vitamin D3, gamma interferon, and control of proliferation of *Mycobacterium tuberculosis* by human monocytes. *Immunology* **57**:159–163.

125. Roussos, A., I. Lagogianni, A. Gonis, I. Ilias, D. Kazi, D. Patsopoulos, and N. Philippou. 2001. Hypercalcaemia in Greek patients with tuberculosis before the initiation of antituberculosis treatment. *Respir. Med.* **95**:187–190.

126. Ruslami, R., H. M. Nijland, I. G. Adhiarta, S. H. Kariadi, B. Alisjahbana, R. E. Aarnoutse, and R. van Crevel. 2010. Pharmacokinetics of antituberculosis drugs in pulmonary tuberculosis patients with type 2 diabetes. *Antimicrob. Agents Chemother.* **54**:1068–1074.

127. Saggese, G., S. Bertelloni, G. I. Baroncelli, and G. Di Nero. 1993. Ketoconazole decreases the serum ionized calcium and 1,25-dihydroxyvitamin D levels in tuberculosis-associated hypercalcemia. *Am. J. Dis. Child.* **147**:270–273.

128. Sanford, J. P., and C. B. Favour. 1956. The interrelationships between Addison's disease and active tuberculosis: a review of 125 cases of Addison's disease. *Ann. Intern. Med.* **45**:56–72.

129. Schatz, M., R. Patterson, R. Kloner, and J. Falk. 1976. The prevalence of tuberculosis and positive tuberculin skin tests in a steroid-treated asthmatic population. *Ann. Intern. Med.* **84**:261–265.

130. Schulte, H. M., H. Monig, G. Benker, H. Pagel, D. Reinwein, and E. E. Ohnhaus. 1987. Pharmacokinetics of aldosterone in patients with Addison's disease: effect of rifampicin treatment on glucocorticoid and mineralocorticoid metabolism. *Clin. Endocrinol.* (Oxford) **27**:655–662.

131. Shai, F., R. K. Baker, J. R. Addrizzo, and S. Wallach. 1972. Hypercalcemia in mycobacterial infection. *J. Clin. Endocrinol. Metab.* **34**:251–256.

132. Shaikh, W. A. 1992. Pulmonary tuberculosis in patients treated with inhaled beclomethasone. *Allergy* **47**:327–330.

133. Sharma, M. C., R. Arora, A. K. Mahapatra, P. Sarat-Chandra, S. B. Gaikwad, and C. Sarkar. 2000. Intrasellar tuberculoma—an enigmatic pituitary infection: a series of 18 cases. *Clin. Neurol. Neurosurg.* **102**:72–77.

134. Sharma, S. C. 1981. Serum calcium in pulmonary tuberculosis. *Postgrad. Med. J.* **57**:694–696.

135. Shek, C. C., A. Natkunam, V. Tsang, C. S. Cockram, and R. Swaminathan. 1990. Incidence, causes and mechanism of hypercalcaemia in a hospital population in Hong Kong. *Q. J. Med.* **77**:1277–1285.

136. Sherman, B. M., P. Gorden, and G. di Chiro. 1971. Postmeningitis selective hypopituitarism with suprasellar calcification. *Arch. Intern. Med.* **128**:600–604.

137. Singh, S., D. Bohn, A. P. Carlotti, M. Cusimano, J. T. Rutka, and M. L. Halperin. 2002. Cerebral salt wasting: truths, fallacies, theories, and challenges. *Crit. Care Med.* **30**:2575–2579.

138. Singla, R., and N. Khan. 2003. Does diabetes predispose to the development of multidrug-resistant tuberculosis? *Chest* **123**:308–309. (Author's reply, **123**:309.)

139. Slavin, R. E., T. J. Walsh, and A. D. Pollack. 1980. Late generalized tuberculosis: a clinical pathologic analysis and comparison of 100 cases in the preantibiotic and antibiotic eras. *Medicine* (Baltimore) **59:**352–366.

140. Sosman, M. C., and J. H. Steidl. 1927. Diabetic tuberculosis. *Am. J. Roentgenol.* **17:**625–629.

141. Stalldecker, G., S. Diez, A. Carabelli, R. Reynoso, R. Rey, N. Hofmann, and A. Beresnak. 2002. Pituitary stalk tuberculoma. *Pituitary* **5:**155–162.

142. Stewart, P. M. 2003. The adrenal cortex, p. 491–551. *In* P. R. Larsen, H. M. Kronenberg, S. Melmed, and K. S. Polonsky (ed.), *Williams Textbook of Endocrinology*, 10th ed. Saunders, Philadelphia, PA.

143. Suarez-Garcia, I., A. Rodriguez-Blanco, J. L. Vidal-Perez, M. A. Garcia-Viejo, M. J. Jaras-Hernandez, O. Lopez, and A. Noguerado-Asensio. 2009. Risk factors for multidrug-resistant tuberculosis in a tuberculosis unit in Madrid, Spain. *Eur. J. Clin. Microbiol. Infect. Dis.* **28:**325–330.

144. Subhash, H. S., I. Ashwin, U. Mukundan, D. Danda, G. John, A. M. Cherian, and K. Thomas. 2003. Drug resistant tuberculosis in diabetes mellitus: a retrospective study from south India. *Trop. Doct.* **33:**154–156.

145. Sullivan, J. N., and W. D. Salmon, Jr. 1987. Hypercalcemia in active pulmonary tuberculosis. *South. Med. J.* **80:**572–576.

146. Swai, A. B., D. G. McLarty, and F. Mugusi. 1990. Tuberculosis in diabetic patients in Tanzania. *Trop. Doct.* **20:**147–150.

147. Tanrikulu, A. C., S. Hosoglu, T. Ozekinci, A. Abakay, and F. Gurkan. 2008. Risk factors for drug resistant tuberculosis in southeast Turkey. *Trop. Doct.* **38:**91–93.

148. Tatar, D., G. Senol, S. Alptekin, C. Karakurum, M. Aydin, and I. Coskunol. 2009. Tuberculosis in diabetics: features in an endemic area. *Jpn. J. Infect. Dis.* **62:**423–427.

149. Ti, L. K., S. C. Kang, and K. F. Cheong. 1998. Acute hyponatraemia secondary to cerebral salt wasting syndrome in a patient with tuberculous meningitis. *Anaesth. Intensive Care* **26:**420–423.

150. Truelove, L. H. 1957. Enhancement of Mantoux reaction coincident with treatment with cortisone and prednisolone. *Br. Med. J.* **2:**1135–1137.

151. Venter, W. D. F., V. R. Panz, C. Feldman, and B. I. Joffe. 2006. Adrenocortical function in hospitalised patients with active pulmonary tuberculosis receiving a rifampicin-based regimen—a pilot study. *S. Afr. Med. J.* **96:**62–66.

152. Vita, J. A., S. J. Silverberg, R. S. Goland, J. H. Austin, and A. I. Knowlton. 1985. Clinical clues to the cause of Addison's disease. *Am. J. Med.* **78:**461–466.

153. Wang, C. S., C. J. Yang, H. C. Chen, S. H. Chuang, I. W. Chong, J. J. Hwang, and M. S. Huang. 2009. Impact of type 2 diabetes on manifestations and treatment outcome of pulmonary tuberculosis. *Epidemiol. Infect.* **137:**203–210.

154. Ward, S., and C. C. Evans. 1985. Sudden death due to isolated adrenal tuberculosis. *Postgrad. Med. J.* **61:**635–636.

155. Weiss, H., and S. Katz. 1965. Hyponatremia resulting from apparently inappropriate secretion of antidiuretic hormone in patients with pulmonary tuberculosis. *Am. Rev. Respir. Dis.* **92:**609–616.

156. Wilkins, E. G., E. Hnizdo, and A. Cope. 1989. Addisonian crisis induced by treatment with rifampicin. *Tubercle* **70:**69–73.

157. Wong, L. L., and J. G. Verbalis. 2002. Systemic diseases associated with disorders of water homeostasis. *Endocrinol. Metab. Clin. N. Am.* **31:**121–140.

158. Wyllie, J. P., A. J. Chippindale, and A. J. Cant. 1993. Miliary tuberculosis and symptomatic hypercalcemia. *Pediatr. Infect. Dis. J.* **12:**780–782.

159. Yokoyama, T., R. Toda, Y. Kimura, M. Mikagi, and H. Aizawa. 2009. Addison's disease induced by miliary tuberculosis and the administration of rifampicin. *Intern. Med.* **48:**1297–1300.

160. Yonemura, K., T. Ohtake, H. Matsushima, Y. Fujigaki, and A. Hishida. 2004. High ratio of 1,25-dihydroxyvitamin D3 to parathyroid hormone in serum of tuberculous patients with end-stage renal disease. *Clin. Nephrol.* **62:**202–207.

161. Zargar, A. H., F. A. Sofi, M. A. Akhtar, M. Salahuddin, S. R. Masoodi, and B. A. Laway. 2001. Adrenocortical reserve in patients with active tuberculosis. *J. Pak. Med. Assoc.* **51:**427–433.

162. Zhang, X. C., Z. G. Yang, Y. Li, P. Q. Min, Y. K. Guo, Y. P. Deng, and Z. H. Dong. 2008. Addison's disease due to adrenal tuberculosis: MRI features. *Abdom. Imaging* **33:**689–694.

Tuberculosis and Nontuberculous Mycobacterial Infections, 6th ed.
Edited by David Schlossberg
© 2011 ASM Press, Washington, DC

Chapter 29

Hematologic Complications of Tuberculosis

RANDALL A. OYER AND DAVID SCHLOSSBERG

Tuberculosis (TB) affects the production and life span of all hematologic cellular components (Table 1). In addition, plasma coagulation factors may be affected. The pharmacological agents used for TB therapy may also cause hematologic changes (Table 2). This chapter reviews and updates known hematologic effects of TB and its therapy.

ERYTHROCYTES

Anemia affects greater than 90% of patients actively infected with TB (52). Anemia associated with TB can be divided into four categories:

1. Anemia of chronic disease
2. Metabolic deficiencies
3. Autoimmune hemolytic anemia
4. Marrow complications

The most common type of anemia in individuals with active TB is the normochromic normocytic anemia associated with chronic disease (69). In this situation, erythrocyte life span is shortened without a compensatory marrow response (21). Fundamental to the anemia of chronic disease is a blockade in the reticuloendothelial transfer of iron to the nucleus of the developing erythrocyte. Additionally, inflammation has been shown to activate reticuloendothelial cells, thus sequestering iron, causing hypoferremia and leading to iron-limited erythropoiesis. In addition to limiting new erythrocyte production, reticuloendothelial activation may also accelerate erythrocyte destruction, promoting a compensatory erythropoietin response. In the setting of anemia of chronic disease, the marrow response to erythropoietin has been shown to be defective, leading to abnormal erythroid colony growth. Furthermore, lactoferrin, which is released from normal white cell granules during phagocytosis, binds iron. This bound iron becomes unavailable for attachment to transferrin, thus impairing normal iron transfer, resulting in

anemia (9). Also reported is a blunted erythropoietin response to anemia in patients with untreated TB. This blunted response is postulated to be due to the release of tumor necrosis factor alpha and other cytokines by TB-activated monocytes, which then impair the compensatory erythropoietin response (22).

There are several metabolic causes of anemia seen in individuals with TB. A macrocytic anemia resulting from folate or B_{12} deficiency is well known. Folate deficiency may occur as a consequence of poor nutritional intake as well as increased utilization of folate in the course of active TB. Much less common is B_{12} deficiency secondary to malabsorption reported for individuals with ileal TB (50). A macrocytic anemia can also be seen during the course of treatment for active TB due to the resumption of normal hematopoiesis. During this time, active inflammation subsides and iron becomes, once again, available for normal hematopoiesis, causing a reticulocytosis (19).

Rarely, a sideroblastic anemia is identified. This is due to abnormal B_6 metabolism and has been reported for individuals genetically predisposed to development of ringed sideroblasts (49).

Anemia is also seen secondary to erythrocyte destruction. A Coombs' positive autoimmune hemolytic anemia has been reported (37). This type of hemolysis occurs while an individual is actively infected with TB and resolves promptly upon successful antimicrobial treatment. As the hemolytic anemia resolves, the Coombs' test reverts to negative. Such accelerated erythrocyte destruction may, however, lead to folate deficiency (46).

Newly described is a series of metabolic events leading to changes in the erythrocyte shape and structure. To begin, active TB infection leads to increased production of reactive oxygen species by neutrophilic granulocytes. These reactive oxygen species diffuse through the erythrocyte membrane and degrade under the effect of catalase located in the erythrocyte membrane. This membrane destruction leads to lysis

Randall A. Oyer • Oncology Program, Lancaster General Hospital, Lancaster, PA 17604-3555. **David Schlossberg** • Department of Medicine, Temple University School of Medicine, Philadelphia, PA 19140.

Table 1. Hematologic changes in TB

Changes in cell lines				Changes in coagulation factors	
Myeloid			Lymphoid (lymphocytes)	Hypercoagulability	Hypocoagulability
Erythrocytes	Granulocytes	Platelets			
Anemia Metabolic deficiencies, marrow complications, chronic disease, hemolysis Polycythemia	Neutrophilia, neutropenia, morphological changes, HPS	Impaired function, thrombocytopenia, thrombocytosis	Lymphocytopenia, lymphocytosis	TTP, DIC	DIC, platelet dysfunction, factor V inhibition, factor VIII inhibition

of both bacterial cells and the erythroid cell itself. Other erythroid changes include structural elongation, microcytosis, and abnormal surface folds. These disruptions in erythroid cellular morphology lead to intensification of the disintegration processes in these cells (36).

There are multiple TB-related bone marrow effects interfering with production of all hematologic cell lines. Anemia may be due to bone marrow fibrosis resulting from proliferation of normal marrow macrophages after they engulf mycobacteria. TB has also been reported to stimulate a direct fibrotic reaction (81). Bone marrow fibrosis may cause impaired production of marrow cellular components, a process referred to as myelophthisis (39). Myelophthisic anemias are characterized by the presence of teardrop erythrocytes, nucleated erythrocytes, and early granulocytes, which can be seen on the peripheral blood smear. These changes have been noted in miliary TB, cavitary pulmonary TB, and granulomatous involvement of the spleen, lymph nodes, and liver (4).

In miliary TB, the bone marrow may become directly infiltrated with tuberculosis. The anemia and pancytopenia seen in this setting are more commonly due to marrow dysfunction rather than marrow aplasia (1).

Table 2. Hematologic toxicity from anti-TB therapy

Cell type	Amikacin	Amoxicillin-clavulanate	Capreomycin	Ciprofloxacin	Clofazimine	Cycloserine	Ethambutol	Ethionamide	Imipenem	Isoniazid	Kanamycin	Levofloxacin	Linezolid	Moxifloxacin	Ofloxacin	PAS	Pyrazinamide	Rifabutin	Rifampin	Rifapentine	Streptomycin	Thiacetazone
Erythrocyte																						
Acute porphyria																		×	×			
Aplastic anemia									×	×		×			×	×		×	×	×	×	
B₁₂-deficient megaloblastosis										×						×						
Folate deficiency						×																
G-6-PD[a] hemolysis																					×	
Immune hemolysis									×	×		×		×	×	×		×	×	×	×	×
Methemoglobinemia																×						
Erythrocyte aplasia										×		×										×
Sideroblastic anemia						×				×						×						
Granulocyte																						
Agranulocystosis		×							×	×						×		×	×	×		×
Eosinophilia	×		×	×	×									×								
Leukemoid reaction																×		×	×			
Leukopenia			×	×	×	×		×	×	×		×		×	×	×		×	×	×	×	
Thrombocyte																						
Thrombocytopenia			×	×			×	×	×	×		×	×	×	×	×	×	×	×	×		×
Thrombocytosis		×								×				×								
TTP												×						×	×	×		

[a]G-6-PD, glucose-6-phosphate dehydrogenase.

The bone marrow may also become infiltrated with granulomata. Amyloidosis of the marrow and bone marrow necrosis have also been reported (31, 55, 70, 72). Marrow necrosis can be accompanied by increased reticulin production, which leads to fibrosis. Anemia, leukopenia, and thrombocytopenia may all result from these marrow fibrotic changes.

Polycythemia has only rarely been reported. Polycythemia appears to be due to tuberculous involvement of the kidney, which causes an elevated erythropoietin level and secondary polycythemia (28).

GRANULOCYTES

Neutrophils, basophils, eosinophils, and the monocyte/macrophage line are all subtypes of granulocytes and all are commonly affected during the course of TB and its treatment. Neutrophils are short-lived cells which are massively released into the bloodstream in response to TB infection. These are subsequently eliminated by macrophage phagocytosis (29). Neutrophilia and neutropenia are both known to occur, with neutrophilia being the more common.

Neutrophils are the predominant cell type affected by TB (24). In this setting, a marked increase in neutrophils is T cell mediated. The neutrophilia then resolves with successful treatment (5). In extreme cases, a leukemoid reaction may be seen. This reaction comprises an outpouring of mature and immature granulocytes in the peripheral blood. The picture may be so profound as to have the appearance of acute leukemia. To differentiate this reaction from true acute leukemia, flow cytometry of the immature granulocytes can demonstrate polyclonality, indicating that these cells are reactive rather than malignant. TB-induced leukemoid reactions occur only in patients who are extremely ill from their TB. Such reactions fully resolve with successful treatment of TB. While true leukemia has also been reported to occur in patients with TB, this leukemia does not resolve with antituberculous therapy and is not considered to be a complication of TB (79).

In addition to quantitative abnormalities, qualitative abnormalities occur as well. Granulocytes may become morphologically abnormal, displaying either increased nuclear segmentation or a dumbbell-shaped nucleus which is two nuclear lobes connected by a thin strand of chromatin. The dumbbell-shaped nuclear morphology is accompanied by blunted chromatin synthesis which may impair chemotaxis. This morphological picture was originally described by Pelger in 1928 and is referred to as the Pelger-Huet

anomaly. When a Pelger-Huet anomaly is acquired during active TB infection, it can be demonstrated to resolve during antituberculous therapy (17, 64). Unrelated to TB, the Pelger-Huet anomaly is also seen in acute leukemia and myelodysplasia. The presence of this morphological anomaly should always prompt a search for its cause, and TB must be included in the differential diagnosis.

Neutropenia occurs secondary to a number of mechanisms, including direct suppression of granulopoiesis by activated T cells (31). Additionally, neutropenia may be caused by many of the factors that cause anemia in individuals infected with TB, including folate and B_{12} deficiency. Marrow fibrosis and marrow dysfunction can be seen. Splenic sequestration can consume neutrophils, just as it does other hematopoietic cell lines.

Basophilia and eosinophilia are normal inflammatory responses which have both been well described for TB (32).

Monocytes and macrophages represent a single cell line central to resistance to many infectious diseases, including TB. The monocyte/macrophage line arises from the myeloid stem cell in the bone marrow. The circulating form is referred to as a monocyte, while "macrophage" is used to identify the cell when it is found in tissue, where it spontaneously transforms in response to inflammation. Circulating monocytosis is well documented in the setting of chronic inflammation (35). Additionally, circulating monocytes may become large and vacuolated. These changes occur along the spectrum of natural transformation from monocyte to macrophage. The monocyte/macrophage cell line is responsible for the formation of granulomata (80). Macrophages acquire functionally active myeloperoxidase by the phagocytosis of apoptotic neutrophils (73). This process allows macrophages to acquire antimicrobial activity from neutrophilic granules. Neutrophils shed cell-like particles which contain myeloperoxidase, lactoferrin, other antimicrobial peptides and nuclear debris. This macrophage ingestion of apoptotic neutrophils results in growth inhibition of intracellular mycobacteria (73).

In the extreme, intensive activation of the macrophage can lead to the pathological hemophagocytic syndrome (HPS). The clinical components of this syndrome include fever, lymphadenopathy, hepatosplenomegaly, liver dysfunction, hypofibrinogenemia, and hyperferritinemia. Hematologic consequences of HPS include anemia, thrombocytopenia, and lymphopenia (11). HPS often responds to effective antituberculous treatment but may also be fatal. Therapeutic plasma exchange has been used as an adjunctive therapeutic modality (14, 44).

PLATELETS

Platelet effects of TB may include thrombocytosis, thrombocytopenia, changes in platelet indices, and impaired functional activity.

Thrombocytosis has been well described for TB. The degree of thrombocytosis is related to the degree of inflammation as estimated by the erythrocyte sedimentation rate. More than 50% of individuals who have active TB are reported to have thrombocytosis (75). Reactive thrombocytosis is mediated by elevated levels of endogenous thrombopoietin produced as an acute-phase reactant (75). Thrombocytosis resolves as inflammation subsides with effective anti-TB treatment.

In the setting of TB, thrombocytopenia is more often a complication of therapy than of the disease itself. However, there are multiple mechanisms leading to decreased platelet counts in individuals with active TB. Immune thrombocytopenia is well described and is postulated to be due to TB-mediated T-cell suppression, which allows development and expression of an antiplatelet antibody (33). An additional factor may be the development of antiplatelet antibodies directed against cryptic antigens which become exposed during active infection. Immunofluorescence studies show an increase in the binding of circulating cytotoxic immunoglobulins to autologous platelets (3, 61). Unlike the usual pattern in immune thrombocytopenia, TB-mediated circulating antiplatelet antibodies do not react with normal donor platelets (34). Therapy with intravenous immunoglobulins rapidly reverses thrombocytopenia by binding to the activated Fc receptor of complement, thus inactivating destructive antibodies (10).

Thrombotic thrombocytopenic purpura (TTP) is a distinct disorder in which thrombocytopenia is seen with microangiopathic hemolytic anemia, renal and neurologic dysfunction, and fever. While this complex has occurred in association with many types of infection, it is rarely reported with TB. There are two case reports of the association of TTP with untreated TB, followed by its resolution with successful antituberculous treatment (54). TTP results from inhibition of the enzyme ADAMTS13, metalloproteinase, which is responsible for cleaving large multimers of von Willebrand factor into smaller functional subunits. Accumulation of large von Willebrand factor multimers leads to pathologic intravascular coagulation, platelet consumption, and the aforementioned complications. Additional mechanisms leading to thrombocytopenia include marrow pathology such as fibrosis, granulomatosis, amyloidosis, and necrosis (27).

Thrombocytopenia may also be due to accelerated platelet destruction by various mechanisms.

Platelet destruction can result from sequestration in the setting of hypersplenism (23). Rapid platelet destruction may also be seen with disseminated intravascular coagulation (DIC) (46, 63). Additionally, thrombocytopenia not attributable to DIC is seen with active TB, as it is with a variety of viral infections (16). When platelet survival is decreased, there may be a compensatory increase in small megakaryocytes in the marrow, and these may demonstrate abnormal nuclear ploidy (43). In addition to their well-known primary hemostatic function, platelets have recently been shown to be an important component of the immune system. Immune functions demonstrated by platelets include chemotaxis, activation of complement factors, and interaction with microorganisms (77). Platelet indices include mean platelet volume (MPV), platelet distribution width (PDW), and plateletcrit. The PDW is a measure of platelet anisocytosis. Plateletcrit is an analog of the hematocrit for platelets which indicates the volume of circulating platelets in a given volume of blood. MPV, PDW, and plateletcrit are significantly elevated in many individuals with active TB. These values return to normal with antituberculous therapy. MPV, PDW, and plateletcrit elevation seem to be specific for active TB. One study shows that the same abnormalities are not seen in individuals with non-TB pneumonia, suggesting that these abnormalities may be used to aid in rapid identification of individuals who should begin anti-TB therapy before diagnostic confirmation (77).

Another platelet abnormality described to occur in individuals with TB is a marked elevation of platelet factor 4 (PF-4), which is a platelet-derived proinflammatory cytokine. This cytokine is stored in the platelet's alpha granules and released upon activation. Plasma concentrations of PF-4 reflect platelet activity. PF-4 activities in patients with active TB have been found to be significantly elevated compared to those in non-TB-infected human immunodeficiency virus (HIV)-seropositive subjects, cancer patients, and healthy individuals (74).

LYMPHOCYTES

Lymphocytopenia and lymphocytosis have both been reported for active TB.

Decreases are reported in total lymphocytes, total T cells, the T4 subset, and B cells. Profound T lymphocytopenia and CD4 counts fewer than 200/ml^3 have been reported for TB-infected HIV-negative patients (26, 83). As with other infections in HIV-negative patients that may result in a transient fall in CD4 count, TB is usually associated with a normal CD4/CD8 ratio greater than 1.0 (40). Impaired production of both interleukin 2 and gamma interferon is noted in T cells of individuals with TB. Other cytokines, including interleukins and tumor necrosis factor, are activated (41). The percentages of CD4-positive T cells were significantly lower in patients with active TB than in healthy subjects (20). Natural killer (NK) cells, a T-cell subset, are relatively increased in individuals with active TB compared to healthy control subjects (59). While lymphocytopenia may be associated with marrow dysfunction, haptoglobin has recently been reported to suppress T-cell proliferation. Haptoglobin is an acute-phase protein which primarily scavenges hemoglobin and exhibits strong inhibition of T-cytokine release (59).

Lymphocyte proliferation is well described to occur in the blood, secondary lymphoid tissues, and organs affected by TB. Lymphadenopathy and splenomegaly are reported to occur (82). Polyclonal increases in immunoglobulin G (IgG), IgA, and IgM are detected. Cryoglobulins are immunoglobulins which precipitate at low temperatures. These have been reported in the setting of many infectious diseases, including TB. Cryoglobulinemia in a TB patient has been reported to cause secondary proteinuria, an elevated sedimentation rate, and anemia. These manifestations resolved with successful treatment of TB (76). Decreases in levels of gamma interferon have been reported (38).

A recent report shows a range of lymphocyte changes suggesting a host-pathogen conflict with variable outcomes even within adjacent tissue in the same organ. An interesting paper describes areas of cavitation showing local neutrophilia with relative lymphopenia. In tissue from nearby areas of pulmonary infiltrate and from radiologically unaffected lobes in the same lung, lymphocytosis with lower levels of neutrophils is described. It is noted that cavitary sites demonstrate a significantly lower mycobacterium-specific T-cell response than do areas of pulmonary infiltrate or areas of radiologically unaffected lung (8).

COAGULATION SYSTEM

Diverse coagulation abnormalities have been reported in the setting of TB. Both hypercoagulability and hypocoagulability have been noted. Hypercoagulability may be a manifestation of a number of TB-induced disorders, including TTP, DIC, and various nonspecific inflammatory responses. Reported mechanisms include increased production of fibrinogen, fibrin degradation products, and tissue plasminogen activator (62, 66). Other biochemical changes resulting in hypercoagulability are activation

of procoagulant factor VIII, depressed levels of the naturally occurring anticoagulants antithrombin and protein C, and increased platelet activation (13, 78).

When the vascular endothelium becomes disrupted due to cytokines released by TB-activated monocytes, the coagulation system may be inappropriately activated, leading to hypercoagulability. This occurs in the setting of DIC, which is a complex disorder with a range of pathological coagulation manifestations. These include both bleeding and thrombosis, sometimes in the same patient. Deep venous thrombosis has been reported to occur in multiple individuals (30, 48, 71). Inferior vena cava thrombosis has been reported as well (60).

In addition to the aforementioned thrombotic manifestations, DIC may also lead to hypocoagulability. In this setting, abnormal bleeding may be due to DIC-induced consumption of clotting factors and platelets. Platelet dysfunction, which is termed acquired platelet storage pool disorder, occurs as hemostatically active platelet granules are depleted in the coagulative process. Coagulation proteins may be negatively affected as well. Acquired factor V dysfunction due to the presence of an immunoglobulin inhibitor has been reported to cause hemorrhage (2). Additionally, abnormal bleeding linked to a TB-associated factor VIII inhibitor has been described. The affected individual presented with an elevated activated partial thromboplastin time, significant factor VIII inhibitor levels, and clinical bleeding. These issues all resolved upon successful treatment of TB (51). Bleeding in TB is also described with direct organ infiltration. Case reports of ileal TB presenting with massive rectal bleeding and endometrial TB presenting as vaginal bleeding have been recently published (7, 45).

EFFECTS OF ANTITUBERCULOUS MEDICATIONS

Despite the fact that nearly all of the antituberculous antimicrobials may produce hematologic side effects, routine hematologic monitoring is recommended by the manufacturer for only three commonly used anti-TB antibiotics—cycloserine, ethambutol, and rifabutin—and the strength of the recommendation varies from drug to drug. For cycloserine, hematologic monitoring is required. For ethambutol, baseline and periodic hematopoietic monitoring is recommended. With rifabutin, monitoring for neutropenia and thrombocytopenia is suggested. However, since nearly all the anti-TB drugs may cause hematologic toxicity, and since they are always used in multiple-drug regimens, the most prudent course is to monitor all patients receiving anti-TB therapy for hematologic toxicity. Five drugs exhibit the widest range of hematologic side effects: isoniazid, p-aminosalicylic acid (PAS), rifampin, rifapentine, and ofloxacin.

Isoniazid can affect all cell lines. Mechanisms of isoniazid-induced anemia include pure erythrocyte aplasia (18), sideroblastic anemia, B_{12} deficiency, and immune hemolysis. Thrombocytopenia and neutropenia are also reported. Isoniazid has also been reported to cause a lupus-like syndrome manifested by hematologic changes and arthralgia (68).

Rifampin is well known to cause thrombocytopenia (6, 57, 58). Among the potential mechanisms, direct drug-dependent binding of antibody to the platelet glycoprotein Ib/IX complex has been demonstrated (57). Rifampin administered on a regular daily basis leads to immune desensitization. Thus, this complication is more likely to occur when rifampin administration is intermittent and sporadic. This thrombocytopenia correlates with the presence of rifampin-dependent antibodies (42). Rifampin has also been described as a cause of TTP. The thrombocytopenia associated with rifampin-induced TTP is reversible upon cessation of the medication (25). Other destructive hematologic complications include PAS-induced hemolytic anemia, which may be further complicated by B_{12}-deficient megaloblastic anemia (12). PAS has also been described as a cause of neutropenia, leukopenia, and thrombocytopenia.

Rifapentine may produce a broad spectrum of hematologic abnormalities. These include neutropenia as well as neutrophilia. It may also produce lymphopenia as well as lymphocytosis.

Ofloxacin causes numerous hematologic abnormalities, particularly in the granulocyte cell line with neutropenia, agranulocytosis, lymphocytosis, and eosinophilia. It can also cause lymphopenia and thrombocytopenia.

Streptomycin has been known to cause a cluster of findings which comprise skin rash, eosinophilia, and systemic symptoms referred to by the acronym DRES (53).

Linezolid, an oxazolidinone active against drug-resistant TB, has been reported to cause mild myelosuppression, resulting in anemia and thrombocytopenia (65). This complication is seen less commonly in patients treated for TB than in patients receiving linezolid for routine bacterial infections, because the anti-TB dosage is 600 mg/day instead of the usual dose of 600 mg twice a day. In fact, the hematologic abnormalities seen in some patients treated for TB have resolved or stabilized when the dosage of linezolid has been reduced even further, to 300 mg/day.

CONCLUSION

The hematologic consequences of TB are varied and complex. Some of the changes are mild and temporary; others can be quite serious and even life-threatening. Additionally, the hematologic and hemostatic side effects of antituberculous therapy warrant special attention and management.

REFERENCES

1. **Adamson, J. W., and A. J. Ersley.** 1990. Aplastic anemia, p. 158–174. *In* W. J. Williams, E. Beutler, A. J. Ersley, et al. (ed.), *Hematology*, 4th ed. McGraw-Hill, New York, NY.
2. **Aliaga, J. L., J. de Gracia, R. Vidal, M. Pico, P. Flores, and G. Sampol.** 1990. Acquired factor V deficiency in a patient with pulmonary tuberculosis. *Eur. Respir. J.* 3:109–110.
3. **Al-Majed, S. A., A. K. Al-Momen, F. A. Al-Kassimi, A. Al-Zeer, A. M. Kambal, and H. Baaqil.** 1995. Tuberculosis presenting as immune thrombocytopenic purpura. *Acta Haematol.* 94:135–138.
4. **Andre, J., R. Schwartz, and W. Dameshek.** 1961. Tuberculosis and myelosclerosis with myeloid metaplasia; report of three cases. *JAMA* 178:1169–1174.
5. **Appleberg, R., and M. T. Silva.** 1989. T-cell-dependent chronic neutrophilia during mycobacterial infections. *Clin. Exp. Immunol.* 78:478–483.
6. **Aquinas, M., W. G. Allan, P. A. Horsfall, P. K. Jenkins, W. Hung-Yan, D. Girling, R. Tall, and W. Fox.** 1972. Adverse reactions to daily and intermittent rifampicin regimens for pulmonary tuberculosis in Hong Kong. *Br. Med. J.* 1(803):765–771.
7. **Balsarkar, D., and M. Joshi.** 2009. Ileal tuberculosis presenting as a case of massive rectal bleeding. Case report. *BHJ* 51:72–74.
8. **Barry, S., R. Breen, M. Lipman, M. Johnson, and G. Janossy.** 2009. Impaired antigen-specific CD4[+] T lymphocyte responses in cavitary tuberculosis. *Tuberculosis* 89:48–53.
9. **Boeser, H. P.** 1974. Iron metabolism in inflammation and malignant disease, p. 605–640. *In* A. Jacobs and M. Worwood (ed.), *Iron in Biochemistry and Medicine, II*. Academic Press, London, England.
10. **Boots, R. J., A. W. Roberts, and D. McEvoy.** 1992. Immune thrombocytopenia complicating pulmonary tuberculosis: case report and investigation of mechanisms. *Thorax* 47:396–397.
11. **Brastianos, P., J. Swanson, M. Torbenson, J. Sperati, and P. C. Karakousis.** 2006. Tuberculosis-associated haemophagocytic syndrome. *Lancet Infect. Dis.* 6:447–454.
12. **Cameron, S. J.** 1974. Tuberculosis and the blood—a special relationship? *Tubercle* 55:55–72.
13. **Casanova-Roman, M. M., J. Rios, A. Sanchez-Porto, et al.** 2004. Deep venous thrombosis associated with pulmonary tuberculosis and transient protein S deficiency. *Am. J. Hematol.* 7:118–119.
14. **Chandra, P., S. A. Chaudhery, F. Rosner, and M. Kagen.** 1975. Transient histiocytosis with striking phagocytosis of platelets, leukocytes, and erythrocytes. *Arch. Intern. Med.* 135:989–991.
15. Reference deleted.
16. **Chia, Y. C., and S. J. Machin.** 1979. Tuberculosis and severe thrombocytopaenia. *Br. J. Clin. Pract.* 33:55–56, 58.
17. **Cicchitto, G., M. Parravicini, S. De Lorenzo, et al.** 1999. Tuberculosis and Pelger-Huet anomaly. Case report. *Panminerva Med.* 41:367–369.

18. Clairborne, R. A., and A. K. Dutt. 1985. Isoniazid-induced pure red cell aplasia. *Am. Rev. Respir. Dis.* **131**:947–949.

19. Das, B. S., U. Devi, C. Mohan Rao, V. K. Srivastava, and P. K. Rath. 2003. Effect of iron supplementation on mild to moderate anaemia in pulmonary tuberculosis. *Br. J. Nutr.* **90**:541–550.

20. Deveci, F., H. H. Akbulut, I. Celik, M. H. Muz, and F. Ilhan. 2006. Lymphocyte subpopulations in pulmonary tuberculosis patients. *Mediators Inflamm.* **6**:1–6.

21. Douglas, S. W., and J. W. Adamson. 1990. The anemia of chronic disorders: studies of marrow regulation and iron metabolism. *Blood* **45**:55–65.

22. Ebrahim, O., P. I. Folb, S. C. Robson, and P. Jacobs. 1995. Blunted erythropoietin response to anaemia in tuberculosis. *Eur. J. Haematol.* **55**:251–254.

23. Ersley, A. J. 1990. Hypersplenism and hyposplenism, p. 695. *In* W. J. Williams, E. Beutler, A. J. Ersley, et al. (ed.), *Hematology*, 4th ed. McGraw-Hill, New York, NY.

24. Eum, S. Y., J. H. Kong, M. S. Hong, Y. J. Lee, J. H. Kim, S. H. Hwang, S. N. Cho, L. Via, and C. Barry III. 2010. Neutrophils are the predominant infected phagocytic cells in the airways of patients with active pulmonary TB. *Chest* **137**:122–128.

25. Fahal, I. H., P. S. Williams, R. E. Clark, and G. M. Bell. 1992. Thrombotic thrombocytopenic purpura due to rifampicin. *BMJ* **304**:882.

26. Fantin, B., V. Joly, C. Elbim, et al. 1996. Lymphocyte subset counts during the course of community-acquired pneumonia: evolution according to age, human immunodeficiency virus status, and etiologic microorganisms. *Clin. Infect. Dis.* **22**:1096–1098.

27. Finch, S. C., and B. Castleman. 1963. Case records of the Massachusetts General Hospital. *N. Engl. J. Med.* **238**:378.

28. Gallagher, N. I., and R. M. Donati. 1968. Inappropriate erythropoietin elaboration. *Ann. N. Y. Acad. Sci.* **149**:528–538.

29. González-Cortés, C., D. Reyes-Ruvalcaba, C. Diez-Tascón, and O. Rivero-Lezcano. 2009. Apoptosis and oxidative burst in neutrophils infected with *Mycobacterium* spp. *Immunol. Lett.* **126**:16–21.

30. Gupta, R., M. Bruteon, J. Fell, and H. Lyall. 2003. An Afghan child with deep vein thrombosis. *J. R. Soc. Med.* **96**:289–291.

31. Huxley, H. M., and H. M. Knox-Macaulay. 1992. Tuberculosis and the haemopoietic system. *Baillier's Clin. Haematol.* **5**:101–129.

32. Juhlin, L. 1963. Basophil and eosinophil leukocytes in various internal disorders. *Acta Med. Scand.* **174**:249–254.

33. Jurak, S. S., R. Aster, and H. Sawaf. 1983. Immune thrombocytopenia associated with tuberculosis. *Clin. Pediatr.* **22**:318–319.

34. Kaufmann, S. H. 1991. The macrophage in tuberculosis: sinner or saint? The T-cell decides. *Pathobiology* **59**:153–155.

35. Kelsey, P. R. 1990. Blood film and marrow, p. 3. *In* I. W. Delamore and J. A. Liu Yin (ed.), *Haematologic Aspects of Systemic Disease*. Bailliere Tindal, London, England.

36. Khvitiya, N., G. Khechinashvili, and S. Sabanadze. 2004. Erythrocyte structure and function in fibrocaverno. *Bull. Exp. Biol. Med.* **138**:613–615.

37. Kuo, P. H., P. C. Yang, S. S. Kuo, and K. T. Luh. 2001. Severe immune hemolytic anemia in disseminated tuberculosis with response to antituberculosis therapy. *Chest* **119**:1961–1963.

38. Kyle, R. A. 1982. Monoclonal gammopathy of undetermined significance (MGUS): a review. *Clin. Haematol.* **1**:123–150.

39. Laszlo, J., and A. T. Huang. 1990. Anemia associated with marrow infiltration, p. 546–548. *In* W. J. Williams, E. Beutler, A. J. Ersley, et al. (ed.), *Hematology*, 4th ed. McGraw-Hill, New York, NY.

40. Laurence, J. 1993. T-cell subsets in health, infectious disease, and idiopathic CD4+ T-lymphocytopenia. *Ann. Intern. Med.* **119**:55–62.

41. Law, K., M. Weiden, T. Harkin, T. Tchou-Wong, C. Chi, and W. N. Rom. 1996. Increased release of interleukin-1 beta, interleukin-6, and tumor necrosis factor-alpha by bronchoalveolar cells lavaged from involved sites in pulmonary tuberculosis. *Am. J. Respir. Crit. Care Med.* **153**:799–804.

42. Lee, C. H., and C. J. Lee. 1989. Thrombocytopenia—a rare but potentially serious side effect of initial daily and interrupted use of rifampicin. *Chest* **96**:202–203.

43. Marchasin, S., R. O. Wallerstein, and P. M. Aggeler. 1964. Variations of the platelet count in disease. *Calif. Med.* **101**:95–100.

44. Mariani, F., D. Goletti, A. Ciaramella, A. Martino, V. Colizzi, and M. Fraziano. 2001. Macrophage response to *Mycobacterium tuberculosis* during HIV infection: relationships between macrophage activation and apoptosis. *Curr. Mol. Med.* **1**:209–216.

45. Mengistu, Z., V. Engh, K. K. Melby, E. von der Lippe, and E. Qvigstad. 2007. Postmenopausal vaginal bleeding caused by endometrial tuberculosis. *Acta Obstet. Gynecol. Scand.* **86**:631–632.

46. Murray, H. W. 1978. Transient autoimmune hemolyctic anemia and pulmonary tuberculosis. *N. Engl. J. Med.* **299**:488.

47. Murray, H. W., C. U. Tuazon, N. Kirmani, and J. N. Sheagren. 1978. The adult respiratory distress syndrome associated with miliary tuberculosis. *Chest* **73**:536–539.

48. Naithani, R., N. Agrawal, and V. Choudhary. 2007. Deep venous thrombosis associated with tuberculosis. *Blood Coagulation Fibrinolysis* **18**:377–380.

49. Nusbaum, N. J. 1990. Concise review: genetic bases for sideroblastic anemia. *Am. J. Hematol.* **37**:41–44.

50. O'Connor, N. J., and A. V. Hotfbrand. 1998. Anaemia in systemic disease, p. 38. *In* I. W. Delamore and J. A. Liu Yin (ed.), *Haematologic Aspects of Systemic Disease*. Bailliere Tindall, London, England.

51. Ogata, H., S. Sakai, F. Koiwa, H. Tayama, E. Kinugasa, T. Ideura, and T. Akizawa. 1999. Plasma exchange for acquired hemophilia: a case report. *Ther. Apher.* **3**:320–322.

52. Olaniyi, J. A., and Y. A. Aken'Ova. 2003. Haemotologic profile of patients with pulmonary tuberculosis in Ibadan, Nigeria. *Afr. J. Med. Sci.* **32**:239–242.

53. Passeron, T., M. C. Ndir, C. Aubron, and P. Hovette. 2004. Drug rash with eosinophilia and systemic symptoms (DRESS) due to streptomycin. *Acta Dermatol. Venereol.* **84**:92–93.

54. Pavithran, K., and N. Vijayalekshmi. 1993. Thrombocytopenic purpura with tuberculous adenitis. *Indian J. Med. Sci.* **4**(10):239–240.

55. Paydas, S., M. Ergin, F. Baslamisli, S. Yavuz, S. Zorludemir, B. Sahin, and F. A. Bolat. 2002. Bone marrow necrosis: clinicopathologic analysis of 20 cases and review of the literature. *Br. J. Haematol.* **70**(4):300–305.

56. Reference deleted.

57. Pereira, J., P. Hidalgo, M. Ocqueteau, M. Blacutt, M. Marchesse, Y. Nien, L. Letelier, and D. Mezzano. 2000. Glycoprotein Ib/IX complex is the target in rifampicin-induced immune thrombocytopenia. *Br. J. Haematol.* **110**(4):907–910.

58. Prasad, R., S. Kant, and D. K. Pandey. 1999. Rifampicin induced thrombocytopenia. *J. Assoc. Physicians India* **47**:252.

59. Quaye, I. 2008. Haptoglobin, inflammation and disease. *Trans. R. Soc. Trop. Med. Hyg.* **102**:735–742.

60. Raj, M., and A. Agrawal. 2006. Inferior vena cava thrombosis complicating tuberculosis. *N. Z. Med. J.* **119**(1244):U2279.

61. **Richards, E. M., J. M. Shneerson, and T. P. Baglin.** 1994. Thrombocyctopenia responding to empirical antituberculous therapy. *Clin. Lab. Haematol.* **16:**89–90.

62. **Robson, S. C., N. W. White, I. Aronson, R. Woollgar, H. Goodman, and P. Jacobs.** 1996. Acute-phase response and the hypercoagulable state in pulmonary tuberculosis. *Br. J. Haematol.* **93:**943–949.

63. **Rosenberg, M. J., and L. W. Rumans.** 1978. Survival of a patient with pancytopenia and disseminated coagulation associated with miliary tuberculosis. *Chest* **73:**536–539.

64. **Savage, P. J., R. P. Dellinger, J. V. Barnes, et al.** 1984. Pelger-Huet anomaly of granulocytes in a patient with tuberculosis. *Chest* **85:**131–132.

65. **Schecter, G. F., C. Scott, L. True, A. Raftery, J. Flood, and S. Mase.** 2010. Linezolid in the treatment of multidrug-resistant tuberculosis. *Clin. Infect. Dis.* **50:**49–55.

66. **Selvaraj, P., N. Venkataprasad, V. K. Vijayan, R. Prabhakar, and P. R. Narayanan.** 1994. Procoagulant activity of bronchoalveolar lavage fluids taken from the site of tuberculosis lesions. *Eur. Respir. J.* **7**(7):1227–1232.

67. **Sharp, R. A., J. G. Lowe, and R. N. Johnston.** 1990. Antituberculous drugs and sideroblastic anaemia. *Br. J. Clin. Pract.* **44**(12):706–707.

68. **Siddiqui, M. A., and I. A. Khan.** 2002. Isoniazid-induced lupus erythematosus presenting with cardiac tamponade. *Am. J. Ther.* **9**(2):163–165.

69. **Singh, K. J., G. Ahluwalia, S. K. Sharma, R. Saxena, V. P. Chaudhary, and M. Anant.** 2001. Significance of haematological manifestations in patients with tuberculosis. *J. Assoc. Physicians India* **49:**790–794.

70. **Singh, R., M. M. Singh, V. L. Lahiri, et al.** 1987. Tuberculosis as a continuing cause of secondary amyloidosis in northern India. *J. Indian Med. Assoc.* **85**(11):328–332.

71. **Suárez Ortega, S., J. Artiles Vizcaino, I. Balda Aguirre, P. Melado Sánchez, M. E. Arkuch Saade, E. Ayala Galán, and P. Betancor León.** 1993. Tuberculosis as risk factor for venous thrombosis. *An. Med. Interna* **10**(8):398–400.

72. **Sunga, M. N., Jr., C. V. Reyes, J. Zvetina, and T. W. Kim.** 1989. Resolution of secondary amyloidosis 14 years after adequate chemotherapy for skeletal tuberculosis. *South. Med. J.* **82:**92–93.

73. **Tan, B., C. Meinken, M. Bastian, H. Bruns, A. Legaspi, M. T. Ochoa, S. Krutzik, B. Bloom, T. Ganz, R. Modlin, and S. Stenger.** 2006. Macrophages acquire neutrophil granules for antimicrobial activity against intracellular pathogens. *J. Immunol.* **177:**1864–1871.

74. **Tarhan, G., F. Gümüşlü, N. Yilmaz, D. Saka, I. Ceyhan, and S. Cesur.** 2006. Serum adenosine deaminase enzyme and plasma platelet factor 4 activities in active pulmonary tuberculosis, HIV-seropositive subjects and cancer patients. *J. Infect.* **52**(4):264–268.

75. **Tengku Muzaffar, T. M. S., A. R. Shalfuzain, Y. Imran, and M. N. Noor Haslina.** 2008. Hematological changes in tuberculous spondylitis patients at the Hospital Universiti Sains Malaysia. *Southeast Asian J. Trop. Med. Public Health* **39**(4):686–689.

76. **Tereul, J. L., R. Matesanz, F. Mampaso, S. Lamas, J. A. Herrero, and J. Ortuño.** 1987. Pulmonary tuberculosis, cryoglobulinemia and immune complex glomerulonephritis. *Clin. Nephrol.* **27:**48–49.

77. **Tozkoparan, E., O. Deniz, E. Ucar, H. Bilgic, and K. Ekiz.** 2007. Changes in platelet count and indices in pulmonary tuberculosis. *Clin. Chem. Lab. Med.* **45:**1009–1013.

78. **Turken, O., E. Kunter, M. Sezer, R. Solmazgul, E. Bozkanat, A. Ozturk, and A. Ilvan.** 2002. Hemostatic changes in active pulmonary tuberculosis. *Int. J. Tuberc. Lung Dis.* **6:**927–932.

79. **Twomey, J. J., and B. S. Leavell.** 1965. Leukemoid reactions to tuberculosis. *Arch. Intern. Med.* **116:**21–28.

80. **Vergne, I., J. Chua, and V. Deretic.** 2003. *Mycobacterium tuberculosis* phagosome maturation arrest: selective targeting of PI3P-dependent membrane trafficking. *Traffic* **4:**600–606.

81. **Viallard, J. F., M. Parren, J. M. Boiron, et al.** 2002. Reversible myelofibrosis induced by tuberculosis. *Clin. Infect. Dis.* **34:**1641–1643.

82. **Williams, W. J.** 1990. Lymph node enlargement, p. 950–955. *In* W. J. Williams, E. Beutler, A. J. Ersley, et al. (ed.), *Hematology*, 4th ed. McGraw-Hill, New York, NY.

83. **Zaharatos, G. J., M. A. Behr, and M. D. Libman.** 2001. Profound T-lymphocytopenia and cryptococcemia in a human immunodeficiency virus-seronegative patient with disseminated tuberculosis. *Clin. Infect. Dis.* **33**(11):E125–E128.

Tuberculosis and Nontuberculous Mycobacterial Infections, 6th ed.
Edited by David Schlossberg
© 2011 ASM Press, Washington, DC

Chapter 30

Tuberculosis in Infants and Children

JEFFREY R. STARKE

The clinical expression of disease caused by *Mycobacterium tuberculosis* is greatly different in infants, children, and adolescents from what it is in adults (70). Much adult pulmonary tuberculosis is caused by a reactivation of dormant organisms which are lodged in the apices of the lungs during hematogenous dissemination at the time of infection. Childhood tuberculosis is usually a complication of the pathophysiologic events surrounding the initial infection. The time interval between infection and disease is usually long (years to decades) in adults but is often only weeks to months in small children. Children are more prone to developing extrapulmonary tuberculosis but rarely develop infectious pulmonary disease. As a result of the basic differences in pathophysiology of tuberculosis between adults and children, the approach to diagnosis, treatment, and prevention of infection and disease in children is necessarily different (107).

Many aspects of the various forms of pediatric tuberculosis have been discussed briefly in other chapters of this book. This chapter will focus on the fundamental nature of exposure, infection, and disease in children, emphasizing how and why children are approached differently from adults. The effects of these differences on the public health approach to tuberculosis control in children will also be explained.

TERMINOLOGY

The terminology used to describe various stages and presentation of childhood tuberculosis often has been a source of confusion for physicians. It follows the pathophysiology, but the stages are sometimes not completely distinct in children.

Exposure means that the child has had significant contact with an adult or adolescent with infectious pulmonary tuberculosis. The contact investigation—examining those individuals close to a suspected case of tuberculosis with a tuberculin skin test (TST), chest radiograph, and physical examination—is the most important activity in a community to prevent cases of tuberculosis in children (57). The most frequent setting for exposure of a child is the household, but it can occur in a school, daycare center, or other closed setting. In this stage, the TST is negative, the chest radiograph is normal, and the child lacks signs or symptoms of disease. Some exposed children may have inhaled droplet nuclei infected with *M. tuberculosis* and have early infection, but the clinician cannot know it because it takes up to 3 months for delayed hypersensitivity to tuberculin, a positive skin test, to develop. The World Health Organization recommends that children younger than 5 years of age in the exposure stage should be treated to prevent the rapid development of disseminated or meningeal tuberculosis, which can occur before the skin test becomes reactive.

Infection occurs when the individual inhales droplet nuclei containing *M. tuberculosis*, which becomes established intracellularly within the lung and associated lymphoid tissue. The hallmark of tuberculosis infection is a reactive TST or gamma interferon release assay (IGRA). In this stage, the child has no signs or symptoms and the chest radiograph is either normal or reveals only granuloma or calcifications in the lung parenchyma and/or regional lymph nodes. In developed countries, virtually all children with tuberculosis infection should receive treatment, usually with isoniazid (INH), to prevent the development of disease in the near or distant future.

Disease occurs when signs or symptoms or radiographic manifestations caused by *M. tuberculosis* become apparent. The word "tuberculosis" refers to disease. Not all infected individuals have the same risk of developing disease. An immunocompetent adult with untreated tuberculosis infection has approximately a 5 to 10% lifetime risk of developing disease; one-half of the risk occurs in the first 2 to 3 years after infection. Historical studies have shown

---

Jeffrey R. Starke • Baylor College of Medicine, One Baylor Plaza, Houston, TX 77030.

that up to 40% of immunocompetent infants with untreated tuberculosis infection develop disease, often serious, life-threatening forms, within 1 to 2 years.

The phrase "primary tuberculosis" has been used to describe childhood pulmonary disease that arises as a complication of the initial infection. Unfortunately, this phrase also has been used to describe the initial infection even in the absence of radiographic or clinical manifestations. Infection and the onset of disease are separated by time in adults and are usually fairly distinct events. In children, however, disease complicates the initial infection, so the two stages are on a continuum, often with indistinct borders (56). This lack of clarity can cause confusion when deciding which treatment regimen—how many drugs—to use. The current consensus in the United States is to consider disease to be present if adenopathy or other chest radiograph manifestations of infection by *M. tuberculosis* can be seen.

EPIDEMIOLOGY

Disease and Infection

Because most children with tuberculosis infection and disease acquired the organism from an adult in their environment, the epidemiology of childhood tuberculosis tends to follow that in adults. The risk of a child acquiring tuberculosis infection is environmental, determined by the likelihood she will be in contact with an adult with contagious tuberculosis. In contrast, the risk of a child developing tuberculosis disease depends more on host immunologic and genetic factors.

It is estimated that the worldwide annual burden of tuberculosis on children is 1.5 million cases and 500,000 deaths (80). Adult tuberculosis case numbers have increased over the past decade in every region of the world except Western Europe. There are no comparable data, but it is likely that childhood tuberculosis has grown in numbers as well.

Between 1953 and 1980, childhood tuberculosis rates in the United States declined about 6% per year. Between 1980 and 1987, the case rates remained relatively flat, but they began to increase in 1988. With improvements in tuberculosis control, rates of childhood tuberculosis started to decline in 1993 and have continued on a downward trend (Fig. 1) (81). In 2008, there were 786 cases in children less than 15 years old (15), a 53% decline since 1993. About 60% of cases occur among infants and children less than 5 years of age. Between the ages of 5 and 14, often called the "favored age," children usually have the lowest rates of tuberculosis disease in any population. The clinical expression of tuberculosis in childhood differs by age (Table 1). Other than meningitis or lymph node disease, other forms of extrapulmonary tuberculosis are more common in older children and adolescents. The gender ratio for tuberculosis in children is about 1:1 in contrast to adults, in whom it predominates in

Table 1. Median age of children (less than 20 years old) with tuberculosis by predominant site, United States, 1988[a]

Site	No. of cases (%)	Median age (yr)
Pulmonary	1,213 (77.5)	6
Lymphatic	209 (13.3)	5
Pleural	49 (3.1)	16
Meningeal	29 (1.9)	2
Bone/joint	19 (1.2)	8
Miliary	14 (0.9)	1
Genitourinary	13 (0.8)	16
Peritoneal	4 (0.3)	13
Other	16 (1.1)	12
Total	1,566 (100)	6

[a]Provided by the Centers of Disease Control and Prevention. Data from reference 81 give similar proportions.

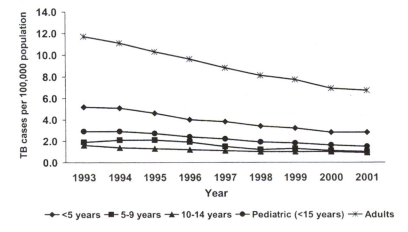

Figure 1. Tuberculosis (TB) case rates by age group for children, 1993–2001. (Data in the public domain, courtesy of the Centers for Disease Control and Prevention).

males. As with adults, immunocompromising conditions and diabetes mellitus increase the risk of tuberculosis in children (125).

Tuberculosis case rates historically have been the highest between January and June in the Northern Hemisphere, possibly because of more extensive indoor contact with infectious adults during the colder months. Childhood tuberculosis is geographically focal in the United States, with several states accounting for 70% of reported cases among children less than 5 years of age (81). As expected, disease rates are highest in cities with more than 250,000 residents.

Childhood tuberculosis case rates in the United States are strikingly higher among ethnic and racial minority groups and the foreign-born than in whites (114). Approximately 88% of cases occur among African American, Hispanic, Asian, and Native American children; this reflects the risk of transmission within the living conditions of these children (81, 119). Although most of these children were born in the United States, the proportion of foreign-born children with tuberculosis rose from 13 to 28% from 1986 to 2001. For all ages, about one-half of cases of tuberculosis in foreign-born persons occur within 5 years of immigration. Foreign-born adoptee children also have high rates of tuberculosis (66, 94).

Most children are infected with *M. tuberculosis* in the home, but outbreaks of childhood tuberculosis centered in elementary and high schools, nursery schools, family daycare homes, churches, school buses, and stores still occur. A high-risk adult working in the area has been the source of the outbreak in most cases.

The recent epidemic of human immunodeficiency virus (HIV) infection has had a profound effect on the epidemiology of tuberculosis among children as a result of two major mechanisms: (i) HIV-infected adults with tuberculosis may transmit *M. tuberculosis* to children, some of whom will develop tuberculosis disease (55), and (ii) children with HIV infection may be at increased risk of progressing from tuberculosis infection to disease (11). Several studies of childhood tuberculosis have demonstrated that increased case rates have been associated with a simultaneous increase among HIV-infected adults in the community. In general, HIV-infected children may be more likely to have contact with HIV-infected adults who are at high risk for tuberculosis. Tuberculosis is probably underdiagnosed among HIV-infected children for three reasons: (i) the similarity of its clinical presentation to other opportunistic infections and AIDS-related conditions, (ii) the difficulty in confirming the diagnosis with positive cultures, and (iii) a high mortality rate in poor countries where tuberculosis may go unrecognized. Children with tuberculosis disease should have HIV serotesting done because the two infections are linked epidemiologically, and HIV-infected children often have more severe manifestations of tuberculosis.

Although data on tuberculosis disease in children are readily available, data concerning tuberculosis infection without disease (positive skin test or IGRA) are lacking. In the United States, tuberculosis infection is a reportable condition in only three states, and national surveys were discontinued in 1971. The most efficient method of finding children infected with *M. tuberculosis* is through contact investigations of adults with infectious pulmonary tuberculosis. On average, 30 to 50% of all household contacts of an index case have a reactive skin test.

In developing countries where tuberculosis is common, tuberculosis infection rates among the young population average 20 to 50%. In most U.S. children, the risk is less than 1%, but in some urban populations, the risk is much higher, as high as 10%. In several surveys, the majority of U.S. children with reactive skin tests were foreign-born. The upward trend in reported pediatric tuberculosis cases among foreign-born children in the United States and the results from these skin test surveys in urban areas imply that the pool of infected children and young adults in the United States is growing in some urban areas.

Transmission

Children usually are infected by an adult or adolescent in the immediate household, most often a parent, grandparent, older sibling, or boarder. Casual extrafamilial contact is the source of infection much less often, but babysitters, schoolteachers, music teachers, school bus drivers, parishioners, nurses, gardeners, and candy storekeepers have been implicated in individual cases and in hundreds of miniepidemics within limited population groups (62). Within the household of an infectious adult, the infants and toddlers almost always are infected. Also at high risk are the older children and teenagers who help the ailing adult, whereas children between 6 and 12 years of age more often escape infection. Adults with pulmonary disease who are receiving regular, appropriate chemotherapy probably rarely infect children; much more dangerous are those with chronic tuberculosis disease that is unrecognized, inadequately treated, or in relapse because of development of resistance.

Wallgren (123), based on studies in orphanages, was the first to point out that children with tuberculosis rarely, if ever, infect other children. Those few children who have transmitted *M. tuberculosis* have the characteristics typical of adult type tuberculosis (27). Many children with tuberculosis have tuberculin-negative siblings and parents. Children with tuberculosis often have been cared for by their families or in hospitals and institutions without infecting their contacts (79). When transmission of *M. tuberculosis* has been documented in children's hospitals, it almost invariably has come from an adult with undiagnosed pulmonary tuberculosis (76, 126). In tuberculous children, tubercle bacilli in endobronchial secretions are relatively sparse, and productive cough is not at all characteristic of endothoracic tuberculosis or of miliary disease (106). When young children cough, they lack the tussive force of adults. Guidelines issued by the Centers for Disease Control and Prevention (CDC) state that most children with typical childhood tuberculosis do not require isolation in the hospital unless they have an uncontrolled productive cough, a cavitary lesion, or acid-fast organism-positive sputum smears (16). Adolescents with typical reactivation-type pulmonary tuberculosis may be as infectious as adults. Children nevertheless play an extremely important role in the transmission of tuberculosis, not so much because they are likely to contaminate their immediate environment but rather because they harbor a partially healed infection that lies dormant, only to reactivate as infectious pulmonary tuberculosis many years later under the social, emotional, and physiologic stresses arising during adolescence, pregnancy, or old age. Thus, children infected with *M. tuberculosis* constitute a long-lasting reservoir of tuberculosis in the population.

The risk of infection for child contacts of adults receiving antituberculosis chemotherapy often is a matter of practical concern. Several studies have revealed that most childhood contacts are infected by the index case before diagnosis and the start of treatment. Although it is not possible to carry out a definitive clinical study, evidence indicates that patients on effective chemotherapy rarely transmit *M. tuberculosis*. Nevertheless, it seems prudent to avoid exposing additional children to adults with positive sputum smears or positive cultures and to assume that adults positive by smear or culture remain infectious for at least 2 weeks after the start of chemotherapy.

PATHOGENESIS IN CHILDREN

The primary complex of tuberculosis consists of local disease at the portal of entry and the regional lymph nodes that drain the area of the primary focus. The portal of entry is the lung in more than 95% of cases. Tubercle bacilli within particles larger than 10 μm usually are caught by the mucociliary mechanisms of the bronchial tree and are expelled. Small particles are inhaled beyond these clearance mechanisms. However, primary infection may occur anywhere in the body. Ingestion of milk infected with bovine tuberculosis can lead to a gastrointestinal primary lesion. Infection of the skin or mucous membrane can occur through an abrasion, cut, or an insect bite. The number of tubercle bacilli required to establish infection in children is unknown, but only several organisms are probably necessary.

The incubation period in children between the time the tubercle bacilli enter the body and the development of cutaneous hypersensitivity is usually 2 to 12 weeks, most often 4 to 8 weeks. The onset of hypersensitivity may be accompanied by a febrile reaction that lasts from 1 to 3 weeks. During this phase of intensified tissue reaction, the primary complex may become visible on chest radiograph. The primary focus grows larger during this time but does not yet become encapsulated. As hypersensitivity develops, the inflammatory response becomes more intense and the regional lymph nodes often enlarge. The parenchymal portion of the primary complex often heals completely by fibrosis or calcification after undergoing caseous necrosis and encapsulation. The parenchymal lesion occasionally enlarges, resulting in focal pneumonitis and thickening of the underlying pleura. If caseation is intense, the center of the lesion may liquefy, empty into the associated bronchus, and leave a residual primary tuberculous cavity.

Tubercle bacilli from the primary complex spread via the bloodstream and lymphatics to many parts of the body during the development of the parenchymal lesion and the accelerated caseation brought on by the development of hypersensitivity. The areas most commonly seeded are the apices of the lungs, liver, spleen, meninges, peritoneum, lymph nodes, pleura, and bone. This dissemination can involve either large numbers of bacilli, which leads to disseminated (miliary) tuberculosis disease, or small numbers of bacilli that leave microscopic tuberculous foci scattered in various tissues. These metastatic foci are clinically inapparent initially, but they are the origin of both extrapulmonary tuberculosis and reactivation pulmonary tuberculosis in some children and many adults.

The tubercle foci in the regional lymph nodes develop some fibrosis and encapsulation, but healing is usually less complete than in the parenchymal lesions. Viable *M. tuberculosis* may persist for decades after calcification of the nodes. The lymph nodes remain normal in size in most cases of primary tuberculosis infection. However, because of their location, hilar and paratracheal lymph nodes that become enlarged by the host inflammatory reaction may encroach upon the regional bronchus. Partial obstruction caused by external compression leads at first to hyperinflation in the distal lung segment.

Such compression may occasionally cause complete obstruction of the bronchus, resulting in atelectasis of the lung segment (69). More often, inflamed caseous nodes attach to the bronchial wall and erode through it, leading to endobronchial tuberculosis or a fistulous tract. The extrusion of infected caseous material into the bronchus can transmit infection to the lung parenchyma and cause bronchial obstruction and atelectasis. The resultant lesion is a combination of pneumonia and atelectasis. The radiographic findings of this process have been referred to as "epituberculosis," "collapse-consolidation," and "segmental" tuberculosis. Rarely, tuberculosis intrathoracic lymph nodes invade other adjacent structures such as the pericardium or esophagus.

A fairly predictable timetable for primary tuberculosis infection and its complications in infants and children is apparent (124). Massive lymphohematogenous dissemination leading to meningitis, miliary, or disseminated disease occurs in 0.5 to 2% of infected children, usually no later than 2 to 6 months after infection. Clinically significant lymph node or endobronchial tuberculosis usually appears within 3 to 9 months. Lesions of the bones and joints usually take at least a year to develop; renal lesions may be evident 5 to 25 years after infection. In general, complications of the primary infection occur within the first year.

Tuberculosis disease that occurs more than a year after the primary infection is thought to be secondary to endogenous regrowth of persistent bacilli from the primary infection and subclinical dissemination. Exogenous reinfection may result in tuberculosis disease, in rare cases, but most cases of postprimary or reactivation tuberculosis in adolescents are believed to be secondary to endogenous organisms. Reactivation tuberculosis is rare in infants and young children. Reactivation tuberculosis among adolescents affects females twice as often as males for unknown reasons. The most common form of reactivation tuberculosis is an infiltrate or cavity in the apex of the lung where oxygen tension is high and there is a heavy concentration of tubercle bacilli deposited during the primary subclinical dissemination of organisms. Dissemination during reactivation tuberculosis is rare among immunocompetent adolescents.

The age of the child at acquisition of tuberculosis infection seems to have a great effect on the occurrence of both primary and reactivation tuberculosis. Hilar lymphadenopathy and subsequent segmental disease complicating the primary infection occur most often in younger children. Approximately 40% of untreated children less than 1 year of age develop radiographically significant lymphadenopathy or segmental lesions, compared with 24% of children 1 to 10 years of age and 16% of children 11 to 15 years of age (75). However, if young children do not suffer early complications, their risk of developing reactivation tuberculosis later in life appears to be quite low. Conversely, older children and adolescents rarely experience complications of the primary infection but have a much higher risk of developing reactivation pulmonary tuberculosis as an adolescent or adult.

CLINICAL MANIFESTATIONS

How Children with Tuberculosis Are Discovered

In the developing world, the only way children with tuberculosis disease are discovered is passively, when they present with a profound illness that is consistent with tuberculosis (95). Having an ill adult contact is an obvious clue to the correct diagnosis. The only available laboratory test usually is an acid-fast smear of sputum, which the child rarely produces. Chest radiography is not available in many high-burden countries. To aid in diagnosis, a variety of clinical scoring systems have been devised based on available tests, clinical signs and symptoms, and known exposures. However, the sensitivity and specificity of these systems can be very low, leading to both over- and underdiagnosis of tuberculosis (43). No clinical scoring system has been validated in a clinical trial.

In industrial countries, children with tuberculosis usually are discovered in one of three ways (6). Obviously, one way is consideration of tuberculosis as the cause of a symptomatic pulmonary or extrapulmonary illness. Discovering an adult contact with infectious tuberculosis is an invaluable aid to diagnosis; the "yield" from contact investigation usually is higher than that from cultures from the child. The second way is discovery of a child with pulmonary tuberculosis during the contact investigation of an adult with tuberculosis. The affected child typically has few or no symptoms, but investigation reveals a positive TST and an abnormal chest radiograph. Up to 50% of children with pulmonary tuberculosis are discovered in this manner in some areas of the United States before significant symptoms have begun. A smaller number of children with tuberculosis disease are found as the result of a community- or school-based tuberculin skin testing program.

Pulmonary Disease

The symptoms and physical signs of intrathoracic tuberculosis in children are surprisingly meager considering the degree of radiographic changes often seen. The physical manifestations of disease tend to differ by the age of onset. Young infants are more likely to have significant signs or symptoms (120).

In the United States, about one-half of infants and children with radiographically moderate to severe pulmonary tuberculosis have no physical findings and are discovered only via contact tracing of an adult with tuberculosis. The chest radiograph typically is "sicker" than the child. Infants are more likely to experience signs and symptoms, probably because of their small airway diameters relative to the parenchymal and lymph node changes in primary tuberculosis (Table 2). Nonproductive cough and mild dyspnea are the most common symptoms. Systemic complaints such as fever, night sweats, anorexia, and decreased activity (malaise) occur less often. Some infants have difficulty gaining weight and develop a failure-to-thrive presentation that often does not improve significantly until after several months of treatment.

Pulmonary signs are even less common. Some infants and young children with bronchial obstruction show signs of air trapping, such as localized wheezing or decreased breath sounds, that may be accompanied by tachypnea or frank respiratory distress. These nonspecific symptoms and signs are occasionally alleviated by antibiotics, suggesting that bacterial superinfection distal to the focus of tuberculous bronchial obstruction contributes to the clinical presentation of disease.

A rare but serious complication of primary tuberculosis in children occurs when the parenchymal focus enlarges and develops a caseous center (41). The radiographic and clinical picture of progressive primary tuberculosis is that of bronchopneumonia with high fever, moderate to severe cough, night sweats, dullness to percussion, rales, and decreased breath sounds. Liquefaction in the center may result in formation of a thin-walled cavity (116).

The enlarging focus may slough debris into adjacent bronchi, leading to intrapulmonary dissemination. Rupture of the cavity into the pleural space may cause a bronchopleural fistula or pyopneumothorax, rupture into the pericardium can cause acute pericarditis with constriction, and rupture into the esophagus can create a tracheoesophageal fistula. Before the advent of antituberculosis chemotherapy, the mortality rate of progressive primary pulmonary tuberculosis was 30 to 50%. Currently, with effective treatment, the prognosis is excellent.

Older children and adolescents, especially those with reactivation-type tuberculosis, are more likely to experience fever, anorexia, malaise, weight loss, night sweats, productive cough, chest pain, and hemoptysis than children with primary pulmonary tuberculosis (67, 82). However, findings on physical examination are usually minor or absent even when cavities or large infiltrates are present. Most signs and symptoms improve within several weeks of starting effective treatment, although cough may last for several months.

As expected, the radiographic findings in childhood tuberculosis reflect the pathophysiology and are quite different from findings in adults (Table 3) (71). The hallmark of primary pulmonary tuberculosis is the relatively large size and importance of the lymphadenitis compared with the less significant size of the initial parenchymal focus. Because of the usual pattern of lymphatic circulation within the lungs, a left-sided parenchymal focus often leads to bilateral hilar adenopathy, while a right-sided focus is associated only with right-sided lymphadenitis. Hilar and/or mediastinal lymphadenopathy is invariably present with childhood tuberculosis but may not be distinct (from the atelectasis and infiltrate) or may be too small to be seen clearly on a plain radiograph. Computed tomography (CT) may reveal small lymph nodes when the chest radiograph is normal, but this finding appears to have no clinical implications (29). It can, however, create a dilemma in deciding on a treatment regimen and reinforces the idea that, in children, infection and disease are on a continuum with often indistinct borders (56).

In most cases of tuberculosis infection in children, the initial mild parenchymal infiltrate and lymphadenitis resolve spontaneously and the chest radiograph

Table 2. Symptoms and signs of childhood pulmonary tuberculosis

Symptom or sign	Infants and young children	Older children and adolescents
Fever	Common	Uncommon
Night sweats	Rare	Uncommon
Cough	Common	Common
Productive cough	Rare	Common
Hemoptysis	Never	Rare
Dyspnea	Common	Rare
Rales	Common	Uncommon
Wheezing	Common	Uncommon
Dullness	Rare	Uncommon
Diminished breath sounds	Common	Uncommon

Table 3. Comparison of chest radiographs of pulmonary tuberculosis in adults and children

Characteristic(s)	Adults	Children
Location	Apical	Anywhere (25% multilobar)
Adenopathy	Rare (except HIV related)	Usual
Cavitation	Common	Rare (except adolescent)
Signs and symptoms	Consistent	Relative paucity

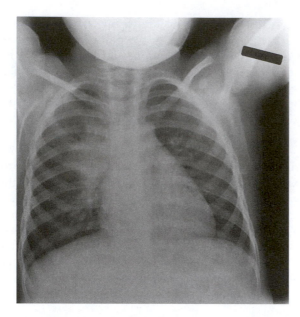

Figure 2. Early collapse-consolidation lesion in a child with tuberculosis. Mediastinal adenopathy also is present on the right side.

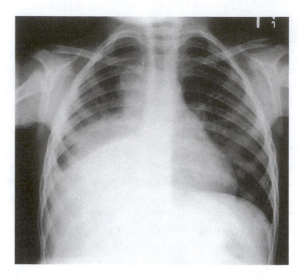

Figure 4. Well-formed collapse-consolidation lesion on the right, with large mediastinal and hilar adenopathy and atelectasis.

is normal. In some children, the hilar or mediastinal lymph nodes continue to enlarge. Partial airway obstruction caused by external compression from the enlarging nodes causes air trapping and hyperinflation. As the nodes attach to and infiltrate the airway, caesium filling the lumen causes complete obstruction, resulting in atelectasis that involves the lobar segment distal to the obstructed lumen (Fig. 2). The resulting radiographic shadows are called collapse-consolidation or segmental lesions (Fig. 3 and 4). These findings resemble those in foreign body aspiration; in the case of tuberculosis, the lymph node is acting as the foreign body. Multiple segmental lesions in different lobes may appear simultaneously, as can atelectasis and hyperinflation.

Other radiographic findings are noted in some children. Occasional children have a lobar pneumonia without distinct hilar adenopathy. In infants and young children, the radiographic appearance can resemble exudative pneumonia, similar to that caused by *Klebsiella pneumoniae* or *Staphylococcus aureus* (Fig. 5). A secondary bacterial pneumonia may contribute to this appearance. When tuberculosis infection is progressively destructive, liquefaction of lung parenchyma leads to formation of a thin-walled primary tuberculosis cavity. Peripheral bullous lesions occur rarely and can lead to pneumothorax (73). Enlargement of subcarinal nodes causes compression of the esophagus, difficulty swallowing, and rarely, a bronchoesophageal fistula. One sign of early

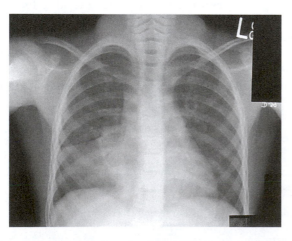

Figure 3. Slightly more extensive right-sided adenopathy with atelectasis in a 2-year-old with tuberculosis.

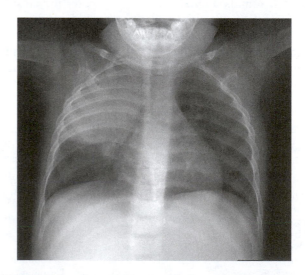

Figure 5. Tuberculous pneumonia with bowing of the horizontal fissure. Children with this finding may have an associated bacterial infection.

subcarinal tuberculosis is horizontal splaying of the mainstem bronchi.

Adolescents with pulmonary tuberculosis may develop segmental lesions with associated adenopathy, but more often, they develop the infiltrates with or without cavitation that are typical of adult reactivation tuberculosis (Fig. 6) (30). The lesions are often smaller in adolescents than adults, and lordotic views, tomograms, or even a CT scan may be necessary to demonstrate small apical foci of disease.

The course of thoracic lymphadenopathy and bronchial obstruction can follow several paths. The segment of lobe reexpands in most cases, and the radiographic abnormalities resolve completely. The resolution occurs slowly, over months to several years, and is not affected greatly by antituberculosis therapy. Of course, children still have infection with *M. tuberculosis* and are at high risk of reactivation tuberculosis in subsequent years if chemotherapy has not been taken. In some cases, the segmental lesion resolves but residual calcification occurs in the primary parenchymal focus or regional lymph nodes. The calcification usually occurs in fine particles creating a stippling effect. Calcification begins 6 months or more after infection. Even with chemotherapy, the enlarged lymph nodes and endobronchial lesions may persist for many months, occasionally resulting in severe airway obstruction. Surgical or endoscopic removal of intraluminal lesions is rarely necessary. Finally, bronchial obstruction may cause scarring and progressive contraction of the lobe or segment, which is often associated with cylindrical bronchiectasis. Complete radiographic and clinical resolution without calcification occur in the vast majority of cases with early institution of adequate treatment for collapse-consolidation lesions.

Pleural Disease

Tuberculous pleural effusions, which can be local or general, usually originate in the discharge of bacilli into the pleural space from a subpleural pulmonary focus or caseated subpleural lymph nodes (63). Asymptomatic local pleural effusion is so frequent in primary tuberculosis that it is basically a component of the primary complex. Most large and clinically significant effusions occur months to years after the primary infection (Fig. 7). Tuberculous pleural effusion is less common in children younger than 6 years of age and rare in those below 2 years of age (26). Such effusions are usually unilateral but can be bilateral. They are virtually never associated with a segmental pulmonary lesion and are rare in miliary tuberculosis.

The clinical onset of tuberculous pleurisy in children is usually fairly sudden, with low to high fever, shortness of breath, chest pain especially on deep inspiration, dullness to percussion, and diminished breath sounds on the affected side. The presentation is similar to that of pyogenic pleurisy. The fever and other symptoms may last for several weeks after the start of antituberculosis chemotherapy. Although corticosteroids may reduce the clinical symptoms, they

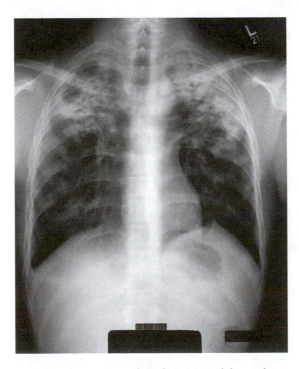

Figure 6. Reactivation-type tuberculosis in an adolescent boy.

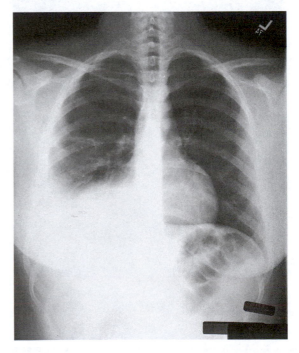

Figure 7. A tuberculous pleural effusion in an adolescent girl.

have little effect on the ultimate outcome. The TST is positive in only 70 to 80% of cases. The prognosis is excellent; radiographic resolution takes months; however, scoliosis rarely complicates recovery of a long-standing effusion.

Extrathoracic Tuberculosis

The various forms of extrapulmonary tuberculosis are reviewed in detail in other chapters. Up to 25 to 35% of childhood tuberculosis cases are extrapulmonary (Table 1), and a careful physical examination is an essential component of the evaluation of a child with tuberculosis exposure or infection. The most common location of extrapulmonary tuberculosis in children is the lymph nodes of the neck (68, 128, 129).

The two forms of extrapulmonary tuberculosis that receive the most attention, because of their life-threatening nature, are disseminated (miliary) disease (Fig. 8) and meningitis. Both forms of disease occur early, often within 2 to 6 months of initial infection. Correct diagnosis requires a high index of suspicion because it is difficult to confirm these diseases microbiologically (101). Acid-fast stains of body fluids are almost always negative; cultures for *M. tuberculosis* are positive in only 50% of cases or fewer and they often take weeks to grow because the initial inoculum of organisms is so low (50, 99, 121). In addition, the TST may be nonreactive initially in up to 50% of

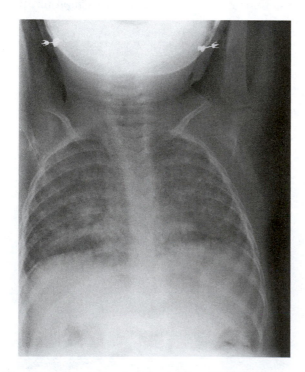

Figure 8. Miliary tuberculosis in an infant. The child presented with fever and respiratory distress.

pediatric patients, and the chest radiograph in both diseases may be normal early on. The key element to correctly diagnose each condition is an epidemiologic history, a search for the adult from whom the child acquired *M. tuberculosis*. Unfortunately, an initial negative history for exposure does not really help. In a study of 31 consecutive infants and children with central nervous system tuberculosis in Houston, TX, the initial family history was negative for tuberculosis in 30 cases, although the adult source case was ultimately identified in over 60% of cases (32). The ill adult often has not yet been diagnosed correctly because the incubation period of disseminated tuberculosis and meningitis in children may be short. An evaluation of the family and other adults and adolescents in close contact with the child should be considered a public health emergency when serious tuberculosis disease is suspected in a child.

The most feared complication of tuberculosis in children is meningitis (93). Although the clinical onset of tuberculous meningitis in children may occur gradually over several weeks, recent studies describe more rapid progression over several days. Early on, the clinical presentation may be similar to that of viral or pyogenic meningitis. However, tuberculous meningitis in children is more likely to be complicated by cranial nerve involvement, basilar leptomeningeal involvement, hydrocephalus, and infarct caused by vasculitis. These findings in any child with meningitis, when no other cause is readily apparent, should prompt immediate initiation of antituberculosis chemotherapy while diagnostic studies and investigation of close contacts for tuberculosis are carried out as quickly as possible.

The widespread use of improved cranial imaging such as CT scan and magnetic resonance imaging have shown that tuberculoma is more common than previously realized, and the distinction in children between tuberculous meningitis and tuberculoma is not as clear as once thought. Tuberculomas account for up to 40% of brain tumors in children in some developing countries. They often occur in children less than 10 years of age, may be single or multiple, and are often located at the base of the brain, near the cerebellum. However, a recently recognized phenomenon is the paradoxical development of intracranial tuberculomas appearing or enlarging during treatment of meningeal, disseminated, and even pulmonary tuberculosis (2). This phenomenon appears to be similar to the well-described worsening of intrathoracic adenopathy seen in many children during the first few months of ultimately successful chemotherapy for tuberculosis. The tuberculomas seem to be mediated immunologically; they respond (slowly) to corticosteroid therapy and a change in antituberculosis therapy is not required.

Some infants with pulmonary tuberculosis and very subtle neurologic signs or symptoms will have one or several tuberculomas, even with a normal cerebrospinal fluid evaluation. Any neurologic abnormality in a child with suspected tuberculosis should be evaluated with a neuroimaging study, when feasible (32).

Tuberculosis in HIV-Infected Children

In adults infected with both HIV and *M. tuberculosis*, the rate of progression from asymptomatic infection to disease is increased greatly (11, 19). The clinical manifestations of tuberculosis in HIV-infected adults tend to be typical when the CD4$^+$ cell count is more than 500 per mm^3 but become "atypical" as the CD4$^+$ cell count falls. Similar correlations have not been reported for dually infected children, though there is some epidemiologic evidence that tuberculosis rates are higher in HIV-infected children in the United States than in the general population. When HIV-infected children develop tuberculosis, the clinical features tend to be fairly typical of disease in immunocompetent children, although the disease often progresses more rapidly and clinical manifestations are more severe (12, 20, 112). There may be an increased tendency for extrapulmonary disease, but the trend is not as dramatic as it is in HIV-infected adults (11). Unfortunately, higher mortality rates have been noted, including those from other AIDS-related conditions, if effective antiretroviral therapy is not also started (44). The diagnosis of tuberculosis in an HIV-infected child can be difficult to establish, as skin test reactivity may be absent, culture confirmation is slow and difficult, and the clinical presentation may be similar to that of other HIV-related infections and conditions (37). A diligent search for an infectious adult in the child's environment often yields the strongest clue to the correct diagnosis.

HIV-infected patients being treated for tuberculosis can experience a worsening of signs and symptoms if concomitant antiretroviral therapy causes a rapid decrease in HIV load and increase in CD4$^+$ counts. The immune reconstitution inflammatory syndrome has been observed in children being treated for tuberculosis and in children who have received a *Mycobacterium bovis* BCG vaccine (7, 45, 46). The most common manifestations are at the anatomic site of the existing tuberculosis, but new onset of tuberculomas, lymphadenopathy, and abdominal manifestations can occur (72, 90). Immune reconstitution inflammatory syndrome should be suspected when an HIV-infected child develops apparent complications of tuberculosis (or BCG vaccination) after starting antiretroviral therapy, though other potential causes should be considered.

DIAGNOSIS

Tuberculin Skin Test (TST)

The TST has been reviewed extensively in a previous chapter. The placement of the Mantoux intradermal skin test, while fairly simple and routine in a cooperative adult, can be a challenge in a squirming, scared child. The technique shown in Fig. 9 allows for better control during placement. The skin tester anchors her hand along the longitudinal axis of the child's arm, which enhances stability and allows the last two fingers to become a fulcrum to guide inoculation of the solution. The tuberculin is injected laterally across the arm. As with adults, a wheal of 6 to 10 mm should be raised after injection. The test is interpreted at 48 to 72 hours after placement. Although recent formal studies are lacking, most experts believe the time course of the reaction and amount of induration produced is similar in children and adults. Infants may make slightly less induration, on average, when infected.

The interpretation of the Mantoux skin test should be similar in children and adults (Table 4) (36, 49, 102). However, most of the "risk factors" for children are actually the risk factors of the adults in their environment, i.e., the likelihood that the child has had significant contact with an adult with contagious pulmonary tuberculosis. Correctly classifying a child's reaction supposes that the risk factors of the adults around the child have been considered. The American Academy of Pediatrics (AAP) has suggested that 10 mm should be the cut-off point for all children less than 4 years of age (4). This recommendation is not based on diminished ability to make an induration reaction in children; it was made to minimize false-negative reactions in

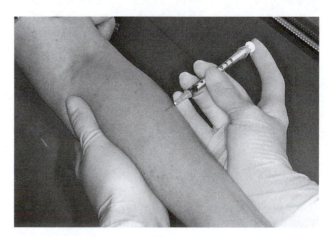

Figure 9. A helpful technique for applying the Mantoux TST on a child. The hand is anchored on the side of the child's arm, providing stability. The tuberculin is injected in a lateral direction.

Table 4. Amount of induration from a
Mantoux TST considered positive in children

Reaction size (mm)	Factor
≥5	Contact with an infectious case
	Abnormal X ray or clinical finding
	HIV infection or immunosuppression
≥10	Birth or previous residence in a high-prevalence country
	Residence in a long-term care facility
	Contact with high-risk adults (when a specific source is not known)
	Age < 4 years
≥15	Absence of risk factors

small children who are at increased risk of developing life-threatening forms of tuberculosis once infected.

The same factors that influence the accuracy of tuberculin skin testing in adults also affect children. About 10 to 20% of children with tuberculosis disease initially have a negative reaction to tuberculin (110). The lack of reactivity may be global or may occur only for tuberculin, so "control" skin tests may be of limited usefulness in children. In most cases (other than those with advanced HIV infection or other ongoing immunosuppression), the reaction becomes positive as the child recovers on chemotherapy. Incubating or manifest viral infections are a frequent cause of false-negative results in children.

Previous inoculation with a BCG vaccination can pose problems with interpretation of a subsequent TST. Although many infants who receive a BCG vaccine never develop a skin test reaction to tuberculin, about 50% will. The reactivity fades over time but can be boosted in children with repeated skin testing (100). Most experts agree that skin test interpretation in children who received a BCG vaccine more than 3 years previously should be the same as if they had never received vaccine, though some false-positive reactions will occur. When skin testing is done sooner after vaccination, interpretation is more difficult. The clinician should have a clear understanding of why the test was placed and realize that a positive reaction most likely represents infection with *M. tuberculosis* if the child had a specific exposure to an infectious adult or adolescent.

IGRAs

QuantiFERON-TB Gold In-Tube and T-SPOT TB are IGRAs. These tests measure ex vivo gamma interferon production from T lymphocytes in response to stimulation with antigens that are fairly specific to *M. tuberculosis* complex. As with TSTs, IGRAs cannot distinguish between latent infection and disease, and a negative result from these tests cannot exclude the possibility of tuberculosis infection or disease in a patient with findings that raise suspicion for these conditions. The sensitivity of these blood tests is similar to that of TSTs for detecting infection in adults and children who have untreated culture-confirmed tuberculosis. The specificity of IGRAs is higher than that for TSTs because the antigens used are not found in BCG or most pathogenic nontuberculous mycobacteria (8, 17, 31). The published experience with testing children with IGRAs is less extensive than for adults, but a number of studies have demonstrated that IGRAs perform well in most children 4 years of age and older (24, 47, 61, 83, 104). Some children who received BCG vaccine may have a false-positive TST result, and latent TB infection (LTBI) is overestimated by use of the TST, even in these circumstances. However, the correct interpretation of a negative IGRA result in a child with a positive TST result remains challenging because of the current absence of longitudinal studies to determine the negative predictive value of the IGRAs (when the TST result is positive and the IGRA result is negative) (60).

At this time, neither an IGRA nor the TST can be considered a gold standard for diagnosis of LTBI. Current recommendations for use of IGRAs in children are as follows (4):

- For immunocompetent children 5 years of age and older, IGRAs can be used in place of a TST to confirm cases of tuberculosis or cases of LTBI and likely will yield fewer false-positive test results.
- Children with a positive result from an IGRA should be considered infected with *M. tuberculosis* complex. A negative IGRA result cannot universally be interpreted as absence of infection.
- Because of their higher specificity and lack of cross-reaction with BCG, IGRAs may be useful in children who have received BCG vaccine. IGRAs may be useful to determine whether a BCG-immunized child with a reactive TST more likely has LTBI or has a false-positive TST reaction caused by the BCG.
- IGRAs cannot be recommended routinely for use in children younger than 5 years of age or for immunocompromised children of any age because of a lack of published data about their utility with these groups (42).
- Indeterminate IGRA results do not exclude tuberculosis infection and should not be used to make clinical decisions.

Diagnostic Mycobacteriology in Children

The demonstration of acid-fast bacilli in stained smears of sputum is presumptive evidence of pulmonary tuberculosis in most patients. However, in children, tubercle bacilli usually are relatively few in number, and sputum cannot be obtained spontaneously from children younger than about 10 years of age. Gastric washings, which often are used in lieu of sputum, can be contaminated with acid-fast organisms from the mouth. However, fluorescence microscopy of gastric washings has been found useful, though the yield is less than 10% (59). Tubercle bacilli in cerebrospinal fluid, pleural fluid, lymph node aspirate, and urine are sparse; thus, only rarely are direct-stained smears for tubercle bacilli positive in pediatric practice. Cultures for tubercle bacilli are of great importance, not only to confirm the diagnosis but increasingly to permit testing for drug susceptibility. However, if culture and drug susceptibility data are available from the associated adult case and the child has a classic presentation of tuberculosis (positive skin test, consistent abnormal chest radiograph, exposure to an adult case), obtaining cultures from the child adds little to the management.

Painstaking collection of specimens is essential for culture diagnosis in children because usually fewer organisms are present than in adults. Gastric lavage should be performed in the very early morning, when the patient has had nothing to eat or drink for 8 hours and before the patient has a chance to wake up and start swallowing saliva, which dilutes the bronchial secretions that were brought up during the night and made their way into the stomach. Inhalation of superheated nebulized saline prior to gastric lavage has been reported to increase the bacteriologic yield (40). The stomach contents should be aspirated first. No more than 50 to 75 ml of sterile distilled water (not saline) should be injected through the stomach tube, and the aspirate should be added to the first collection. The gastric acidity (poorly tolerated by tubercle bacilli) should be neutralized immediately. Concentration and culture should be performed as soon as possible after collection. However, even with optimal, in-hospital collection of three early morning gastric aspirate samples, M. tuberculosis can be isolated from only 30% to 40% of children and 70% of infants with pulmonary tuberculosis (96, 102, 120). The yield from random outpatient gastric aspirate samples is exceedingly low.

Bronchial secretions obtained by stimulating cough with an aerosol solution of propylene glycol in 10% sodium chloride can be used in older children (130, 131). The aerosol is heated in a nebulizer at 46 to 52°C (114.8 to 125.6°F) and administered to the patient for 15 to 30 minutes. This method gives good results and may be superior to gastric lavage both in yield of positive cultures and patient acceptance (52). Bronchial aspirate obtained at bronchoscopy is often thick, and the laboratory will process it using a mucolytic agent, such as N-acetyl-L-cysteine. The yield of M. tuberculosis from bronchoscopy specimens has been lower in most studies than from properly obtained gastric aspirates (1, 18). However, bronchoscopy can help establish the likelihood of tuberculosis in a child with unknown pulmonary disease (13).

Nucleic Acid Amplification

The main form of nucleic acid amplification studied in children with tuberculosis is the PCR, which uses specific DNA sequences as markers for microorganisms. Various PCR techniques, most using the mycobacterial insertion element IS6110 as the DNA marker for M. tuberculosis complex organisms, have a sensitivity and specificity of more than 90% compared with sputum culture for detecting pulmonary tuberculosis in adults. However, test performance varies even among reference laboratories. The test is relatively expensive, requires fairly sophisticated equipment, and requires scrupulous technique to avoid cross-contamination of specimens.

Use of PCR in childhood tuberculosis has been limited. Compared with a clinical diagnosis of pulmonary tuberculosis in children, sensitivity of PCR has varied from 25 to 83% and specificity has varied from 80 to 100% (28, 86, 88, 103). The PCR of gastric aspirates may be positive in a recently infected child even when the chest radiograph is normal, demonstrating the occasional arbitrariness of the distinction between tuberculosis infection and disease in children. The PCR may have a useful but limited role in evaluating children for tuberculosis. A negative PCR never eliminates tuberculosis as a diagnostic possibility, and a positive result does not confirm it. The major use of PCR is evaluating children with significant pulmonary disease when the diagnosis is not established readily by clinical or epidemiologic grounds. PCR may be helpful in evaluating immunocompromised children with pulmonary disease, especially in children with HIV infection, although published reports of its performance in such children are lacking. PCR also may aid in confirming the diagnosis of extrapulmonary tuberculosis.

MANAGEMENT

The first-line drugs, their formulations, and their pediatric doses are listed in Table 5.

Table 5. Commonly used drugs for the treatment of tuberculosis in children

Drug	Dosage forms	Daily dose (mg/kg/day)	Twice-weekly dose (mg/kg/dose)	Maximum daily dose
Ethambutol	Tablets: 100 mg, 400 mg	20–25	50	2.5 g
Isoniazid[a,b]	Scored tablets: 100 mg, 300 mg Syrup,[c] 100 mg/ml	10–15[b]	20–30	Daily, 300 mg; twice weekly, 900 mg
Pyrazinamide	Scored tablets, 500 mg	20–40	50	2 g
Rifampin[a]	Capsules: 150 mg, 300 mg Syrup (formulated in syrup from capsules)	10–20	10–20	Daily, 600 mg; twice weekly, 600 mg
Streptomycin (intramuscular administration)	Vials: 1 g, 4 g	20–40		1 g

[a]Rifamate is a capsule containing 150 mg of isoniazid and 300 mg of rifampin. Two capsules provide the usual adult (>50 kg body weight) daily doses of each drug.
[b]When isoniazid is used in combination with rifampin, the incidence of hepatotoxicity increases if the isoniazid dose exceeds 10 mg/kg/day.
[c]Most experts advise against the use of isoniazid syrup due to instability and a high rate of gastrointestinal adverse reaction (diarrhea, cramps) when more than 5 ml is given.

Exposure

Children exposed to potentially infectious adults with pulmonary tuberculosis should be started on treatment, usually INH only, if the child is younger than 5 years of age or has other risk factors for the rapid development of tuberculosis disease, such as immunocompromise of some kind (87). Failure to do so may result in development of severe tuberculosis disease even before the TST becomes reactive; the "incubation period" of disease may be shorter than that for the skin test. The child is treated for a minimum of 10 to 12 weeks after contact with the infectious case is broken (by physical separation or effective treatment of the case). After 3 months, the TST or IGRA is repeated. If the second test is positive, infection is documented and INH should be continued for a total duration of 9 months; if the second test is negative, the treatment can be stopped. If the exposure was to a case with an INH-resistant but rifampin (RIF)-susceptible isolate, RIF is the recommended treatment.

Two circumstances of exposure deserve special attention. A difficult situation arises when the exposed child is anergic because of immunocompromise. These children are particularly vulnerable to rapid progression of tuberculosis, and it will not be possible to tell if infection has occurred. In general, these children should be treated as if they have tuberculosis infection.

The second situation is exposure of a newborn to a mother (or other adult) with a positive TST or, rarely, a nursery worker with contagious tuberculosis. The management is based on further evaluation of the mother (4).

1. Mother has a normal chest radiograph. No separation of the infant and mother is required. Although the mother should receive treatment for tuberculosis infection and other household members should be evaluated for tuberculosis infection or disease, the infant needs no further work-up or treatment unless a case of disease is found.

2. Mother has an abnormal chest radiograph. The mother and child should be separated until the mother has been evaluated thoroughly. If the radiograph, history, physical examination, and analysis of sputum reveal no evidence of active pulmonary tuberculosis in the mother, it is reasonable to assume the infant is at low risk of infection. However, if the mother remains untreated, she may later develop contagious tuberculosis and expose her infant. Both mother and infant should receive appropriate follow-up care, but the infant does not need treatment. If the radiograph and clinical history are suggestive of pulmonary tuberculosis in the mother, the child and mother should remain separated until both have begun appropriate chemotherapy. The infant should be evaluated for congenital tuberculosis. The placenta should be examined. If the mother has no risk factors for drug-resistant tuberculosis, the infant should receive INH and close follow-up care. The infant should have a TST at 3 or 4 months after the mother is judged no longer to be contagious; evaluation of the infant at this time follows the guidelines for other exposures of children. If no infection is documented at this time, it would be prudent to repeat the TST in 6 to 12 months. If the mother has tuberculosis caused by a multidrug-resistant isolate of *M. tuberculosis* or she has poor adherence to therapy, the child should remain separated from her until she no longer is contagious or the infant can be given a BCG vaccine and be kept separated until the vaccine "takes" (marked by a reactive TST).

Infection

The recommendation for treatment of asymptomatic tuberculin-positive individuals is based on data from several well-controlled studies; it applies particularly to children and adolescents who are at high risk for the development of overt disease but at very low risk for the development of the main toxic manifestation of INH therapy, which is hepatitis (35, 39, 48, 84). The large, carefully controlled U.S. Public Health Study of 1955, followed by others, demonstrated the favorable effect of 12 months of INH on the incidence of complications due to progression of tuberculosis infection. The younger the tuberculin reactor, the greater the benefit (23).

The American Thoracic Society and the CDC (10) recommend that INH treatment of tuberculosis infection be given to all positive tuberculin reactors at risk for developing disease. The question arises as to how long the protective effect can be expected to last. Comstock and associates (22), in their final report on INH prophylaxis in Alaska, demonstrated the protective effect of 1 year of chemoprophylaxis to be at least 19 years. Hsu (48) reported on 2,494 children monitored for up to 30 years and showed that adequate drug treatment prevented reactivation of tuberculosis during adolescence and into young adulthood. It is likely that the decreased risk of tuberculosis after INH therapy may be lifelong in children infected with INH-susceptible tubercle bacilli. Failure of INH after exposure to INH-resistant *M. tuberculosis* has been documented. No controlled study of an alternative regimen has been reported. RIF alone is recommended and widely used.

The dosage of INH to be used has had little study. Most investigators have used a regimen based on 4 to 8 mg/kg of body weight/day, usually taken all at once, for a period of 6 to 12 months. A dose of 5 mg/kg/day was found satisfactory in one study (21). Most clinicians prescribe a dose of 10 to 15 mg/kg/day to a total of 300 mg/day for treatment of infection to be sure of achieving therapeutic levels even among patients who inactivate the drug rapidly by acetylation (74).

The duration of INH treatment initially was set arbitrarily at 12 months. A large trial was conducted on adults in Eastern Europe with old fibrotic lesions caused by tuberculosis, comparing regimens of daily INH taken for 12, 24, and 52 weeks with a placebo for their ability to prevent tuberculosis disease (51). Therapy for 1 year was most effective, especially if patients were adherent. However, therapy for 24 weeks afforded a fairly high level of protection. Subsequently, many health departments accepted 6 months of INH therapy as their standard regimen for

adults. However, the cost-effectiveness analysis does not apply to children.

A duration of 9 months has been recommended for children by the AAP and CDC for many years (105). INH is taken daily under self-supervision or can be taken twice weekly under directly observed therapy (DOT) (87). When the child is infected with an INH-resistant but RIF-susceptible strain of *M. tuberculosis*, 6 months of RIF should be substituted for INH. If the infecting strain is resistant to both INH and RIF, usually two other drugs are used. No combination of drugs is known to be superior to the others; usually two from among pyrazinamide (PZA), ethambutol, ethionamide, cycloserine, or a fluoroquinolone are chosen.

Disease

Clinical trials of antituberculosis drugs in children are difficult to perform, mostly because of the difficulty in obtaining positive cultures at diagnosis or relapse and the need for long-term monitoring (25). Recommendations for treating children with tuberculosis were extrapolated historically from clinical trials of adults with pulmonary tuberculosis. However, during the past 25 years, the results of a large number of clinical trials involving only children have been reported. Patients with only hilar adenopathy can be treated successfully with INH and RIF for 6 months (91). Several major studies of 6-month therapy in children with pulmonary tuberculosis using at least three drugs in the initial phase have been reported (3, 58, 117, 118). The most commonly used regimen was 6 months of INH and RIF supplemented during the first 2 months with PZA. The overall success rate has been greater than 98%, and the incidence of clinically significant adverse reactions is less than 2%. Regimens not using streptomycin were as successful as those that included it. Using twice-weekly medications (under DOT) during the continuation phase was as effective and safe as daily administration. Several studies used twice-weekly therapy throughout the treatment regimen with excellent success (58, 117), and one used daily therapy for only the first 2 weeks. The 6-month, three-drug regimen was successful, tolerated well, and less expensive than the 9-month regimen. It also effects a cure faster, so there is a greater likelihood of successful treatment if the child becomes nonadherent later in therapy. Most experts recommend starting a fourth drug, usually ethambutol, until it can be determined that the child has tuberculosis susceptible to at least INH and RIF (4, 33, 111).

Controlled treatment trials for various forms of extrapulmonary tuberculosis are rare (54). Several of the 6-month, three-drug trials in children included extrapulmonary cases (9, 58). Most non-life-threatening forms of extrapulmonary tuberculosis respond well to a 9-month course of INH and RIF or to a 6-month regimen including INH, RIF, and PZA. One exception may be bone and joint tuberculosis, which may have a high failure rate when 6-month chemotherapy is used, especially when surgical intervention has not taken place; 9 to 12 months of treatment is recommended.

Tuberculous meningitis usually is not included in trials of extrapulmonary tuberculosis therapy because of its serious nature and low incidence. Treatment with INH and RIF for 12 months generally is effective (122). A study from Thailand showed that a 6-month regimen including PZA for serious tuberculous meningitis led to fewer deaths and better outcomes than did longer regimens that did not contain PZA (53). Most children are treated initially with four drugs (INH, RIF, PZA, and ethionamide or streptomycin). The PZA and fourth drug are stopped after 2 months, and INH and RIF are continued for a total of 7 to 12 months.

Drug Resistance

Patterns of drug resistance in children tend to mirror those found in adult patients in the population (14, 98, 109). Outbreaks of drug-resistant tuberculosis in children occurring at schools have been reported (92). The key to determining drug resistance in childhood tuberculosis usually comes from the drug susceptibility results of the infectious adult contact case's isolate.

Therapy for drug-resistant tuberculosis is successful only when at least two bactericidal drugs to which the infecting strain of M. tuberculosis is susceptible are given (108, 115). When INH resistance is considered a possibility, on the basis of epidemiologic risk factors or the identification of an INH-resistant source case isolate, an additional drug, usually ethambutol or streptomycin, should be given initially to the child until the exact susceptibility pattern is determined and a more-specific regimen can be designed. Exact treatment regimens must be tailored to the specific pattern of drug resistance (97). The duration of therapy usually is extended to at least 9 to 12 months if either INH or RIF can be used and to at least 18 to 24 months if resistance to both drugs is present (85). Surgical resection of a diseased lung or lobe is rarely required in children. An expert in tuberculosis always should be involved in the management of children with drug-resistant tuberculosis infection or disease (38).

Adherence and DOT

For many families with a child with tuberculosis, the disease is but one of many social and other problems in the family's life, and at certain times, other problems may supersede the perceived importance of tuberculosis (89). To combat this problem of nonadherence with treatment, most health departments have developed programs of DOT in which a third party, usually but not always a health care worker, is present during the administration of each dose of medication. DOT should be considered standard therapy for children with tuberculosis disease. The clinician should coordinate this treatment with the local health department. In my clinic, all children with tuberculosis are treated exclusively with DOT, which can be given at an office, clinic, home, school, work, or any other setting. It is highly effective and safe, and the patient satisfaction is high if it is offered as a special service to treat tuberculosis. High-risk children with tuberculosis infection are being treated with DOT at schools or in other locations to ensure completion of therapy. DOT also should be considered for all child contacts of adult tuberculosis patients, especially when the adult also is receiving DOT. Although specific controlled studies are lacking, twice-weekly DOT appears to be effective for treating tuberculosis exposure and infection in children and adolescents.

Follow-Up

Follow-up of children treated with antituberculosis drugs has become more streamlined in recent years. The patient should be seen monthly while receiving chemotherapy, both to encourage regular taking of the prescribed drugs and to check, by a few simple questions (concerning appetite and well-being) and a few observations (weight gain, appearance of skin and sclerae, and palpation of liver, spleen, and lymph nodes) that the disease is not spreading and that toxic effects of the drugs are not appearing. Routine biochemical monitoring for hepatitis is not necessary in children, unless they have liver disease or are taking other hepatotoxic drugs. Repeat chest radiographs should be obtained 1 to 2 months after the onset of chemotherapy to ascertain the maximal extent of disease before chemotherapy takes effect; thereafter, they rarely are necessary. Chemotherapy has been so successful that follow-up beyond its termination is not necessary, except for children with serious disease, such as tuberculous meningitis, or those with extensive residual chest radiographic findings at the end of chemotherapy. Chest radiograph findings resolve slowly; it is typical that enlarged lymph nodes take 2 to 3 years to resolve, well beyond the completion of ultimately successful chemotherapy. A normal chest radiograph is not a necessary criterion for stopping therapy.

PUBLIC HEALTH ASPECTS OF PEDIATRIC TUBERCULOSIS

It is hoped that it has become obvious that the control of tuberculosis in children—for a community and for individuals—depends on close cooperation between the clinician and the local health department (34). It is critically important that clinicians report cases of tuberculosis to the health department as soon as possible (127). Public health law in all U.S. states requires that the suspicion of tuberculosis disease in an adult or child be reported immediately to the health department (5). The clinician should not wait for microbiologic confirmation of the diagnosis because it is this reporting that leads to the initiation of the contact investigation that may find infected children and allow them to be treated before disease occurs (64, 65, 113). The child may progress from infection to disease before intervention can occur if the clinician waits for confirmatory laboratory results. The clinician should always feel free to contact the local health department about special issues involving tuberculosis exposure, infection, or disease in a child. Not every clinical situation can be anticipated by normal guidelines, and in some cases, an unusual intervention may be warranted.

It is estimated that about 1 million children in the United States have infection by M. tuberculosis. The major purpose of finding and treating these children is to prevent future cases of tuberculosis. Frequent or periodic skin testing of children, however, will prevent few cases of childhood tuberculosis, especially if the screening is centered on school-aged children (who rarely develop primary disease) (77). The major purpose of testing children is to prevent future cases of tuberculosis in adults. The infection rates are low among young children even in very high risk groups in the United States. The incubation period for childhood tuberculosis is weeks to months, so even annual testing will not prevent many cases. The best way to prevent childhood tuberculosis is via prompt contact investigation centered on adults with suspected contagious tuberculosis (78). This investigation has a high yield—on average, 30 to 50% of childhood household contacts are infected—but also finds the most important individuals, those most recently infected who are in the period of their lives when they are most likely to develop tuberculosis disease. The most important activity in a community to prevent cases of childhood tuberculosis is the contact investigation activity of the public health department.

If perfect contact investigations were performed and foreign-born children coming to the United States received TSTs, there would be virtually no reason to skin test any other children because all infected children would be found. Obviously, these two activities do not occur in a perfect fashion, and testing of certain selected individuals is appropriate. The CDC and AAP have changed and refined their recommendations for tuberculin skin testing of children several times in the past decade. The AAP continues to emphasize that routine tuberculin skin testing of all children, including school-based programs that include populations at low risk, has a low yield of positive results or a large number of false-positive results, representing an inefficient use of limited health care resources (87). Children without specific risk factors who reside in areas with a low prevalence of tuberculosis, therefore, do not need to have any routine tuberculin skin testing. School-based testing may be appropriate only for children with specific risk factors. A child should be considered at increased risk if the child was born in, has resided in, or has traveled (nontourist) to a country with high tuberculosis rates (Central and South America, Africa, Asia, and Eastern Europe); there is a family history of tuberculosis infection or disease; the child is in foster care; or the child is a member of a group identified locally to be at increased risk for tuberculosis infection (examples may include migrant worker families, the homeless, and certain census tracts or neighborhoods).

Much of the focus on tuberculin skin testing should be placed on identification of risk factors for a child being in a group with a high prevalence of infection. Although some risk factors may apply across the country, local health departments must identify those risk factors that are germane to their area. Clinicians and their organizations must work closely with local health departments to establish which children should be tested and which should not. Health departments should advise school districts as to whether any type of school-based skin testing is appropriate and what nature it should take. Social and political problems can occur when selective testing is suggested. What is correct from a public health point of view may not be easy to translate into a workable and generally acceptable policy. Local clinicians can be extremely helpful to health departments in advancing prudent and reasonable tuberculosis control policies, particularly when other government or public agencies are involved.

REFERENCES

1. Abadco, D., and P. Steiner. 1992. Gastric lavage is better than bronchoalveolar lavage for isolation of Mycobacterium tuberculosis in childhood pulmonary tuberculosis. *Pediatr. Infect. Dis. J.* **11**:735–738.

2. Afghani, B., and J. M. Lieberman. 1994. Paradoxical enlargement or development of intracranial tuberculomas during therapy: case report and review. *Clin. Infect. Dis.* **19**:1092–1099.

3. Al-Dossary, F. S., L. T. Ong, A. G. Correa, and J. R. Starke. 2002. Treatment of childhood tuberculosis with a six month directly observed regimen of only two weeks of daily therapy. *Pediatr. Infect. Dis. J.* **21**:91–97.

4. American Academy of Pediatrics. 2009. 2009 *Red Book: Report of the Committee on Infectious Diseases*, 28th ed. American Academy of Pediatrics, Elk Grove Village, IL.

5. American Thoracic Society, Centers for Disease Control and Prevention, and Infectious Disease Society of America. 2005. American Thoracic Society/Centers for Disease Control and Prevention/Infectious Disease Society of America: controlling tuberculosis in the United States. *Am. J. Respir. Crit. Care Med.* **172**:1169–1227.

6. American Thoracic Society. 2000. Diagnostic standards and classification of tuberculosis in adults and children. *Am. J. Respir. Crit. Care Med.* **161**:1376–1395.

7. Azzopardi, P., C. M. Bennett, S. M. Graham, and T. Duke. 2009. Bacille Calmette-Guerin vaccine-related disease in HIV-infected children: a systematic review. *Int. J. Tuberc. Lung Dis.* **13**:1331–1344.

8. Bianchi, L., L. Galli, M. Moriondo, G. Veneruso, L. Becciolini, C. Azzari, E. Chiappini, and M. deMartino. 2009. Interferon-gamma release assay improves the diagnosis of tuberculosis in children. *Pediatr. Infect. Dis. J.* **28**:510–514.

9. Biddulph, J. 1990. Short-course chemotherapy for childhood tuberculosis. *Pediatr. Infect. Dis. J.* **9**:794–801.

10. Blumberg, H. M., W. J. Burman, R. E. Chaisson, C. L. Daley, S. C. Etkind, L. N. Friedman, P. Fujiwara, M. Grzemska, P. C. Hopewell, M. D. Iseman, R. M. Jasmer, V. Koppaka, R. I. Menzies, R. J. O'Brien, R. R. Reves, L. B. Reichman, P. M. Simone, J. R. Starke, A. A. Vernon, American Thoracic Society, Centers for Disease Control and Prevention, and the Infectious Diseases Society. 2003. American Thoracic Society/Centers for Disease Control and Prevention/Infectious Diseases Society of America: treatment of tuberculosis. *Am. J. Respir. Crit. Care Med.* **167**:603–662.

11. Blusse van Oud-Alblas, H. J., M. E. van Vliet, J. L. Kimpen, G. S. deVilliers, H. S. Schaaf, and P. R. Donald. 2002. Human immunodeficiency virus infection in children hospitalized with tuberculosis. *Ann. Trop. Pediatr.* **22**:115–123.

12. Braitstein, P., W. Nyandiko, R. Ureemon, K. Wools-Kaloustian, E. Sang, B. Musick, J. Sidle, C. Yiannoutsos, S. Ayaya, and E. J. Carter. 2009. The clinical burden of tuberculosis among human immunodeficiency virus-infected children in Western Kenya and the impact of combination antiretroviral treatment. *Pediatr. Infect. Dis. J.* **28**:626–632.

13. Cakir, E., Z. S. Uyan, S. Oktem, F. Karakoc, R. Ersu, B. Karadag, and E. Dogli. 2008. Flexible bronchoscopy for diagnosis and follow-up of childhood endobronchial tuberculosis. *Pediatr. Infect. Dis. J.* **27**:783–787.

14. Centers for Disease Control. 1993. Interstate outbreak of drug-resistant tuberculosis involving children: California, Montana, Nevada, Utah. *MMWR Morb. Mortal. Wkly. Rep.* **32**:516–519.

15. Centers for Disease Control and Prevention. 2009. *Reported Tuberculosis in the United States, 2008*. U.S. Department of Health and Human Services, Atlanta, GA.

16. Centers for Disease Control and Prevention. 2005. Guidelines for preventing the transmission of Mycobacterium tuberculosis in health-care facilities. *MMWR Recommend. Rep.* **54**(RR-17):1–141.

17. Centers for Disease Control and Prevention. 2010. Updated guidelines for using interferon gamma release assays to detect Mycobacterium tuberculosis infection---United States, 2010. *MMWR Recommend. Rep.* **59**(RR-5):1–13.

18. Chan, S., D. Abadco, and P. Steiner. 1994. Role of flexible fiber optic bronchoscopy in the diagnosis of childhood endobronchial tuberculosis. *Pediatr. Infect. Dis. J.* **13**:506–509.

19. Chan, S. P., J. Birnbaum, M. Rao, and P. Steiner. 1996. Clinical manifestations and outcome of tuberculosis in children with acquired immunodeficiency syndrome. *Pediatr. Infect. Dis. J.* **15**:443–447.

20. Chintu, C., and P. Mwaba. 2005. Tuberculosis in children with human immunodeficiency virus infection. *Int. J. Tuberc. Lung Dis.* **9**:477–484.

21. Comstock, G. W., L. M. Hammes, and A. Pio. 1969. Isoniazid prophylaxis in Alaskan boarding schools: comparison of two doses. *Am. Rev. Respir. Dis.* **100**:773–779.

22. Comstock, G. W., C. Baum, and D. E. Snider, Jr. 1979. Isoniazid prophylaxis among Alaskan Eskimos: final report of the Bethel isoniazid studies. *Am. Rev. Respir. Dis.* **119**:827–830.

23. Comstock, G. W., V. T. Livesay, and S. F. Woopert. 1974. Prognosis of a positive tuberculin reaction in childhood and adolescence. *Am. J. Epidemiol.* **99**:131–138.

24. Connell, T. G., N. Ritz, G. A. Paxton, J. P. Buttery, N. Curtis, and S. C. Ranganathan. 2008. A three-way comparison of tuberculin skin testing, Quantiferon-TB Gold, and T-SPOT.TB in children. *PLoS One* **3**:e2624–e2631.

25. Cruz, A. T., and J. R. Starke. 2008. Treatment of tuberculosis in children. *Expert Rev. Anti. Infect. Ther.* **6**:939–957.

26. Cruz, A. T., L. T. Ong, and J. R. Starke. 2009. Childhood pleural tuberculosis. A review of 45 cases. *Pediatr. Infect. Dis. J.* **28**:981–984.

27. Curtis, A., R. Ridzon, R. Vogel, S. McDonough, J. Hargreaves, J. Ferry, S. Valway, and I. M. Onerato. 1999. Extensive transmission of Mycobacterium tuberculosis from a child. *N. Engl. J. Med.* **341**:1491–1495.

28. Delacourt, C., J. D. Poveda, C. Chureau, N. Bryden, B. Mahut, J. deBlic, P. Scheinman, and G. Garrigue. 1995. Use of polymerase chain reaction for improved diagnosis of tuberculosis in children. *J. Pediatr.* **126**:703–709.

29. Delacourt, C., T. M. Mani, V. Bonnerot, J. deBlic, N. Soyeg, D. Lallemand, and P. Scheinman. 1993. Computed tomography with normal chest radiograph in tuberculous infection. *Arch. Dis. Child.* **69**:430–432.

30. de Pontual, L., L. Balu, P. Ovetchine, B. Maury-Tisseron, E. Lachassinne, P. Cruaud, V. Jeantis, D. Valeyre, O. Fain, and J. Gaudelus. 2006. Tuberculosis in adolescents: a French retrospective study of 52 cases. *Pediatr. Infect. Dis. J.* **25**:930–932.

31. Detjen, A. K., T. Keili, S. Roll, B. Haver, H. Mauch, U. Wahn, and K. Magdorf. 2007. Interferon-gamma release assays improve the diagnosis of tuberculosis and nontuberculous mycobacterial disease in children in a country with a low incidence of tuberculosis. *Clin. Infect. Dis.* **45**:322–328.

32. Doerr, C. A., J. R. Starke, and L. T. Ong. 1995. Clinical and public health aspects of tuberculous meningitis in children. *J. Pediatr.* **127**:27–33.

33. Donald, P. R., D. Mahan, J. S. Maritz, and S. Qazi. 2006. Ethambutol dosage for the treatment of children: literature review and recommendations. *Int. J. Tuberc. Lung Dis.* **10**:1318–1330.

34. Donald, P. R., D. Maher, and S. Qazi. 2007. A research agenda to promote the management of childhood tuberculosis within

national tuberculosis programs. *Int. J. Tuberc. Lung Dis.* **11:** 327–380.

35. **Dormer, B. A., I. Harrison, J. A. Swart, and S. R. Vidor.** 1959. Prophylactic isoniazid protection of infants in a tuberculosis hospital. *Lancet* **ii:**902–903.

36. **Eamranond, P., and E. Jaramillo.** 2001. Tuberculosis in children: reassessing the need for improved diagnosis in global control strategies. *Int. J. Tuberc. Lung Dis.* **5:**594–603.

37. **Elenga, N., K. A. Kouakoussui, D. Bonard, P. Fassinou, M. F. Anaky, M. L. Wemin, F. Dick-Amon, F. Rovet, V. Vincent, and P. Msellati.** 2005. Diagnosed tuberculosis during the followup of a cohort of human immunodeficiency virus–infected children in Abidjan, Cote d'Ivoire: ANRS 1278 study. *Pediatr. Infect. Dis. J.* **24:**1077–1082.

38. **Feja, K., E. McNelley, C. S. Tran, J. Burzynski, and L. Saimon.** 2008. Management of pediatric multi-drug resistant tuberculosis and latent tuberculosis infections in New York City from 1995 to 2003. *Pediatr. Infect. Dis. J.* **27:**907–912.

39. **Ferebee, S. H.** 1969. Controlled chemoprophylaxis trials in tuberculosis. A general review. *Adv. Tuberc. Res.* **17:**28–106.

40. **Giammona, S. T., and P. S. Zelkowitz.** 1969. The use of superheated nebulized saline and gastric lavage to obtain bacterial cultures in primary pulmonary tuberculosis in children. *Am. J. Dis. Child.* **117:**198–200.

41. **Groussard, P., R. P. Gie, S. Kling, and N. Beyers.** 2004. Expansile pneumonia in children caused by *Mycobacterium tuberculosis*. Clinical, radiological and bronchoscopic appearances. *Pediatr. Pulmonol.* **38:**451–455.

42. **Haustein, T., D. A. Ridout, J. C. Hartley, U. Thaker, D. Shingadia, N. J. Klein, V. Novelli, and G. L. J. Dixon.** 2009. The likelihood of an indeterminate test result from a whole-blood interferon-gamma release assay for the diagnosis of *Mycobacterium tuberculosis* infection in children correlates with age and immune status. *Pediatr. Infect. Dis. J.* **28:**669–673.

43. **Hesseling, A., H. Schaaf, R. Gie, J. R. Starke, and N. Beyers.** 2002. A critical review of diagnostic approaches used in the diagnosis of childhood tuberculosis. *Int. J. Tuberc. Lung Dis.* **6:**1038–1045.

44. **Hesseling, A. C., A. E. Westra, H. Werschkull, P. R. Donald, N. Beyers, G. D. Hussey, W. El-Sadr, and H. S. Schaaf.** 2005. Outcome of HIV-infected children with culture-confirmed tuberculosis. *Arch. Dis. Child.* **90:**1171–1174.

45. **Hesseling, A. C., H. Rabie, B. J. Marais, M. Manders, M. Lips, H. S. Schaaf, R. P. Gie, M. Cotton, P. D. von Helden, R. M. Warren, and N. Beyers.** 2006. Bacille Calmette-Guerin vaccine-induced disease in HIV-infected and HIV-uninfected children. *Clin. Infect. Dis.* **42:**548–558.

46. **Hesseling, A. C., M. F. Cotton, C. F. von Reyn, S. M. Graham, R. P. Gie, and G. D. Hussey.** 2008. Consensus statement on the revised World Health Organization recommendations for BCG vaccination in HIV-infected infants. *Int. J. Tuberc. Lung Dis.* **28:**1376–1379.

47. **Hill, P. C., R. H. Brooks, I. M. O. Adetifa, A. Fox, and D. Jackson-Sillah.** 2006. Comparison of enyzme-linked immunospot assay and tuberculin skin test in healthy children exposed to Mycobacterium tuberculosis. *Pediatrics* **117:**1542–1548.

48. **Hsu, K. H. K.** 1984. Thirty years after isoniazid: its impact on tuberculosis in children and adolescents. *JAMA* **25:**1283–1285.

49. **Huebner, R. E., M. F. Schein, and J. B. Bass.** 1993. The tuberculin skin test. *Clin. Infect. Dis.* **17:**968–975.

50. **Hussey, G., T. Chisholm, and M. Kibel.** 1991. Miliary tuberculosis in children. A review of 94 cases. *Pediatr. Infect. Dis. J.* **10:**832–836.

51. **International Union Against Tuberculosis Committee on Prophylaxis.** 1982. Efficacy of various durations of isoniazid preventive therapy for tuberculosis: five years of follow-up in the IUAT trial. *Bull. W. H. O.* **60:**555–561.

52. **Iriso, R., P. M. Mudido, C. Karamagi, and C. Whalen.** 2005. The diagnosis of childhood tuberculosis in an HIV-endemic setting and the use of induced sputum. *Int. J. Tuberc. Lung Dis.* **9:**16–26.

53. **Jacobs, R. F., P. Sunakorn, T. Chotpitayasunonah, S. Pope, and K. Kelleher.** 1992. Intensive short course chemotherapy for tuberculosis meningitis. *Pediatr. Infect. Dis. J.* **11:**194–198.

54. **Jawahar, M. S., K. Rajaram, S. Sivasubramanian, C. N. Paramasivan, K. Chandrasekar, M. N. Kamaludeen, A. J. Thirithuvathas, V. Ananthalakshmi, and R. Prabhakar.** 2008. Treatment of lymph node tuberculosis: a randomized clinical trial of two 6-month regimens. *Trop. Med. Int. Health* **10:**1090–1098.

55. **Jones, D., J. Malecki, W. Bigler, J. Witte, and M. J. Oxtoby.** 1992. Pediatric tuberculosis and human immunodeficiency virus infection in Palm Beach County, Florida. *Am. J. Dis. Child.* **146:**1166–1170.

56. **Khan, E. A., and J. R. Starke.** 1995. Diagnosis of tuberculosis in children. Increased need for better methods. *Emerg. Infect. Dis.* **1:**115–123.

57. **Kimerling, M., J. Barker, F. Bruce, N. L. Brook and N. E. Dunlap.** 2000. Preventable childhood tuberculosis in Alabama: implications and opportunity. *Pediatrics* **105:**e53.

58. **Kumar, L., R. Dhand, P. D. Singhi, K. L., Rao, and S. Katariya.** 1990. A randomized trial of fully intermittent vs. daily followed by intermittent short-course chemotherapy for childhood tuberculosis. *Pediatr. Infect. Dis. J.* **9:**802–806.

59. **Laven, G. T.** 1977. Diagnosis of tuberculosis in children using fluorescence microscopic examination of gastric washings. *Am. Rev. Respir. Dis.* **115:**743–749.

60. **Lewinsohn, D. A., M. N. Lobato, and J. A. Jereb.** 2010. Interferon-gamma release assays: new diagnostic tests for Mycobacterium tuberculosis infection and their use in children. *Curr. Opin. Pediatr.* **22:**71–76.

61. **Lighter, J., M. Rigaud, R. Eduardo, C. H. Peng, and H. Pollack.** 2009. Latent tuberculosis diagnosis in children by using the QuantiFERON-TB Gold In-Tube test. *Pediatrics* **123:**30–37.

62. **Lincoln, E. M.** 1965. Epidemics of tuberculosis. *Bibl. Tuberc.* **21:**157–201.

63. **Lincoln, E. M., P. A. Davies, and S. Bovornkitti.** 1958. Tuberculous pleurisy with effusion in children. *Am. Rev. Tuberc.* **77:**271–289.

64. **Lobato, M., J. C. Mohle-Boetani, and S. E. Royce.** 2000. Missed opportunities for preventing tuberculosis among children younger than five years of age. *Pediatrics* **106:**e75.

65. **Lobato, M. N., S. J. Sun, P. K. Moonan, S. E. Weis, L. Saiman, A. A. Reichard, K. Feja, and the Zero Tolerance for Pediatric TB Study Group.** 2008. Underuse of effective measures to prevent and manage pediatric tuberculosis in the United States. *Arch. Pediatr. Adolesc. Med.* **162:**426–431.

66. **Mandalakas, A. M., H. L. Kirchner, X. Zhu, K. T. Yeo, and J. R. Starke.** 2008. Interpretation of repeat tuberculin skin testing in international adoptees. *Pediatr. Infect. Dis. J.* **27:**913–919.

67. **Marais, B. J., R. P. Gie, A. C. Hesseling, and N. Beyers.** 2005. Adult-type pulmonary tuberculosis in children aged 10–14 years. *Pediatr. Infect. Dis. J.* **24:**743–744.

68. **Marais, B. J., C. A. Wright, H. S. Schaaf, R. P. Gie, A. C. Hesseling, D. A. Enarson, and N. Beyers.** 2006. Tuberculous lymphadenitis as a cause of persistent cervical lymphadenopathy in children from a tuberculous-endemic area. *Pediatr. Infect. Dis. J.* **25:**142–146.

69. Marais, B. J., R. P. Gie, H. S. Schaaf, A. C. Hesseling, C. C. Obi-hara, J. R. Starke, D. A. Emerson, P. R. Donald, and N. Beyers. 2004. The natural history of childhood intra-thoracic tuberculosis: a critical review of literature from the pre-chemotherapy era. *Int. J. Tuberc. Lung Dis.* 8:278–285.

70. Marais, B. J., R. P. Gie, H. S. Schaaf, N. Beyers, P. R. Donald, and J. R. Starke. 2006. Childhood pulmonary tuberculosis: old wisdom and new challenges. *Am. Rev. Respir. Crit. Care Med.* 173:1078–1090.

71. Marais, B. J., R. P. Gie, H. S. Schaaf, J. R. Starke, A. C. Hesseling, P. R. Donald, and N. Beyers. 2004. A proposed radiological classification of childhood intra-thoracic tuberculosis. *Pediatr. Radiol.* 39:868–894.

72. Martinson, N. A., H. Moultrie, R. van Niekerk, G. Barry, A. Coovadia, M. Cotton, A. Violari, G. E. Gray, R. E. Chaisson, J. A. McIntyre, and T. Meyers. 2009. HAART and the risk of tuberculosis in HIV-infected South African children: a multisite retrospective cohort. *Int. J. Tuberc. Lung Dis.* 13:862–867.

73. Matsaniotis, N., C. Kattamis, C. Economou-Mavrou, and M. Kyriazakou. 1967. Bullous emphysema in childhood tuberculosis. *J. Pediatr.* 71:703–708.

74. McIlleron, H., M. Willemse, C. J. Werely, G. D. Hussey, H. S. Schaaf, P. J. Smith, and P. R. Donald. 2009. Isoniazid plasma concentrations in a cohort of South African children with tuberculosis: implications for international pediatric dosing guidelines. *Clin. Infect. Dis.* 48:1547–1553.

75. Miller, F. J., R. M. E. Seale, and M. D. Taylor. 1963. *Tuberculosis in Children*, p. 214. Little Brown, Boston, MA.

76. Millership, S. E., C. Anderson, A. J. Cummins, S. Bracebridge, and I. Abubakar. 2009. The risk to infant from nosocomial exposure to tuberculosis. *Pediatr. Infect. Dis. J.* 28:915–916.

77. Mohle-Boetani, J. C., B. Miller, M. Halpern, A. Trivedi, J. Lessler, S. L. Soloman, and M. Fenstersheib. 1995. School-based screening for tuberculous infection: a cost-benefit analysis. *JAMA* 274:613–619.

78. Mohle-Boetani, J. C., and J. Flood. 2002. Contact investigations and the continued commitment to control tuberculosis. *JAMA* 287:1040–1042.

79. Munoz, F. M., L. T. Ong, D. Seavy, D. Medina, A. Correa, and J. R. Starke. 2002. Tuberculosis among adult visitors of children with suspected tuberculosis and employees at a children's hospital. *Infect. Control Hosp. Epidemiol.* 23:568–572.

80. Nelson, L. J., and C. D. Wells. 2004. Global epidemiology of childhood tuberculosis. *Int. J. Tuberc. Lung Dis.* 8:636–647.

81. Nelson, L. J., E. Schneider, C. D. Wells, and M. Moore. 2004. Epidemiology of childhood tuberculosis in the United States, 1993-2001: the need for continued vigilance. *Pediatrics* 114:333–341.

82. Nemir, R. L., and K. Krasinski. 1988. Tuberculosis in children and adolescents in the 1980's. *Pediatr. Infect. Dis. J.* 7:375–379.

83. Nicol, M. P., M. A. Danes, K. Wood, N. Dip, M. Hatherill, L. Workman, A. Harkridge, B. Eley, K. A. Wilkinson, R. J. Wilkinson, W. A. Hanekom, O. Beathy, and G. Hussey. 2009. Comparison of T-SPOT. TB assay and tuberculin skin test for the evaluation of young children at high risk for tuberculosis in a community setting. *Pediatrics* 123:38–43.

84. O'Brien, R. J., M. W. Long, F. S. Cross, M. A. Lyle, and D. E. Snider, Jr. 1983. Hepatotoxicity from isoniazid and rifampin among children treated for tuberculosis. *Pediatrics* 72:491–499.

85. Palacios, E., R. Dallman, M. Munoz, R. Hurtado, K. Chalco, D. Guerra, L. Mestanza, K. Llaro, C. Bonilla, P. Drobac, J. Bayona, M. Lygizos, H. Anger, and S. Shin. 2009. Drug-resistant tuberculosis and pregnancy: treatment outcomes of 38 cases in Lima, Peru. *Clin. Infect. Dis.* 48:1413–1419.

86. Pastrana, D. G., R. Torronteras, P. Caro, M. L. Anguita, A. M. Barrio, A. Andres, and J. Navarro. 2001. Comparison of Amplicor, in-house polymerase chain reactions and conventional culture for the diagnosis of tuberculosis in children. *Clin. Infect. Dis.* 32:17–22.

87. Pediatric Tuberculosis Collaborative Group. 2004. Diagnosis and treatment of latent tuberculosis infection in children and adolescents. *Pediatrics* 114:1175–1201.

88. Pierre, C., C. Olivier, D. Lecossier, Y. Boussougont, P. Yeni, and A. J. Hance. 1993. Diagnosis of primary tuberculosis in children by amplification and detection of mycobacterial DNA. *Am. Rev. Respir. Dis.* 147:420–424.

89. Powell, D. A., L. Perkins, D. Scott-Wang, G. Hunt, and N. Ryan-Wenger. 2008. Completion of therapy for latent tuberculosis in children of different nationalities. *Pediatr. Infect. Dis. J.* 28:272–274.

90. Puthanakit, T., P. Oberdorfen, N. Akarathum, P. Wannarit, T. Sirisanthana, and V. Sirisanthana. 2006. Immune reconstitution syndrome after highly active antiretroviral therapy in human immunodeficiency virus-infected Thai children. *Pediatr. Infect. Dis. J.* 25:53–58.

91. Reis, F. J., M. B. Bedran, J. A. Mowra, I. Assis, and M. E. Rodrigues. 1990. Six-month isoniazid-rifampin treatment for pulmonary tuberculosis in children. *Am. Rev. Respir. Dis.* 142:996–999.

92. Ridzon, R., J. H. Kent, S. Valway, P. Weismuller, R. Maxwell, M. Ekock, J. Meador, S. Royce, A. Shefer, P. Smith, C. Woodley, and I. M. Onorato. 1997. Outbreak of drug-resistant tuberculosis with secondary-generation transmission in a high school in California. *J. Pediatr.* 131:863–868.

93. Rock, R. B., M. Olin, C. A. Baker, T. W. Molitor, and P. K. Peterson. 2008. Central nervous system tuberculosis: pathogenesis and clinical aspects. *Clin. Microbiol. Rev.* 21:243–261.

94. Saiman, L., J. Aronson, J. Zhou, C. Gomey-Duarte, P. S. Gabriel, M. Alonso, S. Maloney, and J. Schulte. 2001. Prevalence of infectious diseases among internationally adopted children. *Pediatrics* 109:608–612.

95. Salazar, G. E., T. L. Schmitz, R. Cama, P. Sheen, L. M. Franchi, G. Centano, C. Valera, M. Leyua, S. Montenegro-James, R. Oberhelman, G. H. Gilman, and M. J. Thompson. 2001. Pulmonary tuberculosis in children in a developing country. *Pediatrics* 108:448–453.

96. Schaaf, H. S., B. J. Marais, A. Whitelaw, A. C. Hesseling, B. Eley, G. D. Hussey, and P. R. Donald. 2007. Culture-confirmed childhood tuberculosis in Cape Town, South Africa: a review of 596 cases. *BMC Infect. Dis.* 7:140–147.

97. Schaaf, H. S., M. Willemse, and P. R. Donald. 2009. Long-term linezolid treatment in a young child with extensively drug-resistant tuberculosis. *Pediatr. Infect. Dis. J.* 28:748–750.

98. Schaaf, H. S., R. P. Gie, N. Beyer, F. A. Sirgel, P. J. deKlerk, and P. R. Donald. 2000. Primary drug-resistant tuberculosis in children. *Int. J. Tuberc. Lung Dis.* 4:1149–1156.

99. Schuit, K. E. 1979. Miliary tuberculosis in children. *Am. J. Dis. Child.* 133:583–585.

100. Sepulveda, R. L., C. Burr, X. Ferrer, and R. U. Sorensen. 1988. Booster effect of tuberculosis testing in healthy 6-year-old school children vaccinated with bacilli Calmette-Guérin at birth in Santiago, Chile. *Pediatr. Infect. Dis. J.* 7:578–581.

101. Sharma, S. K., A. Mahan, A. Sharma, and D. K. Mitra. 2005. Miliary tuberculosis: new insights into an old disease. *Lancet Infect. Dis.* 5:415–430.

102. Shingadia, D., and V. Novelli. 2003. Diagnosis and treatment of tuberculosis in children. *Lancet Infect. Dis.* 3:624–632.

103. Smith, K. C., J. R. Starke, K. Eisenach, L. T. Ong and M. Denby. 1996. Detection of *Mycobacterium tuberculosis* in

clinical specimens from children using a polymerase chain reaction. *Pediatrics* 97:155–160.

104. **Soysal, A., O. Turel, D. Toprek, and M. Bakir.** 2008. Comparison of positive tuberculin skin test with an interferongamma based assay in unexposed children. *Jpn. J. Infect. Dis.* 61:192–195.

105. **Spyridis, N. P., P. G. Spyridis, A. Gelesme, V. Sypsa, M. Valianatou, F. Metsou, P. Gourgiotis, and M. N. Tsolic.** 2007. The effectiveness of a 9-month regimen of isoniazid alone versus 3- and 4-month regimens of isoniazid plus rifampin for treatment of latent tuberculosis infection in children: results of an 11-year randomized study. *Clin. Infect. Dis.* 45:715–722.

106. **Starke, J. R.** 2001. Transmission of *Mycobacterium tuberculosis* to and from children and adolescents. *Semin. Pediatr. Infect. Dis.* 12:115–122.

107. **Starke, J. R.** 2007. New concepts in childhood tuberculosis. *Curr. Opin. Pediatr.* 19:306–313.

108. **Steiner, P., and M. Rao.** 1993. Drug-resistant tuberculosis in children. *Semin. Pediatr. Infect. Dis.* 4:275–292.

109. **Steiner, P., M. Rao, M. Mitchell, and M. Steiner.** 1985. Primary drug-resistant tuberculosis in children: correlation of drug-susceptibility patterns of matched patient and sourcecase strains of *Mycobacterium tuberculosis. Am. J. Dis. Child.* 139:780–782.

110. **Steiner, P., M. Rao, M. S. Victoria, H. Jabbar, and M. Steiner.** 1980. Persistently negative tuberculin reactions: their presence among children culture positive for *Mycobacterium tuberculosis. Am. J. Dis. Child.* 134:747–750.

111. **Stop TB Partnership Childhood TB Subgroup.** 2006. Chapter 2: antituberculosis treatment in children. *Int. J. Tuberc. Lung Dis.* 10:1205–1211.

112. **Stop TB Partnership Childhood TB Subgroup.** 2006. Chapter 3: management of TB in the HIV-infected child. *Int. J. Tuberc. Lung Dis.* 10:1331–1336.

113. **Stop TB Partnership Childhood TB Subgroup.** 2007. Chapter 4: childhood contact screening and management. *Int. J. Tuberc. Lung Dis.* 11:12–15.

114. **Stout, J. E., K. K. Saharia, S. Nageswaran, A. Ahmed, and C. D. Hamilton.** 2006. Racial and ethnic disparities in pediatric tuberculosis in North Carolina. *Arch. Pediatr. Adolesc. Med.* 160:631–637.

115. **Swanson, D. S., and J. R. Starke.** 1995. Drug-resistant tuberculosis in pediatrics. *Pediatr. Clin. North Am.* 42:553–581.

116. **Teeratkulpisarn, J., P. Lumbigagnon, S. Pairojkul, and P. Jariyauiladkul.** 1994. Cavitary tuberculosis in a young infant. *Pediatr. Infect. Dis. J.* 13:545–546.

117. **Te Water Naude, J. M., P. R. Donald, D. Hussey, M. A. Kibel, A. Louw, D. R. Perkins, and H. S. Schaaf.** 2000. Twice-weekly vs. daily chemotherapy for childhood tuberculosis. *Pediatr. Infect. Dis. J.* 19:405–410.

118. **Tsakalidis, D., P. Pratsidou, A. Hitoglou-Makedou, G. Tzouvelakis, and I. Sofroniadis.** 1992. Intensive short course chemotherapy for treatment of Greek children with tuberculosis. *Pediatr. Infect. Dis. J.* 11:1036–1042.

119. **Ussery, X. T., S. E. Valway, M. McKenna, G. M. Cauthen, E. McCray, and I. M. Onorato.** 1996. Epidemiology of tuberculosis among children in the United States. *Pediatr. Infect. Dis. J.* 15:697–704.

120. **Vallejo, J., L. Ong, and J. Starke.** 1994. Clinical features, diagnosis and treatment of tuberculosis in infants. *Pediatrics* 94:1–7.

121. **Van der Weert, E. M., N. M. Harters, H. S. Schaaf, B. S. Eley, R. D. Pitcher, N. A. Wierselthaler, R. Laubscher, P. R. Donald, and J. F. Schoeman.** 2006. Comparison of diagnostic criteria for tuberculous meningitis in human immunodeficiency virus-infected and uninfected children. *Pediatr. Infect. Dis. J.* 25:65–69.

122. **Visudhiphan, P., and S. Chiemchanya.** 1989. Tuberculous meningitis in children: treatment with isoniazid and rifampin for twelve months. *J. Pediatr.* 114:875–879.

123. **Wallgren, A.** 1937. On contagiousness of childhood tuberculosis. *Acta Paediatr.* 22:229–241.

124. **Wallgren, A.** 1948. The time-table of tuberculosis. *Tubercle* 29:245–257.

125. **Webb, E. A., A. C. Hesseling, H. S. Schaaf, R. P. Gie, C. J. Lombard, A. Spitaels, S. Delport, B. J. Marais, K. Donald, P. Hindmarsh, and N. Beyers.** 2009. High prevalence of Mycobacterium tuberculosis infection and disease in children and adolescents with type 1 diabetes mellitus. *Int. J. Tuberc. Lung Dis.* 13:868–874.

126. **Weinstein, J., C. Barrett, R. Baltimore, and W. J. Hierlhozer, Jr.** 1995. Nosocomial transmission of tuberculosis from a hospital visitor on a pediatrics ward. *Pediatr. Infect. Dis. J.* 14:232–234.

127. **World Health Organization.** 2006. *Guidance for National Tuberculosis Programmes on the Management of Tuberculosis in Children.* World Health Organization, Geneva, Switzerland.

128. **Wright, C. A., A. C. Hesseling, C. Banford, S. M. Burgess, R. Warren, and B. J. Marais.** 2009. Fine-needle aspiration biopsy: a first-line diagnostic procedure in paediatric tuberculosis suspects with peripheral lymphadenopathy? *Int. J. Tuberc. Lung Dis.* 13:1373–1379.

129. **Wright, C. A., R. M. Warren, and B. J. Marais.** 2009. Fine needle aspiration biopsy–an undervalued diagnostic modality in paediatric mycobacterial disease. *Int. J. Tuberc. Lung Dis.* 13:1467–1475.

130. **Zar, H., E. Tannenbaum, P. Apolles, P. Roux, D. Hanslo, and G. Hussey.** 2000. Sputum induction for the diagnosis of pulmonary tuberculosis in infants and young children in an urban setting in South Africa. *Arch. Dis. Child.* 82:305–308.

131. **Zar, H. J., D. Hanslo, P. Apolles, G. Swingler, and G. Hussey.** 2005. Induced sputum versus gastric lavage for microbiologic confirmation of pulmonary tuberculosis in infants and young children: a prospective study. *Lancet* 365:130–134.

Tuberculosis and Nontuberculous Mycobacterial Infections, 6th ed.
Edited by David Schlossberg
© 2011 ASM Press, Washington, DC

Chapter 31

Pregnancy: Maternal, Fetal, and Neonatal Considerations

DAVID M. FLEECE AND STEPHEN C. ARONOFF

The issue of tuberculosis during pregnancy is not simply an historical inquiry but rather an increasingly familiar clinical problem facing industrial nations as well as the developing countries of the world. This chapter focuses on the maternal aspects of tuberculous infection, as well as transmission to the fetus, and newborn. For discussion of tuberculosis in infants and children, the reader is referred to chapter 30.

EPIDEMIOLOGY

The epidemiology of tuberculosis in pregnancy reflects that of tuberculosis at large. Worldwide, the number of cases of tuberculosis appears to have peaked in 2004, with declining rates in Western and Central Europe, Latin America, the Eastern Mediterranean, Southeast Asia, and the Western Pacific. High prevalence rates have yet to decline substantially in Africa and Eastern Europe (35). For the United States, the rising incidence of tuberculosis seen during the late 1980s and early 1990s appears to have ended. The U.S. case rate (per 100,000 total population) of 10.4 in 1992 declined to 4.4 in 2007. Different ethnic groups have widely different rates, however. The 2008 tuberculosis case rates for women of childbearing age from various ethnic groups are found in Table 1 (10).

For women of childbearing age, infection with human immunodeficiency virus (HIV) represents a significant risk factor for tuberculosis infection. Of 16 pregnant women with tuberculosis in New York City reported by Margono and coworkers, 7 of 11 (64%) tested were HIV positive (21). Another study of a cohort of HIV-infected women in the United States found that 5 out of 46 (11%) of the pregnant women were coinfected with tuberculosis (24). In sub-Saharan Africa, where the burden of HIV and tuberculosis is among the largest worldwide, HIV infection has been correlated with a 10-fold-higher incidence of tuberculosis infection (1).

EFFECT OF PREGNANCY ON TUBERCULOSIS

Hippocrates believed that pregnancy had a salutary effect on tuberculosis. This belief persisted until the middle of the 19th century, when case reports of accelerated progression of disease during pregnancy surfaced (14). Osler recommended that physicians veto the marriage of any girl "whose family history is bad, whose chest expansion is slight, and whose physique is below the standard" (27). By the early 20th century, physicians began to advocate sterilization for women suffering from a variety of health problems, including tuberculosis. J. Edgar Clifton, a physician writing in 1918, stated, "A candidate for tuberculosis runs very great risk of becoming consumptive through childbirth" (20).

A number of reports from the 1950s, however, showed that pregnancy did not predispose women to progressive disease (17, 29). In a report of 250 women with active tuberculosis in the pretreatment era, 83.9% remained stable during pregnancy and 9.1% improved. Although only 7% had evidence of progressive disease during pregnancy, an additional 8.2% experienced progression in the year following pregnancy (17). A study from New York published two decades later, in the era of chemotherapy, had similar results, with a progression rate of only 2% in the cohort of pregnant and postpartum women who had received antitubercular chemotherapy. As with the earlier study, most of the relapses occurred in the postpartum period (31). These findings were similar to other studies of nonpregnant women, thus showing that pregnancy does not adversely impact the course of tuberculosis infection. Pregnancy does not alter the site of disease; most studies report 5 to 10% of patients with extrapulmonary disease, similar to the rate in nonpregnant patients (5, 34).

Pregnancy itself, however, may mimic and thus mask the symptoms of early tuberculosis, such as tachypnea and fatigue; this in turn may delay diagnosis and treatment. Of pregnant women screened for

---

David M. Fleece and Stephen C. Aronoff • Department of Pediatrics, Temple University School of Medicine, Philadelphia, PA 19140.

Table 1. Tuberculosis case rates per 100,000 population for women of children bearing age, United States, 2008[a]

Ethnic group	Case rate for:	
	15–24-yr-olds	25–44-yr-olds
White, non-Hispanic	0.3	0.7
Black, non-Hispanic	5.7	8.1
Hispanic	5.5	6.9
Asian	20.7	24.7
Native Hawaiian/Pacific Islander	23.6	17.5
American Indian/Alaskan Native	3.5	4.3

[a]Source: reference 10.

and diagnosed with tuberculosis, the majority have been shown to be asymptomatic and unaware of their disease (5, 34). Failure to recognize and treat the infection in the pregnant woman may lead to congenital infection in the infant. As evidence of this, in some series of congenital tuberculosis, the mother was evaluated and tuberculosis was diagnosed only after the disease was diagnosed in the infant.

EFFECT OF TUBERCULOSIS ON PREGNANCY

Tuberculosis can impact all phases of female reproduction, including fertility and birth outcomes. Infection of the reproductive organs may result in infertility as well as abdominal or tubal pregnancy (25). In the prechemotherapy era, prematurity rates in tuberculous women ranged from 23 to 44%, with the higher rates in the most severely affected mothers (30). Studies from Mexico and India have shown that infants born to mothers with tuberculosis have a two- to threefold increase in rates of prematurity and low birth weight and an increase in perinatal death as high as sixfold (12, 19). Adverse perinatal outcome was associated with late diagnosis, inadequate treatment, and advanced disease (19). With early recognition and effective chemotherapy, however, there is no evidence of an adverse effect on pregnancy (23, 31).

PATHOGENESIS AND CONGENITAL INFECTION

The pathogenesis of tuberculosis in the pregnant woman begins as in all other patients. After exposure, usually by inhalation, and local replication, there is dissemination of the organism by lymphatic spread, hematogenous spread, or both. If the organism affects the placenta or genital tract, the child may be congenitally infected. The mycobacterium may be delivered to the infant directly via the umbilical vein or through aspiration of infected amniotic fluid (15).

Congenital infection, or infection of the fetus, must be distinguished from disease in the newborn acquired postnatally. The original standardized criteria for distinguishing between the two were proposed by Beitzke (3) in 1935 and were as follows:

- Infant has proven tuberculous lesions, and one of the following:
- Lesions in the first few days of life
- A primary hepatic complex
- Exclusion of postnatal transmission by separation at birth of the infant from the mother and other potential sources

Cantwell et al. (4) reviewed congenital tuberculosis in 1994, including all published case reports since 1980. They concluded that the original diagnostic criteria had limited use, based, in part, on overreliance on autopsy or liver biopsy data as well as the now uncommon practice of isolating the newborn. Therefore, they proposed modified diagnostic criteria, more compatible with modern practice. These consist of the following:

- Infant has proven tuberculous lesions and one of the following:
- Lesions in the first week of life
- A primary hepatic complex or caseating hepatic granulomas
- Tuberculous infection of the placenta or maternal genital tract
- Exclusion of postnatal transmission by a thorough investigation of contacts and adherence to current infection control guidelines

The authors showed these criteria to have increased diagnostic sensitivity when applied to the cases reported in the literature.

CLINICAL MANIFESTATIONS

The clinical manifestations of tuberculosis in pregnancy are similar to those in nonpregnant women. Good and associates (13) reported that among 27 pregnant women with active disease, cough (71%), weight loss (41%), fever (30%), and malaise and fatigue (30%) were the most common symptoms. However, 20% of the women in their cohort were asymptomatic.

The lungs are the most common site affected and account for approximately 90% of all cases (16, 34). Lymph node, bone, and kidney disease affect most of the remaining patients. HIV infection modifies the type of tuberculosis disease to more serious forms. In a study of 16 patients with tuberculosis in an area of high HIV prevalence, there were 10 cases of pulmonary disease (5 cavitary), 2 meningeal, 1 mediastinal, 1 renal, 1 gastrointestinal, and 1 pleural (21).

DIAGNOSIS

The tuberculin skin test (Mantoux) is the test of choice for diagnosing tuberculosis infection in pregnant women. In recent years, blood tests have been developed which measure T-cell gamma interferon release in response to specific tuberculin antigens. These tests have potential advantages in terms of logistics (only one visit needed) and accuracy (not subjectively interpreted and not affected by previous *Mycobacterium bovis* BCG vaccination). However, there is currently insufficient data on the use of these tests in pregnant women to recommend them as the method of choice.

Although pregnant women have suppressed cell-mediated immunity to tuberculin in in vitro studies (11, 33), this does not appear to be clinically relevant (28). While pregnancy does not alter the response to a tuberculin skin test, 10 to 25% of immunocompetent persons with active tuberculosis, pregnant or not, will have a negative test result (18). Because the nonspecific symptoms of tuberculosis (increased respiratory rate and fatigue) mimic the physiologic changes in pregnancy and therefore may be missed, tuberculosis skin testing should be pursued in high-risk populations. These include minority urban communities, recent immigrants from countries with a high prevalence of tuberculosis, intravenous drug users, populations at high risk for HIV infection, and persons already infected with HIV (6).

HIV-infected persons with active tuberculosis have a negative skin test result in 40 to 60% of cases (6, 21). Skin test negativity is highly correlated with CD4 count and not with pregnancy. A study of pregnant and nonpregnant women infected with HIV showed that the anergy rate to tetanus toxin and mumps was 14 of 46 (30%) in pregnant women and 38 of 78 (49%) in nonpregnant women. Anergy was associated with lower CD4 counts in both groups in this study, and although the nonpregnant women were more likely to be anergic, the CD4 counts were similar in both groups (24).

A thorough investigation to detect tuberculosis should be pursued for all persons with clinical features compatible with tuberculosis. To rule out active disease, routine chest radiographs (with proper shielding of the abdomen after the 12th week of gestation) should be performed in women with a positive tuberculin skin test result. Chest radiographs should be performed sooner if symptoms suggest pulmonary tuberculosis, even if the skin test result is negative. In addition, examination of specimens for mycobacteria should be performed in all patients with HIV infection and pulmonary symptoms. A complete review of systems and physical examination should be conducted to exclude extrapulmonary tuberculosis (6, 7).

TREATMENT

Preventive Therapy

Isoniazid (INH) effectively prevents the progression of latent infection to active disease in individuals infected with susceptible strains. There is no evidence of teratogenic effects on the fetus. The major side effect of INH is hepatitis, which occurs most frequently in persons over 35 years of age. Pregnancy and the postpartum period, however, are also considered independent risk factors for INH toxicity. In a report of 20 deaths due to INH toxicity, 4 were of women who began taking INH in pregnancy and continued after delivery. The incidence of death was estimated to be 1 in 2,000 postpartum women taking INH (26).

The American Thoracic Society states that, for most pregnant women, preventive therapy should generally be delayed until after delivery. The exception is for women with recent infection. In this case, preventive therapy should begin when tuberculosis is documented but not until after the first trimester. The recommendation to begin therapy after delivery is based on the increased risk of active tuberculosis during the postpartum period, notwithstanding the increased toxicity of INH during this period (2). Because of the high risk of development of active disease in the tuberculosis-infected, HIV-positive woman, preventive therapy should be given to all patients who demonstrate purified protein derivative conversion. Preventive therapy should also be considered for HIV-positive women who have negative test results but are anergic and live in high-incidence areas.

In all cases, preventive therapy should consist of 300 mg of INH in a single daily dose. Pyridoxine supplementation (25 mg/day) should be given to all pregnant and breast-feeding women taking INH (9). In addition, because nursing infants receive approximately 20% of a therapeutic dosage of INH through breast milk, these infants should also receive pyridoxine supplementation (8). Although neurotoxicity, including seizures, has been reported in nursing children of mothers taking INH (22), treatment with first-line agents should not be considered a contraindication to nursing (32). Breast-feeding mothers may take their medication immediately after breast-feeding and consider substituting a bottle for the next feeding if feasible.

Active Disease

Pregnant women with active tuberculosis should begin therapy as soon as the diagnosis is established. The risk of transmission of the organism to the infant outweighs the risks of the drugs to the mother's own health. The preferred initial treatment for pregnant women is the combination of INH, rifampin, and ethambutol. Pyrazinamide is recommended for routine use in pregnant women by the WHO but has not received such approval in the United States due to a paucity of safety data. Streptomycin should not be used because there is a risk of sensorineural hearing loss in the infant (9).

If resistance to the first-line drugs is encountered, the risks and benefits of second-line drugs should be weighed and their use considered. Unfortunately, most second-line medications may have deleterious effects on the fetus. Ethionamide use has been associated with teratogenic effects in animals. Aminoglycosides including kanamycin, capreomycin, and amikacin presumably share streptomycin's ototoxic potential. The fluoroquinolones have been shown to damage growing cartilage and thus should be avoided in pregnancy if at all possible (9). Treatment duration should be 9 months.

REFERENCES

1. Adhikari, M. 2009. Tuberculosis and tuberculosis/HIV co-infection in pregnancy. *Semin. Fetal Neonatal Med.* 14:234–240.
2. American Thoracic Society. 1986. Treatment of tuberculosis and tuberculosis infection in adults and children. *Am. Rev. Respir. Dis.* 134:355–363.
3. Beitzke, H. 1935. Ueber die angeborene tuberkuloese infection. *Ergeb. Ges. Tuberk. Forsch.* 7:1–30.
4. Cantwell, M. F., Z. M. Shehab, A. M. Costello, L. Sands, W. F. Green, E. P. Ewing, Jr., S. E. Valway, and I. M. Onorato. 1994. Brief report: congenital tuberculosis. *N. Engl. J. Med.* 330:1051–1054.
5. Carter, E. J., and S. Mates. 1994. Tuberculosis during pregnancy. The Rhode Island experience, 1987 to 1991. *Chest* 106:1466–1470.
6. Centers for Disease Control. 1990. Screening for tuberculosis and tuberculous infection in high-risk populations. Recommendations of the Advisory Committee for Elimination of Tuberculosis. *MMWR Recommend. Rep.* 39(RR-8):1–7.
7. Centers for Disease Control. 1990. The use of preventive therapy for tuberculous infection in the United States. Recommendations of the Advisory Committee for Elimination of Tuberculosis. *MMWR Recommend. Rep.* 39(RR-8):9–12.
8. Centers for Disease Control and Prevention. 2000. Targeted tuberculin testing and treatment of latent tuberculosis infection. American Thoracic Society. *MMWR Recommend. Rep.* 49(RR-6):1–51.
9. Centers for Disease Control and Prevention. 2003. Treatment of tuberculosis, American Thoracic Society. CDC and Infectious Diseases Society of America. *MMWR Recommend. Rep.* 52(RR-11):1–77.
10. Centers for Disease Control and Prevention. 2009. *Reported Tuberculosis in the United States, 2008.* U.S. Department of Health and Human Services, Atlanta, GA.
11. Covelli, H. D., and R. T. Wilson. 1978. Immunologic and medical considerations in tuberculin-sensitized pregnant patients. *Am. J. Obstet. Gynecol.* 132:256–259.
12. Figueroa-Damian, R., and J. L. Arredondo-Garcia. 2001. Neonatal outcome of children born to women with tuberculosis. *Arch. Med. Res.* 32:66–69.
13. Good, J. T., Jr., M. D. Iseman, P. T. Davidson, S. Lakshminarayan, and S. A. Sahn. 1981. Tuberculosis in association with pregnancy. *Am. J. Obstet. Gynecol.* 140:492–498.
14. Grisolle, A. 1850. De l'influence que la grossesse et la phthisie pulmonaire exercent reciproquement l'une sur l'autre. *Arch. Gen. Med.* 22:41.
15. Hamadeh, M. A., and J. Glassroth. 1992. Tuberculosis and pregnancy. *Chest* 101:1114–1120.
16. Hammer, G. S., and S. Z. Hirshman. 1985. Infections in pregnancy, p. 14–15. *In* S. H. Cherry, R. L. Berkowitz, and N. G. Kase (ed.), *Medical, Surgical, and Gynecological Complications of Pregnancy,* 3rd ed. Williams and Wilkins, Baltimore, MD.
17. Hedvall, E. 1953. Pregnancy and tuberculosis. *Acta Med. Scand. Suppl.* 286:1–101.
18. Huebner, R. E., M. F. Schein, and J. B. Bass, Jr. 1993. The tuberculin skin test. *Clin. Infect. Dis.* 17:968–975.
19. Jana, N., K. Vasishta, S. K. Jindal, B. Khunnu, and K. Ghosh. 1994. Perinatal outcome in pregnancies complicated by pulmonary tuberculosis. *Int. J. Gynaecol. Obstet.* 44:119–124.
20. Lerner, B. H. 1994. Constructing medical indications: the sterilization of women with heart disease or tuberculosis, 1905-1935. *J. Hist. Med. Allied Sci.* 49:362–379.
21. Margono, F., J. Mroueh, A. Garely, D. White, A. Duerr, and H. L. Minkoff. 1994. Resurgence of active tuberculosis among pregnant women. *Obstet. Gynecol.* 83:911–914.
22. McKenzie, S. A., A. J. Macnab, and G. Katz. 1976. Neonatal pyridoxine responsive convulsions due to isoniazid therapy. *Arch. Dis. Child.* 51:567–568.
23. Mehta, B. R. 1961. Pregnancy and tuberculosis. *Dis. Chest* 39:505–511.
24. Mofenson, L. M., E. M. Rodriguez, R. Hershow, H. E. Fox, S. Landesman, R. Tuomala, C. Diaz, E. Daniels, and D. Brambilla. 1995. Mycobacterium tuberculosis infection in pregnant and nonpregnant women infected with HIV in the Women and Infants Transmission Study. *Arch. Intern. Med.* 155:1066–1072.
25. Mondal, S. K., and T. K. Dutta. 2009. A ten year clinicopathological study of female genital tuberculosis and impact on fertility. *JNMA J. Nepal Med. Assoc.* 48:52–57.
26. Moulding, T. S., A. G. Redeker, and G. C. Kanel. 1989. Twenty isoniazid-associated deaths in one state. *Am. Rev. Respir. Dis.* 140:700–705.
27. Osler, W. 1897. *The Principles and Practice of Medicine.* Appleton, New York, NY.
28. Present, P. A., and G. W. Comstock. 1975. Tuberculin sensitivity in pregnancy. *Am. Rev. Respir. Dis.* 112:413–416.

29. **Pugh, D. L.** 1955. The relation of child-bearing and child-rearing to pulmonary tuberculosis. *Br. J. Tuberc. Dis. Chest* **49:**206–216.

30. **Ratner, B., A. E. Rostler, and P. S. Salgado.** 1951. Care, feeding and fate of premature and full term infants born of tuberculous mothers. *Am. J. Dis. Child.* **81:**471–482.

31. **Schaefer, G., I. A. Zervoudakis, F. F. Fuchs, and S. David.** 1975. Pregnancy and pulmonary tuberculosis. *Obstet. Gynecol.* **46:** 706–715.

32. **Snider, D. E., Jr., and K. E. Powell.** 1984. Should women taking antituberculosis drugs breast-feed? *Arch. Intern. Med.* **144:** 589–590.

33. **Tanaka, A., K. Hirota, K. Takahashi, and Y. Numazaki.** 1983. Suppression of cell mediated immunity to cytomegalovirus and tuberculin in pregnancy employing the leukocyte migration inhibition test. *Microbiol. Immunol.* **27:**937–943.

34. **Wilson, E. A., T. J. Thelin, and P. V. Dilts, Jr.** 1973. Tuberculosis complicated by pregnancy. *Am. J. Obstet. Gynecol.* **115:** 526–529.

35. **World Health Organization.** 2009. *Global Tuberculosis Control: Epidemiology, Strategy, Financing. WHO Report 2009.* World Health Organization, Geneva, Switzerland.

Chapter 32

Tuberculosis Associated with HIV Infection

MIDORI KATO-MAEDA, ANNIE LUETKEMEYER, AND PETER M. SMALL

INTRODUCTION

Tuberculosis and human immunodeficiency virus (HIV) infection are two major global public health threats that undermine the development of societies because of their high morbidity and mortality. This is especially evident in sub-Saharan Africa, where more than 20 million of the global estimated 33 million patients with HIV type 1 infection live (124). Tuberculosis is an opportunistic infection in patients infected with HIV. In persons infected with *Mycobacterium tuberculosis* (MTB) alone, the risk of developing tuberculosis is approximately 10% during their lifetime (127). In contrast, in patients infected with both HIV and MTB, the overall risk of developing tuberculosis is 10% per year (104). The association of HIV and MTB coinfection is explained by the synergic interaction of MTB and HIV. HIV induces immunosuppression and therefore is an important risk factor for the progression of MTB infection to disease and for death by tuberculosis. Conversely, MTB accelerates the progression of HIV infection. In this chapter, we review the pathogenesis of the coinfection of HIV and MTB, the epidemiology, and the clinical aspects of tuberculosis associated with HIV infection.

PATHOGENESIS OF THE COINFECTION OF MTB-HIV

Patients infected with HIV are 20 to 37 times more likely than people not infected with HIV to develop tuberculosis (133). This is because patients infected with HIV have a high risk of getting infected by patients with active tuberculosis, and those that are infected have a high risk to progress rapidly to active tuberculosis (38).

The principal effect of the HIV is immune dysfunction and immune depletion. HIV enters macrophages facilitated by the attachment of its glycoprotein GP120 to the CD4 receptor and the chemokine receptor CCR5, which is critical in the initial establishment of HIV infection (111). Recently, a defective MTB-mediated alveolar macrophage apoptosis (which is considered a critical mechanism to eliminate MTB [14]) was described among patients infected with HIV. This defect decreased the killing of MTB and increased the susceptibility to active tuberculosis, even among patients infected with HIV that have relatively preserved $CD4^+$ T lymphocytes (94). HIV also infects T-lymphocyte helper cells facilitated by the CD4 receptor in conjunction with the chemokine receptor CXCR4 (111). Eventually, HIV causes profound immunosuppression, at some point manifested as an opportunistic infection, neoplasm, or other life-threatening complications.

Tuberculosis is observed in all stages of the HIV infection. At $CD4^+$ T cell counts of greater than 350 cells/mm^3, the inflammatory response and the clinical and histopathologic characteristics of tuberculosis are similar to those of persons who are not infected with HIV, with the presence of granuloma with or without central caseation (22). However, with the progression of the immunosuppression, granulomas are either not well formed or absent. Instead, abundant tubercle bacilli and abscess formation in soft tissues are frequently observed (102) and disseminated tuberculosis is more frequent. Antiretroviral therapy (ART) greatly reduces the risk of tuberculosis in HIV infection, but it appears that in most populations, even after effective treatment with ART, the risk of tuberculosis is still on average 5- to 10-fold higher than in the HIV-uninfected population (74, 86). This may be explained in part by an incomplete

Midori Kato-Maeda • San Francisco General Hospital, University of California San Francisco, Francis J. Curry National Tuberculosis Center, Division of Pulmonary and Critical Care Medicine, 1001 Potrero Ave., Building 100, Room 109, Mailbox 0841, San Francisco, CA 94110.   **Annie Luetkemeyer** • San Francisco General Hospital, University of California San Francisco, HIV/AIDS Division, 995 Potrero Ave., Box 0874, San Francisco, CA 94110.   **Peter M. Small** • Institute for Systems Biology, 1441 N. 34th St., Seattle, WA 98103-8904.

reconstitution of tuberculosis-specific immune response (73, 101, 115).

MTB induces progression of HIV immunosuppression by several mechanisms (122). Clinical studies have demonstrated increased HIV RNA in patients with tuberculosis (39, 52). This has been confirmed in laboratory studies where MTB induces replication of HIV in monocytes (24) and in acutely infected macrophages (123). This phenomenon has been attributed to proinflammatory cytokines such as tumor necrosis factor alpha which is induced in mononuclear cells by MTB. HIV replication is also accelerated by the presence of monocyte chemoattractant protein-1 and is considered a critical agent for the activation of HIV at sites where MTB is present (82). MTB activates transcriptionally latent HIV in alveolar macrophages or in monocytes newly recruited to sites of MTB infection (122). Interestingly, there is also a clinical study that showed that MTB infection decreased HIV RNA (110), and in vitro data that suggest that MTB has an inhibitory effect of HIV replication in monocyte-derived macrophages (51). The inconsistent finding about the effect of tuberculosis on HIV replication may be due to variation between patients and due to host and viral factors.

The result of the complex immunological interaction of MTB and HIV is progressive immunosuppression that increases the risk of tuberculosis both by reactivation of a latent tuberculosis infection (LTBI) and by recent infection and rapid evolution to tuberculosis. HIV is the strongest risk factor, independent of the number of CD4$^+$ T cells, for reactivation of LTBI. Among intravenous drug users with positive tuberculin skin tests (TST), 7 of 49 (14%) persons infected with HIV developed active tuberculosis within 2 years compared with 0 of 62 not infected with HIV, which was higher than the lifetime risk of reactivation in patients without HIV infection (104). HIV is also a risk factor for tuberculosis due to recent transmission. A study performed in New York City demonstrated that 40% of the cases of tuberculosis were the result of recent transmission, with HIV being an independent risk factor (3). The immunosuppression by HIV accelerates the progression of recently acquired infection to active tuberculosis. In Italy, 7 of 18 (35%) patients with HIV exposed to MTB in a nosocomial outbreak developed tuberculosis within 60 days (41). In San Francisco, 37% of the contacts of a smear-positive tuberculosis patient in a residential facility of patients with AIDS developed active tuberculosis by the same strain within 3 months of diagnosis of the first case (38). However, the role of HIV infection in the infectiousness of MTB from individual patients with tuberculosis is not very clear. A recent study found that the infectiousness of patients

with tuberculosis associated with HIV was highly variable but, on average, was six times greater than the average infectiousness recorded in the 1950s. The authors hypothesized that this difference could be because of the HIV infection, although in their study, the smear positivity was an important factor for infectiousness (45).

EPIDEMIOLOGY

The interaction of MTB and HIV/AIDS has consequences at the population level, both in the United States as well as in other parts of the world, by increasing the number of cases of tuberculosis, which has compromised the possibility of controlling this epidemic.

In the United States, by the end of 2008, 479,868 persons were living with AIDS (prevalence of 157.7 per 100,000 population) and 263,936 were living with HIV infection but not AIDS (prevalence of 154.2 per 100,000 adolescents and adults) (34). From 2006 to 2009, the estimated rate of diagnosis of HIV infection remained stable in the 40 states with a confidential name-based HIV infection reporting system. These 40 states represent approximately 75% of the cases of AIDS diagnosed in the 50 states and the District of Columbia. The mortality rate due to AIDS decreased 7% from 2006 to 2008. At the end of 2006, it was estimated that approximately 232,700 (95% confidence interval [CI] = 221,200 to 244,200) persons were infected with HIV but were unaware of their infection (the last year for which these data are available) (23).

The epidemic of HIV/AIDS was temporally associated with the resurgence of tuberculosis in the United States and other industrialized countries. The increase in tuberculosis case rates was more dramatic in the geographic areas and populations such as the homeless population (88) that have been most severely affected by AIDS. Although it is clear that the increased susceptibility of patients infected with HIV greatly contributed to the increase in tuberculosis rates in the United States and worldwide (61), it must be stressed that this increase was also in part due to waning attention to and decreased funding of control efforts. Indirect evidence for this is the fact that after peaking in 1992, tuberculosis rates in the United States began a steady decline despite the increase in the number of cases of HIV/AIDS (91). The average percent decline of cases of tuberculosis was 7.3% per year from 1993 to 2000 and 3.8% from 2000 to 2008 (31). From 2008 to 2009, there was a decrease of 11.4% in cases of tuberculosis, the greatest single-year decrease ever recorded in the United States (27).

In 2009, in the United States there were 11,540 cases of tuberculosis reported (3.8 cases per 100,000 inhabitants) (27). From these patients, the HIV test result was known in 6,743 (58%) persons and 690 (10.2%) were infected with HIV (the data did not include information from California and Vermont) (27). As the overall rate of tuberculosis decreased, the frequency of tuberculosis associated with HIV also decreased from 15% in 2003 to 12.4% in 2006, although the percentage with unknown HIV status increased from 28.7% in 2005 to 31.7% in 2006 (17). The decrease in the cases of tuberculosis associated with HIV is attributed to (i) tuberculosis control measures, such as improvements in the completion of therapy against tuberculosis with direct observed therapy short course and an increase in the detection of cases and (ii) the increase in the use of ART which has reduced the incidence of tuberculosis (RH = 0.6; 95% CI, 0.4 to 1.0) (89). ART has also decreased the mortality due to tuberculosis associated with HIV; those receiving both ART and antituberculosis therapy had one-sixth of the risk of death compared with patients not receiving ART (44, 99). However, tuberculosis is still a risk factor for AIDS-related deaths in the United States (76, 77).

Although the frequency of tuberculosis associated with HIV is decreasing in the United States, there are an estimated 11 million persons with LTBI (113) and more than 700,000 persons living with AIDS and HIV (34). Moreover, recent studies estimated that among those infected with HIV, the risk to develop active tuberculosis increases linearly up to at least 11 years from the moment of HIV seroconversion (50).

Globally, the impact of the HIV infection on the epidemiology of tuberculosis is staggering. In 2009, there were approximately 9.4 million new cases of tuberculosis in the world, 1.0 to 1.2 million among people infected with HIV, and approximately 380,000 deaths (range, 320,000 to 450,000) have been attributed to HIV-tuberculosis (133a). The distribution of tuberculosis associated with HIV is heterogeneous around the world; 79% of the cases occurred in Africa, with 28% of the global burden occurring in South Africa (133b). The incident cases of tuberculosis associated with HIV peaked at 1.39 million in 2005 and are now decreasing (133b). However, tuberculosis is still the leading cause of death among patients infected with HIV (138).

There are several aspects of the epidemiology of tuberculosis that are specifically associated with HIV. The first one is the high frequency of recurrent tuberculosis compared with patients without HIV, both in areas where tuberculosis is not endemic (90) and in areas where it is endemic (93), including recurrent tuberculosis due to reinfection with drug-resistant MTB

strains (6). The second one is the association of HIV and drug-resistant tuberculosis. HIV infection is associated with tuberculosis resistant to rifamycin in two situations: (i) patients that used rifapentine once a week (currently contraindicated in patients with HIV) (126) and (ii) patients with fewer than 100 CD4$^+$ T cells/mm^3 who received rifamycin twice weekly during the maintenance phase (19). The acquired resistance has been attributed to poor adherence to treatment, advanced immunosuppression, and suboptimal levels of the drug (120). HIV has been also associated with resistance to other antituberculosis drugs in institutional outbreaks (128), where the delay in diagnosis and inadequate treatment of tuberculosis led to an increase in transmission as well as mortality. A recent survey showed that HIV was associated with drug-resistant tuberculosis with odds ratios of 2.1 (95% CI, 1.4 to 3.0; $P < 0.01$) (132) and 1.7 (95% CI, 1.3 to 2.3) (42) in Latvia and Ukraine, respectively. Interestingly, a review of publications about HIV infection and multidrug-resistant (MDR; defined as resistance to at least isoniazid and rifampin) tuberculosis, specifically in areas with ≥2% overall prevalence of MDR and ≥1% prevalence of HIV infection, did not demonstrate a clear association between HIV infection and MDR tuberculosis in the community. However, the authors did find that MDR tuberculosis associated with HIV had a high mortality (128). The study also demonstrated the presence of a geographic overlap of the epidemics of HIV and MDR tuberculosis and the potential of these epidemics to fuel each other (128). In fact, this situation was recently observed in KwaZulu Natal, South Africa, where an outbreak of extensively drug-resistant (XDR) tuberculosis (defined as MDR organisms that are also resistant to fluoroquinolones and at least one of the injectable second-line agents) occurred among patients infected with HIV (48). These patients had exceptionally high mortality rates of 51% within 30 days of sputum collection and 83% at 1 year (49). In the United States, 53% of the XDR cases occurred among patients with HIV (105). Therefore, the strategies for the control of tuberculosis and HIV should also consider interventions to control drug-resistant tuberculosis (106).

CLINICAL PRESENTATION

HIV does not alter the symptoms classically associated with tuberculosis such as fatigue, weight loss, fevers, sweats, cough, and anorexia. However, the symptoms are less specific because other conditions, such as HIV-associated fever and weight loss, lymphoma, and disseminated histoplasmosis produce symptoms consistent with tuberculosis. Also, the use of ART in severely immunosuppressed patients may lead to unusual manifestations of pulmonary disease as a result of the immune reconstitution inflammatory syndrome (IRIS) (see below and reviewed elsewhere in this book).

Given that much of the pathology of tuberculosis results from the host's response to the infection, it is not surprising that the signs of tuberculosis vary considerably with the severity of HIV-induced immunosuppression (Table 1). With mild immunosuppression, MTB causes disease that closely resembles that in patients without HIV infection. As immunosuppression becomes progressively severe, the clinical presentation of tuberculosis becomes more "atypical," with unusual radiographic manifestations and nonreactive TST, as well as disseminated and extrapulmonary tuberculosis (108, 114).

Tuberculosis in patients with HIV can affect any organ. In a prospective study of tuberculosis in patients without and with HIV infection (81% with ≤200 $CD4^+$ T cells/mm^3), the lung was involved similarly in both groups: 78.3% and 74.3%, respectively (4). The majority of patients with pulmonary involvement had positive cultures for MTB, but the direct sputum examination was positive in only 54.3% of patients infected with HIV as opposed to nearly 75% in patients without HIV infection. Interestingly, this discrepancy persisted even when only those patients who had either focal infiltrates or cavities apparent on chest radiographs were analyzed. The incidence of pleural effusion is variable (from 15 to 90% of patients with tuberculosis) and usually more common in patients with high $CD4^+$ T cell counts (54). Extrapulmonary tuberculosis, either as the sole presentation or concomitant with pulmonary involvement, is more frequent in patients infected with HIV (56.5%

versus 35.7%) and HIV is a strong risk factor for this type of tuberculosis (odds ratio, 4.93; 95% CI, 1.95 to 12.46) (136). The most common location of extrapulmonary tuberculosis among 85 patients in Arkansas was bone and/or joint tuberculosis (27%), followed by cervical lymphatic tuberculosis (17.7%) (136). Other forms seen were genitourinary, peritoneal, noncervical lymphatic, meningeal, and disseminated disease. Tuberculosis bacteremia, which is extremely rare in patients without HIV infection, was observed in 20 to 40% of patients (9), and tuberculous meningitis was observed in up to 10% of patients with tuberculosis associated with HIV (104). The clinical presentation of extrapulmonary tuberculosis is similar to that of immunocompetent patients (136). However, tuberculous meningitis in patients infected with HIV has more ventricular dilatation and infarcts (103), and abdominal tuberculosis has more visceral lesions and intra-abdominal lymphadenopathy (instead of the ascites and omental thickening observed in patients without HIV infection) (46).

DIAGNOSIS

Because of the high frequency of coinfection of MTB and HIV, all patients infected with HIV should be screened for LTBI and tuberculosis (66). Also, all patients with tuberculosis should be advised to undergo voluntary counseling and testing for HIV infection (13). The methods used to diagnose LTBI and tuberculosis are the same as in patients without HIV infection and are reviewed elsewhere is this book. However, the interpretation of the tests is complicated by the possibility of false-negative results as well as the lack of specificity of the symptoms.

Diagnosis of LTBI

At the time of diagnosis of HIV, all patients should be tested for LTBI (66). Persons that have a negative result and fewer than 200 $CD4^+$ T cells/mm^3 without indication for treatment for LTBI should be retested for LTBI when starting ART and their $CD4^+$ T cell counts are ≥200 cells/mm^3. If negative, an annual testing is recommended for patients that have repeated exposure to patients with active tuberculosis. Patients with a positive test for LTBI should be evaluated for active tuberculosis through a clinical and microbiological examination and chest radiography (66).

There are several approaches to diagnose LTBI. The first is the TST with 0.1 ml of purified protein derivative (PPD). In patients infected with HIV, any induration greater than 5 mm after 48 to 72 hours

Table 1. Clinical characteristics of tuberculosis in patients coinfected with HIV

During early HIV infection (typical features of tuberculosis are frequent)
    Usually pulmonary disease with involvement of the upper lobe and presence of cavitation
    PPD positive in >50% of cases
    Good response to therapy

During advanced HIV infection
    Any organ can be affected
    Extrapulmonary involvement is common (bone and/or joint, lymphatic, meningeal, pleural, hepatic, renal, splenic, spinal, cutaneous, and miliary dissemination), with manifestations similar to those seen in patients without HIV infection
    Unusual radiographic findings (diffuse infiltration, mid- and lower-lung zone infiltrates, intrathoracic adenopathy, pleural effusion, or normal)
    PPD test results positive in <40% of cases
    Good response to therapy but early mortality may be high

should be classified as a positive test (29). Anergy is common with progression of HIV disease. Unfortunately, there is no reliable method to evaluate anergy, and simultaneous testing with candida and mumps antigens is not recommended (28, 107).

The second approach is the use of gamma interferon release assays (IGRAs) (71). There are three IGRAs currently approved for marketing in the United States, QuantiFERON-TB Gold test (QFT) and QuantiFERON-TB Gold In-tube (QFT In-tube) (Cellestis Limited, Carnegie, Victoria, Australia) and the T.SPOT.*TB* test (Oxford Immunotec, Abingdon, United Kingdom), all of which are reviewed elsewhere in this book. In contrast to TST, which has variable cutoffs based on the tuberculosis risk category and immune suppression, IGRAs use the same cutoff values for all individuals, including those with HIV infection.

There are few studies analyzing the performance of IGRA in patients infected with HIV, and the results are heterogeneous. Several studies showed poor concordance between TST and IGRA in patients with HIV (79, 119). A recent study performed in the United States compared TST, QFT In-Tube and the T.SPOT. *TB* in 336 patients with HIV infection (119). Twenty-seven (8%) had at least one positive diagnostic test, 7 (2.5%) were positive to the TST, 9 (2.7%) to the QFT In-tube, and 14 (4.2%) to the T.SPOT. *TB*. Only two patients had positive results with two diagnostic tests, and just one patient had positive results for all three diagnostic tests. In contrast, a study in Senegal comparing an in-house enzyme-linked immunospot IGRA with TST in 247 patients with HIV infection demonstrated that both tests were concordant for 151 patients (61%; kappa, 0.230) (67). In a recent systematic review and meta-analysis, the authors concluded that IGRAs performed similarly to TST at identifying LTBI among HIV-infected individuals (26a). In most of the studies, patients with $CD4^+$ T-cell counts of less than 200 cells/mm^3 were more likely to have IGRAs with indeterminate results (67, 79, 119). However, in a study performed in Uganda, the valid results of the T.SPOT.*TB* assay were independent of the level of $CD4^+$ T cells (75). Although indeterminate results may be more common with advanced immunosuppression, patients with low $CD4^+$ T-cell counts will still frequently have valid IGRA results, and therefore, IGRA can be used to diagnose LTBI in patients with HIV across the spectrum of immunosuppression (66). TST can be used to diagnose LTBI in patients when IGRA is not available (66). In fact, recently the CDC suggested that, in patients with HIV, both tests together (a TST and an IGRA) might be useful to diagnose LTBI (82a). In patients infected with HIV, a positive result to any of the diagnostic tests should be considered a diagnosis of infection with MTB (66).

The third approach for the diagnosis of LTBI is the chest radiography. The presence of fibrotic lesions is an indication to rule out active tuberculosis. After ruling out active tuberculosis, patients with HIV infection should be considered to have LTBI (independent of the results of TST and IGRA) if they have fewer than 200 $CD4^+$ T cells/mm^3 and do not have prior history of LTBI treatment or tuberculosis treatment (66).

Diagnosis of Tuberculosis

The approach to diagnose tuberculosis is similar to that for patients without HIV infection. The definitive diagnosis of tuberculosis is established with the isolation of MTB in the specimens of the site suspected of being infected.

Sputum should be submitted for mycobacterial smear examination and culture. The sensitivity of the sputum smear examination is lower in patients with advanced HIV infection than in patients without HIV infection (43, 64). A recent systematic review demonstrated that smear examination using fluorescence microscopy is more sensitive than conventional microscopy and has similar specificity in patients without HIV infection (112). Although this systematic review could not address the performance in individuals with HIV infection (as there were not enough studies to evaluate), the available data suggest that fluorescence-based staining techniques may increase the sensitivity of the smear examination (84) but may decrease the specificity (26). If the sputum smear examination is negative or if the patient does not produce sputum, it is recommended to obtain samples through sputum induction by the inhalation of a hypertonic (3% to 5%) saline mist generated by an ultrasonic nebulizer, which increases the diagnostic yield in patients with a negative smear (84). Bronchoscopic procedures have been especially helpful in the diagnostic evaluations of patients with HIV infection unable to expectorate sputum (10).

The use of species testing to confirm whether the acid-fast bacilli (AFB) observed in a smear are MTB is particularly important in patients infected with HIV, as they may be infected with nontuberculous mycobacteria. Nucleic acid amplification testing is one method of rapid species identification (positive predictive value, >95%) (32). A study in Kenya demonstrated that the sensitivity of the nucleic acid amplification method was 89% in patients with HIV infection and 95% in patients without HIV infection when using culture in Lowenstein-Jensen media as the gold standard (69). More recently, a fully automated molecular test for tuberculosis and rifampin resistance detection called Xpert MTB/RIF was described. The method has been tested under research conditions in two South African sites that included more than 70% of individuals infected with HIV. The sensitivity of the test was >99% in smear- and culture-positive tuberculosis cases and >86% in smear-negative and culture-positive cases. The specificity was >97%. The method is described elsewhere in this book.

Culture for mycobacterium is considered the gold standard for the diagnosis of tuberculosis and is reviewed extensively elsewhere in this book. If the clinical suspicion of tuberculosis is high and the smear examination and culture are negative, it is advisable to continue the patient evaluation, including invasive diagnostic procedures to obtain samples for histopathological and microbiological studies or to perform a treatment trial.

The chest radiograph during the early stages of HIV infection may demonstrate upper-lobe involvement and cavitation, as in patients without HIV infection. During later stages where the immunosuppression is more severe, it is possible to find involvement of the mid- and lower lung lobes, lymphadenopathy (Fig. 1), pleural effusion (Fig. 2), and diffuse infiltrates (Fig. 3). The chest radiograph may be also normal in patients with advanced HIV, despite the presence of AFB upon direct sputum examination

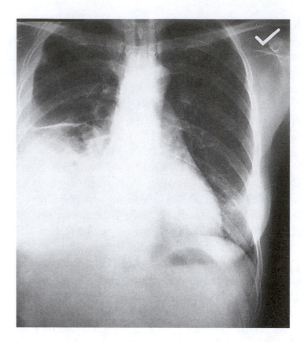

Figure 2. Posteroanterior chest radiograph demonstrating extensive right lower infiltrate associated with pleural effusion.

(95). A recent study demonstrated that 8% of chest radiographs were normal despite the presence of AFB in the smear examination and a positive culture for *M. tuberculosis* (35).

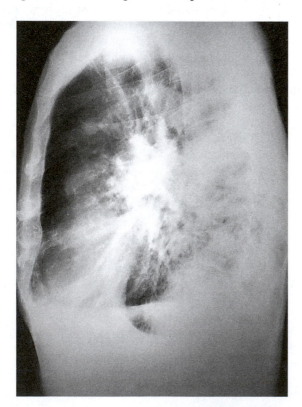

Figure 1. Lateral chest radiograph showing extensive mid- and lower-lung field involvement and associated lymphadenopathy in a man with AIDS.

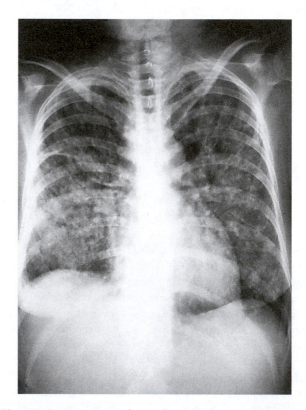

Figure 3. Posteroanterior chest radiograph showing extensive bilateral diffuse infiltrate in a young woman with advanced HIV infection.

IGRA can be used when there is a high suspicion of active tuberculosis and the microbiological studies are negative; however, similar to TST, the sensitivity for detection of active tuberculosis with IGRA is limited. A recent study performed in India with 112 patients (50% with culture-confirmed MTB and 50% with culture-negative tuberculosis) demonstrated that QFT In-tube was positive in 65%, negative in 18%, and indeterminate in 17% (118). In Zambia, 37 of 59 (63%) HIV-positive patients with smear-positive tuberculosis had a positive QFT In-tube results (97). In addition, a reactive IGRA does not differentiate LTBI from tuberculosis, limiting the utility of IGRAs for active tuberculosis diagnosis in regions with endemic tuberculosis.

The diagnosis of extrapulmonary tuberculosis is challenging because of the difficulty of obtaining an appropriate sample. The histopathologic findings will depend on the degree of immunodeficiency. Patients with relatively normal immunological function will have the typical granulomatous inflammation; in contrast, patients with severe immunodeficiency will have poorly formed or no granulomatous inflammation (21, 65). Culture and nucleic acid amplification testing are less sensitive and specific for the diagnosis of extrapulmonary tuberculosis. Sometimes the diagnosis relies on epidemiological data, clinical manifestations, and the response to antituberculosis drugs (22, 100).

Because of the high mortality rate among patients with HIV infection and drug-resistant tuberculosis, drug susceptibility testing to the primary antituberculous drugs (isoniazid, rifampin, ethambutol, and pyrazinamide) should be performed for all patients with HIV infection (134), and treatment should be adjusted based on the results. Drug susceptibility testing should be repeated if the cultures remain positive after 3 months of treatment or become positive after being negative for 1 month or more (66). The drug susceptibility test to second-line drugs should be performed in reference laboratories for patients with (i) previous antituberculosis therapy, (ii) history of contact with drug-resistant tuberculosis, (iii) disease due to a strain that is resistant to first-line drugs, or (iv) positive cultures after 3 months of treatment or (v) for patients from regions with a high prevalence of MDR or XDR tuberculosis (66).

TREATMENT

Treatment of LTBI

HIV infection increases the risk of reactivation of LTBI by 20-fold (133), but this can be reduced by using ART and isoniazid preventive therapy. ART itself is a potent means of tuberculosis prevention,

reducing tuberculosis incidence by more than half (47, 53). The efficacy of treatment of LTBI in persons with HIV is highest in those with reactive TST, with a reduction in relative risk of active tuberculosis of 0.38 (95% CI, 0.25 to 0.85) (2). Several studies have shown a trend toward decreased risk of active tuberculosis with negative diagnostic tests for LTBI (98, 116), but this has not been demonstrated in all studies (2) and may depend on the TB prevalence and epidemiology of a particular site. Treatment of LTBI has demonstrated a mortality benefit in some studies (62), but this has also not been consistently demonstrated (2).

Although the risk for tuberculosis has decreased considerably with ART, it is still 5- to 10-fold higher than among individuals without HIV infection (74). Therefore, an attempt should be made to identify and treat all dually infected persons (25, 109). The current indications for LTBI treatment for the general population apply to patients infected with HIV: (i) persons with a positive diagnostic test for LTBI without previous history of treatment for LTBI or tuberculosis, (ii) close contacts of persons with infectious pulmonary tuberculosis regardless of the LTBI diagnostic test results, and (iii) persons with untreated or inadequately treated, healed tuberculosis regardless of the LTBI diagnostic test results (66). Individuals that come from geographic areas with a high prevalence of tuberculosis may receive treatment for LTBI based on their CD4$^+$ T-cell count (66).

The medications used for LTBI treatment are the same as those used for patients without HIV infection. The treatment should be started after excluding the presence of active tuberculosis with a medical history, physical examination, chest X ray, and microbiological evaluation, if indicated. The recommended regimens are isoniazid daily or twice a week for 9 months together with pyridoxine (25 mg/day) to minimize the risk of developing peripheral neuropathy (66). Longer courses or even indefinite treatment with isoniazid may be more efficacious in regions of the world with high rates of tuberculosis and therefore, where HIV patients are constantly exposed to tuberculosis (i.e., sub-Saharan Africa). These strategies of lengthy and indefinite LTBI treatment are under active investigation (98). If isoniazid cannot be used because of the high possibility of contact with an isoniazid-resistant MTB or other contraindication, it is possible to use rifampin or rifabutin for 4 months (66). In this case, it is important to make the adequate adjustments, as rifamycin interacts with the metabolism of the antiretroviral drugs (see below). Treatment with rifampin and pyrazinamide is not recommended regardless of HIV status due to the high toxicity (30). Although there are no data on treatment for LTBI by MDR MTB, experts suggest treatment with either pyrazinamide and ethambutol or pyrazinamide and quinolone (e.g., ofloxacin) for 12 months (5).

Children infected with HIV have a high risk of developing primary tuberculosis and high mortality (59). A randomized controlled trial demonstrated that preventive therapy with isoniazid reduced the incidence of tuberculosis and death; however, the long-term efficacy and the duration of the protective effect are unknown (137). A recent systematic review concluded that there was insufficient information to guide the duration of prophylaxis and to support its use in children using ART and living in areas of low tuberculosis prevalence (56).

Treatment of Tuberculosis

Tuberculosis in patients infected with HIV responds well to therapy, and their treatment has been reviewed recently (66, 134). The treatment should be initiated when tuberculosis is suspected in a patient infected with HIV (66, 134). Because of the difficulty in distinguishing MTB from *M. avium* complex, it is prudent to empirically initiate antituberculosis therapy when sputum samples demonstrate AFB while awaiting mycobacterial species identification. The drugs for the treatment of pulmonary tuberculosis and follow-up of the patient are similar to those for patients without HIV infection, independent of the degree of immunodeficiency (13, 66, 134), and they are reviewed extensively elsewhere in this book. However, patients with HIV should receive daily treatment in the intensive and continuation phases (134). This recommendation is based on a recent systematic review that showed 2 to 3 times higher incidence of relapse and failure when using intermittent therapy (68). In cases where daily treatment in the continuation phase is not possible, intermittent administration three times a week is an acceptable alternative (134). The recommended therapy is summarized in Table 2. Because peripheral neuropathies are common in patients infected with HIV, pyridoxine (25 mg/day) should be prescribed for all patients receiving isoniazid.

The recommended rifamycin for use with ART has been rifabutin, which has fewer drug interactions than rifampin and therefore can be coadministered with antiretrovirals from the protease inhibitor (PI), nonnucleoside reverse transcriptase inhibitor (NNRTI), and nucleoside reverse transcriptase inhibitor classes. However, there have been reports of acquired rifamycin resistance during coadministration of rifabutin with ritonavir-boosted PI, raising questions of whether standard rifabutin dosing should be increased when coadministered with PI (15, 63). In addition, because rifabutin dosing should be increased with NNRTIs and be decreased with PIs, interruption of HIV treatment without prompt adjustment of rifabutin can lead to toxicity or inadequate levels, respectively. Because treatment of patients infected with HIV is a rapidly evolving field, we advise the readers to review updates at the WHO and CDC websites.

Rifampin can be used but requires the appropriate adjustment to ART (see below) and cannot be given safely with many antiretrovirals. Rifapentine is not recommended because the once-a-week dose was associated with the development of acquired rifamycin resistance (126). Thiacetazone (a drug used in areas where rifampin is not available) is not recommended due to the risk of severe and sometimes fatal skin reaction in patients infected with HIV (92).

Patients with pulmonary tuberculosis may be monitored with sputum smear examination and culture at the end of the intensive phase of treatment (if the smear examination is positive, obtain a sputum sample at month 3, and if positive, obtain culture and drug susceptibility test), and at the fifth and sixth months of treatment (60, 134). It is also important to monitor the HIV viral load to assess the efficacy of the ART. The current guidelines recommend that patients should be treated at least for the same duration as HIV-negative patients (134). However, a recent systematic review found lower relapse rates when patients with HIV were treated with 8 or more months of rifampin-containing regimens, although the authors commented that the quality of the studies was low (68). At the completion of the

Table 2. Recommended regimen for tuberculosis treatment

Intensive phase drugs (dose)	Maintenance phase drugs (dose)	Comments
Isoniazid (300 mg/day)	Isoniazid (300 mg/day)	If sputum remains smear positive after completion of 2 mo of treatment, request new sputum after the 3rd mo. If the sputum remains positive, perform culture to determine susceptibility of MTB.
Rifampin (450 mg/day if less than 50 kg or 600 mg/day if more than 50 kg) or rifabutin (300 mg/day)	Rifampin (450 mg/day if less than 50 kg or 600 mg/day if more than 50 kg)	
Pyrazinamide (25 mg/kg/day)		
Ethambutol (25 mg/kg/day)		
Pyridoxine (25 mg/day)[a]		

[a]To decrease the risk of peripheral neuropathies associated with isoniazid.

intensive phase, patients with cavitary disease and positive cultures for a fully susceptible MTB should receive maintenance phase drugs (isoniazid and rifamycin) for an additional 3 or 4 months after cultures become negative (66). Directly observed therapy should be the standard of care for all HIV-infected patients (66).

Patients with highly infectious tuberculosis (i.e., smear-positive pulmonary disease) should be cautioned about the possibility of transmitting tuberculosis to other persons. Patients should not go back to a congregate living setting or any setting with persons susceptible to tuberculosis until their sputum smear examination is negative (66). If the patients have MDR, the current recommendation is that culture of sputum should be negative before returning to a congregate setting (66).

Patients with extrapulmonary tuberculosis should receive 2 months of intensive therapy, followed by 4 to 7 months of isoniazid and rifampin (66). The exceptions are patients with tuberculosis with central nervous system disease and bone and joint infection, which should be treated with regimens containing rifamycin for 9 to 12 months (66). The indications for adjuvant corticosteroids are similar to those for patients without HIV infection, including tuberculosis in the central nervous system (96) and pericardium (66). The recommended regimens are dexamethasone, 0.3 to 0.4 mg/kg of body weight tapered over 6 to 8 weeks (121), or prednisone, 1 mg/kg for 3 weeks then tapered for 3 to 5 weeks (96).

The management of treatment failure, relapse, MDR tuberculosis, and tuberculosis in children infected with HIV is similar to that for patients without HIV infection and can be reviewed elsewhere in this book and in several reviews (13, 66, 85). The possibility that patients are infected with organisms that are resistant to multiple antituberculosis drugs should be considered for all patients infected with HIV as well as those who have resided in areas that have a high incidence of drug resistance or who have been previously treated for tuberculosis.

Timing of Antiretroviral Initiation Relative to Tuberculosis Treatment

Patients already receiving ART at the time of tuberculosis diagnosis should start antituberculosis drugs as soon as possible, and drugs for both infections should be adjusted based on drug interaction and side effects (11, 13). Frequently, patients with tuberculosis have advanced HIV disease and have not yet started antiretroviral drugs at the time of tuberculosis diagnosis. Randomized controlled trials of patients with CD4$^+$ T-cell counts of <500 cells/mm^3

have demonstrated that waiting until after the completion of maintenance tuberculosis therapy was associated with a twofold-higher risk of death across all CD4$^+$ T-cell strata (1). Initiation of ART during TB therapy has been addressed by three randomized controlled trials to date. A study in Cambodia found a mortality benefit to starting ART 2 weeks compared with 8 weeks after TB treatment in a population with advanced HIV disease (median CD4$^+$, 25 cells/mm^3) (IQR 10-56) (12a). Two additional studies have demonstrated reduced mortality or AIDS progression for patients with CD4$^+$ cell counts of <50 cells/mm^3 when ART was started within 2 to 4 weeks, compared with 8 to 12 weeks, after starting TB treatment (1, 56a). HIV suppression was not negatively impacted with early initiation of ART. However, starting ART shortly after TB treatment initiation is associated with an approximately two- to fourfold-higher incidence of TB IRIS than those who deferred ART for 8 weeks or longer and should be anticipated as a common complication of early initiation of ART. The WHO now recommends that ART be initiated in all HIV-MTB coinfected patients as soon as possible after tuberculosis treatment is started, regardless of CD4$^+$ T-cell count (131). Tuberculosis meningitis merits special consideration as the optimal timing of ART initiation in this case is not clear. Unlike non-CNS TB, one study has indicated a slightly increased mortality as well as an increase in grade 4 adverse events with immediate ART initiation compared with deferred ART (123a). Given that IRIS to CNS infections can be severe and potentially fatal, close monitoring is required when ART is initiated in CNS meningitis and additional data are needed to inform optimal timing of ART.

Drug Interactions

There are complex interactions between rifamycins and most of the drugs used to treat HIV infection. Only the nucleoside analogues other than zidovudine and enfuvirtide (an intramuscularly injected entry inhibitor) do not have significant drug interactions with rifamycins (33). Rifamycins induce the activity of the isoenzymes CYP3A4 and CYP2C8/9 of the cytochrome P450 system. Rifampin is the most potent inducer, followed by rifapentine (which is not recommended for patients infected with HIV in the current once-weekly dosing). Rifabutin is the least powerful inducer and is recommended for the treatment of tuberculosis in patients with HIV infection, especially if protease inhibitors are required to treat HIV (66). Here we summarize the interaction of rifampin and rifabutin with approved antiretroviral drugs (Table 3).

Table 3. Dose adjustment required when coadministering rifamycin (rifampin or rifabutin) and antiretroviral drugs (33)

Antiretroviral drug	Coadministration with: Rifampin		Rifabutin	
	Recommended changes	Comments	Recommended changes	Comments
NNRTI				
Efavirenz	None	No change in rifampin concn	Increase rifabutin to 450–600 mg/day	No change in efavirenz concn
Nevirapine		No changes		No changes
Etravirine		Do not use together		No change recommended but limited clinical experience
PI				
Nelfinavir		Do not use together	Decrease rifabutin to 150 mg/day	
Saquinavir-ritonavir	Use 400 mg–saquinavir, 400 mg ritonavir twice a day	No changes to rifampin, but use with caution because of hepatitis risk		
Lopinavir-ritonavir	Increase to 800 mg lopinavir–200 mg ritonavir (double dosed)	Use with caution; it caused hepatitis in healthy volunteers	Decrease rifabutin to 150 mg every other day or 3 times/week	
Super-boosted lopinavir-ritonavir	Use 400 mg lopinavir–100 mg ritonavir plus 300 mg of ritonavir (as super boost)	Use with caution because of hepatitis risk	Decrease rifabutin to 150 mg every other day or 3 times/week	
CCR-5 receptor antagonist maraviroc	Increase maraviroc to 600 mg twice a day	No clinical experience		No change recommended but no clinical experience
Integrase inhibitor raltegravir	Increase to 800 mg twice daily	No clinical experience		No change recommended but no clinical experience

Rifampin

The preferred antiretroviral combination in a patient receiving rifampin is efavirenz (an NNRTI) and two nucleoside reverse transcriptase inhibitors. Although rifampin decreases the serum concentration of efavirenz by 20% in patients receiving rifampin, most studies suggest that efavirenz doses do not need to be increased with rifampin coadministration or adjusted based on patient weight (36). Efavirenz has appeared to be superior to nevirapine virologically in several studies, particularly when ART is started after rifampin-containing tuberculosis treatment (16, 70, 117). When efavirenz cannot be used (because of pregnancy, intolerance, and HIV-2 resistance), the alternative is to use a combination of rifampin-based antituberculosis therapy with nevirapine. Although rifampin reduces the serum concentration of nevirapine and increased doses of nevirapine increase the toxicity, the recommendation is to use nevirapine at standard doses (7, 33, 70). Similarly, there is concern that nevirapine levels may be inadequate during the recommended lead-in

phase of nevirapine (200 mg daily rather than twice a day) when rifampin is already being coadministered (7, 117), but starting with 200 mg twice daily despite rifampin coadministration may be associated with more nevirapine hypersensitivity. Optimal dosing of nevirapine with rifampin coadministration is under active investigation.

The use of non-ritonavir-boosted protease inhibitors is contraindicated in patients receiving rifampin, as this drug decreases the serum concentration of most of the protease inhibitors by more than 90% (18, 20). The use of 100 to 200 mg of ritonavir (boosted regimens) also results in inadequate protease inhibitor concentrations and therefore should not be used. More recently, "super-boosted protease inhibitors" (400 mg of ritonavir twice a day) or double doses (800 mg of lopinavir and 200 of mg ritonavir twice daily) have been shown to overcome the effect of rifampin on the serum concentration of the protease inhibitors in healthy volunteers, but it is associated with high rates of hepatotoxicity and gastrointestinal toxicity. Therefore, this combination should be used only in settings where close monitoring is possible.

The use of regimens with only nucleosides cannot be recommended as preferred therapy, but it is an acceptable alternative in patients in whom NNRTIs cannot be used (33). There are limited data for other HIV agents. The integrase inhibitor raltegravir may need to be increased to 800 mg twice daily when administered with rifampin (129); however, standard dosing of raltegravir (400 mg twice daily) with rifampin is under active investigation. The CCR5 antagonist maraviroc should be increased to 600 mg twice daily when coadministered with rifampin. However, insufficient clinical data exist to determine the efficacy of maraviroc, raltegravir, and etravirine when given in conjunction with rifampin (33).

Rifabutin

Although rifabutin has less effect on the cytochrome P450 system, it is more expensive than rifampin and has complex interactions with antiretrovirals. Rifabutin-based antituberculosis therapy with protease-inhibitor-based ART is the preferred therapy in patients unable to take NNRTI-based ART. Protease inhibitors increase the serum concentration and toxicity of rifabutin; therefore, the rifabutin dose should be decreased for coadministration with ritonavir-boosted protease inhibitors. However, there are concerns that this dosage may be associated with the development of acquired rifamycin resistance (15, 63), and monitoring of rifabutin levels (if available) is a consideration to ensure adequate levels. The adherence of the protease inhibitor should be assessed together with the antituberculosis drugs because, if the protease inhibitor is suspended, the normal dose of rifabutin should be used, otherwise the dose of rifabutin will be suboptimal (33).

There is not enough clinical experience on the treatment of tuberculosis and HIV in pregnant women, in children, and those with MDR tuberculosis. The possible treatment alternatives are described in the guidelines published by CDC (33).

Drug Side Effects

The treatment of both tuberculosis and HIV infection will require, on average, seven drugs. Therefore, it is not surprising to observe a high frequency of adverse drug reactions. In a study of 188 patients, 45% started ART while on tuberculosis treatment. Adverse reactions occurred in 54% of these patients, and one-third changed or interrupted their treatment. The most frequent side effects were peripheral neuropathy (21%), rash (17%), and gastrointestinal upset (10%). Most of the side effects occurred during the first 2 months (39). Compared with patients without HIV infection, hepatitis due to antituberculosis

drugs is 4-fold more frequent in patients with HIV and 14-fold more frequent in patients infected with HIV and hepatitis C virus (125). Therefore, patients infected with HIV and receiving treatment for LTBI or tuberculosis should have a baseline laboratory evaluation of the hepatic function (if receiving isoniazid) and blood count, including platelets (if receiving rifampin or rifabutin). Patients should be monitored at least monthly (66). In patients with adverse events, determining the responsible agent can be difficult and the management of the patient can be complicated. Therefore, consultation with a specialist in treating HIV and tuberculosis is recommended, particularly for complex cases (66).

Tuberculosis-Associated IRIS

IRIS is a complication observed in the early phases of ART, as the result of the recovery of the immune response to previously recognized MTB antigens, and is reviewed extensively elsewhere is this book. Briefly, there are two main syndromes (83). The first syndrome is the paradoxical tuberculosis-associated IRIS, which usually occurs within 3 months of initiation, reinitiation, or regimen change of the ART in patients receiving tuberculosis treatment. The syndrome is characterized by the clinical deterioration of the preexisting tuberculosis, with new or worsening of symptoms or signs, including worsening of the radiological manifestations. The risk factors for the development of this syndrome include advanced HIV disease, disseminated and extrapulmonary tuberculosis, and a shorter delay between the start of tuberculosis treatment and ART. Paradoxical IRIS is a diagnosis of exclusion. A new infectious or malignant condition, poor adherence to tuberculosis treatment, or the presence of drug-resistant tuberculosis must be excluded before the diagnosis of paradoxical IRIS can be made. There are currently no reliable diagnostic tests for this condition. The treatment of mild cases includes the continuation of ART and symptomatic treatment. Moderate to severe IRIS may require corticosteroids (1 mg/kg of body weight) for several weeks with a gradual reduction (66). Interruption of ART is only recommended if severe or life-threatening manifestations of IRIS are present, such as a space-occupying intracranial lesion.

The second syndrome is the ART-associated tuberculosis in which tuberculosis is diagnosed (or "unmasked") during ART, with the restoration of previously acquired tuberculosis antigen-specific functional immune responses (80, 83). Initiation of tuberculosis therapy is the main treatment for unmasking IRIS, with use of anti-inflammatory agents and corticosteroids as needed. Detailed information can be found elsewhere in this book.

PREVENTION

There are several interventions that can reduce the frequency of tuberculosis among patients infected with HIV. (i) The use of antiretroviral drugs for the treatment of HIV infection has reduced the incidence and recurrence of tuberculosis (53, 87, 89). However, the rates of tuberculosis remain 5- to 10-fold higher than in patients without HIV infection, in spite of ART for 3 years (74). (ii) The use of isoniazid preventive therapy has an additive effect when used together with ART (53). Unfortunately, isoniazid preventive therapy is used by just 5% of patients with HIV in the world, most of them in developed countries (135). (iii) Infection control measures can be used to decrease transmission of MTB in health care facilities, such as increasing ventilation and informing patients infected with HIV about the settings where MTB can be transmitted (66). (iv) Case finding for active tuberculosis can be intensified, so patients can be adequately treated and, therefore, sources of infections can be decreased. The last three activities are part of the strategy known as "the three I's," isoniazid preventive treatment, intensified case finding for active tuberculosis, and tuberculosis infection control, which were recently implemented by WHO to decrease the impact of tuberculosis on people living with HIV and for a better integration of tuberculosis and HIV care and treatment (130).

The current recommendation is not to use *Mycobacterium bovis* BCG vaccination in patients infected with HIV (8, 57). This is based on the results of a recent study in South Africa, where approximately 992 per 100,000 BCG-vaccinated HIV-infected children developed disseminated BCG disease (58). This is extremely higher than the 5 per million estimated in the general population (78). Also, it was demonstrated that the CD4$^+$ and CD8$^+$ T-cell response to BCG of children infected with HIV was severely impaired, providing little or no benefit (81).

FINAL REMARKS

It is remarkable how difficult it has been to control the epidemic of tuberculosis, a curable disease. HIV is the most important factor contributing to the increase of cases of tuberculosis, but tuberculosis is both preventable and treatable even in persons with HIV infection. We need to accelerate the development of new diagnostic tools, new antituberculosis drugs, and a new effective vaccine. Currently, there are new diagnostic methods, but none of them are point-of-care diagnostic tests (55). For the first time

in decades, there are several promising drugs, such as moxifloxacin, which may reduce the duration of treatment (37); rifalazil (12), which has less interaction with antiretroviral drugs; and TMC-207, an antimycobacterial drug from the diarylquinoline class with a novel anti-ATPase mechanism of action (40). However, we are still far from having drugs that can cure tuberculosis in weeks and not in months. Multiple candidate vaccines have shown promising results in preclinical studies and are now being tested in clinical trials (72). However, until new tools are available, the current strategies to treat and control tuberculosis and HIV should be used and used more efficiently, including improved efforts to integrate HIV and tuberculosis care.

REFERENCES

1. **Abdool Karim, S. S., K. Naidoo, A. Grobler, N. Padayatchi, C. Baxter, A. Gray, T. Gengiah, G. Nair, S. Bamber, A. Singh, M. Khan, J. Pienaar, W. El-Sadr, G. Friedland, and Q. Abdool Karim.** 2010. Timing of initiation of antiretroviral drugs during tuberculosis therapy. *N. Engl. J. Med.* **362:**697–706.

2. **Akolo, C., I. Adetifa, S. Shepperd, and J. Volmink.** 2010. Treatment of latent tuberculosis infection in HIV infected persons. *Cochrane Database Syst. Rev.* **2010:**CD000171.

3. **Alland, D., G. E. Kalkut, A. R. Moss, R. A. McAdam, J. A. Hahn, W. Bosworth, E. Drucker, and B. R. Bloom.** 1994. Transmission of tuberculosis in New York City. An analysis by DNA fingerprinting and conventional epidemiologic methods. *N. Engl. J. Med.* **330:**1710–1716.

4. **Alpert, P. L., S. S. Munsiff, M. N. Gourevitch, B. Greenberg, and R. S. Klein.** 1997. A prospective study of tuberculosis and human immunodeficiency virus infection: clinical manifestations and factors associated with survival. *Clin. Infect. Dis.* **24:**661–668.

5. **American Thoracic Society.** 2000. Targeted tuberculin testing and treatment of latent tuberculosis infection. This official statement of the American Thoracic Society was adopted by the ATS Board of Directors, July 1999. This is a Joint Statement of the American Thoracic Society (ATS) and the Centers for Disease Control and Prevention (CDC). This statement was endorsed by the Council of the Infectious Diseases Society of America. (IDSA), September 1999, and the sections of this statement. *Am. J. Respir. Crit. Care Med.* **161:**S221–S247.

6. **Andrews, J. R., N. R. Gandhi, P. Moodley, N. S. Shah, L. Bohlken, A. P. Moll, M. Pillay, G. Friedland, and A. W. Sturm.** 2008. Exogenous reinfection as a cause of multidrug-resistant and extensively drug-resistant tuberculosis in rural South Africa. *J. Infect. Dis.* **198:**1582–1589.

7. **Avihingsanon, A., W. Manosuthi, P. Kantipong, C. Chuchotaworn, S. Moolphate, W. Sakornjun, M. Gorowara, N. Yamada, H. Yanai, S. Mitarai, N. Ishikawa, D. A. Cooper, P. Phanuphak, D. Burger, and K. Ruxrungtham.** 2008. Pharmacokinetics and 48-week efficacy of nevirapine: 400 mg versus 600 mg per day in HIV-tuberculosis coinfection receiving rifampicin. *Antivir. Ther.* **13:**529–536.

8. **Bannister, C., L. Bennett, A. Carville, and P. Azzopardi.** 2009. Evidence behind the WHO guidelines: hospital care for children: what is the evidence that BCG vaccination should not be used in HIV-infected children? *J. Trop. Pediatr.* **55:**78–82.

9. **Barber, T. W., D. E. Craven, and W. R. McCabe.** 1990. Bacteremia due to *Mycobacterium tuberculosis* in patients with human immunodeficiency virus infection. A report of 9 cases and a review of the literature. *Medicine* (Baltimore) **69:**375–383.

10. **Barnes, P. F.** 1993. Role of fiberoptic bronchoscopy in diagnosis of pulmonary tuberculosis in patients at risk for AIDS. *Chest* **103:**1923–1924.

11. **Benson, C. A., J. E. Kaplan, H. Masur, A. Pau, and K. K. Holmes.** 2004. Treating opportunistic infections among HIV-infected adults and adolescents: recommendations from CDC, the National Institutes of Health, and the HIV Medicine Association/Infectious Diseases Society of America. *MMWR Recommend. Rep.* **53:**1–112.

12. **Biava, M., G. C. Porretta, D. Deidda, and R. Pompei.** 2006. New trends in development of antimycobacterial compounds. *Infect. Disord. Drug Targets* **6:**159–172.

12a.**Blanc, F. X., T. Sok, D. Laureillard, L. Borand, C. Rekacewicz, E. Nerrienet, Y. Madec, O. Marcy, S. Chan, N. Prak, C. Kim, K. K. Lak, C. Hak, B. Dim, C. I. Sin, S. Sun, B. Guillard, B. Sar, S. Vong, M. Fernandez, L. Fox, J. F. Delfraissy, and A. E. Goldfeld.** 2010. Significant enhancement in survival with early (2 weeks) vs. late (8 weeks) initiation of highly active antiretroviral treatment (HAART) in severely immunosuppressed HIV-infected adults with newly diagnosed tuberculosis, abstr. THLBB106. Presented at the International AIDS Conference, Vienna, Austria.

13. **Blumberg, H. M., W. J. Burman, R. E. Chaisson, C. L. Daley, S. C. Etkind, L. N. Friedman, P. Fujiwara, M. Grzemska, P. C. Hopewell, M. D. Iseman, R. M. Jasmer, V. Koppaka, R. I. Menzies, R. J. O'Brien, R. R. Reves, L. B. Reichman, P. M. Simone, J. R. Starke, and A. A. Vernon.** 2003. American Thoracic Society/Centers for Disease Control and Prevention/Infectious Diseases Society of America: treatment of tuberculosis. *Am. J. Respir. Crit. Care Med.* **167:**603–662.

13a.**Boehme, C. C., P. Nabeta, D. Hillemann, M. P. Nicol, S. Shenai, F. Krapp, J. Allen, R. Tahirli, R. Blakemore, R. Rustomjee, A. Milovic, M. Jones, S. M. O'Brien, D. H. Persing, S. Ruesch-Gerdes, E. Gotuzzo, C. Rodrigues, D. Alland, and M. D. Perkins.** 2010. Rapid molecular detection of tuberculosis and rifampin resistance. *N. Engl. J. Med.* **363:**1005–1015.

14. **Bocchino, M., D. Galati, A. Sanduzzi, V. Colizzi, E. Brunetti, and G. Mancino.** 2005. Role of mycobacteria-induced monocyte/macrophage apoptosis in the pathogenesis of human tuberculosis. *Int. J. Tuberc. Lung Dis.* **9:**375–383.

15. **Boulanger, C., E. Hollender, K. Farrell, J. J. Stambaugh, D. Maasen, D. Ashkin, S. Symes, L. A. Espinoza, R. O. Rivero, J. J. Graham, and C. A. Peloquin.** 2009. Pharmacokinetic evaluation of rifabutin in combination with lopinavir-ritonavir in patients with HIV infection and active tuberculosis. *Clin. Infect. Dis.* **49:**1305–1311.

16. **Boulle, A., G. Van Cutsem, K. Cohen, K. Hilderbrand, S. Mathee, M. Abrahams, E. Goemaere, D. Coetzee, and G. Maartens.** 2008. Outcomes of nevirapine- and efavirenz-based antiretroviral therapy when coadministered with rifampicin-based antitubercular therapy. *JAMA* **300:**530–539.

17. **Branson, B. M., H. H. Handsfield, M. A. Lampe, R. S. Janssen, A. W. Taylor, S. B. Lyss, and J. E. Clark.** 2006. Revised recommendations for HIV testing of adults, adolescents, and pregnant women in health-care settings. *MMWR Recommend. Rep.* **55:**1–17.

18. **Burger, D. M., S. Agarwala, M. Child, A. Been-Tiktak, Y. Wang, and R. Bertz.** 2006. Effect of rifampin on steady-state pharmacokinetics of atazanavir with ritonavir in healthy volunteers. *Antimicrob. Agents Chemother.* **50:**3336–3342.

18a.**Burman, W. J.** 2010. Rip Van Winkle wakes up: development of tuberculosis treatment in the 21st century. *Clin. Infect. Dis.* **50**(Suppl. 3):S165–S172.

19. **Burman, W., D. Benator, A. Vernon, A. Khan, B. Jones, C. Silva, C. Lahart, S. Weis, B. King, B. Mangura, M. Weiner, and W. El-Sadr.** 2006. Acquired rifamycin resistance with twice-weekly treatment of HIV-related tuberculosis. *Am. J. Respir. Crit. Care Med.* **173:**350–356.

20. **Burman, W. J., K. Gallicano, and C. Peloquin.** 1999. Therapeutic implications of drug interactions in the treatment of human immunodeficiency virus-related tuberculosis. *Clin. Infect. Dis.* **28:**419–430.

21. **Burman, W. J., and B. E. Jones.** 2001. Treatment of HIV-related tuberculosis in the era of effective antiretroviral therapy. *Am. J. Respir. Crit. Care Med.* **164:**7–12.

22. **Burman, W. J., and B. E. Jones.** 2003. Clinical and radiographic features of HIV-related tuberculosis. *Semin. Respir. Infect.* **18:**263–271.

23. **Campsmith, M. L., P. H. Rhodes, H. I. Hall, and T. A. Green.** 2010. Undiagnosed HIV prevalence among adults and adolescents in the United States at the end of 2006. *J. Acquir. Immune Defic. Syndr.* **53:**619–624.

24. **Canaday, D. H., M. Wu, S. Lu, H. Aung, P. Peters, J. Baseke, W. Mackay, H. Mayanja-Kizza, and Z. Toossi.** 2009. Induction of HIV type 1 expression correlates with T cell responsiveness to mycobacteria in patients coinfected with HIV type 1 and *Mycobacterium tuberculosis*. *AIDS Res. Hum. Retrovir.* **25:**213–216.

25. **Casado, J. L., S. Moreno, J. Fortun, A. Antela, C. Quereda, E. Navas, A. Moreno, and F. Dronda.** 2002. Risk factors for development of tuberculosis after isoniazid chemoprophylaxis in human immunodeficiency virus-infected patients. *Clin. Infect. Dis.* **34:**386–389.

26. **Cattamanchi, A., J. L. Davis, W. Worodria, S. den Boon, S. Yoo, J. Matovu, J. Kiidha, F. Nankya, R. Kyeyune, P. Byanyima, A. Andama, M. Joloba, D. H. Osmond, P. C. Hopewell, and L. Huang.** 2009. Sensitivity and specificity of fluorescence microscopy for diagnosing pulmonary tuberculosis in a high HIV prevalence setting. *Int. J. Tuberc. Lung Dis.* **13:**1130–1136.

26a.**Cattamanchi, A., R. Smith, K. R. Steingart, J. Z. Metcalfe, A. Date, C. Coleman, B. J. Marston, L. Huang, P. C. Hopewell, and M. Pai.** 2010. Interferon-gamma release assays for the diagnosis of latent tuberculosis infection in HIV-infected individuals: a systematic review and meta-analysis. *J. Acquir. Immune Defic. Syndr.* **56:**230–238.

27. **Centers for Disease Control and Prevention.** 2010. Decrease in reported tuberculosis cases—United States, 2009. *MMWR Morb. Mortal. Wkly. Rep.* **59:**289–294.

28. **Centers for Disease Control and Prevention.** 1997. Anergy skin testing and tuberculosis [corrected] preventive therapy for HIV-infected persons: revised recommendations. *MMWR Recommend. Rep.* **46:**1–10.

29. **Centers for Disease Control and Prevention.** 2000. Targeted tuberculin testing and treatment of latent tuberculosis infection. American Thoracic Society. *MMWR Recommend. Rep.* **49:**1–51.

30. **Centers for Disease Control and Prevention.** 2003. Update: adverse event data and revised American Thoracic Society/CDC recommendations against the use of rifampin and pyrazinamide for treatment of latent tuberculosis infection—United States, 2003. *MMWR Morb. Mortal. Wkly. Rep.* **52:**735–739.

31. **Centers for Disease Control and Prevention.** 2009. Trends in tuberculosis—United States, 2008. *MMWR Morb. Mortal. Wkly. Rep.* **58:**249–253.

32. Centers for Disease Control and Prevention. 2009. Updated guidelines for the use of nucleic acid amplification tests in the diagnosis of tuberculosis. *MMWR Morb. Mortal. Wkly. Rep.* **58:**7–10.

33. Centers for Disease Control and Prevention. 2007. *Managing Drug Interactions in the Treatment of HIV-Related Tuberculosis.* Centers for Disease Control and Prevention, Atlanta, GA.

34. Centers for Disease Control and Prevention. 2010. Diagnoses of HIV infection and AIDS in the United States and dependent areas, 2009. HIV Surveillance Report, vol. 21. Centers for Disease Control and Prevention, Atlanta, GA.

35. Chamie, G., A. Luetkemeyer, M. Walusimbi-Nanteza, A. Okwera, C. C. Whalen, R. D. Mugerwa, D. V. Havlir, and E. D. Charlebois. 2010. Significant variation in presentation of pulmonary tuberculosis across a high resolution of CD4 strata. *Int. J. Tuberc. Lung Dis.* **14:**1295–1302.

35a. Charalambous, S., A. D. Grant, C. Innes, C. J. Hoffmann, R. Dowdeswell, J. Pienaar, K. L. Fielding, and G. J. Churchyard. 2010. Association of isoniazid preventive therapy with lower early mortality in individuals on antiretroviral therapy in a workplace programme. *AIDS* **24**(Suppl 5):S5–13.

36. Cohen, K., A. Grant, C. Dandara, H. McIlleron, L. Pemba, K. Fielding, S. Charalombous, G. Churchyard, P. Smith, and G. Maartens. 2009. Effect of rifampicin-based antitubercular therapy and the cytochrome P450 2B6 516G>T polymorphism on efavirenz concentrations in adults in South Africa. *Antivir. Ther.* **14:**687–695.

37. Conde, M. B., A. Efron, C. Loredo, G. R. De Souza, N. P. Graca, M. C. Cezar, M. Ram, M. A. Chaudhary, W. R. Bishai, A. L. Kritski, and R. E. Chaisson. 2009. Moxifloxacin versus ethambutol in the initial treatment of tuberculosis: a double-blind, randomised, controlled phase II trial. *Lancet* **373:**1183–1189.

38. Daley, C. L., P. M. Small, G. F. Schecter, G. K. Schoolnik, R. A. McAdam, W. R. Jacobs, Jr., and P. C. Hopewell. 1992. An outbreak of tuberculosis with accelerated progression among persons infected with the human immunodeficiency virus. An analysis using restriction-fragment-length polymorphisms. *N. Engl. J. Med.* **326:**231–235.

39. Dean, G. L., S. G. Edwards, N. J. Ives, G. Matthews, E. F. Fox, L. Navaratne, M. Fisher, G. P. Taylor, R. Miller, C. B. Taylor, A. de Ruiter, and A. L. Pozniak. 2002. Treatment of tuberculosis in HIV-infected persons in the era of highly active antiretroviral therapy. *AIDS* **16:**75–83.

40. Diacon, A. H., A. Pym, M. Grobusch, R. Patientia, R. Rustomjee, L. Page-Shipp, C. Pistorius, R. Krause, M. Bogoshi, G. Churchyard, A. Venter, J. Allen, J. C. Palomino, T. De Marez, R. P. van Heeswijk, N. Lounis, P. Meyvisch, J. Verbeeck, W. Parys, K. de Beule, K. Andries, and D. F. Mc Neeley. 2009. The diarylquinoline TMC207 for multidrug-resistant tuberculosis. *N. Engl. J. Med.* **360:**2397–2405.

41. Di Perri, G., M. Cruciani, M. C. Danzi, R. Luzzati, G. De Checchi, M. Malena, S. Pizzighella, R. Mazzi, M. Solbiati, E. Concia, et al. 1989. Nosocomial epidemic of active tuberculosis among HIV-infected patients. *Lancet* **ii:**1502–1504.

42. Dubrovina, I., K. Miskinis, S. Lyepshina, Y. Yann, H. Hoffmann, R. Zaleskis, P. Nunn, and M. Zignol. 2008. Drug-resistant tuberculosis and HIV in Ukraine: a threatening convergence of two epidemics? *Int. J. Tuberc. Lung Dis.* **12:**756–762.

43. Elliott, A. M., K. Namaambo, B. W. Allen, N. Luo, R. J. Hayes, J. O. Pobee, and K. P. McAdam. 1993. Negative sputum smear results in HIV-positive patients with pulmonary tuberculosis in Lusaka, Zambia. *Tuber. Lung Dis.* **74:**191–194.

44. Eng, B., K. P. Cain, K. Nong, V. Chhum, E. Sin, S. Roeun, S. Kim, S. Keo, T. A. Heller, and J. K. Varma. 2009. Impact of a public antiretroviral program on TB/HIV mortality: Banteay Meanchey, Cambodia. *Southeast Asian J. Trop. Med. Public Health* **40:**89–92.

45. Escombe, A. R., D. A. Moore, R. H. Gilman, W. Pan, M. Navincopa, E. Ticona, C. Martinez, L. Caviedes, P. Sheen, A. Gonzalez, C. J. Noakes, J. S. Friedland, and C. A. Evans. 2008. The infectiousness of tuberculosis patients coinfected with HIV. *PLoS Med.* **5:**e188.

46. Fee, M. J., M. M. Oo, A. E. Gabayan, D. R. Radin and P. F. Barnes. 1995. Abdominal tuberculosis in patients infected with the human immunodeficiency virus. *Clin. Infect. Dis.* **20:**938–944.

47. Fitzgerald, D., et al. 2009. Early versus delayed ART: results from Haiti, abstract WESY201. Presented at the Fifth IAS Conference on HIV Pathogenesis, Treatment, and Prevention.

48. Gandhi, N. R., A. Moll, A. W. Sturm, R. Pawinski, T. Govender, U. Lalloo, K. Zeller, J. Andrews, and G. Friedland. 2006. Extensively drug-resistant tuberculosis as a cause of death in patients co-infected with tuberculosis and HIV in a rural area of South Africa. *Lancet* **368:**1575–1580.

49. Gandhi, N. R., N. S. Shah, J. R. Andrews, V. Vella, A. P. Moll, M. Scott, D. Weissman, C. Marra, U. G. Lalloo, and G. H. Friedland. 2010. HIV coinfection in multidrug- and extensively drug-resistant tuberculosis results in high early mortality. *Am. J. Respir. Crit. Care Med.* **181:**80–86.

50. Glynn, J. R., J. Murray, A. Bester, G. Nelson, S. Shearer, and P. Sonnenberg. 2008. Effects of duration of HIV infection and secondary tuberculosis transmission on tuberculosis incidence in the South African gold mines. *AIDS* **22:**1859–1867.

51. Goletti, D., S. Carrara, D. Vincenti, E. Giacomini, L. Fattorini, A. R. Garbuglia, M. R. Capobianchi, T. Alonzi, G. M. Fimia, M. Federico, G. Poli, and E. Coccia. 2004. Inhibition of HIV-1 replication in monocyte-derived macrophages by *Mycobacterium tuberculosis*. *J. Infect. Dis.* **189:**624–633.

52. Goletti, D., D. Weissman, R. W. Jackson, N. M. Graham, D. Vlahov, R. S. Klein, S. S. Munsiff, L. Ortona, R. Cauda, and A. S. Fauci. 1996. Effect of *Mycobacterium tuberculosis* on HIV replication. Role of immune activation. *J. Immunol.* **157:**1271–1278.

53. Golub, J. E., V. Saraceni, S. C. Cavalcante, A. G. Pacheco, L. H. Moulton, B. S. King, A. Efron, R. D. Moore, R. E. Chaisson, and B. Durovni. 2007. The impact of antiretroviral therapy and isoniazid preventive therapy on tuberculosis incidence in HIV-infected patients in Rio de Janeiro, Brazil. *AIDS* **21:**1441–1448.

54. Gopi, A., S. M. Madhavan, S. K. Sharma, and S. A. Sahn. 2007. Diagnosis and treatment of tuberculous pleural effusion in 2006. *Chest* **131:**880–889.

55. Grandjean, L., and D. A. Moore. 2008. Tuberculosis in the developing world: recent advances in diagnosis with special consideration of extensively drug-resistant tuberculosis. *Curr. Opin. Infect. Dis.* **21:**454–461.

56. Gray, D. M., H. Zar, and M. Cotton. 2009. Impact of tuberculosis preventive therapy on tuberculosis and mortality in HIV-infected children. *Cochrane Database Syst. Rev.* **2009:**CD006418

56a. Havlir, D., P. Ive, M. Kendall, et al. 2011. International Randomized Trail of Immediate vs. Early ART in HIV+ patients treated for TB: ACTG 5221 STRIDE study, abstr. #38. Presented at the 18th Conference on Retroviruses and Opportunistic Infections, Boston, MA.

57. Hesseling, A. C., M. F. Cotton, C. Fordham von Reyn, S. M. Graham, R. P. Gie, and G. D. Hussey. 2008. Consensus state-

ment on the revised World Health Organization recommendations for BCG vaccination in HIV-infected infants. *Int. J. Tuberc. Lung Dis.* **12:**1376–1379.

58. **Hesseling, A. C., L. F. Johnson, H. Jaspan, M. F. Cotton, A. Whitelaw, H. S. Schaaf, P. E. Fine, B. S. Eley, B. J. Marais, J. Nuttall, N. Beyers, and P. Godfrey-Faussett.** 2009. Disseminated bacille Calmette-Guerin disease in HIV-infected South African infants. *Bull. W. H. O.* **87:**505–511.

59. **Hesseling, A. C., A. E. Westra, H. Werschkull, P. R. Donald, N. Beyers, G. D. Hussey, W. El-Sadr, and H. S. Schaaf.** 2005. Outcome of HIV infected children with culture confirmed tuberculosis. *Arch. Dis. Child.* **90:**1171–1174.

60. **Hopewell, P. C., M. Pai, D. Maher, M. Uplekar, and M. C. Raviglione.** 2006. International standards for tuberculosis care. *Lancet Infect. Dis.* **6:**710–725.

61. **Iademarco, M. F., and K. G. Castro.** 2003. Epidemiology of tuberculosis. *Semin. Respir. Infect.* **18:**225–240.

62. Reference deleted.

63. **Jenny-Avital, E. R., and K. Joseph.** 2009. Rifamycin-resistant *Mycobacterium tuberculosis* in the highly active antiretroviral therapy era: a report of 3 relapses with acquired rifampin resistance following alternate-day rifabutin and boosted protease inhibitor therapy. *Clin. Infect. Dis.* **48:**1471–1474.

64. **Johnson, J. L., M. J. Vjecha, A. Okwera, E. Hatanga, F. Byekwaso, K. Wolski, T. Aisu, C. C. Whalen, R. Huebner, R. D. Mugerwa, and J. J. Ellner.** 1998. Impact of human immunodeficiency virus type-1 infection on the initial bacteriologic and radiographic manifestations of pulmonary tuberculosis in Uganda. Makerere University-Case Western Reserve University Research Collaboration. *Int. J. Tuberc. Lung Dis.* **2:**397–404.

65. **Jones, B. E., S. M. Young, D. Antoniskis, P. T. Davidson, F. Kramer, and P. F. Barnes.** 1993. Relationship of the manifestations of tuberculosis to CD4 cell counts in patients with human immunodeficiency virus infection. *Am. Rev. Respir. Dis.* **148:**1292–1297.

66. **Kaplan, J. E., C. Benson, K. H. Holmes, J. T. Brooks, A. Pau, and H. Masur.** 2009. Guidelines for prevention and treatment of opportunistic infections in HIV-infected adults and adolescents: recommendations from CDC, the National Institutes of Health, and the HIV Medicine Association of the Infectious Diseases Society of America. *MMWR Recommend. Rep.* **58:**1–207.

67. **Karam, F., F. Mbow, H. Fletcher, C. S. Senghor, K. D. Coulibaly, A. M. LeFevre, N. F. Ngom Gueye, T. Dieye, P. S. Sow, S. Mboup, and C. Lienhardt.** 2008. Sensitivity of IFN-gamma release assay to detect latent tuberculosis infection is retained in HIV-infected patients but dependent on HIV/AIDS progression. *PLoS One* **3:**e1441.

68. **Khan, F. A., J. Minion, M. Pai, S. Royce, W. Burman, A. D. Harries, and D. Menzies.** 2010. Treatment of active tuberculosis in HIV co-infected patients: a systematic review and meta-analysis. *Clin. Infect. Dis.* **50:**1288–1299.

69. **Kivihya-Ndugga, L., M. van Cleeff, E. Juma, J. Kimwomi, W. Githui, L. Oskam, A. Schuitema, D. van Soolingen, L. Nganga, D. Kibuga, J. Odhiambo, and P. Klatser.** 2004. Comparison of PCR with the routine procedure for diagnosis of tuberculosis in a population with high prevalences of tuberculosis and human immunodeficiency virus. *J. Clin. Microbiol.* **42:**1012–1015.

70. **Kwara, A., G. Ramachandran, and S. Swaminathan.** 2010. Dose adjustment of the non-nucleoside reverse transcriptase inhibitors during concurrent rifampicin-containing tuberculosis therapy: one size does not fit all. *Expert Opin. Drug Metab. Toxicol.* **6:**55–68.

71. **Lalvani, A., and M. Pareek.** 2010. Interferon gamma release assays: principles and practice. *Enferm. Infecc. Microbiol. Clin.* **28:**245–252.

72. **Lambert, P. H., T. Hawkridge, and W. A. Hanekom.** 2009. New vaccines against tuberculosis. *Clin. Chest Med.* **30:**811–826.

73. **Lawn, S. D., L. G. Bekker, and R. Wood.** 2005. How effectively does HAART restore immune responses to *Mycobacterium tuberculosis*? Implications for tuberculosis control. *AIDS* **19:**1113–1124.

74. **Lawn, S. D., L. Myer, L. G. Bekker, and R. Wood.** 2006. Burden of tuberculosis in an antiretroviral treatment programme in sub-Saharan Africa: impact on treatment outcomes and implications for tuberculosis control. *AIDS* **20:**1605–1612.

75. **Leidl, L., H. Mayanja-Kizza, G. Sotgiu, J. Baseke, M. Ernst, C. Hirsch, D. Goletti, Z. Toossi, and C. Lange.** 2010. Relationship of immunodiagnostic assays for tuberculosis and numbers of circulating CD4+ T-cells in HIV-infection. *Eur. Respir. J.* **35:**619–626.

76. **Lopez-Gatell, H., S. R. Cole, N. A. Hessol, A. L. French, R. M. Greenblatt, S. Landesman, S. Preston-Martin, and K. Anastos.** 2007. Effect of tuberculosis on the survival of women infected with human immunodeficiency virus. *Am. J. Epidemiol.* **165:**1134–1142.

77. **Lopez-Gatell, H., S. R. Cole, J. B. Margolick, M. D. Witt, J. Martinson, J. P. Phair, and L. P. Jacobson.** 2008. Effect of tuberculosis on the survival of HIV-infected men in a country with low tuberculosis incidence. *AIDS* **22:**1869–1873.

78. **Lotte, A., O. Wasz-Hockert, N. Poisson, H. Engbaek, H. Landmann, U. Quast, B. Andrasofszky, L. Lugosi, I. Vadasz, P. Mihailescu, et al.** 1988. Second IUATLD study on complications induced by intradermal BCG-vaccination. *Bull. Int. Union Tuberc. Lung Dis.* **63:**47–59.

79. **Luetkemeyer, A. F., E. D. Charlebois, L. L. Flores, D. R. Bangsberg, S. G. Deeks, J. N. Martin, and D. V. Havlir.** 2007. Comparison of an interferon-gamma release assay with tuberculin skin testing in HIV-infected individuals. *Am. J. Respir. Crit. Care Med.* **175:**737–742.

80. **Manabe, Y. C., R. Breen, T. Perti, E. Girardi, and T. R. Sterling.** 2009. Unmasked tuberculosis and tuberculosis immune reconstitution inflammatory disease: a disease spectrum after initiation of antiretroviral therapy. *J. Infect. Dis.* **199:**437–444.

81. **Mansoor, N., T. J. Scriba, M. de Kock, M. Tameris, B. Abel, A. Keyser, F. Little, A. Soares, S. Gelderbloem, S. Mlenjeni, L. Denation, A. Hawkridge, W. H. Boom, G. Kaplan, G. D. Hussey, and W. A. Hanekom.** 2009. HIV-1 infection in infants severely impairs the immune response induced by Bacille Calmette-Guerin vaccine. *J. Infect. Dis.* **199:**982–990.

82. **Mayanja-Kizza, H., M. Wu, H. Aung, S. Liu, H. Luzze, C. Hirsch, and Z. Toossi.** 2009. The interaction of monocyte chemoattractant protein-1 and tumour necrosis factor-alpha in *Mycobacterium tuberculosis*-induced HIV-1 replication at sites of active tuberculosis. *Scand. J. Immunol.* **69:**516–520.

82a. **Mazurek, G. H., J. Jereb, A. Vernon, P. LoBue, S. Goldberg, and K. Castro.** 2010. Updated guidelines for using interferon gamma release assays to detect *Mycobacterium tuberculosis* infection—United States. *MMWR Recomm. Rep.* **59:**1–25.

83. **Meintjes, G., S. D. Lawn, F. Scano, G. Maartens, M. A. French, W. Worodria, J. H. Elliott, D. Murdoch, R. J. Wilkinson, C. Seyler, L. John, M. S. van der Loeff, P. Reiss, L. Lynen, E. N. Janoff, C. Gilks, and R. Colebunders.** 2008. Tuberculosis-associated immune reconstitution inflammatory syndrome: case definitions for use in resource-limited settings. *Lancet Infect. Dis.* **8:**516–523.

84. Mendelson, M. 2007. Diagnosing tuberculosis in HIV-infected patients: challenges and future prospects. *Br. Med. Bull.* 81-82:149–165.

85. Mofenson, L. M., M. T. Brady, S. P. Danner, K. L. Dominguez, R. Hazra, E. Handelsman, P. Havens, S. Nesheim, J. S. Read, L. Serchuck, and R. Van Dyke. 2009. Guidelines for the prevention and treatment of opportunistic infections among HIV-exposed and HIV-infected children: recommendations from CDC, the National Institutes of Health, the HIV Medicine Association of the Infectious Diseases Society of America, the Pediatric Infectious Diseases Society, and the American Academy of Pediatrics. *MMWR Recommend. Rep.* 58:1–166.

86. Moore, D., C. Liechty, P. Ekwaru, W. Were, G. Mwima, P. Solberg, G. Rutherford, and J. Mermin. 2007. Prevalence, incidence and mortality associated with tuberculosis in HIV-infected patients initiating antiretroviral therapy in rural Uganda. *AIDS* 21:713–719.

87. Moreno, S., I. Jarrin, J. A. Iribarren, M. J. Perez-Elias, P. Viciana, J. Parra-Ruiz, J. L. Gomez-Sirvent, J. Lopez-Aldeguer, F. Gutierrez, J. R. Blanco, F. Vidal, M. Leal, M. A. Rodriguez Arenas, and J. Del Amo. 2008. Incidence and risk factors for tuberculosis in HIV-positive subjects by HAART status. *Int. J. Tuberc. Lung Dis.* 12:1393–1400.

88. Moss, A. R., J. A. Hahn, J. P. Tulsky, C. L. Daley, P. M. Small, and P. C. Hopewell. 2000. Tuberculosis in the homeless. A prospective study. *Am. J. Respir. Crit. Care Med.* 162:460–464.

89. Muga, R., I. Ferreros, K. Langohr, P. G. de Olalla, J. Del Romero, M. Quintana, I. Alastrue, J. Belda, J. Tor, S. Perez-Hoyos, and J. Del Amo. 2007. Changes in the incidence of tuberculosis in a cohort of HIV-seroconverters before and after the introduction of HAART. *AIDS* 21:2521–2527.

90. Nahid, P., L. C. Gonzalez, I. Rudoy, B. C. de Jong, A. Unger, L. M. Kawamura, D. H. Osmond, P. C. Hopewell, and C. L. Daley. 2007. Treatment outcomes of patients with HIV and tuberculosis. *Am. J. Respir. Crit. Care Med.* 175:1199–1206.

91. National Center for HIV STD and TB Prevention. 2003. Estimated numbers of diagnoses of HIV/AIDS, by year of diagnosis and selected characteristics of persons, 1999–2002—30 areas with confidential name-based HIV infection reporting, p. 10. *HIV/AIDS Surveillance Report*, vol. 14. National Center for HIV STD and TB Prevention, Atlanta, GA.

92. Okwera, A., J. L. Johnson, M. J. Vjecha, K. Wolski, C. C. Whalen, D. Hom, R. Huebner, R. D. Mugerwa, and J. J. Ellner. 1997. Risk factors for adverse drug reactions during thiacetazone treatment of pulmonary tuberculosis in human immunodeficiency virus infected adults. *Int. J. Tuberc. Lung Dis.* 1:441–445.

93. Panjabi, R., G. W. Comstock, and J. E. Golub. 2007. Recurrent tuberculosis and its risk factors: adequately treated patients are still at high risk. *Int. J. Tuberc. Lung Dis.* 11:828–837.

94. Patel, N. R., K. Swan, X. Li, S. D. Tachado, and H. Koziel. 2009. Impaired *M. tuberculosis*-mediated apoptosis in alveolar macrophages from HIV+ persons: potential role of IL-10 and BCL-3. *J. Leukoc. Biol.* 86:53–60.

95. Perlman, D. C., W. M. el-Sadr, E. T. Nelson, J. P. Matts, E. E. Telzak, N. Salomon, K. Chirgwin, R. Hafner, et al. 1997. Variation of chest radiographic patterns in pulmonary tuberculosis by degree of human immunodeficiency virus-related immunosuppression. The Terry Beirn Community Programs for Clinical Research on AIDS (CPCRA). *Clin. Infect. Dis.* 25:242–246.

96. Prasad, K., and M. B. Singh. 2008. Corticosteroids for managing tuberculous meningitis. *Cochrane Database Syst. Rev.* 2008:CD002244.

97. Raby, E., M. Moyo, A. Devendra, J. Banda, P. De Haas, H. Ayles, and P. Godfrey-Faussett. 2008. The effects of HIV on the sensitivity of a whole blood IFN-gamma release assay in Zambian adults with active tuberculosis. *PLoS One* 3:e2489.

98. Samandari, T., B. Mosimaneotsile, T. Agizew, S. Nyirenda, Z. Tedla, T. Sibanda, O. Motsamai, N. Shang, P. Kilmarx, and C. Wells. 2010. Randomized, placebo-controlled trial of 6 vs 36 months isoniazid TB preventive therapy for HIV-infected adults in Botswana, abstr. 104LB. *17th Conf. Retrovir. Oppor. Infect.*

99. Sanguanwongse, N., K. P. Cain, P. Suriya, S. Nateniyom, N. Yamada, W. Wattanaamornkiat, S. Sumnapan, W. Sattayawuthipong, S. Kaewsa-ard, S. Ingkaseth, and J. K. Varma. 2008. Antiretroviral therapy for HIV-infected tuberculosis patients saves lives but needs to be used more frequently in Thailand. *J. Acquir. Immune Defic. Syndr.* 48:181–189.

100. Schluger, N. W. 2003. The diagnosis of tuberculosis: what's old, what's new. *Semin. Respir. Infect.* 18:241–248.

101. Schluger, N. W., D. Perez, and Y. M. Liu. 2002. Reconstitution of immune responses to tuberculosis in patients with HIV infection who receive antiretroviral therapy. *Chest* 122:597–602.

102. Schluger, N. W., and W. N. Rom. 1998. The host immune response to tuberculosis. *Am. J. Respir. Crit. Care Med.* 157:679–691.

103. Schutte, C. M. 2001. Clinical, cerebrospinal fluid and pathological findings and outcomes in HIV-positive and HIV-negative patients with tuberculous meningitis. *Infection* 29:213–217.

104. Selwyn, P. A., D. Hartel, V. A. Lewis, E. E. Schoenbaum, S. H. Vermund, R. S. Klein, A. T. Walker, and G. H. Friedland. 1989. A prospective study of the risk of tuberculosis among intravenous drug users with human immunodeficiency virus infection. *N. Engl. J. Med.* 320:545–550.

105. Shah, N. S., R. Pratt, L. Armstrong, V. Robison, K. G. Castro, and J. P. Cegielski. 2008. Extensively drug-resistant tuberculosis in the United States, 1993-2007. *JAMA* 300:2153–2160.

106. Shenoi, S., S. Heysell, A. Moll, and G. Friedland. 2009. Multidrug-resistant and extensively drug-resistant tuberculosis: consequences for the global HIV community. *Curr. Opin. Infect. Dis.* 22:11–17.

107. Slovis, B. S., J. D. Plitman, and D. W. Haas. 2000. The case against anergy testing as a routine adjunct to tuberculin skin testing. *JAMA* 283:2003–2007.

108. Small, P. M., G. F. Schecter, P. C. Goodman, M. A. Sande, R. E. Chaisson, and P. C. Hopewell. 1991. Treatment of tuberculosis in patients with advanced human immunodeficiency virus infection. *N. Engl. J. Med.* 324:289–294.

109. Sonnenberg, P., J. R. Glynn, K. Fielding, J. Murray, P. Godfrey-Faussett, and S. Shearer. 2004. HIV and pulmonary tuberculosis: the impact goes beyond those infected with HIV. *AIDS* 18:657–662.

110. Srikantiah, P., J. K. Wong, T. Liegler, M. Walusimbi, H. Mayanja-Kizza, H. K. Kayanja, R. D. Mugerwa, E. D. Charlebois, W. H. Boom, C. C. Whalen, and D. V. Havlir. 2008. Unexpected low-level viremia among HIV-infected Ugandan adults with untreated active tuberculosis. *J. Acquir. Immune Defic. Syndr.* 49:458–460.

111. Stebbing, J., B. Gazzard, and D. C. Douek. 2004. Where does HIV live? *N. Engl. J. Med.* 350:1872–1880.

112. Steingart, K. R., M. Henry, V. Ng, P. C. Hopewell, A. Ramsay, J. Cunningham, R. Urbanczik, M. Perkins, M. A. Aziz, and M. Pai. 2006. Fluorescence versus conventional sputum

smear microscopy for tuberculosis: a systematic review. *Lancet Infect. Dis.* **6:**570–581.

113. Sterling, T. R., J. Bethel, S. Goldberg, P. Weinfurter, L. Yun, and C. R. Horsburgh. 2006. The scope and impact of treatment of latent tuberculosis infection in the United States and Canada. *Am. J. Respir. Crit. Care Med.* **173:**927–931.

114. Sunderam, G., R. J. McDonald, T. Maniatis, J. Oleske, R. Kapila, and L. B. Reichman. 1986. Tuberculosis as a manifestation of the acquired immunodeficiency syndrome (AIDS). *JAMA* **256:**362–366.

115. Sutherland, R., H. Yang, T. J. Scriba, B. Ondondo, N. Robinson, C. Conlon, A. Suttill, H. McShane, S. Fidler, A. McMichael, and L. Dorrell. 2006. Impaired IFN-gamma-secreting capacity in mycobacterial antigen-specific CD4 T cells during chronic HIV-1 infection despite long-term HAART. *AIDS* **20:**821–829.

116. Swaminathan, S., P. Menon, V. Perumal, R. K. Santhanakrishnan, R. Ramachandran, P. Chinnaiah, S. Iliayas, N. Gopalan, P. Chandrasekaran, and P. Narayanan. 2010. Efficacy of a 6-month vs a 36-month regimen for prevention of TB in HIV-infected persons in India: a randomized clinical trial, abstr. 103. *17th Conf. Retrovir. Oppor. Infect.*

117. Swaminathan, S., P. Venkatesan, et al. 2009. Once-daily nevirapine vs efavirenz in the treatment of HIV-infected patients with TB: a randomized clinical trial, abstr. 35. *16th Conf. Retrovir. Oppor. Infect.*

118. Syed Ahamed Kabeer, B., R. Sikhamani, S. Swaminathan, V. Perumal, P. Paramasivam, and A. Raja. 2009. Role of interferon gamma release assay in active TB diagnosis among HIV infected individuals. *PLoS One* **4:**e5718.

119. Talati, N. J., U. Seybold, B. Humphrey, A. Aina, J. Tapia, P. Weinfurter, R. Albalak, and H. M. Blumberg. 2009. Poor concordance between interferon-gamma release assays and tuberculin skin tests in diagnosis of latent tuberculosis infection among HIV-infected individuals. *BMC Infect. Dis.* **9:**15.

120. Tappero, J. W., W. Z. Bradford, T. B. Agerton, P. Hopewell, A. L. Reingold, S. Lockman, A. Oyewo, E. A. Talbot, T. A. Kenyon, T. L. Moeti, H. J. Moffat, and C. A. Peloquin. 2005. Serum concentrations of antimycobacterial drugs in patients with pulmonary tuberculosis in Botswana. *Clin. Infect. Dis.* **41:**461–469.

121. Thwaites, G. E., D. B. Nguyen, H. D. Nguyen, T. Q. Hoang, T. T. Do, T. C. Nguyen, Q. H. Nguyen, T. T. Nguyen, N. H. Nguyen, T. N. Nguyen, N. L. Nguyen, N. T. Vu, H. H. Cao, T. H. Tran, P. M. Pham, T. D. Nguyen, K. Stepniewska, N. J. White, and J. J. Farrar. 2004. Dexamethasone for the treatment of tuberculous meningitis in adolescents and adults. *N. Engl. J. Med.* **351:**1741–1751.

122. Toossi, Z. 2003. Virological and immunological impact of tuberculosis on human immunodeficiency virus type 1 disease. *J. Infect. Dis.* **188:**1146–1155.

123. Toossi, Z., H. Mayanja-Kizza, C. S. Hirsch, K. L. Edmonds, T. Spahlinger, D. L. Hom, H. Aung, P. Mugyenyi, J. J. Ellner, and C. W. Whalen. 2001. Impact of tuberculosis (TB) on HIV-1 activity in dually infected patients. *Clin. Exp. Immunol.* **123:**233–238.

123a.Torok, M. Y. N., T. Chau, N. Mai, N. Phu, P. Mai, and J. Farrar. 2009. Randomised controlled trial of immediate versus deferred antiretroviral therapy in HIV-associated tuberculosis meningitis, abstr. H-1224. Presented at the 49th Interscience Conference on Antimicrobial Agents and Chemotherapy, San Francisco, CA.

124. UNAIDS. 2010. *UNAIDS Report On the Global AIDS Epidemic.* UNAIDS, Geneva, Switzerland.

125. Ungo, J. R., D. Jones, D. Ashkin, E. S. Hollender, D. Bernstein, A. P. Albanese, and A. E. Pitchenik. 1998. Antituberculosis drug-induced hepatotoxicity. The role of hepatitis C virus and the human immunodeficiency virus. *Am. J. Respir. Crit. Care Med.* **157:**1871–1876.

126. Vernon, A., W. Burman, D. Benator, A. Khan, L. Bozeman, et al. 1999. Acquired rifamycin monoresistance in patients with HIV-related tuberculosis treated with once-weekly rifapentine and isoniazid. *Lancet* **353:**1843–1847.

127. Vynnycky, E., and P. E. Fine. 1997. The natural history of tuberculosis: the implications of age-dependent risks of disease and the role of reinfection. *Epidemiol. Infect.* **119:**183–201.

128. Wells, C. D., J. P. Cegielski, L. J. Nelson, K. F. Laserson, T. H. Holtz, A. Finlay, K. G. Castro, and K. Weyer. 2007. HIV infection and multidrug-resistant tuberculosis: the perfect storm. *J. Infect. Dis.* **196**(Suppl. 1):S86–S107.

129. Wenning, L. A., W. D. Hanley, D. M. Brainard, A. S. Petry, K. Ghosh, B. Jin, E. Mangin, T. C. Marbury, J. K. Berg, J. A. Chodakewitz, J. A. Stone, K. M. Gottesdiener, J. A. Wagner, and M. Iwamoto. 2009. Effect of rifampin, a potent inducer of drug-metabolizing enzymes, on the pharmacokinetics of raltegravir. *Antimicrob. Agents Chemother.* **53:**2852–2856.

130. WHO. 2008. *WHO Three I's Meeting.* World Health Organization, Geneva, Switzerland.

131. WHO. 2009. *Antiretroviral Therapy for HIV Infection In Adults and Adolescents.* World Health Organization, Geneva, Switzerland.

132. World Health Organization. 2008. *Anti-Tuberculosis Drug Resistance In the World. Fourth Global Report.* World Health Organization, Geneva, Switzerland.

133. World Health Organization. 2009. *Global Tuberculosis Control 2009: Epidemiology, Strategy, Financing.* World Health Organization, Geneva, Switzerland.

133a.World Health Organization. 2010. *Global Tuberculosis Control 2010.* World Health Organization, Geneva, Switzerland.

134. World Health Organization. 2009. *Treatment of Tuberculosis: Guidelines.* World Health Organization, Geneva, Switzerland.

135. World Health Organization Europe. 2003. *HIV/AIDS Treatment: Antiretroviral Therapy. Fact Sheet EURO/06/03.* World Health Organization, Geneva, Switzerland.

136. Yang, Z., Y. Kong, F. Wilson, B. Foxman, A. H. Fowler, C. F. Marrs, M. D. Cave, and J. H. Bates. 2004. Identification of risk factors for extrapulmonary tuberculosis. *Clin. Infect. Dis.* **38:**199–205.

137. Zar, H. J., M. F. Cotton, S. Strauss, J. Karpakis, G. Hussey, H. S. Schaaf, H. Rabie, and C. J. Lombard. 2007. Effect of isoniazid prophylaxis on mortality and incidence of tuberculosis in children with HIV: randomised controlled trial. *BMJ* **334:**136.

138. Zwang, J., M. Garenne, K. Kahn, M. Collinson, and S. M. Tollman. 2007. Trends in mortality from pulmonary tuberculosis and HIV/AIDS co-infection in rural South Africa (Agincourt). *Trans. R. Soc. Trop. Med. Hyg.* **101:**893–898.

Chapter 33

Tuberculosis and Organ Transplantation

José M. Aguado and Nina Singh

EPIDEMIOLOGY AND RISK FACTORS

Mycobacterium tuberculosis is a significant opportunistic pathogen in solid organ transplant (SOT) recipients (2, 54, 66, 69) due to its high morbidity and mortality. The frequency of tuberculosis in SOT recipients ranges from 1.2 to 15% (2, 54, 66), which is 20 to 74 times higher than that in the general population in a given geographic area, but the exact incidence of tuberculosis in SOT recipients is not well known. Table 1 sets out the prevalence and incidence rates of tuberculosis in SOT recipients in the most numerous series in the literature (2, 17, 54, 62, 66, 69, 75, 81) and compares them with information available by the Spanish Network of Infection in Transplantation (RESITRA) (75). These data reveal a considerably higher risk of tuberculosis among SOT recipients than in the general population

SOT recipients should be considered a high-risk group for tuberculosis, although incidence differences have been shown among different types of organs. For example, tuberculosis incidence is particularly high in lung transplant recipients (14, 52). Receiving a pulmonary graft instead of another organ increases the risk of tuberculosis up to 5.6 times, and these patients have 73.3 times more risk of tuberculosis than a patient from the general population (75). In the RESITRA series, overall tuberculosis incidence in SOT recipients was 25 times higher than in the general population, 4 times higher than in recipients of allogeneic hematopoietic stem cell transplants (21), and more than 6 times higher than in candidates for transplant (75).

Most cases of tuberculosis in SOT recipients are caused by reactivation of a latent infection after immunosuppressive therapy is started. However, few risk factors have been clearly defined in these patients (9, 76), primarily because most series are retrospective or small and lack control-transplant recipients without tuberculosis (9, 34, 36, 62). Furthermore, most of the available information refers to kidney recipients, and this cannot necessarily be applied to other transplant recipients.

Risk factors previously described in the literature (Table 2) include a history of previous exposure to *M. tuberculosis* (positive purified protein derivative [PPD] and/or residual tuberculosis lesions in pretransplant chest X-ray). Other recognized risk factors are certain pretransplant clinical conditions (recipient's age, dialysis, diabetes, cirrhosis, hepatitis C virus infection, or other coexisting infections) and the intensity of immunosuppression (use of antilymphocyte antibodies, type of basal immunosuppression, and intensification of immunosuppressive treatment as a result of rejection) (9, 10, 35, 66, 75, 76). The role of intensification of immunosuppression for a failing graft appears to be important (28). In fact, 65% of patients in some series were considered to be overimmunosuppressed, as they required treatment for rejection (2). Although some authors have suggested that the use of antilymphocyte antibodies (especially OKT3) increases the risk of tuberculosis dissemination (30, 47), as occurs in mice (53), the crude mortality does not appear to increase when these drugs are used (2). The use of new immunosuppressive drugs such as sirolimus, everolimus, or monoclonal antibodies (daclizumab or basiliximab) does not appear to increase the risk of tuberculosis in SOT recipients (75). It seems reasonable to assume that other factors associated with increased risk of tuberculosis in the general population can also be applied to transplant recipients. These include smoking, malnutrition, or human immunodeficiency virus (HIV) infection.

José M. Aguado • University Hospital 12 de Octubre, Unit of Infectious Diseases, Avda. de Andalucía Km 5,400, 28041 Madrid, Spain. **Nina Singh** • University of Pittsburgh Medical Center, 2A 137 Infectious Diseases Section, VA Pittsburgh Healthcare System and University of Pittsburgh, University Drive C, Pittsburgh, PA 15240.

Table 1. Prevalence and incidence of tuberculosis in SOT

Frequency measure	Type of SOT					
	Overall	Pulmonary	Cardiac	Renal	Hepatic	Renal-pancreatic
Prevalence						
Literature[a]	1.2–6.4%[c] 15%[d]	2–6.5%	1–1.5%	0.5–15%	0.7–2.3%	
RESITRA[b]	0.48%	1.32%	0.25%	0.34%	0.53%	0.82%
Incidence (cases/10^5 transplants/yr) (range)[b]	512 (317–783)	2,072 (565–5,306)	255 (6.5–1,421)	358 (144–728)	541 (269–1,065)	1,204 (30.5–6,710)

[a]Data were taken from references 2, 54, 62, 66, 69, 75, and 81.
[b]Data were from RESITRA (75).
[c]In developed countries.
[d]In areas where tuberculosis is highly endemic.

CLINICAL PRESENTATION: CHRONOLOGY AND CLINICAL SYMPTOMS

The time of onset of symptoms of tuberculosis after transplantation varies. Some authors have observed a bimodal distribution (2, 28, 32). Most SOT recipients developed tuberculosis in the first year after transplant, with a median time of onset of symptoms of 9 months (75), but up to a third of patients may develop symptoms of tuberculosis after the first year of transplantation (2). In our experience, renal transplant patients have a later onset of symptoms than other SOT recipients (75). This may be due in part to the lower grade of immunosuppression received by these patients.

Although it has been suggested that patients developing *early* (during the first year of transplantation) tuberculosis were more severely immunosuppressed than patients with *late* tuberculosis (33), we and other authors (2, 28) did not confirm this observation. However, patients with prior clinical or radiological

Table 2. Risk factors for tuberculosis

History of previous exposure to *Mycobacterium tuberculosis*
  Positive PPD result (degree of evidence III)
  Radiological evidence of untreated previous TB (degree of evidence III)
Pretransplant clinical conditions
  Receptor's age
  Chronic renal insufficiency or hemodialysis (kidney transplant) (degree of evidence II)
  Diabetes mellitus (degree of evidence II)
  Hepatitis C virus (kidney transplant) (degree of evidence III)
  Chronic liver disease (degree of evidence III)
  Other coexisting infections: profound mycoses, cytomegalovirus, *Pneumocystis jirovecii* or *Nocardia* pneumonia (degree of evidence III)
Immunosuppressive therapy
  OKT3 or anti-T-lymphocyte antibodies (degree of evidence III)
  Intensification of immunosuppression associated with graft rejection (degree of evidence II)
  Mycophenolate mofetil and tacrolimus vs azathioprine-cyclosporine-prednisone (degree of evidence III)

evidence of tuberculosis did appear to develop the disease earlier than patients without these antecedents. These data suggest that patients with a history of tuberculosis have a higher risk of reactivation during the first months after transplantation, independent of the type of immunosuppression received.

In general, most patients develop pulmonary forms of tuberculosis, but the percentage of patients who develop extrapulmonary or disseminated forms of tuberculosis is higher than in the general population (42), with incidence rates as high as 38 to 64% (42, 59). These extrapulmonary or disseminated forms are more frequent in the first six months after transplantation, coinciding with the peak of maximum pharmacological immunosuppression.

The most common symptoms are fever, cough, dyspnea, musculoskeletal pain, night sweats, and weight loss, along with lymphadenopathy (2). Unlike the general population, tuberculosis in SOT recipients is often asymptomatic, and diagnosis is established by routine surveillance cultures; not infrequently, the diagnosis is made at necropsy. Up to one-third of patients may have a normal chest radiograph (74).

Pulmonary tuberculosis usually manifests with cough, fever, tachypnea, hemoptysis, and radiological images of parenchymal involvement in upper lobes, diffuse involvement, or miliary dissemination. It is rare to find images of cavitation, as seen in very immunosuppressed HIV patients. The most common symptoms of presentation of gastrointestinal tuberculosis are fever, gastrointestinal bleeding, and abdominal pain (19). The ileocecal area is most frequently affected. Patients with urological tuberculosis will develop urinary symptoms, back pain, and fever accompanied by sterile pyuria.

The most common presenting symptom of disseminated tuberculosis is fever. Some have reported patients with miliary tuberculosis who develop initial symptoms resembling life-threatening sepsis or adverse drug reactions (2). In SOT recipients, the chance of disseminated tuberculosis should be considered when there is indirect evidence of involvement of organs other than those initially affected. For example, the presence of osteoarticular and cutaneous forms is often a result of tuberculosis dissemination. No relationship has been found between factors such as age, type of organ transplanted, type of immunosuppressive therapy, rejection, and history of exposure to mycobacteria and the development of disseminated tuberculosis. In particular, patients receiving overimmunosuppression (boluses of steroids or antilymphocyte antibodies) do not appear to be at higher risk for the development of disseminated disease.

DIAGNOSIS CONSIDERATIONS

It is quite common for the diagnosis of tuberculosis in SOT recipients to be delayed for weeks, due to absence of clinical suspicion. The possibility of tuberculosis in a transplant patient should always be taken into account, especially in areas of high endemicity. In these patients, the diagnosis is particularly difficult because, as noted, the disease is often asymptomatic or scarcely symptomatic and only about one-quarter of patients have clinical or radiological data suggestive of tuberculosis. In addition, a large proportion of patients have a negative tuberculosis skin test because of cutaneous anergy secondary to pharmacological immunosuppression.

Therefore, the presence of fever, night sweats, weight loss, lymphadenopathy, or radiographic abnormalities should raise suspicion of the possibility of tuberculosis, especially in patients with a history of contact with *M. tuberculosis* (PPD positive). Tuberculosis should be particularly considered early in patients with lung transplantation. In these patients, the candidate's PPD and pretransplant thorax imaging have little value, since tuberculosis can appear through the reactivation of latent infection in the graft (75).

Once tuberculosis is suspected, it is necessary to perform various examinations to confirm the diagnosis. It is very important to collect specimens (sputum, urine, or feces, etc.) for culture using specific media for mycobacteria. If the diagnosis is not made with the usual techniques and clinical suspicion remains high, it would be justified to use more aggressive diagnostic measures (bronchoscopy, mediastinoscopy, or laparoscopy with biopsy, etc.)

After transplant, the diagnostic yield of tuberculin skin test (PPD) is very low but nevertheless remains the first step in posttransplant evaluation of suspected tuberculosis. Unfortunately, in spite of being widely recommended, PPD was carried out in only 40.6% of patients in a recent series (75). Moreover, prophylaxis was prescribed in less than half of patients with positive PPD.

Positive PPD should be defined as induration over or equal to 5 mm in diameter 48 to 72 hours after the administration of 2 IU of strain RT-23, equivalent to 5 IU of PPD tuberculin. T-cell gamma interferon release assays QuantiFERON-Gold (Cellestis) and T-SPOT.TB (Oxford Immunotec Ltd.) may have a role in detecting latent tuberculosis infection (18, 22) but are not yet included for the management of these patients in most centers.

EVALUATION OF CANDIDATES AND DONORS

Evaluation of Candidates for SOT

What follows are some considerations on the evaluation of donors and recipients of SOT regarding tuberculosis infection contained in the Consensus Statement of the Group for the Study of Infection in Transplant Recipients (GESITRA) of the Spanish Society of Infectious Diseases and Clinical Microbiology (3). In parentheses is the degree of evidence for each recommendation based on the strength and quality of the evidence analyzed.

Evaluation of an SOT candidate—as far as tuberculosis is concerned—must involve a study of any history of infection or disease and, if this is the case, whether treatment was administered, with which drugs, and for how long. It is important to know if there has been contact with cases of active tuberculosis in the family or workplace and if the patient has undergone PPD skin testing (BIII). History should include possible institutional exposure and travel to areas of high endemicity.

All candidates should undergo PPD testing, even those who have been vaccinated against *Mycobacterium bovis* BCG (AII). This test should be repeated at 7 to 10 days (booster effect). The only reason for not carrying out PPD testing would be if the patient had already had a positive PPD result or previous tuberculosis (69). Correct interpretation of the PPD test necessarily involves knowing whether the transplant candidate has received treatment against latent tuberculosis infection. The PPD result should be interpreted independent of the BCG vaccination status (3).

Active tuberculosis should always be ruled out by a chest radiograph. In symptomatic patients, active tuberculosis must be ruled out, as it is a contraindication for transplant. A patient with active pulmonary tuberculosis could be considered a candidate for nonpulmonary SOT, as long as the patient is receiving antituberculosis treatment and stains for the detection of acid-fast bacilli in sputum are negative when the transplant is to be performed.

Management of Candidates with a Positive PPD Result

It is extremely important to rule out active tuberculosis in these patients (AII). If clinical or radiological data suggest tuberculosis, sputum smears and culture must be carried out and, if this is not possible, bronchoscopy and culture of the bronchoalveolar aspirate/lavage fluid should be performed. Clinically guided additional examinations may be necessary, such as abdominal ultrasound to detect enlarged abdominal lymph nodes or biopsy and lymph node culture. In asymptomatic patients whose chest radiograph reveals residual lesions, sputum should be cultured and, in specific cases, bronchoscopy and culture of aspirate or lavage fluid performed. Once active tuberculosis has been ruled out, the transplantation candidate could start treatment of latent tuberculosis infection while on the waiting list (except in case of liver transplantation, see below) and, if possible, continue treatment after the transplant.

Management of Candidates with a Negative PPD Result

If the initial PPD test result is negative, PPD testing should be repeated at 7 to 10 days after the initial test (booster effect). Following the recommendations of the American Society of Transplantation (69), an induration of 5 mm or more indicates that the test result is positive (BIII). Patients awaiting an SOT often have cutaneous anergy due to their underlying disease. Cellular immune testing (multitest or specific testing for selected antigens, such as *Candida albicans* or tetanus toxoid) could be performed at the time of the second PPD skin test to determine the presence of anergy. Unfortunately, there are not enough data on the use of these tests in SOT recipients. The real risk of developing tuberculosis in patients with cutaneous anergy is unknown. It is probable that not all anergic patients require treatment, particularly if they have a low risk for acquiring primary infection. If there is a high risk for primary infection, they should be managed as if they had a positive PPD test until more data are available (3).

New techniques, such as measurement of the release of gamma interferon in response to *M. tuberculosis* antigens, including QuantiFERON-Gold (Cellestis) and T-SPOT.TB (Oxford Immunotec Ltd.), are being developed and validated, and these could help improve the diagnosis of latent tuberculosis infection in transplantation candidates.

Evaluation of Solid Organ Donors

Tuberculosis has been transmitted through kidney, lung, and liver grafts (38). Latent infection by *M. tuberculosis* in the donor could be reactivated in the transplant recipient. Therefore, all living donors should undergo PPD skin testing. If the result is positive, active tuberculosis should be ruled out (AII) (69). The situation is more complex in cadaveric donors, since there is often not enough information to rule out the existence of latent tuberculosis infection or active tuberculosis. Therefore, in principle, not only active tuberculosis but also a well-founded suspicion of it should contraindicate SOT (AII). Biopsy samples from local lymph nodes must be obtained during surgery and cultures must be performed at the time of transplantation to rule out active tuberculosis in the donor.

Residual pulmonary lesions in the donor contraindicate lung transplant; however, this is not true for other organs. For lung transplantation, a histopathological and microbiological study of the donor lung should be performed to rule out active infection. Techniques that amplify the nucleic acids of *M. tuberculosis* are highly sensitive and specific in respiratory samples and may prove to be useful in the evaluation of donors (12). Disseminated tuberculosis is an absolute contraindication for the use of any organ for transplantation (3).

When the transplant is urgent, respiratory and urine samples must be obtained for culture for *M. tuberculosis*. Similarly, samples should be obtained from both the donor and the recipient during surgery if any enlarged lymph node is found in the surgical bed. A positive culture would indicate the need to start specific treatment (73).

TREATMENT OF LATENT TUBERCULOSIS INFECTION IN SOT RECIPIENTS OR CANDIDATES

Indications for Treatment of Latent Tuberculosis Infection

The recommendations that follow have been taken in part from the Consensus Statement of the Spanish GESITRA recently published (3).

In SOT recipients, tuberculosis usually develops from a site of latent infection in the recipient. Ideally, treatment of latent tuberculosis infection should start before transplantation. If this cannot be completed before the procedure, it should be completed afterwards. Treatment of latent tuberculosis infection should be provided for all patients on the waiting list or recipients who have one or more of the following conditions: (i) a PPD skin test (initial or after a booster effect) with an induration ≥5 mm, (ii) a history of untreated tuberculosis, or (iii) a history of contact with a patient with active tuberculosis. Patients with chest radiograph findings compatible with untreated tuberculosis (apical fibronodular lesions, calcified solitary nodule, calcified lymph nodes, or pleural thickening) should also receive therapy for latent tuberculosis infection (AII) (13). The value of such radiological data as an indication of a history of tuberculosis is greater in areas such as Europe, where there are no regional mycoses (histoplasmosis, coccidioidomycosis, or blastomycosis) that could cause similar lesions.

Transmission of active tuberculosis from a donor is less common, although it has been reported (27). In general, except in the case of living donors (29), clinical data indicating whether the donor had tuberculosis may not be available. Therefore, as stated above, biopsies and cultures of lymph nodes must be performed at the time of transplantation to rule out active tuberculosis in the donor. Treatment of latent tuberculosis infection must be administered to recipients of an organ whose donor has a history of or data that suggest untreated tuberculosis (66). There are no data addressing prophylaxis if the recipient is tuberculin negative and receives an organ from a PPD-positive donor, but some authors suggest that a course of isoniazid (INH) should be considered (26, 59, 68) .

Before initiation of treatment of latent tuberculosis infection, patients should undergo an exhaustive study to rule out active tuberculosis (culture and PCR for mycobacteria in blood, sputum, and urine samples). For patients with radiological alterations who are unable to expectorate, sputum should be induced with hypertonic saline or fiber optic bronchoscopy should be performed (11). Patients whose previous tuberculosis was properly treated do not require treatment of latent tuberculosis infection (60).

Recommendations for the Treatment of Latent Tuberculosis Infection

The American Thoracic Society (5) and the American Society of Transplantation Infectious Disease Guidelines (69) recommend routine administration of INH to tuberculin-positive transplant recipients with healed pulmonary tuberculosis. The drug of choice for treatment of latent tuberculosis infection is INH (300 mg/day) supplemented with vitamin B_6 for 9 months (3, 23, 37, 61, 66). Prophylaxis with INH was proven to prevent tuberculosis in randomized studies involving kidney recipients (1, 37, 78) (AI).

The ideal approach is to treat latent tuberculosis infection before transplant, except possibly in the case of liver transplantation. The duration and dose of INH therapy are the same, irrespective of whether it is administered before or after transplant. Patients who have completed therapy before transplantation do not need to repeat it after the procedure.

The possibility of INH-induced hepatotoxicity should be borne in mind for these patients. Tolerance to INH is generally good (7, 46) and the interaction with calcineurin inhibitors is very limited (70); however, in a series of renal patients receiving INH prophylaxis, 11% had evidence of hepatic dysfunction attributable solely to INH and 2.5% developed major hepatic dysfunction, with 2 deaths related to liver failure (72). Results like these prompt many authors to recommend that INH chemoprophylaxis be limited to patients with a positive tuberculin skin test who fall into high-risk categories (patients born in areas of endemicity, with chronic advanced underlying illness, rejection, and/or adjunctive immunosuppression), demonstrating abnormal chest X ray or documented recent skin conversion (47).

All patients should have baseline hepatic measurements of serum aspartate aminotransferase, alanine aminotransferase, and bilirubin. They should receive follow-up evaluations at least monthly. Patients should be educated about the side effects associated with treatment of latent tuberculosis and advised to stop treatment and promptly seek medical evaluation when they occur. Treatment of latent tuberculosis infection must be suspended if aspartate aminotransferase or alanine aminotransferase values increase threefold in patients with symptoms or fivefold in patients with no accompanying symptoms (80).

Alternatives to INH include rifampin (with or without INH) for 4 months (72) (BII) or rifampin and pyrazinamide for 2 months (31) (CIII). However, this last combination has been associated with severe liver toxicity and is generally not recommended (except when prophylaxis must be completed over a short period) and must always be administered under expert supervision (80). This regimen is not recommended for patients with previous liver disease, consumers of alcohol, or patients who have developed INH-induced hepatotoxicity (13). The regimens that include rifampin are only recommended for pretransplant treatment of latent tuberculosis infection due to the medication interactions that affect this drug.

In cases of severe toxicity, a liver biopsy is only recommended when there is a doubtful diagnosis or when laboratory values do not return to normal when treatment is suspended. When suspension of treatment of latent tuberculosis infection is necessary because of toxicity, the patient should be closely monitored and treatment of latent tuberculosis infection should be completed with drugs other than INH, although only in patients at high risk of tuberculosis, such as those who recently had a positive PPD result after having a negative result. For patients at high risk of tuberculosis, we recommend levofloxacin and ethambutol for at least 6 months (BIII).

When active tuberculosis cannot be ruled out in a transplant recipient, it is recommended that treatment is initiated with 3 drugs (INH, ethambutol, and pyrazinamide); a fourth drug, e.g., a fluoroquinolone, should be added if the disease is severe or until susceptibilities are known. Treatment can be completed with only INH if, after 8 weeks of incubation of samples, cultures are negative for *M. tuberculosis* and the chest radiograph findings remain normal.

Exclusions from Treatment of Latent Tuberculosis Infection and Precautions

Liver transplant recipients present special problems when receiving treatment for latent tuberculosis infection due to the high risk of hepatotoxicity. Some authors consider that this risk outweighs any potential benefits, since the frequency of reactivation is not excessively high (11). However, other authors have not observed increased toxicity with INH in liver transplant recipients (67). The GESITRA Consensus Statement (3) recommends delaying the administration of treatment for latent tuberculosis disease in liver recipients until after the transplant, when liver function is stable, since administration of therapy when the patient is still on the waiting list (which is recommended for recipients of other organs) can cause liver dysfunction and require an emergency transplant (BIII). The advisability of treating latent tuberculosis infection in liver recipients is clearer when there are high-risk factors such as recent change in PPD results from negative to positive, a history of incorrectly treated tuberculosis, direct contact with an untreated person with tuberculosis, residual tuberculosis lesions on the chest radiograph, and added immunosuppression factors (e.g., treatment of graft rejection episodes in patients with a positive PPD result who have not received treatment of latent tuberculosis infection).

TREATMENT OF TUBERCULOSIS IN SOT RECIPIENTS

Treatment of tuberculosis in transplant patients is complicated especially by the high risk of developing toxicity, particularly in liver recipients. The recommendations for treatment of tuberculosis in transplant recipients are similar to those for the general population (13), with 2 differences: (i) the interaction between rifamycins (rifampin, rifabutin, or rifapentine) and immunosuppressors of the calcineurin inhibitor family (cyclosporine and tacrolimus), rapamycin, and corticosteroids; and (ii) the duration of treatment. It should be noted that recommendations for the diagnosis and treatment of active tuberculosis disease in SOT recipients are made based on consensus guidelines formulated by experts in the field (3, 6, 13, 69, 75, 79).

The decision to use specific regimens in SOT recipients is driven by the rate of resistance in each country and based on the epidemiology in individual cases. Mycobacterial susceptibility testing is currently critical for designing the treatment of tuberculosis in SOT recipients, especially in the eventuality of multidrug-resistant and extensively drug-resistant tuberculosis. Although rifampin has been widely used in SOT recipients (mainly kidney recipients), the need for the drug in all cases is controversial (4, 63). The recently published Consensus Statement of the Spanish GESITRA (3) recommends avoiding rifamycins in patients with localized, nonsevere forms of tuberculosis, without suspicion or evidence of resistance to INH. The use of rifamycins is recommended for patients with severe or disseminated forms of tuberculosis or with suspicion or evidence of resistance to INH (Table 3).

Rifampin reduces the serum levels of tacrolimus, cyclosporine, rapamycin (sirolimus), everolimus, and corticosteroids. The reductions in these levels have been associated with a high risk of graft rejection (56); therefore, the dose of calcineurin inhibitors should be increased three- to fivefold, and levels should be closely monitored (2, 54). Even with suitable monitoring, combining rifampin and cyclosporine increases the frequency of graft rejection, graft loss, and overall tuberculosis-related mortality (2, 54, 66). Rifabutin could be an alternative, since it is a weaker inducer of cytochrome P450 than rifampin. There have been favorable experiences with rifabutin in kidney recipients (41, 44), but data are limited. Some studies have reported that these drugs may be safe with rigorous control of immunosuppressor levels in spite of the fact that they have increased rejection and mortality in certain cases (77). In our experience, we have not observed higher crude mortality among patients who received rifamycins (17.6 versus 25%) (75).

INH and pyrazinamide have been widely used in transplant recipients with tuberculosis. Given the risk of hepatotoxicity, a close follow-up of liver enzyme values is necessary, especially in patients undergoing

Table 3. Recommendations of the GESITRA (75) for treatment of tuberculosis in SOT

Situation	Initial treatment	Maintenance treatment
Patients with localized, nonsevere forms of TB without suspicion or evidence of resistance to isoniazid	Isoniazid, ethambutol, and pyrazinamide (or levofloxacin) Avoid the use of rifamycins; if rifamycins are used, the levels of immunosuppressors should be closely monitored and the doses of cyclosporine or tacrolimus increased (AII) If treatment is started early, it is not necessary to reduce immunosuppression (CIII)	Isoniazid and ethambutol (or pyrazinamide) are recommended for 12 to 18 mo (CIII) Incorporation of a third drug, such as pyrazinamide or levofloxacin,[a] could reduce this period to 12 mo (CIII)
Severe, mainly disseminated, forms of TB or suspicion or evidence of resistance to isoniazid[c] In cases of multiresistance or when there is some limitation for the use of the above-mentioned drugs	Consider adding rifampin or rifabutin to isoniazid, ethambutol, and pyrazinamide (or levofloxacin) (BIII)[b] If isoniazid and rifamycins cannot be used, induction treatment should include 4–6 drugs, including injectable antimicrobials—such as streptomycin,[d] amikacin, kanamycin, or capreomycin, linezolid, or other second-line drugs (CIII)[e]	Complete treatment with isoniazid and rifampin or rifabutin until complete at least 9 mo of treatment Absence of isoniazid and rifamycin in initial treatment makes it difficult to calculate duration of treatment and types of drugs to be used; therapy should be individualized

[a]It is necessary to remember that prolonged use of fluoroquinolones can be associated with arthralgias, and the combination of pyrazinamide and levofloxacin is poorly tolerated by the digestive system.

[b]The use of rifampin or rifabutin would require increased doses of cyclosporine or tacrolimus and closer monitoring of the levels of these drugs (AII). Resistance to rifampin is almost systematically associated with cross-resistance to rifabutin and rifapentine; therefore, these are not suitable alternatives (DII).

[c]If isoniazid cannot be used, we must use induction and maintenance treatment that includes 4 drugs for at least 18 months (CIII).

[d]In cases of resistance to streptomycin, there is no cross-resistance with other injectable drugs (amikacin, kanamycin, capreomycin); however, cross-resistance between amikacin and kanamycin is universal. The combination of injectable drugs is not recommended, given their intolerance and the association of side effects (DII).

[e]There is no experience with the use of intermittent regimens, which in any case, are not recommended in the management of multiresistant tuberculosis, except for the use of injectable drugs once a period of at least 2 to 3 months of daily administration has been completed (DII).

liver transplant. The administration of streptomycin and aminoglycosides to transplant recipients should be considered carefully because of the risk of boosting the nephrotoxicity of these drugs with calcineurin inhibitors. Fluoroquinolones are an alternative for these patients because of the disadvantages associated with rifamycins and aminoglycosides, and they can sometimes be used as first-line agents (55). Nevertheless, indiscriminate use of fluoroquinolones in the general population has been associated with an increase in resistance of *M. tuberculosis* to these drugs in recent years (25). Combined and prolonged use of levofloxacin and pyrazinamide has been associated with poor tolerance in SOT recipients, mainly gastrointestinal (45). In special cases of resistance or toxicity, linezolid has proven to be effective in patients with tuberculosis (24). However, prolonged use of this drug is associated with frequent development of thrombopenia and anemia and, in some cases, polyneuropathy, especially in patients with other associated conditions such as diabetes or kidney disease. Therefore, use of linezolid in transplant recipients is limited.

In liver recipients, the development of liver toxicity is a particular concern during the treatment of tuberculosis (64). In recipients of other organs, INH is generally well tolerated, although the risk of hepatotoxicity has also been reported in kidney recipients

(48). As mentioned above, rifampin must be used with extreme caution when treating tuberculosis in transplant recipients. When combined with INH, it has led to a considerable increase in hepatotoxicity, especially in liver recipients. Initial treatment with INH, rifampin, and pyrazinamide in liver recipients with tuberculosis has been associated with histologically confirmed hepatotoxicity in 88% of cases (39). A particularly high risk of hepatotoxicity has also been reported with the combination of rifampin and pyrazinamide for the treatment of latent tuberculosis infection (39).

Special Considerations in HIV-Infected Transplant Recipients

More than 200 liver transplantations have been performed in HIV-infected patients, and the risk of tuberculosis does not seem to be significantly greater after transplantation than it is before transplantation (50). The main problems that can occur after transplantation are the drug interactions and the recurrence of hepatitis C virus infection, which may increase the risk of tuberculosis and favor toxicity (76).

Although reported experience is scant, the standard regimen used for treatment of tuberculosis in HIV-infected transplant recipients seems to be as effective as in other HIV-infected patients (49). Rifamycins may lead to greater hepatotoxicity in HIV-infected patients (compared with HIV-uninfected patients) and jeopardize antiretroviral therapy because of their interaction with protease inhibitors and nonnucleoside reverse transcriptase inhibitors. All 3 groups of drugs can inhibit or induce the isoenzyme family of cytochrome P450, thus leading to interactions that are difficult to manage. A combination of INH, pyrazinamide, ethambutol, and a quinolone is recommended in these patients. The use of aminoglycosides is limited by the risk of nephrotoxicity induced by calcineurin inhibitors.

Risk of Immune Reconstitution Syndrome

It is worth remembering that, as in HIV-infected patients, SOT recipients with tuberculosis can develop an immune reconstitution syndrome related to changes in immunosuppressive treatment and to interactions with immunosuppressors and the medications used to treat tuberculosis, especially the rifamycins (8, 58). The precise frequency with which it occurs, who are the patients at high risk, and its appropriate management are not known. Immune reconstitution syndrome in SOT recipients could be interpreted as failure of therapy or a relapse, often leading to unnecessary changes in therapy and inappropriate management decisions (65). The most common manifestations of tuberculosis-associated immune reconstitution syndrome are fever, lymphadenopathy, and worsening respiratory symptoms (40).

Duration of Antituberculosis Treatment in Transplant Recipients

The duration of treatment and type of drugs to be used after the first 2 months are very controversial issues, especially if rifampin is not used in the first 2 months or must be suspended due to intolerance. The Guidelines of the Expert Group in Renal Transplantation (23) and the American Society of Transplantation Infectious Disease Guidelines (69) recommend 2 months of INH, rifampin, and pyrazinamide therapy (with the addition of ethambutol when there is >4% INH resistance), followed by INH and rifampin for an additional 4 months (BIII). However, one Spanish study (2) observed that administering treatment for less than 9 months was associated with greater mortality. Another study observed that the only factor that was significantly associated with greater recurrence in tuberculosis was duration of treatment: no recurrence was observed in patients who received more than 12 months of treatment, irrespective of whether

the treatment regimen included rifampin (57). Experience in the general population with antituberculosis regimens that do not include rifampin should be considered. Most patients who receive suitably managed rifamycin therapy and who experience relapse are usually infected with a rifamycin-susceptible strain. However, in rifamycin-sparing regimens, especially if these are not supervised, drug resistance occurs more frequently (13).

In the general population, INH, pyrazinamide, and streptomycin have proven to be effective when the regimen is administered for 9 months (13), although it is difficult to maintain injected drugs over long periods because of the risk of ototoxicity and renal toxicity. Furthermore, the use of injectable drugs in transplant recipients should be avoided because of the risk of nephrotoxicity. There are no studies on the use of ethambutol instead of streptomycin in these circumstances. Nevertheless, in the general population, and therefore in transplant recipients, oral regimens should be maintained for 12 to 18 months (CIII) and the benefit of injectable agents should be evaluated during the first 2 to 3 months in extensive or cavitary forms.

OUTCOME AND RISK FACTORS INFLUENCING MORTALITY

Tuberculosis has important implications in the outcome of transplant patients. The overall mortality rate in solid organ recipients with tuberculosis is as high as 29% (1). Disseminated tuberculosis, prior rejection, and receipt of antilymphocyte antibodies portend a poor prognosis in these patients (66). The average percentage of mortality directly related to tuberculosis in several large series of transplant recipients reviewed was 15% (2). Tuberculosis causes tremendous mortality in these patients as compared to mortality in the general population and in transplant patients without tuberculosis (43, 68, 71). This high mortality rate has decreased only partially in the more recently published series. In comparison with a previous retrospective study conducted by the GESITRA in the last decade (period, 1980 to 1994) (2), we have ascertained a reduction of crude mortality (31 versus 19%) and related mortality (20 versus 9.5%) in a more recent experience within the period 2003 to 2006 (75).

The important drug interactions associated with antimycobacterial therapy in SOT recipients are relatively unique and play a considerable role in the poor outcome of tuberculosis in this population. In our experience, up to 25% of our patients lost their grafts due to rejection, and in the majority of cases, rejection was due to the interference of rifampin with cyclosporine. Other authors have reported similar findings (15, 16, 20, 51); rejection following interference with cyclosporine or tacrolimus by rifampin was one of the most significant risk factors for both crude and tuberculosis-related mortality.

REFERENCES

1. Agarwal, S. K., S. Gupta, S. C. Dash, D. Bhowmik, and S. C. Tiwari. 2004. Prospective randomised trial of isoniazid prophylaxis in renal transplant recipient. *Int. Urol. Nephrol.* **36:** 425–431.
2. Aguado, J. M., J. A. Herrero, J. Gavaldá, J. Torre-Cisneros, M. Blanes, G. Rufí, A. Moreno, M. Gurguí, M. Hayek, C. Lumbreras, C. Cantarell, et al. 1997. Clinical presentation and outcome of tuberculosis in kidney, liver, and heart transplant recipients in Spain. *Transplantation* **63:**1278–1286.
3. Aguado, J. M., J. Torre-Cisneros, J. Fortún, N. Benito, Y. Meije, A. Doblas, and P. Muñoz. 2009. Tuberculosis in solid-organ transplant recipients: consensus statement of the group for the study of infection in transplant recipients (GESITRA) of the Spanish Society of Infectious Diseases and Clinical Microbiology. *Clin. Infect. Dis.* **48:**1276–1284.
4. al-Sulaiman, M. H., J. M. Dhar, and A. A. al-Khader. 1990. Successful use of rifampicin in the treatment of tuberculosis in renal transplant patients immunosuppressed with cyclosporine. *Transplantation* **50:**597–598.
5. American Thoracic Society. 1974. Preventive therapy of tuberculous infection. *Am. Rev. Respir. Dis.* **110:**371–374.
6. American Thoracic Society, Centers for Disease Control and Prevention, and Infectious Diseases Society of America. 2005. American Thoracic Society/Centers for Disease Control and Prevention/Infectious Diseases Society of America: controlling tuberculosis in the United States. *Am. J. Respir. Crit. Care Med.* **172:**1169–1227.
7. Antony, S. J., C. Ynares, and J. S. Dummer. 1997. Isoniazid hepatotoxicity in renal transplant recipients. *Clin. Transplant.* **11:**34–37.
8. Asano, T., H. Kawamoto, J. Asakuma, T. Tanimoto, H. Kobayashi, and M. Hayakawa. 2000. Paradoxical worsening of tuberculosis after anti-TB therapy in a kidney transplant recipient. *Transplant. Proc.* **32:**1960–1962.
9. Basiri, A., S. M. Moghaddam, N. Simforoosh, B. Einollahi, M. Hosseini, A. Foirouzan, F. Pourrezagholi, M. Nafar, M. A. Zargar, G. Pourmand, A. Tara, H. Mombeni, M. R. Moradi, A. Taghizadeh, H. R. Gholamrezaee, A. Bohlouli, H. Nezhadgashti, A. Amirzadehpasha, E. Ahmad, M. Salehipour, M. Yazdani, A. Nasrollahi, K. Falaknazi, M. R. Mahdavi, A. Shamsa, B. Feizzadeh, M. J. Mojahedi, N. Oghbaee, R. E. Azad, and Z. Mohammadi. 2005. Preliminary report of a nationwide case-control study for identifying risk factors of tuberculosis following renal transplantation. *Transplant. Proc.* **37:**3041–3044.
10. Basiri, A., S. M. Hosseini-Moghaddam, N. Simforoosh, B. Einollahi, M. Hosseini, A. Foirouzan, F. Pourrezagholi, M. Nafar, M. A. Zargar, G. Pourmand, A. Tara, H. Mombeni, M. R. Moradi, A. T. Afshar, H. R. Gholamrezaee, A. Bohlouli, H. Nezhadgashti, A. Akbarzadehpasha, E. Ahmad, M. Salehipour, M. Yazdani, A. Nasrollahi, N. Oghbaee, R. E. Azad, Z. Mohammadi, and Z. Razzaghi. 2008. The risk factors and laboratory diagnostics for post renal transplant tuberculosis: a case-control, country-wide study on definitive cases. *Transpl. Infect. Dis.* **10:**231–235.
11. Benito, N., O. Sued, A. Moreno, J. P. Horcajada, J. González, M. Navasa, and A. Rimola. 2002. Diagnosis and treatment of latent tuberculosis infection in liver transplant recipients in an endemic area. *Transplantation* **74:**1381–1386.
12. Blanes, M., D. Gomez, M. J. Giménez, and M. Salavert. 2009. Evaluación de la infección en el donante y en el receptor de trasplante de órgano sólido y de progenitors hematopoyéticos, p. 131–158. *In* J. M. Aguado, J. Fortún, J. Gavaldà, A. Pahissa, and J. Torre-Cisneros (ed.), *Infecciones en Pacientes Trasplantados*, 3a ed. Elsevier, Madrid, Spain.
13. Blumberg, H. M., W. J. Burman, R. E. Chaisson, C. L. Daley, S. C. Etkind, L. N. Friedman, P. Fujiwara, M. Grzemska, P. C. Hopewell, M. D. Iseman, R. M. Jasmer, V. Koppaka, R. I. Menzies, R. J. O'Brien, R. R. Reves, L. B. Reichman, P. M. Simone, J. R. Starke, and A. A. Vernon. 2003. American Thoracic Society/Centers for Disease Control and Prevention/Infectious Diseases Society of America: treatment of tuberculosis. *Am. J. Respir. Crit. Care Med.* **167:**603–662.
14. Bravo, C., J. Roldán, A. Roman, J. Degracia, J. Majo, J. Guerra, V. Monforte, R. Vidal, and F. Morell. 2005. Tuberculosis in lung transplant recipients. *Transplantation* **79:**59–64.
15. Buffington, G. A., J. H. Dominguez, W. F. Piering, L. A. Hebert, H. M. Kauffman, Jr., and J. Lemann, Jr. 1976. Interaction of rifampicin and glucocorticoids. Adverse effect on renal allograft function. *JAMA* **236:**1958–1960.
16. Chan, G. L., J. T. Sinnott, P. J. Emmanuel, S. Cyanle, and S. S. Weinstein. 1992. Drug interactions with cyclosporine: focus on antimicrobial agents. *Clin. Transpl.* **6:**141–153.
17. Chou, N. K., J. L. Wang, N. H. Chi, I. H. Wu, S. C. Huang, Y. S. Chen, H. Y. Yu, C. I. Tsao, W. J. Ko, H. Y. Su, S. C. Chang, S. H. Chu, and S. S. Wang. 2008. Tuberculosis after heart transplantation: twenty years of experience in a single center in Taiwan. *Transplant. Proc.* **40:**2631–2633.
18. Codeluppi, M., S. Cocchi, G. Guaraldi, F. Di Benedetto, N. De Ruvo, M. Meacci, B. Meccugni, R. Esposito, and G. E. Gerunda. 2006. Posttransplant Mycobacterium tuberculosis disease following liver transplantation and the need for cautious evaluation of Quantiferon TB GOLD results in the transplant setting: a case report. *Transplant. Proc.* **38:**1083–1085.
19. Costa, J. M. N., A. M. Meyers, J. R. Botha, A. A. Conlan, and A. Myburgh. 1998. Mycobacterial infections in recipients of kidney allografts. A seventeen-year experience. *Acta Med. Port.* **1:**51–57.
20. Daniels, N. J., J. S. Dover, and R. K. Schachter. 1984. Interaction between cyclosporin and rifampin. *Lancet* **ii:**639.
21. de la Cámara, R., R. Martino, E. Granados, F. J. Rodriguez-Salvanés, M. Rovira, R. Cabrera, J. López, R. Parody, J. Sierra, J. M. Fernández-Rañada, E. Carreras, et al. 2000. Tuberculosis after hematopoietic stem cell transplantation: incidence, clinical characteristics and outcome. *Bone Marrow Transplant.* **26:** 291–298.
22. Dheda, K., Z. F. Udwadia, J. F. Huggett, M. A. Johnson, and G. A. Rook. 2005. Utility of the antigen-specific interferon-gamma assay for the management of tuberculosis. *Curr. Opin. Pulm. Med.* **11:**195–202.
23. EBPG Expert Group on Renal Transplantation. 2002. European best practice guidelines for renal transplantation. Section IV: long-term management of the transplant recipient. IV.7.2. Late infections. Tuberculosis. *Nephrol. Dial. Transplant.* **17**(Suppl. 4):39–43.
24. Fortún, J., P. Martín-Dávila, E. Navas, M. J. Pérez-Elías, J. Cobo, M. Tato, E. G. De la Pedrosa, E. Gómez-Mampaso, and S. Moreno. 2005. Linezolid for the treatment of multidrug-resistant tuberculosis. *J. Antimicrob. Chemother.* **56:**180–185.

25. Ginsburg, A. S., J. H. Grosset, and W. R. Bishai. 2003. Fluoro-quinolones, tuberculosis, and resistance. *Lancet Infect. Dis.* 3:432–442.

26. Gottesdiener, K. M. 1989. Transplanted infections: donor-to-host transmission with the allograft. *Ann. Intern. Med.* 110:1001–1016.

27. Graham, J. C., A. M. Kearns, J. G. Magee, M. F. El-Sheikh, M. Hudson, D. Manas, F. K. Gould, K. E. Orr, and R. Freeman. 2001. Tuberculosis transmitted through transplantation. *J. Infect.* 43:251–254.

28. Hall, C. M., P. A. Willcox, C. R. Swanepoel, D. Kahn, and R. Van Zyl-Smit. 1994. Mycobacterial infection in renal transplant recipients. *Chest* 106:435–439.

29. Hernandez-Hernandez, E., J. Alberu, L. Gonzalez-Michaca, M. Bobadilla-del Valle, R. Correa-Rotter, and J. Sifuentes-Osornio. 2006. Screening for tuberculosis in the study of the living renal donor in a developing country. *Transplantation* 81:290–292.

30. Higgins, R. S. D., S. Kusne, J. Reyes, S. Yousem, R. Gordon, and R. Van Thiel. 1992. *Mycobacterium tuberculosis* after liver transplantation: management and guidelines for prevention. *Clin. Transplant.* 6:81–90.

31. Horsburgh, C. R., Jr., S. Feldman, and R. Ridzon. 2000. Practice guidelines for the treatment of tuberculosis. *Clin. Infect. Dis.* 31:633–639.

32. Hsu, M. S., J. L. Wang, W. J. Ko, P. H. Lee, N. K. Chou, S. S. Wang, S. H. Chu, and S. C. Chang. 2007. Clinical features and outcome of tuberculosis in solid organ transplant recipients. *Am. J. Med. Sci.* 334:106–110.

33. Jereb, J. A., D. R. Burwen, S. W. Dooley, W. H. Haas, J. T. Crawford, and L. J. Geiter. 1993. Nosocomial outbreak of tuberculosis in a renal transplant unit: application of a new technique for restriction fragment polymorphism analysis of *Mycobacterium tuberculosis* isolates. *J. Infect. Dis.* 168:1219–1224.

34. Jie, T., A. J. Matas, K. J. Gillingham, D. E. Sutherland, D. L. Dunn, and A. Humar. 2005. Mycobacterial infections after kidney transplant. *Transplant. Proc.* 37:937–939.

35. John, G. T., V. Shankar, A. M. Abraham, U. Mukundan, P. P. Thomas, and C. K. Jacob. 2001. Risk factors for post-transplant tuberculosis. *Kidney Int.* 60:1148–1153.

36. John, G. T., and V. Shankar. 2002. Mycobacterial infections in organ transplant recipients. *Semin. Respir. Infect.* 17:274–283.

37. John, G. T., P. P. Thomas, M. Thomas, L. Jeyaseelan, C. K. Jacob, and J. C. Shastry. 1994. A double-blind random-ized controlled trial of primary isoniazid prophylaxis in dialysis and transplant patients. *Transplantation* 57:1683–1684.

38. Kiuchi, T., Y. Inomata, S. Uemoto, K. Satomura, H. Egawa, H. Okajima, Y. Yamaoka, and K. Tanaka. 1997. A hepatic graft tuberculosis transmitted from a living-related donor. *Transplantation* 63:905–907.

39. Kunimoto, D., A. Warman, A. Beckon, D. Doering, and L. Melenka. 2003. Severe hepatotoxicity associated with rifampin-pyrazinamide preventative therapy requiring transplantation in an individual at low risk for hepatotoxicity. *Clin. Infect. Dis.* 36:e158–e161.

40. Lawn, S. D., L. G. Bekker, and R. F. Miller. 2005. Immune re-constitution disease associated with mycobacterial infections in HIV-infected individuals receiving antiretrovirals. *Lancet Infect. Dis.* 5:361–373.

41. Lee, J., W. W. Yew, C. F. Wong, P. C. Wong, and C. S. Chiu. 2003. Multidrug-resistant tuberculosis in a lung transplant re-cipient. *J. Heart Lung Transplant.* 22:1168–1173.

42. Lichtenstein, I. H., and R. R. MacGregor. 1983. Mycobacterial infections in renal transplant recipients: report of five cases and review of the literature. *Rev. Infect. Dis.* 5:216–226.

43. Lloveras, J., P. K. Peterson, R. L. Simmons, and J. S. Najarian. 1982 Mycobacterial infections in renal transplant recipients. *Arch. Intern. Med.* 142:888–892.

44. Lopez-Montes, A., E. Gallego, E. Lopez, J. Perez, I. Lorenzo, F. Llamas, A. Serrano, E. Andres, L. Illescas, and C. Gomez. 2004. Treatment of tuberculosis with rifabutin in a renal transplant recipient. *Am. J. Kidney Dis.* 44:e59–e63.

45. Lou, H. X., M. A. Shullo, and T. P. McKaveney. 2002. Limited tolerability of levofloxacin and pyrazinamide for multidrug-resistant tuberculosis prophylaxis in a solid organ transplant population. *Pharmacotherapy* 226:701–704.

46. Lui, S. L., F. K. Li, B. Y. Choy, T. M. Chan, W. K. Lo, and K. N. Lai. 2004. Long-term outcome of isoniazid prophylaxis against tuberculosis in Chinese renal transplant recipients. *Transpl. Infect. Dis.* 6:55–56.

47. Meyers, B. R., M. Halpern, P. Sheiner, M. H. Mendelson, E. Neibart, and C. Miller. 1994. Tuberculosis in liver transplant patients. *Transplantation* 58:301–306.

48. Meyers, B. R., G. A. Papanicolaou, P. Sheiner, S. Emre, and C. Miller. 2000. Tuberculosis in orthotopic liver transplant patients: increased toxicity of recommended agents; cure of disseminated infection with nonconventional regimens. *Transplantation* 69:64–69.

49. Miró, J. M., F. Aguero, M. Laguno, M. Tuset, C. Cervera, A. Moreno, J. C. Garcia-Valdecasas, A. Rimola, and Hospital Clinic OLT in HIV Working Group. 2007. Liver transplanta-tion in HIV/hepatitis co-infection. *J. HIV Ther.* 12:24–35.

50. Miró, J. M., J. Torre-Cisnero, A. Moreno, M. Tuset, C. Que-reda, M. Laguno, E. Vidal, A. Rivero, J. Gonzalez, C. Lum-breras, J. A. Iribarren, J. Fortún, A. Rimola, A. Rafecas, G. Barril, M. Crespo, J. Colom, J. Vilardell, J. A. Salvador, R. Polo, G. Garrido, L. Chamorro, and B. Miranda. 2005. GESIDA/GESITRA-SEIMC, PNS and ONT consensus document on solid organ transplant (SOT) in HIV-infected patients in Spain (March, 2005). *Enferm. Infecc. Microbiol. Clin.* 23:353–362.

51. Modry, D. L., E. B. Stinson, P. E. Oyer, S. W. Jamieson, J. C. Baldwin, and N. E. Shumway. 1985. Acute rejection and mas-sive cyclosporine requirements in heart transplant recipients treated with rifampin. *Transplantation* 39:313–314.

52. Morales, P., A. Briones, J. J. Torres, A. Sole, D. Perez, and A. Pastor. 2005. Pulmonary tuberculosis in lung and heart-lung transplantation: fifteen years of experience in a single center in Spain. *Transplant. Proc.* 37:4050–4055.

53. Mullerova, M., J. Pekarek, and J. Nouzak. 1974. Immunosup-pression and experimental tuberculosis. *Biomed* 20:390–397.

54. Muñoz, P., C. Rodriguez, and E. Bouza. 2005. Mycobacterium tuberculosis infection in recipients of solid organ transplants. *Clin. Infect. Dis.* 40:581–587.

55. O'Brien, R. J. 2003. Development of fluoroquinolones as first-line drugs for tuberculosis--at long last! *Am. J. Respir. Crit. Care Med.* 168:1266–1268.

56. Offermann, G., F. Keller, and M. Molzahn. 1985. Low cyclo-sporin A blood levels and acute graft rejection in a renal trans-plant recipient during rifampin treatment. *Am. J. Nephrol.* 5:385–387.

57. Park, Y. S., J. Y. Choi, C. H. Cho, K. H. Chang, Y. G. Song, Y. S. Kim, and J. M. Kim. 2004. Clinical outcomes of tuberculosis in renal transplant recipients. *Yonsei Med. J.* 45:865–872.

58. Place, S., C. Knoop, M. Remmelink, S. Baldassarre, J. P. Van Vooren, F. Jacobs, F. Mascart, and M. Estenne. 2007. Para-doxical worsening of tuberculosis in a heart-lung transplant recipient. *Transpl. Infect. Dis.* 9:219–224.

59. Qunibi, W. Y., M. B. Al-Sibai, S. Taher, E. J. Harder, E. De Vol, O. Al-Furayh, and H. E. Ginn. 1990. Mycobacterial infection after renal transplantation-report of 14 cases and review of the literature. *Q. J. Med.* **77:**1039–1060.

60. Riska, H., C. Gronhagen-Riska, and J. Ahonen. 1987. Tuberculosis and renal allograft transplantation. *Transplant. Proc.* **19:**4096–4097.

61. Roman, A., C. Bravo, G. Levy, V. Monforte, R. Vidal, J. Sole, J. Maestre, and F. Morell. 2000. Isoniazid prophylaxis in lung transplantation. *J. Heart Lung Transplant.* **19:**903–906.

62. Rungruanghiranya, S., C. Ekpanyaskul, S. Jirasiritum, C. Nilthong, K. Pipatpanawong, and V. Mavichak. 2008. Tuberculosis in Thai renal transplant recipients: a 15-year experience. *Transplant. Proc.* **40:**2376–2379.

63. Sayiner, A., T. Ece, S. Duman, A. Yildiz, M. Ozkahya, Z. Kilicaslan, and Y. Tokat. 1990. Tuberculosis in renal transplant recipients. *Transplantation* **68:**1268–1271.

64. Schluger, L. K., P. A. Sheiner, M. Jonas, J. V. Guarrera, I. M. Fiel, B. Meyers, and P. D. Berk. 1996. Isoniazid hepatotoxicity after orthotopic liver transplantation. *Mt. Sinai J. Med.* **63:**364–369.

65. Singh, N., O. Lortholary, B. D. Alexander, K. L. Gupta, G. T. John, K. Pursell, P. Munoz, G. B. Klintmalm, V. Stosor, R. del Busto, A. P. Limaye, J. Somani, M. Lyon, S. Houston, A. A. House, T. L. Pruett, S. Orloff, A. Humar, L. Dowdy, J. Garcia-Diaz, A. C. Kalil, R. A. Fisher, and S. Husain. 2005. An immune reconstitution syndrome-like illness associated with Cryptococcus neoformans infection in organ transplant recipients. *Clin. Infect. Dis.* **40:**1756–1761.

66. Singh, N., and D. L. Paterson. 1998. *Mycobacterium tuberculosis* infection in solid-organ transplant recipients: impact and implications for management. *Clin. Infect. Dis.* **27:**1266–1277.

67. Singh, N., M. M. Wagener, and T. Gayowski. 2002. Safety and efficacy of isoniazid chemoprophylaxis administered during liver transplant candidacy for the prevention of posttransplant tuberculosis. *Transplantation* **74:**892–895.

68. Sinnott, J. T, and P. J. Emmanuel. 1990. Mycobacterial infections in the transplant patient. *Semin. Respir. Infect.* **5:**65–73.

69. Subramanian, A., S. Dorman, and AST Infectious Diseases Community of Practice. 2009. Mycobacterium tuberculosis in solid organ transplant recipients. *Am. J. Transplant.* **9**(Suppl. 4)**:**S57–S62.

70. Sud, K., T. Muthukumar, B. Singh, S. K. Garg, H. S. Kohli, V. Jha, K. L. Gupta, and V. Sakhuja. 2000. Isoniazid does not affect bioavailability of cyclosporine in renal transplant recipients. *Methods Find. Exp. Clin. Pharmacol.* **22:**647–649.

71. Sundberg, R., R. Shapiro, F. Darras, C. Jensen, V. Scantlebury, M. Jordan, J. McCauley, S. Kusne, M. B. Edmond, and M. Ho. 1991. A tuberculosis outbreak in a renal transplant program. *Transpl. Proc.* **23:**3091–3092.

72. Thomas, P. A., and M. A. Manko. 1975. Chemoprophylaxis for the prevention of the tuberculosis in the immunosuppressed renal allograft recipient. *Transplantation* **20:**76–77.

73. Torre-Cisneros, J., J. J. Castón, J. Moreno, A. Rivero, E. Vidal, R. Jurado, and J. M. Kindelán. 2004. Tuberculosis in the transplant candidate: importance of early diagnosis and treatment. *Transplantation* **77:**1376–1380.

74. Torre-Cisneros, J., M. De la Mata, S. Rufian, J. L. Villanueva-Marcos, J. Gutiérrez-Aroca, M. Casal, G. Miño, and C. Pera. 1995. Importance of surveillance mycobacterial cultures after liver transplantation. *Transplantation* **60:**1054–1055.

75. Torre-Cisneros, J., A. Doblas, J. M. Aguado, R. San Juan, M. Blanes, M. Montejo, C. Cervera, O. Len, J. Carratala, J. M. Cisneros, G. Bou, P. Muñoz, A. Ramos, M. Gurgui, N. Borrell, J. Fortún, A. Moreno, J. Gavalda, and Spanish Network for Research in Infectious Diseases. 2009. Tuberculosis after solid-organ transplant: incidence, risk factors, and clinical characteristics in the RESITRA (Spanish Network of Infection in Transplantation) cohort. *Clin. Infect. Dis.* **48:**1657–1665.

76. Torres, J., J. M. Aguado, R. San Juan, A. Andrés, P. Sierra, F. López-Medrano, and J. M. Morales. 2008. Hepatitis C virus, an important risk factor for tuberculosis in immunocompromised: experience with kidney transplantation. *Transpl. Int.* **21:**873–878.

77. Vandevelde, C., A. Chang, D. Andrews, W. Riggs, and P. Jewesson. 1991. Rifampin and ansamycin interactions with cyclosporine after renal transplantation. *Pharmacotherapy* **11:**88–89.

78. Vikrant, S., S. K. Agarwal, S. Gupta, D. Bhowmik, S. C. Tiwari, S. C. Dash, S. Guleria, and S. N. Mehta. 2005. Prospective randomized control trial of isoniazid chemoprophylaxis during renal replacement therapy. *Transpl. Infect. Dis.* **7:**99–108.

79. Weisdorf, D. 2003. Typical and atypical Mycobacterium infections after hemopoietic stem cell or solid organ transplantation, p. 250–258 *In* R. A. Bowden, P. Ljungman, and C. V. Paya (ed.), *Transplant Infections*, 2nd ed. Lippincott Williams & Wilkins, Philadelphia, PA.

80. Yee, D., C. Valiquette, M. Pelletier, I. Parisien, I. Rocher, and D. Menzies. 2003. Incidence of serious side effects from first-line antituberculosis drugs among patients treated for active tuberculosis. *Am. J. Respir. Crit. Care Med.* **167:**1472–1477.

81. Zhang, X. F., Y. Lv, W. J. Xue, B. Wang, C. Liu, P. X. Tian, L. Yu, X. Y. Chen, and X. M. Liu. 2008. Mycobacterium tuberculosis infection in solid organ transplant recipients: experience from a single center in China. *Transplant. Proc.* **40:**1382–1385.

Chapter 34

Paradoxical Reactions and the Immune Reconstitution Inflammatory Syndrome

PRESTON CHURCH AND MARC A. JUDSON

INTRODUCTION

The immune response to mycobacterial infection is complex, involving several arms of the immune system. Organs are damaged by mycobacteria directly and also by the necrotic granulomatous immune response of the host to this pathogen. Ideally, mycobacterial infection is met with a balanced immune response that is sufficient to kill organisms but not so severe as to cause excessive tissue injury. Immunosuppression may promote growth of mycobacteria while decreasing tissue injury by the host response to the infection. Conversely, enhancement of the host's immune response may kill more organisms but may also result in more organ damage.

An example may be seen with highly active antiretroviral therapy (HAART) for human immunodeficiency virus (HIV)-infected individuals with mycobacterial infection. HAART may result in a heightened granulomatous response that helps rid mycobacterial organisms, but the granulomatous inflammation may cause considerable damage. Such paradoxical injurious reactions have been defined as transient worsening or appearance of new signs, symptoms, or radiographic manifestations of tuberculosis (TB) that occur after initiation of treatment and are not the result of treatment failure or a second process (13). In HIV-infected individuals, paradoxical reactions after the initiation of HAART are associated with a variety of underlying infections and have been called "the immune reconstitution inflammatory syndrome" (IRIS) (89). In cases of IRIS associated with TB, two distinct patterns of disease are recognized: (i) the progression of subclinical TB to clinical disease after the initiation of HAART, referred to as "unmasking"; and (ii) the progression or appearance of new clinical and/or radiographic disease in patients with previously recognized TB after the initiation of

HAART, the classic TB IRIS (42, 57). The following is a review of the basic clinical and immunological aspects of these phenomena.

HOST RESPONSE TO MYCOBACTERIA

TB infection is initiated via inhalation of airborne droplet nuclei containing mycobacteria into the terminal airspaces of the lung. The organisms are engulfed by alveolar macrophages with subsequent release of proinflammatory cytokines including tumor necrosis factor, interleukin-1 (IL-1), and IL-12 (63). This leads to an early inflammatory reaction that includes the recruitment of monocytes from the bloodstream into the infected area of the lung (63). Eventually, a population of specific T lymphocytes is stimulated to proliferate and participate in a cell-mediated immune reaction (63). However, prior to the development of a specific immune response, the organisms are poorly contained and mycobacteremia occurs with systemic seeding of organisms (63). The acquired specific immunity to the organism follows: antigen-presenting cells (APC) (alveolar macrophages and dendritic cells), having engulfed mycobacterial proteins, then process them into small peptides so that these peptides can be presented to naive CD4$^+$ cells via major histocompatibility complex class II molecules (63). The APC produce cytokines IL-12 and IL-1 that drive a specific immune response. IL-12 biases the immune reaction by causing additional cytokines to be released to cause a T helper 1 (Th1) response (63). IL-1 stimulates CD4$^+$ lymphocytes to produce IL-2 and upregulate lymphocyte IL-2 surface receptors, resulting in a rapid clonal expansion of specific CD4$^+$ Th1 lymphocytes. These produce gamma interferon (IFN-γ), a cytokine that activates the macrophages that have engulfed mycobacteria to produce

Preston Church • Ralph H. Johnson VAMC, Charleston, SC 29425.   **Marc A. Judson** • Division of Pulmonary and Critical Care Medicine, CSB-812, Medical University of South Carolina, Charleston, SC 29425.

a variety of substances, such as reactive oxygen and nitrogen species that are involved in growth inhibition and killing of mycobacteria (85). The central role of IFN-γ secretion by lymphocytes in mycobacterial containment is evidenced by animal models of fatal infections in the absence of this cytokine (22, 31). In addition, disseminated disease has been reported in humans with genetic abnormalities in the IFN-γ receptor (47, 77).

Although the intended effect of this immune response is eradication of mycobacteria, viable organisms persist in the lung (63). Therefore, over the next 7 to 14 days, an ongoing Th1 response results in further accumulation of macrophages and lymphocytes, culminating in granuloma formation (48, 63). The granuloma represents the manifestation of cell-mediated immunity to wall off the focus of infection and further limit the spread of TB. Viable bacteria persist within the cells of the granuloma although they fail to progressively replicate, and thereby, latent infection is established (63). These sites of latent infection could become foci of active infection both in the lungs and at distant sites.

TB AND THE "PARADOXICAL REACTION"

In the 1950s, following introduction of effective antituberculous chemotherapy, physicians noted that some patients developed a recrudescence of their illness during the first few months of therapy. Initial reports described fever and increased pulmonary infiltrates on chest radiograph in 22 of 43 newly treated children (20). Symptoms often occurred during the second or third week of isoniazid and streptomycin and persisted for a week before gradually resolving without modification or discontinuation of therapy.

Subsequent case reports in adults described worsening of pulmonary disease with paradoxical reactions, including new pleural effusions (64) and acute respiratory failure (76), although substantiation of an enhanced inflammatory response in these cases is clouded by persistent positive cultures for *M. tuberculosis*, leaving open the possibility of disease progression. A retrospective review of tuberculous pleural effusions demonstrated paradoxical worsening in 10 of 61 (16%) patients (3) with six of these patients requiring thoracentesis and five requiring corticosteroids.

Paradoxical reactions may occur in up to 25% of patients treated for tuberculous lymphadenitis, characterized by new or enlarging lymphadenopathy, which may be tender or painful (11, 14, 17). Suppuration or cutaneous fistula formation may occur, requiring surgical extirpation (14, 17). New or enlarging mass lesions (tuberculomas) are well recognized complications of antituberculous chemotherapy of central nervous system (CNS) TB (both meningitis and tuberculomas) (2, 52, 93) and pose significant management problems. The frequency of paradoxical reactions in this setting is unknown but was 50% (4 of 8) in one series (52). The time to presentation is unpredictable, ranging from 1 week to 27 months after the initiation of antituberculous chemotherapy. Corticosteroids, often used in the first 3 months of CNS TB, may contribute to a delay in the development of this complication.

The clinical features of paradoxical reaction in adults treated for TB are outlined in Table 1. Considerable variability exists due to differences in study populations (U.S. adults versus adults and children from Africa and Southeast Asia) and the spectrum of TB under treatment. In the report by Breen et al. (8), only 6 of 50 patients had disseminated TB, yet

Table 1. Clinical features: TB, paradoxical reaction and IRIS

Clinical features	Paradoxical reaction ($n = 143$)[a]	IRIS ($n \leq 417$)[b]
Median time to onset (range), days	60 (20–157)	14 (2–114)
% with CD4 ≤ 100 cells/μl		45–90
Extrapulmonary TB (%)	50–80	20–100
Disseminated TB (≥2 sites) (%)	12–30	Up to 40
Reaction at site of primary infection (%)	75	65–100
Reaction at new site (%)	25	Up to 35
Fever (%)	14	65
New or increased pulmonary signs/symptoms (%)	35	40
New or increased lymphadenopathy (%)	4–25	67
New or increased GI signs/symptoms[c] (%)	2	Up to 60
New or increased CNS signs/symptoms (%)	46	0–15
Mortality rate, all	Rare	0–9.5
Mortality rate, CNS disease (%)		Up to 30

[a]Data are from references 8, 18, and 19.
[b]Data are from references 5, 8, 9, 12, 45, 51, 53, 56, 61, 62, 65, 66, 73, 74, 79, 86, 88, 92, and 95.
[c]GI, gastrointestinal.

4 of the 5 cases of paradoxical reaction occurred in these 6 patients. Although fever at 2 to 3 weeks was prominent in the original report by Choremis, lower rates of fever and longer intervals to disease onset are characteristic of series dominated by cases of extrapulmonary TB (20).

Distinguishing paradoxical reactions from disease progression, drug fever, or secondary complications remains an important issue in TB management. Fever in conjunction with new foci of disease or worsening of preexisting disease excludes a drug reaction as the cause. In pulmonary and pleural disease, paradoxical reactions follow a typical time course, with a period of definite improvement followed by transient worsening 2 to 4 weeks later (3, 20). This temporal pattern would not be expected with progressive disease unless concomitant corticosteroids are used, which could also cause transient amelioration. In CNS and lymphatic TB, the time to presentation of a paradoxical reaction may occur 2 weeks to 8 months after the initiation of antituberculous therapy, with most episodes presenting by week 12 (2, 11, 52, 93). Initial improvement may be absent in these patients, necessitating aspiration or biopsy to distinguish paradoxical reaction from treatment failure. Most presentations of paradoxical reaction can be managed palliatively with continuation of antituberculous therapy. Corticosteroids are probably indicated for severe pleural and most CNS paradoxical reactions to manage symptoms and CNS edema. The optimum dose and duration has not been established; published recommendations for initial corticosteroid management of pleural and CNS disease are reasonable guidelines (28).

EFFECT OF HIV AND HAART ON THE GRANULOMATOUS RESPONSE

The importance of CD4$^+$ lymphocytes in the control of mycobacteria has been demonstrated in several animal models in which rapidly progressive, fatal infection has occurred when this class of lymphocytes has been depleted (69, 82, 83).

It is logical to suspect that HIV infection would hamper the granulomatous response to mycobacteria by depleting the number of circulating CD4$^+$ lymphocytes. It has been demonstrated that HIV-infected individuals with low CD4$^+$ counts have a decreased secretion of IFN-γ and decreased proliferation of peripheral blood mononuclear cells in response to mycobacterial antigens (84). This most probably explains the impaired granulomatous response to *Mycobacterium tuberculosis* that is seen in HIV-infected individuals (55) and also accounts for the high rate of active TB that is seen in this population (7, 39).

HAART has been associated with an increase in the proliferation of peripheral blood mononuclear cells and IFN-γ in response to specific mycobacterial antigens (84). These increases occur over several months and do not reach levels seen in healthy control subjects. Therefore, HAART would be expected to improve immunity to *Mycobacterium tuberculosis* by increasing the function and number of CD4$^+$ lymphocytes, thereby augmenting the Th1 response to mycobacterial antigens and improving the granulomatous response to the organism (48). Although the heightened granulomatous response from HAART would help clear mycobacterial organisms, the granulomatous inflammation itself may cause significant damage, thus resulting in IRIS.

TB IRIS CASE PRESENTATION

A 48-year-old man presented with fever and thrush. His chest radiograph showed an interstitial infiltrate proven to be due to *Pneumocystis jirovecii* pneumonia, and he responded to therapy with trimethoprim-sulfamethoxazole. HIV enzyme-linked immunosorbent assay and Western blot were positive, and his CD4 cell count was 75 cells/microliter. A purified protein derivative TB skin test was negative.

One month later, his chest radiograph was normal (Fig. 1A). His HIV viral load was 442,000 copies/ml and antiretroviral therapy was initiated with zidovudine, lamivudine, and indinavir. After three months on this antiretroviral regimen, his CD4 count had increased to 167 and his viral load had decreased to <400 copies/ml. He then presented with wheezing and cough when lying on his left side. Auscultation of the chest was normal. Radiologic studies demonstrated a mass in the left hilum (Fig. 1B and C). Bronchoscopy revealed an endobronchial mass at the orifice of the left upper lobe and biopsy specimens revealed caseating granulomata. Special stains and cultures for acid-fast bacilli and fungi were negative. A purified protein derivative test result was now 12 mm. A diagnosis of pulmonary TB was made, and antituberculous therapy was administered. His symptoms resolved completely and he remains well 7 years later.

COMMENT ON CASE: "UNMASKING" IRIS

Two distinct presentations of IRIS are currently recognized with *M. tuberculosis*. This case is typical of "unmasking" TB IRIS, defined as the appearance of symptomatic TB in a patient not on antituberculous medications within 3 months after the initiation of HAART (60), a period that generally coincides

A

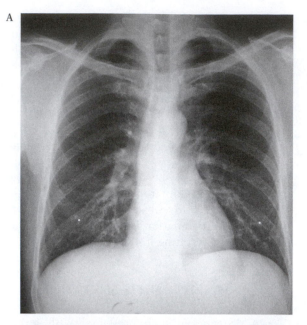

B

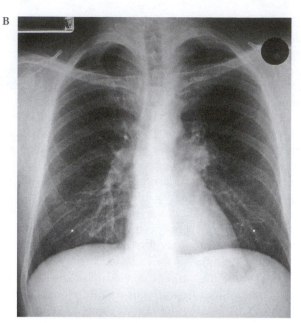

C

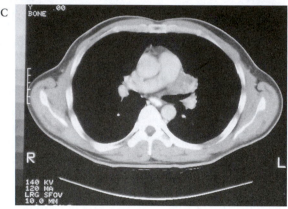

Figure 1. Chest X ray before (A) and 3 months after (B) initiation of antiretroviral therapy, demonstrating a new left hilar mass (arrow). Chest computed tomography scan (C) demonstrates a 2.0- by 2.0- by 2.5-cm heterogeneous mass just anterior to the left upper lobe bronchus. The lung parenchyma is normal, and no mediastinal adenopathy is present.

with a rise in the absolute CD4 count and a decline in HIV viremia. During this time period, TB incidence rates are higher than the period prior to the initiation of HAART, suggesting that the occurrence of cases during this period is more than just TB reactivation due to immune suppression. These cases often display disease manifestations beyond what would be expected by reactivation alone and suggest a strong inflammatory component to the disease (24, 37, 60). Unmasking presentations have been more commonly associated with infection by low-virulence organisms such as *Mycobacterium avium* complex (89). Because of the more virulent nature of *M. tuberculosis* and the greater likelihood of progression to symptomatic disease when CD4 counts are low, the window of time where infection is subclinical would appear to be small. It is also clear, however, that a substantial number of HIV-infected patients with low CD4 counts may harbor latent infection, as shown by tuberculin skin test conversion after restoration of CD4 counts above 200 (36), or are asymptomatically infected, as

demonstrated by screening studies from South Africa with rates of asymptomatic, culture-proven infection of 5% (97).

Patients with unmasking TB IRIS respond to usual antituberculous therapy as expected, although corticosteroids have been used in cases presenting with either miliary disease or severe lung injury (37). The key to reducing the occurrence of this syndrome rests with improved TB screening and diagnostics in patients at risk to identify candidates for antituberculous therapy prior to clinical illness.

One important distinction in *M. tuberculosis*-associated IRIS is the importance of immune reconstitution due to antiretroviral therapy versus the reversal of immunosuppressive effects attributable to TB alone (the "paradoxical reaction" described previously). The occurrence of IRIS in the absence of antituberculous therapy suggests that antiretroviral therapy is important in the pathogenesis of IRIS and that the paradoxical reaction and IRIS are not the same.

TYPICAL (OR "PARADOXICAL") TB-ASSOCIATED IRIS

The more common presentation of IRIS occurs after initiating antiretroviral therapy in HIV patients already on treatment for *M. tuberculosis*. This situation commonly arises when patients present with symptomatic TB and are diagnosed with HIV infection as part of the initial evaluation. Four case series from the United States compare the incidence of IRIS in HIV-infected patients simultaneously or subsequently assigned to HAART to the incidence of paradoxical reactions in patients with (73, 74, 95) or without (74) HIV. Incidence rates were 11 to 36% in the patients receiving HAART and 0 to 10% in the various control groups. When one patient cohort (73) was reassessed on the basis of radiographic changes alone, the incidence of IRIS was 45% (30). Three of these studies concluded that the incidence of IRIS in patients receiving HAART was significantly greater than the incidence of paradoxical reactions (8, 73, 74,) Although the frequency of IRIS was not statistically different in one study (95), patients receiving HAART required hospitalization because of fever, weight loss, and lymphadenitis or psoas abscess within 4 weeks of initiating antiretroviral therapy (95). By contrast, the patients with TB and HIV but not receiving HAART who developed paradoxical worsening had only new or enlarging lymphadenopathy which occurred in the setting of weight gain and resolving pulmonary infiltrates (95).

Tables 1 and 2 outline the clinical characteristics and incidence of IRIS, respectively. Recent prospective studies confirm TB IRIS rates of 12 to 20% when HAART is initiated during the first 10 weeks of antituberculous therapy (1, 29). The median time to onset of IRIS is 14 days in most series, although the time of presentation may range widely (8, 29, 56, 62, 65, 73, 92). Fever and new or increasing lymphadenopathy are the most common presenting symptoms. Radiographic findings usually include new or worsening lymphadenopathy and worsening localized pulmonary infiltrates (30, 73). Newly recognized foci of infection occur in up to 25% of patients and may include cervical adenopathy (8, 73, 95); visceral, musculoskeletal (95), or subcutaneous abscesses (73); pleural effusions (8, 34, 73); ascites (8, 34, 36, 73); hepatitis (34); epididymitis and orchitis (34); CNS tuberculomas (8, 45); ileitis with intestinal perforation (41); or granulomatous nephritis (46). Recently, there has been an increasing appreciation of intra-abdominal presentations of IRIS, and frequencies of

Table 2. Incidence: TB, paradoxical reaction, and IRIS

Reference	Incidence (no. with response/total no. [%])			
	HIV positive on HAART (IRIS)	HIV positive on HAART (unmasking)	HIV positive, no HAART (paradoxical reaction)	HIV negative (paradoxical reaction)
73	12/33 (36)		2/28 (7)	1/55 (2)
45	6/69 (9)			
95	3/28 (11)		3/44 (7)	
74	6/17 (35)		0/59	
19				16/104 (15.4)
8	14/50 (28)			5/50 (10)
9	16/37 (43)			
51	11/144 (7.6)			
88	26/86 (30)			
66	14/55 (26)			
61	21/167 (12.6)			
56	19/160 (12)			
86	10/84 (12)			
92	15/101 (15)			
12	19/109 (17)	6/21 (29)		
5	13/45 (29)			
62	23/126 (18)			
29	15/75 (20)	11/231 (4.8)		
87	0/70 (0)			
1	53/429 (12.4)[a]			
42	18/102 (18)	19/396 (4.8)		
79[b]	22/109 (20)		17/100 (17)	4/83 (4.8)

[a]Early therapy group only.
[b]Incidence of IRIS may be underestimated and incidence of paradoxical reaction in HIV-positive patients may be overestimated due to the nature of data presentation.

35 to 60% have been reported (56, 65). Up to half of these presentations may include hepatic involvement that is difficult to distinguish from antituberculous and antiretroviral drug toxicity, exacerbations of hepatitis as a frequent comorbid condition, or disease progression. It remains a key challenge in all IRIS presentations to distinguish TB IRIS from treatment failure and disease progression due to antituberculous drug resistance, overwhelming disease, comorbid conditions, or even IRIS to other coexisting pathogens (78).

Risk factors for developing IRIS have yet to be fully defined. In many reports, absolute CD4 counts have been lower and viral loads higher at baseline in the group developing IRIS, but the values overlap considerably. IRIS is more frequently identified in patients with disseminated infection (8, 9, 95) and is more likely to occur when antiretroviral therapy is started within 4 to 6 weeks of antituberculous therapy (8, 29). In most studies, the absolute increase in CD4 count is not a risk factor. Breton et al. (9) found a strong correlation with the change in CD4 percentages (median of +11% in patients with IRIS versus 2% in controls; $P < 0.001$; odds ratio, 1.34 [1.08 to 1.56]), suggesting that changes in the quality of the immune response on antiretroviral therapy is a major determinant in the occurrence of IRIS. An even stronger predictive risk factor was an increase in the CD4 percentage by $\geq 12\%$ in the first 30 days on HAART. Efforts to define this further through evaluation of specific immune responses to *M. tuberculosis* antigens have yielded inconclusive results (29). Differences in antiretroviral therapy have not proven to be risk factors, although one study (87) using a triple nucleoside regimen saw no cases of IRIS in 70 patients with HIV and TB. Less-potent suppression of HIV viral load and a less-robust rate of rise of CD4 counts may explain this observation but require further study. In the absence of reliable biomarkers to predict which patients are at risk for IRIS, it would appear on the surface that the best prevention scheme would be to delay the initiation of antiretroviral therapy until the risk period has passed. A large, randomized trial to compare early (within the first 10 weeks of antituberculous therapy) versus late (after completion of antituberculous therapy) initiation of antiretrovirals clearly demonstrated a survival advantage in the early administration group (1). Although a greater benefit to early antiretroviral administration was seen in patients with CD4 counts below 200 cells/μl, there was still a favorable trend in patients with CD4 counts between 200 and 500 cells/μl. TB IRIS occurred in 12.4% of the early treatment groups; however, no deaths were attributable to IRIS. Given the low mortality attributable to IRIS and the significant mortality incurred by delaying antiretroviral therapy, some experts now recommend that all patients on antituberculous therapy with HIV be started on antiretroviral therapy as early as possible and preferably within the first 2 months of antituberculous therapy (see also chapter 32). However, this is an area of active investigation, and recommendations are likely to evolve as relevant studies are performed.

IRIS has been successfully managed with corticosteroids in several series, and this therapy has now been validated in a randomized, placebo-controlled trial involving 109 patients using prednisone at 1.5 mg/kg of body weight/day for 2 weeks followed by 0.75 mg/kg/day for 2 weeks in the study arm (65). Although the overall mortality was too low to show a benefit, patients treated with prednisone required fewer hospital days and fewer invasive procedures. The use of prednisone in this setting does not appear to be associated with TB treatment failure (26, 34, 40, 44). Discontinuation of antiretroviral therapy is not recommended as a management strategy for IRIS; second episodes have been reported with resumption of treatment (73).

MYCOBACTERIUM AVIUM COMPLEX IRIS CASE PRESENTATION

A 40-year-old man with AIDS presented with several months' history of watery diarrhea, weight loss, night sweats, and low-grade fevers. His physical examination revealed oral candidiasis and multiple nontender, mobile, 1-cm nodes in the axillae and posterior cervical chains. Cultures of blood and stool, including cultures for mycobacteria, were negative. A chest radiograph was normal; an abdominal computed tomography scan showed 1-cm periaortic and retroperitoneal adenopathy. His CD4 count was 42 cells/microliter, and viral load was >100,000 copies/ml. HAART was initiated.

Four weeks later, the patient complained of a painful mass in his neck. Exam revealed a warm, tender, and fluctuant 3- by 5-cm mass in the right posterior neck. His CD4 count was now 200 cells/μl, and viral load was 2,800 copies/ml. Aspiration of the mass yielded 15 ml of pus; Gram stain revealed many neutrophils and gram-positive rods which were also acid-fast. Cultures were ultimately positive for *M. avium* complex. Clarithromycin and ethambutol were initiated, and antiretrovirals were continued. His neck pain gradually subsided over the next several weeks, and no new lymphadenopathy appeared.

COMMENT ON CASE: *M. AVIUM* COMPLEX IRIS

This case is typical of IRIS associated with *M. avium* complex disease occurring after the initiation of HAART. Patients usually have no prior symptoms of *M. avium* infection and have very low CD4 counts. Weeks to months after HAART is initiated, symptoms emerge, most commonly lymphadenitis. CD4 counts have usually increased, and a prominent inflammatory response with neutrophils is common.

M. AVIUM COMPLEX IRIS

Disseminated *M. avium* complex infections were first recognized in patients with AIDS in 1982 (98). Typical findings of such infections included fever, weight loss, and malaise. In addition, *M. avium* complex was usually recovered from blood or bone marrow culture. A new presentation of *M. avium* complex was first reported in 1989 (6) in three patients started on zidovudine monotherapy. One to three months after initiation of zidovudine, all 3 patients developed acute, localized lymphadenitis characterized by swelling, erythema, pain, and tenderness, with subsequent isolation of *M. avium* complex from the mass. Systemic illness, including fever, was notably absent, and in all cases, cultures of blood and bone marrow were negative. French et al. (33) observed localized *M. avium* complex disease developing 1 to 2 weeks after initiation of zidovudine in 4 patients. In all 4 patients, anergy to tuberculin had been documented prior to zidovudine monotherapy, with subsequent tuberculin reactivity appearing at the time of symptom onset. Interestingly, all 4 patients lost tuberculin reactivity by 28 weeks of zidovudine, and this was associated with the resolution of focal symptoms in all patients and subsequent mycobacteremia in 2 patients.

In contrast with *M. tuberculosis*, *M. avium* complex infection is often subclinical in the HIV-infected individual due to the low virulence of the organism. In patients with (59, 80) or without (6, 15, 80) evidence of disseminated infection, focal disease, most commonly lymphadenitis, may ensue with the initiation of HAART. Lymphadenitis is characterized by superficial or deep lymph node enlargement, frequently with erythema and tenderness and occasionally by suppuration and formation of draining sinuses (6, 15, 89). These findings characteristically present during the first 8 weeks of antiretroviral therapy. Fever may or may not be present, but the characteristic wasting seen in disseminated *M. avium* complex is absent at the time of IRIS. Disease onset correlates with a rapid

rise in CD4 count (median, 120 cells/microliter) (80, 90) and significant reductions in HIV RNA in the majority of cases. Focal extranodal disease has included granulomatous hepatitis (90), pneumonitis (81), pyomyositis with cutaneous abscesses (54), enteritis (21), colitis (90), a paravertebral abscess (25), and a CNS mass (71). The majority of extranodal cases also present within the first 8 weeks of antiretroviral therapy. Three reported cases of extranodal IRIS due to *M. avium* occurred 1 to 2 years after initiation of antiretroviral therapy (21, 25, 71). In each of these cases, the patient had been on one or more drugs for the treatment of *M. avium* complex at the time of initiation of HAART, possibly delaying or abrogating the onset of IRIS. The frequency of IRIS due to *M. avium* complex is unknown, but in patients with CD4 counts less than 200 cells/microliter at the time HAART is initiated, the overall rate of IRIS may be as high as 25%.

Biopsy specimens of lymph nodes or other involved organs show granulomatous inflammation with caseous necrosis, features not seen in patients with untreated HIV and *M. avium* infection. Acid-fast smears are frequently positive, and the organism is usually recovered from cultures of tissue. Blood and bone marrow cultures are usually negative. Management of IRIS due to *M. avium* complex disease should be directed at treating the infection and managing symptoms. The antimicrobial therapy of *M. avium* complex infection is discussed in detail in chapter 36 and has been reviewed elsewhere (49). For symptom management, a trial of nonsteroidal anti-inflammatory drugs should be considered, but no data exist to document their efficacy in this setting. Corticosteroids are effective in reducing fever and local symptoms and are useful for more serious or disabling cases (27). Although symptoms will resolve with cessation of antiretrovirals, discontinuation of these drugs is discouraged, as relapses frequently occur with the resumption of HAART (27).

THE GRANULOMATOUS RESPONSE IN SARCOIDOSIS

Our current understanding of sarcoidosis is that its development requires three major events: exposure to antigen, acquired cellular immunity directed against the antigen mediated through APC and antigen-specific T-lymphocytes, and the appearance of immune effector cells that promote a nonspecific inflammatory response (75). More specifically, alveolar macrophages from patients with pulmonary sarcoidosis show enhanced antigen-presenting capacity by the enhanced expression of HLA (major histocompatibility complex) class II molecules. This is probably induced by interaction with the sarcoidosis antigen(s) and possibly IFN-γ (23). These macrophages recognize, process, and present the putative antigen to CD4$^+$ T cells of the Th1 type (23). These activated macrophages produce IL-12 that induces a lymphocyte shift toward a Th1 profile and causes T lymphocytes to secrete IFN-γ. These activated T cells release IL-2 and chemotactic factors that recruit monocytes and macrophages to the site of disease activity. IL-2 is also activated and expands various T-cell clones (50). IFN-γ is able to further activate macrophages and to transform them into giant cells, which are important building blocks of the granuloma (50, 91).

Thus, the immunopathogenesis of granuloma formation in sarcoidosis is similar to that seen with pulmonary TB. The major difference is that the antigens responsible for granulomatous inflammation in TB are peptides resulting from digestion and processing of the microorganism, whereas in sarcoidosis the putative antigens are unknown. Like TB, CD4$^+$ cells are essential to granuloma formation.

SARCOIDOSIS IRIS CASE PRESENTATION

A 39-year-old African-American woman was admitted to the hospital after a 2-week history of increasing dyspnea, productive cough, and wheezing. Prior history included a diagnosis of sarcoidosis confirmed 9 years previously by transbronchial lung biopsy. She also had clinical evidence of sarcoidosis involvement of the skin, eye, and liver. She was receiving 20 mg of prednisone/day upon admission. On admission, her spirometry showed a 350-ml decline in forced vital capacity to 2.10 liters (67% predicted) and a 100-ml decline in forced expiratory volume in 1 s to 1.28 liters (50% predicted).

She had a history of HIV infection thought to be the result of sexual transmission. She had been receiving antiretroviral therapy with lamivudine, zidovudine, and efavirenz for a year, although for financial reasons she discontinued this therapy 5 months prior to admission and restarted it 2 months prior to admission. Three months before admission, her CD4 count was 386 cells/microliter and it had increased to 639 cells/microliter on admission. Her HIV RNA viral load decreased from 57,440 to undetectable over this period of time.

On physical examination, she was afebrile. She had indurated skin papules consistent with sarcoidosis on her left arm. Auscultation of the chest revealed minimal crackles in both posterior bases. A chest radiograph revealed fibrotic changes that were most prominent in the right upper lobe that were unchanged from previous films. A bronchoalveolar lavage was performed, and a cell count revealed 790 red blood cells/cubic mm and 289 nucleated cells/cubic mm, with 70% lymphocytes, 21% macrophages, 3% neutrophils, 3% basophils, and 2% eosinophils. Stains and cultures for mycobacteria and fungi were negative. Cytology and stains for pneumocystis were also negative. Her daily prednisone dose was increased to 40 mg/day, and she was discharged after a 3-day hospitalization. Her pulmonary symptoms slowly improved over the subsequent 2 weeks. Spirometry performed 2 weeks after discharge showed a significant improvement in forced vital capacity (2.41 liters), although the forced expiratory volume in 1 s was minimally improved at 1.33 liters.

COMMENT ON CASE

This patient had reactivation of sarcoidosis following institution of HAART, which is an uncommon presentation. This scenario has occurred more than 15 years after the diagnosis of sarcoidosis in patients who had not previously required treatment (58). The CD4 count is usually greater than 200 cells/microliter at the time of sarcoidosis reactivation (58).

TYPICAL IRIS IN SARCOIDOSIS: CLINICAL ASPECTS

New-onset sarcoidosis is rare in HIV-infected patients (44). This can probably be explained by the HIV-induced alteration in cell-mediated immunity described above (40, 67). However, several cases of sarcoidosis have been reported after initiation of HAART (Table 3) (4, 16, 32, 38, 44, 58, 67, 68, 72, 94, 96). The pathogenesis of this condition is likely to be very similar to the paradoxical reactions seen in HAART-treated HIV-infected patients with TB. It is likely that the antigen(s) that cause sarcoidosis are present in the HIV-infected individual with a low CD4$^+$ count. However, CD4$^+$ lymphocyte number and function are inadequate to mount a significant Th1-induced granulomatous response until HAART is given. Once HAART induces a granulomatous response, all of the clinical manifestations of sarcoidosis may be seen.

Sarcoidosis has developed in as little as 3 months and as long as 4 years after starting HAART (4, 72) and has developed with several different antiretroviral regimens (32). At the time of the diagnosis of sarcoidosis, the CD4$^+$ count has risen in all cases, has always exceeded 150 cells/mm^3, and is usually above 200 cells/mm^3 (32, 44, 58, 94).

Table 3. Sarcoidosis and IRIS case reports

Time of sarcoidosis onset	Reference	n	Time from sarcoidosis diagnosis to sarcoidosis exacerbation	1st documented CD$_4$ count (cells/μl)	CD$_4$ count (cells/μl) at sarcoidosis exacerbation	Organ(s) involved	Chest radiograph findings
Prior to	67	2	15–30+ yr	178, unknown	250, 371	Lung, liver	Bilateral infiltrates
HAART	68	1	3 yr	194	341	Lung, ear	Focal nodules
After HAART	68	2	4 yr	26, 11	199, 126	Lung	Hilar adenopathy, cavitary nodules
	71	2	3/15 mo	19, 275	219, 318	Lung, salivary gland	Bilateral infiltrates
	73	1	16 mo		550	Lung	Bilateral infiltrates
	70	1	Unknown	200	503	Lung	Hilar adenopathy
	67	8	29 ± 16 mo	<300 (in all)	418 ± 234 (increased in all)	Lung (all), salivary glands, liver, spleen	Scadding stages: I (2), II (2), III (4)
	74	1	20 mo	130	510	Lung, skin	Scadding stage II
	72	1	14 mo	5	235	Lung	Scadding stage I
	76	1	3 mo	151	Unknown	Joints	Unknown
	77	1	4 yr	228	435	Lung, peripheral lymph nodes	Scadding stage III
	78	5	Not reported	123–686	260–916	Lung (all), skin, peripheral lymph nodes	Scadding stages: I (2), II (1), III (2)

Sarcoidosis from immune reconstitution mirrors sarcoidosis that is not related to this entity. It most commonly occurs in the lungs, but the liver, spleen, skin, parotid glands, salivary glands, peripheral lymph nodes, and muscle may be involved (4, 16, 32, 38, 44, 58, 67, 68, 72, 94, 96). The patient may present without symptoms and with only a chest radiographic abnormality (58, 72) or with symptoms of dyspnea, cough, wheezing, or chest pain (32, 58, 94). Chest radiographs typically reveal bilateral interstitial infiltrates with or without hilar lymphadenopathy (4, 16, 32, 38, 44, 58, 67, 68, 72, 94, 96). Spirometry reveals predominantly a restrictive ventilatory defect (58, 72). The serum angiotensin-converting enzyme level is often, although not always, increased (32, 67, 72, 94). Bronchoalveolar lavage reveals a lymphocytosis in the bronchoalveolar lavage fluid (BALF). Analysis of lymphocytes in blood and BALF show a movement of CD4$^+$ lymphocytes out of the blood compartment and into the lung compartment, with a low CD4/CD8 ratio in the blood (<1.0) and a high CD4/CD8 ratio in the BALF (>5.0) (72).

The diagnosis of sarcoidosis in HIV-infected patients must be made with caution, as infectious causes of granulomatous disease must be rigorously excluded. Tuberculin skin testing is not sufficient to exclude TB, as it may be negative for up to 25% of patients with miliary disease (35, 70). All patients should undergo a diagnostic biopsy, which will show granulomatous inflammation. The specimens need to be examined appropriately for mycobacteria

and fungi. The presence of caseating granulomas suggests a diagnosis of TB and not sarcoidosis (10). However, the finding of noncaseating granulomas does not exclude TB, as this is seen with TB in 20% of cases (10).

Treatment with prednisone must be undertaken with caution, as such therapy may cause significant morbidity (or death) if the granulomatous inflammation is truly the result of infection. On occasion, the sarcoidosis IRIS will remit on its own without therapy (32, 67), and this should be considered if the patient is asymptomatic. Corticosteroids in doses of 20 to 50 mg/day have been successful in inducing a clinical response (32, 58, 94).

SUMMARY

The IRIS represents an augmentation of the patient's ability to mount a granulomatous response to specific antigens. For the patient with HIV, this occurs via a HAART-induced increase in the number and function of CD4$^+$ cells. Such cells are a key element in the granulomatous response. Although the heightened granulomatous response may effectively clear TB antigens and the unknown antigens of sarcoidosis, this inflammatory response may be directly injurious to the host. In these cases, the clinician faces the difficult clinical dilemma of balancing the benefits of an improved host response while trying to avoid its potential injurious consequences.

REFERENCES

1. **Abdool Karim, S. S., K. Naidoo, A. Grobler, N. Padayatchi, C. Baxter, A. Gray, T. Gengiah, G. Nair, S. Bamber, A. Singh, M. Khan, J. Pienaar, W. El-Sadr, G. Friedland, and Q. Abdool Karim.** 2010. Timing of initiation of antiretroviral drugs during tuberculosis therapy. *N. Engl. J. Med.* **362:**697–706.

2. **Afghani, B., and J. M. Lieberman.** 1994. Paradoxical enlargement or development of intracranial tuberculomas during therapy: case report and review. *Clin. Infect. Dis.* **19:**1092–1099.

3. **Al-Majed, S. A.** 1996. Study of paradoxical response to chemotherapy in tuberculous pleural effusion. *Respir. Med.* **90:**211–214.

4. **Almeida, F. A., Jr., J. S. Sager, and G. Eiger.** 2006. Coexistent sarcoidosis and HIV infection: an immunological paradox? *J. Infect.* **52:**195–201.

5. **Baalwa, J., H. Mayanja-Kizza, M. R. Kamya, L. John, A. Kambugu, and R. Colebunders.** 2008. Worsening and unmasking of tuberculosis in HIV-1 infected patients after initiating highly active anti-retroviral therapy in Uganda. *Afr. Health Sci.* **8:**190–195.

6. **Barbaro, D. J., V. L. Orcutt, and B. M. Coldiron.** 1989. Mycobacterium avium-Mycobacterium intracellulare infection limited to the skin and lymph nodes in patients with AIDS. *Rev. Infect. Dis.* **11:**625–628.

7. **Barnes, P. F., A. B. Bloch, P. T. Davidson, and D. E. Snider, Jr.** 1991. Tuberculosis in patients with human immunodeficiency virus infection. *N. Engl. J. Med.* **324:**1644–1650.

8. **Breen, R. A., C. J. Smith, H. Bettinson, S. Dart, B. Bannister, M. A. Johnson, and M. C. Lipman.** 2004. Paradoxical reactions during tuberculosis treatment in patients with and without HIV co-infection. *Thorax* **59:**704–707.

9. **Breton, G., X. Duval, and C. Estellat.** 2004. Factors associated with immune reconstitution inflammatory syndrome during tuberculosis in HIV-1 infected patients, abstr. 757. *11th Conf. Retrovir. Oppor. Infect.*, San Francisco, CA.

10. **Brice, E. A., W. Friedlander, E. D. Bateman, and R. E. Kirsch.** 1995. Serum angiotensin-converting enzyme activity, concentration, and specific activity in granulomatous interstitial lung disease, tuberculosis, and COPD. *Chest* **107:**706–710.

11. **British Thoracic Society Research Committee.** 1985. Short course chemotherapy for tuberculosis of lymph nodes: a controlled trial. *Br. Med. J. (Clin. Res. Ed.)* **290:**1106–1108.

12. **Burman, W., S. Weis, A. Vernon, A. Khan, D. Benator, B. Jones, C. Silva, B. King, C. LaHart, B. Mangura, M. Weiner, and W. El-Sadr.** 2007. Frequency, severity and duration of immune reconstitution events in HIV-related tuberculosis. *Int. J. Tuberc. Lung Dis.* **11:**1282–1289.

13. **Burman, W. J., and B. E. Jones.** 2001. Treatment of HIV-related tuberculosis in the era of effective antiretroviral therapy. *Am. J. Respir. Crit. Care Med.* **164:**7–12.

14. **Byrd, R. B., R. K. Bopp, D. R. Gracey, and E. M. Puritz.** 1971. The role of surgery in tuberculous lymphadenitis in adults. *Am. Rev. Respir. Dis.* **103:**816–820.

15. **Cabie, A., S. Abel, A. Brebion, N. Desbois, and G. Sobesky.** 1998. Mycobacterial lymphadenitis after initiation of highly active antiretroviral therapy. *Eur. J. Clin. Microbiol. Infect. Dis.* **17:**812–813.

16. **Calabrese, L. H., E. Kirchner, and R. Shrestha.** 2005. Rheumatic complications of human immunodeficiency virus infection in the era of highly active antiretroviral therapy: emergence of a new syndrome of immune reconstitution and changing patterns of disease. *Semin. Arthritis Rheum.* **35:**166–174.

17. **Campbell, I. A., and A. J. Dyson.** 1977. Lymph node tuberculosis: a comparison of various methods of treatment. *Tubercle* **58:**171–179.

18. **Cheng, V. C., P. L. Ho, R. A. Lee, K. S. Chan, K. K. Chan, P. C. Woo, S. K. Lau, and K. Y. Yuen.** 2002. Clinical spectrum of paradoxical deterioration during antituberculosis therapy in non-HIV-infected patients. *Eur. J. Clin. Microbiol. Infect. Dis.* **21:**803–809.

19. **Cheng, V. C., W. C. Yam, P. C. Woo, S. K. Lau, I. F. Hung, S. P. Wong, W. C. Cheung, and K. Y. Yuen.** 2003. Risk factors for development of paradoxical response during antituberculosis therapy in HIV-negative patients. *Eur. J. Clin. Microbiol. Infect. Dis.* **22:**597–602.

20. **Choremis, C. B., C. Padiatellis, D. Zou Mbou Lakis, and D. Yannakos.** 1955. Transitory exacerbation of fever and roentgenographic findings during treatment of tuberculosis in children. *Am. Rev. Tuberc.* **72:**527–536.

21. **Cinti, S. K., D. R. Kaul, P. E. Sax, L. R. Crane, and P. H. Kazanjian.** 2000. Recurrence of Mycobacterium avium infection in patients receiving highly active antiretroviral therapy and antimycobacterial agents. *Clin. Infect. Dis.* **30:**511–514.

22. **Cooper, A. M., D. K. Dalton, T. A. Stewart, J. P. Griffin, D. G. Russell, and I. M. Orme.** 1993. Disseminated tuberculosis in interferon gamma gene-disrupted mice. *J. Exp. Med.* **178:**2243–2247.

23. **Costabel, U.** 2001. Sarcoidosis: clinical update. *Eur. Respir. J. Suppl.* **32:**56S–68S.

24. **Crump, J. A., M. J. Tyrer, S. J. Lloyd-Owen, L. Y. Han, M. C. Lipman, and M. A. Johnson.** 1998. Miliary tuberculosis with paradoxical expansion of intracranial tuberculomas complicating human immunodeficiency virus infection in a patient receiving highly active antiretroviral therapy. *Clin. Infect. Dis.* **26:**1008–1009.

25. **Currier, J. S., P. L. Williams, S. L. Koletar, S. E. Cohn, R. L. Murphy, A. E. Heald, R. Hafner, E. L. Bassily, H. M. Lederman, C. Knirsch, C. A. Benson, H. Valdez, J. A. Aberg, J. A. McCutchan, et al.** 2000. Discontinuation of Mycobacterium avium complex prophylaxis in patients with antiretroviral therapy-induced increases in CD4+ cell count. A randomized, double-blind, placebo-controlled trial. *Ann. Intern. Med.* **133:**493–503.

26. **de Jong, B. C., D. M. Israelski, E. L. Corbett, and P. M. Small.** 2004. Clinical management of tuberculosis in the context of HIV infection. *Annu. Rev. Med.* **55:**283–301.

27. **Desimone, J. A., Jr., T. J. Babinchak, K. R. Kaulback, and R. J. Pomerantz.** 2003. Treatment of Mycobacterium avium complex immune reconstitution disease in HIV-1-infected individuals. *AIDS Patient Care STDS* **17:**617–622.

28. **Dooley, D. P., J. L. Carpenter, and S. Rademacher.** 1997. Adjunctive corticosteroid therapy for tuberculosis: a critical reappraisal of the literature. *Clin. Infect. Dis.* **25:**872–887.

29. **Elliott, J. H., K. Vohith, S. Saramony, C. Savuth, C. Dara, C. Sarim, S. Huffam, R. Oelrichs, P. Sophea, V. Saphonn, J. Kaldor, D. A. Cooper, M. Chhi Vun, and M. A. French.** 2009. Immunopathogenesis and diagnosis of tuberculosis and tuberculosis-associated immune reconstitution inflammatory syndrome during early antiretroviral therapy. *J. Infect. Dis.* **200:**1736–1745.

30. **Fishman, J. E., E. Saraf-Lavi, M. Narita, E. S. Hollender, R. Ramsinghani, and D. Ashkin.** 2000. Pulmonary tuberculosis in AIDS patients: transient chest radiographic worsening after initiation of antiretroviral therapy. *AJR Am. J. Roentgenol.* **174:**43–49.

31. **Flynn, J. L., J. Chan, K. J. Triebold, D. K. Dalton, T. A. Stewart, and B. R. Bloom.** 1993. An essential role for interferon gamma

in resistance to Mycobacterium tuberculosis infection. *J. Exp. Med.* **178:**2249–2254.

32. Foulon, G., M. Wislez, J. M. Naccache, F. X. Blanc, A. Rabbat, D. Israel-Biet, D. Valeyre, C. Mayaud, and J. Cadranel. 2004. Sarcoidosis in HIV-infected patients in the era of highly active antiretroviral therapy. *Clin. Infect. Dis.* **38:**418–425.

33. French, M. A., S. A. Mallal, and R. L. Dawkins. 1992. Zidovudine-induced restoration of cell-mediated immunity to mycobacteria in immunodeficient HIV-infected patients. *AIDS* **6:**1293–1297.

34. Furrer, H., and R. Malinverni. 1999. Systemic inflammatory reaction after starting highly active antiretroviral therapy in AIDS patients treated for extrapulmonary tuberculosis. *Am. J. Med.* **106:**371–372.

35. Geppert, E. F., and A. Leff. 1979. The pathogenesis of pulmonary and miliary tuberculosis. *Arch. Intern. Med.* **139:**1381–1383.

36. Girardi, E., F. Palmieri, M. Zaccarelli, V. Tozzi, M. P. Trotta, C. Selva, P. Narciso, N. Petrosillo, A. Antinori, and G. Ippolito. 2002. High incidence of tuberculin skin test conversion among HIV-infected individuals who have a favourable immunological response to highly active antiretroviral therapy. *AIDS* **16:**1976–1979.

37. Goldsack, N. R., S. Allen, and M. C. Lipman. 2003. Adult respiratory distress syndrome as a severe immune reconstitution disease following the commencement of highly active antiretroviral therapy. *Sex. Transm. Infect.* **79:**337–338.

38. Gomez, V., P. R. Smith, J. Burack, R. Daley, and U. Rosa. 2000. Sarcoidosis after antiretroviral therapy in a patient with acquired immunodeficiency syndrome. *Clin. Infect. Dis.* **31:**1278–1280.

39. Graham, N. M., and R. E. Chaisson. 1993. Tuberculosis and HIV infection: epidemiology, pathogenesis, and clinical aspects. *Ann. Allergy* **71:**421–433.

40. Granieri, J., J. J. Wisnieski, R. C. Graham, H. Smith, P. Gogate, and J. N. Aucott. 1995. Sarcoid myopathy in a patient with human immunodeficiency virus infection. *South. Med. J.* **88:**591–595.

41. Guex, A. C., H. C. Bucher, N. Demartines, U. Fluckiger, and M. Battegay. 2002. Inflammatory bowel perforation during immune restoration after one year of antiretroviral and antituberculous therapy in an HIV-1-infected patient: report of a case. *Dis. Colon Rectum* **45:**977–978.

42. Haddow, L. J., P. J. Easterbrook, A. Mosam, N. G. Khanyile, R. Parboosing, P. Moodley, and M. Y. Moosa. 2009. Defining immune reconstitution inflammatory syndrome: evaluation of expert opinion versus 2 case definitions in a South African cohort. *Clin. Infect. Dis.* **49:**1424–1432.

43. Haddow, L. J., M. Y. Moosa, and P. J. Easterbrook. 2010. Validation of a published case definition for tuberculosis-associated immune reconstitution inflammatory syndrome. *AIDS* **24:**103–108.

44. Haramati, L. B., G. Lee, A. Singh, P. L. Molina, and C. S. White. 2001. Newly diagnosed pulmonary sarcoidosis in HIV-infected patients. *Radiology* **218:**242–246.

45. Hollender, E., M. Narita, and D. Ashkin. 2000. CNS manifestations of paradoxical reaction in HIV+ TB patients on HAART, abstr. 258. *7th Conf. Retrovir. Oppor. Infect.,* San Francisco, CA.

46. Jehle, A. W., N. Khanna, J. P. Sigle, K. Glatz-Krieger, M. Battegay, J. Steiger, M. Dickenmann, and H. H. Hirsch. 2004. Acute renal failure on immune reconstitution in an HIV-positive patient with miliary tuberculosis. *Clin. Infect. Dis.* **38:**e32–e35.

47. Jouanguy, E., F. Altare, S. Lamhamedi, P. Revy, J. F. Emile, M. Newport, M. Levin, S. Blanche, E. Seboun, A. Fischer, and J. L.

Casanova. 1996. Interferon-gamma-receptor deficiency in an infant with fatal bacille Calmette-Guerin infection. *N. Engl. J. Med.* **335:**1956–1961.

48. Judson, M. A. 2002. Highly active antiretroviral therapy for HIV with tuberculosis: pardon the granuloma. *Chest* **122:**399–400.

49. Karakousis, P. C., R. D. Moore, and R. E. Chaisson. 2004. Mycobacterium avium complex in patients with HIV infection in the era of highly active antiretroviral therapy. *Lancet Infect. Dis.* **4:**557–565.

50. Konishi, K., D. R. Moller, C. Saltini, M. Kirby, and R. G. Crystal. 1988. Spontaneous expression of the interleukin 2 receptor gene and presence of functional interleukin 2 receptors on T lymphocytes in the blood of individuals with active pulmonary sarcoidosis. *J. Clin. Investig.* **82:**775–781.

51. Kumarasamy, N., S. Chaguturu, K. H. Mayer, S. Solomon, H. T. Yepthomi, P. Balakrishnan, and T. P. Flanigan. 2004. Incidence of immune reconstitution syndrome in HIV/tuberculosis-coinfected patients after initiation of generic antiretroviral therapy in India. *J. Acquir. Immune Defic. Syndr.* **37:**1574–1576.

52. Labhard, N., L. Nicod, and J. P. Zellweger. 1994. Cerebral tuberculosis in the immunocompetent host: 8 cases observed in Switzerland. *Tuber. Lung Dis.* **75:**454–459.

53. Lawn, S. D., L. G. Bekker, and R. F. Miller. 2005. Immune reconstitution disease associated with mycobacterial infections in HIV-infected individuals receiving antiretrovirals. *Lancet Infect. Dis.* **5:**361–373.

54. Lawn, S. D., T. A. Bicanic, and D. C. Macallan. 2004. Pyomyositis and cutaneous abscesses due to Mycobacterium avium: an immune reconstitution manifestation in a patient with AIDS. *Clin. Infect. Dis.* **38:**461–463.

55. Lawn, S. D., S. T. Butera, and T. M. Shinnick. 2002. Tuberculosis unleashed: the impact of human immunodeficiency virus infection on the host granulomatous response to Mycobacterium tuberculosis. *Microbes Infect.* **4:**635–646.

56. Lawn, S. D., L. Myer, L. G. Bekker, and R. Wood. 2007. Tuberculosis-associated immune reconstitution disease: incidence, risk factors and impact in an antiretroviral treatment service in South Africa. *AIDS* **21:**335–341.

57. Lawn, S. D., R. J. Wilkinson, M. C. Lipman, and R. Wood. 2008. Immune reconstitution and "unmasking" of tuberculosis during antiretroviral therapy. *Am. J. Respir. Crit. Care Med.* **177:**680–685.

58. Lenner, R., Z. Bregman, A. S. Teirstein, and L. DePalo. 2001. Recurrent pulmonary sarcoidosis in HIV-infected patients receiving highly active antiretroviral therapy. *Chest* **119:**978–981.

59. Mallal, S. A., I. R. James, and M. A. French. 1994. Detection of subclinical Mycobacterium avium intracellulare complex infection in immunodeficient HIV-infected patients treated with zidovudine. *AIDS* **8:**1263–1269.

60. Manabe, Y. C., R. Breen, T. Perti, E. Girardi, and T. R. Sterling. 2009. Unmasked tuberculosis and tuberculosis immune reconstitution inflammatory disease: a disease spectrum after initiation of antiretroviral therapy. *J. Infect. Dis.* **199:**437–444.

61. Manosuthi, W., S. Kiertiburanakul, T. Phoorisri, and S. Sungkanuparph. 2006. Immune reconstitution inflammatory syndrome of tuberculosis among HIV-infected patients receiving antituberculous and antiretroviral therapy. *J. Infect.* **53:**357–363.

62. Manosuthi, W., H. Van Tieu, W. Mankatitham, A. Lueangniyomkul, J. Ananworanich, A. Avihingsanon, U. Siangphoe, S. Klongugkara, S. Likanonsakul, U. Thawornwan, B. Suntisuk-

lappon, and S. Sungkanuparph. 2009. Clinical case definition and manifestations of paradoxical tuberculosis-associated immune reconstitution inflammatory syndrome. *AIDS* **23:**2467–2471.

63. Mason, C. M., and J. Ali. 2004. Immunity against mycobacteria. *Semin. Respir. Crit. Care Med.* **25:**53–61.

64. Matthay, R. A., T. A. Neff, and M. D. Iseman. 1974. Tuberculous pleural effusions developing during chemotherapy for pulmonary tuberculosis. *Am. Rev. Respir. Dis.* **109:**469–472.

65. Meintjes, G., R. Wilkinson, C. Morroni, D. Pepper, K. Rebe, M. Rangakal, T. Oni, and G. Martens. 2009. Randomized placebo-controlled trial of prednisone for the TB reconstitution inflammatory syndrome, abstr. 34. *16th Conf. Retrovir. Oppor. Infect.*, Montreal, Canada.

66. Michailidis, C., A. L. Pozniak, S. Mandalia, S. Basnayake, M. R. Nelson, and B. G. Gazzard. 2005. Clinical characteristics of IRIS syndrome in patients with HIV and tuberculosis. *Antivir. Ther.* **10:**417–422.

67. Mirmirani, P., T. A. Maurer, B. Herndier, M. McGrath, M. D. Weinstein, and T. G. Berger. 1999. Sarcoidosis in a patient with AIDS: a manifestation of immune restoration syndrome. *J. Am. Acad. Dermatol.* **41:**285–286.

68. Morris, D. G., R. M. Jasmer, L. Huang, M. B. Gotway, S. Nishimura, and T. E. King, Jr. 2003. Sarcoidosis following HIV infection: evidence for CD4+ lymphocyte dependence. *Chest* **124:**929–935.

69. Muller, I., S. P. Cobbold, H. Waldmann, and S. H. Kaufmann. 1987. Impaired resistance to *Mycobacterium tuberculosis* infection after selective in vivo depletion of L3T4+ and Lyt-2+ T cells. *Infect. Immun.* **55:**2037–2041.

70. Munt, P. W. 1972. Miliary tuberculosis in the chemotherapy era: with a clinical review in 69 American adults. *Medicine* (Baltimore) **51:**139–155.

71. Murray, R., S. Mallal, C. Heath, and M. French. 2001. Cerebral Mycobacterium avium infection in an HIV-infected patient following immune reconstitution and cessation of therapy for disseminated Mycobacterium avium complex infection. *Eur. J. Clin. Microbiol. Infect. Dis.* **20:**199–201.

72. Naccache, J. M., M. Antoine, M. Wislez, J. Fleury-Feith, E. Oksenhendler, C. Mayaud, and J. Cadranel. 1999. Sarcoid-like pulmonary disorder in human immunodeficiency virus-infected patients receiving antiretroviral therapy. *Am. J. Respir. Crit. Care Med.* **159:**2009–2013.

73. Narita, M., D. Ashkin, E. S. Hollender, and A. E. Pitchenik. 1998. Paradoxical worsening of tuberculosis following antiretroviral therapy in patients with AIDS. *Am. J. Respir. Crit. Care Med.* **158:**157–161.

74. Navas, E., P. Martin-Davila, L. Moreno, V. Pintado, J. L. Casado, J. Fortun, M. J. Perez-Elias, E. Gomez-Mampaso, and S. Moreno. 2002. Paradoxical reactions of tuberculosis in patients with the acquired immunodeficiency syndrome who are treated with highly active antiretroviral therapy. *Arch. Intern. Med.* **162:**97–99.

75. Newman, L. S., C. S. Rose, and L. A. Maier. 1997. Sarcoidosis. *N. Engl. J. Med.* **336:**1224–1234.

76. Onwubalili, J. K., G. M. Scott, and H. Smith. 1986. Acute respiratory distress related to chemotherapy of advanced pulmonary tuberculosis: a study of two cases and review of the literature. *Q. J. Med.* **59:**599–610.

77. Ottenhoff, T. H., D. Kumararatne, and J. L. Casanova. 1998. Novel human immunodeficiencies reveal the essential role of type-I cytokines in immunity to intracellular bacteria. *Immunol. Today* **19:**491–494.

78. Pepper, D. J., S. Marais, G. Maartens, K. Rebe, C. Morroni, M. X. Rangaka, T. Oni, R. J. Wilkinson, and G. Meintjes. 2009. Neurologic manifestations of paradoxical tuberculosis-associated immune reconstitution inflammatory syndrome: a case series. *Clin. Infect. Dis.* **48:**e96–e107.

79. Pepper, D. J., S. Marais, R. J. Wilkinson, F. Bhaijee, G. Maartens, H. McIlleron, V. De Azevedo, H. Cox, C. McDermid, S. Sokhela, J. Patel, and G. Meintjes. 2010. Clinical deterioration during antituberculosis treatment in Africa: incidence, causes and risk factors. *BMC Infect Dis.* **10:**83.

80. Phillips, P., M. B. Kwiatkowski, M. Copland, K. Craib, and J. Montaner. 1999. Mycobacterial lymphadenitis associated with the initiation of combination antiretroviral therapy. *J. Acquir. Immune Defic. Syndr. Hum. Retrovirol.* **20:**122–128.

81. Salama, C., M. Policar, and M. Venkataraman. 2003. Isolated pulmonary Mycobacterium avium complex infection in patients with human immunodeficiency virus infection: case reports and literature review. *Clin. Infect. Dis.* **37:**e35–e40.

82. Saunders, B. M., A. A. Frank, I. M. Orme, and A. M. Cooper. 2002. CD4 is required for the development of a protective granulomatous response to pulmonary tuberculosis. *Cell. Immunol.* **216:**65–72.

83. Scanga, C. A., V. P. Mohan, K. Yu, H. Joseph, K. Tanaka, J. Chan, and J. L. Flynn. 2000. Depletion of CD4(+) T cells causes reactivation of murine persistent tuberculosis despite continued expression of interferon gamma and nitric oxide synthase 2. *J. Exp. Med.* **192:**347–358.

84. Schluger, N. W., D. Perez, and Y. M. Liu. 2002. Reconstitution of immune responses to tuberculosis in patients with HIV infection who receive antiretroviral therapy. *Chest* **122:**597–602.

85. Schluger, N. W., and W. N. Rom. 1998. The host immune response to tuberculosis. *Am. J. Respir. Crit. Care Med.* **157:**679–691.

86. Serra, F. C., D. Hadad, R. L. Orofino, F. Marinho, C. Lourenco, M. Morgado, and V. Rolla. 2007. Immune reconstitution syndrome in patients treated for HIV and tuberculosis in Rio de Janeiro. *Braz. J. Infect. Dis.* **11:**462–465.

87. Shao, H. J., J. A. Crump, H. O. Ramadhani, L. O. Ulso, S. Ole-Nguyaine, A. M. Moon, R. A. Kuwera, C. W. Woods, J. F. Shao, H. A. Bartlett, and N. M. Thielman. 2009. Early versus delayed fixed dose combination abacavir/lamivudine/zidovudine in patients with HIV and tuberculosis in Tanzania. *AIDS Res. Hum. Retrovir.* **25:**1277–1285.

88. Shelburne, S. A., F. Visnegarwala, J. Darcourt, E. A. Graviss, T. P. Giordano, A. C. White, Jr., and R. J. Hamill. 2005. Incidence and risk factors for immune reconstitution inflammatory syndrome during highly active antiretroviral therapy. *AIDS* **19:**399–406.

89. Shelburne, S. A., III, and R. J. Hamill. 2003. The immune reconstitution inflammatory syndrome. *AIDS Rev.* **5:**67–79.

90. Shelburne, S. A., III, R. J. Hamill, M. C. Rodriguez-Barradas, S. B. Greenberg, R. L. Atmar, D. W. Musher, J. C. Gathe, Jr., F. Visnegarwala, and B. W. Trautner. 2002. Immune reconstitution inflammatory syndrome: emergence of a unique syndrome during highly active antiretroviral therapy. *Medicine* (Baltimore) **81:**213–227.

91. Steffen, M., J. Petersen, M. Oldigs, A. Karmeier, H. Magnussen, H. G. Thiele, and A. Raedler. 1993. Increased secretion of tumor necrosis factor-alpha, interleukin-1-beta, and interleukin-6 by alveolar macrophages from patients with sarcoidosis. *J. Allergy Clin. Immunol.* **91:**939–949.

92. Tansuphasawadkul, S., W. Saito, J. Kim, B. Phonrat, J. Dhitavat, S. Chamnachanan, and P. Pitisuttihum. 2007. Outcomes in

HIV-infected patients on antiretroviral therapy with tuberculosis. *Southeast Asian J. Trop. Med. Public Health* **38**:1053–1060.

93. Teoh, R., M. J. Humphries, and G. O'Mahony. 1987. Symptomatic intracranial tuberculoma developing during treatment of tuberculosis: a report of 10 patients and review of the literature. *Q. J. Med.* **63**:449–460.

94. Trevenzoli, M., A. M. Cattelan, F. Marino, U. Marchioro, and P. Cadrobbi. 2003. Sarcoidosis and HIV infection: a case report and a review of the literature. *Postgrad. Med. J.* **79**:535–538.

95. Wendel, K. A., K. S. Alwood, R. Gachuhi, R. E. Chaisson, W. R. Bishai, and T. R. Sterling. 2001. Paradoxical worsening of tuberculosis in HIV-infected persons. *Chest* **120**:193–197.

96. Wittram, C., J. Fogg, and H. Farber. 2001. Immune restoration syndrome manifested by pulmonary sarcoidosis. *AJR Am. J. Roentgenol.* **177**:1427.

97. Wood, R., K. Middelkoop, L. Myer, A. D. Grant, A. Whitelaw, S. D. Lawn, G. Kaplan, R. Huebner, J. McIntyre, and L. G. Bekker. 2007. Undiagnosed tuberculosis in a community with high HIV prevalence: implications for tuberculosis control. *Am. J. Respir. Crit. Care Med.* **175**:87–93.

98. Zakowski, P., S. Fligiel, G. W. Berlin, and L. Johnson, Jr. 1982. Disseminated Mycobacterium avium-intracellulare infection in homosexual men dying of acquired immunodeficiency. *JAMA* **248**:2980–2982.

III. NONTUBERCULOUS MYCOBACTERIA

Tuberculosis and Nontuberculous Mycobacterial Infections, 6th ed.
Edited by David Schlossberg
© 2011 ASM Press, Washington, DC

Chapter 35

Nontuberculous Mycobacteria—Introduction

HENRY YEAGER

INTRODUCTION

Microorganisms related to the bacteria that cause tuberculosis and leprosy are abundant in our environment and have been known since the discovery of the tubercle bacillus in the late 1800s. These organisms have been variously described by the terms "atypical," "anonymous," "mycobacteria other than tuberculosis," "environmental," "environmental opportunistic," and most commonly, "nontuberculous," or "NTM." It was not until the development of effective antibiotics for tuberculosis, however, in the 1940s and 1950s, that widespread culturing of mycobacteria was done, and the diseases associated with NTM began to be appreciated (4). Since the last edition of this book, there has been a considerable increase in the literature on NTM. The American Thoracic Society and Infectious Disease Society of America issued a joint document on the topic in 2007: "An official ATS/IDSA statement: diagnosis, treatment, and prevention of nontuberculous mycobacterial diseases" (7). A not-for-profit foundation has been established to further research on NTM disease, NTM Info and Research, Coral Gables, FL (http://www.ntminfo.org). Ongoing research and clinical trials are posted on their website. Another resource with a major interest in NTM is The Laboratory of Clinical Infectious Diseases at the NIH (Steven M. Holland, NIAID, NIH, CRC B3-4141, MSC 1684, Bethesda, MD, 20892-1684). The American Society for Microbiology has available pertinent reference publications, such as the *Manual of Clinical Microbiology*, 10th ed., available in print or in an electronic format (http://estore.asm.org).

TAXONOMY

Four groups of human pathogens are recognized in the *Mycobacterium* genus: *M. tuberculosis* complex, *M. leprae*, slowly growing NTM (includes all species of NTM except "rapid growers"), and rapidly growing mycobacteria ("RGM," as they are called in the ATS/IDSA statement mentioned above). Early on, NTM were classified by Timpe and Runyon according to their growth rate and pigment formation (16) (Fig. 1). Types I, II, and III, slow growers, took 7 days or more to grow and were told apart by their coloration. If pigment was produced only on exposure to light, they were photochromogens (type I); if pigment was produced even if grown in the dark, they were scotochromogens (type II); if they were not strongly pigmented, they were nonphotochromogens (type III). Rapid growers (type IV) grew in less than 7 days but more slowly than most bacteria. Now, species identification is recommended to be done in all cases, since this influences the choice of treatment. There are well over 125 species recognized now, and a significant portion of all NTM isolates are not presently assigned to a species.

Nucleic acid probes are now available for the most frequently seen mycobacterial species, *M. tuberculosis* complex, *M. avium* complex, *M. kansasii*, and *M. gordonae*. These tests use acridium-ester-labeled DNA probes specific for the above species and are based on release of target 16S rRNA from the microorganisms (Accuprobe; Gen-Probe, Inc., San Diego, CA). In some laboratories, high-performance liquid chromatography is used for help in identifying some members of the slowly growing NTM, by evaluating mycolic acid patterns in acid-fast bacillus (AFB) smear-positive subjects. Another promising technique is genotypic identification of NTM species by nucleic acid sequence determination (7, 9).

EPIDEMIOLOGY

Joseph Falkinham and associates at Virginia Polytechnic University, and scientists concerned with environmental biology elsewhere, have done careful

Henry Yeager • Pulmonary, Critical Care, and Sleep Medicine Division, Department of Medicine, Georgetown University Medical Center, Washington, DC 20007.

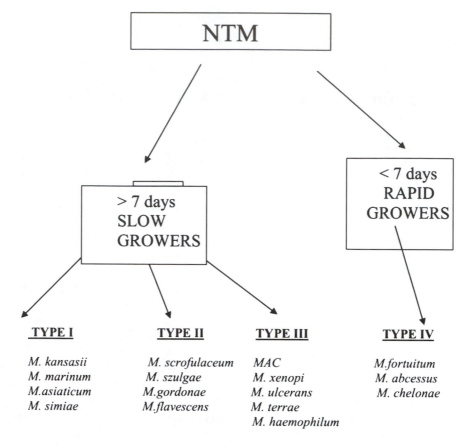

Figure 1. Classification according to Timpe and Runyon. Reprinted from *Tuberculosis & Nontuberculous Mycobacterial Infections*, 5th ed., edited by D. Schlossberg, with permission of McGraw-Hill, New York, NY.

studies of NTM in nature. Falkinham has found NTM in coastal swamps and adjoining streams and in forests, especially those rich in peat. In addition, NTM also are present in high concentrations in potting soil (5). Most recently, NTM have been reported as present in substantial concentrations in biofilms taken from showerheads (6). Feazel et al. did nucleic acid studies on material taken from showerheads in use in nine U.S. cities in different parts of the United States and compared the results from the fixtures with results obtained from water feeding into those showerheads. They amplified rRNA genes from sample DNA by PCR, using nominally universal primers, then cloned the amplicons and determined their sequences. Sequences typical of NTM were enriched to greater than 100-fold more than above background water contents in numerous showerhead biofilms. Health risks associated with this phenomenon remain to be elucidated; however, the authors in their discussion made a cautious suggestion that shower usage may be "contraindicated in persons with compromised immune or pulmonary systems."

It has seemed as if there is an increase in NTM disease in the United States and other developed countries in recent years, but it has not been clear whether this is a true increase or just better detection. There are data now that suggest that there has been an increase both in exposure and in disease. Khan et al. (11) compared the frequency of positive skin tests to the prototypical NTM species, *Mycobacterium intracellulare*, in the 1971–1972 and 1999–2000 U.S. National Health and Nutrition Examination Surveys (NHANES). The included cohorts consisted of 1,480 and 7,384 persons, respectively. Between the two surveys, there was an increase in skin positivity from 11.2 to 16.6%. Important risk factors for this sensitization included male sex, non-Hispanic black race, and birth outside the United States. The highest prevalence was in subjects in the 20- to 39-year age range. Male sex predominance was seen and was postulated to be due to greater occupational exposure.

A George Washington University/NIH group reviewed hospitalization data for pulmonary NTM admission in 11 states in the United States with data from 1998 through 2005 (2). Cases increased 3.2% per year for men and 6.5% for women in Florida and 4.6% for women in New York, with no change for men in New York and both genders in California. Hospitalization rates increased with age in both sexes. Many factors may have contributed to this rise: better clinical awareness of NTM disease and improved laboratory techniques, to be sure, but also there seems to have been a genuine increase in pulmonary NTM disease that is severe enough to warrant hospitalization (8). It is interesting that, contrary to the situation in environmental exposure, female sex and elderly persons predominate among the subjects seen with NTM disease, unless there is marked immunologic compromise, in which case all bets are off.

Cassidy et al. reported prevalence rates of NTM lung disease in Oregon in 2005–2006, using the 2007 ATS/IDSA criteria for NTM lung disease. They found that more than half of NTM isolates came from subjects who met the stated criteria for true disease. Eighty-five percent of subjects with NTM lung disease were over 50; 58% were female. There were many more subjects from the wetter, more populated western part of the state (3).

Iseman and Marras, in a 2008 editorial in the *American Journal of Respiratory and Critical Care Medicine*, suggested that in a number of industrialized countries new cases of NTM lung disease approach or exceed those of pulmonary tuberculosis (10). Furthermore, while tuberculosis is successfully treated in compliant subjects most of the time in 6 to 9 months, NTM lung disease takes 18 months to treat at best, and there is about a 50% chance of relapse and a need for retreatment.

A recent review from India suggests that increasing NTM disease is a worldwide phenomenon and not confined to the more highly industrialized nations, as has often been thought (1). It had been reported years ago that the highest pulmonary NTM rates in the world had been found in gold miners in South Africa (13), but these data seem to have been neglected.

The most common NTM cause of pulmonary disease in the United States and worldwide is the *Mycobacterium avium* complex (MAC), made up of *M. avium* and *M. intracellulare. M. kansasii*, the second most common cause of pulmonary disease, is found in the United States, Europe, South Africa, and coal-mining regions elsewhere. *M. abscessus* is worldwide in distribution and may be found alongside MAC. *M. malmoense* lung disease is common in the United Kingdom and northern Europe but not common in the United States. *M. xenopi* is common in Europe and Canada but not common in the United States (7).

It has been speculated that infection with tuberculosis and *M. bovis* bacillus-Calmette-Guérin (BCG) may provide immune protection against NTM infection; in fact, many investigations have observed decreasing rates of tuberculosis concomitant with the increase of NTM. Consistent with this idea, studies from Sweden, since the end of compulsory BCG vaccination in infants, have shown a marked rise in NTM cervical lymphadenitis (15). In addition to pulmonary infection, other sites of disease are commonly associated with specific NTM, as outlined in Table 1.

PATHOGENESIS

Early on, pulmonary NTM infections seemed to occur mainly in persons who had previous structural lung disease, such as chronic obstructive pulmonary disease, tuberculosis, histoplasmosis, or other causes of bronchiectasis. In that period, cystic fibrosis patients with bronchiectasis usually succumbed to other causes before they became infected with NTM. Disseminated NTM infections, almost always fatal, occurred in persons with profoundly suppressed cell-mediated immunity, such as those with neoplastic disease on chemotherapy or immunosuppressed because of an organ transplant. In the 1980s, with the human immunodeficiency virus/AIDS era, the occurrence of widespread abdominal and hematogenous MAC and other infections with NTM greatly increased the medical community's awareness of these pathogens. A clear-cut increase in disseminated NTM infections occurred in AIDS patients when their CD4 lymphocyte counts dropped to less than 50.

In 2008, Sexton and Harrison reviewed the range of conditions predisposing to NTM respiratory disease that had come to light in the preceding 20 or so years (17). A "distinct preexisting syndrome predisposing to NTM lung disease" of a series of thoracic connective tissue abnormalities has been reported from the NIH (12). Patients are middle-aged and older, mostly female and white or Asian, mostly nonsmokers, and taller and thinner than matched NHANES control subjects, with bronchiectasis and a striking amount of scoliosis, pectus excavatum, and mitral valve prolapse. Thirty-six percent have mutations in the cystic fibrosis transmembrane conductance regulator gene. Immunologic function is not substantially different from normal, with only a few exceptions. Impaired mucociliary clearance has been suggested as an explanation, but the relationship of NTM to the underlying body habitus is not well understood.

Persons with certain uncommon, genetically based cell-mediated immune system abnormalities are also at risk for NTM disease in general. In particular, defects in the interleukin-12/gamma interferon/STAT1 axis have been documented. There usually is more disseminated or extrapulmonary NTM disease than pulmonary NTM disease in this category of

Table 1. Features of the common species[a]

Clinical disease	Species with common etiology	Geography[b]	Morphologic features
Pulmonary disease	M. avium complex	Worldwide	Usually not pigmented, slow growth (>7 days)
	M. kansasii	USA, coal-mining regions, Europe	Pigmented; often large and beaded on acid-fast stain
	M. abscessus	Worldwide but mostly USA	Rapid growth (<7 days); not pigmented
	M. xenopi	Europe, Canada	Slow growth; pigmented
	M. malmoense	UK, northern Europe	Slow growth; not pigmented
Lymphadenitis	M. avium complex	Worldwide	Usually not pigmented
	M. scrofulaceum	Worldwide	Pigmented
	M. malmoense	UK, northern Europe (especially Scandinavia)	Slow growth
Cutaneous disease	M. marinum	Worldwide	Photochromogen; requires low temperatures (28–30°C) for isolation
	M. fortuitum	Worldwide, mostly USA	Rapid growth; not pigmented
	M. chelonae		
	M. abscessus		
	M. ulcerans	Australia, tropics, Africa, Southeast Asia	Grows slowly; pigmented
Disseminated disease	M. avium complex	Worldwide	Isolates from patients with AIDS usually pigmented (80%)
	M. kansasii	USA	Photochromogen
	M. chelonae	USA	Not pigmented
	M. haemophilum	USA, Australia	Not pigmented; requires hemin, often low temperatures, and CO_2 to grow

[a]Reprinted from *Tuberculosis & Nontuberculous Mycobacterial Infections*, 5th ed., edited by D. Schlossberg, with permission of McGraw-Hill, New York, NY.
[b]USA, United States; UK, United Kingdom.

patients. Also, among the congenital or inherited predispositions to NTM lung disease are persons born with certain human leukocyte antigen alleles, polymorphisms of the N-RAMP protein gene (also known as "soluble carrier 11A1") and polymorphisms of the vitamin D receptor.

As far as acquired causes of NTM lung disease susceptibility, human immunodeficiency virus/AIDS and immune suppression due to either malignancies or the treatments given for malignancies, or given in the course of organ transplantation, are well known. It can be speculated that certain factors that put patients at risk for pulmonary tuberculosis, such as diabetes mellitus, chronic renal failure, and oral corticosteroid treatment, may be risk factors for NTM pulmonary disease as well. Gastroesophageal reflux disease, and its treatment by acid suppressive therapy, has been speculated to be a risk factor, but there does not seem to be a lot of evidence for this contention.

A more recent cause of immune-suppression-triggered NTM lung diseases (and NTM disease generally) has been the introduction of biologic agents, especially tumor necrosis factor alpha inhibitors. In 2009, Winthrop et al. collected 239 case reports of NTM infections in patients being treated with these agents. Most patients were women, with a median age of 63 years, and had pulmonary infections. Many were taking methotrexate or steroids concurrently. Nine patients had died by the time their cases were reported (18).

The likely cellular pathogenesis of the most common NTM infections was outlined by McGarvey and Bermudez (14). NTM strains can get into the body either through the gastrointestinal or respiratory mucosal membranes, or less commonly, by inoculation. MAC can withstand normal gastric acidity and tends to be taken up by the lining cells of the small intestine, especially the enterocytes of the terminal ileum. The receptor(s) by which MAC gets into the intestinal cell is unknown. There is a change in MAC phenotype inside the epithelial cell, whereby after it exits these cells, it is better able to withstand the antimicrobial properties of the macrophage. In the respiratory tract, NTM are inhaled, from water, dirt, dust, or other aerosols, and most of the time are handled by innate host defenses, mainly mucociliary clearance and cough, and do not cause disease.

NONTUBERCULOUS MYCOBACTERIA RESEARCH FUNDING

The 2007 ATS/IDSA Statement (7) includes a section in which the authors conclude that "more fundamental information is needed to improve understanding in essentially all areas of NTM disease." This author can only agree: the greatest hindrance to research in the area may be the fact that NTM-caused illnesses are not officially reportable in all sectors of our country. Without good data about the total burden of disease caused by these organisms, it is hard to persuade those in charge of biomedical research funding to devote more funds to NTM research.

DIAGNOSIS OF DISEASE

The last ATS/IDSA Statement on Nontuberculous Mycobacterial Disease summarized criteria for diagnosis of NTM disease (7) (Table 2). For extrapulmonary disease, a combination of clinical and bacteriologic criteria (such as isolation of organisms from normally sterile sites), sometimes helped

Table 2. Clinical and microbiologic criteria for diagnosing nontuberculous mycobacterial lung disease[a]

Clinical criteria (both required)
  Pulmonary symptoms, nodular or cavitary opacities on chest radiograph, or an HRCT scan that shows multifocal bronchiectasis with multiple small nodules
  and
  Appropriate exclusion of other diagnoses

Microbiologic criteria
  Positive culture results from at least 2 separate expectorated sputum samples; if the results from 1 are nondiagnostic, consider repeat sputum AFB smears and cultures
  or
  Positive culture result from at least 1 bronchial wash or lavage
  or
  Transbronchial or other lung biopsy specimen with mycobacterial histopathologic features (granulomatous inflammation or AFB) and positive culture for NTM or biopsy specimen showing mycobaterial histopathologic features (granulomatous inflammation or AFB) and one or more sputum samples or bronchial washings that are culture positive for NTM
  Expert consultation should be obtained when NTM are recovered that are either infrequently encountered or that usually represent environmental contamination
  Patients who are suspected of having NTM lung disease but do not meet the diagnostic criteria should be monitored until the diagnosis is firmly established or excluded
  Making the diagnosis of NTM lung disease does not, per se, necessitate the institution of therapy, which is a decision based on potential risk and benefits of therapy for individual patients

[a]Adapted from reference 7, with permission.

by pathologic confirmation, is used. For diagnosis of pulmonary disease, it has been difficult to tell whether a positive culture represents only laboratory contamination, respiratory tract colonization, or true disease. A combination of clinical, radiologic, and bacteriologic features has been suggested for diagnosis of true pulmonary NTM disease.

Evaluation should include, beside appropriate history and physical, chest imaging using high-resolution computed tomography (HRCT), unless there is obvious cavitation by chest X ray. HRCT views may show scattered areas of bronchiectasis and often mixed nodular and cavitary infiltrates, with an occasional "tree in bud" pattern. At least three sputum samples need to be collected for AFB smear and culture, and other disorders excluded, in particular, *M. tuberculosis* disease. These criteria are established the best for disease caused by MAC, *M. kansasii,* and *M. abscessus.*

If possible, NTM should be identified at the species level. To repeat, DNA probes are available for the *M. tuberculosis* complex, MAC, *M. kansasii,* and *M. gordonae.*

Patients suspected of having NTM disease should be monitored closely until the diagnosis is made or excluded. Making a diagnosis of NTM disease does not automatically dictate that treatment should be started; the risk/benefit ratio must be weighed in each situation.

REFERENCES

1. Alvarez-Uria, G. 2010. Lung disease caused by nontuberculous mycobacteria. *Curr. Opin. Pulm. Med.* **16**:251–256.
2. Billinger, M. E., K. N. Olivier, C. Viboud, R. M. de Oca, C. Steiner, S. M. Holland, and D. R. Prevots. 2009. Hospitalizations for nontuberculous mycobacteria-associated lung disease, United States, 1998-2005. *Emerg. Infect. Dis.* **15**:1562–1569.
3. Cassidy, P. M., K. Hedberg, A. Saulson, E. McNelly, and K. L. Winthrop. 2009. Nontuberculous mycobacterial disease prevalence and risk factors: a changing epidemiology. *Clin. Infect. Dis.* **49**:e124–e129.
4. Chapman, J. S. 1977. *The Atypical Mycobacteria and Human Mycobacterioses.* Plenum Publishing Co., New York, NY.
5. Falkinham, J. O., III. 2009. The biology of environmental mycobacteria. *Environ. Microbiol. Rep.* **1**:477–487.
6. Feazel, L. M., L. K. Baumgartner, K. L. Peterson, D. N. Frank, J. K. Harris, and N. R. Pace. 2009. Opportunistic pathogens enriched in showerhead biofilms. *Proc. Natl. Acad. Sci. USA* **106**:16393–16399.
7. Griffith, D. E., T. Aksamit, B. A. Brown-Elliott, A. Catanzaro, C. Daley, F. Gordin, S. M. Holland, R. Horsburgh, G. Huitt, M. F. Iademarco, M. Iseman, K. Olivier, S. Ruoss, C. F. Von Reyn, R. J. Wallace, Jr., and K. Winthrop, on behalf of the ATS Mycobacterial Diseases Subcommittee. 2007. An official ATS/IDSA statement: diagnosis, treatment, and prevention of nontuberculous mycobacterial diseases. *Am. J. Respir. Crit. Care Med.* **175**:367–416.
8. Griffith, D. E. 2010. Nontuberculous mycobacterial disease. *Curr. Opin. Infect. Dis.* **23**:185–190.

9. Hall, L., K. A. Doerr, S. L. Wohlfiel, and G. D. Roberts. 2003. Evaluation of the MicroSeq system for identification of mycobacteria by 16S ribosomal DNA sequencing and its integration into a routine clinical mycobacteriology laboratory. *J. Clin. Microbiol.* **41:**1447–1453.

10. Iseman, M. D., and T. K. Marras. 2008. The importance of nontuberculous mycobacterial disease. *Am. J. Respir. Crit. Care Med.* **178:**999–1000.

11. Khan K., K. J. Wang, and T. K. Marras. 2010. Nontuberculous mycobacterial sensitization in the United States. *Am. J. Respir. Crit. Care Med.* **176:**306–311.

12. Kim, R. D., D. E. Greenberg, M. E. Ehrmantraut, S. V. Guide, L. Ding, Y. Shea, M. R. Brown, M. Chernick, W. K. Steagall, C. G. Glasgow, J. Lin, C. Jolley, L. Sorbara, M. Raffeld, S. Hill, N. Avila, V. Sachdev, L. A. Barnhart, V. L. Anderson, R. Claypool, D. Hilligoss, M. Garofalo, S. Anaya-O'Brien, D. Darnell, R. DeCastro, H. M. Menning, S. M. Ricklefs, S. F. Porcella, K. N. Olivier, J. Moss, and S. M. Holland. 2008. Pulmonary nontuberculous mycobacterial disease: prospective study of a distinct preexisting syndrome. *Am. J. Respir. Crit. Care Med.* **178:**1066–1074.

13. Marras, T. K., and C. L. Daley. 2002. Epidemiology of human pulmonary infection with nontuberculous mycobacteria. *Clin. Chest Med.* **23:**553–567.

14. McGarvey J., and L. E. Bermudez. 2002. Pathogenesis of nontuberculous mycobacteria infections. *Clin. Infect. Dis.* **23:**569–583.

15. Romanus, V., H. O. Hollander, P. Wahlen, A. M. Olinder-Nielson, P. H. W. Magnusson, and I. Juhlin. 1995. Atypical mycobacteria in extrapulmonary disease among children. Incidence in Sweden from 1969 to 1980, related to changing BCG-vaccination coverage. *Tuber. Lung Dis.* **76:**300–310.

16. Runyon, E. H. 1959. Anonymous mycobacteria in pulmonary disease. *Med. Clin. N. Am.* **43:**273–290.

17. Sexton, P., and A. C. Harrison. 2008. Susceptibility to nontuberculous mycobacterial lung disease. *Eur. Respir. J.* **31:**1322–1333.

18. Winthrop, K. L., E. Chang, S. Yamashita, M. F. Iadomarco, and P. A. LoBue. 2009. Nontuberculous mycobacteria infections and anti-tumor necrosis factor-alpha therapy. *Emerg. Infect. Dis.* **15:**1556–1560.

Tuberculosis and Nontuberculous Mycobacterial Infections, 6th ed.
Edited by David Schlossberg
© 2011 ASM Press, Washington, DC

Chapter 36

Mycobacterium avium Complex Disease

JASON E. STOUT AND CAROL D. HAMILTON

ECOLOGY AND EPIDEMIOLOGY OF MAC

Ecology and Transmission

Robert Koch announced the studies that proved that the tubercle bacillus caused tuberculosis (TB) in 1882. Investigators identified other mycobacterial species in the ensuing years by examining environmental as well as human and animal materials. It was not until the TB epidemic began to wane in the United States and Europe, however, that the pathogenic nature of some of these nontuberculous mycobacteria (NTM) began to be recognized and characterized. In 1979, Emanuel Wolinsky published a summary of the early recognition of NTM and the extensive ecologic and epidemiologic studies performed after 1950 (314). As is true today, *Mycobacterium kansasii* and *M. avium-M. intracellulare-M. scrofulaceum* complex were the organisms most commonly associated with diseases in humans. United States-based studies have found significant geographic variability in the frequency with which *M. avium-M. intracellulare* and other NTM are isolated in the environment. Soil characteristics in certain regions may favor the growth of *M. avium* complex (MAC), leading to regional differences in epidemiology. A survey of U.S. state public health laboratories in 1979 showed that the highest laboratory MAC isolation rates (>4.8 per 100,000 population) were in Florida, North Carolina, Maryland, Connecticut, Kansas, and Arizona. All of the Gulf states had rates between 3.3 and 4.8 per 100,000 population (Fig. 1 and 2) (97). *M. tuberculosis* case rates at the same time were 9.7 per 100,000 population.

Organisms belonging to the MAC (Table 1) are commonly isolated from water (151, 221, 303), house dust (139), and soil (28, 160). They are relatively resistant to chemical disinfection by chlorine, chloramines, and ozone (74, 284); as a result, the organisms can often be found in water distribution systems (75, 128). One recent molecular analysis of the communities of organisms living within showerhead assemblies showed that, compared to the chlorine-treated municipal water feeding into the system, density of NTM and, in particular, *M. avium*, was enriched 100-fold in the showerhead. Speculation that NTM resistance to chlorine gives them a selective advantage in their microenvironment was supported when the authors found that in a limited sampling of untreated well water, no mycobacterial species were isolated (77). It has also recently been shown that *M. avium* forms biofilms on plasticized polyvinyl chloride catheter tubing, and like other catheter-associated infections, organisms associated with the biofilm were significantly more resistant to clarithromycin and rifampin than non-catheter-associated organisms (73).

HIV-infected populations

There are laboratory and clinical data suggesting that *M. avium*, which is by far the most common species to infect patients with human immunodeficiency virus (HIV), is probably acquired via the gastrointestinal tract (51). MAC strains isolated from hospital water have been described as very similar to strains isolated from AIDS patients with MAC disease treated in those hospitals (13, 63, 288, 302). In a separate study, gastrointestinal inoculation of *M. avium* into immunosuppressed rodents resulted in bacteremic dissemination of the organism to the spleen and bone marrow, analogous to human disease (23, 30, 216). The predominance of *M. avium* in disseminated disease may be partially explained by the fact that *M. avium* is somewhat more resistant to gastric acid than *M. intracellulare*, and *M. avium* invades intestinal cells in both cell culture and a mouse model significantly more efficiently than *M. intracellulare* (190). In addition, gastrointestinal colonization with strains that demonstrate greater invasion

Jason E. Stout • Division of Infectious Diseases and International Health, Duke University Medical Center, Durham, NC 27710.
Carol D. Hamilton • Family Health International and Duke University Medical Center, Durham, NC 27710.

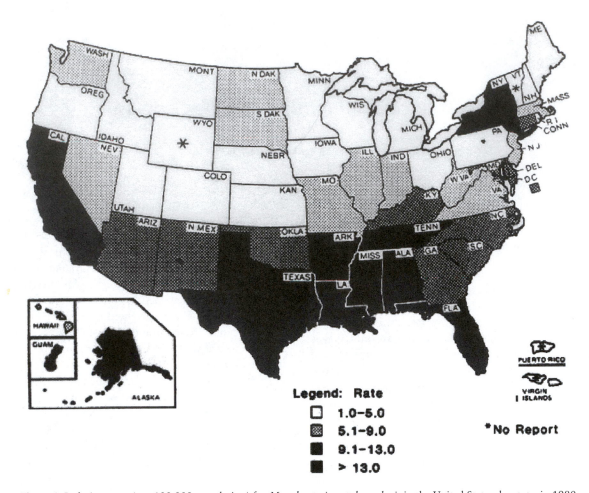

Figure 1. Isolation rates (per 100,000 population) for *Mycobacterium tuberculosis* in the United States, by state, in 1980.

of gastrointestinal cells and macrophages in vitro is associated with disseminated MAC disease (210). While it is often assumed that disease occurs as a result of relatively recent exposure, a recent study with rhesus macaques suggested that latent infection may occur, with subsequent reactivation causing disseminated MAC disease (188).

General populations

In contrast to HIV-associated disseminated MAC disease, MAC pulmonary disease in immunocompetent patients is usually caused by *M. intracellulare* (111, 304, 308) and is most likely acquired by the respiratory route. *M. intracellulare* is preferentially isolated from environmental aerosols (221, 312), and studies have found associations with contaminated hospital water and subsequent MAC respiratory colonization among hospitalized patients with chronic lung disease (173). Furthermore, patients with pulmonary MAC were significantly more likely than a comparison group of healthy volunteers to have MAC isolated from their bathrooms (205). Potting soil used

by patients referred to a specialty respiratory hospital in the United States yielded both *M. avium* and *M. intracellulare* by culture of aerosolized soil samples. In addition, investigators found one patient-soil isolate matching pair using pulsed-field gel electrophoresis (55). The predilection for MAC pulmonary disease to involve the right middle lobe and lingula (233, 279), which are common anatomic sites of aspiration, implies that aspiration may also be an important mechanism for infection.

Person-to-person transmission of MAC does not seem to occur. When clusters of patients infected with

Table 1. Organisms belonging to the
Mycobacterium avium complex

M. arosiense
M. avium
M. bouchedurhonense
M. chimaera (MAC-A sequevar)
M. colombiense (MAC-X sequevar)
M. intracellulare
M. marseillense
M. timonense

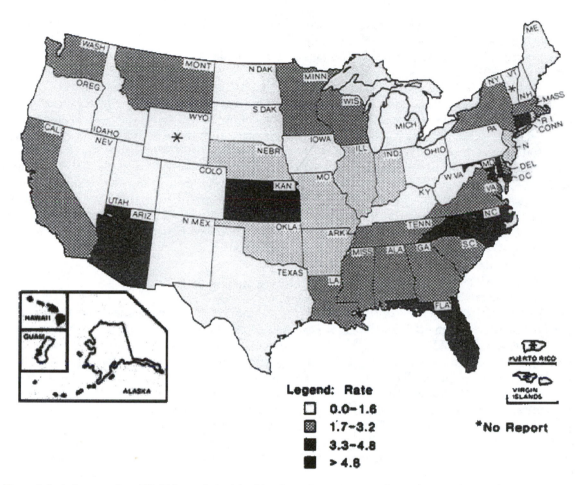

Figure 2. Isolation rates (per 100,000 population) for *Mycobacterium avium complex* in the United States, by state, in 1980.

similar isolates are found, the link is usually a common water source (168, 177, 285, 302). Although the organisms have been recovered from cigarettes (66) before and after smoking, no cases of MAC disease have been associated with shared cigarettes. Most disease is sporadic, not associated with a common source. Indeed, a detailed analysis looking for space-time clustering of cases in northern England was unable to detect environmental or population-based clusters (249).

Inhalation of infectious aerosols is most clearly responsible for disease among persons with a particular syndrome of diffuse pulmonary infiltrates and granulomatous inflammation, termed "hot tub lung." The syndrome has been associated with exposure to poorly cleaned and maintained hot tubs (9) or after introduction into the hot tub by contaminated soil on the skin of persons who did not shower prior to using the hot tub (69, 186). In several reported series, multiple family members have developed disease from the same hot tub (186). In these clusters, MAC is usually isolated from both the hot tub water and from the patients' lungs, and molecular strain typing has confirmed that the strains from the hot tub and patients' lungs are identical (69, 185, 234).

Humans appear to be exposed to MAC at an early age. Studies in the United States and Europe have shown that humoral and cell-mediated immune recognition of MAC antigens increases with age, and there are striking differences between those <6 years of age and the older age groups (72, 171).

Epidemiology

HIV-infected populations

In 1984, NIH investigators reported findings from 30 men with a clinical diagnosis of AIDS, 16 of whom were investigated because of unremitting fevers and weight loss. They found 8 patients with disseminated MAC (DMAC) and found that over time they remained persistently bacteremic (184). This and other early studies of AIDS defined DMAC as an important AIDS-associated opportunistic infection (76). It became evident that DMAC occurred at the extreme of CD4 lymphopenia and was highly associated with mortality within the following year (36, 42, 134, 136, 143). The Swiss HIV Cohort Study specifically looked at DMAC in a prospectively monitored cohort of 6,290 HIV-infected subjects between 1987 and 1995. They found 2-year probabilities of developing DMAC to be 22% among those whose first CD4 count was <50 cells/mm^3 and 11% if their CD4 count was 50 to 99 cells/mm^3 (182). Furthermore, they found that the cumulative probability of MAC disease after 2 years of follow-up increased from 9.8% (95% confidence interval [CI], 4.4 to 15.2%) to 29.8% (95% CI, 20.8 to 38.8%) among those entering the cohort in later years (1993 to 1995 compared to 1987 to 1989). There was no improvement in survival over the same time period, with the median survival following diagnosis of DMAC being 7.9 months. As AIDS reports accumulated in the 1980s, the percentage of AIDS cases with DMAC reported to the Centers for Disease Control and Prevention (CDC) increased from 4.7% in 1987 (257) to 7.6% by the end of 1990 (132).

There has clearly been a change in the epidemiology of DMAC over the life of the AIDS epidemic in the United States and Europe (191). Potent combination antiretroviral therapy (ART) came into widespread use between 1995 and 1997, and overall HIV-associated mortality rates began declining by 1996 (83, 142, 218). Data from a multicenter study, the HIV Outpatient Study Cohort, noted a dramatic increase in the use of protease-inhibitor-containing regimens, from 2% of patients taking HIV therapy in mid-1995 to 82% by mid-1997 (218). Though the rates of prophylaxis for DMAC remained the same over the time period of the study, the incidence of DMAC declined from as high as 20 per 100 person-years to <5 per 10 person-years between 1994 and 1997. DMAC in Atlanta, GA, decreased from a peak of 198 cases in 1995 to only 66 cases in 2000. Rates in Sao Paulo, Brazil, decreased from >20% in 1995 to 1996 to <7% by 1998 and correlated with increased availability of ART (113). In a multicohort collaborative study of European and North American patients, the impact of various AIDS-defining events on mortality was assessed prospectively in patients initiating ART. Of 31,620 patients monitored for a median of 43 months, DMAC had an adjusted mortality hazard rate (aMHR) of 4.1, putting it in a "moderate" category for mortality risk, midway between non-Hodgkin's lymphoma with an aMHR of 17.6 and herpes simplex virus disease with an aMHR of 1.1.

Once a person is diagnosed with DMAC, the greatest correlation with subsequent survival is initiation of ART; treatment with a macrolide-containing DMAC treatment regimen is also associated with improved survival (133, 148, 149). In low-income settings, the highly virulent pathogen *M. tuberculosis* is the single most common cause of death in HIV/AIDS patients and can occur relatively early during HIV infection. How much DMAC contributes to morbidity and mortality in the poorest, hardest hit countries of Africa and Asia is unclear, as mycobacterial culture is unavailable except in a few highly specialized and high-resource settings. In one study of 723 consecutive patients presenting to the hospital with fever in northern Tanzania, investigators found mycobacterial bloodstream infections in only 30 (4.1%). Only 1 isolate was determined to be MAC, and this patient was confirmed to have HIV infection (49).

General populations

Evidence of environmental exposure to NTM has been known since the 1960s when U.S. Navy recruits were studied for skin test reactivity to antigens prepared from *M. intracellulare* (PPD-B) and *M. scrofulaceum* (PPD-G). There was a pronounced clustering of reactors in the southeastern United States (67). Subsequently, Von Reyn and colleagues confirmed these findings using dual skin testing with *M. avium* sensitin and *M. tuberculosis* purified protein derivative (PPD), testing asymptomatic health care workers and medical students from northern and southern U.S. sites. They found that *M. avium* sensitin-dominant reactions, indicating exposure to MAC and possibly other NTM, were significantly more common among subjects in the South than in subjects in the North (46% versus 33%; $P < 0.001$) (301). In follow-up, several of the authors performed a cross-sectional study in western Palm Beach, FL, between 1998 and 2000 and found that 33% of that particular population had positive *M. avium* sensitin skin test results but did not find an association with water exposure, food, or pets (232).

A more recent U.S. study examined findings from the most recent (1999 to 2000) National Health and Nutrition Examination Surveys (NHANES) and compared them to the 1971 to 1972 cohort. The prevalence of *M. avium* sensitin reactivity increased by ~50%, from 11.2% (95% CI, 9.2 to 13.5%) to 16.6% (95% CI, 13.2 to 20.6%). On multivariate analysis, the highest prevalence of sensitization was in the age group 20 to 39 years, in males, among non-Hispanic blacks, and among those born outside the United States, especially Mexico (155).

Numerous studies from around the world describe NTM and MAC incidence among the general population, and some note increasing rates of disease, roughly correlating with declining incidence of tuberculosis. Incidence of NTM disease in New Zealand, during 2004, was estimated at 1.92 per 100,000 population, with MAC being the predominately isolated pathogen (85). In France, NTM pulmonary infection in HIV-negative populations has been estimated at 0.7 per 100,000 population between 2001 and 2003 (50), with MAC the most commonly isolated pathogen. Incidence of NTM disease in Denmark is estimated at 1.08 per 100,000, remaining steady over the previous 12 years (11). A study in Japan between 1971 and 1984 reported an annual incidence of 1.29 cases of MAC pulmonary disease per 100,000 population, with no secular trend. Similar to patients in the United States, patients were primarily male (64%) and over 60 years of age (298). A study of pulmonary MAC in the Northern Territory, Australia, between 1989 and 1997 revealed an annual incidence of 2.1 cases per 100,000 population, with an increase in the number of cases over time (208). Patients were predominantly male and over 50 years of age.

It does appear that NTM sensitization and disease are on the increase, though speculation remains about whether disease incidence is truly increasing, or whether the apparent increase is related to better detection. Investigators in British Columbia, Canada, evaluated the apparent rise in reported MAC and found that the increase of 35.4% in overall MAC incidence coincided with the introduction of more-sensitive liquid broth culture and rapid detection systems across the province in 1999 and 2000 (126).

Several epidemiologic studies of MAC and other NTM in developing countries have recently been published. One study from Zambia found that of 180 patients with chronic cough recruited from a hospital, only 4 had MAC or other NTM cultured more than once; all were HIV positive and died within weeks of culture-positive findings (31). Another study has been reported out of Karamoja, Uganda, where a large proportion of the population lives in pastoral communities in close contact with cattle herds known to have high prevalence of bovine tuberculosis (*Mycobacterium bovis*). Surprisingly, of 43 cervical lymph node biopsies performed in patients coming for initiation of TB therapy, MAC was the most commonly isolated pathogen, followed by *M. tuberculosis* and *M. bovis* (214).

The demographics of patients with MAC pulmonary disease in recent case series have also shifted from primarily older males with tobacco-related lung disease to older females, many of whom have no underlying pulmonary disease (52, 106, 228, 281). The magnitude and significance of this demographic shift are unclear, but it may partially reflect greater awareness of the different clinical manifestations of MAC pulmonary disease in women.

MAC is currently the most common etiology of NTM-related extrapulmonary disease in HIV-uninfected hosts, causing 60 to 85% of cases in the United States, though prior to 1970 *M. scrofulaceum* dominated (209, 313). Cervical lymphadenitis is the most common manifestation of MAC in immunocompetent hosts, occurring most commonly in young children. In Sweden, where NTM infection has been a reportable condition since 1989, in a study of 183 children <7 years of age with culture-proven MAC lymphadenopathy, investigators found significant seasonal variation, with a peak in October and nadir in April, and noted a higher incidence in children living close to water (287). They calculated an incidence rate of 4.5/100,000 children. Of note, previous studies from Sweden showed that the incidence of NTM disease in children increased from 0.06/100,000 to 5.7 per 100,000 children after discontinuation of the country's general *M. bovis* BCG vaccination program in 1975 (243). MAC can also infect other organ systems, causing diverse syndromes including intrathoracic adenopathy (84), osteomyelitis, septic arthritis, skin and soft tissue infections, and middle ear disease (see clinical section below).

HOST AND PATHOGEN FACTORS ASSOCIATED WITH MAC DISEASE

Once they gain entry into the host, MAC organisms may produce a range of clinical manifestations from asymptomatic colonization to severe, disseminated disease. Any clinical manifestations resulting from MAC infection depend significantly on the interaction between the particular organism and the host. Both parameters will be explored.

Host Factors

MAC and other NTM are common in the environment, yet few people develop clinical disease. Thus, susceptibility to MAC is the exception rather than the rule. The first line of defense is clearly the lung macrophage, which must be activated to effectively phagocytose and destroy the organism. The complex networks of activating and modulating influences within the immune system determine the effectiveness of these effector cells. HIV-associated acquired immunodeficiency helped demonstrate the critical role that CD4-positive T-helper lymphocytes (CD4 cells) have in maintaining host resistance to MAC. Disseminated MAC occurs almost exclusively among patients with profound depletion of CD4$^+$ T lymphocytes; almost all patients with disseminated MAC have CD4$^+$ T lymphocyte counts of <100 cells/mm^3, with the median T-cell count in many studies in the 20 to 40 range (41, 98, 299). HIV-infected patients with disseminated MAC disease have higher HIV RNA levels than similar patients without disseminated MAC (296). This observation can be partially explained by a reciprocal interaction between HIV and MAC in human monocytes. In vitro MAC infection enhances replication of HIV in human monocytes through NF-κB-dependent mechanisms that are independent of cytokine induction (94). Conversely, HIV infection of human macrophages increases intracellular growth of MAC organisms inside these macrophages (146).

CD4 cell decline is also associated with a cascade of dysfunction within the cell-mediated immune, or TH1, pathway, including alterations in cytokine levels and responsiveness. Mouse models have been used to investigate disseminated BCG, *M. tuberculosis*, and MAC, and these studies have shown the importance of CD4 and CD8 T cells and their associated cytokines in controlling infection, again because of their proactivating effect on macrophages and monocytes. Studies of Toll-like receptors (TLR) show they are important players in innate host defense, and some may have pathogen-specific importance for mycobacterial infections (96, 252). Investigators in Korea have shown that in a local population, comparing patients with nodular bronchiectatic NTM disease to controls, guanine-thymine (GT) repeat microsatellite polymorphisms in intron II of the TLR2 gene is associated with disease (318), while TLR2 Arg753Gln and Arg677Trp polymorphisms were not associated with disease (250). Interleukin-12 (IL-12) (265), gamma interferon (IFN-γ), and tumor necrosis factor alpha are important in macrophage activation and regulation, and nitric oxide is an important mediator of lethality for the intracellular pathogen (25, 68).

In addition to acquired host vulnerability to MAC, there are likely genetically determined differences in humans. By analogy, certain inbred mice are particularly vulnerable to mycobacteria, and this vulnerability has been mapped to a gene called the *bcg* locus (268). The human correlate, previously termed *NRAMP1*, now called "the solute carrier family 11" (SLC11A1), has been examined for association with *M. tuberculosis* disease in large populations. While at least one group in Japan has found an association of NRAMP1 polymorphisms in a cohort of individuals with MAC disease compared to controls (282), the results have otherwise been mixed, depending on the population studied, leading most to believe that susceptibility/resistance to MAC is a complex interplay between multiple genes, modulated by other host and pathogen factors (Fig. 3) (80).

Experiments of nature have contributed to our understanding of genetic determinants of immunity to mycobacteria. There are a series of Mendelian immune disorders that predispose humans to mycobacterial infections due to either absence or dysfunction

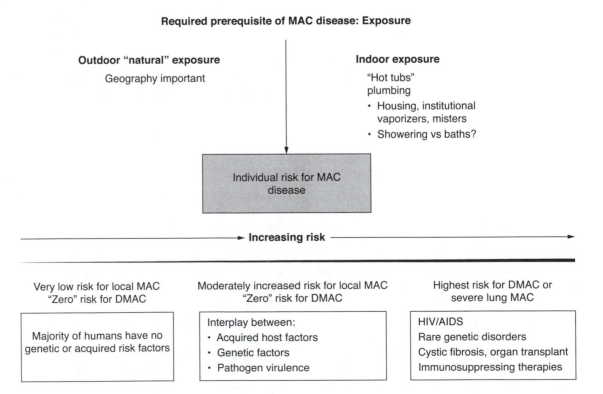

Figure 3. Interplay between environmental exposure, host susceptibility, and pathogen virulence.

of T cells, altered NF-κB signaling, or disorders of the IL-12/IFN-γ axis. "Mendelian susceptibility to mycobacterial disease" comprises several disorders related to IFN-γ production deficits or poor responsiveness to IFN-γ due to receptor abnormalities or deficiencies (33, 267). While informative, these Mendelian disorders account for a very small number of cases of MAC (95, 138, 271, 280). On the other hand, investigators in Japan found two HLA antigens associated with having MAC disease compared to control Japanese populations. They found HLA-DR6 in 50.8% of cases versus 20.2% of controls and HLA-A33 in 28.8% of cases versus 12.5% of controls (278). In a different analysis among Japanese patients with pulmonary MAC, HLA-A26 antigen was associated with pulmonary deterioration (166). More recently, other investigators in Japan used haplotype tag single-nucleotide polymorphism analyses, identified polymorphisms in the major histocompatibility complex class I chain-related A (MICA) gene that are associated with pulmonary MAC, and demonstrated increased expression of MICA in bronchiolar epithelium, alveolar macrophages, and granulomatous lesions (264).

Because patients with cystic fibrosis are often colonized and frequently become ill with MAC, there has been interest in whether a polymorphism or mutation in the cystic fibrosis transmembrane conductance regulator (CFTR) might also be a host susceptibility factor for development of MAC disease among individuals without other signs or symptoms of cystic fibrosis. Investigators in Japan examined CFTR variants poly-T, TG repeats, and M470V and found an association between the intron 8 (IVS8) T5 allele and MAC disease (185). Another study, in the United States, of HIV-seronegative women referred for severe pulmonary MAC disease found no defects in any of the cytokines measured and showed that T-cell responses to mitogens were entirely normal. However, 36.5% had at least one mutation in the CFTR gene compared to 15.6% in an age-matched control group. Most were heterozygotes, and all had normal sweat chloride levels. The authors conclude that pulmonary NTM among a certain population of women with a discernible complex morphotype—being relatively tall, lean, and with high rates of scoliosis, pectus excavatum, and mitral valve prolapse—is associated with high rates of a single mutation in CFTR.

In summary, the critical effector cell for controlling MAC is the lung macrophage, which ingests the mycobacteria (244). Once engulfed by the macrophage, the bacteria's fate—destruction, persistence, or replication—is determined by the cell's state of immune activation, which is determined by interactions between cells in the TH1 pathway and their associated cytokines, particularly the IL-12/IFN-γ

axis. Numerous other cytokines (e.g., IL-18, IL-23, and IL-29), receptors (e.g., vitamin D receptor), and unidentified cofactors (82) may also be important. Perturbations in cytokine production, protein conformation, or receptors increase the likelihood that the bacteria will replicate and cause disease. A mutation found in the CFTR gene that has been associated with severe pulmonary NTM in women is of great interest and may help contribute to a greater understanding of MAC disease in this and the cystic fibrosis population. A number of excellent reviews are available that focus on host immunity to MAC and other mycobacteria, to which the reader is referred (217).

Pathogen Factors

Different subgroups of organisms within the *Mycobacterium avium* complex are associated with different manifestations of disease; whether these clinical differences represent differential pathogenicity of the organisms, differences in environmental niches, or differences in host susceptibilities is unclear. It is becoming increasingly clear that species and subspecies differences within MAC have clinical importance.

The *M. avium* complex consists of a growing number of species as defined by molecular techniques. In the past decade, *M. avium* and *M. intracellulare* have been joined by *M. chimaera* (also known as MAC-A sequevar), *M. colombiense* (MAC-X) (197), *M. arosiense*, *M. bouchedurhonense*, *M. marseillense*, and *M. timonense*. Two commercially available DNA probes (Gen-Probe, San Diego, CA) are available to specifically identify *M. avium* and *M. intracellulare*, although these probes can misidentify some of the newer MAC species (251, 294). Other methods employed to differentiate MAC strains include phage typing (47), multilocus enzyme electrophoresis analysis (78, 310), restriction fragment length polymorphism analysis of insertion elements such as IS*1245* (109) and others (222, 242), and nucleotide sequencing of regions of the 65-kilodalton heat shock protein (*hsp65*) (274, 300), the *rpoB* gene, and the internal transcribed spacer located between the genes encoding 16S and 23S rRNAs (89).

Agreement between these various methods has not always been consistent. In studies examining human and animal MAC isolates from Australia (78) and the United States (310), there was no clear correspondence between the results of serotyping and multienzyme electrophoresis. However, subgroups obtained by sequencing *hsp65* and the internal transcribed spacer located between the genes encoding 16S and 23S rRNAs have correlated reasonably well (274). Newer methods using a consensus of multiple gene loci have been used to assign species to some rapidly growing mycobacteria (320), and similar methods are starting to be applied to assigning species and sequevars within MAC (197).

Substrain identification of MAC isolates is important for exploring pathogenetic mechanisms underlying different forms of disease. Disseminated MAC disease is predominantly (80 to 95%) caused by *M. avium*, while isolates from patients with pulmonary disease tend to more commonly be *M. intracellulare* (15, 32, 58, 111, 230, 292). The relative proclivity of different substrains to cause pulmonary disease is debated; one case-control study of patients with MAC in respiratory specimens suggested that *M. avium* was less frequently isolated from respiratory specimens but more likely to be causing pulmonary disease when present (272), but another study in a cohort of cancer patients suggested that *M. avium* was often isolated from patients with hematologic malignancy but rarely caused lung disease (116). Some recent work has suggested that certain genetically clustered subgroups of MAC may be associated with progressive (as opposed to stable) disease; these findings may be potentially useful to decide which patients require more aggressive management but require confirmation (157). The dominance of *M. avium* in disseminated disease is considerably clearer. In particular, the most common *M. avium* strain isolated from AIDS patients with disseminated MAC is Mav-B (79 to 90%), followed by Mav-A (5 to 16%) and Mav-E (0 to 5%) (58, 87, 88, 124). These three strains were also the most common isolates found in HIV-uninfected children with MAC lymphadenitis in two studies (58, 87, 88, 124), although in another study, the majority of isolates (69%) belonged to the species *M. intracellulare* (275).

M. avium, particularly the Mav-A/Mav-B strains, may be more likely to cause disseminated disease in AIDS patients because of specific virulence factors. Two putative virulence factors have been identified in *M. avium*: *mig* (225) and hemolysin (189). Expression of the *mig*, or macrophage-induced gene, occurs only when the organisms are replicating within macrophages (225). Secretion of the 30-kilodalton Mig protein is induced by the acid environment present inside the macrophage. While the exact function of the protein is unknown, variation in the *mig* gene correlates with the ability of *M. avium* to replicate in human macrophages (193), and survival of *mig*-transfected *M. smegmatis* inside macrophages (224) is enhanced compared to wild-type *M. smegmatis* strains. In at least one study, the *mig* gene was present in *M. avium* strains but absent from *M. intracellulare* strains (15), which correlates with the proclivity of these two species to cause disseminated disease.

The role of the *mig* gene in lung disease is unclear. A study of 45 HIV-negative patients with MAC isolated from respiratory specimens found the *mig* gene in 100% of isolates (22 of which were *M. intracellulare*) and found no correlation between *mig* sequence and presence of lung disease (319). Hemolysin is a magnesium-dependent, cell-wall-associated protein that may be important for intracellular survival. Expression of hemolysin has been strongly associated with *M. avium* strains responsible for disseminated disease in both AIDS and other immunosuppressed patients (189); *M. avium* and *M. intracellulare* strains associated with pulmonary disease generally did not express hemolysin. More recent data have demonstrated that human isolates of Mav-A and Mav-B obtained from patients with both disseminated and pulmonary disease are strong producers of hemolysin, while animal isolates in the Mav-A and Mav-C groups were significantly less hemolytic (238).

A key component of the virulence of MAC organisms may be the ability of the organisms to invade human epithelial cells (24). This invasion likely occurs by MAC proteins that adhere to fibronectin and other extracellular matrix proteins (231). Colonial morphology on solid media has been traditionally correlated with the relative invasiveness of MAC organisms. MAC strains with smooth, flat, and transparent colonial morphology seem to be more virulent than strains with domed and opaque morphology in some studies (48, 256, 263). Colonial morphology appears to be determined by the glycopeptidolipid content of the mycobacterial wall, and differences in glycopeptidolipid seem to be associated with differential inhibition of intracellular killing of *M. avium* (283). The less-virulent *M. avium* strains, as identified by colony morphology, appear to induce more IL-18 expression by the infected monocyte, resulting in more IFN-γ production and greater inhibition of mycobacterial growth, than more virulent strains (262). The resulting milieu, rich in IFN-γ, also may explain why these less-virulent strains appear to be phagocytosed by human monocytes more readily than more-virulent strains (263).

CLINICAL SYNDROMES ASSOCIATED WITH MAC

MAC in the Setting of HIV/AIDS

Pulmonary: colonization versus disease

Pulmonary parenchymal disease caused by MAC is uncommon among patients with AIDS (129). However, prospective studies have examined whether pulmonary or gastrointestinal colonization with MAC might predict subsequent DMAC. One study showed that in patients with CD4 counts of <50, 67% of those who had MAC in sputum or stool developed DMAC within 1 year, though few developed pulmonary disease per se. However, of those who developed DMAC, only about a third had preceding positive stool or sputum cultures. Tuberculosis, not MAC, should be the greatest concern for the clinician who receives a report showing acid-fast bacilli on the sputum smear from a patient with HIV/AIDS. While the finding of MAC in sputum might cause concern for future dissemination, TB is an imminent threat to the patient, and to those in his or her home, clinic, hospital, or work environment. In settings where highly active antiretroviral therapy (HAART) is available, the cost-effectiveness of checking for MAC in sputum or stool is dwarfed by the benefits of starting HAART to prevent the emergence of DMAC. If HAART is ineffective, due to HIV multidrug resistance, for example, or CD4 lymphocyte improvement is delayed in a particular individual, MAC prophylaxis is still an important adjunct to care and is cost-effective (131).

Disseminated MAC

Initially, there was confusion about whether MAC was causative of symptoms and eventual death among those suffering from AIDS. MAC was easily cultured from lymph nodes, bone marrow, sputum, and other organ systems when looked for in patients with late-stage AIDS (100). However, the frequent finding of concurrent pathogens, such as cytomegalovirus, and the paucity of typical granulomatous inflammatory response made its role in symptomatology and clinical deterioration unclear. When investigators used newer broth culture techniques to look for the organism in the blood, they found that the patients were almost uniformly mycobacteremic, illustrating the overwhelming nature of their infection (184).

It became clear that DMAC was one of the entities that could cause the end-of-life event known as "wasting syndrome." In an attempt to tease out the impact of DMAC itself from the generalized immune deterioration in advanced AIDS, one group performed a case control study of patients with one episode of *Pneumocystis carinii* pneumonia as well as respiratory and sterile body cultures for mycobacteria. Survival of cases (with DMAC) and controls was indexed to their first episode of *P. carinii* pneumonia. Median survival was shorter in those with DMAC (107 days; 95% CI, 55 to 179) compared to those with negative MAC cultures (275 days; 95% CI, 230 to 319; $P < 0.01$) (143). Other studies confirmed this finding and also found that poor survival was associated with

lack of antiretroviral therapy, the level of anemia, and lack of antimycobacterial chemotherapy (136). A prospective observational study examined the impact of treatment of DMAC on survival among patients with AIDS in the pre-HAART era and confirmed earlier findings that patients with AIDS who developed DMAC were more likely to die, but that those receiving antimycobacterial therapy had improved survival (median, 263 compared to 139 days; $P < 0.001$) (42). Unfortunately, 23% of those with DMAC died within 29 days of diagnosis, and most of these persons had not yet had time to initiate DMAC therapy.

Clinically, patients who have DMAC in the setting of AIDS have persistent, high-grade fevers, profound night sweats, weight loss, anorexia, fatigue, and diarrhea often associated with cramping abdominal pain (136). Laboratory abnormalities classically have reflected the disseminated nature of the disease with profound anemia out of proportion to neutropenia or thrombocytopenia, and elevated transaminases and alkaline phosphatase. Either because of improved diagnosis or concurrent antiretroviral therapy, these laboratory abnormalities may be less common among patients with DMAC diagnosed in the present day than among those diagnosed earlier in the HIV/AIDS epidemic. For example, a recent study found that over the period 1991 to 1997, patients presenting with DMAC were significantly less likely to have anemia or an elevated alkaline phosphatase (133). Radiographic findings frequently demonstrate diffuse adenopathy on chest or abdominal CT scans. Bone marrow biopsy may show granulomas, though these may be poorly formed, and acid-fast stain of the bone marrow often shows evidence of unchecked mycobacterial replication, easily confirmed by microbiologic culture. Culture of blood is the easiest diagnostic method and reflects the high-level bacteremia, with a projected sensitivity of 90% with a single blood culture (102). Autopsy results in one series of 44 patients with documented MAC bacteremia showed that 31 (70%) also had histologic findings of MAC in other organs, and this was associated with elevated hepatocellular enzymes to a statistically significant degree (293). The organism can be cultured from essentially every body site at autopsy in those with DMAC at death (123).

Profound anemia frequently accompanies patients with HIV/AIDS and DMAC, while the other cell lines remain relatively intact. Investigators found that bone marrow cellularity and appearance, as well as erythropoietin levels, were indistinguishable between patients with AIDS with and without DMAC. However, bone marrow mononuclear cells were able to generate fewer erythroid progenitor colonies, and sera from patients with DMAC were markedly inhibitory to the erythroid progenitors as compared to sera from patients with AIDS but without DMAC (93). One study seeking a model to predict DMAC in patients with AIDS found in a multivariate analysis that among those whose CD4 count was <50 cells/mm³, there were 3 independent predictors of DMAC: fever on >30 days in the preceding 3 months, hematocrit of <30%, and a serum albumin concentration of <3.0 g/dl (41).

MAC In General Populations

Pulmonary: colonization versus disease

In persons without HIV/AIDS, the most common site of MAC infection is the respiratory tract. MAC pulmonary infection has a wide spectrum of clinical manifestations, ranging from asymptomatic colonization to progressive, symptomatic disease (Table 2). Understanding of this spectrum has increased significantly during the past 50 years. Seminal work by Ernest Runyon and others published in the 1940s and 1950s described both asymptomatic colonization and a chronic pulmonary disease with clinical manifestations similar to tuberculosis (248). This chronic pulmonary disease, now often called "classic" MAC pulmonary disease, primarily affected white males over the age of 50 with underlying pulmonary diseases such as silicosis, prior pneumonia, or a history of pulmonary tuberculosis (Fig. 4). The clinical syndrome was often insidious in onset; prominent manifestations included chronic cough, hemoptysis, weight loss, and low-grade fever (14, 159, 179). The disease was generally slowly progressive, frequently did not respond well to available antituberculous agents (14, 79, 179, 245, 297), and

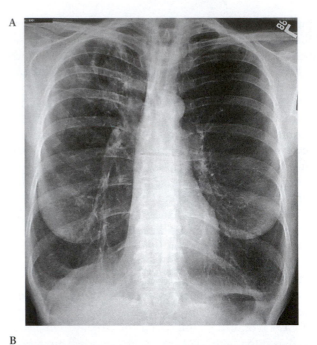

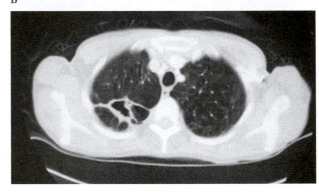

Figure 4. Chest radiograph (A) and CT scan (B) from a patient with "classic" type pulmonary MAC. The chest radiograph demonstrates fibronodular upper lobe opacities, and cavitation is evident on the CT scan.

Table 2. Spectrum of pulmonary disease caused by MAC

Type of disease	Host characteristics	Demographics	Radiographic features
Cavitary	Underlying lung disease, especially chronic obstructive pulmonary disease	Males over 50 yr	Cavitation, often upper lobes involved, fibronodular infiltrates
Nodular/bronchiectatic	No underlying lung disease, possibly associated with thoracic deformities	Elderly females	Multiple nodules associated with areas of bronchiectasis; predilection for right middle lobe/lingual
Pediatric	Healthy children	Usually under 5 yr of age, no gender/racial proclivity	Intrathoracic lymphadenopathy, focal atelectasis
Pulmonary/disseminated	Late-stage HIV infection, bone marrow transplants, other immunodeficiency (severe combined immunodeficiency, IL-12 or IFN-γ deficiency)	No age/gender/racial proclivity	Multiple nodules, diffuse interstitial infiltrate, cavitation in setting of disseminated MAC
Hot tub lung	Generally immunocompetent	No age/gender/racial proclivity	Bilateral interstitial with or without alveolar infiltrates, ground-glass appearance on CT scan

frequently was treated with adjunctive surgical resection. Most of these patients had positive tuberculin skin tests, but when concurrent testing with PPD-B antigen (derived from the "Battey bacillus," i.e., *M. intracellulare*) was performed, the reaction to PPD-B was generally larger than to the PPD-S tuberculin reagent (79, 179). No distinctive physical examination findings were reported. Cavitation was present on chest radiographs in most cases; calcification and pleural effusions were also occasionally observed (159, 179, 248). The disease generally ran an indolent course despite ineffective therapy, and patients usually died from other underlying illnesses. In one series of 100 patients evaluated between 1968 and 1972 with 10 years of longitudinal follow-up, 26 patients demonstrated improvement, 55 were clinically stable, and 19 had progressive symptoms and radiographic findings. Twenty-nine of the 100 patients died during follow-up, but only 4 persons were felt to have died directly because of MAC pulmonary disease (245, 246). Dyspnea on initial presentation and presence of coexisting lung disease have been associated with increased mortality among patients with MAC pulmonary disease (70).

During the late 1970s and 1980s, understanding of the range of reported clinical manifestations of MAC in the lung significantly increased. In one series of 20 patients with solitary, granulomatous pulmonary nodules, 12 (60%) grew MAC from the resected nodule, whereas only 1 grew *M. tuberculosis* (101). Most of these patients were asymptomatic. Nontuberculous mycobacteria grew from open-lung biopsy specimens obtained from 40 patients at the same medical center during the same time period (1969 to 1980); 24 grew MAC, and 16 of these 24 biopsy specimens were solitary pulmonary nodules. Thirteen of these 16 patients had no other medical problems, and only 1 of the 16 had a prior history of any predisposing lung disease (187). In a more recent series of 41 patients from South Korea (a medium-incidence country for tuberculosis) with solitary pulmonary nodules attributable to mycobacteria, 15/41 (37%) grew MAC (115). A report by Prince et al. (228) in 1989 described a series of 21 patients with pulmonary MAC disease who had no predisposing medical conditions. Unlike previous series, these patients were overwhelmingly (86%) female. They presented with an indolent cough that had been present for a long period (average, 25.6 weeks) prior to diagnosis. Most of the patients had no other symptoms. The radiographic pattern of disease was also different than what had previously been described. Most of the patients had multiple pulmonary nodules, and only 24% had cavities on chest radiographs (Fig. 5). In most patients, the disease was very slowly

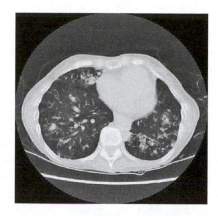

Figure 5. Chest CT scan from a patient with "new" type pulmonary MAC, demonstrating multiple pulmonary nodules throughout both lungs.

progressive, and often 2 to 3 years passed before radiographic progression was noted. Four of the 21 patients died directly of MAC pulmonary disease.

Subsequent reports from the past 2 decades have confirmed that elderly, primarily Caucasian females constitute a majority of patients with MAC pulmonary disease (137, 234). These female patients often have no known underlying pulmonary disease and often are nonsmokers (137, 228, 276, 311). Two small studies have noted that these patients tend to be relatively tall and thin, with higher rates of scoliosis, pectus excavatum, and mitral valve prolapse than in either a comparison group with tuberculosis or the general population (141, 158). A subset of these patients have isolated involvement of the right middle lobe and lingula, often with associated bronchiectasis (Fig. 6). This pattern has been named the Lady Windermere Syndrome, after a fastidious character in the play *Lady Windermere's Fan* by Oscar Wilde (233). The presumption is that patients with this syndrome voluntarily suppress the cough reflex, resulting in aspiration and damage to the right middle lobe and/or lingula. Despite anecdotal connections

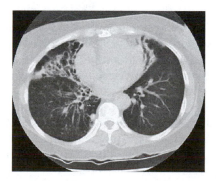

Figure 6. "Lady Windermere" pattern of MAC pulmonary disease, with prominent bronchiectasis affecting the right middle lobe and lingula.

between cough suppression and this syndrome (60), the pathogenesis of MAC pulmonary disease in these patients is unclear.

As awareness of MAC as a respiratory pathogen has increased among clinicians, more affected populations with unique disease manifestations have been identified. Patients with cystic fibrosis are one such population. These patients almost always have bronchiectasis and frequently have nodular infiltrates on chest computed tomography (CT) presumed to be due to mucus impaction. Because of the overwhelming respiratory manifestations of cystic fibrosis and associated superinfections, it is very difficult to tease out what part of the clinical picture might be attributable to MAC infection. Recent data have demonstrated that a significant proportion of these patients' lungs are at least colonized with MAC. In a large, multicenter, cross-sectional study of patients with cystic fibrosis, 13% had pulmonary colonization with at least one nontuberculous mycobacterium, and 72% of these mycobacteria were MAC (213). Interestingly, in this study, MAC colonization was associated with older age, higher forced expiratory volume in 1 s, higher rates of colonization by *Staphylococcus aureus*, lower rates of colonization by *Pseudomonas aeruginosa*, and overall, a better prognosis. In a nested-cohort study, the same authors found that cystic fibrosis patients with positive sputum cultures for nontuberculous mycobacteria (primarily MAC) had the same rate of decline in higher forced expiratory volume in 1 s as cystic fibrosis patients without positive sputum cultures for nontuberculous mycobacteria. However, cystic fibrosis patients who met the American Thoracic Society criteria for nontuberculous mycobacterial pulmonary disease were significantly more likely to have progressive high-resolution chest CT changes over time, consistent with progression of nontuberculous mycobacterial pulmonary disease (212). Studies from France and Israel have found that 6.6% and 22.6% of cystic fibrosis patients, respectively, have at least one respiratory culture that grows nontuberculous mycobacteria, but in these studies, MAC was significantly less common than *M. abscessus* group organisms (178, 247). Interestingly, recurrent pulmonary nontuberculous mycobacterial infection in an otherwise healthy 54-year-old man was recently reported as the presenting manifestation of adult cystic fibrosis (39). Further research is needed in this area to better understand the role of MAC and other nontuberculous mycobacteria in deterioration of lung function and symptomatology among patients with cystic fibrosis.

Until recently, MAC was not reported to be a significant cause of pulmonary disease among immunocompetent, healthy children. However, an increasing number of case reports describe a syndrome of subacute respiratory symptoms associated with mediastinal adenopathy and/or endobronchial lesions with frequent partial lung collapse. Immunologic evaluation of these children has not revealed any underlying immunodeficiency or cystic fibrosis gene mutations (84). Two percent of children in a 2-year prospective surveillance study in The Netherlands with nontuberculous mycobacterial infection had mediastinal lymphadenopathy, and 3% had pulmonary abnormalities (121). A recent review of the literature found 43 published cases of intrathoracic disease caused by nontuberculous mycobacteria among otherwise healthy children between 1930 and 2003 (206). Of these, 29 patients were infected by MAC organisms. Interestingly, over half the cases were published after 1990, suggesting either an increasing prevalence of MAC pulmonary disease in children or increased awareness of this clinical entity. Most children with intrathoracic MAC disease are under 5 years of age, but children up to 14 years old have been affected. Children with intrathoracic MAC disease generally present with cough, wheezing (due to bronchial obstruction), and sometimes respiratory distress. Approximately half these children will have constitutional symptoms, including fever, night sweats, anorexia, and weight loss. Radiographs frequently demonstrate hilar lymphadenopathy, air trapping, or focal infiltrates. Bronchoscopy or surgical biopsy is often required to make the diagnosis, although gastric lavage has been useful in some cases.

Finally, an entirely different form of MAC pulmonary disease has been described since the late 1990s (69, 145). This disease, usually termed "hot tub lung," occupies a gray area between infection and a hypersensitivity reaction to the organism. Patients with hot tub lung are usually immunocompetent persons who have repeated exposures to indoor hot tubs. In one consecutive series of patients with hypersensitivity pneumonitis, hot tub lung was the second most common etiology of hypersensitivity pneumonitis, afflicting 21% of patients for whom an etiology was found (117). These patients develop progressive dyspnea, often accompanied by nonproductive cough, fever, and chills (69, 156, 186). Chest radiography demonstrates diffuse infiltrates with a ground-glass appearance; multiple small nodules may be seen as well. Lung biopsy reveals granulomatous inflammation with or without acid-fast bacilli. Sputum or lung biopsy cultures usually are positive for MAC; in a minority of cases, other nontuberculous mycobacteria such as *M. fortuitum* may be responsible (156, 186). Outbreaks of hot tub lung affecting multiple family members and/or close associates have been reported (69, 186), so detection of one case should prompt evaluation of other persons who have had consistent exposure to the same hot tub. Whether the hot tub lung syndrome actually represents infection, hypersensitivity pneumonitis, or both is a subject of active debate (9), as many patients recover spontaneously once exposure to the hot tub ceases, in the absence of antimycobacterial therapy (118).

Extrapulmonary disease

In addition to pulmonary disease, MAC has been reported to cause symptomatic disease at a number of other sites. The lymph nodes are by far the most common extrapulmonary site of disease. MAC lymphadenitis primarily afflicts healthy children with normal immune systems. Studies from Europe, Australia, and New Zealand have reported similar incidence rates of nontuberculous mycobacterial lymphadenitis among children under 15 (between 0.42 to 0.88 cases/100,000), with MAC by far the most common species isolated (26, 85, 121). Even in developing countries with a high incidence of tuberculosis, MAC has been demonstrated to be an underrecognized cause of lymphadenitis in young children (10, 214). In general, MAC lymphadenitis affects the anterior cervical lymph nodes, is unilateral, affects primarily children between the ages of 1 and 4, and has a tendency to occur more often in the winter than in other seasons (26, 219, 255, 287, 313). Most affected children have positive tuberculin skin tests, which makes the syndrome difficult to differentiate from tuberculosis (121, 229, 313). However, at least one study has suggested that IFN-γ release assays, which do not cross-react with MAC, may be useful to make the distinction between nontuberculous mycobacterial lymphadenitis (59). The majority of children in this and other series (81, 219, 229) have presented with an enlarging neck mass with no systemic symptoms and no evidence of MAC infection elsewhere in the body. Without treatment, the lymph nodes often spontaneously regress, but on occasion they will suppurate and erode through the overlying skin, creating chronic fistulas and scarring (255, 277, 313, 314).

Focal extrapulmonary MAC disease outside the lymph nodes is relatively rare but increasingly reported. Among these uncommon manifestations, musculoskeletal and cutaneous infections are the most frequently reported. In particular, MAC can cause a chronic tenosynovitis, usually of the hand or arm. Patients with this syndrome usually present with stiffness, swelling, and pain of the affected extremity. A history of prior trauma to the affected extremity can sometimes be elicited, but often the source of the infection is unclear. Systemic symptoms are uncommon,

and laboratory studies are frequently unrevealing. Patients often experience significant diagnostic delays and frequently receive multiple empiric corticosteroid injections, which may exacerbate the underlying infection. Mycobacterial culture of synovial biopsies is essential for diagnosis, as pathology frequently demonstrates granulomatous inflammation but no acid-fast bacilli (12, 125, 176, 215). In addition to tenosynovitis, MAC may cause septic arthritis (27, 110, 198) and osteomyelitis (192); these manifestations are quite rare and usually occur in immunocompromised hosts or in patients who have had prior trauma to the affected area (37). Bursitis, particularly of the olecranon bursa, has been reported in a number of cases. Many of these patients are immunocompetent individuals who present with a painless or minimally painful swollen, enlarged bursa in the absence of systemic symptoms (92). Prior trauma may or may not be reported, and if reported, is often minimal. MAC can also cause primary cutaneous disease without evidence of systemic dissemination in both immunocompetent and immunocompromised hosts. The clinical manifestations have included papulonodular lesions on the trunk and thighs (165), erythematous patches with pustules on the abdomen, legs, and buttock (254), Sweet's syndrome (286), and plaques on the face resembling lupus vulgaris (167). An outbreak of cutaneous MAC disease has been reported in 3 immunocompetent family members, associated with common exposure to a circulating, constantly heated bath water system (273). Cutaneous MAC disease is chronic and very slowly progressive in all cases, with onset ranging from 4 months to 10 years prior to diagnosis. Biopsies usually demonstrate granulomatous inflammation, but acid-fast bacilli are usually not seen, and culture is required for diagnosis.

DIAGNOSTIC CONSIDERATIONS

Microbiologic

The diagnosis of MAC pulmonary disease can be difficult because the signs and symptoms are frequently subtle and nonspecific. A combination of clinical, radiographic, and microbiologic data is necessary to make the diagnosis with confidence. The American Thoracic Society published revised criteria for diagnosis of MAC pulmonary disease in 2007 (Table 3) (102). These criteria emphasize the importance of establishing the chronicity of symptoms associated with microbiologic or radiographic evidence of parenchymal damage. Unfortunately, these criteria are based on expert opinion, and most experts would agree that clinical studies are needed to assess their validity and long-term patient outcomes.

Table 3. The 2007 American Thoracic Society diagnostic criteria for nontuberculous mycobaterial lung disease (taken from reference 102)

Clinical criterial (both required)
  Pulmonary symptoms, nodular or cavitary opacities on chest radiograph, or a high-resolution CT scan that shows multifocal bronchiectasis with multiple small nodules *and*
  Appropriate exclusion of other diagnoses

Microbiologic criteria
  Positive culture from at least 2 separate expectorated sputum samples (consider repeat sputum acid-fast smears/cultures if nondiagnostic) *or*
  Positive culture from at least 1 bronchial wash or lavage *or*
  Transbronchial or other lung biopsy specimen with mycobacterial histopathologic features (granulomatous inflammation or acid-fast bacilli) and positive culture for nontuberculous mycobacteria or biopsy specimen showing mycobacterial histologic features (granulomatous inflammation or acid-fast bacilli) and 1 or more sputum samples or bronchial washings that are culture positive for nontuberculous mycobacteria
  Biopsy specimen showing mycobacterial histopathologic features (granulomatous inflammation and/or acid-fast bacilli) and 1 or more sputum samples or bronchial washings that are positive for a nontuberculous mycobacterium, even in low numbers

Radiographic

High-resolution chest CT is vital to diagnosis and management of MAC pulmonary disease, particularly in patients with nodular/bronchiectatic disease. In one study of 26 consecutive patients with chest CT scans demonstrating clusters of small nodules in the lung periphery associated with bronchiectasis, 13 (50%) were eventually diagnosed with MAC pulmonary disease (279). Furthermore, 8 of these patients had cavities noted on CT that were not readily apparent on plain radiographs. Notably, only 6 of these patients had MAC grow from sputum; bronchoscopy and/or open-lung biopsy was necessary to make the diagnosis in the others. Cavitation on CT has been associated with positive sputum cultures; patients without cavities may require more invasive procedures to obtain microbiologic confirmation of MAC pulmonary disease (46). Another study of 100 unselected patients with bronchiectasis on chest CT reported that this constellation of radiographic findings—bronchiectasis plus peripheral parenchymal nodules—was 80% sensitive and 87% specific for the diagnosis of MAC pulmonary disease (276). In recent years, this constellation has been the most common radiographic presentation of MAC pulmonary disease; for example, in two series published in the early 1990s, bronchiectasis and nodules were seen in 70 to 94% of patients, while cavities were seen in 0 to 28% (119, 227). Areas of the lung affected by MAC

pulmonary disease generally have high uptake of 18F-fluorodeoxyglucose, so distinguishing MAC disease from lung cancer is not possible using currently available positron emission tomography; interestingly, at least one group found that this technique could be used to monitor treatment response among patients with MAC pulmonary disease (56).

In light of the difficulties in obtaining a clear-cut diagnosis of MAC pulmonary disease, particularly given the propensity for this disease to afflict relatively elderly and frail patients, less invasive diagnostic methods are needed. Immunologic testing of blood specimens, either examining cellular or humoral responses, may offer one such method. A group of Japanese investigators have studied an enzyme immunoassay system that detects antibody responses to glycopeptidolipid antigens specific for MAC. In an early study of this technique among a mixed group of healthy patients and patients with mycobacterial infections, this test had a sensitivity of 92% and a specificity of 97% for diagnosis of MAC pulmonary disease. Furthermore, the level of these antibodies declined significantly among patients with MAC who converted sputum cultures from positive to negative (162). A second group, also in Japan, found that serologic responses to two MAC lipid antigens (trehalose monomycolate and apolar-glycopeptidolipid) successfully distinguished patients with pulmonary MAC from patients with pulmonary tuberculosis, *M. kansasii*, or healthy volunteers, with sensitivity of 89.2% and specificity of 94 to 97% at the optimized cutoff level (204). Subsequent work using an enzyme-linked immunosorbent assay for immunoglobulin A antibodies to the MAC glycopetidolipid core antigen also reported good discrimination of patients with MAC pulmonary disease from other groups of patients with lung disease, including patients with MAC isolated from respiratory specimens who did not have lung disease (sensitivity, 84.3%; specificity, 100% at the optimum cutoff). Furthermore, antibody titers correlated with the radiographic extent of disease (161). At the time of this writing, these assays are available for research purposes only, but hopefully with further validation and data, this type of assay may become available for clinical use.

THERAPY FOR MAC DISEASE

Basic Principles

MAC organisms are resistant to many antibiotic agents, and treatment is complicated by the need for long-term therapy in frequently frail patients who are often taking multiple other medications concurrently.

Table 4. Antimicrobial agents useful for treatment of MAC infection[a]

Drugs	Common side effects
Likely useful	
Macrolides	
Azithromycin	Diarrhea, nausea, abdominal pain, rash, elevated hepatic transaminases, tinnitus, hearing loss
Clarithromycin	Diarrhea, nausea, abnormal taste, dyspepsia, abdominal pain, headache, rash, hearing loss, elevated hepatic transaminases, QT prolongation
Ethambutol	Decreased visual acuity (optic neuritis), rash
Rifamycins	
Rifabutin	Abdominal pain, nausea, rash, abnormal taste, arthralgias, uveitis, leukopenia, thrombocytopenia, "flu-like syndrome," elevated hepatic transaminases, orange secretions
Rifampin	Abdominal pain, nausea, rash, elevated hepatic transaminases, hyperbilirubinemia, "flu-like syndrome," leukopenia, thrombocytopenia, interstitial nephritis, orange secretions
Aminoglycosides	
Amikacin	Both drugs: vestibulotoxicity (particularly streptomycin), cochlear toxicity (hearing loss),
Streptomycin	nephrotoxicity (less so with streptomycin than amikacin), rash, fever, muscle weakness (neuromuscular blockage)
Fluoroquinolones	
Ciprofloxacin	Nausea, vomiting, abdominal pain, rash, abnormal liver transaminases, central nervous system
Gatifloxacin	effects (delirium, dizziness, insomnia), tendonitis/tendon rupture, QT prolongation
Levofloxacin	
Moxifloxacin	
Potentially useful	
Clofazimine	Abdominal pain, diarrhea, nausea, vomiting, skin discoloration, rash, dry skin, conjunctival and corneal pigmentation, eye irritation
IFN-γ	Fever, myalgias, elevated hepatic transaminases, neutropenia, thrombocytopenia, delirium, gait disturbances
Linezolid	Diarrhea, nausea, headache, myelosuppression, lactic acidosis, optic neuropathy, peripheral neuropathy
Mefloquine	Dizziness, myalgias, nausea, vomiting, headache, rash, hair loss, sleep disorders, psychosis, cardiac conduction abnormalities, elevated hepatic transaminases
Telithromycin	Diarrhea, nausea, dizziness, visual disturbances, QT prolongation, elevated hepatic transaminases, exacerbation of myasthenia gravis

[a]Data are from references 29, 86, 108, and 147 and from package inserts for Biaxin (http://www.accessdata.fda.gov/drugsatfda_docs/label/2009/050662s042,050698s024,050775s0131b1.pdf), Ketek (http://www.accessdata.fda.gov/drugsatfda_docs/label/2007/021144s012lbl.pdf), Myambutol (http://www.fda.gov/medwatch/SAFETY/2004/mar_PI/Myambutol_PI.pdf), Mycobutin (http://www.pfizer.com/dowload/uspi_mycobutin.pdf), rifampin (http://www.fda.gov/cder/foi/label/2000/50662S291b1.pdf), and Zithromax (http://www.fda.gov/cder/foi/label/2000/50662S291b1.pdf).

Agents with proven or potential clinical utility for MAC treatment are listed in Table 4. In general, it is advisable to administer an expanded-spectrum macrolide (clarithromycin or azithromycin) in combination with one or more other agents to reduce the likelihood that drug-resistant MAC strains will emerge on therapy. Monitoring for side effects and long-term toxicity related to antimicrobial agents is essential. Many of the drugs used for MAC therapy have potentially significant drug interactions with other commonly used medications; some of the most common of these interactions are noted in Table 5.

Drug Susceptibility Testing

The use of susceptibility testing to guide treatment of MAC disease is controversial. Correlation between in vitro drug susceptibility and clinical outcomes has been clearly demonstrated only for macrolides (34, 281). Furthermore, treatment of clarithromycin-resistant MAC with clarithromycin does result in reduced levels of mycobacteremia, at least in mice (22). Studies attempting to correlate results of antimicrobial susceptibility testing of MAC to other drugs with clinical outcomes have described mixed results (135, 266). The latest recommendation from the National Committee for Clinical Laboratory Standards advises that antimicrobial susceptibility testing for MAC should be performed only for the macrolides and only in the following circumstances (269):

1. The patient has received prior macrolide therapy
2. The patient developed MAC bacteremia while receiving macrolide prophylaxis
3. The patient developed a relapse of MAC disease while receiving macrolide therapy
4. The MAC isolate is an initial, clinically significant isolate used to determine baseline drug resistance

Table 5. Common drug interactions for drugs used to treat MAC infection

Primary drug	Second drug	Interaction
Clarithromycin (inhibits cytochrome P450 3A4 enzyme)	Rifabutin	↑ Rifabutin AUC, higher risk for uveitis ↓ Clarithromycin AUC
	Rifampin	↓ Clarithromycin concentrations
	Fluoroquinolones	Both classes cause QT prolongation; use with caution
	Protease inhibitors	↑ Clarithromycin AUC
	Efavirenz	↑ Clarithromycin AUC, possible ↑ risk of rash
	Nevirapine	↓ Clarithromycin AUC
Rifabutin	Protease inhibitors	↑ Rifabutin AUC; decrease in AUC of some protease inhibitors (indinavir, saquinavir)
	Efavirenz	↓ Rifabutin AUC (rifabutin dose increase to 450–600 mg daily recommended)
	Clarithromycin	See above
Rifampin	Protease inhibitors	↓ Protease inhibitor AUC; coadministration generally not recommended
	Efavirenz	↓ Efavirenz AUC
	Nevirapine	↓ Nevirapine AUC
	Clarithromycin	See above
	Mefloquine	↓ Mefloquine AUC
	Telithromycin	↓ Telithromycin AUC
Linezolid	Antidepressants, particularly serotonin reuptake inhibitors	Possible serotonin syndrome due to monoamine oxidase inhibition by linezolid

[a]Data are from references 29, 86, 147, and 305 and from package inserts for Biaxin, Ketek, Myambutol, Mycobutin, rifampin, and Zithromax (see footnote *a* to Table 4 for source information). AUC, area under the concentration-time curve; ↑, increased; ↓, decreased.

Drug susceptibility testing of MAC isolates should be performed at a laboratory with significant experience in these techniques, as the reproducibility of these results is lower at inexperienced laboratories (316).

Treatment in the Setting of HIV/AIDS

Treatment of disseminated MAC

The most important component of treatment of disseminated MAC infection in persons with advanced HIV disease is control of the underlying HIV disease. Median survival among patients in one study who received macrolide-based antimycobacterial therapy for MAC in the pre-HAART era was 8.6 months (259). Mortality rates in other studies of disseminated MAC with low rates of concurrent HAART use were also very high (45, 64). Since the introduction of HAART, survival after diagnosis of disseminated MAC has improved significantly (149). This improvement in survival has been independently associated with prescription of HAART (133).

Initial therapy for disseminated MAC should include at least a macrolide (clarithromycin or azithromycin) plus ethambutol (Table 6). Macrolide-based therapy has been associated with significant improvements in survival after diagnosis of disseminated MAC (259). Clarithromycin monotherapy has been associated with emergence of clarithromycin-resistant organisms (34), and the addition of ethambutol at a dose of 15 mg/kg of body weight daily significantly reduces relapses and emergence of clarithromycin resistance (62). Clarithromycin should be used at a dose of 500 mg twice daily (or 1,000 mg of the extended-release formulation once daily), as higher doses have been associated with increased mortality (45). Azithromycin, at a dose of 600 mg daily, may also be used (64), although this agent may be less effective at sterilizing blood cultures than clarithromycin (309). The primary consideration for which macrolide to use will be driven by tolerability and possible drug-drug interactions.

Many clinicians use a third drug in addition to a macrolide and ethambutol for treatment of disseminated MAC. Rifabutin has been most commonly used as this third drug. In one randomized, placebo-controlled trial, bacteriologic response and survival were no different between patients treated with or without rifabutin (300 mg daily) added to a regimen of clarithromycin 500 mg twice daily and ethambutol 1,200 mg once daily (99). However, a more recent three-arm, randomized, controlled trial reported that survival among patients assigned to a 3-drug regimen consisting of clarithromycin, ethambutol, and rifabutin was better than among patients assigned to either clarithromycin plus ethambutol or clarithromycin plus rifabutin (17). However, microbiologic and clinical responses to therapy were not statistically different among the 3 arms. Drug interactions

Table 6. Recommendations for medical treatment of MAC disease (102)

Type of disease	Recommended therapy[a]
Prophylaxis for disseminated MAC	Azithromycin 1,200 mg p.o. once weekly *or* clarithromycin 500 mg p.o. QD or BID
Disseminated MAC	Clarithromycin 1,000 mg p.o.[b] *or* azithromycin 500–600 mg p.o. QD *plus* Ethambutol 15 mg/kg p.o. QD *plus* Rifabutin 300–450 mg p.o. QD *or* fluoroquinolone (ciprofloxacin 750 mg p.o. BID, levofloxacin 750 mg p.o. QD, moxifloxacin 400 mg p.o. QD, gatifloxacin 400 mg p.o. QD) Plus antiretroviral therapy for patients with HIV
Pulmonary MAC	
Nodular/bronchiectatic disease, mild to moderate, initial treatment	Clarithromycin 1,000 mg thrice weekly[b] *or* azithromycin 500–600 mg p.o. thrice weekly *plus* Ethambutol 25 mg p.o. thrice weekly *plus* Rifampin 600 mg p.o. thrice weekly
Cavitary disease, initial treatment	Clarithromycin 1,000 mg daily[b] *or* azithromycin 250–300 mg p.o. QD *plus* Ethambutol 15 mg/kg p.o. QD *plus* Rifampin 450–600 mg p.o. QD *plus or minus* Aminoglycoside (streptomycin 500–1,000 mg or amikacin 15 mg/kg 2–3 times weekly) for the first 2 mo
Severe or previously treated disease	Clarithromycin 1,000 mg daily[b] *or* azithromycin 250–300 mg p.o. QD *plus* Ethambutol 15 mg/kg p.o. QD *plus* Rifampin 450–600 mg p.o. QD *or* rifabutin 150–300 mg p.o. QD *plus* Aminoglycoside (streptomycin 500–1,000 mg or amikacin 15 mg/kg 2–3 times weekly) for the first 2 mo or longer

[a] p.o., orally; QD, once a day; BID, twice a day.
[b] Clarithromycin may be administered as 1,000 mg of the extended release formulation instead of 500 mg twice daily of the usual formulation.

between rifabutin and other components of therapy are a significant consideration (Table 5). In particular, a high rate of rifabutin-associated uveitis has been reported when clarithromycin and high-dose rifabutin (600 mg daily) were coadministered (259). Uveitis was noted at a much lower rate when the rifabutin dose was lowered to 300 mg daily (99, 258). A fluoroquinolone is also a reasonable choice as a third agent, and one retrospective study suggested a survival advantage when ciprofloxacin was added to clarithromycin and ethambutol for treatment of disseminated MAC (154). The newer fluoroquinolones, moxifloxacin and gatifloxacin, have demonstrated in vitro activity against MAC that is superior to that of ciprofloxacin or levofloxacin (19, 239, 290, 291), but published clinical experience with these compounds is lacking and in vitro antagonism has been noted in at least one study (164). Amikacin, at a dose of 15 mg/kg of body weight daily, may also be useful as part of a multidrug regimen to treat disseminated MAC (43, 220, 241), but no large studies have been performed to validate its utility. Addition of clofazimine to clarithromycin and ethambutol has been associated with an increase in mortality compared to no clofazimine, so clofazimine should generally not be used for treatment of disseminated MAC (35). Other compounds have in vitro activity against MAC, but clinical experience with these has been very limited. IFN-γ as adjunctive therapy was tried in 2 HIV-infected patients with disseminated MAC but produced only transient clinical improvement (172). Both linezolid and mefloquine have in vitro activity against MAC (21, 240), and addition of these 2 drugs to clarithromycin, moxifloxacin, granulocyte-macrophage colony-stimulating factor (GM-CSF), and ethambutol resulted in successful treatment of a patient with chronic lymphocytic leukemia and disseminated MAC (199).

Other adjunctive therapies that have been used in very limited numbers of patients include GM-CSF and corticosteroids. GM-CSF augments MAC phagocytosis and intracellular killing of MAC by macrophages in vitro and in vivo and was associated with delayed time to blood culture positivity in one HIV-infected patient (153). A study of GM-CSF added to azithromycin in a group of 8 patients with advanced HIV demonstrated enhanced mycobacterial killing by these patients' macrophages but nonsignificant decreases in mycobacteremia (169). Corticosteroids have been studied in small, uncontrolled series; one study of 5 patients with advanced HIV and refractory MAC demonstrated clinical improvement when 2 mg of dexamethasone was given daily in addition to antimycobacterial therapy (317).

Disseminated MAC is a relatively rare disease in persons without HIV, and there are no large studies to direct therapy in HIV-seronegative persons. It is reasonable to apply the same general principles of therapy to HIV-seronegative patients with disseminated MAC. IFN-γ may have a particular role in treatment of disseminated MAC among patients with certain types of congenital and acquired immunodeficiencies. In a study of 7 patients with refractory, disseminated nontuberculous mycobacterial infection, the addition of IFN-γ produced significant clinical benefit (130). One case report described a good clinical response to IL-2 in a patient with idiopathic $CD4^+$ lymphopenia (295). Among patients who have disseminated MAC in the setting of bone marrow or solid organ transplantation, reduction of the level of immunosuppression may also be helpful (61, 196). In this patient population, the use of rifamycins is often problematic due to multiple drug interactions with immunosuppressive medications, and a fluoroquinolone may be preferable as a third agent.

Treatment of patients with refractory disease or relapse is difficult, and the elements of management will differ depending on the underlying disease. In the setting of advanced HIV infection, aggressive HIV treatment is the most important element, and improving HIV control alone may suffice to control disseminated MAC. Susceptibility testing of the MAC isolate can be helpful, keeping the above caveats in mind. In the setting of failure or relapse, therapeutic drug monitoring to ensure adequate absorption of orally administered antimicrobial agents may be helpful (114). Addition of 2 new agents with activity against MAC, if possible, is a reasonable approach to these patients, but data to support this approach are lacking.

For patients with advanced HIV who have a good response to antiretroviral therapy, treatment of disseminated MAC disease may be discontinued in some cases. Cure of disseminated MAC infection has been reported with concurrent effective antiretroviral therapy (7, 112). Patients who have a sustained increase in the CD4 count to over 100 cells/mm^3 for at least 6 months, and who have completed at least 12 months of antimycobacterial therapy, may be considered for discontinuation of MAC therapy (7, 147). The patient should be asymptomatic, with documentation of a negative mycobacterial blood culture, prior to discontinuation of therapy. Caution should be used when considering discontinuation of therapy in patients whose immune reconstitution has not been robust, as relapses in this setting have been reported (44). These patients should be closely monitored for relapse, particularly if the CD4 count falls below 100 cells/mm^3.

Management of IRIS

Clinicians are increasingly recognizing that HIV-infected patients may develop new focal manifestations or clinical deterioration of MAC disease associated with immune reconstitution. These clinical manifestations have been termed immune reconstitution inflammatory syndromes (IRIS) and have been described in association with multiple pathogens including tuberculosis (91, 200), cytomegalovirus (150), *Pneumocystis jirovecii*, aspergillus, hepatitis B, and hepatitis C, among others (40). The incidence of IRIS associated with disseminated MAC is unknown, but MAC accounts for a significant proportion of IRIS cases among HIV-infected persons (40, 174). The manifestations of MAC-associated IRIS are diverse; many patients experience new onset of fever and malaise, but focal manifestations vary widely. Common manifestations include lymphadenopathy in the abdomen or mediastinum, new focal lung infiltrates, or nodules (183). Other reports have described focal cervical lymphadenitis with spontaneous drainage (226), pyomyositis with cutaneous abscesses (175), and brain abscess (18). The syndrome usually occurs within the first 3 months after the initiation of effective antiretroviral therapy and usually is associated with significant increases in the CD4 count and rapid decline in HIV RNA after initiation of antiretrovirals (40, 260). There are no firm data to guide management of the syndrome. Case reports have described good outcomes with focal drainage of localized abscesses (175, 226), surgical excision of a focal brain lesion (18), and systemic corticosteroids (40); in all cases, concurrent MAC therapy was prescribed. In our experience and that of others (57), symptomatic therapy with nonsteroidal inflammatory agents, corticosteroids, and drainage of focal collections in addition to antimycobacterial therapy is sufficient for most patients. Resolution of MAC IRIS may take a long time; in one cohort of 20 patients with MAC IRIS, the median time to resolution was 19.5 months among the 16 patients who responded to treatment (antimycobacterials ± corticosteroids), and one patient required over 5 years for complete resolution (237). In a few cases with severe symptoms, temporary discontinuation of antiretroviral therapy while attempting to reduce the MAC burden with antimycobacterial agents may be necessary, but there are no data to demonstrate the efficacy or safety of this approach.

Prophylaxis for disseminated MAC in patients with advanced HIV disease

Persons with advanced HIV are at significant risk to develop disseminated MAC. The incidence of disseminated MAC among HIV-infected patients with CD4 counts of less than 100/mm^3 is approximately 20% per year without antiretroviral therapy or prophylactic antibiotics (202). Azithromycin, clarithromycin, and rifabutin have all been clearly effective in reducing the risk of disseminated MAC in patients with such low CD4 counts. Two randomized, double-blind, placebo-controlled trials of rifabutin 300 mg daily versus placebo demonstrated an approximately 50% reduction of the risk of development of disseminated MAC (203). There was a nonsignificant trend toward improved survival in the rifabutin arms of these studies. A randomized, double-blind study comparing clarithromycin 500 mg twice daily to placebo demonstrated a 69% reduction in the incidence of disseminated MAC disease and a significant 25% reduction in mortality (223). Clarithromycin both at this dosing schedule and at a dose of 500 mg once daily was superior to rifabutin, and adding rifabutin to clarithromycin was no more effective than using clarithromycin alone (16, 127). Azithromycin at a dose of 1,200 mg once weekly was also more effective than rifabutin (122), and although no direct comparisons have been performed, it appears to be approximately as effective as clarithromycin in prevention of disseminated MAC. When once-weekly azithromycin was compared to placebo, patients in the azithromycin arm had a 66% reduction in the incidence of disseminated MAC (211). Adding rifabutin 300 mg daily to azithromycin 1,200 mg weekly further reduced the incidence of disseminated MAC over either drug alone but was associated with an increase in drug-associated toxicity (122). The current U.S. Public Health Service/Infectious Diseases Society of America guidelines recommend either azithromycin 1,200 mg once weekly or clarithromycin 500 mg twice daily as first-line therapy for disseminated MAC prophylaxis among HIV-infected patients with CD4 counts of less than 50/mm^3 (Table 6) (147). Clarithromycin 500 mg once daily or rifabutin 300 mg once daily are reasonable second-line alternatives. Prophylaxis may be discontinued safely in patients whose CD4 counts rise to consistently over 100 cells/mm^3 for at least 3 months.

Treatment in General Populations

Treatment of pulmonary MAC

The data for treatment of pulmonary MAC in HIV-seronegative patients are limited by the paucity of randomized, controlled trials. Older, noncomparative studies in which patients were treated with combinations of conventional antituberculous agents reported highly variable outcomes. Patients in these studies did not necessarily have uniform definitions of disease, radiographic response, or cure. In most cases, conversion of sputum cultures to negative was the primary outcome. Sputum conversion rates using standard

antituberculous agents, primarily in populations with classic MAC pulmonary disease, ranged from 38 to 91% across studies published between 1967 and 1988 (8, 53, 65, 71, 79, 297). A more recent randomized, controlled trial compared 2 years of isoniazid, rifampin, and ethambutol to 2 years of rifampin plus ethambutol in 75 patients from the United Kingdom and Scandinavia (235, 236). Study patients primarily had classic MAC pulmonary disease; 61% had pre-existing lung disease and 61% had cavitary disease. Cure was defined as having negative sputum cultures in the last 3 months of treatment, with persistently negative sputum cultures during 3 years of follow-up. At the end of 5 years, 10/37 (27%) patients in the rifampin-ethambutol arm were cured, compared with 13/38 (34%) in the isoniazid-rifampin-ethambutol arm ($P = 0.67$). Of note, 27 (36%) patients had died at the end of 5-year follow-up, and 21 (28%) were considered treatment failures or relapses. Only 3 of the deaths were directly attributed to MAC disease. In vitro susceptibility testing of the MAC organisms to multiple antituberculous agents was performed using the modal resistance method but had no significant correlation with treatment outcome.

Subsequently, the new macrolides (azithromycin and clarithromycin) were found to possess significant activity against MAC. Furthermore, in the United States, rifabutin is often used as a component of pulmonary MAC treatment instead of rifampin because of better in vitro activity and somewhat less induction of cytochrome P450 metabolism (315). An early study of 30 patients with MAC pulmonary disease reported that 58% of patients who completed a 4-month course of clarithromycin monotherapy 500 mg twice daily converted sputum cultures to negative, and another 21% had a significant reduction in the number of MAC colonies grown in sputum culture (307). A majority of these patients had classic MAC pulmonary disease: 60% were male and 65% had fibrocavitary disease on chest radiographs. Of note, only 20 of the initial 30 patients completed the study and were assessed for sputum conversion. Isolates obtained after relapse or end of therapy from 3 (16%) of these 20 patients had developed high-level clarithromycin resistance. A similar study examined azithromycin monotherapy, 600 mg once daily for 4 months. Twenty-nine patients entered the study, and 23 (79%) completed the full course of treatment. Among these 23 patients, 38% converted sputum cultures to negative and another 38% had a significant reduction in the number of MAC colonies in their sputum (107). Again, the majority of patients in this study were male (52%), 48% had fibrocavitary disease on chest radiographs, and 65% were former or current smokers. Acquired macrolide resistance was not noted in this study. In both of these studies, gastrointestinal side effects were common, and changes in hearing were not infrequent.

These two studies strongly suggested that clarithromycin and azithromycin have clinical utility for treatment of pulmonary MAC. An open-label study of high-dose clarithromycin (30 mg/kg daily) with or without other medications in 45 French patients reported a 71% sputum culture conversion rate, but treatment regimens were heterogeneous and 49% of patients had received other antimycobacterial treatment (52). Richard Wallace and colleagues published the results of the first 50 patients they treated with a clarithromycin-based regimen consisting of clarithromycin 500 mg twice daily, rifampin or rifabutin, ethambutol, and initial streptomycin in 1996 (306). Eleven (22%) of these patients dropped out of the study in the first 3 months, but of the remaining 39, 36 (92%) converted sputum cultures to negative. Relapse occurred in 4 of these patients, and isolates from 6 of the 39 (15%) patients became clarithromycin resistant. Of note, one or more drugs were discontinued in 16 of 39 (41%) patients because of side effects. A second study performed in Japan enrolled sequential HIV-seronegative patients with pulmonary MAC disease between 1992 and 1997 (281). Patients were treated with clarithromycin 10 mg/kg, ethambutol 15 mg/kg, and rifampin 10 mg/kg daily. For the first 2 to 6 months, kanamycin 20 mg/kg was administered intramuscularly 3 times weekly, followed by either ofloxacin 10 mg/kg daily or levofloxacin 5 mg/kg daily thereafter. Patients were treated for 24 months total, and if patients had difficulty with the planned treatment regimen, other antituberculous agents including enviomycin, isoniazid, or ethionamide could be used in place of one or more of the drugs in the standard regimen. Forty-six patients participated in the study, of whom 32 (70%) were female, 22 (48%) had underlying pulmonary conditions, and only 18 (39%) had cavitary disease. Only 29 of the 46 patients were actually begun on the planned treatment regimen; the remainder used a modified regimen because of preexisting conditions or refusal to take the standard regimen. Thirty-nine (85%) patients completed at least 6 months of treatment, and only 21 (54%) completed a full 24 months. Twenty-two (48%) of the original 46 patients converted their sputum cultures to negative and remained culture negative at the end of the study. Both of these studies enrolled patients whose pretreatment MAC isolates demonstrated in vitro resistance to clarithromycin, and patients in both studies infected with clarithromycin-resistant MAC had significantly lower culture conversion rates than patients infected with clarithromycin-susceptible MAC.

Subsequently, a number of different studies have examined macrolide-based, multidrug regimens for treatment of pulmonary MAC. All of these studies have been small, with heterogeneous treatments and outcomes. Table 7 contains a concise summary of these studies. In general, tolerability is a significant issue with all of these regimens, but if patients can tolerate the drugs, microbiologic outcomes are reasonably good. Most studies do not attempt to distinguish relapse from reinfection, and since reinfection is thought to occur with some frequency, this distinction may be important in understanding the effect of antimicrobials on the disease. While current guidelines (102) recommend intermittent therapy for nodular/bronchiectatic disease and daily therapy for cavitary disease, this recommendation has never been tested in a randomized, controlled trial. The use of aminoglycosides (streptomycin or amikacin) should be considered for cavitary or severe disease, although the randomized trial by Kobashi et al. (163) did not demonstrate overwhelming benefit.

Despite these seminal contributions to understanding of the medical management of MAC pulmonary disease, much remains to be learned. Radiographic and clinical outcomes in most of these studies were not standardized, and loss to follow-up was a significant problem. Furthermore, correlations among radiographic, clinical, and microbiologic outcomes during treatment of MAC pulmonary disease are relatively weak, and the most relevant of these outcomes to long-term morbidity is unclear (170). Notably, reported mortality associated with MAC pulmonary disease is markedly different in European studies (over 40% 5-year mortality) than in U.S. or Japanese studies (very low mortality, 2.7% in one study) (Table 7). These differences in mortality may be partially explained by the difference in disease spectrum among these studies (more cavitary disease in the European studies, more nodular/bronchiectatic disease in U.S./Japan studies), but other factors, as yet not understood, are likely contributory. Many patients with MAC pulmonary disease only receive microbiologic confirmation by use of bronchoscopy or other invasive procedures because they do not effectively produce sputum (279, 281), so sputum conversion is not always an outcome that can be effectively used to assess treatment efficacy. As noted above, drug intolerance in the generally frail, elderly group of patients with pulmonary MAC is a major barrier to effective therapy. Interactions between other medications that patients are taking and antimycobacterial agents, particularly clarithromycin and rifabutin, also present significant challenges to medical therapy (Table 5). Despite these caveats, recommendations for first-line therapy of pulmonary MAC are presented in Table 6.

Table 7. Summary of macrolide-based, multiple-drug treatment studies for MAC pulmonary disease[a]

Reference	Design	Regimen(s)	Outcome	Success, intention to treat (%) (n/total)	Dropout rate (%) (n/total)
106	Cohort	Azi 300–600, RBT 150–300, EMB 25/kg (daily, decreased to 15/kg after 2 mo), SM 500–1,000 2–3 times/wk for 2 mo (n = 32)	Culture conversion with 12 mo of negative cultures	59 (17/32)	9 (3/32)
		Azi 600 (3 times/wk), RBT 150–300 daily, EMB 25/kg (daily, decreased to 15/kg after 2 mo), SM 500–1,000 2–3 times/wk for 2 mo (n = 22)		55 (11/22)	9 (2/22)
		Azi 600, RBT 300–600, EMB 25/kg (all 3 times/wk), plus SM 500–1,000 3 times/wk for 2 mo (n = 49)		65 (28/49)	12 (6/49)
105	Cohort	Clari 1,000, RBT 300–600, EMB 25/kg 3 times/wk (n = 59)	Sputum conversion at 6 mo	54 (32/59)	31 (18/59)
120	Cohort	Clari 400, RIF 450, EMB 750 (daily for 18 mo) (n = 9)	Sputum conversion by end of treatment	55.6 (5/9)	11 (1/9)
		Clari 800, RIF 450, EMB 750 (daily for 18 mo) (n = 12)		91.7 (11/12)	8 (1/12)
		Clari 800, RIF 600, EMB 1,000 (daily for 18 mo) (n = 13)		92.3 (12/13)	15 (2/13)
194	RTC, double blind, placebo controlled	Azi 500, Cip 1,000, RIF 600, EMB 2,000, placebo (daily for 6 mo) (n = 14)	Combined clinical/microbiological endpoint at 6 and 18 mo	36 (5/14) at 6 mo; 29 (4/14) at 18 mo	29 (4/14)
		Azi 500, Cip 1,000, RIF 600, EMB 2,000, IFN-γ (1 million units SQ) (daily for 6 mo) (n = 18)		72 (13/18) at 6 mo; 67 (12/18) at 18 mo	11 (2/18)
163	RCT, double blind	Clari 15 mg/kg, RIF 10 mg/kg, EMB 15 mg/kg (all daily for 24 mo) plus SM 15 mg/kg IM (3 times/wk for 3 mo) (n = 73)	3 separate: clinical improvement, sputum culture conversion, relapse	Clinical, 42.5; Culture, 71.2; Relapse, 30.8	2.7 (1/73, died)
		Clari 15 mg/kg, RIF 10 mg/kg, EMB 15 mg/kg (all daily for 24 mo) plus placebo (3 times/wk for 3 mo) (n = 73)		Clinical, 28.8; Culture, 50.7; Relapse, 35.1	2.7 (1/73, died)
170	Secondary analysis of RCT (groups combined)	Clari 750–1,000 (or Azi 375–600 if Clari not tolerated), EMB 25 mg/kg, RIF 450–600 (3 times/wk for 52 wk) (n = 91)	3 separate: clinical radiographic, microbiologic (sputum culture conversion)	Clinical, 53; Radiographic, 60; Microbiologic, 11 (12/91)	36 (33/91)
90	Cohort	Clari 400–600, RIF 450, EMB 750 (all daily for 24+ mo) (n = 38)	Sputum culture conversion without relapse	75% (not separated by treatment group, but no significant difference between groups)	6 (7/111) failed to complete 6 mo; 23 (25/111) changed regimen due to side effects
		Clari 400–600, RIF 450, EMB 750 (all daily for 24+ mo) + SM 1g IM 2 times/wk (for 6 mo) (n = 73)			
144	RCT	RIF 450–600, EMB 15 kg (both daily), Clari 500 BID (n = 66)	Mortality at 5 yr; treatment failure/relapse (defined as positive sputum cultures and/or clinical deterioration)	Mortality was 48% in combined Clari arms vs 29% in combined Cip arms	35% of all Clari patients deviated from protocol vs 43% of Cip patients (about half of deviations due to drug intolerance but not broken down by group)
		RIF 450–600, EMB 15 kg (both daily), Clari 500 BID plus M. vaccae immunotherapy (n = 17)		13 (11/83) (failure/relapse in Clari group)	
		RIF 450–600, EMB 15/kg (both daily), Cip 750 BID (n = 68)		23 (20/87) (failure/relapse in Cip group)	
		RIF 450–600, EMB 15/kg (both daily), Cip 750 BID plus M. vaccae immunotherapy (n = 19)		No effect of M. vaccae immunotherapy	

[a]Abbreviations: Azi, azithromycin; Cip, ciprofloxacin; Clari, clarithromycin; EMB, ethambutol; RBT, rifabutin; RCT, randomized, controlled trial; RIF, rifampin; SM, streptomycin; IM, intramuscularly; BID, twice a day. Numbers next to medication abbreviations indicate dosages, in milligrams, unless otherwise specified.

Lung resection surgery has been used as an adjunct to medical treatment. Surgery may be useful in the setting of patients with localized pulmonary disease who are refractory to medical therapy or who do not tolerate medical therapy. The largest published series described 236 patients who underwent resection surgery for nontuberculous mycobacterial lung disease between 1983 and 2006, 189 (80%) of whom had MAC. Of these, 126 had lobectomies, 55 segmentectomies, 44 pneumonectomies, and 40 mixed procedures. Operative mortality was 2.6%, with another 18.5% of patients having significant perioperative complications. The most common complications included bronchopleural fistula (4.2%) and respiratory failure/nosocomial pneumonia (3.4%). A positive sputum culture at the time of surgery and right pneumonectomy seemed to be risk factors for postoperative bronchopleural fistula (195). Long-term outcomes were unfortunately not reported in that study. Another series of 28 patients who had pulmonary resection for MAC reported perioperative complications in 9 (32%) (201). Complications included persistent air leak requiring repeat operation (5 patients), bronchopleural fistula (1 patient), atelectasis (1 patient), and postoperative death (2 patients). Of 26 surviving patients, 24 (92%) had persistently negative postoperative sputum cultures. In another series of 21 patients, postoperative complications occurred in 6 (29%), but no perioperative deaths were reported. Eighty-seven percent of patients were considered disease free at 3 years of follow-up (261). Patients described in these series are carefully selected, and surgery was performed at referral centers with extensive experience in treatment of pulmonary MAC. One scenario in which surgical intervention seems to be important is in the setting of macrolide-resistant MAC lung disease. The largest published series of patients with macrolide-resistant MAC ($n = 51$) reported that among 14 patients treated with lung resection surgery plus prolonged aminoglycosides, high-dose ethambutol, and rifabutin, 11 (79%) converted sputum cultures to negative. Conversely, among 35 patients who received medical therapy without surgery, only 2 (5.7%) converted sputum cultures to negative (103).

Several other classes of drugs have promise for treatment of pulmonary MAC, but clinical evidence for their use is limited. Perhaps the most promising class of drugs is the fluoroquinolones, particularly the new agents moxifloxacin and gatifloxacin. Fluoroquinolones have good in vitro activity against MAC (19, 152, 253, 289, 290), and a retrospective study of treatment of patients with disseminated MAC suggested that the addition of ciprofloxacin to clarithromycin and ethambutol was associated with improved survival (154). A single randomized trial compared a ciprofloxacin-based regimen to a clarithromycin-based regimen for pulmonary MAC and found no significant difference in outcomes between groups (Table 7) (144). In our clinical experience, the fluoroquinolones represent a reasonable alternative as the third drug (in addition to a macrolide and ethambutol) for patients who have intolerance or unacceptable drug interactions with the rifamycins. Other drugs with good in vitro activity against MAC, but limited published data to support their use in treatment of pulmonary MAC disease, include linezolid (199, 240), mefloquine (21, 199), and telithromycin (20). Such therapies must be used with care and close monitoring for toxicity; for example, a recent review of long-term linezolid used for treatment of mycobacterial infections (only 1/24 had pulmonary MAC, the others had tuberculosis) reported a high rate of anemia (41.7%) and neuropathy (45.8%, either peripheral or optic) (207). Inhaled antibiotics represent an interesting approach to treatment of pulmonary MAC, with potential for high drug concentrations at the site of disease but low systemic toxicity. Inhaled amikacin has been used by some experts in addition to oral medications (140), and a small case series of six patients with pulmonary MAC treated with aerosolized amikacin (15 mg/kg daily) reported that five of six responded favorably to treatment (54). Inhaled IFN-γ has produced transient improvement in a few patients (38), but a randomized, placebo-controlled phase II trial of aerosolized IFN-γ-1b three times weekly in addition to standard antimycobacterial therapy was stopped early due to lack of efficacy (170).

We generally use a multifaceted treatment strategy for our patients with MAC pulmonary disease. Many of these patients are elderly, frail, and intolerant of multiple medications. In our experience, many patients tolerate rifabutin poorly and have underlying diseases that make parenteral aminoglycosides unattractive. Initial daily therapy with azithromycin, rifampin, and ethambutol is a reasonable choice for many patients, with modification to thrice-weekly therapy for patients who do not tolerate these medications on a daily basis. Treatment is recommended to continue for 12 months after sputum culture conversion to negative, again in the absence of data to support this recommendation (102). Adjunctive therapy with bronchodilators, mucus clearance devices, and pulmonary rehabilitation is helpful for many patients, particularly patients with bronchiectasis and chronic, productive cough. Baseline hearing and vision testing is important to monitor potential toxicity from long-term use of the macrolides and ethambutol, respectively. However, patient education regarding optic neuropathy is probably more important than medical monitoring, as most patients present due to symptoms and are not detected with routine monitoring (104). For patients with significant comorbidities, poor drug tolerance, and limited projected life span, suppressive therapy with two drugs (macrolide plus ethambutol) or close observation with symptomatic therapy is reasonable.

Treatment of extrapulmonary MAC

Extrapulmonary MAC infection is relatively uncommon, and no large trials exist to guide treatment of most forms. Children with lymphadenitis usually do well with surgical excision alone, so excisional biopsy is the first-line treatment for cervical lymphadenitis due to MAC (81, 255, 270, 313). A randomized, controlled trial clearly demonstrated the superiority of surgery alone (96% cure) over medical therapy with clarithromycin plus rifabutin (66% cure) (180), with better esthetic outcomes in the surgical group (181). For other sites of disease, the same general principles of therapy used to treat disseminated MAC are reasonable. First-line therapy should include at least a macrolide plus ethambutol, with a third drug (rifabutin, fluoroquinolone) added for extensive disease. An aminoglycoside, particularly amikacin or streptomycin, also may be helpful in the initial stages of therapy. Patients with tenosynovitis often require extensive debridement in addition to medical therapy for cure of their disease (12, 176). Patients with extrapulmonary MAC disease (apart from cervical lymphadenitis) have often been treated with 12 to 24 months of multidrug therapy, depending on the site of disease, underlying immunosuppression, and clinical response.

CONCLUSION

MAC organisms are commonly found in the environment but cause disease in relatively few of those who are infected. *M. avium*, the most common species to infect patients with HIV/AIDS, is probably acquired via the gastrointestinal tract, while *M. intracellulare* is likely acquired by the respiratory tract. DMAC is almost exclusively seen in patients with late-stage AIDS and can be treated with the combination of either clarithromycin or azithromycin in combination with ethambutol, with or without rifabutin or a fluoroquinolone. The most important intervention in this setting, however, is to gain HIV viral control with the use of potent antiretroviral therapy. Pulmonary MAC is seen most often in elderly patients, and the epidemiology has shifted from primarily older men

to a demographic that includes women with underlying bronchiectasis. Differentiating colonization from MAC pulmonary disease can be challenging, and successful treatment requires a multipronged approach that includes antibiotics, aggressive pulmonary hygiene, and sometimes resection of the diseased lung. More data are urgently needed to address the key clinical questions surrounding MAC infection. (i) Which host factors accurately predict susceptibility to MAC? (ii) Which patients with MAC pulmonary disease should be treated with antimicrobials, and which should be observed without treatment? (iii) Which treatments, given for what duration, are most effective for MAC infection?

REFERENCES

1. Reference deleted.
2. Reference deleted.
3. Reference deleted.
4. Reference deleted.
5. Reference deleted.
6. Reference deleted.
7. Aberg, J. A., D. M. Yajko, and M. A. Jacobson. 1998. Eradication of AIDS-related disseminated Mycobacterium avium complex infection after 12 months of antimycobacterial therapy combined with highly active antiretroviral therapy. *J. Infect. Dis.* **178:**1446–1449.
8. Ahn, C. H., S. S. Ahn, R. A. Anderson, D. T. Murphy, and A. Mammo. 1986. A four-drug regimen for initial treatment of cavitary disease caused by Mycobacterium avium complex. *Am. Rev. Respir. Dis.* **134:**438–441.
9. Aksamit, T. R. 2003. Hot tub lung: infection, inflammation, or both? *Semin. Respir. Infect.* **18:**33–39.
10. Al-Mahruqi, S. H., J. van-Ingen, S. Al-Busaidy, M. J. Boeree, S. Al-Zadjali, A. Patel, P. N. Richard-Dekhuijzen, and D. van-Soolingen. 2009. Clinical relevance of nontuberculous Mycobacteria, Oman. *Emerg. Infect. Dis.* **15:**292–294.
11. Andrejak, C., V. O. Thomsen, I. S. Johansen, A. Riis, T. L. Benfield, P. Duhaut, H. T. Sorensen, F. X. Lescure, and R. W. Thomsen. 2010. Nontuberculous pulmonary mycobacteriosis in Denmark: incidence and prognostic factors. *Am. J. Respir. Crit. Care Med.* **181:**514–521.
12. Anim-Appiah, D., B. Bono, E. Fleegler, N. Roach, R. Samuel, and A. R. Myers. 2004. Mycobacterium avium complex tenosynovitis of the wrist and hand. *Arthritis Rheum.* **51:**140–142.
13. Aronson, T., A. Holtzman, N. Glover, M. Boian, S. Froman, O. G. Berlin, H. Hill, and G. Stelma, Jr. 1999. Comparison of large restriction fragments of *Mycobacterium avium* isolates recovered from AIDS and non-AIDS patients with those of isolates from potable water. *J. Clin. Microbiol.* **37:**1008–1012.
14. Bates, J. H. 1967. A study of pulmonary disease associated with mycobacteria other than Mycobacterium tuberculosis: clinical characteristics. *Am. Rev. Respir. Dis.* **96:**1151–1157.
15. Beggs, M. L., R. Stevanova, and K. D. Eisenach. 2000. Species identification of *Mycobacterium avium* complex isolates by a variety of molecular techniques. *J. Clin. Microbiol.* **38:**508–512.
16. Benson, C. A., P. L. Williams, D. L. Cohn, S. Becker, P. Hojczyk, T. Nevin, J. A. Korvick, L. Heifets, C. C. Child, M. M. Lederman, R. C. Reichman, W. G. Powderly, G. F. Notario, B. A. Wynne, R. Hafner, et al. 2000. Clarithromycin or rifabutin

alone or in combination for primary prophylaxis of Mycobacterium avium complex disease in patients with AIDS: a randomized, double-blind, placebo-controlled trial. *J. Infect. Dis.* **181:**1289–1297.

17. Benson, C. A., P. L. Williams, J. S. Currier, F. Holland, L. F. Mahon, R. R. MacGregor, C. B. Inderlied, C. Flexner, J. Neidig, R. Chaisson, G. F. Notario, and R. Hafner. 2003. A prospective, randomized trial examining the efficacy and safety of clarithromycin in combination with ethambutol, rifabutin, or both for the treatment of disseminated Mycobacterium avium complex disease in persons with acquired immunodeficiency syndrome. *Clin. Infect. Dis.* **37:**1234–1243.

18. Berger, P., H. Lepidi, M. P. Drogoul-Vey, I. Poizot-Martin, and M. Drancourt. 2004. Mycobacterium avium brain abscess at the initiation of highly active antiretroviral therapy. *Eur. J. Clin. Microbiol. Infect. Dis.* **23:**142–144.

19. Bermudez, L. E., C. B. Inderlied, P. Kolonoski, M. Petrofsky, P. Aralar, M. Wu, and L. S. Young. 2001. Activity of moxifloxacin by itself and in combination with ethambutol, rifabutin, and azithromycin in vitro and in vivo against Mycobacterium avium. *Antimicrob. Agents Chemother.* **45:**217–222.

20. Bermudez, L. E., C. B. Inderlied, P. Kolonoski, M. Wu, P. Aralar, and L. S. Young. 2001. Telithromycin is active against *Mycobacterium avium* in mice despite lacking significant activity in standard in vitro and macrophage assays and is associated with low frequency of resistance during treatment. *Antimicrob. Agents Chemother.* **45:**2210–2214.

21. Bermudez, L. E., P. Kolonoski, M. Wu, P. A. Aralar, C. B. Inderlied, and L. S. Young. 1999. Mefloquine is active in vitro and in vivo against *Mycobacterium avium* complex. *Antimicrob. Agents Chemother.* **43:**1870–1874.

22. Bermudez, L. E., K. Nash, M. Petrofsky, L. S. Young, and C. B. Inderlied. 2000. Clarithromycin-resistant *Mycobacterium avium* is still susceptible to treatment with clarithromycin and is virulent in mice. *Antimicrob. Agents Chemother.* **44:**2619–2622.

23. Bermudez, L. E., M. Petrofsky, P. Kolonoski, and L. S. Young. 1992. An animal model of Mycobacterium avium complex disseminated infection after colonization of the intestinal tract. *J. Infect. Dis.* **165:**75–79.

24. Bermudez, L. E., K. Shelton, and L. S. Young. 1995. Comparison of the ability of Mycobacterium avium, M. smegmatis and M. tuberculosis to invade and replicate within HEp-2 epithelial cells. *Tuber. Lung Dis.* **76:**240–247.

25. Bhattacharyya, A., S. Pathak, M. Kundu, and J. Basu. 2002. Mitogen-activated protein kinases regulate Mycobacterium avium-induced tumor necrosis factor-alpha release from macrophages. *FEMS Immunol. Med. Microbiol.* **34:**73–80.

26. Blyth, C. C., E. J. Best, C. A. Jones, C. Nourse, P. N. Goldwater, A. J. Daley, D. Burgner, G. Henry, and P. Palasanthiran. 2009. Nontuberculous mycobacterial infection in children: a prospective national study. *Pediatr. Infect. Dis. J.* **28:**801–805.

27. Bridges, M. J., and F. McGarry. 2002. Two cases of Mycobacterium avium septic arthritis. *Ann. Rheum. Dis.* **61:**186–187.

28. Brooks, R. W., B. C. Parker, H. Gruft, and J. O. Falkinham III. 1984. Epidemiology of infection by nontuberculous mycobacteria. V. Numbers in eastern United States soils and correlation with soil characteristics. *Am. Rev. Respir. Dis.* **130:**630–633.

29. Brown, B. A., R. J. Wallace, Jr., D. E. Griffith, and W. Girard. 1995. Clarithromycin-induced hepatotoxicity. *Clin. Infect. Dis.* **20:**1073–1074.

30. Brown, S. T., F. F. Edwards, E. M. Bernard, Y. Niki, and D. Armstrong. 1991. Progressive disseminated infection with Mycobacterium avium complex after intravenous and oral challenge in cyclosporine-treated rats. *J. Infect. Dis.* **164:**922–927.

31. Buijtels, P. C., M. A. van-der-Sande, C. S. de-Graaff, S. Parkinson, H. A. Verbrugh, P. L. Petit, and D. van-Soolingen. 2009. Nontuberculous mycobacteria, Zambia. *Emerg. Infect. Dis.* **15:**242–249.

32. Cangelosi, G. A., R. J. Freeman, K. N. Lewis, D. Livingston-Rosanoff, K. S. Shah, S. J. Milan, and S. V. Goldberg. 2004. Evaluation of a high-throughput repetitive-sequence-based PCR system for DNA fingerprinting of *Mycobacterium tuberculosis* and *Mycobacterium avium* complex strains. *J. Clin. Microbiol.* **42:**2685–2693.

33. Casanova, J. L., and L. Abel. 2002. Genetic dissection of immunity to mycobacteria: the human model. *Annu. Rev. Immunol.* **20:**581–620.

34. Chaisson, R. E., C. A. Benson, M. P. Dube, L. B. Heifets, J. A. Korvick, S. Elkin, T. Smith, J. C. Craft, and F. R. Sattler. 1994. Clarithromycin therapy for bacteremic Mycobacterium avium complex disease. A randomized, double-blind, dose-ranging study in patients with AIDS. *Ann. Intern. Med.* **121:**905–911.

35. Chaisson, R. E., P. Keiser, M. Pierce, W. J. Fessel, J. Ruskin, C. Lahart, C. A. Benson, K. Meek, N. Siepman, and J. C. Craft. 1997. Clarithromycin and ethambutol with or without clofazimine for the treatment of bacteremic Mycobacterium avium complex disease in patients with HIV infection. *AIDS* **11:**311–317.

36. Chaisson, R. E., R. D. Moore, D. D. Richman, J. Keruly, T. Creagh, et al. 1992. Incidence and natural history of Mycobacterium avium-complex infections in patients with advanced human immunodeficiency virus disease treated with zidovudine. *Am. Rev. Respir. Dis.* **146:**285–289.

37. Chan, E. D., P. M. Kong, K. Fennelly, A. P. Dwyer, and M. D. Iseman. 2001. Vertebral osteomyelitis due to infection with nontuberculous Mycobacterium species after blunt trauma to the back: 3 examples of the principle of locus minoris resistentiae. *Clin. Infect. Dis.* **32:**1506–1510.

38. Chatte, G., G. Panteix, M. Perrin-Fayolle, and Y. Pacheco. 1995. Aerosolized interferon gamma for Mycobacterium avium-complex lung disease. *Am. J. Respir. Crit. Care Med.* **152:**1094–1096.

39. Chbeir, E., L. Casas, N. Toubia, M. Tawk, and B. Brown. 2006. Adult cystic fibrosis presenting with recurrent nontuberculous mycobacterial infections. *Lancet* **367:**1952.

40. Cheng, V. C., K. Y. Yuen, W. M. Chan, S. S. Wong, E. S. Ma, and R. M. Chan. 2000. Immunorestitution disease involving the innate and adaptive response. *Clin. Infect. Dis.* **30:**882–892.

41. Chin, D. P., A. L. Reingold, C. R. Horsburgh, Jr., D. M. Yajko, W. K. Hadley, E. P. Elkin, E. N. Stone, E. M. Simon, P. C. Gonzalez, and S. M. Ostroff. 1994. Predicting Mycobacterium avium complex bacteremia in patients infected with human immunodeficiency virus: a prospectively validated model. *Clin. Infect. Dis.* **19:**668–674.

42. Chin, D. P., A. L. Reingold, E. N. Stone, E. Vittinghoff, C. R. Horsburgh, Jr., E. M. Simon, D. M. Yajko, W. K. Hadley, S. M. Ostroff, and P. C. Hopewell. 1994. The impact of Mycobacterium avium complex bacteremia and its treatment on survival of AIDS patients--a prospective study. *J. Infect. Dis.* **170:**578–584.

43. Chiu, J., J. Nussbaum, S. Bozzette, J. G. Tilles, L. S. Young, J. Leedom, P. N. Heseltine, J. A. McCutchan, et al. 1990. Treatment of disseminated Mycobacterium avium complex infection in AIDS with amikacin, ethambutol, rifampin, and ciprofloxacin. *Ann. Intern. Med.* **113:**358–361.

44. Cinti, S. K., D. R. Kaul, P. E. Sax, L. R. Crane, and P. H. Kazanjian. 2000. Recurrence of Mycobacterium avium infection in patients receiving highly active antiretroviral therapy and antimycobacterial agents. *Clin. Infect. Dis.* **30:**511–514.

45. Cohn, D. L., E. J. Fisher, G. T. Peng, J. S. Hodges, J. Chesnut, C. C. Child, B. Franchino, C. L. Gibert, W. El Sadr, R. Hafner, J. Korvick, M. Ropka, L. Heifets, J. Clotfelter, D. Munroe, C. R. Horsburgh, Jr., et al. 1999. A prospective randomized trial of four three-drug regimens in the treatment of disseminated Mycobacterium avium complex disease in AIDS patients: excess mortality associated with high-dose clarithromycin. *Clin. Infect. Dis.* **29:**125–133.

46. Corbett, E. L., L. Blumberg, G. J. Churchyard, N. Moloi, K. Mallory, T. Clayton, B. G. Williams, R. E. Chaisson, R. J. Hayes, and K. M. De Cock. 1999. Nontuberculous mycobacteria: defining disease in a prospective cohort of South African miners. *Am. J. Respir. Crit. Care Med.* **160:**15–21.

47. Crawford, J. T., and J. H. Bates. 1985. Phage typing of the Mycobacterium avium-intracellulare-scrofulaceum complex. A study of strains of diverse geographic and host origin. *Am. Rev. Respir. Dis.* **132:**386–389.

48. Crowle, A. J., A. Y. Tsang, A. E. Vatter, and M. H. May. 1986. Comparison of 15 laboratory and patient-derived strains of *Mycobacterium avium* for ability to infect and multiply in cultured human macrophages. *J. Clin. Microbiol.* **24:**812–821.

49. Crump, J. A., J. van Ingen, A. B. Morrissey, M. J. Boeree, D. R. Mavura, B. Swai, N. M. Thielman, J. A. Bartlett, H. Grossman, V. P. Maro, and D. van Soolingen. 2009. Invasive disease caused by nontuberculous mycobacteria, Tanzania. *Emerg. Infect. Dis.* **15:**53–55.

50. Dailloux, M., M. L. Abalain, C. Laurain, L. Lebrun, C. Loos-Ayav, A. Lozniewski, and J. Maugein. 2006. Respiratory infections associated with nontuberculous mycobacteria in non-HIV patients. *Eur. Respir. J.* **28:**1211–1215.

51. Damsker, B., and E. J. Bottone. 1985. Mycobacterium avium-Mycobacterium intracellulare from the intestinal tracts of patients with the acquired immunodeficiency syndrome: concepts regarding acquisition and pathogenesis. *J. Infect. Dis.* **151:**179–181.

52. Dautzenberg, B., D. Piperno, P. Diot, C. Truffot-Pernot, J. P. Chauvin, et al. 1995. Clarithromycin in the treatment of Mycobacterium avium lung infections in patients without AIDS. *Chest* **107:**1035–1040.

53. Davidson, P. T., V. Khanijo, M. Goble, and T. S. Moulding. 1981. Treatment of disease due to Mycobacterium intracellulare. *Rev. Infect. Dis.* **3:**1052–1059.

54. Davis, K. K., P. N. Kao, S. S. Jacobs, and S. J. Ruoss. 2007. Aerosolized amikacin for treatment of pulmonary Mycobacterium avium infections: an observational case series. *BMC Pulm. Med.* **7:**2.

55. De Groote, M. A., N. R. Pace, K. Fulton, and J. O. Falkinham III. 2006. Relationships between *Mycobacterium* isolates from patients with pulmonary mycobacterial infection and potting soils. *Appl. Environ. Microbiol.* **72:**7602–7606.

56. Demura, Y., T. Tsuchida, D. Uesaka, Y. Umeda, M. Morikawa, S. Ameshima, T. Ishizaki, Y. Fujibayashi, and H. Okazawa. 2009. Usefulness of 18F-fluorodeoxyglucose positron emission tomography for diagnosing disease activity and monitoring therapeutic response in patients with pulmonary mycobacteriosis. *Eur. J. Nucl. Med. Mol. Imaging* **36:**632–639.

57. Desimone, J. A., Jr., T. J. Babinchak, K. R. Kaulback, and R. J. Pomerantz. 2003. Treatment of Mycobacterium avium complex immune reconstitution disease in HIV-1-infected individuals. *AIDS Patient Care STDS* **17:**617–622.

58. De Smet, K. A., I. N. Brown, M. Yates, and J. Ivanyi. 1995. Ribosomal internal transcribed spacer sequences are identical among Mycobacterium avium-intracellulare complex isolates from AIDS patients, but vary among isolates from elderly pulmonary disease patients. *Microbiology* **141**(Pt. 10):2739–2747.

59. Detjen, A. K., T. Keil, S. Roll, B. Hauer, H. Mauch, U. Wahn, and K. Magdorf. 2007. Interferon-gamma release assays improve the diagnosis of tuberculosis and nontuberculous mycobacterial disease in children in a country with a low incidence of tuberculosis. *Clin. Infect. Dis.* **45:**322–328.

60. Dhillon, S. S., and C. Watanakunakorn. 2000. Lady Windermere syndrome: middle lobe bronchiectasis and Mycobacterium avium complex infection due to voluntary cough suppression. *Clin. Infect. Dis.* **30:**572–575.

61. Doucette, K., and J. A. Fishman. 2004. Nontuberculous mycobacterial infection in hematopoietic stem cell and solid organ transplant recipients. *Clin. Infect. Dis.* **38:**1428–1439.

62. Dube, M. P., F. R. Sattler, F. J. Torriani, D. See, D. V. Havlir, C. A. Kemper, M. G. Dezfuli, S. A. Bozzette, A. E. Bartok, J. M. Leedom, J. G. Tilles, J. A. McCutchan, et al. 1997. A randomized evaluation of ethambutol for prevention of relapse and drug resistance during treatment of Mycobacterium avium complex bacteremia with clarithromycin-based combination therapy. *J. Infect. Dis.* **176:**1225–1232.

63. du Moulin, G. C., K. D. Stottmeier, P. A. Pelletier, A. Y. Tsang, and J. Hedley-Whyte. 1988. Concentration of Mycobacterium avium by hospital hot water systems. *JAMA* **260:**1599–1601.

64. Dunne, M., J. Fessel, P. Kumar, G. Dickenson, P. Keiser, M. Boulos, M. Mogyros, A. C. White, Jr., P. Cahn, M. O'Connor, D. Lewi, S. Green, J. Tilles, C. Hicks, J. Bissett, M. M. Schneider, and R. Benner. 2000. A randomized, double-blind trial comparing azithromycin and clarithromycin in the treatment of disseminated Mycobacterium avium infection in patients with human immunodeficiency virus. *Clin. Infect. Dis.* **31:**1245–1252.

65. Dutt, A. K., and W. W. Stead. 1979. Long-term results of medical treatment in Mycobacterium intracellulare infection. *Am. J. Med.* **67:**449–453.

66. Eaton, T., J. O. Falkinham III, and C. F. von Reyn. 1995. Recovery of *Mycobacterium avium* from cigarettes. *J. Clin. Microbiol.* **33:**2757–2758.

67. Edwards, L. B., F. A. Acquaviva, V. T. Livesay, F. W. Cross, and C. E. Palmer. 1969. An atlas of sensitivity to tuberculin, PPD-B, and histoplasmin in the United States. *Am. Rev. Respir. Dis.* **99**(Suppl.):1–132.

68. Ehlers, S. 1999. Immunity to tuberculosis: a delicate balance between protection and pathology. *FEMS Immunol. Med. Microbiol.* **23:**149–158.

69. Embil, J., P. Warren, M. Yakrus, R. Stark, S. Corne, D. Forrest, and E. Hershfield. 1997. Pulmonary illness associated with exposure to Mycobacterium-avium complex in hot tub water. Hypersensitivity pneumonitis or infection? *Chest* **111:**813–816.

70. Engbaek, H. C., B. Vergmann, and M. W. Bentzon. 1981. Lung disease caused by Mycobacterium avium/Mycobacterium intracellulare. An analysis of Danish patients during the period 1962-1976. *Eur. J. Respir. Dis.* **62:**72–83.

71. Etzkorn, E. T., S. Aldarondo, C. K. McAllister, J. Matthews, and A. J. Ognibene. 1986. Medical therapy of Mycobacterium avium-intracellulare pulmonary disease. *Am. Rev. Respir. Dis.* **134:**442–445.

72. Fairchok, M. P., J. H. Rouse, and S. L. Morris. 1995. Age-dependent humoral responses of children to mycobacterial antigens. *Clin. Diagn. Lab. Immunol.* **2:**443–447.

73. Falkinham, J. O., III. 2007. Growth in catheter biofilms and antibiotic resistance of Mycobacterium avium. *J. Med. Microbiol.* **56:**250–254.

74. Falkinham, J. O., III. 2003. Factors influencing the chlorine susceptibility of Mycobacterium avium, Mycobacterium intracellulare, and Mycobacterium scrofulaceum. *Appl. Environ. Microbiol.* **69:**5685–5689.

75. Falkinham, J. O., III, C. D. Norton, and M. W. LeChevallier. 2001. Factors influencing numbers of *Mycobacterium avium*, *Mycobacterium intracellulare*, and other *Mycobacteria* in drinking water distribution systems. *Appl. Environ. Microbiol.* 67:1225–1231.

76. Fauci, A. S., A. M. Macher, D. L. Longo, H. C. Lane, A. H. Rook, H. Masur, and E. P. Gelmann. 1984. NIH conference. Acquired immunodeficiency syndrome: epidemiologic, clinical, immunologic, and therapeutic considerations. *Ann. Intern. Med.* 100:92–106.

77. Feazel, L. M., L. K. Baumgartner, K. L. Peterson, D. N. Frank, J. K. Harris, and N. R. Pace. 2009. Opportunistic pathogens enriched in showerhead biofilms. *Proc. Natl. Acad. Sci. USA* 106:16393–16399.

78. Feizabadi, M. M., I. D. Robertson, D. V. Cousins, D. Dawson, W. Chew, G. L. Gilbert, and D. J. Hampson. 1996. Genetic characterization of Mycobacterium avium isolates recovered from humans and animals in Australia. *Epidemiol. Infect.* 116:41–49.

79. Fischer, D. A., W. Lester, and W. B. Schaefer. 1968. Infections with atypical mycobacteria. Five years' experience at the National Jewish Hospital. *Am. Rev. Respir. Dis.* 98:29–34.

80. Fitness, J., S. Floyd, D. K. Warndorff, L. Sichali, S. Malema, A. C. Crampin, P. E. Fine, and A. V. S. Hill. 2004. Large-scale candidate gene study of tuberculosis susceptibility in the Karonga district of northern Malawi. *Am. J. Trop. Med. Hyg.* 71:341–349.

81. Flint, D., M. Mahadevan, C. Barber, D. Grayson, and R. Small. 2000. Cervical lymphadenitis due to non-tuberculous mycobacteria: surgical treatment and review. *Int. J. Pediatr. Otorhinolaryngol.* 53:187–194.

82. Florido, M., A. S. Goncalves, R. A. Silva, S. Ehlers, A. M. Cooper, and R. Appelberg. 1999. Resistance of virulent *Mycobacterium avium* to gamma interferon-mediated antimicrobial activity suggests additional signals for induction of mycobacteriostasis. *Infect. Immun.* 67:3610–3618.

83. Forrest, D. M., E. Seminari, R. S. Hogg, B. Yip, J. Raboud, L. Lawson, P. Phillips, M. T. Schechter, M. V. O'Shaughnessy, and J. S. G. Montaner. 1998. The incidence and spectrum of AIDS-defining illnesses in persons treated with antiretroviral drugs. *Clin. Infect. Dis.* 27:1379–1385.

84. Freeman, A. F., K. N. Olivier, T. T. Rubio, G. Bartlett, J. W. Ochi, R. J. Claypool, L. Ding, D. B. Kuhns, and S. M. Holland. 2009. Intrathoracic nontuberculous mycobacterial infections in otherwise healthy children. *Pediatr. Pulmonol.* 44:1051–1056.

85. Freeman, J., A. Morris, T. Blackmore, D. Hammer, S. Munroe, and L. McKnight. 2007. Incidence of nontuberculous mycobacterial disease in New Zealand, 2004. *N. Z. Med. J.* 120:U2580.

86. Frothingham, R. 2001. Rates of torsades de pointes associated with ciprofloxacin, ofloxacin, levofloxacin, gatifloxacin, and moxifloxacin. *Pharmacotherapy* 21:1468–1472.

87. Frothingham, R., W. A. Meeker-O'Connell, A. J. Cobb, and S. M. Holland. 2000. Association of Mycobacterium avium sequevars Mav-B and Mav-E with disseminated disease in immunodeficient hosts. *Clin. Infect. Dis.* 31:309.

88. Frothingham, R., and K. H. Wilson. 1994. Molecular phylogeny of the Mycobacterium avium complex demonstrates clinically meaningful divisions. *J. Infect. Dis.* 169:305–312.

89. Frothingham, R., and K. H. Wilson. 1993. Sequence-based differentiation of strains in the *Mycobacterium avium* complex. *J. Bacteriol.* 175:2818–2825.

90. Fujikane, T., S. Fujiuchi, Y. Yamazaki, M. Sato, Y. Yamamoto, A. Takeda, Y. Nishigaki, Y. Fujita, and T. Shimizu. 2005. Efficacy and outcomes of clarithromycin treatment for pulmonary MAC disease. *Int. J. Tuberc. Lung Dis.* 9:1281–1287.

91. Furrer, H., and R. Malinverni. 1999. Systemic inflammatory reaction after starting highly active antiretroviral therapy in AIDS patients treated for extrapulmonary tuberculosis. *Am. J. Med.* 106:371–372.

92. Garrigues, G. E., J. M. Aldridge III, A. P. Toth, and J. E. Stout. 2009. Nontuberculous mycobacterial olecranon bursitis: case reports and literature review. *J. Shoulder Elbow Surg.* 18:e1–e5.

93. Gascon, P., S. S. Sathe, and P. Rameshwar. 1993. Impaired erythropoiesis in the acquired immunodeficiency syndrome with disseminated Mycobacterium avium complex. *Am. J. Med.* 94:41–48.

94. Ghassemi, M., F. K. Asadi, B. R. Andersen, and R. M. Novak. 2000. Mycobacterium avium induces HIV upregulation through mechanisms independent of cytokine induction. *AIDS Res. Hum. Retrovir.* 16:435–440.

95. Glosli, H., A. Stray-Pedersen, A. C. Brun, L. W. Holtmon, T. Tonjum, A. Chapgier, J. L. Casanova, and T. G. Abrahamsen. 2008. Infections due to various atypical mycobacteria in a Norwegian multiplex family with dominant interferon-gamma receptor deficiency. *Clin. Infect. Dis.* 46:e23–e27.

96. Gomes, M. S., M. Florido, J. V. Cordeiro, C. M. Teixeira, O. Takeuchi, S. Akira, and R. Appelberg. 2004. Limited role of the Toll-like receptor-2 in resistance to Mycobacterium avium. *Immunology* 111:179–185.

97. Good, R. C., and D. E. Snider, Jr. 1982. Isolation of nontuberculous mycobacteria in the United States, 1980. *J. Infect. Dis.* 146:829–833.

98. Gordin, F. M., D. L. Cohn, P. M. Sullam, J. R. Schoenfelder, B. A. Wynne, and C. R. Horsburgh, Jr. 1997. Early manifestations of disseminated Mycobacterium avium complex disease: a prospective evaluation. *J. Infect. Dis.* 176:126–132.

99. Gordin, F. M., P. M. Sullam, S. D. Shafran, D. L. Cohn, B. Wynne, L. Paxton, K. Perry, and C. R. Horsburgh, Jr. 1999. A randomized, placebo-controlled study of rifabutin added to a regimen of clarithromycin and ethambutol for treatment of disseminated infection with Mycobacterium avium complex. *Clin. Infect. Dis.* 28:1080–1085.

100. Greene, J. B., G. S. Sidhu, S. Lewin, J. F. Levine, H. Masur, M. S. Simberkoff, P. Nicholas, R. C. Good, S. B. Zolla-Pazner, A. A. Pollock, M. L. Tapper, and R. S. Holzman. 1982. Mycobacterium avium-intracellulare: a cause of disseminated life-threatening infection in homosexuals and drug abusers. *Ann. Intern. Med.* 97:539–546.

101. Gribetz, A. R., B. Damsker, E. J. Bottone, P. A. Kirschner, and A. S. Teirstein. 1981. Solitary pulmonary nodules due to non-tuberculous mycobacterial infection. *Am. J. Med.* 70:39–43.

102. Griffith, D. E., T. Aksamit, B. A. Brown-Elliott, A. Catanzaro, C. Daley, F. Gordin, S. M. Holland, R. Horsburgh, G. Huitt, M. F. Iademarco, M. Iseman, K. Olivier, S. Ruoss, C. F. von Reyn, R. J. Wallace, Jr., and K. Winthrop. 2007. An official ATS/IDSA statement: diagnosis, treatment, and prevention of nontuberculous mycobacterial diseases. *Am. J. Respir. Crit. Care Med.* 175:367–416.

103. Griffith, D. E., B. A. Brown-Elliott, B. Langsjoen, Y. Zhang, X. Pan, W. Girard, K. Nelson, J. Caccitolo, J. Alvarez, S. Shepherd, R. Wilson, E. A. Graviss, and R. J. Wallace, Jr. 2006. Clinical and molecular analysis of macrolide resistance in Mycobacterium avium complex lung disease. *Am. J. Respir. Crit. Care Med.* 174:928–934.

104. Griffith, D. E., B. A. Brown-Elliott, S. Shepherd, J. McLarty, L. Griffith, and R. J. Wallace, Jr. 2005. Ethambutol ocular toxicity in treatment regimens for Mycobacterium avium complex lung disease. *Am. J. Respir. Crit. Care Med.* 172:250–253.

105. Griffith, D. E., B. A. Brown, P. Cegielski, D. T. Murphy, and R. J. Wallace, Jr. 2000. Early results (at 6 months) with intermittent clarithromycin-including regimens for lung disease due to Mycobacterium avium complex. *Clin. Infect. Dis.* 30:288–292.

106. Griffith, D. E., B. A. Brown, W. M. Girard, B. E. Griffith, L. A. Couch, and R. J. Wallace, Jr. 2001. Azithromycin-containing regimens for treatment of Mycobacterium avium complex lung disease. *Clin. Infect. Dis.* 32:1547–1553.

107. Griffith, D. E., B. A. Brown, W. M. Girard, D. T. Murphy, and R. J. Wallace, Jr. 1996. Azithromycin activity against Mycobacterium avium complex lung disease in patients who were not infected with human immunodeficiency virus. *Clin. Infect. Dis.* 23:983–989.

108. Griffith, D. E., B. A. Brown, W. M. Girard, and R. J. Wallace, Jr. 1995. Adverse events associated with high-dose rifabutin in macrolide-containing regimens for the treatment of Mycobacterium avium complex lung disease. *Clin. Infect. Dis.* 21:594–598.

109. Guerrero, C., C. Bernasconi, D. Burki, T. Bodmer, and A. Telenti. 1995. A novel insertion element from Mycobacterium avium, IS1245, is a specific target for analysis of strain relatedness. *J. Clin. Microbiol.* 33:304–307.

110. Gupta, A., and H. Clauss. 2009. Prosthetic joint infection with Mycobacterium avium complex in a solid organ transplant recipient. *Transpl. Infect. Dis.* 11:537–540.

111. Guthertz, L. S., B. Damsker, E. J. Bottone, E. G. Ford, T. F. Midura, and J. M. Janda. 1989. Mycobacterium avium and Mycobacterium intracellulare infections in patients with and without AIDS. *J. Infect. Dis.* 160:1037–1041.

112. Hadad, D. J., D. S. Lewi, A. C. Pignatari, M. C. Martins, W. Vitti Junior, and R. D. Arbeit. 1998. Resolution of Mycobacterium avium complex bacteremia following highly active antiretroviral therapy. *Clin. Infect. Dis.* 26:758–759.

113. Hadad, D. J., M. Palaci, A. C. Pignatari, D. S. Lewi, M. A. Machado, M. A. Telles, M. C. Martins, S. Y. Ueki, G. M. Vasconcelos, and M. C. Palhares. 2004. Mycobacteraemia among HIV-1-infected patients in Sao Paulo, Brazil: 1995 to 1998. *Epidemiol. Infect.* 132:151–155.

114. Hafner, R., J. A. Cohn, D. J. Wright, N. E. Dunlap, M. J. Egorin, M. E. Enama, K. Muth, C. A. Peloquin, N. Mor, L. B. Heifets, et al. 1997. Early bactericidal activity of isoniazid in pulmonary tuberculosis. Optimization of methodology. *Am. J. Respir. Crit. Care Med.* 156:918–923.

115. Hahm, C. R., H. Y. Park, K. Jeon, S. W. Um, G. Y. Suh, M. P. Chung, H. Kim, O. J. Kwon, and W. J. Koh. 2010. Solitary pulmonary nodules caused by Mycobacterium tuberculosis and Mycobacterium avium complex. *Lung* 188:25–31.

116. Han, X. Y., J. J. Tarrand, R. Infante, K. L. Jacobson, and M. Truong. 2005. Clinical significance and epidemiologic analyses of *Mycobacterium avium* and *Mycobacterium intracellulare* among patients without AIDS. *J. Clin. Microbiol.* 43:4407–4412.

117. Hanak, V., J. M. Golbin, and J. H. Ryu. 2007. Causes and presenting features in 85 consecutive patients with hypersensitivity pneumonitis. *Mayo Clin. Proc.* 82:812–816.

118. Hanak, V., S. Kalra, T. R. Aksamit, T. E. Hartman, H. D. Tazelaar, and J. H. Ryu. 2006. Hot tub lung: presenting features and clinical course of 21 patients. *Respir. Med.* 100:610–615.

119. Hartman, T. E., S. J. Swensen, and D. E. Williams. 1993. Mycobacterium avium-intracellulare complex: evaluation with CT. *Radiology* 187:23–26.

120. Hasegawa, N., T. Nishimura, S. Ohtani, K. Takeshita, K. Fukunaga, S. Tasaka, T. Urano, K. Ishii, M. Miyairi, and A. Ishizaka. 2009. Therapeutic effects of various initial combinations of chemotherapy including clarithromycin against Mycobacterium avium complex pulmonary disease. *Chest* 136:1569–1575.

121. Haverkamp, M. H., S. M. Arend, J. A. Lindeboom, N. G. Hartwig, and J. T. van Dissel. 2004. Nontuberculous mycobacterial infection in children: a 2-year prospective surveillance study in the Netherlands. *Clin. Infect. Dis.* 39:450–456.

122. Havlir, D. V., M. P. Dube, F. R. Sattler, D. N. Forthal, C. A. Kemper, M. W. Dunne, D. M. Parenti, J. P. Lavelle, A. C. White, Jr., M. D. Witt, S. A. Bozzette, J. A. McCutchan, et al. 1996. Prophylaxis against disseminated Mycobacterium avium complex with weekly azithromycin, daily rifabutin, or both. *N. Engl. J. Med.* 335:392–398.

123. Hawkins, C. C., J. W. Gold, E. Whimbey, T. E. Kiehn, P. Brannon, R. Cammarata, A. E. Brown, and D. Armstrong. 1986. Mycobacterium avium complex infections in patients with the acquired immunodeficiency syndrome. *Ann. Intern. Med.* 105:184–188.

124. Hazra, R., S. H. Lee, J. N. Maslow, and R. N. Husson. 2000. Related strains of Mycobacterium avium cause disease in children with AIDS and in children with lymphadenitis. *J. Infect. Dis.* 181:1298–1303.

125. Hellinger, W. C., J. D. Smilack, J. L. Greider, Jr., S. Alvarez, S. D. Trigg, N. S. Brewer, and R. S. Edson. 1995. Localized soft-tissue infections with Mycobacterium avium/ Mycobacterium intracellulare complex in immunocompetent patients: granulomatous tenosynovitis of the hand or wrist. *Clin. Infect. Dis.* 21:65–69.

126. Hernandez-Garduno, E., M. Rodrigues, and R. K. Elwood. 2009. The incidence of pulmonary non-tuberculous mycobacteria in British Columbia, Canada. *Int. J. Tuberc. Lung Dis.* 13:1086–1093.

127. Hewitt, R. G., G. D. Papandonatos, M. J. Shelton, C. B. Hsiao, B. J. Harmon, S. R. Kaczmarek, and D. Amsterdam. 1999. Prevention of disseminated Mycobacterium avium complex infection with reduced dose clarithromycin in patients with advanced HIV disease. *AIDS* 13:1367–1372.

128. Hilborn, E. D., T. C. Covert, M. A. Yakrus, S. I. Harris, S. F. Donnelly, E. W. Rice, S. Toney, S. A. Bailey, and G. N. Stelma, Jr. 2006. Persistence of nontuberculous mycobacteria in a drinking water system after addition of filtration treatment. *Appl. Environ. Microbiol.* 72:5864–5869.

129. Hocqueloux, L., P. Lesprit, J. L. Herrmann, A. de La Blanchardiere, A. M. Zagdanski, J. M. Decazes, and J. Modai. 1998. Pulmonary Mycobacterium avium complex disease without dissemination in HIV-infected patients. *Chest* 113:542–548.

130. Holland, S. M., E. M. Eisenstein, D. B. Kuhns, M. L. Turner, T. A. Fleisher, W. Strober, and J. I. Gallin. 1994. Treatment of refractory disseminated nontuberculous mycobacterial infection with interferon gamma. A preliminary report. *N. Engl. J. Med.* 330:1348–1355.

131. Holmes, C. B., E. Losina, R. P. Walensky, Y. Yazdanpanah, and K. A. Freedberg. 2003. Review of human immunodeficiency virus type 1-related opportunistic infections in sub-Saharan Africa. *Clin. Infect. Dis.* 36:652–662.

132. Horsburgh, C. R., Jr. 1991. Mycobacterium avium complex infection in the acquired immunodeficiency syndrome. *N. Engl. J. Med.* 324:1332–1338.

133. Horsburgh, C. R., Jr., J. Gettings, L. N. Alexander, and J. L. Lennox. 2001. Disseminated Mycobacterium avium complex disease among patients infected with human immunodeficiency virus, 1985-2000. *Clin. Infect. Dis.* 33:1938–1943.

134. Horsburgh, C. R., Jr., J. A. Havlik, D. A. Ellis, E. Kennedy, S. A. Fann, R. E. Dubois, and S. E. Thompson. 1991. Survival of patients with acquired immune deficiency syndrome and disseminated Mycobacterium avium complex infection

with and without antimycobacterial chemotherapy. *Am. Rev. Respir. Dis.* **144**:557–559.

135. Horsburgh, C. R., Jr., U. G. Mason III, L. B. Heifets, K. Southwick, J. Labrecque, and M. D. Iseman. 1987. Response to therapy of pulmonary Mycobacterium avium-intracellulare infection correlates with results of in vitro susceptibility testing. *Am. Rev. Respir. Dis.* **135**:418–421.

136. Horsburgh, C. R., Jr., B. Metchock, S. M. Gordon, J. A. Havlik, Jr., J. E. McGowan, Jr., and S. E. Thompson III. 1994. Predictors of survival in patients with AIDS and disseminated Mycobacterium avium complex disease. *J. Infect. Dis.* **170**:573–577.

137. Huang, J. H., P. N. Kao, V. Adi, and S. J. Ruoss. 1999. Mycobacterium avium-intracellulare pulmonary infection in HIV-negative patients without preexisting lung disease: diagnostic and management limitations. *Chest* **115**:1033–1040.

138. Huang, J. H., P. J. Oefner, V. Adi, K. Ratnam, S. J. Ruoss, E. Trako, and P. N. Kao. 1998. Analyses of the NRAMP1 and INF-gammaR1 genes in women with Mycobacterium avium-intracellulare pulmonary disease. *Am. J. Respir. Crit. Care Med.* **157**:377–381.

139. Ichiyama, S., K. Shimokata, and M. Tsukamura. 1988. The isolation of Mycobacterium avium complex from soil, water, and dusts. *Microbiol. Immunol.* **32**:733–739.

140. Iseman, M. D. 2002. Medical management of pulmonary disease caused by Mycobacterium avium complex. *Clin. Chest Med.* **23**:633–641.

141. Iseman, M. D., D. L. Buschman, and L. M. Ackerson. 1991. Pectus excavatum and scoliosis. Thoracic anomalies associated with pulmonary disease caused by Mycobacterium avium complex. *Am. Rev. Respir. Dis.* **144**:914–916.

142. Ives, N. J., B. G. Gazzard, and P. J. Easterbrook. 2001. The changing pattern of AIDS-defining illnesses with the introduction of highly active antiretroviral therapy (HAART) in a London clinic. *J. Infect.* **42**:134–139.

143. Jacobson, M. A., P. Bacchetti, A. Kolokathis, R. E. Chaisson, S. Szabo, B. Polsky, G. T. Valainis, D. Mildvan, D. Abrams, and J. Wilber. 1991. Surrogate markers for survival in patients with AIDS and AIDS related complex treated with zidovudine. *BMJ* **302**:73–78.

144. Jenkins, P. A., I. A. Campbell, J. Banks, C. M. Gelder, R. J. Prescott, and A. P. Smith. 2008. Clarithromycin vs ciprofloxacin as adjuncts to rifampicin and ethambutol in treating opportunist mycobacterial lung diseases and an assessment of Mycobacterium vaccae immunotherapy. *Thorax* **63**:627–634.

145. Kahana, L. M., J. M. Kay, M. A. Yakrus, and S. Waserman. 1997. Mycobacterium avium complex infection in an immunocompetent young adult related to hot tub exposure. *Chest* **111**:242–245.

146. Kallenius, G., T. Koivula, K. J. Rydgard, S. E. Hoffner, A. Valentin, B. Asjo, C. Ljungh, U. Sharma, and S. B. Svenson. 1992. Human immunodeficiency virus type 1 enhances intracellular growth of *Mycobacterium avium* in human macrophages. *Infect. Immun.* **60**:2453–2458.

147. Kaplan, J. E., C. Benson, K. H. Holmes, J. T. Brooks, A. Pau, and H. Masur. 2009. Guidelines for prevention and treatment of opportunistic infections in HIV-infected adults and adolescents: recommendations from CDC, the National Institutes of Health, and the HIV Medicine Association of the Infectious Diseases Society of America. *MMWR Recomm. Rep.* **58**:1–207.

148. Kaplan, J. E., D. Hanson, M. S. Dworkin, T. Frederick, J. Bertolli, M. L. Lindegren, S. Holmberg, and J. L. Jones. 2000. Epidemiology of human immunodeficiency virus-associated opportunistic infections in the United States in the era of highly active antiretroviral therapy. *Clin. Infect. Dis.* **30**(Suppl. 1):S5–S14.

149. Karakousis, P. C., R. D. Moore, and R. E. Chaisson. 2004. Mycobacterium avium complex in patients with HIV infection in the era of highly active antiretroviral therapy. *Lancet Infect. Dis.* **4**:557–565.

150. Karavellas, M. P., C. Y. Lowder, C. Macdonald, C. P. Avila, Jr., and W. R. Freeman. 1998. Immune recovery vitritis associated with inactive cytomegalovirus retinitis: a new syndrome. *Arch. Ophthalmol.* **116**:169–175.

151. Katila, M. L., E. Iivanainen, P. Torkko, J. Kauppinen, P. Martikainen, and P. Vaananen. 1995. Isolation of potentially pathogenic mycobacteria in the Finnish environment. *Scand. J. Infect. Dis. Suppl.* **98**:9–11.

152. Kaur, D., and G. K. Khuller. 2001. In vitro, ex-vivo and in vivo activities of ethambutol and sparfloxacin alone and in combination against mycobacteria. *Int. J. Antimicrob. Agents* **17**:51–55.

153. Kedzierska, K., J. Mak, A. Mijch, I. Cooke, M. Rainbird, S. Roberts, G. Paukovics, D. Jolley, A. Lopez, and S. M. Crowe. 2000. Granulocyte-macrophage colony-stimulating factor augments phagocytosis of Mycobacterium avium complex by human immunodeficiency virus type 1-infected monocytes/macrophages in vitro and in vivo. *J. Infect. Dis.* **181**:390–394.

154. Keiser, P., N. Nassar, D. Skiest, S. Rademacher, and J. W. Smith. 1999. A retrospective study of the addition of ciprofloxacin to clarithromycin and ethambutol in the treatment of disseminated Mycobacterium avium complex infection. *Int. J. STD AIDS* **10**:791–794.

155. Khan, K., J. Wang, and T. K. Marras. 2007. Nontuberculous mycobacterial sensitization in the United States: national trends over three decades. *Am. J. Respir. Crit. Care Med.* **176**:306–313.

156. Khoor, A., K. O. Leslie, H. D. Tazelaar, R. A. Helmers, and T. V. Colby. 2001. Diffuse pulmonary disease caused by nontuberculous mycobacteria in immunocompetent people (hot tub lung). *Am. J. Clin. Pathol.* **115**:755–762.

157. Kikuchi, T., A. Watanabe, K. Gomi, T. Sakakibara, K. Nishimori, H. Daito, S. Fujimura, R. Tazawa, A. Inoue, M. Ebina, Y. Tokue, M. Kaku, and T. Nukiwa. 2009. Association between mycobacterial genotypes and disease progression in Mycobacterium avium pulmonary infection. *Thorax* **64**:901–907.

158. Kim, R. D., D. E. Greenberg, M. E. Ehrmantraut, S. V. Guide, L. Ding, Y. Shea, M. R. Brown, M. Chernick, W. K. Steagall, C. G. Glasgow, J. Lin, C. Jolley, L. Sorbara, M. Raffeld, S. Hill, N. Avila, V. Sachdev, L. A. Barnhart, V. L. Anderson, R. Claypool, D. M. Hilligoss, M. Garofalo, A. Fitzgerald, S. Anaya-O'Brien, D. Darnell, R. DeCastro, H. M. Menning, S. M. Ricklefs, S. F. Porcella, K. N. Olivier, J. Moss, and S. M. Holland. 2008. Pulmonary nontuberculous mycobacterial disease: prospective study of a distinct preexisting syndrome. *Am. J. Respir. Crit. Care Med.* **178**:1066–1074.

159. Kim, T. C., N. S. Arora, T. K. Aldrich, and D. F. Rochester. 1981. Atypical mycobacterial infections: a clinical study of 92 patients. *South. Med. J.* **74**:1304–1308.

160. Kirschner, R. A., Jr., B. C. Parker, and J. O. Falkinham III. 1992. Epidemiology of infection by nontuberculous mycobacteria. Mycobacterium avium, Mycobacterium intracellulare, and Mycobacterium scrofulaceum in acid, brown-water swamps of the southeastern United States and their association with environmental variables. *Am. Rev. Respir. Dis.* **145**:271–275.

161. Kitada, S., K. Kobayashi, S. Ichiyama, S. Takakura, M. Sakatani, K. Suzuki, T. Takashima, T. Nagai, I. Sakurabayashi, M.

Ito, and R. Maekura. 2008. Serodiagnosis of Mycobacterium avium-complex pulmonary disease using an enzyme immunoassay kit. *Am. J. Respir. Crit. Care Med.* **177:**793–797.

162. Kitada, S., R. Maekura, N. Toyoshima, N. Fujiwara, I. Yano, T. Ogura, M. Ito, and K. Kobayashi. 2002. Serodiagnosis of pulmonary disease due to Mycobacterium avium complex with an enzyme immunoassay that uses a mixture of glyco-peptidolipid antigens. *Clin. Infect. Dis.* **35:**1328–1335.

163. Kobashi, Y., T. Matsushima, and M. Oka. 2007. A double-blind randomized study of aminoglycoside infusion with combined therapy for pulmonary Mycobacterium avium complex disease. *Respir. Med.* **101:**130–138.

164. Kohno, Y., H. Ohno, Y. Miyazaki, Y. Higashiyama, K. Yanagihara, Y. Hirakata, K. Fukushima, and S. Kohno. 2007. In vitro and in vivo activities of novel fluoroquinolones alone and in combination with clarithromycin against clinically isolated *Mycobacterium avium* complex strains in Japan. *Antimicrob. Agents Chemother.* **51:**4071–4076.

165. Komatsu, H., A. Terunuma, N. Tabata, and H. Tagami. 1999. Mycobacterium avium infection of the skin associated with lichen scrofulosorum: report of three cases. *Br. J. Dermatol.* **141:**554–557.

166. Kubo, K., Y. Yamazaki, M. Hanaoka, H. Nomura, K. Fujimoto, T. Honda, M. Ota, and Y. Kamijou. 2000. Analysis of HLA antigens in Mycobacterium avium-intracellulare pulmonary infection. *Am. J. Respir. Crit. Care Med.* **161:**1368–1371.

167. Kullavanijaya, P., S. Sirimachan, and S. Surarak. 1997. Primary cutaneous infection with Mycobacterium avium intracellulare complex resembling lupus vulgaris. *Br. J. Dermatol.* **136:**264–266.

168. Kunimoto, D. Y., M. S. Peppler, J. Talbot, P. Phillips, S. D. Shafran, and Canadian HIV Trials Network Protocol 010 Study Group. 2003. Analysis of *Mycobacterium avium* complex isolates from blood samples of AIDS patients by pulsed-field gel electrophoresis. *J. Clin. Microbiol.* **41:**498–499.

169. Lalezari, J. P., G. N. Holland, F. Kramer, G. F. McKinley, C. A. Kemper, D. V. Ives, R. Nelson, W. D. Hardy, B. D. Kuppermann, D. W. Northfelt, M. Youle, M. Johnson, R. A. Lewis, D. V. Weinberg, G. L. Simon, R. A. Wolitz, A. E. Ruby, R. J. Stagg, and H. S. Jaffe. 1998. Randomized, controlled study of the safety and efficacy of intravenous cidofovir for the treatment of relapsing cytomegalovirus retinitis in patients with AIDS. *J. Acquir. Immune Defic. Syndr. Hum. Retrovirol.* **17:**339–344.

170. Lam, P. K., D. E. Griffith, T. R. Aksamit, S. J. Ruoss, S. M. Garay, C. L. Daley, and A. Catanzaro. 2006. Factors related to response to intermittent treatment of Mycobacterium avium complex lung disease. *Am. J. Respir. Crit. Care Med.* **173:**1283–1289.

171. Larsson, L. O., B. E. Skoogh, M. W. Bentzon, M. Magnusson, J. Olofson, J. Taranger, and A. Lind. 1991. Sensitivity to sensitins and tuberculin in Swedish children. II. A study of preschool children. *Tubercle* **72:**37–42.

172. Lauw, F. N., J. T. Der Meer, J. de Metz, S. A. Danner, and P. T. van Der. 2001. No beneficial effect of interferon-gamma treatment in 2 human immunodeficiency virus–infected patients with Mycobacterium avium complex infection. *Clin. Infect. Dis.* **32:**e81–e82.

173. Lavy, A., R. Rusu, and S. Shaheen. 1990. Mycobacterium avium-intracellulare in clinical specimens: etiological factor or contaminant? *Isr. J. Med. Sci.* **26:**374–378.

174. Lawn, S. D., L. G. Bekker, and R. F. Miller. 2005. Immune reconstitution disease associated with mycobacterial infections in HIV-infected individuals receiving antiretrovirals. *Lancet Infect. Dis.* **5:**361–373.

175. Lawn, S. D., T. A. Bicanic, and D. C. Macallan. 2004. Pyomyositis and cutaneous abscesses due to Mycobacterium avium: an immune reconstitution manifestation in a patient with AIDS. *Clin. Infect. Dis.* **38:**461–463.

176. Lefevre, P., P. Gilot, H. Godiscal, J. Content, and M. Fauville-Dufaux. 2000. Mycobacterium intracellulare as a cause of a recurrent granulomatous tenosynovitis of the hand. *Diagn. Microbiol. Infect. Dis.* **38:**127–129.

177. Legrand, E., C. Sola, B. Verdol, and N. Rastogi. 2000. Genetic diversity of Mycobacterium avium recovered from AIDS patients in the Caribbean as studied by a consensus IS1245-RFLP method and pulsed-field gel electrophoresis. *Res. Microbiol.* **151:**271–283.

178. Levy, I., G. Grisaru-Soen, L. Lerner-Geva, E. Kerem, H. Blau, L. Bentur, M. Aviram, J. Rivlin, E. Picard, A. Lavy, Y. Yahav, and G. Rahav. 2008. Multicenter cross-sectional study of nontuberculous mycobacterial infections among cystic fibrosis patients, Israel. *Emerg. Infect. Dis.* **14:**378–384.

179. Lewis, A. G., Jr., E. M. Lasche, A. L. Armstrong, and F. P. Dunbar. 1960. A clinical study of the chronic lung disease due to nonphotochromogenic acid-fast bacilli. *Ann. Intern. Med.* **53:**273–285.

180. Lindeboom, J. A., E. J. Kuijper, E. S. Bruijnesteijn van Coppenraet, R. Lindeboom, and J. M. Prins. 2007. Surgical excision versus antibiotic treatment for nontuberculous mycobacterial cervicofacial lymphadenitis in children: a multicenter, randomized, controlled trial. *Clin. Infect. Dis.* **44:**1057–1064.

181. Lindeboom, J. A., R. Lindeboom, E. S. Bruijnesteijn van Coppenraet, E. J. Kuijper, J. Tuk, and J. M. Prins. 2009. Esthetic outcome of surgical excision versus antibiotic therapy for nontuberculous mycobacterial cervicofacial lymphadenitis in children. *Pediatr. Infect. Dis. J.* **28:**1028–1030.

182. Low, N., D. Pfluger, M. Egger, M. Battegay, E. Bernasconi, P. Burgisser, P. Erb, W. Fierz, M. Flepp, P. Francioli, P. Grob, U. Gruninger, B. Hirschel, L. Jeannerod, B. Ledergerber, R. Luthy, R. Malinverni, L. Matter, M. Opravil, F. Paccaud, L. Perrin, W. Pichler, G. C. Piffaretti, M. Rickenbach, O. Rutschmann, P. Vernazza, and J. vonOverbeck. 1997. Disseminated Mycobacterium avium complex disease in the Swiss HIV cohort study: increasing incidence, unchanged prognosis. *AIDS* **11:**1165–1171.

183. Maas, J. J., N. A. Foudraine, P. T. Schellekens, M. E. Mensen, J. Veenstra, M. T. Roos, R. van Leeuwen, and R. A. Coutinho. 1999. Reliability of tuberculin purified derivative skin testing and delayed-type hypersensitivity skin test anergy in HIV-infected homosexual men, at risk of tuberculosis. *AIDS* **13:**1784–1785.

184. Macher, A. M., J. A. Kovacs, V. Gill, G. D. Roberts, J. Ames, C. H. Park, S. Straus, H. C. Lane, J. E. Parrillo, A. S. Fauci, et al. 1983. Bacteremia due to Mycobacterium avium-intracellulare in the acquired immunodeficiency syndrome. *Ann. Intern. Med.* **99:**782–785.

185. Mai, H. N., M. Hijikata, Y. Inoue, K. Suzuki, M. Sakatani, M. Okada, K. Kimura, N. Kobayashi, E. Toyota, K. Kudo, H. Nagai, A. Kurashima, A. Kajiki, N. Oketani, H. Hayakawa, G. Tanaka, J. Shojima, I. Matsushita, S. Sakurada, K. Tokunaga, and N. Keicho. 2007. Pulmonary Mycobacterium avium complex infection associated with the IVS8-T5 allele of the CFTR gene. *Int. J. Tuberc. Lung Dis.* **11:**808–813.

186. Mangione, E. J., G. Huitt, D. Lenaway, J. Beebe, A. Bailey, M. Figoski, M. P. Rau, K. D. Albrecht, and M. A. Yakrus. 2001. Nontuberculous mycobacterial disease following hot tub exposure. *Emerg. Infect. Dis.* **7:**1039–1042.

187. Marchevsky, A., B. Damsker, A. Gribetz, S. Tepper, and S. A. Geller. 1982. The spectrum of pathology of nontuberculous

mycobacterial infections in open-lung biopsy specimens. *Am. J. Clin. Pathol.* **78:**695–700.

188. Maslow, J. N., I. Brar, G. Smith, G. W. Newman, R. Mehta, C. Thornton, and P. Didier. 2003. Latent infection as a source of disseminated disease caused by organisms of the Mycobacterium avium complex in simian immunodeficiency virus-infected rhesus macaques. *J. Infect. Dis.* **187:**1748–1755.

189. Maslow, J. N., D. Dawson, E. A. Carlin, and S. M. Holland. 1999. Hemolysin as a virulence factor for systemic infection with isolates of *Mycobacterium avium* complex. *J. Clin. Microbiol.* **37:**445–446.

190. McGarvey, J. A., and L. E. Bermudez. 2001. Phenotypic and genomic analyses of the *Mycobacterium avium* complex reveal differences in gastrointestinal invasion and genomic composition. *Infect. Immun.* **69:**7242–7249.

191. McNaghten, A. D., D. L. Hanson, J. L. Jones, M. S. Dworkin, J. W. Ward, et al. 1999. Effects of antiretroviral therapy and opportunistic illness primary chemoprophylaxis on survival after AIDS diagnosis. *AIDS* **13:**1687–1695.

192. Mehta, J. B., M. W. Emery, M. Girish, R. P. Byrd, Jr., and T. M. Roy. 2003. Atypical Pott's disease: localized infection of the thoracic spine due to Mycobacterium avium-intracellulare in a patient without human immunodeficiency virus infection. *South. Med. J.* **96:**685–688.

193. Meyer, M., P. W. von Grunberg, T. Knoop, P. Hartmann, and G. Plum. 1998. The macrophage-induced gene mig as a marker for clinical pathogenicity and in vitro virulence of *Mycobacterium avium* complex strains. *Infect. Immun.* **66:**4549–4552.

194. Milanes-Virelles, M. T., I. Garcia-Garcia, Y. Santos-Herrera, M. Valdes-Quintana, C. M. Valenzuela-Silva, G. Jimenez-Madrigal, T. I. Ramos-Gomez, I. Bello-Rivero, N. Fernandez-Olivera, R. B. Sanchez-de la Osa, C. Rodriguez-Acosta, L. Gonzalez-Mendez, G. Martinez-Sanchez, and P. A. Lopez-Saura. 2008. Adjuvant interferon gamma in patients with pulmonary atypical Mycobacteriosis: a randomized, double-blind, placebo-controlled study. *BMC Infect. Dis.* **8:**17.

195. Mitchell, J. D., A. Bishop, A. Cafaro, M. J. Weyant, and M. Pomerantz. 2008. Anatomic lung resection for nontuberculous mycobacterial disease. *Ann. Thorac. Surg.* **85:**1887–1892.

196. Munoz, R. M., L. Alonso-Pulpon, M. Yebra, J. Segovia, J. C. Gallego, and R. M. Daza. 2000. Intestinal involvement by nontuberculous mycobacteria after heart transplantation. *Clin. Infect. Dis.* **30:**603–605.

197. Murcia, M. I., E. Tortoli, M. C. Menendez, E. Palenque, and M. J. Garcia. 2006. Mycobacterium colombiense sp. nov., a novel member of the Mycobacterium avium complex and description of MAC-X as a new ITS genetic variant. *Int. J. Syst. Evol. Microbiol.* **56:**2049–2054.

198. Murdoch, D. M., and J. R. McDonald. 2007. Mycobacterium avium-intracellulare cellulitis occurring with septic arthritis after joint injection: a case report. *BMC Infect. Dis.* **7:**9.

199. Nannini, E. C., M. Keating, P. Binstock, G. Samonis, and D. P. Kontoyiannis. 2002. Successful treatment of refractory disseminated Mycobacterium avium complex infection with the addition of linezolid and mefloquine. *J. Infect.* **44:**201–203.

200. Narita, M., D. Ashkin, E. S. Hollender, and A. E. Pitchenik. 1998. Paradoxical worsening of tuberculosis following antiretroviral therapy in patients with AIDS. *Am. J. Respir. Crit. Care Med.* **158:**157–161.

201. Nelson, K. G., D. E. Griffith, B. A. Brown, and R. J. Wallace, Jr. 1998. Results of operation in Mycobacterium avium-intracellulare lung disease. *Ann. Thorac. Surg.* **66:**325–330.

202. Nightingale, S. D., L. T. Byrd, P. M. Southern, J. D. Jockusch, S. X. Cal, and B. A. Wynne. 1992. Incidence of Mycobac-

terium avium-intracellulare complex bacteremia in human immunodeficiency virus-positive patients. *J. Infect. Dis.* **165:**1082–1085.

203. Nightingale, S. D., D. W. Cameron, F. M. Gordin, P. M. Sullam, D. L. Cohn, R. E. Chaisson, L. J. Eron, P. D. Sparti, B. Bihari, D. L. Kaufman, J. J. Stern, D. D. Pearce, W. G. Weinberg, A. LaMarca, and F. P. Siegal. 1993. Two controlled trials of rifabutin prophylaxis against Mycobacterium avium complex infection in AIDS. *N. Engl. J. Med.* **329:**828–833.

204. Nishimura, T., N. Hasegawa, Y. Fujita, I. Yano, and A. Ishizaka. 2009. Serodiagnostic contributions of antibody titers against mycobacterial lipid antigens in Mycobacterium avium complex pulmonary disease. *Clin. Infect. Dis.* **49:**529–535.

205. Nishiuchi, Y., R. Maekura, S. Kitada, A. Tamaru, T. Taguri, Y. Kira, T. Hiraga, A. Hirotani, K. Yoshimura, M. Miki, and M. Ito. 2007. The recovery of Mycobacterium avium-intracellulare complex (MAC) from the residential bathrooms of patients with pulmonary MAC. *Clin. Infect. Dis.* **45:**347–351.

206. Nolt, D., M. G. Michaels, and E. R. Wald. 2003. Intrathoracic disease from nontuberculous mycobacteria in children: two cases and a review of the literature. *Pediatrics* **112:**e434.

207. Ntziora, F., and M. E. Falagas. 2007. Linezolid for the treatment of patients with [corrected] mycobacterial infections [corrected] a systematic review. *Int. J. Tuberc. Lung Dis.* **11:**606–611.

208. O'Brien, D. P., B. J. Currie, and V. L. Krause. 2000. Nontuberculous mycobacterial disease in northern Australia: a case series and review of the literature. *Clin. Infect. Dis.* **31:**958–967.

209. O'Brien, R. J., L. J. Geiter, and D. E. Snider, Jr. 1987. The epidemiology of nontuberculous mycobacterial diseases in the United States. Results from a national survey. *Am. Rev. Respir. Dis.* **135:**1007–1014.

210. Ohkusu, K., L. E. Bermudez, K. A. Nash, R. R. MacGregor, and C. B. Inderlied. 2004. Differential virulence of Mycobacterium avium strains isolated from HIV-infected patients with disseminated M. avium complex disease. *J. Infect. Dis.* **190:**1347–1354.

211. Oldfield, E. C., III, W. J. Fessel, M. W. Dunne, G. Dickinson, M. R. Wallace, W. Byrne, R. Chung, K. F. Wagner, S. F. Paparello, D. B. Craig, G. Melcher, M. Zajdowicz, R. F. Williams, J. W. Kelly, M. Zelasky, L. B. Heifets, and J. D. Berman. 1998. Once weekly azithromycin therapy for prevention of Mycobacterium avium complex infection in patients with AIDS: a randomized, double-blind, placebo-controlled multicenter trial. *Clin. Infect. Dis.* **26:**611–619.

212. Olivier, K. N., D. J. Weber, J. H. Lee, A. Handler, G. Tudor, P. L. Molina, J. Tomashefski, and M. R. Knowles. 2003. Nontuberculous mycobacteria. II: nested-cohort study of impact on cystic fibrosis lung disease. *Am. J. Respir. Crit. Care Med.* **167:**835–840.

213. Olivier, K. N., D. J. Weber, R. J. Wallace, Jr., A. R. Faiz, J. H. Lee, Y. Zhang, B. A. Brown-Elliott, A. Handler, R. W. Wilson, M. S. Schechter, L. J. Edwards, S. Chakraborti, and M. R. Knowles. 2003. Nontuberculous mycobacteria. I. Multicenter prevalence study in cystic fibrosis. *Am. J. Respir. Crit. Care Med.* **167:**828–834.

214. Oloya, J., J. Opuda-Asibo, R. Kazwala, A. B. Demelash, E. Skjerve, A. Lund, T. B. Johansen, and B. Djonne. 2008. Mycobacteria causing human cervical lymphadenitis in pastoral communities in the Karamoja region of Uganda. *Epidemiol. Infect.* **136:**636–643.

215. Olsen, R. J., P. L. Cernoch, and G. A. Land. 2006. Mycobacterial synovitis caused by slow-growing nonchromogenic

species: eighteen cases and a review of the literature. *Arch. Pathol. Lab. Med.* **130**:783–791.

216. Orme, I. M., S. K. Furney, and A. D. Roberts. 1992. Dissemination of enteric *Mycobacterium avium* infections in mice rendered immunodeficient by thymectomy and CD4 depletion or by prior infection with murine AIDS retroviruses. *Infect. Immun.* **60**:4747–4753.

217. Ottenhoff, T. H. M., F. A. W. Verreck, E. G. R. Lichtenauer-Kaligis, M. A. Hoeve, O. Sanal, and J. T. van Dissel. 2002. Genetics, cytokines and human infectious disease: lessons from weakly pathogenic mycobacteria and salmonellae. *Nat. Genet.* **32**:97–104.

218. Palella, F. J., Jr., K. M. DeLaney, A. C. Moorman, M. O. Loveless, J. Fuhrer, G. A. Satten, D. J. Aschman, S. D. Holmberg, et al. 1998. Declining morbidity and mortality among patients with advanced human immunodeficiency virus infection. *N. Engl. J. Med.* **338**:853–860.

219. Panesar, J., K. Higgins, H. Daya, V. Forte, and U. Allen. 2003. Nontuberculous mycobacterial cervical adenitis: a ten-year retrospective review. *Laryngoscope* **113**:149–154.

220. Parenti, D. M., P. L. Williams, R. Hafner, M. R. Jacobs, P. Hojczyk, T. M. Hooton, T. W. Barber, G. Simpson, C. van der Horst, J. Currier, W. G. Powderly, M. Limjoco, J. J. Ellner, et al. 1998. A phase II/III trial of antimicrobial therapy with or without amikacin in the treatment of disseminated Mycobacterium avium infection in HIV-infected individuals. *AIDS* **12**:2439–2446.

221. Parker, B. C., M. A. Ford, H. Gruft, and J. O. Falkinham III. 1983. Epidemiology of infection by nontuberculous mycobacteria. IV. Preferential aerosolization of Mycobacterium intracellulare from natural waters. *Am. Rev. Respir. Dis.* **128**:652–656.

222. Pavlik, I., P. Svastova, J. Bartl, L. Dvorska, and I. Rychlik. 2000. Relationship between IS*901* in the *Mycobacterium avium* complex strains isolated from birds, animals, humans, and the environment and virulence for poultry. *Clin. Diagn. Lab. Immunol.* **7**:212–217.

223. Pierce, M., S. Crampton, D. Henry, L. Heifets, A. LaMarca, M. Montecalvo, G. P. Wormser, H. Jablonowski, J. Jemsek, M. Cynamon, B. G. Yangco, G. Notario, and J. C. Craft. 1996. A randomized trial of clarithromycin as prophylaxis against disseminated Mycobacterium avium complex infection in patients with advanced acquired immunodeficiency syndrome. *N. Engl. J. Med.* **335**:384–391.

224. Plum, G., M. Brenden, J. E. Clark-Curtiss, and G. Pulverer. 1997. Cloning, sequencing, and expression of the *mig* gene of *Mycobacterium avium*, which codes for a secreted macrophage-induced protein. *Infect. Immun.* **65**:4548–4557.

225. Plum, G., and J. E. Clark-Curtiss. 1994. Induction of *Mycobacterium avium* gene expression following phagocytosis by human macrophages. *Infect. Immun.* **62**:476–483.

226. Price, L. M., and C. O'Mahony. 2000. Focal adenitis developing after immune reconstitution with HAART. *Int. J. STD AIDS* **11**:685–686.

227. Primack, S. L., P. M. Logan, T. E. Hartman, K. S. Lee, and N. L. Muller. 1995. Pulmonary tuberculosis and Mycobacterium avium-intracellulare: a comparison of CT findings. *Radiology* **194**:413–417.

228. Prince, D. S., D. D. Peterson, R. M. Steiner, J. E. Gottlieb, R. Scott, H. L. Israel, W. G. Figueroa, and J. E. Fish. 1989. Infection with Mycobacterium avium complex in patients without predisposing conditions. *N. Engl. J. Med.* **321**:863–868.

229. Rahal, A., A. Abela, P. H. Arcand, M. C. Quintal, M. H. Lebel, and B. F. Tapiero. 2001. Nontuberculous mycobacterial adenitis of the head and neck in children: experience from a tertiary care pediatric center. *Laryngoscope* **111**:1791–1796.

230. Raszka, W. V., Jr., L. P. Skillman, P. L. McEvoy, and M. L. Robb. 1995. Isolation of nontuberculous, non-avium mycobacteria from patients infected with human immunodeficiency virus. *Clin. Infect. Dis.* **20**:73–76.

231. Ratliff, T. L., R. McCarthy, W. B. Telle, and E. J. Brown. 1993. Purification of a mycobacterial adhesin for fibronectin. *Infect. Immun.* **61**:1889–1894.

232. Reed, C., C. F. von Reyn, S. Chamblee, T. V. Ellerbrock, J. W. Johnson, B. J. Marsh, L. S. Johnson, R. J. Trenschel, and C. R. Horsburgh, Jr. 2006. Environmental risk factors for infection with Mycobacterium avium complex. *Am. J. Epidemiol.* **164**:32–40.

233. Reich, J. M., and R. E. Johnson. 1992. Mycobacterium avium complex pulmonary disease presenting as an isolated lingular or middle lobe pattern. The Lady Windermere syndrome. *Chest* **101**:1605–1609.

234. Reich, J. M., and R. E. Johnson. 1991. Mycobacterium avium complex pulmonary disease. Incidence, presentation, and response to therapy in a community setting. *Am. Rev. Respir. Dis.* **143**:1381–1385.

235. Research Committee of the British Thoracic Society. 2001. First randomised trial of treatments for pulmonary disease caused by M avium intracellulare, M malmoense, and M xenopi in HIV negative patients: rifampicin, ethambutol and isoniazid versus rifampicin and ethambutol. *Thorax* **56**:167–172.

236. Research Committee of the British Thoracic Society. 2002. Pulmonary disease caused by Mycobacterium avium-intracellulare in HIV-negative patients: five-year follow-up of patients receiving standardised treatment. *Int. J. Tuberc. Lung Dis.* **6**:628–634.

237. Riddell, J. T., D. R. Kaul, P. C. Karakousis, J. E. Gallant, J. Mitty, and P. H. Kazanjian. 2007. Mycobacterium avium complex immune reconstitution inflammatory syndrome: long term outcomes. *J. Transl. Med.* **5**:50.

238. Rindi, L., D. Bonanni, N. Lari, and C. Garzelli. 2003. Most human isolates of *Mycobacterium avium* Mav-A and Mav-B are strong producers of hemolysin, a putative virulence factor. *J. Clin. Microbiol.* **41**:5738–5740.

239. Rodriguez, J. C., L. Cebrian, M. Lopez, M. Ruiz, and G. Royo. 2005. Usefulness of various antibiotics against Mycobacterium avium-intracellulare, measured by their mutant prevention concentration. *Int. J. Antimicrob. Agents* **25**:221–225.

240. Rodriguez Diaz, J. C., M. Lopez, M. Ruiz, and G. Royo. 2003. In vitro activity of new fluoroquinolones and linezolid against non-tuberculous mycobacteria. *Int. J. Antimicrob. Agents* **21**:585–588.

241. Roger, P. M., M. Carles, I. Agussol-Foin, L. Pandiani, O. Keita-Perse, V. Mondain, F. De Salvador, and P. Dellamonica. 1999. Efficacy and safety of an intravenous induction therapy for treatment of disseminated Mycobacterium avium complex infection in AIDS patients: a pilot study. *J. Antimicrob. Chemother.* **44**:129–131.

242. Roiz, M. P., E. Palenque, C. Guerrero, and M. J. Garcia. 1995. Use of restriction fragment length polymorphism as a genetic marker for typing *Mycobacterium avium* strains. *J. Clin. Microbiol.* **33**:1389–1391.

243. Romanus, V., H. O. Hallander, P. Wahlen, A. M. Olinder-Nielsen, P. H. Magnusson, and I. Juhlin. 1995. Atypical mycobacteria in extrapulmonary disease among children. Incidence in Sweden from 1969 to 1990, related to changing BCG-vaccination coverage. *Tuber. Lung Dis.* **76**:300–310.

244. Rook, G. A. W. 1994. Macrophages and Mycobacterium tuberculosis: the key to pathogenesis. *Immunol. Ser.* **60**:249–261.

245. Rosenzweig, D. Y. 1979. Pulmonary mycobacterial infections due to Mycobacterium intracellulare- avium complex. Clinical features and course in 100 consecutive cases. *Chest* **75:** 115–119.

246. Rosenzweig, D. Y., and D. P. Schlueter. 1981. Spectrum of clinical disease in pulmonary infection with Mycobacterium avium-intracellulare. *Rev. Infect. Dis.* **3:**1046–1051.

247. Roux, A. L., E. Catherinot, F. Ripoll, N. Soismier, E. Macheras, S. Ravilly, G. Bellis, M. A. Vibet, E. Le Roux, L. Lemonnier, C. Gutierrez, V. Vincent, B. Fauroux, M. Rottman, D. Guillemot, and J. L. Gaillard. 2009. Multicenter study of prevalence of nontuberculous mycobacteria in patients with cystic fibrosis in France. *J. Clin. Microbiol.* **47:**4124–4128.

248. Runyon, E. H. 1959. Anonymous mycobacteria in pulmonary disease. *Med. Clin. N. Am.* **43:**273–290.

249. Rushton, S. P., M. Goodfellow, A. G. O'Donnell, and J. G. Magee. 2007. The epidemiology of atypical mycobacterial diseases in northern England: a space-time clustering and generalized linear modelling approach. *Epidemiol. Infect.* **135:**765–774.

250. Ryu, Y. J., E. J. Kim, W. J. Koh, H. Kim, O. J. Kwon, and J. H. Chang. 2006. Toll-like receptor 2 polymorphisms and nontuberculous mycobacterial lung diseases. *Clin. Vaccine Immunol.* **13:**818–819.

251. Saito, H., H. Tomioka, K. Sato, H. Tasaka, and D. J. Dawson. 1990. Identification of various serovar strains of *Mycobacterium avium* complex by using DNA probes specific for *Mycobacterium avium* and *Mycobacterium intracellulare*. *J. Clin. Microbiol.* **28:**1694–1697.

252. Sampaio, E. P., H. Z. Elloumi, A. Zelazny, L. Ding, M. L. Paulson, A. Sher, A. L. Bafica, Y. R. Shea, and S. M. Holland. 2008. Mycobacterium abscessus and M. avium trigger Toll-like receptor 2 and distinct cytokine response in human cells. *Am. J. Respir. Cell Mol. Biol.* **39:**431–439.

253. Sato, K., H. Tomioka, T. Akaki, and S. Kawahara. 2000. Antimicrobial activities of levofloxacin, clarithromycin, and KRM-1648 against Mycobacterium tuberculosis and Mycobacterium avium complex replicating within Mono Mac 6 human macrophage and A-549 type II alveolar cell lines. *Int. J. Antimicrob. Agents* **16:**25–29.

254. Satta, R., G. Retanda, and F. Cottoni. 1999. Mycobacterium avium complex: cutaneous infection in an immunocompetent host. *Acta Derm. Venereol.* **79:**249–250.

255. Schaad, U. B., T. P. Votteler, G. H. McCracken, Jr., and J. D. Nelson. 1979. Management of atypical mycobacterial lymphadenitis in childhood: a review based on 380 cases. *J. Pediatr.* **95:**356–360.

256. Schaefer, W. B., C. L. Davis, and M. L. Cohn. 1970. Pathogenicity of transparent, opaque, and rough variants of Mycobacterium avium in chickens and mice. *Am. Rev. Respir. Dis.* **102:**499–506.

257. Selik, R. M., E. T. Starcher, and J. W. Curran. 1987. Opportunistic diseases reported in AIDS patients: frequencies, associations, and trends. *AIDS* **1:**175–182.

258. Shafran, S. D., J. Singer, D. P. Zarowny, J. Deschenes, P. Phillips, F. Turgeon, F. Y. Aoki, E. Toma, M. Miller, R. Duperval, C. Lemieux, W. F. Schlech III, et al. 1998. Determinants of rifabutin-associated uveitis in patients treated with rifabutin, clarithromycin, and ethambutol for Mycobacterium avium complex bacteremia: a multivariate analysis. *J. Infect. Dis.* **177:**252–255.

259. Shafran, S. D., J. Singer, D. P. Zarowny, P. Phillips, I. Salit, S. L. Walmsley, I. W. Fong, M. J. Gill, A. R. Rachlis, R. G. Lalonde, M. M. Fanning, C. M. Tsoukas, et al. 1996. A comparison of two regimens for the treatment of Mycobacterium avium complex bacteremia in AIDS: rifabutin, ethambutol, and clarithromycin versus rifampin, ethambutol, clofazimine, and ciprofloxacin. *N. Engl. J. Med.* **335:**377–383.

260. Shelburne, S. A., F. Visnegarwala, J. Darcourt, E. A. Graviss, T. P. Giordano, A. C. White, Jr., and R. J. Hamill. 2005. Incidence and risk factors for immune reconstitution inflammatory syndrome during highly active antiretroviral therapy. *AIDS* **19:**399–406.

261. Shiraishi, Y., Y. Nakajima, K. Takasuna, T. Hanaoka, N. Katsuragi, and H. Konno. 2002. Surgery for Mycobacterium avium complex lung disease in the clarithromycin era. *Eur. J. Cardiothorac. Surg.* **21:**314–318.

262. Shiratsuchi, H., and J. J. Ellner. 2001. Expression of IL-18 by Mycobacterium avium-infected human monocytes; association with M. avium virulence. *Clin. Exp. Immunol.* **123:** 203–209.

263. Shiratsuchi, H., J. L. Johnson, H. Toba, and J. J. Ellner. 1990. Strain- and donor-related differences in the interaction of Mycobacterium avium with human monocytes and its modulation by interferon-gamma. *J. Infect. Dis.* **162:**932–938.

264. Shojima, J., G. Tanaka, N. Keicho, G. Tamiya, S. Ando, A. Oka, Y. Inoue, K. Suzuki, M. Sakatani, M. Okada, N. Kobayashi, E. Toyota, K. Kudo, A. Kajiki, H. Nagai, A. Kurashima, N. Oketani, H. Hayakawa, T. Takemura, K. Nakata, H. Ito, T. Morita, I. Matsushita, M. Hijikata, S. Sakurada, T. Sasazuki, and H. Inoko. 2009. Identification of MICA as a susceptibility gene for pulmonary Mycobacterium avium complex infection. *J. Infect. Dis.* **199:**1707–1715.

265. Silva, R. A., M. Florido, and R. Appelberg. 2001. Interleukin-12 primes CD4+ T cells for interferon-gamma production and protective immunity during Mycobacterium avium infection. *Immunology* **103:**368–374.

266. Sison, J. P., Y. Yao, C. A. Kemper, J. R. Hamilton, E. Brummer, D. A. Stevens, and S. C. Deresinski. 1996. Treatment of Mycobacterium avium complex infection: do the results of in vitro susceptibility tests predict therapeutic outcome in humans? *J. Infect. Dis.* **173:**677–683.

267. Skamene, E. 1998. Genetic control of susceptibility to infections with intracellular pathogens. *Pathol. Biol.* **46:**689–692.

268. Skamene, E., E. Schurr, and P. Gros. 1998. Infection genomics: Nramp1 as a major determinant of natural resistance to intracellular infections. *Annu. Rev. Med.* **49:**275–287.

269. Smith, M. B., M. C. Boyars, S. Veasey, and G. L. Woods. 2000. Generalized tuberculosis in the acquired immune deficiency syndrome. *Arch. Pathol. Lab. Med.* **124:**1267–1274.

270. Starke, J. R. 2000. Management of nontuberculous mycobacterial cervical adenitis. *Pediatr. Infect. Dis. J.* **19:**674–675.

271. Storgaard, M., K. Varming, T. Herlin, and N. Obel. 2006. Novel mutation in the interferon-gamma-receptor gene and susceptibility to mycobacterial infections. *Scand. J. Immunol.* **64:**137–139.

272. Stout, J. E., G. W. Hopkins, J. R. McDonald, A. Quinn, C. D. Hamilton, L. B. Reller, and R. Frothingham. 2008. Association between 16S-23S internal transcribed spacer sequence groups of *Mycobacterium avium* complex and pulmonary disease. *J. Clin. Microbiol.* **46:**2790–2793.

273. Sugita, Y., N. Ishii, M. Katsuno, R. Yamada, and H. Nakajima. 2000. Familial cluster of cutaneous Mycobacterium avium infection resulting from use of a circulating, constantly heated bath water system. *Br. J. Dermatol.* **142:**789–793.

274. Swanson, D. S., V. Kapur, K. Stockbauer, X. Pan, R. Frothingham, and J. M. Musser. 1997. Subspecific differentiation of Mycobacterium avium complex strains by automated sequencing of a region of the gene (hsp65) encoding a 65-kilodalton heat shock protein. *Int. J. Syst. Bacteriol.* **47:** 414–419.

275. Swanson, D. S., X. Pan, M. W. Kline, R. E. McKinney, Jr., R. Yogev, L. L. Lewis, M. T. Brady, G. D. McSherry, W. M. Dankner, and J. M. Musser. 1998. Genetic diversity among Mycobacterium avium complex strains recovered from children with and without human immunodeficiency virus infection. *J. Infect. Dis.* **178:**776–782.

276. Swensen, S. J., T. E. Hartman, and D. E. Williams. 1994. Computed tomographic diagnosis of Mycobacterium avium-intracellulare complex in patients with bronchiectasis. *Chest* **105:**49–52.

277. Taha, A. M., P. T. Davidson, and W. C. Bailey. 1985. Surgical treatment of atypical mycobacterial lymphadenitis in children. *Pediatr. Infect. Dis.* **4:**664–667.

278. Takahashi, M., A. Ishizaka, H. Nakamura, K. Kobayashi, M. Nakamura, M. Namiki, T. Sekita, and S. Okajima. 2000. Specific HLA in pulmonary MAC infection in a Japanese population. *Am. J. Respir. Crit. Care Med.* **162:**316–318.

279. Tanaka, E., R. Amitani, A. Niimi, K. Suzuki, T. Murayama, and F. Kuze. 1997. Yield of computed tomography and bronchoscopy for the diagnosis of Mycobacterium avium complex pulmonary disease. *Am. J. Respir. Crit. Care Med.* **155:**2041–2046.

280. Tanaka, E., T. Kimoto, H. Matsumoto, K. Tsuyuguchi, K. Suzuki, S. Nagai, M. Shimadzu, H. Ishibatake, T. Murayama, and R. Amitani. 2000. Familial pulmonary Mycobacterium avium complex disease. *Am. J. Respir. Crit. Care Med.* **161:**1643–1647.

281. Tanaka, E., T. Kimoto, K. Tsuyuguchi, I. Watanabe, H. Matsumoto, A. Niimi, K. Suzuki, T. Murayama, R. Amitani, and F. Kuze. 1999. Effect of clarithromycin regimen for Mycobacterium avium complex pulmonary disease. *Am. J. Respir. Crit. Care Med.* **160:**866–872.

282. Tanaka, G., J. Shojima, I. Matsushita, H. Nagai, A. Kurashima, K. Nakata, E. Toyota, N. Kobayashi, K. Kudo, and N. Keicho. 2007. Pulmonary Mycobacterium avium complex infection: association with NRAMP1 polymorphisms. *Eur. Respir. J.* **30:**90–96.

283. Tassell, S. K., M. Pourshafie, E. L. Wright, M. G. Richmond, and W. W. Barrow. 1992. Modified lymphocyte response to mitogens induced by the lipopeptide fragment derived from *Mycobacterium avium* serovar-specific glycopeptidolipids. *Infect. Immun.* **60:**706–711.

284. Taylor, R. H., J. O. Falkinham III, C. D. Norton, and M. W. LeChevallier. 2000. Chlorine, chloramine, chlorine dioxide, and ozone susceptibility of Mycobacterium avium. *Appl. Environ. Microbiol.* **66:**1702–1705.

285. Telles, M. A., M. D. Yates, M. Curcio, S. Y. Ueki, M. Palaci, D. J. Hadad, F. A. Drobniewski, and A. L. Pozniak. 1999. Molecular epidemiology of Mycobacterium avium complex isolated from patients with and without AIDS in Brazil and England. *Epidemiol. Infect.* **122:**435–440.

286. Teraki, Y., S. Ono, and S. Izaki. 2008. Sweet's syndrome associated with Mycobacterium avium infection. *Clin. Exp. Dermatol.* **33:**599–601.

287. Thegerstrom, J., V. Romanus, V. Friman, L. Brudin, P. D. Haemig, and B. Olsen. 2008. Mycobacterium avium lymphadenopathy among children, Sweden. *Emerg. Infect. Dis.* **14:**661–663.

288. Tobin-D'Angelo, M. J., M. A. Blass, C. del Rio, J. S. Halvosa, H. M. Blumberg, and C. R. Horsburgh, Jr. 2004. Hospital water as a source of Mycobacterium avium complex isolates in respiratory specimens. *J. Infect. Dis.* **189:**98–104.

289. Tomioka, H. 2000. Prospects for development of new antimycobacterial drugs, with special reference to a new benzoxazinorifamycin, KRM-1648. *Arch. Immunol. Ther. Exp.* **48:**183–188.

290. Tomioka, H., C. Sano, K. Sato, and T. Shimizu. 2002. Antimicrobial activities of clarithromycin, gatifloxacin and sitafloxacin, in combination with various antimycobacterial drugs against extracellular and intramacrophage Mycobacterium avium complex. *Int. J. Antimicrob. Agents* **19:**139–145.

291. Tomioka, H., K. Sato, H. Kajitani, T. Akaki, and S. Shishido. 2000. Comparative antimicrobial activities of the newly synthesized quinolone WQ-3034, levofloxacin, sparfloxacin, and ciprofloxacin against *Mycobacterium tuberculosis* and *Mycobacterium avium* complex. *Antimicrob. Agents Chemother.* **44:**283–286.

292. Torrelles, J. B., D. Chatterjee, J. G. Lonca, J. M. Manterola, V. R. Ausina, and P. J. Brennan. 2000. Serovars of Mycobacterium avium complex isolated from AIDS and non-AIDS patients in Spain. *J. Appl. Microbiol.* **88:**266–279.

293. Torriani, F. J., J. A. McCutchan, S. A. Bozzette, M. R. Grafe, and D. V. Havlir. 1994. Autopsy findings in AIDS patients with Mycobacterium avium complex bacteremia. *J. Infect. Dis.* **170:**1601–1605.

294. Tortoli, E., M. Pecorari, G. Fabio, M. Messino, and A. Fabio. 2010. Commercial DNA probes for mycobacteria incorrectly identify a number of less frequently encountered species. *J. Clin. Microbiol.* **48:**307–310.

295. Trojan, T., R. Collins, and D. A. Khan. 2009. Safety and efficacy of treatment using interleukin-2 in a patient with idiopathic CD4(+) lymphopenia and Mycobacterium avium-intracellulare. *Clin. Exp. Immunol.* **156:**440–445.

296. Tsukaguchi, K., T. Yoneda, H. Okamura, S. Tamaki, H. Takenaka, Y. Okamoto, and N. Narita. 2000. Defective T cell function for inhibition of growth of Mycobacterium avium-intracellulare complex (MAC) in patients with MAC disease: restoration by cytokines. *J. Infect. Dis.* **182:**1664–1671.

297. Tsukamura, M., and S. Ichiyama. 1988. Comparison of antituberculosis drug regimens for lung disease caused by Mycobacterium avium complex. *Chest* **93:**821–823.

298. Tsukamura, M., N. Kita, H. Shimoide, H. Arakawa, and A. Kuze. 1988. Studies on the epidemiology of nontuberculous mycobacteriosis in Japan. *Am. Rev. Respir. Dis.* **137:**1280–1284.

299. Tumbarello, M., E. Tacconelli, K. G. de Donati, S. Bertagnolio, B. Longo, F. Ardito, G. Fadda, and R. Cauda. 2001. Changes in incidence and risk factors of Mycobacterium avium complex infections in patients with AIDS in the era of new antiretroviral therapies. *Eur. J. Clin. Microbiol. Infect. Dis.* **20:**498–501.

300. Turenne, C. Y., M. Semret, D. V. Cousins, D. M. Collins, and M. A. Behr. 2006. Sequencing of hsp65 distinguishes among subsets of the *Mycobacterium avium* complex. *J. Clin. Microbiol.* **44:**433–440.

301. von Reyn, C. F., C. R. Horsburgh, K. N. Olivier, P. F. Barnes, R. Waddell, C. Warren, S. Tvaroha, A. S. Jaeger, A. D. Lein, L. N. Alexander, D. J. Weber, and A. N. Tosteson. 2001. Skin test reactions to Mycobacterium tuberculosis purified protein derivative and Mycobacterium avium sensitin among health care workers and medical students in the United States. *Int. J. Tuberc. Lung Dis.* **5:**1122–1128.

302. von Reyn, C. F., J. N. Maslow, T. W. Barber, J. O. Falkinham III, and R. D. Arbeit. 1994. Persistent colonisation of potable water as a source of Mycobacterium avium infection in AIDS. *Lancet* **343:**1137–1141.

303. von Reyn, C. F., R. D. Waddell, T. Eaton, R. D. Arbeit, J. N. Maslow, T. W. Barber, R. J. Brindle, C. F. Gilks, J. Lumio, J. Lahdevirta, A. Ranki, D. Dawson, and J. O. Falkinham III. 1993. Isolation of Mycobacterium avium complex from water in the United States, Finland, Zaire, and Kenya. *J. Clin. Microbiol.* **31:**3227–3230.

304. Wallace, R. J., Jr., Y. Zhang, B. A. Brown-Elliott, M. A. Yakrus, R. W. Wilson, L. Mann, L. Couch, W. M. Girard, and D. E. Griffith. 2002. Repeat positive cultures in Mycobacterium intracellulare lung disease after macrolide therapy represent new infections in patients with nodular bronchiectasis. *J. Infect. Dis.* **186:**266–273.

305. Wallace, R. J., Jr., B. A. Brown, D. E. Griffith, W. Girard, and K. Tanaka. 1995. Reduced serum levels of clarithromycin in patients treated with multidrug regimens including rifampin or rifabutin for Mycobacterium avium-M. intracellulare infection. *J. Infect. Dis.* **171:**747–750.

306. Wallace, R. J., Jr., B. A. Brown, D. E. Griffith, W. M. Girard, and D. T. Murphy. 1996. Clarithromycin regimens for pulmonary Mycobacterium avium complex. The first 50 patients. *Am. J. Respir. Crit. Care Med.* **153:**1766–1772.

307. Wallace, R. J., Jr., B. A. Brown, D. E. Griffith, W. M. Girard, D. T. Murphy, G. O. Onyi, V. A. Steingrube, and G. H. Mazurek. 1994. Initial clarithromycin monotherapy for Mycobacterium avium-intracellulare complex lung disease. *Am. J. Respir. Crit. Care Med.* **149:**1335–1341.

308. Wallace, R. J., Jr., Y. Zhang, B. A. Brown, D. Dawson, D. T. Murphy, R. Wilson, and D. E. Griffith. 1998. Polyclonal Mycobacterium avium complex infections in patients with nodular bronchiectasis. *Am. J. Respir. Crit. Care Med.* **158:**1235–1244.

309. Ward, T. T., D. Rimland, C. Kauffman, M. Huycke, T. G. Evans, L. Heifets, et al. 1998. Randomized, open-label trial of azithromycin plus ethambutol vs. clarithromycin plus ethambutol as therapy for Mycobacterium avium complex bacteremia in patients with human immunodeficiency virus infection. *Clin. Infect. Dis.* **27:**1278–1285.

310. Wasem, C. F., C. M. McCarthy, and L. W. Murray. 1991. Multilocus enzyme electrophoresis analysis of the *Mycobacterium avium* complex and other mycobacteria. *J. Clin. Microbiol.* **29:**264–271.

311. Watanabe, K., M. Fujimura, K. Kasahara, M. Yasui, S. Myou, A. Watanabe, and S. Nakao. 2003. Characteristics of pulmonary Mycobacterium avium-intracellulare complex (MAC) infection in comparison with those of tuberculosis. *Respir. Med.* **97:**654–659.

312. Wendt, S. L., K. L. George, B. C. Parker, H. Gruft, and J. O. Falkinham III. 1980. Epidemiology of infection by nontuberculous Mycobacteria. III. Isolation of potentially pathogenic mycobacteria from aerosols. *Am. Rev. Respir. Dis.* **122:**259–263.

313. Wolinsky, E. 1995. Mycobacterial lymphadenitis in children: a prospective study of 105 nontuberculous cases with long-term follow-up. *Clin. Infect. Dis.* **20:**954–963.

314. Wolinsky, E. 1979. Nontuberculous mycobacteria and associated diseases. *Am. Rev. Respir. Dis.* **119:**107–159.

315. Woodley, C. L., and J. O. Kilburn. 1982. In vitro susceptibility of Mycobacterium avium complex and Mycobacterium tuberculosis strains to a spiro-piperidyl rifamycin. *Am. Rev. Respir. Dis.* **126:**586–587.

316. Woods, G. L., N. Williams-Bouyer, R. J. Wallace, Jr., B. A. Brown-Elliott, F. G. Witebsky, P. S. Conville, M. Plaunt, G. Hall, P. Aralar, and C. Inderlied. 2003. Multisite reproducibility of results obtained by two broth dilution methods for susceptibility testing of *Mycobacterium avium* complex. *J. Clin. Microbiol.* **41:**627–631.

317. Wormser, G. P., H. Horowitz, and B. Dworkin. 1994. Low-dose dexamethasone as adjunctive therapy for disseminated *Mycobacterium avium* complex infections in AIDS patients. *Antimicrob. Agents Chemother.* **38:**2215–2217.

318. Yim, J. J., H. J. Kim, O. J. Kwon, and W. J. Koh. 2008. Association between microsatellite polymorphisms in intron II of the human Toll-like receptor 2 gene and nontuberculous mycobacterial lung disease in a Korean population. *Hum. Immunol.* **69:**572–576.

319. Yoon, J. H., E. C. Kim, J. S. Kim, E. Y. Song, J. Yi, and S. Shin. 2009. Possession of the macrophage-induced gene by isolates of the Mycobacterium avium complex is not associated with significant clinical disease. *J. Med. Microbiol.* **58:**256–260.

320. Zelazny, A. M., J. M. Root, Y. R. Shea, R. E. Colombo, I. C. Shamputa, F. Stock, S. Conlan, S. McNulty, B. A. Brown-Elliott, R. J. Wallace, Jr., K. N. Olivier, S. M. Holland, and E. P. Sampaio. 2009. Cohort study of molecular identification and typing of *Mycobacterium abscessus, Mycobacterium massiliense*, and *Mycobacterium bolletii*. *J. Clin. Microbiol.* **47:**1985–1995.

Tuberculosis and Nontuberculous Mycobacterial Infections, 6th ed.
Edited by David Schlossberg
© 2011 ASM Press, Washington, DC

Chapter 37

Rapidly Growing Mycobacteria

BARBARA A. BROWN-ELLIOTT AND RICHARD J. WALLACE, JR.

TAXONOMY

Historical Background

The history of the major pathogenic species of rapidly growing mycobacteria (RGM) can be traced back to the early 20th century beginning with Friedmann's recovery of *Mycobacterium chelonae* from the lungs of two sea turtles (hence, the name *chelonae* from the Latin "of a turtle") (16). Almost 50 years later, the closely related *Mycobacterium abscessus* was first reported as a cause of human skin and soft tissue infection in a patient with multiple soft tissue abscesses of a lower extremity (51).

Another RGM species, *Mycobacterium fortuitum* (formerly *Mycobacterium ranae*), was originally recovered from frogs in 1905. However, in 1938, da Costa Cruz gave the name *M. fortuitum* to an isolate that he thought was a new mycobacterial species isolated from a patient with a skin abscess following local vitamin injections (21). Subsequently, the two organisms were proven to be the same, with the illegitimate name *M. fortuitum* retained as the species name on the request of Ernest Runyon (64).

Early taxonomic studies that utilized phenotypic analysis concluded that the two species *M. fortuitum* and *M. chelonae* were composed of several "subspecies" (i.e., *M. chelonae* subsp. *chelonae* and *M. chelonae* subsp. *abscessus*) or "biovariants" (*M. fortuitum* biovariant *fortuitum*, *M. fortuitum* biovariant *peregrinum*, and *M. fortuitum* third biovariant complex) (43).

More recent taxonomic studies that utilized molecular analysis with DNA-DNA hybridization and 16S ribosomal sequencing have shown that these "biovars" and "subspecies" are in fact separate species, and most have been renamed without the subgroup designation (67).

One exception is the recent subgroup reclassification of isolates previously identified as *Mycobacterium*

massiliense and *Mycobacterium bolletii*. A proposal has been made to the *International Journal of Systematic and Evolutionary Microbiology* that these two taxa originally described as unique species in 2004 and 2006, respectively (1, 3), should be reclassified as *M. abscessus* subsp. *bolletii* based on low intraspecies variability by multilocus gene sequencing (46). Likewise, *M. abscessus* would be revised to *M. abscessus* subsp. *abscessus*. Thus, with these new taxonomic changes within the *M. chelonae*/*M. abscessus* group, only three species, including *M. chelonae*, *Mycobacterium immunogenum*, and *M. abscessus* now would be recognized (46, 97).

Current Classification

Currently, the RGM are grouped into six major taxonomic groups according to pigmentation and genetic relatedness. The major groups are the *M. fortuitum* group, the *M. chelonae*/*M. abscessus* group, the *Mycobacterium smegmatis* group (*M. smegmatis* and *Mycobacterium goodii*), the *Mycobacterium mucogenicum* group, the *Mycobacterium mageritense*/*Mycobacterium wolinskyi* group, and the pigmented RGM. There are now more than 70 recognized species, representing approximately 50% of all recognized mycobacterial species. The three most important clinical pathogenic species that represent more than 80% of clinical isolates of RGM are *M. fortuitum*, *M. chelonae*, and *M. abscessus* (10). Since 2004, 18 new species or subspecies have been described. These include rare or unproven human pathogens: *M. aubagnense*, *M. insubricum*, *M. phocaicum*, *M. setense*, *M. monacense*, *M. novacastrense*, *M. barrassiae*, and as noted previously, the species proposed to be reclassified as *M. abscessus* subsp. *bolletii* (1, 4, 34, 45, 46). One new species, *M. canariasense*, has been isolated in 17 patients with suspected nosocomial infection from infected central venous catheters (39). Additionally, one species (pathogenic for fish), *M. salmoniphilum*,

Barbara A. Brown-Elliott and Richard J. Wallace, Jr. • Department of Microbiology, The University of Texas Health Science Center, 11937 U.S. Hwy. 271, Tyler, TX 75708.

originally described in 1960 has been recently revived (90). Nine environmental species, including *M. fluoroanthenivorans, M. llatzerense, M. aromaticivorans, M. crocinum, M. pallens, M. poriferae, M. pyrenivorans, M. rufum,* and *M. rutilum,* have also been described (Table 1) (38, 73, 74).

EPIDEMIOLOGY

Community-Acquired Disease

The RGM are ubiquitous in the environment (10, 25). Human infections have been reported from most developed areas of the world, and RGM have been isolated from 30% to 78% of soil samples from various geographical regions in the United States (10, 94). Until recently, most reported cases of disease have been from the United States, with most clustered outbreaks and studies of selected diseases having shown a strong disease localization in the southern United States (10, 35). Community-acquired localized skin, soft tissue, and/or bone disease often follows a traumatic injury with potential soil contamination (e.g., stepping on a nail, motor vehicle accident with an open fracture, etc.). The reservoir for RGM pulmonary disease is unknown (35).

Nail Salon/Footbath-Associated Folliculitis

Recently, RGM lower extremity skin infections involving *M. fortuitum, M. mageritense,* and a newly described species, *M. cosmeticum,* associated with the use of contaminated nail salon whirlpool footbaths has also been described (17, 33, 92). Patients were defined as salon customers with persistent skin infections below the knee (92). Most often the infections involve a furunculosis of the lower leg hair follicles (33). The disease pathogenesis likely results from microtrauma caused by shaving the legs prior to pedicures and footbath water that is heavily contaminated with RGM due to failure to routinely clear the footbath filters (92).

Anti-TNF-α Therapy-Associated Infections

Tuberculosis and NTM infections associated with the use of biologic therapies that inhibit tumor necrosis factor alpha (TNF-α) have been reported. Patients receiving anti-TNF-α therapy are at high risk for activation of tuberculosis. They appear to have some increase in disease risk or difference in clinical manifestation for NTM as well, although little is known about the disease (93). A recent review of the

Table 1. Currently recognized species of RGM

Pathogen type	Nonpigmented species	Pigmented species
Common	*M. abscessus* subsp. *abscessus*[a], *M. chelonae, M. fortuitum*	None
Infrequent but proven	*M. fortuitum* group (*M. boenickei, M. houstonense, M. peregrinum, M. porcinum, M. senegalense*) *M. abscessus* subsp. *bolletii*[e], *M. immunogenum, M. mucogenicum*[b], *M. mageritense, M. wolinskyi, M. canariasense*	*M. goodii*[d], *M. smegmatis* (formerly sensu stricto)[d], *M. neoaurum, M. cosmeticum, M. bacteremicum*
Rare or unproven	*M. agri*[f], *M. alvei*[f], *M. aubagnense*[b], *M. barrassiae*[e], *M. brisbanense*[e], *M. brumae*[f], *M. chitae*[f], *M. confluentis*[f,b], *M. diernhoferi, M. fallax*[f], *M. fluoranthenivorans*[f], *M. insubricum*[f,g], *M. llatzerense*[f], *M. moriokaense*[f], *M. neworleansense*[e], *M. phocaicum*[b], *M. salmoniphilum*[g], *M. septicum*[e], *M. setense*[e]	*M. aichiense*[f], *M. aromaticivorans*[f], *M. aurum*[f], *M. austroafricanum*[f], *M. chlorophenicolicum*[f], *M. chubuense*[f], *M. crocinum*[f], *M. duvalii*[f], *M. elephantis*[e], *M. flavescens*[f], *M. frederiksbergense*[f], *M. gadium*[f], *M. gilvum*[f], *M. hassiacum*[f], *M. hodleri*[f], *M. holsaticum*[f], *M. komossense*[f], *M. madagascariense*[f], *M. monacense*[e], *M. murale*[f], *M. novocastrense*[e], *M. obuense*[f], *M. pallens*[f], *M. parafortuitum*[f], *M. phlei*[f], *M. poriferae*[f], *M. psychrotolerans*[f], *M. pyrenivorans*[f], *M. rhodesiae*[f], *M. rufum*[f], *M. rutilum*[f], *M. sphagni*[f], *M. thermoresistible, M. tokaiense*[f], *M. vaccae*[f], *M. vanbaalenii*[f]

[a]Formerly *M. abscessus* (46).
[b]*M. mucogenicum* group is composed of *M. mucogenicum, M. aubagnense,* and *M. phocaicum.*
[c]Formerly *M. massiliense, M. bolletii* (46).
[d]Late pigmentation.
[e]Associated with human disease, but fewer than 5 cases.
[f]No established clinical significance in humans.
[g]Associated with disease in fish.
[h]Late brown/black pigment develops after several weeks.

U.S. Food and Drug Administration Med Watch database reports identified 239 possible cases of NTM disease associated with TNF-α inhibitor use from 1999 to 2006 of which 105 cases (44%) met NTM disease criteria. NTM infections were associated with immunosuppressive therapies including infliximab, etanercept, and adalmumab. The most common underlying condition was rheumatoid arthritis (75%), and 65% and 55% of patients in this study were also taking prednisone and methotrexate, respectively. Infections with M. avium complex were most commonly reported, while 20/105 cases (20%) involved RGM species. Species involved were M. abscessus, M. chelonae, and M. fortuitum (93).

Nosocomial/Health Care-Associated Disease

Exposure to tap water appears to be the major risk factor for nosocomial (health care-associated) disease (10, 19, 58). Most outbreaks of health care-associated infections or pseudoinfections have been associated epidemiologically with various water sources, including water-based solutions, distilled water, tap water, ice, and ice water (10, 36, 72). One study of hemodialysis centers in the United States showed that 55% of incoming city water contained mycobacteria, of which rapidly growing species were the most common (12). Biofilms, which are the slimy layers that occur at water-solid interfaces, appear to be present in most pipes and tubings, and up to 90% of these from community-piped water systems contain mycobacteria (68). Compared with free-living mycobacteria, mycobacteria associated with biofilms are more resistant to water treatment and biofilms play a role in the persistence of the mycobacteria (31). The utilization of pulsed-field gel electrophoresis and randomly amplified polymorphic DNA PCR methods for analyzing genomic DNA large restriction fragment patterns has made possible the identification of specific strains of RGM and thus improved the investigation of nosocomial outbreaks (10, 37, 98). DNA fingerprinting for some of these outbreaks has confirmed molecular identity between water and human isolates. Water or water-based solutions may also be responsible for sporadic health care-associated infections due to M. fortuitum, M. chelonae, and M. abscessus. These include catheter-related infections, sternal wound infections following cardiac bypass surgery, and infected augmentation mammaplasty sites (10).

Infections following insertion of prosthetic devices, including prosthetic heart valves, lens implants, artificial knees and hips, and metal rods inserted to stabilize bones following fractures have also been reported (10, 24). A combination of resection arthroplasty and antimicrobial therapy is the preferred treatment for joint infections (24).

Outbreaks involving RGM have been described for more than 30 years and continue to be problematic (10, 44, 72, 98). Large outbreaks of postinjection abscesses involving M. abscessus have also been reported by Villanueva and colleagues from Colombia (80), Zhibang et al. in China (99), Kim et al. (42) in Korea, and Tiwari et al. (72) and Galil et al. (32) from the United States. An unusual outbreak of catheter-associated bacteremia caused by the newly described species, M. phocaicum, was reported in a Texas hospital in 2006 (18).

Infections with RGM species including M. chelonae and M. fortuitum and, most recently, M. immunogenum appear to have a special association with cosmetic surgery procedures, especially liposuction, breast augmentation, and recently, mesotherapy (13, 14, 22, 50, 60, 66, 78). A recent outbreak following breast augmentation procedures and liposuction has been reported from the Dominican Republic (14). Additional similar outbreaks involving M. abscessus have been reported from U.S. tourists ("lipotourists") who underwent abdominoplasty in the Dominican Republic (30). Outbreaks involving infection with RGM following acupuncture treatment have also been detailed previously (10, 95). Case reports and outbreaks of lower extremity furunculosis involving M. fortuitum, M. abscessus, and less common species such as M. mageritense have also been recently reported associated with contaminated whirlpool water baths at nail salons (33, 79, 81, 93).

The largest epidemic of post-video laparoscopy infections caused by RGM was reported with M. abscessus subsp. massiliense from 2006 to 2007 in Brazil (23). Of special interest was the isolates' consistent tolerance to 2% glutaraldehyde disinfectants. Other RGM postsurgical outbreaks involving laparoscopic, arthroscopic, plastic surgery or cosmetic interventions in 63 hospitals in Brazil have been ongoing since 2004 (46, 79).

Additionally, pseudo-outbreaks of M. abscessus or M. immunogenum related to contaminated automated bronchoscope disinfection machines, contaminated gastric endoscopes, and laboratory contamination have been described (10, 44, 91).

LABORATORY IDENTIFICATION

Phenotypic Methods, High-Performance Liquid Chromatography (HPLC)

Phenotypic laboratory identification of RGM as the M. fortuitum complex (includes the three major pathogenic species of M. fortuitum, M. chelonae, and

M. abscessus) previously has been primarily based on growth in less than 7 days, typical Gram stain and colony morphology, acid-fastness, the absence of pigmentation, and a positive arylsulfatase at 3 days (10). However, the recent introduction of multiple new species has emphasized the fact that definitive identification to the species level is no longer possible without molecular techniques. Moreover, identification to the species level is needed for most clinical isolates to access differences in treatment regimens (10, 69).

HPLC of mycolic acids that may be used in large reference laboratories can identify only a few species adequately. HPLC may be useful for separating organisms into complexes or groups but lacks the specificity needed for full species-level identification (10).

Molecular Methods

PRA

Restriction fragment length polymorphism analysis of selected gene targets such as *hsp65* are currently used in some larger reference laboratories (69, 73, 74, 97). Previous studies using PCR restriction fragment analysis (PRA) of a 441-bp portion (Telenti fragment) of the 65-kilodalton heat shock protein (*hsp65*) gene sequence have shown single unique restriction fragment length polymorphism patterns for most of the common species of RGM (69, 71), although PRA has not been evaluated extensively in the identification of the pigmented RGM and newly described species. Some modifications may be necessary to implement this technology for species identification of the RGM into a clinical laboratory; however, it is readily adaptable to a reference laboratory. PRA seems particularly adaptable to the clinical laboratory for identifying isolates that yield equivocal results when nonmolecular identification techniques are used (69). Because there is no commercial system available for the *hsp* PRA, in-house validation coupled with regular organism database updates are necessary.

16S rRNA gene sequencing

Since the advent of molecular technology, the primary gene target of molecular taxonomic studies has been the 16S rRNA gene. The 16S rRNA gene is composed of approximately 1,500 nucleotides encoded by the 16S rRNA gene, a highly conserved gene composed of two major sequences known as regions A and B.

For mycobacterial species identification, sequencing of region A, which contains most of the species-specific sequence variations ("signature sequences"), is often adequate, while region B may be confirmatory. All of the RGM (except for *M. chelonae* and *M. abscessus*, which each contain two copies) contain one copy of the 16S rRNA gene (73). Generally, members of the genus *Mycobacterium* are closely related to each other and may differ by only a few base pairs or none.

However, differentiation of *M. chelonae* and *M. abscessus* and some species within the *M. fortuitum* group requires sequencing of 16S rRNA gene sites outside regions A and B. *M. chelonae* and *M. abscessus* differ by only 4 bp in the 16S gene, so complete 16S rRNA sequence analysis is required for species identification unless other gene targets are sequenced.

Commercial gene sequencing (MicroSeq 500 16S rRNA gene; Applied Biosystems, Foster City, CA), which is more widely used in clinical and research laboratories, employs analysis of the first 500 bp sequences of the 16S rRNA gene which are subsequently compared to a commercial database. However, this database usually contains only a single entry (usually the type strain) and is often inadequate for species-level identification, especially with isolates of *M. chelonae*, *M. abscessus*, and some species within the *M. fortuitum* group. Therefore, many laboratories that use the system choose to supplement the commercial database with additional sequences from their own libraries or other public databases such as GenBank or Ribosomal Differentiation of Medical Microorganisms (RIDOM). Careful in-house validation and strict quality control measures are necessary to verify the accuracy and reliability of this procedure (77).

Recently, the Clinical and Laboratory Standards Institute (CLSI) has proposed standards for identification of nontuberculous mycobacteria based on sequence probabilities (57). The CLSI recommends that a minimum of "300 bp of quality sequence should be compared between the reference and query sequences and cover at least one region of the gene where variations are to be expected" to ensure accuracy (57).

Although commercial sequencing has benefited many laboratories, sequencing remains a complex and often cost-prohibitive method unless the laboratory handles a sufficient volume of testing to develop expertise with the method. Therefore, the general consensus of opinion has been that for laboratories for whom in-house sequencing is not available or justifiable, samples should be referred to a qualified reference laboratory with expertise and knowledge of mycobacterial sequencing (28).

hsp65 gene sequencing

The 65-kDa heat shock protein gene (*hsp65*) also presents hypervariable regions whose sequences may be used for identification to species level. Like the *hsp65* PRA, most sequence analysis of this 65-kDa gene involves the same 441-bp segment (71).

hsp65 is less well conserved than the 16S rRNA gene sequence and has proven useful for species-level identification of closely related isolates such as *M. abscessus* and *M. chelonae*. These two species differ by 0 bp in the first 500 bases of the 16S rRNA gene and by only 3 bp of approximately 1,500, while the two species differ by almost 30 bp in the 441-bp *hsp65* Telenti fragment. Additionally, species such as *M. fortuitum*, *M. septicum*, *M. peregrinum*, *M. houstonense*, and *M. senegalense* are more readily discriminated with the *hsp65* gene analysis than by 16S rRNA gene analysis (49).

As with all gene sequence methods, the integrity and updating of the database for *hsp65* gene sequences remain the major limitation for this method of identification.

rpoβ gene sequencing

The *rpoβ* gene is a single-copy gene that encodes the β subunit of RNA polymerase and has been used recently in the identification of RGM, including the identification of several new species (1–4, 41). Sequencing of the *rpoβ* gene is advantageous when compared to 16S rRNA sequencing in that a single site without a deletion or insertion is usually small enough to be sequenced directly in both directions at one time and contains enough information to identify many of the RGM to species (2, 41). Recent studies have shown that the complete *rpoβ* sequences vary from 84.3 to 96.6% for most species compared to a 95.7 to 99.7% variation by sequencing of the 16S rRNA gene (2). The most commonly used sequence for RGM is a 723-bp fragment in region V (2, 3).

Just as for other sequence databases, a sufficient, updated and quality-controlled database is necessary for accurate identification of RGM to species.

Sequencing of other genes

Other gene targets including the *dnaJ* gene, the 32-kDa protein gene, the superoxide dismutase (*sod*) gene, the 16S-23S rRNA internal transcribed spacer, the *secA1* gene, and the *recA* gene have been proposed as useful for identification of the RGM. However, data on the utility of these genes are only preliminary primarily due to lack of sufficient databases (3).

Recently multilocus gene sequencing (i.e., sequencing portions of multiple genes) has been recommended. Although this approach may be impractical for clinical laboratories, it has been proposed for the evaluation of species definition and identification of new species (48).

Nucleic acid probes

Currently, the only nucleic acid probe available for identification of the RGM but not yet cleared by the Food and Drug Administration in the United States is the INNO-LiPA multiplex probe assay (Innogenetics, Ghent, Belgium). The assay can identify members of the genus *Mycobacterium* including slowly growing and rapidly growing species. The principle of the method is based on biotinylation of DNA obtained by PCR amplification of the 16S-23S internal transcribed spacer region which is subsequently hybridized with specific oligonucleotide probes immobilized as parallel lines on a membrane strip. The major advantage is that a large variety of species can be identified by a single probe without necessitating the selection of a specific probe for each species. However, some cross-reactivity among closely related species (most notably the *M. fortuitum* group) and the inability to differentiate isolates of *M. chelonae* from *M. abscessus* have been disadvantages of the method (75, 76).

The INNO-LiPA and a similar commercial system which targets the 23 rRNA gene, the Genotype Mycobacterium assay (Hain Lifescience, GmbH, Nehren, Germany), have been widely used in Europe for identification of RGM (62, 76).

ANTIMICROBIAL SUSCEPTIBILITY

Current antimicrobial regimens for treatment of disease caused by the RGM are based upon their unique in vitro susceptibility patterns (10, 84, 85, 87). Isolates of RGM are not susceptible to the first-line antituberculous drugs and require susceptibility testing in specialized mycobacterial laboratories. Laboratory guidelines for susceptibility testing of the RGM have recently been published, including definitions of susceptible and resistant MIC breakpoints for the recommended drugs (96). The nine current drugs which should be tested for susceptibility include amikacin, cefoxitin, imipenem, sulfamethoxazole or trimethoprim-sulfamethoxazole, clarithromycin, ciprofloxacin, doxycycline, linezolid, and tobramycin (the latter only for isolates of *M. chelonae*). Additional agents such as minocycline, moxifloxacin, meropenem, and tigecycline have been proposed but are not yet included in the CLSI document (96).

Isolates of the *M. fortuitum* group, *M. smegmatis* group, and *M. mucogenicum* group are generally the most susceptible of the more commonly encountered species of RGM (7, 10). They are usually susceptible or intermediate to amikacin, cefoxitin, imipenem, ciprofloxacin, sulfonamides, and moxifloxacin, with about 50% of the isolates of *M. fortuitum* susceptible to doxycycline (Table 2). Both minocycline and doxycycline are preferred over tetracycline because of greater in vitro activity of the former two antimicrobials in previous studies of the RGM (83).

Clarithromycin inhibits all isolates of *M. chelonae* and *M. abscessus* and approximately 80% of *M. fortuitum* at a concentration of 4 µg/ml at 3 days (8). However, all isolates of the *M. smegmatis* group, *M. houstonense*, and *M. mageritense* are macrolide resistant at 3 days (7, 8, 10, 67). The MICs for several species are in the susceptible range with 3 days of incubation but become resistant with an incubation of 14 days (e.g., most isolates of *M. fortuitum* and *M. abscessus*). Recent studies have shown that RGM species that have early or late intrinsic resistance to clarithromycin (e.g., *M. fortuitum* [*erm*39], *M. smegmatis* [*erm*38], *M. mageritense* [*erm*40], and *M. wolinskyi* [*erm*40]) contain an inducible erythromycin methylase (*erm*) gene that methylates the 23S rRNA macrolide binding site (52–55). Furthermore, species within the *M. fortuitum* group (*M. boenickei*, *M. houstonense*, *M. neworleansense*, and *M. porcinum*) also have this gene along with *M. abscessus* (*erm*41). Multiple different genes have been recognized, including *erm*38 (*M. smegmatis*), *erm*39 (*M.*

fortuitum), *erm*40 (*M. mageritense* and *M. houstonense*), and *erm*41 (*M. abscessus*). Some species have no detectable *erm* gene (e.g., *M. chelonae* and *M. peregrinum*), and these species show little or no change in clarithromycin MICs with prolonged incubation.

The recent finding of the presence of the *erm* gene raises questions regarding macrolide effectiveness for therapy despite susceptible routine in vitro MICs with standard (3 days) incubation times. A recent clinical study in Korea showed that patients with *M. bolletii* (formerly *M. massiliense*) responded more favorably than patients with *M. abscessus* (formerly *M. abscessus* subsp. *abscessus*) (42a). Thus results of routine in vitro macrolide susceptibility testing should be interpreted judiciously and should be considered when assessing macrolides for potential efficacy (53). A proposal to the CLSI for final reading of the clarithromycin MICs for RGM at 14 days, to detect inducible resistance, has been submitted but not yet accepted.

In general, isolates of *M. abscessus* and *M. chelonae* are more drug resistant than other RGM species and generally susceptible or intermediate only to amikacin, imipenem, and clarithromycin (10). Isolates of *M. abscessus* are moderately susceptible (intermediate) to cefoxitin (MIC ≤ 64 µg/ml), whereas isolates of *M. chelonae* are highly resistant (MIC ≥ 256 µg/ml). Additionally, for isolates of *M. chelonae*, MICs of tobramycin are lower than those of amikacin, and *M. chelonae* is the only species of RGM for which amikacin is not the preferred aminoglycoside. Approximately 20% of the strains of *M. chelonae* are also susceptible to achievable serum levels of ciprofloxacin and/or doxycycline or minocycline (10, 83) (Tables 2 and 3).

Among a new class of antimicrobials, known as the oxazolidinones, linezolid has been shown to have in vitro activity against the *M. fortuitum* group (modal MIC was 4 µg/ml) and *M. chelonae* (modal MIC was 8 µg/ml) (86). Linezolid has been used subsequently in the treatment of infections due to RGM, including disseminated *M. chelonae* with acquired mutational resistance to clarithromycin (11). Isolates of *M. abscessus* have variable susceptibility to linezolid.

Finally, tigecycline, a new glycylcycline derivative of minocycline, has shown excellent in vitro activity with all MICs of ≤1 µg/ml against all species of RGM tested, including *M. chelonae*, *M. abscessus*, and tetracycline-susceptible and -resistant isolates of the *M. fortuitum* group (83). However, MIC breakpoints for this agent with the RGM have not been proposed.

Table 2. Antimicrobials used for treatment of commonly encountered species of RGM

Species	Drugs[a]
M. fortuitum	Parenteral: amikacin, cefoxitin, imipenem,[b] tigecycline[c]
	Oral: ciprofloxacin, levofloxacin, sulfonamide or trimethoprim-sulfamethoxazole, moxifloxacin, clarithromycin[d] (80%), doxycycline (50%), linezolid (86%)
M. abscessus	Parenteral: amikacin, tigecycline,[c] cefoxitin (70%), imipenem,[e] tigecycline[c]
	Oral: clarithromycin or azithromycin,[d] doxycycline (<5%), ciprofloxacin (<5%), moxifloxacin (~15%), linezolid (23%)
M. chelonae	Parenteral: tobramycin, amikacin (70%), imipenem,[e] tigecycline[c]
	Oral: doxycycline (25%), ciprofloxacin (25%), linezolid (54%), clarithromycin or azithromycin

[a]Untreated strains are 100% susceptible unless otherwise noted.
[b]Susceptible or intermediate.
[c]No breakpoints are currently available for tigecycline with RGM, but all MICs for *M. fortuitum*, *M. abscessus*, and *M. chelonae* have been ≤1 µg/ml.
[d]3-day readings; does not include inducible (*erm*) resistance.
[e]At the present time, susceptibility testing of these species by current methods is not reproducible (96).

Table 3. General principles of therapy of RGM disease

Clinical setting	Drug treatment[a]
Pulmonary disease	
M. fortuitum..	Short-term i.v. treatment (2–4 wk), then multiple p.o. medicines for minimum of 6 mo
M. abscessus..	May be incurable with antimicrobials; clinical improvement with clarithromycin or short-term low-dose amikacin (single daily dose with peaks in low- to mid-20 range), cefoxitin, and/or tigecycline or imipenem
	Best oral antimicrobials are clarithromycin or azithromycin and linezolid with addition of pyridoxine (to potentially reduce risk of peripheral neuropathy)
Localized skin/soft tissue/bone disease	
M. fortuitum, M. chelonae, M. abscessus.........	i.v. treatment for extensive disease (2–4 wk), followed by p.o. medicines; p.o. medicines only for minor disease. Remove catheter or foreign body. Treat 6 mo total for significant disease, including all cases with osteomyelitis.
	Linezolid (oral or i.v.) with addition of pyridoxine (to potentially reduce risk of peripheral neuropathy) has also been successful for M. chelonae
Disseminated (cutaneous) disease	
M. chelonae..	Once-daily low-dose tobramycin or intermittent imipenem plus clarithromycin for first 2–4 wk, then clarithromycin only to complete 6 mo; linezolid with addition of pyridoxine (to potentially reduce risk of peripheral neuropathy)
M. abscessus..	Same as for M. chelonae except use amikacin in place of tobramycin and cefoxitin may replace imipenem

[a]i.v., intravenous; p.o., oral.

CLINICAL DISEASE

Localized Posttraumatic Wound Infections

The best-known clinical disease syndrome due to RGM is a localized wound infection following accidental trauma (10). Table 4 shows a list of the types of injury responsible for infections due to RGM. All involve some form of penetrating trauma such as open fracture and stepping on a nail, often followed by osteomyelitis. Patients with this type of infection are generally healthy, and drug-induced immune suppression does not appear to be a risk factor. After an incubation period of 3 to 6 weeks, local redness and swelling with spontaneous drainage usually occurs. Systemic symptoms such as fever, chills, malaise, and fatigue are usually absent. The drainage is usually thin and watery but occasionally may be thick and purulent. Sinus tract formations with intermittent drainage are common.

The most common pathogens in these settings are the M. fortuitum group including M. fortuitum, M. porcinum, and M. houstonense, but almost any of

the pathogenic species may cause disease in patients with infected open fractures (10, 67, 87). Furthermore, these infections frequently are often polymicrobial, reflecting environmental contamination with more than one species of mycobacteria or a combination of bacteria and mycobacteria.

Surgical Wound Infections

Surgical wound infections, including cataract excision, corneal graft (70), laser surgery (61), extremity amputations, dacrocystorhinostomy, plastic surgery of the face (10), prosthetic hip or knee insertions, coronary artery bypass (10), excision of basal cell carcinoma (65), and as previously mentioned, augmentation mammaplasty and cosmetic surgeries including liposuction and liposculpture (10, 13, 50), present in a similar fashion to accidental trauma. After an incubation period of 2 to 8 weeks, the healing wound will develop serous drainage and redness. Localized nodular areas adjacent to the incision may develop which are often painful and may require incision and drainage. Low-grade fever of 99 to 101°F

Table 4. Species or taxonomic group and their common clinical diseases

M. fortuitum group	M. chelonae	M. abscessus
Localized posttraumatic infections	Disseminated skin infections	Chronic lung infections
Catheter infections	Localized posttraumatic wound infections	Localized posttraumatic wound infections
Surgical wound infections	Catheter infections	Catheter infections
Augmentation mammaplasty	Sinusitis	Disseminated skin infections
Cardiac surgery	Corneal infections	Corneal infections

may also be present if the infection is extensive. Isolates of the *M. fortuitum* group are most commonly recovered in these settings, but other species may also be involved (10, 29).

Catheter-Related Infections

The most common health care-associated disease since the 1990s has been central venous catheter infections. These may manifest as occult bacteremia, granulomatous hepatitis, septic lung infiltrates, tunnel infections, or exit site infections (10). The timing of these infections has not been established, but they involve catheters that have been in place at least several months. The usual etiologic agent is *M. fortuitum*, although pigmented species such as *M. neoaurum* and *M. bacteremicum* have also been associated with catheter sepsis recently (10a, 59, 89). Other long-term catheters, including chronic peritoneal dialysis catheters, hemodialysis catheters, nasolacrimal duct catheters, and ventriculoperitoneal shunts also have been associated with RGM infection (5, 47, 67).

Disseminated Cutaneous Infections

Two basic types of cutaneous disease unique to the RGM have been described. The first is marked by the presence of multiple noncontiguous nodular draining skin lesions on one or more extremities. In patients with chronic diseases that require chronic steroid therapy, multiple skin lesions develop and tend to be a nuisance rather than life-threatening. These almost always involve the lower extremity and are most often due to *M. chelonae* (10). Steroid doses may be as low as 5 to 10 mg of prednisone daily. The most common underlying disease is rheumatoid arthritis but may also include organ transplants and chronic

autoimmune disorders (10). The patients are often asymptomatic except for the local discomfort of the lesions.

The second type of disseminated skin disease is seen in patients with rapidly fatal disorders, especially poorly controlled leukemias and lymphoma (10, 47). This infection tends to be systemic, with positive cultures of blood and bone marrow. A portal of entry for the organism is rarely identified, although central catheters may be involved. It is usually caused by *M. abscessus* and, combined with the underlying disease, was often fatal in the era before adequate antimicrobial therapy was available. Interestingly, members of the *M. fortuitum* and *M. smegmatis* groups are rarely associated with either type of disseminated disease (10, 15).

Chronic Pulmonary Infections

Chronic pulmonary infections are most often associated with *M. abscessus* (10, 35) (Table 5). These infections are typically found in elderly nonsmoking females who present with chronic cough and fatigue. By high-resolution computerized tomography of the chest, most patients have patchy cylindrical bronchiectasis and small nodules of <5 mm involving the right middle lobe and lingula. This radiographic pattern is referred to as nodular bronchiectasis, was first recognized in patients with *M. avium* complex, and also may be present in patients with *M. abscessus*. The disease tends to be very slowly progressive, with minimal morbidity. Hemoptysis may be present, and fever may occur with more advanced disease (35). Another pulmonary syndrome following infection with *Mycobacterium tuberculosis* involves the portion of the lung previously damaged and most often is associated with *M. abscessus*.

Table 5. Pulmonary syndromes associated with positive respiratory cultures for RGM

Finding	Interpretation	Most common RGM involved
Single AFB smear-negative culture-positive specimen	Transient colonization or specimen with low organism colony count contamination	
Multiple culture-positive specimens		
Elderly nonsmoking patients, no risk factors, bilateral streaky infiltrates on chest radiograph	Probable nodular bronchiectasis (confirm by HRCT)[a]	*M. abscessus*
Prior tuberculosis, now with increased infiltrate in same area	Posttuberculous infection	*M. abscessus*
Achalasia with chronic vomiting and bilateral interstitial/alveolar infiltrates or known lipoid pneumonia	Chronic pneumonitis	*M. fortuitum*
Cystic fibrosis	Focal pneumonitis or colonization (HRCT may be helpful in determination)	*M. abscessus*

[a]HRCT, high-resolution computerized tomography.

In contrast, the *M. fortuitum* group is most often seen in patients with achalasia and chronic vomiting who manifest a relatively acute respiratory syndrome associated with high fevers, striking leucocytosis of 20,000 to 40,000 white blood cells/mm³, and alveolar infiltrates. Histopathologically, lipoid pneumonia is usually present and may be the major risk factor.

Chronic pulmonary infections with *M. abscessus* also are seen in patients with cystic fibrosis (CF) (20, 26, 56). Some patients have unremitting fever and some have increased hemoptysis or shortness of breath, while others show no apparent change in their clinical symptoms (6). Recent multicenter studies have emphasized infections with RGM in CF lung disease. The most common pathogens associated with CF lung disease have been members of the *M. abscessus*/*M. chelonae* group. One-half of the 104 isolates of NTM recovered in a multicenter study involving 1,582 CF patients (mean age, 18.9 years) in France were identified as *M. abscessus* subsp. *abscessus* and *M. abscessus* subsp. *bolletii* (formerly *M. massiliense* and *M. bolletii*) (63). A previous large study over a 6-year period of CF centers in the United States reviewed older CF patients (average age, 23 years) and found that isolates of *M. abscessus* were second in prevalence to those of the *M. avium* complex (56). Although some patients appear to have transient carriage, other patients remain culture positive, with significant symptoms and high morbidity and mortality (56).

Patients with CF have accompanying bronchiectasis in addition to chronic recurrent airway and parenchymal infections due to *Pseudomonas aeruginosa* and other bacterial pathogens that may be the primary risk factors for development of RGM disease (40, 56).

Central Nervous System Infections

Only a small number of cases of central nervous system infection due to the RGM have been documented (27, 82). These cases include those associated with infection with a foreign body following a motor vehicle accident, lumbar disectomy, chronic otitis media, brain abscess, chronic mastoiditis, deep wound infection, and infection of a ventriculoatrial shunt. The majority of these cases are related to infections with *M. fortuitum* (82).

Ophthalmic Infections

A recent study of 100 patients with ophthalmic infections showed that 95% of the infections were due to RGM. The most commonly isolated RGM were *M. chelonae* and *M. abscessus*, and 33% of the cases with known sources were from corneal infections (9).

DRUG THERAPY/DRUG RESISTANCE

Therapy for RGM infections has not been established by clinical trials except for clarithromycin monotherapy for infections due to *M. chelonae* (10, 35). Current recommendations are based on uncontrolled case series and individual experience. Mutational drug resistance that develops on therapy is a concern for ribosomal active drugs, such as clarithromycin and amikacin, for *M. chelonae* and *M. abscessus*, which have only one chromosomal copy of the ribosome (all other RGM have two copies) (88). Mutational resistance is also a concern for all single-copy genes, especially the quinolones. Hence, therapy with these agents should include combination therapy when possible for extensive disease with presumed large numbers of organisms. Acquired mutational resistance with the tetracyclines and sulfonamide monotherapy has not been described.

The general recommendation for serious wound infections is combination therapy with initial parenteral therapy for *M. chelonae* and *M. abscessus* until clinically improved, followed by oral therapy for a total treatment duration of 6 months. Development of new lesions on therapy is not necessarily indicative of treatment failure. Cultures should be obtained, and antibiotic therapy should be continued. In most cases, cultures are sterile following approximately 6 to 8 weeks of proper treatment, but treatment should be continued for a minimum of 4 months for less serious infections and 6 months for more serious infections. Abscess drainage and surgical debridement is important. Treatment of *M. abscessus* lung disease is limited by the complexity, expense, and toxicity of the required intravenous antibiotics, such as amikacin and imipenem. The disease is treatable, but many cases are currently incurable with drugs. Therefore, intermittent therapy to produce disease suppression is generally recommended (35). See Tables 2 and 3 for a summary of drugs and therapeutic approaches.

REFERENCES

1. Adékambi, T., P. Berger, D. Raoult, and M. Drancourt. 2006. *rpoB* gene sequence-based characterization of emerging nontuberculous mycobacteria with descriptions of *Mycobacterium bolletii* sp. nov., *M. phocaicum* sp. nov. and *Mycobacterium aubagnense* sp. nov. *Int. J. Syst. Evol. Microbiol.* **56:**133–143.

2. Adékambi, T., P. Colson, and M. Drancourt. 2003. *rpoB*-based identification of nonpigmented and late pigmented rapidly growing mycobacteria. *J. Clin. Microbiol.* **41:**5699–5708.

3. Adékambi, T., and M. Drancourt. 2004. Dissection of phylogenetic relationships among nineteen rapidly growing mycobacterium species by 16S rRNA, *hsp65*, *sodA*, *recA*, and *rpoB* gene sequencing. *Int. J. Syst. Evol. Microbiol.* **54:**2095–2105.

4. Adékambi, T., M. Reynaud-Gaubert, G. Greub, M. J. Gevaudan, B. La Scola, D. Raoult, and M. Drancourt. 2004. Amoebal coculture of "*Mycobacterium massiliense*" sp. nov. from the sputum of a patient with hemoptoic pneumonia. *J. Clin. Microbiol.* **42:**5493–5501.

5. Al Shaalan, M., B. J. Law, S. J. Israels, P. Pianosi, A. G. Lacson, and R. Higgins. 1997. *Mycobacterium fortuitum* interstitial pneumonia with vasculitis in a child with Wilms tumor. *Pediatr. Infect. Dis. J.* **16:**996–1000.

6. Bange, F.-C., B. A. Brown, C. Smaczny, R. J. Wallace, Jr., and E. C. Böttger. 2001. Lack of transmission of *Mycobacterium abscessus* among patients with cystic fibrosis attending a single clinic. *Clin. Infect. Dis.* **32:**1648–1650.

7. Brown, B. A., B. Springer, V. A. Steingrube, R. W. Wilson, G. E. Pfyffer, M. J. Garcia, M. C. Menendez, B. Rodriguez-Salgado, K. C. Jost, S. H. Chiu, G. O. Onyi, E. C. Böttger, and R. J. Wallace, Jr. 1999. *Mycobacterium wolinskyi* sp. nov. and *Mycobacterium goodii* sp. nov., two new rapidly growing species related to *Mycobacterium smegmatis* and associated with human wound infections: a cooperative study from the International Working Group on Mycobacterial Taxonomy. *Int. J. Syst. Bacteriol.* **49:**1493–1511.

8. Brown, B. A., R. J. Wallace, Jr., G. Onyi, V. DeRosas, and R. J. Wallace III. 1992. Activities of four macrolides including clarithromycin against *Mycobacterium fortuitum*, *Mycobacterium chelonae*, and *Mycobacterium chelonae*-like organisms. *Antimicrob. Agents Chemother.* **36:**180–184.

9. Brown-Elliott, B. A., M. McGlasson, P. Painter, L. Mann, D. Hall, L. Battee, and R. J. Wallace, Jr. 2009. Comparison of antimicrobials including besifloxacin, ciprofloxacin, gatifloxacin, moxifloxacin, levofloxacin, azithromycin, clarithromycin, amikacin, imipenem, and tobramycin against ophthalmic isolates of nontuberculous mycobacteria, abstr. U-041, p. 583. *109th Gen. Meet. Am. Soc. Microbiol.*, Philadelphia, PA.

10. Brown-Elliott, B. A., and R. J. Wallace, Jr. 2002. Clinical and taxonomic status of pathogenic nonpigmented or late-pigmenting rapidly growing mycobacteria. *Clin. Microbiol. Rev.* **15:**716–746.

10a. Brown-Elliott, B. A., R. J. Wallace, C. A. Petti, L. B. Mann, M. McGlasson, S. Chihara, G. L. Smith, P. Painter, D. Hail, R. Wilson, and K. E. Simmon. 2010. *Mycobacterium neoaurum* and *Mycobacterium bacteremicum* sp. nov. as causes of bacteremia. *J. Clin. Microbiol.* **48:**4377–4385.

11. Brown-Elliott, B. A., R. J. Wallace, Jr., R. Blinkhorn, C. J. Crist, and L. M. Mann. 2001. Successful treatment of disseminated *Mycobacterium chelonae* infection with linezolid. *Clin. Infect. Dis.* **33:**1433–1434.

12. Carson, L. A., L. A. Bland, L. B. Cusick, M. S. Favero, G. A. Bolan, A. L. Reingold, and R. C. Good. 1988. Prevalence of nontuberculous mycobacteria in water supplies of hemodialysis centers. *Appl. Environ. Microbiol.* **54:**3122–3125.

13. Centers for Disease Control and Prevention. 1998. Rapidly growing mycobacterial infection following liposuction and liposculpture—Caracas, Venezuela, 1996-1998. *MMWR Morb. Mortal. Wkly. Rep.* **47:**1065.

14. Centers for Disease Control and Prevention. 2004. Nontuberculous mycobacterial infections after cosmetic surgery—Santo Domingo, Dominican Republic, 2003-2004. *MMWR Morb. Mortal. Wkly. Rep.* **53:**509.

15. Chetchotisakd, P., P. Mootsikapun, S. Anunnatsiri, K. Jirarattanapochai, C. Choonhakarn, A. Chaiprasert, P. N. Ubol, L. J. Wheat, and T. E. Davis. 2000. Disseminated infection due to rapidly growing mycobacteria in immunocompetent hosts presenting with chronic lymphadenopathy: a previously unrecognized clinical entity. *Clin. Infect. Dis.* **32:**29–34.

16. Cobbett, L. 1918. An acid-fast bacillus obtained from a pustular eruption. *Br. Med. J.* **2:**158.

17. Cooksey, R. C., J. H. de Waard, M. A. Yakrus, I. Rivera, M. Chopite, S. R. Toney, G. P. Morlock, and W. R. Butler. 2004. *Mycobacterium cosmeticum* sp. nov., a novel rapidly growing species isolated from a cosmetic infection and from a nail salon. *Int. J. Syst. Evol. Microbiol.* **54:**2385–2391.

18. Cooksey, R. C., M. A. Jhung, M. A. Yakrus, W. R. Butler, T. Adékambi, G. P. Morlock, M. Williams, A. M. Shams, B. J. Jensen, R. E. Morey, N. Charles, S. R. Toney, K. C. Jost, Jr., D. F. Dunbar, V. Bennett, M. Kuan, and A. Srinivasan. 2008. Multiphasic approach reveals genetic diversity of environmental and patient isolates of *Mycobacterium mucogenicum* and *Mycobacterium phocaicum* associated with an outbreak of bacteremias at a Texas Hospital. *Appl. Environ. Microbiol.* **74:**2480–2487.

19. Covert, T. C., M. R. Rodgers, A. L. Reyes, and G. N. Stelma, Jr. 1999. Occurrence of nontuberculous mycobacteria in environmental samples. *Appl. Environ. Microbiol.* **65:**2492–2496.

20. Cullen, A. R., C. L. Cannon, E. J. Mark, and A. A. Colin. 2000. *Mycobacterium abscessus* infection in cystic fibrosis. *Am. J. Respir. Crit. Care Med.* **161:**641–645.

21. da Costa Cruz, J. C. 1938. *Mycobacterium fortuitum*: um novo bacilo acido-resistente patogenico para o homen (new acid fast bacillus pathogenic for man). *Acta Med.* (Rio de Jâneiro) **1:**298–301.

22. del Castillo, M., D. J. Palmero, B. Lopez, R. Paul, V. Ritacco, P. Bonvehi, L. Clara, M. Ambroggi, L. Barrera, and C. Vay. 2009. Mesotherapy-associated outbreak caused by *Mycobacterium immunogenum*. *Emerg. Infect. Dis.* **15:**357–358.

23. Duarte, R. S., M. C. Silva Lourenço, L. de Souza Fonseca, S. C. Leão, E. D. L. T. Amorim, I. L. L. Rocha, F. S. Coelho, C. Viana-Niero, K. M. Gomes, M. G. da Silva, N. S. de Oliveira Lorena, M. B. Pitombo, R. M. C. Ferreira, M. H. de Oliveira Garcia, G. P. de Oliveira, O. Lupi, B. R. Vilaça, L. R. Serradas, A. Chebato, E. A. Marques, L. M. Teixeira, M. Dalcolmo, S. G. Senna, and J. L. M. Sampaio. 2009. Epidemic of postsurgical infections caused by *Mycobacterium massiliense*. *J. Clin. Microbiol.* **47:**2149–2155.

24. Eid, A. J., F. Bergari, I. G. Sia, N. L. Wengenack, D. R. Osmon, and R. R. Razonable. 2007. Prosthetic joint infection due to rapidly growing mycobacteria: report of 8 cases and review of the literature. *Clin. Infect. Dis.* **45:**687–694.

25. Falkinham, J. O., III. 2003. The changing pattern of nontuberculous mycobacterial disease. *Can. J. Infect. Dis.* **14:**281–286.

26. Fauroux, B., B. Delaisi, A. Clément, C. Saizou, D. Moissenet, C. Truffot-Pernot, G. Tournier, and H. Vu Thien. 1997. Mycobacterial lung disease in cystic fibrosis: a prospective study. *Pediatr. Infect. Dis. J.* **16:**354–358.

27. Flor, A., J. A. Capdevila, N. Martin, J. Gavaldà, and A. Pahissa. 1996. Nontuberculous mycobacterial meningitis: report of two cases and review. *Clin. Infect. Dis.* **23:**1266–1273.

28. Forbes, B. A., N. Banaiee, K. G. Beavis, B. A. Brown-Elliott, P. Della Latta, L. B. Elliott, G. S. Hall, B. Hanna, M. D. Perkins, S. H. Siddiqi, R. J. Wallace, Jr., and N. G. Warren. 2008. *Laboratory Detection and Identification of Mycobacteria; Approved Guideline. CLSI Document M48-A.* CLSI, Wayne, PA.

29. Friedman, N. D., and D. J. Sexton. 2001. Bursitis due to *Mycobacterium goodii*, a recently described, rapidly growing mycobacterium. *J. Clin. Microbiol.* **39:**404–405.

30. Furuya, E. Y., A. Paez, A. Srinivasan, R. Cooksey, M. Augenbraun, M. Baron, K. Brudney, P. Della-Latta, C. Estivariz, S. Fischer, M. Flood, P. Kellner, C. Roman, M. Yakrus, D. Weiss, and E. V. Granowitz. 2008. Outbreak of *Mycobacterium abscessus* wound infections among "lipotourists" from the United States who underwent abdominoplasty in the Dominican Republic. *Clin. Infect. Dis.* **46:**1181–1188.

31. Galassi, L., R. Donato, E. Tortoli, D. Burrini, D. Santianni, and R. Dei. 2003. Nontuberculous mycobacteria in hospital water systems: application of HPLC for identification of environmental mycobacteria. *J. Water Health* **1:**133–139.

32. Galil, K., L. A. Miller, M. A. Yakrus, R. J. Wallace, Jr., D. G. Mosley, B. England, G. Huitt, M. M. McNeill, and B. A. Perkins. 1999. Abscesses due to *Mycobacterium abscessus* linked to injection of unapproved alternative medication. *Emerg. Infect. Dis.* **5:**681–687.

33. Gira, A. K., H. Reisenauer, L. Hammock, U. Nadiminti, J. T. Macy, A. Reeves, C. Burnett, M. A. Yakrus, S. Toney, B. J. Jensen, H. M. Blumberg, S. W. Caughman, and F. S. Nolte. 2004. Furunculosis due to *Mycobacterium mageritense* associated with footbaths at a nail salon. *J. Clin. Microbiol.* **42:**1813–1817.

34. Gomila, M., A. Ramirez, J. Gascó, and J. Lalucat. 2008. *Mycobacterium llatzerense* sp. nov., a facultatively autotrophic, hydrogen-oxidizing bacterium isolated from haemodialysis water. *Int. J. Syst. Evol. Microbiol.* **58:**2769–2773.

35. Griffith, D. E., T. Aksamit, B. A. Brown-Elliott, A. Catanzaro, C. Daley, F. Gordin, S. M. Holland, R. Horsburgh, G. Huitt, M. F. Iademarco, M. Iseman, K. Olivier, S. Ruoss, C. F. von Reyn, R. J. Wallace, Jr., and K. Winthrop. 2007. An official ATS/IDSA statement: diagnosis, treatment and prevention of nontuberculous mycobacterial diseases. American Thoracic Society statement. *Am. J. Respir. Crit. Care Med.* **175:**367–416.

36. Gubler, J. G. H., M. Salfinger, and A. von Graevenitz. 1992. Pseudoepidemic of nontuberculous mycobacteria due to a contaminated bronchoscope cleaning machine: report of an outbreak and review of the literature. *Chest* **101:**1245–1249.

37. Hector, J. S. R., Y. Pang, G. H. Mazurek, Y. Zhang, B. A. Brown, and R. J. Wallace, Jr. 1992. Large restriction fragment patterns of genomic *Mycobacterium fortuitum* DNA as strain-specific markers and their use in epidemiologic investigation of four nosocomial outbreaks. *J. Clin. Microbiol.* **30:**1250–1255.

38. Hennessee, C. T., J.-S. Seo, A. M. Alvarez, and Q. X. Li. 2009. Polycyclic aromatic hydrocarbon-degrading species isolates from Hawaiian soils: *Mycobacterium crocinum* sp. nov., *Mycobacterium pallens* sp. nov., *Mycobacterium rutilum* sp. nov., *Mycobacterium rufum* sp. nov., and *Mycobacterium aromaticivorans* sp. nov. *Int. J. Syst. Evol. Microbiol.* **59:**378–387.

39. Jiménez, M. S., M. I. Campos-Herrero, D. García, M. Luquin, L. Herrera, and M. J. García. 2004. *Mycobacterium canariasense* sp. nov. *Int. J. Syst. Evol. Microbiol.* **54:**1729–1734.

40. Jönsson, B. E., M. Gilljam, A. Landblad, M. Ridell, A. E. Wold, and C. Welinder-Olsson. 2007. Molecular epidemiology of *Mycobacterium abscessus* with focus on cystic fibrosis. *J. Clin. Microbiol.* **45:**1497–1504.

41. Kim, H.-Y., Y. Kook, Y.-J. Yun, C. G. Park, N. Y. Lee, T. S. Shim, B.-J. Kim, and Y.-H. Kook. 2008. Proportion of *Mycobacterium massiliense* and *Mycobacterium bolletii* in strains among Korean *Mycobacterium chelonae-Mycobacterium abscessus* group isolates. *J. Clin. Microbiol.* **46:**3384–3390.

42. Kim, H.-Y., Y.-J. Yun, C. G. Park, D. H. Lee, Y. K. Cho, B. J. Park, S.-I. Joo, E.-C. Kim, Y. J. Hur, B.-J. Kim, and Y. H. Kook.
2007. Outbreak of *Mycobacterium massiliense* infection associated with intramuscular injections. *J. Clin. Microbiol.* **45:**3127–3130.

42a. Koh, W.-J., J. Kyeongman, N.-Y. Lee, B.-J. Kim, Y.-H. Kook, S.-H. Lee, Y. K. Park, C. K. Kim, S. J. Shin, G. A. Huitt, C. L. Daley, and D. J. Kwon. 2011. Clinical significance of differentiation of *Mycobacterium massiliense* from *Mycobacterium abscessus*. *Am. J. Respir. Crit. Care Med.* **183:**405–410.

43. Kusunoki, S., and T. Ezaki. 1992. Proposal of *Mycobacterium peregrinum* sp. nov., nom. rev., and elevation of *Mycobacterium chelonae* subsp. *abscessus* (Kubica et al.) to species status: *Mycobacterium abscessus* comb. nov. *Int. J. Syst. Bacteriol.* **42:**240–245.

44. Lai, K. K., B. A. Brown, J. A. Westerling, S. A. Fontecchio, Y. Zhang, and R. J. Wallace, Jr. 1998. Long-term laboratory contamination by *Mycobacterium abscessus* resulting in two pseudo-outbreaks: recognition with use of random amplified polymorphic DNA (RAPD) polymerase chain reaction. *Clin. Infect. Dis.* **27:**169–175.

45. Lamy, B., H. Marchandin, K. Hamitouche, and F. Laurent. 2008. *Mycobacterium setense* sp. nov., a *Mycobacterium fortuitum* group organism isolated from a patient with soft tissue infection and osteitis. *Int. J. Syst. Evol. Microbiol.* **58:**486–490.

46. Leao, S. C., E. Tortoli, C. Viana-Niero, S. Y. M. Ueki, K. V. B. Lima, M. L. Lopes, J. Yubero, M. C. Menendez, and M. J. Garcia. 2009. Characterization of mycobacteria from a major Brazilian outbreak suggests a revision of the taxonomic status of members of the *Mycobacterium chelonae-abscessus* group. *J. Clin. Microbiol.* **47:**2691–2698.

46a. Leao, S. C., E. Tortoli, J. P. Euzeby, and M. J. Garcia. 2010 (Epub ahead of print). Proposal that the two species *Mycobacterium massiliense* and *Mycobacterium bolletii* be reclassified as *Mycobacterium abscessus* subsp. *bolletii* comb. nov., designation of *Mycobacterium abscessus* subsp. *abscessus* subsp. nov., and emendation of *Mycobacterium abscessus*. *Int. J. Syst. Evol. Microbiol.* doi:10.1099/ijs.0.023770-0.

47. Levendoglu-Tugal, O., J. Munoz, A. Brudnicki, M. F. Ozkaynak, C. Sandoval, and S. Jayabose. 1998. Infections due to nontuberculous mycobacteria in children with leukemia. *Clin. Infect. Dis.* **27:**1227–1230.

48. Macheras, E., A.-L. Roux, F. Ripoll, V. Sivadon-Tardy, C. Gutierrez, J.-L. Gaillard, and B. Heym. 2009. Inaccuracy of single-target sequencing for discriminating species of the *Mycobacterium abscessus* group. *J. Clin. Microbiol.* **47:**2596–2600.

49. McNabb, A., D. Eisler, K. Adie, M. Amos, M. Rodrigues, G. Stephens, W. A. Black, and J. Isaac-Renton. 2004. Assessment of partial sequencing of the 65-kilodalton heat shock protein gene (*hsp65*) for routine identification of *Mycobacterium* species isolated from clinical sources. *J. Clin. Microbiol.* **42:**3000–3011.

50. Meyers, H., B. A. Brown-Elliott, D. Moore, J. Curry, C. Truong, Y. Zhang, and R. J. Wallace, Jr. 2002. An outbreak of *Mycobacterium chelonae* infection following liposuction. *Clin. Infect. Dis.* **34:**1500–1507.

51. Moore, M., and J. B. Frerichs. 1953. An unusual acid fast infection of the knee with subcutaneous, abscess-like lesions of the gluteal region: report of a case study with a study of the organism, *Mycobacterium abscessus*. *J. Investig. Dermatol.* **20:**133–169.

52. Nash, K. A. 2003. Intrinsic macrolide resistance in *Mycobacterium smegmatis* is conferred by a novel *erm* gene, *erm*(38). *Antimicrob. Agents Chemother.* **47:**3053–3060.

53. Nash, K. A., N. Andini, Y. Zhang, B. A. Brown-Elliott, and R. J. Wallace, Jr. 2006. Intrinsic macrolide resistance in rapidly

growing mycobacteria. *Antimicrob. Agents Chemother.* 50: 3476–3478.

54. Nash, K. A., B. A. Brown-Elliott, and R. J. Wallace, Jr. 2009. A novel gene, *erm*(41), confers inducible macrolide resistance to clinical isolates of *Mycobacterium abscessus* but is absent from *Mycobacterium chelonae. Antimicrob. Agents Chemother.* 53:1367–1376.

55. Nash, K. A., Y. Zhang, B. A. Brown-Elliott, and R. J. Wallace, Jr. 2005. Molecular basis of intrinsic macrolide resistance in clinical isolates of *Mycobacterium fortuitum. J. Antimicrob. Chemother.* 55:170–177.

56. Olivier, K. N., D. J. Weber, R. J. Wallace, Jr., A. R. Faiz, J.-H. Lee, Y. Zhang, B. A. Brown-Elliott, A. Handler, R. W. Wilson, M. S. Schechter, L. J. Edwards, S. Chakraborti, and M. R. Knowles for the Nontuberculous Mycobacteria in Cystic Fibrosis Study Group. 2003. Nontuberculous mycobacteria. I. Multicenter prevalence study in cystic fibrosis. *Am. J. Respir. Crit. Care Med.* 167:828–834.

57. Petti, C. A., P. P. Bosshard, M. E. Brandt, J. E. Clarridge III, T. V. Feldblyum, P. Foxall, M. R. Furtado, N. Pace, and G. Procop. 2007. *Interpretive Criteria for Microorganism Identification by DNA Target Sequencing: Proposed Guideline. CLSI Document MM18-P.* Clinical and Laboratory Standards Institute, Wayne, PA.

58. Phillips, M. S., and C. F. von Reyn. 2001. Nosocomial infections due to nontuberculous mycobacteria. *Clin. Infect. Dis.* 33:1363–1374.

59. Raad, I. I., S. Vartivarian, A. Khan, and G. P. Bodey. 1991. Catheter-related infections caused by the *Mycobacterium fortuitum* complex: 15 cases and review. *Rev. Infect. Dis.* 13: 1120–1125.

60. Regnier, S., E. Cambau, J.-P. Meningaud, A. Guihot, L. Deforges, A. Carbonne, F. Bricaire, and E. Caumes. 2009. Clinical management of rapidly growing mycobacterial cutaneous infections in patients after mesotherapy. *Clin. Infect. Dis.* 49: 1358–1364.

61. Reviglio, V., M. L. Rodriguez, G. S. Picotti, M. Paradello, J. D. Luna, and C. P. Juárez. 1998. *Mycobacterium chelonae* keratitis following laser in situ keratomileusis. *J. Refract. Surg.* 14: 357–360.

62. Richter, E., S. Rüsch-Gerdes, and D. Hillemann. 2006. Evaluation of the GenoType Mycobacterium assay for identification of mycobacterial species from cultures. *J. Clin. Microbiol.* 44: 1769–1775.

63. Roux, A.-L., E. Catherinot, F. Ripoll, N. Soismier, E. Macheras, S. Ravilly, G. Bellis, M.-A. Vibet, E. Le Roux, L. Lemonnier, C. Gutierrez, V. Vincent, B. Fauroux, M. Rottman, D. Guillemot, J.-L. Gaillard, and J.-L. Herrman for the OMA Group. 2009. Multicenter study of prevalence of nontuberculous mycobacteria in patients with cystic fibrosis in France. *J. Clin. Microbiol.* 47:4124–4128.

64. Runyon, H. 1972. Conservation of the specific epithet *fortuitum* in the name of the organism known as *Mycobacterium fortuitum* da Costa Cruz. *Int. J. Syst. Bacteriol.* 22:50–51.

65. Saluja, A., N. T. Peters, L. Lowe, and T. M. Johnson. 1997. A surgical wound infection due to *Mycobacterium chelonae* successfully treated with clarithromycin. *Dermatol. Surg.* 23: 539–543.

66. Sampaio, J. L., E. Chimara, L. Ferrazoli, M. A. da Silva Telles, V. M. Del Guercio, Z. V. Jericó, K. Miyashiro, C. M. Fortaleza, M. C. Padoveze, and S. C. Leão. 2006. Application of four molecular typing methods for analysis of *Mycobacterium fortuitum* group strains causing post-mammaplasty infections. *Clin. Microbiol. Infect.* 12:142–149.

67. Schinsky, M. F., R. E. Morey, A. G. Steigerwalt, M. P. Douglas, R. W. Wilson, M. M. Floyd, W. R. Butler, M. I. Daneshvar, B. A. Brown-Elliott, R. J. Wallace, Jr., M. M. McNeil, D. J. Brenner, and J. M. Brown. 2004. Taxonomic variation in the *Mycobacterium fortuitum* third-biovariant complex: description of *Mycobacterium boenickei* sp. nov., *Mycobacterium houstonense* sp. nov., *Mycobacterium neworleanense* sp. nov., *Mycobacterium brisbanense* sp. nov., and recognition of *Mycobacterium porcinum* from human clinical isolates. *Int. J. Syst. Evol. Microbiol.* 54:1653–1667.

68. Schulze-Röbbecke, R., B. Janning, and R. Fischeder. 1992. Occurrence of mycobacteria in biofilm samples. *Tuberc. Lung Dis.* 73:141–144.

69. Steingrube, V. A., J. L. Gibson, B. A. Brown, Y. Zhang, R. W. Wilson, M. Rajagopalan, and R. J. Wallace, Jr. 1995. PCR amplification and restriction endonuclease analysis of a 65-kilodalton heat shock protein gene sequence for taxonomic separation of rapidly growing mycobacteria. *J. Clin. Microbiol.* 33:149–153. (Erratum, 33:1686.)

70. Sudesh, S., E. J. Cohen, L. W. Schwartz, and J. S. Myers. 2000. *Mycobacterium chelonae* infection in a corneal graft. *Arch. Ophthalmol.* 118:294–295.

71. Telenti, A., F. Marchesi, M. Balz, F. Bally, E. C. Böttger, and T. Bodmer. 1993. Rapid identification of mycobacteria to the species level by polymerase chain reaction and restriction enzyme analysis. *J. Clin. Microbiol.* 31:175–178.

72. Tiwari, T. S. P., B. Ray, K. C. Jost, Jr., M. K. Rathod, Y. Zhang, B. A. Brown-Elliott, K. Hendricks, and R. J. Wallace, Jr. 2003. Forty years of disinfectant failure: outbreak of postinjection *Mycobacterium abscessus* infection caused by contamination of benzalkonium chloride. *Clin. Infect. Dis.* 36:954–962.

73. Tortoli, E. 2003. Impact of genotypic studies on mycobacterial taxonomy: the new mycobacteria of the 1990s. *Clin. Microbiol. Rev.* 16:319–354.

74. Tortoli, E. 2006. The new mycobacteria: an update. *FEMS Immunol. Med. Microbiol.* 48:159–178.

75. Tortoli, E., A. Nanetti, C. Piersimoni, P. Cichero, C. Farina, G. Mucignat, C. Scarparo, L. Bartolini, R. Valentini, D. Nista, G. Gesu, C. Passerini Tosi, M. Crovatto, and G. Brusarosco. 2001. Performance assessment of new multiplex probe assay for identification of mycobacteria. *J. Clin. Microbiol.* 39: 1079–1084.

76. Tortoli, E., M. Pecorari, G. Fabio, M. Messinò, and A. Fabio. 2010. Commercial DNA probes for mycobacteria incorrectly identify a number of less frequently encountered species. *J. Clin. Microbiol.* 48:307–310.

77. Turenne, C. Y., L. Tschetter, J. Wolfe, and A. Kabani. 2001. Necessity of quality-controlled 16S rRNA gene sequence databases: identifying nontuberculous *Mycobacterium* species. *J. Clin. Microbiol.* 39:3637–3648.

78. van Dissel, J. T., and E. J. Kuijper. 2009. Rapidly growing mycobacteria: emerging pathogens in cosmetic procedures of the skin. *Clin. Infect. Dis.* 49:1365–1368.

79. Viana-Nicro, C., K. V. B. Lima, M. L. Lopes, M. C. da Silva Rabello, L. R. Marsola, V. C. R. Brilhante, A. M. Durham, and S. C. Leão. 2008. Molecular characterization of *Mycobacterium massiliense* and *Mycobacterium bolletii* in isolates collected from outbreaks of infections after laparoscopic surgeries and cosmetic procedures. *J. Clin. Microbiol.* 46:850–855.

80. Villanueva, A., R. V. Calderon, B. A. Vargas, F. Ruiz, S. Aguero, Y. Zhang, B. A. Brown, and R. J. Wallace, Jr. 1997. Report on an outbreak of post-injection abscesses due to *Mycobacterium abscessus*, including management with surgery and clarithromycin therapy and comparison of strains by random amplified polymorphic DNA polymerase chain reaction. *Clin. Infect. Dis.* 24:1147–1153.

81. Vugia, D. J., Y. Jang, C. Zizek, J. Ely, K. L. Winthrop, and E. Desmond. 2005. Mycobacteria in nail salon whirlpool footbaths, California. *Emerg. Infect. Dis.* **11:**616–618.

82. Wallace, R. J., Jr. 2004. Infections due to nontuberculous mycobacteria, p. 461–478. *In* W. M. Scheld, R. J. Whitley, and C. M. Marra (ed.), *Infections of the Central Nervous System*, 3rd ed. Lippincott Williams & Wilkins, Philadelphia, PA.

83. Wallace, R. J., Jr., B. A. Brown-Elliott, C. J. Crist, L. Mann, and R. W. Wilson. 2002. Comparison of the in vitro activity of the glycylcycline tigecycline (formerly GAR-936) with those of tetracycline, minocycline, and doxycycline against isolates of nontuberculous mycobacteria. *Antimicrob. Agents. Chemother.* **46:**3164–3167.

84. Wallace, R. J., Jr., B. A. Brown-Elliott, J. M. Brown, A. G. Steigerwalt, L. Hall, G. Woods, J. Cloud, L. Mann, R. W. Wilson, C. Crist, K. C. Jost, Jr., D. E. Byrer, J. Tang, J. Cooper, E. Stamenova, B. Campbell, J. Wolfe, and C. Turenne. 2005. Polyphasic characterization reveals that the human pathogen *Mycobacterium peregrinum* type II belongs to the bovine pathogen species *Mycobacterium senegalense*. *J. Clin. Microbiol.* **43:**5925–5935.

85. Wallace, R. J., Jr., B. A. Brown-Elliott, L. Hall, G. Roberts, R. W. Wilson, L. B. Mann, C. J. Crist, S. H. Chiu, R. Dunlap, M. J. Garcia, J. T. Bagwell, and K. C. Jost, Jr. 2002. Clinical and laboratory features of *Mycobacterium mageritense*. *J. Clin. Microbiol.* **40:**2930–2935.

86. Wallace, R. J., Jr., B. A. Brown-Elliott, S. C. Ward, C. J. Crist, L. B. Mann, and R. W. Wilson. 2001. Activities of linezolid against rapidly growing mycobacteria. *Antimicrob. Agents Chemother.* **45:**764–767.

87. Wallace, R. J., Jr., B. A. Brown-Elliott, R. W. Wilson, L. Mann, L. Hall, Y. Zhang, K. C. Jost, Jr., J. M. Brown, A. Kabani, M. F. Schinsky, A. G. Steigerwalt, C. J. Crist, G. D. Roberts, Z. Blacklock, M. Tsukamura, and V. Silcox, and C. Turenne. 2004. Clinical and laboratory features of *Mycobacterium porcinum*. *J. Clin. Microbiol.* **42:**5689–5697.

88. Wallace, R. J., Jr., A. Meier, B. A. Brown, Y. Zhang, P. Sander, G. O. Onyi, and E. C. Böttger. 1996. Genetic basis for clarithromycin resistance among isolates of *Mycobacterium chelonae* and *Mycobacterium abscessus*. *Antimicrob. Agents Chemother.* **40:**1676–1681.

89. Washer, L. L., J. Riddell IV, J. Rider, and C. E. Chenoweth. 2007. *Mycobacterium neoaurum* bloodstream infection: report of 4 cases and review of the literature. *Clin. Infect. Dis.* **45:**e10–e13.

90. Whipps, C. M. W. R. Butler, F. Pourahmad, V. G. Watral, and M. L. Kent. 2007. Molecular systematics support the revival of *Mycobacterium salmoniphilum* (ex Ross 1960) sp. nov., nom. rev., a species closely related to *Mycobacterium chelonae*. *Int. J. Syst. Evol. Microbiol.* **57:**2525–2531.

91. Wilson, R. W., V. A. Steingrube, E. C. Böttger, B. Springer, B. A. Brown-Elliott, V. Vincent, K. C. Jost, Jr., Y. Zhang, M. J. Garcia, S. H. Chiu, G. O. Onyi, H. Rossmoore, D. R. Nash, and R. J. Wallace, Jr. 2001. *Mycobacterium immunogenum* sp. nov., a novel species related to *Mycobacterium abscessus* and associated with clinical disease, pseudo-outbreaks, and contaminated metalworking fluids: an international cooperative study on mycobacterial taxonomy. *Int. J. Syst. Evol. Microbiol.* **51:**1751–1764.

92. Winthrop, K. L., K. Albridge, D. South, P. Albrecht, M. Abrams, M. C. Samuel, W. Leonard, J. Wagner, and D. J. Vugia. 2004. The clinical management and outcome of nail salon-acquired *Mycobacterium fortuitum* skin infection. *Clin. Infect. Dis.* **38:**38–44.

93. Winthrop, K. L., E. Chang, S. Yamashita, M. F. Iademarco, and P. A. LoBue. 2009. Nontuberculous mycobacteria infections and anti-tumor necrosis factor-alpha therapy. *Emerg. Infect. Dis.* **15:**1556–1561.

94. Wolinsky, E. 1979. State of the art: nontuberculous mycobacterial and associated disease. *Am. Rev. Respir. Dis.* **119:**107–159.

95. Woo, P. C. Y., K.-W. Leung, S. S. Y. Wong, K. T. K. Chong, E. Y. L. Cheung, and K.-Y. Yuen. 2002. Relatively alcohol-resistant mycobacteria are emerging pathogens in patients receiving acupuncture treatment. *J. Clin. Microbiol.* **40:**1219–1224.

96. Woods, G. L., B. A. Brown-Elliott, E. P. Desmond, G. S. Hall, L. Heifets, G. E. Pfyffer, M. R. Ridderhof, R. J. Wallace, Jr., N. G. Warren, and F. G. Witebsky. 2003. *Susceptibility Testing of Mycobacteria, Nocardia, and Other Aerobic Actinomycetes; Approved Standard M24-A*. NCCLS, Wayne, PA.

97. Zelazny, A. M., J. M. Root, Y. R. Shea, R. E. Colombo, I. C. Shamputa, F. Stock, S. S. Conlan, S. McNulty, B. A. Brown-Elliott, R. J. Wallace, Jr., K. N. Olivier, S. M. Holland, and E. P. Sampaio. 2009. Cohort study of molecular identification and typing of *Mycobacterium abscessus*, *Mycobacterium massiliense* and *Mycobacterium bolletii*. *J. Clin. Microbiol.* **47:**1985–1995.

98. Zhang, Y., M. Rajagopalan, B. A. Brown, and R. J. Wallace, Jr. 1997. Randomly amplified polymorphic DNA PCR for comparison of *Mycobacterium abscessus* strains from nosocomial outbreaks. *J. Clin. Microbiol.* **35:**3132–3139.

99. Zhibang, Y., Z. Bixia, L. Qishan, C. Lihao, L. Xiangquan, and L. Huaping. 2002. Large-scale outbreak of infection with *Mycobacterium chelonae* subsp. *abscessus* after penicillin injection. *J. Clin. Microbiol.* **40:**2626–2628.

Tuberculosis and Nontuberculous Mycobacterial Infections, 6th ed.
Edited by David Schlossberg
© 2011 ASM Press, Washington, DC

Chapter 38

Mycobacterium kansasii

JAMES C. JOHNSTON AND KEVIN ELWOOD

BACKGROUND

Mycobacterium kansasii was first isolated in Kansas City in 1953 by Buhler and Pollack (13). The species was initially characterized by the formation of "yellow colonies" when exposed to light, a phenomenon resulting from the deposition of beta carotene and later termed photochromogenicity (18, 57). In his classification of "atypical" mycobacteria, Runyon divided nontuberculous mycobacteria into four groups based on growth rate and pigmentation. *M. kansasii* was classified into group I along with other photochromogens such as *M. marinum* (57).

Soon after Runyon's characterization, *M. kansasii* was recognized as one of the most frequently isolated nontuberculous mycobacteria in the United States and Europe (3, 29, 47). The organism has been known primarily as a pulmonary pathogen, but cases of extrapulmonary and disseminated disease also occur. Most authors consider this to be the most pathogenic nontuberculous mycobacterium, with the majority of culture-positive cases presenting with clinical disease (28, 44).

In contrast to other common nontuberculous mycobacteria, *M. kansasii* is infrequently isolated from natural water sources or soil (63). The major reservoir appears to be tap water. Infection is likely acquired through the aerosol route, with low infectivity in regions of endemicity. Human-to-human transmission is not thought to occur despite two case reports of familial clustering (48, 51). Clustering more likely reflects a shared environment or susceptibility rather than human-to-human transmission.

EPIDEMIOLOGY

True epidemiological estimates of the *M. kansasii* disease rates are difficult to determine. Unlike *Mycobacterium tuberculosis*, a positive *M. kansasii* culture is not a reportable health event, which makes unbiased population-based measurements difficult. Moreover, laboratory-based rate estimates may be misleading as *M. kansasii* growth can represent host colonization or laboratory contamination. When compared with other nontuberculous mycobacteria, however, laboratory estimates may better represent true community rates as positive *M. kansasii* cultures more often reflect disease (28).

Estimates of *M. kansasii* incidence vary widely by region and have varied over time. In North America, rates are highest in the central and southern United States, giving rise to an "inverted T" distribution (23). In Europe, high rates have been consistently reported in England, Spain, and the Czech Republic (36, 37, 38, 56). Likewise, Japan, South Africa, and Brazil have reported high rates of infection (47), leading some to suggest links with industrialization. Accordingly, several publications have noted an urban predominance or an association with mining practices (3, 30, 36, 38). But no systematic sampling of rural and underdeveloped regions has been performed to buttress these claims.

Temporal changes in *M. kansasii* rates are more difficult to discern from the published literature. Longitudinal prevalence studies have yielded conflicting results, likely representing marked regional variability (28, 30, 43, 47, 50). Disease rates have also been influenced by the human immunodeficiency virus (HIV) epidemic, as rates of infection are markedly higher in this population. The annual *M. kansasii* infection rate in HIV-positive patients may be as high as 532 per 100,000, compared to 0.5 per 100,000 in a survey of 44 U.S. states prior to the HIV epidemic (23, 45). Unlike other nontuberculous mycobacteria, however, such as *Mycobacterium xenopi* and *Mycobacterium avium*, there has been no clear increase in *M. kansasii* prevalence over time. In fact, data from some centers suggest decreasing prevalence (28, 47).

James C. Johnston and Kevin Elwood • Division of Tuberculosis Control, British Columbia Centre for Disease Control, 655 West 12th Ave., Vancouver, British Columbia, Canada V5Z 4R4.

MICROBIOLOGY

M. kansasii is a slow-growing, acid-fast, photo-chromogenic mycobacterium. The organism grows readily in several mediums, including Bactec broth, Middlebrook 7H10 agar, and Lowenstein-Jensen agar, but may take up to 6 weeks to grow. As a slowly growing mycobacterium, *M. kansasii* takes more than 7 days to form colonies (65). Culture colonies appear smooth or rough with the yellow pigmentation and characteristic photochromogenicity. With prolonged incubation, cultures will turn reddish-orange. On microscopy, *M. kansasii* appears longer and broader than *M. tuberculosis*, often with a beaded or cross-barred appearance with Ziehl-Neelsen or Kinyoun staining. Species can be identified through characteristic culture findings, biochemical testing, or high performance liquid chromatography. More recently, a species-specific DNA probe has been developed and is in commercial use.

Through molecular analysis, five subtypes of *M. kansasii* have been identified (53, 68). Subtype I is responsible for most human infection in Europe, the United States, and Japan. Clinical isolates appear to be highly clonal, with the same genotypes present in most human infections (65). This may point to highly conserved virulence factors and may complicate efforts to discriminate infecting strains.

CLINICAL CHARACTERISTICS

M. kansasii infection often presents with a clinical syndrome indistinguishable from that of *M. tuberculosis*. Most patients present with pulmonary disease that is symptomatic for several months prior to diagnosis (5). The most common presenting symptoms are cough, chest pain, nonmassive hemoptysis, and dyspnea (5, 42). Clinically significant disease is occasionally discovered incidentally on radiology, but these patients are often symptomatic and represent less than 20% of cases in most published series (5, 8, 22, 42, 62). Disseminated disease is an uncommon presentation in HIV-negative patients and is usually associated with severe immunosuppression (40). Patients present over a wide range of ages, with a peak prevalence in the fifth to sixth decade of life, and with male predominance. Ethnic, racial, and socioeconomic discrepancies have not been consistently identified (1).

The majority of patients with *M. kansasii* pulmonary disease have underlying pulmonary comorbidities, such as smoking, chronic obstructive pulmonary disease, bronchiectasis, and prior or concurrent *M. tuberculosis* infection. In patients with pneumoconioses, such as silicosis, *M. kansasii* is the most common

cause of nontuberculous mycobacterial infection. Other common comorbidities include alcohol abuse, HIV, and malignancies (22, 40, 41, 42, 54). Defects in cell-mediated immunity in HIV-negative patients have not been identified (5).

The apparent similarities between *M. tuberculosis* and *M. kansasii* have prompted several clinical and radiological comparisons (14, 16, 21, 22, 62, 69). Results have been inconsistent, but clinical presentations appear to be quite similar with no reliable distinctions in terms of presenting signs or symptoms. Patients infected with *M. kansasii* are more likely to have underlying lung disease such as chronic obstructive pulmonary disease, while patients with tuberculosis may have more immunocompromising comorbidities (22, 62). Given their similarities in clinical presentation, physicians should rely on local epidemiology and prompt microbiological confirmation to distinguish these infections.

HIV-positive patients present with significantly higher disease rates and severity of presentation, and are often severely immunocompromised, with an average CD4 count of $<50/mm^3$ in most studies (7, 11, 15, 34, 39, 41, 46, 58, 64, 67). In a systematic review by Marras et al., 92% of culture-positive patients had clinically important disease, compared to an estimated 50% in HIV-negative populations (44, 45). Patients can present earlier, with CD4 counts exceeding $400/mm^3$, particularly when pulmonary comorbidities are present (17). Disseminated disease is more common at lower CD4 counts and is considered an AIDS-defining diagnosis (60, 64). Accordingly, rates of infection and disseminated disease appear to have decreased since the introduction of highly active antiretroviral therapy (HAART).

EXTRAPULMONARY DISEASE

M. kansasii extrapulmonary disease is relatively infrequent in most regions. In a large study by Kaustova et al. only 0.6% of *M. kansasii*-infected patients presented with extrapulmonary manifestations (34). A survey in Great Britain, however, noted higher rates, with 9% of *M. kansasii* infections presenting with extrapulmonary disease (37). Common sites of extrapulmonary disease include lymph nodes, skin, musculoskeletal, and genitourinary systems.

Compared with other nontuberculous mycobacteria, *M. kansasii* is a relatively infrequent cause of lymphadenopathy. Affected patients present with painless swelling, without associated constitutional symptoms. In contrast, skin and soft tissue infections can present a number of ways (12, 55). Generally, immunocompetent patients present with localized lesions and a history of dermatological disease, corticosteroid injection, or skin injury. Immunosuppressed patients present with more diffuse disease or abscess formation. The natural history of *M. kansasii* skin infection appears to be one of slow progression (12).

Musculoskeletal manifestations include tenosynovitis and monoarticular septic arthritis. These are often associated with recent trauma or corticosteroid use, while approximately half of patients have underlying systemic disease (10). Patients with septic arthritis often have mild symptoms such as stiffness in the wrist, knee, or elbow for several months. Arthrocentesis is often ineffective for diagnosis, as the majority of samples will have negative smear and cultures. Synovial biopsy is usually necessary for diagnosis.

RADIOLOGY

Classically, the radiological findings of *M. kansasii* pulmonary disease in HIV-negative patients are similar to those of reactivation pulmonary tuberculosis, with unilateral, upper lobe airspace opacification and cavitary disease. Although bilateral disease or lower lobe involvement is commonly observed (16, 21, 62, 69), less common manifestations of *M. kansasii* pulmonary disease include pleural thickening, pleural effusions, nodules, and hilar adenopathy. Less than 10% of cases have normal chest X rays (16, 21). Reliable radiological findings that differentiate *M. kansasii* from *M. tuberculosis* have not been demonstrated.

The minority of HIV-positive patients present with cavitary disease. When present, this finding is associated with high mortality (14, 15). Hilar lymphadenopathy and miliary patterns are more common in HIV-positive populations, particularly with declining CD4 counts (24).

DIAGNOSIS

The signs and symptoms of *M. kansasii* disease are variable and nonspecific. Patients often present in middle age with vague pulmonary or constitutional symptoms and a history of comorbid lung disease, making clinical and radiological evaluation difficult. Moreover, there are no reliable indicators distinguishing *M. kansasii* disease from tuberculosis and other mycobacterial infections. Thus, culture results along with a thorough clinical and radiological evaluation are essential for accurate diagnosis.

The most recent American Thoracic Society/ Infectious Disease Society of America (ATS/IDSA) guidelines recommend a minimal radiological evaluation with chest X ray (or high-resolution computed tomography in the absence of cavitation), combined with "positive" cultures and clinical exclusion of other diagnoses (25). Cultures are considered positive when two consecutive positive sputum cultures, one positive culture from bronchoscopy specimens, or one positive sputum culture with compatible pathology is present. Although relaxed since the 1997 guidelines, these microbiological criteria remain somewhat stringent. The ATS/IDSA guidelines apply to all nontuberculous mycobacteria and reflect the need to differentiate disease from contamination and colonization. *M. kansasii* is rarely a colonizing organism and can rapidly progress in immunocompromised patients. This has led some authors to consider a lower diagnostic threshold for patients with positive *M. kansasii* cultures, particularly in those patients with HIV (17).

IGRAs

Recently gamma interferon release assays (IGRAs) have been identified as sensitive and specific tools for diagnosing *M. tuberculosis* infection (49). The specificity of IGRAs for *M. tuberculosis* may be reduced by *M. kansasii* infection, as *M. kansasii* encodes for CFP-10 and ESAT-6, two antigens targeted by IGRAs (6). Some authors have suggested that IGRAs may prove useful for rapid diagnosis of *M. kansasii* infection. Indeed, a recent publication demonstrated the potential utility of IGRAs in smear-positive, PCR probe-negative patients with suspected *M. kansasii* disease (35). We feel, however, that the utility of IGRA in this context is questionable in the face of rapid, highly sensitive and specific DNA probes.

TREATMENT OF HIV-NEGATIVE PATIENTS

M. kansasii infection in HIV-negative patients typically responds well to medical therapy. With susceptible organisms, sputum is usually cleared within 4 months of therapy, and most patients have low rates of relapse. Perhaps reflecting this success, there is limited high-quality evidence to guide the treatment of *M. kansasii* disease. There are few prospective studies and only one published randomized controlled trial (26, 32, 59). The current ATS/IDSA guidelines recommend daily therapy with isoniazid, rifampin, and ethambutol for fully sensitive disease (Table 1). Alternative medications that are active against *M. kansasii* include streptomycin, clarithromycin, amikacin, ethionamide, sulfamethoxazole, rifabutin, linezolid, and fluoroquinolones.

Table 1. ATS/IDSA recommended regimens

Regimen type	Medication	Dose	Frequency	Comments
Rifampin-sensitive disease (25)	Rifampin	10 mg/kg (maximum, 600 mg)	Daily	Treat with the 4-drug regimen (including pyridoxine) until sputum is culture negative for at least 12 mo. An initial dose of ethambutol 25 mg/kg for the first 2 mo is no longer recommended.
	Isoniazid	5 mg/kg (maximum, 300 mg)	Daily	
	Ethambutol	15 mg/kg	Daily	
	Pyridoxine	50 mg/day	Daily	
Alternative treatment (26, 61, 62)	Rifampin	10 mg/kg (maximum, 600 mg)	Thrice weekly or daily	Treat with 3 drugs until culture negative for 12 mo. Ethambutol is dosed at 15 mg/kg. Some authors recommend 25 mg/kg for the first 2–3 mo then 15 mg/kg for the duration of therapy; consider this strategy with thrice-weekly therapy.
	Ethambutol	15–25 mg/kg	Thrice weekly or daily	
	Clarithromycin	500–1,000 mg	Thrice weekly or daily	
Rifampin-resistant disease (66)	Rifabutin	300 mg	Daily	In vitro susceptibilities should be performed. Treat with a minimum of 3 drugs based on culture susceptibilities. Treatment should continue until sputum is culture negative for 12–15 mo. If an aminoglycoside is necessary, dosing should be established by following drug levels. Aminoglycosides can be administered 5 days/week for the first 3 mo. If further aminoglycoside therapy is required in the continuation phase, dose frequency should be decreased to 3 days/week.
	Clarithromycin	1,000 mg	Daily	
	Ethambutol	15–25 mg/kg	Daily	
	Moxifloxacin	400 mg	Daily	
	Isoniazid	300–900 mg	Daily	
	Streptomycin	15 mg/kg (maximum, 1,000 mg)	3–5 days/week	
	Amikacin	15 mg/kg (maximum, 1,000 mg)	3–5 days/week	
	Sulfamethoxazole	1,000 mg	Thrice daily	

Prior to the introduction of rifampin in 1968, retrospective series showed high levels of treatment failure and relapse rates close to 10% (33). Surgical interventions were also common, with 20 to 54% of patients subjected to surgery (9, 33). The introduction of rifampin-enhanced sputum clearance decreased surgical interventions and reduced relapse rates (19, 27, 34). In this context, the value of so-called companion drugs such as isoniazid and ethambutol is less clear. These drugs may not enhance efficacy but may instead act to prevent the emergence of rifampin resistance (24). In particular, the efficacy of isoniazid has come into question. In a British Thoracic Society (BTS) trial examining the efficacy of rifampin/ethambutol, early empiric treatment with isoniazid did not improve outcomes (32). Moreover, isoniazid resistance does not appear to affect outcomes in rifampin-sensitive strains (1).

Given the importance of rifampin to current regimens, ATS/IDSA guidelines recommend routine susceptibility testing of rifampin alone (25). Only when rifampin resistance is present should extended susceptibility testing be employed. Reported rates of rifampin resistance are generally low, with most series reporting rates less than 5% (8, 22, 66). Acquired resistance has been reported and should be of particular concern in noncompliant patients (52). In

contrast, depending on the cutoff used, rates of isoniazid resistance exceed 70% in many series (38, 58).

More recently, clarithromycin and fluoroquinolones have been promoted as effective therapies. The efficacy of clarithromycin has been demonstrated in three published series. In a prospective study of 18 patients with *M. kansasii* disease, Griffith et al. demonstrated the efficacy of intermittent therapy with clarithromycin, ethambutol, and rifampin; most patients cleared their sputum within 2 months and there were no cases of relapse despite an average treatment duration of 13 months (26). Shitrit et al. treated 62 patients with rifampin, ethambutol, and clarithromycin until sputum cultures were negative for 12 months. All patients survived with no cases of relapse (61, 62). Based on these data, clarithromycin appears to be a safe and possibly preferable alternative to isoniazid. Fluoroquinolones, on the other hand, appear quite effective in vitro, but reliable patient data are lacking.

TREATMENT OF EXTRAPULMONARY DISEASE

There are limited data on treatment of extrapulmonary disease. Generally, a first episode of *M.*

kansasii lymphadenopathy is best treated with surgical excision and close clinical follow-up. With recurrent disease, surgical excision followed by medical therapy should be considered. When treating septic arthritis, one should consider surgical debridement, along with 12 to 18 months of antimycobacterial therapy (10). In terms of other sites of infection, there are limited data to guide treatment; standard therapy for 12 months would seem reasonable in most contexts.

TREATMENT IN HIV-POSITIVE PATIENTS

Prior to the introduction of HAART, the prognosis of HIV-associated disease was poor, with a median survival of 12 months (45). The majority of deaths were not attributed to *M. kansasii* infection and were likely secondary to advanced HIV disease. Survival has improved since the introduction of HAART (46, 58, 64). *M. kansasii* patients, however, tend to present with advanced immunosuppression, so 1-year mortality remains high (58, 64). Current evidence supports the use of standard antimycobacterial regimens for HIV-positive patients. Choosing an appropriate regimen, however, can be complicated by drug interactions with HAART, as several rifamycin derivatives interact with most protease inhibitors and nonnucleoside reverse transcriptase inhibitors. This can result in subtherapeutic drug levels which may in turn facilitate the development of HIV drug resistance. Rifabutin, a rifamycin derivative and less potent cytochrome inducer, has shown promise based on in vitro data. Limited in

vivo data on 12 HAART patients from Santin and Alcaide show that rifabutin may be an acceptable alternative (58).

Clarithromycin appears to be an attractive alternative to rifamycin derivatives. In a small series of 38 patients with *M. kansasii*-HIV coinfection, clarithromycin improved average survival from 2 to 10 months (64). However, five of the clarithromycin-treated patients in this series also received fluoroquinolones. Recommendations on HIV-antimycobacterial drug interactions can be found on the United States Center for Disease Control website (www.cdc.gov). At present, there is no evidence to support *M. kansasii* prophylaxis (25).

TREATMENT OF RIFAMPIN-RESISTANT DISEASE

Therapy for rifampin-resistant *M. kansasii* disease should be tailored to sensitivity profiles, with at least three drugs as part of the regimen (Table 1). Wallace et al. evaluated therapy in rifampin-resistant disease (66). Patients with acquired rifampin resistance were treated with daily high-dose ethambutol, isoniazid, sulfamethoxazole, and pyridoxine combined with aminoglycoside therapy. This regimen was relatively effective with 90% sputum conversion in those completing therapy; however, 38% of patients discontinued therapy prior to completing the regimen. Given the potential toxicities, particularly with aminoglycoside therapy, clarithromycin and/or moxifloxacin therapy could be considered as alternatives.

Table 2. Duration of therapy and relapse rate in patients completing rifampin-containing regimens

Treatment duration	Source (reference)	Population (n)	Treatment duration (mo [range])	Sputum conversion (%)	Length of follow-up (mo [range])	Relapse (n [%])
≤12 mo	Ahn et al. (2)	40	12 (0)	100	31 (6–68)	1 (3)
	Banks et al. (8)[a]	7	(6–12)	100	>49	0 (0)
	Evans et al. (22)	39	10 (0–22)	NA[b]	37 (5–108)	0 (0)
	Jenkins et al. (32)	154	9	100	51	15 (10)
	Santin and Alcaide (58)	75	12	100	41.5 (11–48)	5 (7)
	Sauret et al. (59)[a]	14	12	100	(11–25)	1 (7)
	Total (mean)	329				22 (7)
>12 mo	Ahn et al. (1)	64	≥18	100	16 (6–38)	0 (0)
	Banks et al. (8)[a]	22	(13–24)	100	>30	0 (0)
	Griffith et al. (26)	14	13	100	46	0 (0)
	Sauret et al. (59)[a]	14	18	100	(12–24)	0 (0)
	Shitrit et al. (61)	62	>12	NA	39 (28–108)	0 (0)
	Total (mean)	176				0 (0)

[a]Data are included for both treatment duration categories.
[b]NA, not applicable.

DURATION OF THERAPY

In patients with susceptible strains taking a rifampin-containing regimen, sputum usually converts within the first 4 months of therapy, although lengthy treatment regimens are still required to prevent relapse. Several studies have examined "short course chemotherapy" in *M. kansasii* disease with variable results (1, 8, 32, 34, 58, 59). In six series involving 329 patients receiving 6 to 12 months of a rifampin-containing regimen, the relapse rate was 7% (Table 2) (1, 8, 22, 32, 58, 59). This high rate of relapse was driven by data from a BTS trial that treated 154 patients with 9 months of rifampin and ethambutol. The relapse rate in the BTS trial was 10%, while in 176 patients treated for over 12 months with a rifampin-containing regimen there were no cases of relapse (1, 8, 26, 59, 61). Further investigation is needed, but the current published data support the most recent ATS/IDSA recommendations, which require 12 months of sputum smear negativity (4).

REFERENCES

1. Ahn, C. H., J. R. Lowell, S. S. Ahn, S. Ahn, and G. A. Hurst. 1981. Chemotherapy for pulmonary disease due to *Mycobacterium kansasii*: efficacies of some individual drugs. *Rev. Infect. Dis.* 3:1028–1034.

2. Ahn, C. H., J. R. Lowell, S. S. Ahn, S. I. Ahn, and G. A. Hurst. 1983. Short-course chemotherapy for pulmonary disease caused by *Mycobacterium kansasii*. *Am. Rev. Respir. Dis.* 128: 1048–1050.

3. Ahn, C. H., J. R. Lowell, G. D. Onstad, E. H. Shuford, and G. A. Hurst. 1979. A demographic study of disease due to *Mycobacterium kansasii* or *M. intracellulare-avium* in Texas. *Chest* 75:120–125.

4. American Thoracic Society. 1997. Diagnosis and treatment of disease caused by nontuberculous mycobacteria. *Am. J. Respir. Crit. Care Med.* 156:S1–S25.

5. Arend, S. M., E. Cerda de Palou, P. de Haas, R. Janssen, M. A. Hoeve, E. M. Verhard, T. H. M. Ottenhoff, D. van Soolingen, and J. T. van Dissel. 2004. Pneumonia caused by *Mycobacterium kansasii* in a series of patients without recognised immune defect. *Clin. Microbiol. Infect.* 10:738–748.

6. Arend, S. M., K. E. van Meijgaarden, K. de Boer, E. C. de Palou, D. van Soolingen, T. H. M. Ottenhoff, and J. T. van Dissel. 2002. Tuberculosis skin testing and in vitro T cell responses to ESAT-6 and CFP-10 after infection with *Mycobacterium marinum* or *M. kansasii*. *J. Infect. Dis.* 186:1797–1807.

7. Bamberger, D. M., M. R. Driks, M. R. Gupta, M. C. O'Connor, P. M. Jost, R. E. Neihart, D. S. McKinsey, and L. A. Moore. 1994. *Mycobacterium kansasii* among patients infected with human immunodeficiency virus in Kansas City. *Clin. Infect. Dis.* 18:398–400.

8. Banks, J., A. M. Hunter, I. A. Campbell, P. A. Jenkins, and A. P. Smith. 1983. Pulmonary infection with *Mycobacterium kansasii* in Wales, 1970-9: review of treatment and response. *Thorax* 38:271–274.

9. Bates, J. H. 1967. A study of pulmonary disease associated with mycobacteria other than *Mycobacterium tuberculosis*: clinical characteristics. *Am. Rev. Respir. Dis.* 96:1151–1157.

10. Bernard, L., V. Vincent, O. Lortholary, L. Raskine, C. Vettier, D. Colaitis, D. Mechali, F. Bricaire, E. Bouvet, F. Bani Sadr, V. Lalande, and C. Perronne. 1999. *Mycobacterium kansasii* septic arthritis: French retrospective study of 5 years and review. *Clin. Infect. Dis.* 29:1455–1460.

11. Bloch, K. C., L. Zwerling, M. J. Pletcher, J. A. Hahn, J. L. Gerberding, S. M. Ostroff, D. J. Vugia, and A. L. Reingold. 1998. Incidence and clinical implications of isolation of *Mycobacterium kansasii*: results of a 5-year population study. *Ann. Intern. Med.* 129:698–704.

12. Breathnach, A., N. Levell, C. Munro, S. Natarajan, and S. Pedler. 1995. Cutaneous *Mycobacterium kansasii* infection: case report and review. *Clin. Infect. Dis.* 20:812–817.

13. Buhler, V. B., and A. Pollack. 1953. Human infection with atypical acid fast organisms: report of two cases with pathologic findings. *Am. J. Clin. Pathol.* 23:363–374.

14. Canueto-Quintero, J., F. J. Caballero-Granado, M. Herrero-Romero, A. Dominguez- Castellano, P. Martin-Rico, E. Vidal Verdu, D. S. Santamaria, R. C. Cerquera, and M. Torres-Tortosa. 2003. Epidemiological, clinical, and prognostic differences between the diseases caused by *Mycobacterium kansasii* and *Mycobacterium tuberculosis* in patients infected with human immunodeficiency virus: a multicenter study. *Clin. Infect. Dis.* 37:584–590.

15. Cattamanchi, A., P. Nahid, T. K. Marras, M. B. Gotway, T. J. Lee, L. C. Gonzalez, A. Morris, W. R. Webb, D. H. Osmond, and C. L. Daley. 2008. Detailed analysis of the radiographic presentation of *Mycobacterium kansasii* lung disease in patients with HIV infection. *Chest* 133:875–880.

16. Christensen, E. E., G. W. Dietz, C. H. Ahn, J. S. Chapman, R. C. Murry, and G. A. Hurst. 1978. Radiographic manifestations of pulmonary *Mycobacterium kansasii* infections. *AJR Am. J. Roentgenol.* 131:985–993.

17. Corbett, E. L., M. Hay, G. J. Churchyard, P. Herselman, T. Clayton, B. G. Williams, R. Hayes, D. Mulder, and K. M. de Cock. 1999. *Mycobacterium kansasii* and *M. scrofulaceum* isolates from HIV-negative South African gold miners: incidence, clinical significance and radiology. *Int. J. Tuberc. Lung Dis.* 3:501–507.

18. David, H. L. 1974. Biogenesis of beta-carotene in *Mycobacterium kansasii*. *J. Bacteriol.* 119:527–533.

19. Davidson, P. T., M. Goble, and W. Lester. 1972. The antituberculosis efficacy of rifampin in 136 patients. *Chest* 61:574–578.

20. Reference deleted.

21. Evans, A. J., A. J. Crisp, R. B. Hubbard, A. Colville, S. A. Evans, and I. D. A. Johnston. 1996. Pulmonary *Mycobacterium kansasii* infection: comparison of radiological appearances with pulmonary tuberculosis. *Thorax* 51:1243–1247.

22. Evans, S. A., A. Colville, A. J. Evans, A. J. Crisp, and I. D. A. Johnston. 1996. Pulmonary *Mycobacterium kansasii* infection: comparison of the clinical features, treatment and outcome with pulmonary tuberculosis. *Thorax* 51:1248–1252.

23. Good, R. C. 1980. Isolation of nontuberculous mycobacteria in the United States, 1979. *J. Infect. Dis.* 142:779–783.

24. Griffith, D. E. 2002. Management of disease due to *Mycobacterium kansasii*. *Clin. Chest Med.* 23:613–621.

25. Griffith, D. E., T. Aksamit, B. A. Brown-Elliot, A. Catanzaro, C. Daley, F. Gordin, S. M. Holland, R. Horsburgh, G. Huitt, M. F. Iademarco, M. Iseman, K. Oliver, S. Ruoss, C. F. von Reyn, R. J. Wallace, Jr., and K. Withrop. 2007. An official ATS/IDSA statement: diagnosis, treatment and prevention of non-

tuberculosis mycobacterial diseases. *Am. J. Respir. Crit. Care Med.* **175:**367–416.

26. Griffith, D. E., B. A. Brown-Elliott, and R. J. Wallace, Jr. 2003. Thrice-weekly clarithromycin-containing regimen for treatment of *Mycobacterium kansasii* lung disease: results of a preliminary study. *Clin. Infect. Dis.* **37:**1178–1182.

27. Harris, G. D., W. G. Johanson, Jr., and D. P. Nicholson. 1975. Response to chemotherapy of pulmonary infection due to *Mycobacterium kansasii. Am. Rev. Respir. Dis.* **112:**31–36.

28. Hernandez-Garduno, E., M. Rodrigues, and R. K. Elwood. 2009. The incidence of pulmonary non-tuberculous mycobacteria in British Columbia, Canada. *Int. J. Tuberc. Lung Dis.* **13:**1086–1093.

29. Hobby, G. L., W. B. Redmond, E. H. Runyon, W. B. Schaefer, L. G. Wayne, and R. H. Wichelhausen. 1967. A study of pulmonary disease associated with mycobacteria other than *Mycobacterium tuberculosis*: identification and characterization of the mycobacteria. *Am. Rev. Respir. Dis.* **95:**954–971.

30. Isaac-Renton, J. L., E. A. Allen, C. W. Chao, S. Grzybowski, E. I. Whittaker, and W. A. Black. 1985. Isolation and geographic distribution of mycobacterium other than *M. tuberculosis* in British Columbia, 1972-1981. *Can. Med. Assoc. J.* **133:**573–576.

31. Reference deleted.

32. Jenkins, P. A., J. Banks, I. A. Campbell, and A. P. Smith. 1994. *Mycobacterium kansasii* pulmonary infection: a prospective study of the results of nine months of treatment with rifampicin and ethambutol. *Thorax* **49:**442–445.

33. Johanson, W. G., Jr., and D. P. Nicholson. 1969. Pulmonary disease due to *Mycobacterium kansasii*: an analysis of some factors affecting prognosis. *Am. Rev. Respir. Dis.* **99:**73–85.

34. Kaustova, J., M. Chmelik, D. Ettlova, V. Hudec, H. Lazarcva, and S. Richtrova. 1995. Disease due to *Mycobacterium kansasii* in the Czech Republic: 1984-1989. *Tuberc. Lung Dis.* **76:**205–209.

35. Kobashi, Y., K. Mouri, N. Miyashita, and M. Oka. 2009. Clinical usefulness of QuantiFERON TB-2G test for the early diagnosis of pulmonary *Mycobacterium kansasii* disease. *Jpn. J. Infect. Dis.* **62:**239–241.

36. Kubin, M., E. Svandova, B. Medek, S. Chobot, and Z. Olsovsky. 1980. *Mycobacterium kansasii* infection in an endemic area of Czechoslovakia. *Tubercle* **51:**207–212.

37. Lambden, K., J. M. Watson, G. Knerer, M. J. Ryan, and P. A. Jenkins. 1996. Opportunist mycobacteria in England and Wales 1982–1994. *CDR Rev.* **11:**147–151.

38. Leal Arranz, M. V., A. Gaafar, M. J. Unzaga Baranano, J. A. Crespo Notario, R. Cisterna Cancer, and F. Gardia Cebrian. 2005. Clinical and epidemiological study of disease caused by *Mycobacterium kansasii* in the metropolitan area of Bilbao, Spain. *Arch. Bronconeumol.* **41:**189–196.

39. Levine, B., and R. E. Chaisson. 1991. *Mycobacterium kansasii*: a cause of treatable pulmonary disease associated with advanced human immunodeficiency virus (HIV) infection. *Ann. Intern. Med.* **114:**861–868.

40. Lillo, M., S. Orengo, P. Cernoch, and R. L. Harris. 1990. Pulmonary and disseminated infection due to *Mycobacterium kansasii*: a decade of experience. *Rev. Infect. Dis.* **12:**760–767.

41. Lortholary, O., F. Deniel, P. Boudon, M. P. Le Pennec, M. Mathieu, M. Soilleux, C. Le Pendeven, P. Loiseau, V. Vincent, D. Valeyre, and Groupe d'Etude des Mycobacteries de la Seine-Saint-Denis. 1999. *Mycobacterium kansasii* infection in a Paris suburb: comparison of disease presentation and outcome according to human immunodeficiency virus status. *Int. J. Tuberc. Lung Dis.* **3:**68–73.

42. Maliwan, N., and J. R. Zvetina. 2005. Clinical features and follow up of 302 patients with *Mycobacterium kansasii* pulmonary infection: a 50 year experience. *Postgrad. Med. J.* **81:**530–533.

43. Marras, T. K., P. Chedore, A. M. Ying, and F. Jamieson. 2007. Isolation prevalence of pulmonary non-tuberculous mycobacteria in Ontario, 1997-2003. *Thorax* **62:**661–666.

44. Marras, T. K., and C. L. Daley. 2002. Epidemiology of human pulmonary infection with nontuberculous mycobacteria. *Clin. Chest Med.* **23:**553–567.

45. Marras, T. K., and C. L. Daley. 2004. A systematic review of the clinical significance of pulmonary *Mycobacterium kansasii* isolates in HIV infection. *J. Acquir. Immune Defic. Syndr.* **36:**883–889.

46. Marras, T. K., A. Morris, L. C. Gonzalez, and C. L. Daley. 2004. Mortality prediction in pulmonary *Mycobacterium kansasii* infection and human immunodeficiency virus. *Am. J. Respir. Crit. Care Med.* **170:**793–798.

47. Martín-Casabona, N., A. R. Bahrmand, J. Bennedsen, V. Østergaard Thomsen, M. Curcio, M. Fauville-Dufaux, K. Feldman, M. Havelkova, M.-L. Katila, K. Köksalan, M. F. Pereira, F. Rodrigues, G. E. Pfyffer, F. Portaels, J. Rosselló Urgell, and S. Rüsch-Gerdes. 2004. Non-tuberculous mycobacteria: patterns of isolation. A multi-country retrospective survey. *Int. J. Tuberc. Lung Dis.* **8:**1186–1193.

48. Onstad, G. D. 1969. Familial aggregations of group I atypical mycobacterial disease. *Am. Rev. Respir. Dis.* **99:**426–429.

49. Pai, M., A. Zwerling, and D. Menzies. 2008. Systematic review: T-cell-based assays for the diagnosis of latent tuberculosis infection: an update. *Ann. Intern. Med.* **149:**177–184.

50. Pang, S. M. 1991. *Mycobacterium kansasii* infections in Western Australia (1962-1987). *Respir. Med.* **85:**213–218.

51. Penny, M. E., R. B. Cole, and J. Gray. 1982. Two cases of *Mycobacterium kansasii* infection occurring in the same household. *Tubercle* **63:**129–131.

52. Pezzia, W., J. W. Raleigh, M. C. Bailey, E. A. Toth, and J. Silverblatt. 1981. Treatment of pulmonary disease due to *Mycobacterium kansasii*: recent experience with rifampin. **3:**1035–1039.

53. Picardeau, M., G. Prod'hom, L. Raskine, M. P. LePennec, and V. Vincent. 1997. Genotypic characterization of five subspecies of *Mycobacterium kansasii. J. Clin. Microbiol.* **35:**25–32.

54. Rauscher, C. R., G. Kerby, and W. E. Ruth. 1974. *Mycobacterium kansasii* in Kansas: saprophyte or infection? *Chest* **66:**162–164.

55. Razavi, B., and M. G. Cleveland. 2000. Cutaneous infection due to *Mycobacterium kansasii. Diagn. Microbiol. Infect. Dis.* **38:**173–175.

56. Research Committee of the British Thoracic and Tuberculosis Association and the British Medical Research Council's Pneumoconiosis Unit. 1975. Opportunist mycobacterial pulmonary infection and occupational dust exposure: an investigation in England and Wales. *Tubercle* **56:**295–313.

57. Runyon, E. H. 1959. Anonymous mycobacteria in pulmonary disease. *Med. Clin. N. Am.* **43:**273–290.

58. Santin, M., and F. Alcaide. 2003. *Mycobacterium kansasii* disease among patients infected with human immunodeficiency virus type 1: improved prognosis in the era of highly active antiretroviral therapy. *Int. J. Tuberc. Lung Dis.* **7:**670–677.

59. Sauret, J., S. Hernandez-Flix, E. Castro, L. Hernandez, V. Ausina, and P. Coll. 1995. Treatment of pulmonary disease caused by *Mycobacterium kansasii*: results of 18 vs 12 months' chemotherapy. *Tuberc. Lung Dis.* **76:**104–108.

60. Schneider, E., S. Whitmore, K. M. Glynn, K. Dominguez, A. Mitsch, M. T. McKenna, and Centers for Disease Control and Prevention. 2008. Revised surveillance case definitions for HIV infection among adults, adolescents, and children aged <18 months and for HIV infection and AIDS among children aged 18 months to <13 years—United States, 2008. *MMWR Recommend. Rep.* **57:**1–12.

61. Shitrit, D., N. Peled, J. Bishara, R. Priess, S. Pitlik, Z. Samra, and M. R. Kramer. 2008. Clinical and radiological features of *Mycobacterium kansasii* infection and *Mycobacterium simiae* infection. *Respir. Med.* **102:**1598–1603.

62. Shitrit, D., R. Priess, N. Peled, G. Bishara, D. Shlomi, and M. R. Kramer. 2007. Differentiation of *Mycobacterium kansasii* infection from *Mycobacterium tuberculosis* infection: comparison of clinical features, radiological appearance, and outcome. *Eur. J. Clin. Microbiol. Infect. Dis.* **26:**679–684.

63. Steadham, J. E. 1980. High-catalase strains of *Mycobacterium kansasii* isolated from water in Texas. *J. Clin. Microbiol.* **11:**496–498.

64. Tomkins, J. C., and R. S. Witzig. 2007. *Mycobacterium kansasii* in HIV patients: clarithromycin and antiretroviral effects. *Int. J. Tuberc. Lung Dis.* **11:**331–337.

65. Vincent, V., and M. C. Gutierrez. 2007. *Mycobacterium*: laboratory characteristics of slowly growing mycobacteria, p. 573–588. *In* P. R. Murray, E. J. Baron, J. H. Jorgensen, M. L. Landry, and M. A. Pfaller (ed.), *Manual of Clinical Microbiology*, 9th ed. ASM Press, Washington, DC.

66. Wallace, R. J., Jr., D. Dunbar, B. A. Brown, G. Onyi, R. Dunlap, C. H. Ahn, and D. T. Murphy. 1994. Rifampin-resistant *Mycobacterium kansasii*. *Clin. Infect. Dis.* **18:**736–743.

67. Witzig, R. S., B. A. Fazal, R. M. Mera, D. M. Mushatt, P. M. J. T. Dejace, D. L. Greer, and N. E. Hyslop, Jr. 1995. Clinical manifestations and implications of coinfection with *Mycobacterium kansasii* and human immunodeficiency virus type 1. *Clin. Infect. Dis.* **21:**77–85.

68. Zhang, Y., L. B. Mann, R. W. Wilson, B. A. Brown-Elliott, V. Vincent, Y. Iinuma, and R. J. Wallace, Jr. 2004. Molecular analysis of *Mycobacterium kansasii* isolates from the United States. *J. Clin. Microbiol.* **42:**119–125.

69. Zvetina, J. R., T. C. Demos, N. Maliwan, M. Van Drunen, W. Frederick, J. Lentino, and A. M. Modh. 1984. Pulmonary cavitations in *Mycobacterium kansasii*: distinctions from *M. tuberculosis*. *Am. J. Radiol.* **143:**127–130.

Chapter 39

Mycobacterium marinum

EMMANUELLE CAMBAU AND ALEXANDRA AUBRY

INTRODUCTION AND HISTORY

The first report of a mycobacterium isolated in fish, thought to be *Mycobacterium marinum*, has been attributed to Bataillon et al. (1897) who isolated acid-fast bacilli named *Mycobacterium piscium* from a tuberculous lesion in a common carp (*Cyprinus carpio*) (10). *M. marinum* was then originally isolated and identified from marine fish at Philadelphia Aquarium (3). *M. marinum* was initially thought to infect marine fishes only and was named accordingly, but it is now known to be a ubiquitous species. The above-mentioned original freshwater isolate of *M. piscium* was quite possibly an *M. marinum* variant. In the early literature, other marine *Mycobacterium* species were described, such as *M. platypoecilus*, *M. anabanti*, and *M. balnei*. Comparative sugar fermentative reactions together with published morphological, cultural, and pathogenic data suggested that they were all synonymous with *M. marinum* (7) even if *M. piscium* has not been recognized as a valid species, since its type culture was no longer available.

Human infection due to *M. marinum* was reported as a tuberculoid infection in people using public swimming pools in Sweden (1939) and in the United States (1951) (61). Linell and Norden identified the causative organism in 1954 after 80 persons had showed the same granulomatous skin lesions (61). These early findings led to the disease's once-common name of "swimming pool granuloma." Today, however, due to sanitary chlorination practices, these kinds of outbreaks have largely disappeared. The names "fish tank granuloma" and "fish handler's disease" are now used because of the association with home aquariums and water-related activities such as swimming, fishing, and boating (1).

Scientific interest for *M. marinum* is mainly due to its genetic relatedness with *M. tuberculosis* and because experimental infection of *M. marinum* in the goldfish (*Carassius auratus*) mimics tuberculosis pathogenesis (76). More recently, *M. marinum* interest was linked with the emergence and burden of *M. ulcerans* infection. However, clinical interest for *M. marinum* infections may eventually reemerge due to the expansion of aquarium-related activities.

FUNDAMENTAL BIOLOGY OF *M. MARINUM*

Taxonomy

M. marinum is one of the 120 species of the genus *Mycobacterium* (11, 106), the only genus of the *Mycobacteriaceae* family. *M. marinum* is a nontuberculous mycobacterium (NTM), atypical mycobacterial, or one of the mycobacteria other than *M. tuberculosis*. According to Runyon's classification, it belongs to group I, photochromogenic species. Although it can grow in fewer than 7 days, its characteristics are far different from the so-called rapidly growing species of mycobacteria, such as *M. chelonae* or *M. fortuitum*. Since it carries a single rRNA operon (43) and its 16S rRNA sequence contains the molecular signature of slowly growing mycobacteria (81), it definitely belongs to the slow-growing group of mycobacteria.

M. marinum is a pathogenic mycobacterium, which makes it, along with its related species *M. ulcerans*, distinct from the other NTM that are opportunistic pathogens (108). From phylogenetic analysis based on the 16S rRNA, *M. marinum* lies on a branch of the genus that is close to the branch containing members of the *M. tuberculosis* complex. DNA-DNA hybridization and mycolic acid studies confirm that *M. marinum* is one of the two species (still along with *M. ulcerans*) most closely related to the *M. tuberculosis* complex (75, 95).

Emmanuelle Cambau • Centre National de Référence pour la résistance des Mycobactéries aux antituberculeux, Laboratoire de Bactériologie, Université Paris Diderot, AP-HP Hôpital Saint Louis-Lariboisière, Paris, France. **Alexandra Aubry** • Centre National de Référence pour la résistance des Mycobactéries aux antituberculeux, Université Pierre et Marie Curie, AP-HP Hôpital Pitié-Salpêtrière, Paris, France.

Genetics

The *M. marinum* genome (strain M) was one of the major mycobacteria sequenced. The length of *M. marinum* genome is 6.5 Mb, which is larger than that of *M. tuberculosis* (4.4 Mb), that of *M. leprae* (3.3 Mb), and that of *M. ulcerans* (5.8 Mb) (for specific searches, see http://mycobrowser.epfl.ch/marinolist.html). The *M. marinum* genome compares with the *M. ulcerans* (86) and *M. tuberculosis* (85) genomes.

M. marinum shares more than 98% nucleotide sequence identity with the *M. ulcerans* genome. On the basis of sequences of the housekeeping and structural genes used for identification, such as those coding for the ribosomal operon, RNA polymerase (*rpoB*), DNA gyrase (*gyrA* and *gyrB*), and the heat shock protein 65 kDa (*hsp*), *M. marinum* cannot be differentiated from *M. ulcerans*, the minor nucleotide differences observed in some of these genes being related to strain variation (27, 52, 85). The major conclusion is that *M. marinum* seems to be an *M. ulcerans* ancestor (83, 85). Divergence would have occurred along with the gain by *M. ulcerans* of genes (grouped on the virulence plasmid, pMUM001) encoding the virulence factor mycolactone (84) and of copies of the insertion sequences IS2404 and IS2606 (19, 83).

Mycobacteria that contain genes for the production of mycolactone were designated as mycolactone-producing mycobacteria. These strains are all closely related, and there is some justification for considering them forming the *M. marinum* complex (109). *M. pseudoshottsii* and *M. liflandii* are mycolactone-producing mycobacteria described in fishes only (88). Although *M. marinum* is devoid of the mycolactone-producing coding sequences as the one found in *M. ulcerans*, another mycolactone (mycolactone F) has been isolated from strains of *M. marinum* that have produced disease in fishes of the Red Sea (73, 99).

Molecular biology of *M. marinum* has been developed because it is less pathogenic and grows faster than *M. tuberculosis*; it is a suitable model for tuberculosis pathogenesis (68, 76). Genetic manipulations such as transformation and transposition have been successful (69, 92). Virulence genes have been brought up by gene expression either in cultured macrophages or in granuloma (18, 69, 76). Mutations in the virulence genes were often complemented by the corresponding gene of *M. tuberculosis* that demonstrated the high relatedness of the genome of the two species. Genome sequencing revealed that the region of difference 1, which contains the ESAT-6 and CFP-10 encoding genes in *M. tuberculosis*, does exist also in *M. marinum* (102). The ESAT-6-like secretion system is probably a major secretion pathway for *M. marinum*, and this system is responsible for the secretion of recently evolved PE_PGRS and PPE proteins, which are especially abundant in *M. marinum*. The Esx secretion system is critical for virulence of both *M. tuberculosis* and *M. marinum* and is highly conserved between the two species (85).

Pathogenesis

The availability of fish models (goldfish, zebrafish) mimicking a natural mycobacterial infection (68, 91, 97) enables the study of the pathogen-host interaction. New models of infection have been described: *Drosophila melanogaster*, where *M. marinum* infection is lethal at a low dose (29); intraperitoneal infection of adult leopard frogs (*Rana pipiens*); and infection of embryonic zebrafish (*Danio rerio*) (22). However, these models were mostly used for studying tuberculosis physiopathology and rarely *M. marinum* infection itself.

Both *M. tuberculosis* and *M. marinum* are intracellular pathogens that proliferate within macrophages in a nonacid (pH 6.1 to 6.5) phagosome that does not fuse with the lysosome (9). Taking into account that both species are also genetically related, it is probable that analogous molecular mechanisms are involved in the survival of these organisms in a hostile cell environment. *M. marinum* is therefore a very useful model system for studying intracellular survival of mycobacteria and possible other host-pathogen interactions associated with tuberculosis (35, 97), including innate susceptibility (94). Ultrastructure studies have shown that *M. marinum* stays within activated macrophages in granulomas. Some of the genes that seem important in the capacity to replicate in macrophages and to explain the persistence in granulomas are homologous to the PE-PGRS family of genes discovered in the *M. tuberculosis* genome (18).

The organism is able to survive and replicate in macrophages and even escape from the phagosomes into the cytoplasm where it can induce actin polymerization, leading to direct cell spread (8, 82). It was shown recently that *M. marinum* bacteria are ejected from the cell through the ejectosome, an actin-based structure-spreading mechanism that requires a cytoskeleton regulator from the host and an intact mycobacterial ESX-1 secretion system (40, 82).

Infection experiments with zebrafish with different strains of *M. marinum* showed that strains can be divided into two distinct types based on genetic diversity and virulence. Cluster I contained predominantly strains isolated from humans with fish tank granuloma, whereas the majority of the cluster II strains were isolated from poikilothermic species. Acute disease progression was noted only with strains belonging to cluster I, whereas chronic-disease-causing isolates belonged to cluster II (101).

MICROBIOLOGICAL CHARACTERS OF *M. MARINUM*

Microscopy and Cell Wall

Under the microscope, *M. marinum* cannot be distinguished from *M. tuberculosis*. It is a pleiomorphic rod (1.0 to 4.0 μm by 0.2 to 0.6 μm), not motile, true branching, difficult to stain by usual methods but appears as an acid-fast bacillus after staining by the reference carbol fuchsin or Ziehl-Neelsen method (17).

The formation of microscopic cords has been described in *M. marinum* as it is classically described with *M. tuberculosis*, and a link between cording and virulence was observed in both species (37, 51).

The cell wall of *M. marinum* is mainly composed of keto-mycolates and methoxy-mycolates that differentiate from those of *M. tuberculosis* and of other mycobacteria except *M. ulcerans* (23, 95).

Specific Characters of *M. marinum*

Culture

Like other mycobacteria, *M. marinum* is a strict aerobe. Its preferred carbon sources are glycerol, pyruvate, and glucose, but ethanol can be also used by *M. marinum*. *M. marinum* has an optimal growth temperature of 30°C, whereas small colonies or no growth is observed at 37°C.

In primary culture, the growth rate might be slow and positive culture may be obtained only after several weeks' incubation. In subculture, the growth rate is between 1 and 2 weeks but can reach 4 to 5 days because of its rapid ability to adapt to laboratory conditions.

M. marinum is less exigent than *M. tuberculosis* for growth. It grows in all the media used for mycobacterial growth (egg based, broth, and agar based), without any additives or only 2 to 5% oxalic acid-albumin-dextrose-catalase instead of the 10% used for *M. tuberculosis*, and also on blood-containing agar. After subcultures, some of the strains may even grow on ordinary culture media.

Although its growth is dependent on oxygen, such as other mycobacteria, 2% to 5% carbon dioxide in the gas phase above the medium improves the growth of *M. marinum*.

Phenotypic characters

Colonies of *M. marinum* are typically smooth or intermediate, white or beige when the media are kept in obscurity and yellow to orange after exposure to

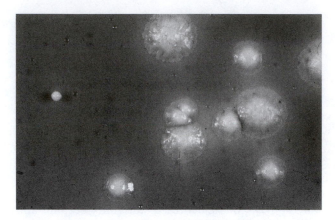

Figure 1. Typical photochromogenic colonies of *Mycobacterium marinum* grown on Löwenstein-Jensen solid medium.

light (photochromogenic) (17) (Fig. 1). It is included in group I of Runyon's classification along with *M. kansasii*. Differentiation between these two pathogenic NTM is done classically on the basis of biochemical characteristics. The absence of production of nitrate reductase and growth on medium containing thiacetazone is in favor of *M. marinum*. Photochromogenicity is due to the active production of beta carotene mediated by the gene *crtB* and can be inhibited by chloramphenicol (70).

Molecular identification

Molecular biology techniques have been successfully applied to identification of mycobacteria. Molecular methods are an alternative for identification offering the advantages of being rapid and accurate. Although nucleic acid probes such as Accuprobe, used for *M. tuberculosis* complex identification, are not available for *M. marinum*, PCR-based methods have been developed. Two of these methods are commercially available: INNOLiPA Mycobacteria v2 (Innogenetics), based on the amplification of the ribosomal gene spacer (16S-23S), and GenoType mycobacteria CM/AS (Hain Lifescience), based on the amplification of a 23S rRNA gene (77, 96). Both use PCR coupled with reverse hybridization. So far, they cannot differentiate *M. marinum* from *M. ulcerans*, since the rRNA sequences are similar (see "Genetics" above). Specific PCR protocols have been described for detection in fishes (78).

Genotyping

Although infection due to *M. marinum* is not contagious between humans, strain genotyping has been undertaken for three reasons: first, to relate environmental strains to strains isolated in infected humans; second, to differentiate strains in aquaculture isolated among fishes or water-living animals (99); and third, to demonstrate relapse or reinfection (46). The technique used was mainly pulsed-field gel electrophoresis, since PCR based methods showed low discriminative properties (80).

Mycobacterial interspersed repetitive-unit variable-number tandem repeat typing, which is one of the reference typing methods for *M. tuberculosis*, was applied to *M. marinum* and *M. ulcerans*. Unlike *M. ulcerans*, the *M. marinum* genotypes could not be clearly related to the geographic origins of the isolates or discriminated between recurrence and reinfection (87).

Multilocus sequence analysis applied to 22 *M. marinum* strains showed that the level of intraspecies nucleotide sequence divergence was higher than in *M. ulcerans* strains (83). *M. marinum* isolates from humans and fish have been also compared by sequencing of the 16S rRNA and *hsp65* genes, restriction mapping, and amplified fragment length polymorphism analysis (98). In this study, significant molecular differences separated clinical isolates from the piscine isolates.

M. MARINUM INFECTION

Manifestations of *M. marinum* Disease

Fish disease

M. marinum disease in fish is very common, especially in aquarium fish. Some evidence suggests the gastrointestinal tract as the primary route of infection (41), and it has been demonstrated that poor diets and stress exacerbate mycobacterial infections in zebrafish (41, 49, 72). The severity of the infection ranges from chronic infection associated with a low mortality to a more acute form in which the entire population died. The acute, fulminating disease is rare and is characterized by rapid morbidity and mortality with few clinical signs. *M. marinum* infection is more often a chronic progressive infection that may take years to develop into a noticeable illness. Affected fishes show behavioral changes such as separating from other fish and refusing food. They may have skin ulcerations or pigment alterations and develop spinal curvature. Unilateral or bilateral exophthalmia is also a typical feature. In fish, *M. marinum* infection is a systemic disease that can affect virtually any organ system, but especially the spleen, kidney, and liver (28).

Human disease

Due to the optimal growth at 30°C and poor growth at 37°C, human infections with *M. marinum* are localized primarily to the skin. Infection in human immunodeficiency virus-positive patients is usually not different from infection in human immunodeficiency virus-negative patients. Scarce cases of *M. marinum* infection occurring in patients treated with tumor necrosis factor alpha inhibitor therapy have been reported since 2002. Therefore, it is not possible yet to draw any conclusions regarding the frequency or the severity of *M. marinum* infection in this population (25, 26, 44, 71). We recommend preventive strategies (see below) especially for those patients.

M. marinum infection has different clinical presentations (Table 1). Most commonly (about 60% of the cases in reference 5), *M. marinum* is a cutaneous disease as a solitary papulonodular lesion on a finger or hand. In 25% of cases, *M. marinum* disease takes on a "sporotrichoid" form (5, 38) (Fig. 2). This occurs when the infection spreads along the lymphatic vessels to the regional lymph nodes, producing multiple nodules resembling sporotrichosis. Occasionally, skin

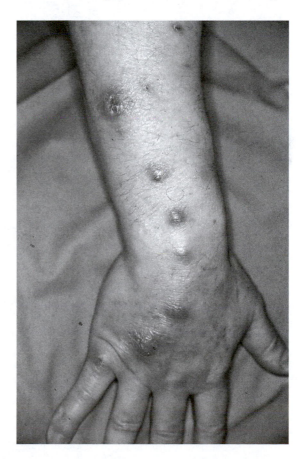

Figure 2. Sporotrichoid form of skin lesions typical of *M. marinum* infection. (Courtesy of Hervé Darie, Noisy le Grand, France.)

Table 1. Published studies of *M. marinum* infections that include more than 10 patients

| Reference | No. patients (no. with deep infection) | Fish exposure (%) | Cure (%) | Duration (mo) (mean) | Antibiotic treatment[a] | | | Surgery (% cured) |
| | | | | | Monotherapy | | Combination therapy (no.) | |
					No. of patients	Antibiotic and no. of patients (% cured)		
Even-Paz 1976[b]	10 (0)	0	44	NA	NA		NA	NA
Chow 1987	24 (24)	87.5	83	9	0		24	10 (70%)
Bonafe 1992	27 (1)	93	>74	3.8	NA		NA	NA
Kozin 1994	12 (6)	100	100	6	7	D = 5 (100%), Co = 2 (100%), R = 1 (100%)	5	12 (100%)
Edelstein 1994	31 (0)	NA	81	4	19[e]	M = 14 (71%), D = 3 (67%), T = 1 (100%), Co = 1 (100%)	10[e]	NA
Ang 2000[c]	38 (NA)	45	81	3.5	22[d]	Co = 19 (93%), M = 3 (100%)	12[d]	1 (100%)
Casal 2001	39	90	99	2–4	20	M = 12 (NA), R = 8 (NA)	7	NA
Aubry 2002	63 (18)	84	87	3.5	23	M = 19 (100%), C = 4 (100%)	40	30 (16%)
Ho 2006	17 (NA)	24	94	4.5	16	D = 4 (NA), Co = 1 (NA), M = 11 (NA)	1	0

[a]NA, not available; M, minocycline; C, clarithromycin; R, rifampin; D, doxycycline; T, tetracycline; Co, co-trimoxazole.
[b]100% swimming pool exposure.
[c]Only one culture-confirmed case.
[d]One was treated with surgery, and one defaulted treatment.
[e]One was treated with excision, and three defaulted treatment.

lesions appear as pustular, nodulo-ulcerative, granu-lomatous, or verrucous plaques.

Deep infections such as tenosynovitis (the most frequent), osteomyelitis, arthritis, and bursitis occur in 20 to 40% of cases (5, 21, 31, 38, 111). They result from the extension of a cutaneous infection or direct inoculation of the organism. Systemic dissemination is exceptional and has been reported to occur only in immunocompromised patients (56, 89, 93), and general symptoms are usually absent. Localized adenopathy is rare (15% of the cases in reference 5), and infection of deep organs, such as the lungs, is exceptional (57).

There is often a several-month delay between the onset of the lesions and the patient seeking medical care (66) because the lesions are subacute or chronic and usually painless. Moreover, the lesions can be self-limited and may heal spontaneously, though healing can take months to several years. Initial misdiagnosis of the osteoarticular form of *M. marinum* infection can lead to intralesional injection of corticosteroid that favors local dissemination (31). These forms are often associated with a poor prognosis (106).

Distal aspects of the upper limbs, such as the finger or hand, are the most common sites of infection in relation to fish or water animal exposure. The patients who have skin lesions on the lower limbs are swimming pool cases or indirect cases. *M. marinum* is assumed to be introduced in the skin accidentally through preexisting wounds or abrasion. History of preceding minor trauma is common, and an occupation or hobby that resulted in a likely environmental water exposure is the rule. However, since the incubation period is very long, on average 3 weeks up to 9 months (5, 50), minor abrasions or wounds that preceded the contact are usually not remembered at the time of diagnosis.

Immunity

Tuberculin skin testing is usually positive because of cross-reaction with *M. tuberculosis* (60). It may suggest a mycobacterial infection but will not distinguish *M. marinum* from tuberculosis or other mycobacterial infections and is therefore of little utility in the workup.

False positivity of the gamma interferon release assays, performed today for the diagnosis of latent tuberculosis infection, have been also reported with *M. marinum* infection. Indeed, as said above, *M. marinum* shares with *M. tuberculosis* the specific antigens (ESAT-6 and CFP-10) used in these tests. However, gamma interferon release assays were not found useful as a diagnostic method for *M. marinum* infection (2, 54).

Diagnosis can be difficult for the clinician (111) because the presentation is often insidious and non-specific. If key historical information, such as fish exposure, is not obtained, the diagnosis is commonly delayed (50). Diagnosing an infection due to *M. marinum* requires a high index of suspicion, a properly obtained exposure history, and knowledge of the laboratory growth characteristics of the organism.

Differential diagnosis includes infection due to other atypical mycobacteria known to cause cutaneous infection, such as *M. chelonae*, *M. ulcerans*, *M. ulcerans* subspecies, *M. shinshuense* (34), *M. haemophilum*, *M. fortuitum*, and *M. tuberculosis*, and other noninfectious diseases such as sporotrichosis, sarcoidosis, skin tumors, and foreign body reactions.

Though the diagnosis can be suspected clinically, especially when exposure is established, the diagnosis relies on isolation of a mycobacterium subsequently identified as *M. marinum*.

Clinical significance

Isolation of *M. marinum* has clinical significance regardless of the number of colonies or the smear positivity of the specimen, since it usually does not grow from the laboratory environment or from the uninfected human body. This important point differentiates *M. marinum* infection from infections due to other NTM such as *M. fortuitum* or *M. chelonae* (104). Thus correct identification is required (17, 106).

Bacteriological findings

Microscopic examination of the specimen after Ziehl-Neelsen staining is positive in only 30% of cases. Even when positive, smear microscopy cannot distinguish *M. marinum* from other mycobacteria including species of the *M. tuberculosis* complex.

A definite diagnosis is obtained by a positive culture. Cultures are reported as positive in 70 to 80% of cases, but this number could be increased with attention to specimen collection and proper temperature for incubation. The microbiologist should be made aware of suspicion of *M. marinum* infection to perform appropriate cultures at 30°C.

Collection of specimens. The majority of specimens containing *M. marinum* are from the skin, either skin biopsy specimens or aspirates of pus. Swabs should be avoided for many reasons (38). Other specimens are articular fluids or subcutaneous tissues and exudates, often obtained at surgery. Specimens must be collected before chemotherapy begins. The container should be sterile and should not contain any fixative or preservative. The collected specimen should be kept at 4°C if delays are encountered in delivery to the laboratory. Since *M. marinum* infection is not a multibacillary infection, it is necessary to collect the largest possible specimen volume, especially in the case of skin biopsy or surgery.

Isolation procedures. Laboratory processing for *M. marinum* disease diagnosis is not an emergency. A level 2 laboratory might be sufficient for isolation and identification, although level 3 might be required for studies requiring large-volume subcultures (17).

Safety measures are required for handling specimens and cultures: wearing gloves, disinfection of the material and benches, and avoiding the use of needles, so accidental inoculation does not occur.

Skin biopsy or wound fluids might be contaminated with skin flora, such as staphylococci, and consequently require a decontamination procedure (standard NALC–2% NaOH procedure or 4% HCl decontamination) prior to culture. Specimens from sterile deep structures (i.e., articular fluid) might be inoculated directly without decontamination (17, 65).

Since *M. marinum* grows poorly at 37°C, the aspirate or biopsy specimen should be cultured at 30 to 32°C. Colonies grow within 5 to 14 days, but cultures should be kept for 6 to 12 weeks. Because of other possible mycobacterial diagnoses, specimens should also be incubated at 37°C.

After successful isolation of photochromogenic mycobacteria, further differentiation between *M. marinum* and other organisms in Runyon group I is required (see above).

Methods based on molecular biology are limited by the high homology between *M. marinum* and *M. ulcerans* (see "Molecular Identification" above). Neither the commercial INNO-LiPA v2 assay kits nor the GenoType mycobacteria CM/AS allows differentiation between *M. marinum*, *M. ulcerans*, *M. ulcerans* subspecies, *M. shinshuense*, *M. shottsii*, and *M. pseudoshottsii* (67).

Molecular identification using the analysis of 16S rRNA or another conserved gene (*hsp65*, *gyrA*, *rpoB*, 16-23S internal transcribed spacer) associated with a 7-day growth of photochromogenic colonies easily identifies *M. marinum*. However, in the case of absence of photochromogen colonies or culture in broth, a gene sequence belonging to *M. marinum* or *M. ulcerans* (27, 52) coupled with the absence of IS*2404* and IS*2606* (19) may indicate *M. marinum* (36). We recommend waiting for the colony morphology to confirm the identification result. In the past few years, a mycolactone-producing subgroup of the *M. marinum* complex has been identified and analyzed. These IS*2404*-positive strains cause pathology in frogs and fish but so far not in humans (88).

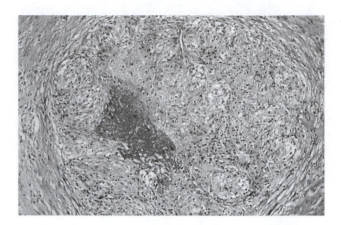

Figure 3. Active disease histopathologic section of tissue from a patient with an *M. marinum* infection. The lesion shows granulomatous infiltrate with epithelioid and giant cells. (Courtesy of Bernard Cribier, Strasbourg, France.)

Histological findings

Tissue biopsy for histopathology is important but supports the diagnosis of mycobacteriosis in only half of cases, since histological changes depend on the age of the lesion.

Granulomas suggest the diagnosis but are not pathognomonic and are also present in other mycobacterial infections. They are often absent or poorly formed. During the first months, there is a nonspecific inflammatory infiltrate. Later, granulomata with multinucleated giant cells are common findings (Fig. 3). Fibrinoid necrosis, but not true caseation, can be observed. Langhans giant cells are seen only occasionally. Hyperkeratosis with focal parakeratosis, hyperplasia, and liquefaction degeneration of the basal layer can be observed (32).

Although acid-fast bacilli are seldom seen in the histological sections (28), staining should be attempted.

ANTIMICROBIAL SUSCEPTIBILITIES AND TREATMENT

Mode of Action and Resistance Mechanisms in *M. marinum*

The permeability of the *M. marinum* cell wall has not been investigated but has been demonstrated to vary at least 10-fold between mycobacterial species, with that of *M. tuberculosis* being 10-fold more permeable than that of *M. chelonae* (62). Considering the natural multidrug resistance of *M. marinum* (see below), permeability of its cell wall could be close to that of *M. chelonae*. This low permeability probably allows survival in unfavorable environments.

In the genome, several genes encoding antibiotic resistance mechanisms were reported. Genes encoding enzymes known to hydrolyze antibiotics were found for β-lactams (*blaC*), aminoglycosides (*aac2'*), and chloramphenicol (*cph*). Many potential efflux pumps and ABC transporters have been also described, including potential extruders for cyclines, macrolides, and aminoglycosides.

In Vitro Susceptibility to Antibiotics

From the studies dealing with a large number of strains and applying a standard method of testing, *M. marinum* has a natural multidrug resistance pattern (6, 100). Indeed, *M. marinum* is resistant to the antituberculous drugs isoniazid, ethambutol, and pyrazinamide in most studies. Rifampin and rifabutin are the most active drugs in terms of MICs. MICs of minocycline, doxycycline, clarithromycin, linezolid, sparfloxacin, moxifloxacin, imipenem, sulfamethoxazole, and amikacin are close to the susceptibility breakpoints, and thus, these drugs may have moderate activity. MICs of trimethoprim, azithromycin, telithromycin, quinupristin-dalfopristin, ciprofloxacin, gemifloxacin, ofloxacin, and levofloxacin are above the concentrations usually obtained in vivo, and consequently, *M. marinum* may be considered resistant to them (14, 15, 74, 103).

All the strains have a similar susceptibility pattern, since for each drug, the MIC_{50}, geometric mean MIC, and modal MIC are very close (6, 14). This constitutes the natural or intrinsic susceptibility pattern of *M. marinum* (Table 2).

Acquired resistance has not been described for *M. marinum* so far for any of those antibiotics, even in relapsed cases. Slight differences with the above pattern of natural antibiotic susceptibility that might be observed are usually due to differences in the method or the technique of susceptibility testing.

Susceptibility Testing

Etest has been demonstrated to be an accurate and precise method of MIC determination for bacteria other than mycobacteria, for rapidly growing mycobacterial species, and even for some of the slowly growing mycobacterial species (33, 58, 105). Different authors questioned the reliability of the Etest for *M. marinum* and also for other mycobacteria, claiming it may cause reports of false resistance (6, 14). Agreement between MICs, yielded by either the Etest method or the agar dilution method used as a reference, depends on the antibiotic and was 83% for minocycline, 59% for rifampin, 43% for clarithromycin, and 24% for sparfloxacin (6, 107). Moreover, reproducibility with the Etest was low, in contrast to that with the agar dilution method. In conclusion, Etest is not recommended for *M. marinum* antibiotic susceptibility testing, and the agar dilution method remains the method recommended.

Broth microdilution susceptibility testing is recommended by CLSI and may use the commercially available Sensititre MIC plates. Although it may be recommended to use the slow-growing mycobacteria MIC plate for *M. marinum*, we think that testing antibiotics contained in the rapidly growing mycobacteria MIC plate may be more appropriate with regard to the antibiotics for which MICs are low (Table 2).

Since no primary resistance has been described so far, routine susceptibility testing seems unnecessary except for relapsed cases, as recommended for other atypical mycobacteria (5, 104).

Table 2. MICs of 17 antibiotics against 54 strains of *Mycobacterium marinum* determined by the agar dilution method

Antibiotic	MIC_{50} (μg/ml)	MIC_{90} (μg/ml)	Modal MIC (μg/ml)	Geometric mean ± SD (μg/ml)	Range (μg/ml)
Rifampin	0.25	0.5	0.25	0.24 ± 1.7	0.125–4
Rifabutin	0.06	0.06	0.06	0.06 ± 1.8	0.015–1
Isoniazid	4	8	4	5.6 ± 1.5	4–16
Ethambutol	2	4	2	1.7 ± 1.6	1–4
Amikacin	2	4	4	1 ± 1.7	1–8
Doxycycline	8	16	8	5.7 ± 2	0.5–16
Minocycline	2	4	2	2.9 ± 1.7	0.5–8
Clarithromycin	1	4	2	1.2 ± 2.3	0.5–4
Azithromycin	32	128	32	NA[a]	8–>128
Ofloxacin	4	16	4	6.1 ± 1.7	2–32
Ciprofloxacin	4	8	4	3.8 ± 1.8	1–16
Levofloxacin	4	8	4	4.5 ± 1.7	2–32
Sparfloxacin	1	2	1	1 ± 1.8	0.5–4
Moxifloxacin	0.5	1	0.5	0.6 ± 1.7	0.25–4
Sulfamethoxazole	8	128	8	NA	4–>128
Trimethoprim	64	128	128	67.4 ± 2.3	16–512
Imipenem	2	8	2	2.6 ± 2.6	0.5–16

[a]NA, not applicable (upper MICs above the highest concentration tested; from reference 6).

Antimicrobial Therapy of *M. marinum* Infections

Patients infected with *M. marinum* are usually treated with antibiotics (Table 1). Different antibiotic regimens have been reported (31). The choice of the regimen appeared to be based more on personal experience and preference of individual authors than on the demonstrated efficacy. Antibiotic efficacy is unknown, since (i) cases are reported separately in the literature, (ii) no therapeutic trial has been carried out, and (iii) *M. marinum* infection may resolve spontaneously (32, 47, 108).

A variety of antibiotics have been used, including tetracyclines, co-trimoxazole, rifampin plus ethambutol, and more rarely clarithromycin, levofloxacin, and amikacin (20, 31, 47, 48). Cure as well as failure has been described with all of these drugs (31, 47, 55). Overall, most patients are cured after therapy that included tetracyclines or clarithromycin and rifampin, but failures have been also observed. Failures were rarely observed with tetracyclines, but most of the patients treated by tetracyclines, and especially by tetracyclines alone, had mild infection limited to skin and soft tissue. On the other hand, rifampin and rifabutin, which are the only antibiotics with low MICs close to those found for *M. tuberculosis*, were usually given in complicated cases with extension of the infection to deeper structures such as tenosynovitis and osteoarthritis and failed to cure all cases. In our study, failure was related to deep infections (72% only were cured) and to ulcerated lesions (5).

The in vivo activity of the new fluoroquinolones, moxifloxacin and gatifloxacin, whose MICs are lower than classical fluoroquinolones and which are very potent antituberculous drugs, has yet to be demonstrated. The efficacy of linezolid, which shows low MICs, needs also to be tested in vivo.

We currently need results of in vivo experiments in the animal model or therapeutic trials in humans showing evidence of efficacy of some antibiotics. Until this is obtained, it is reasonable to recommend tetracyclines for *M. marinum* infection limited to the skin and the combination of rifampin and clarithromycin for infection extended to deeper structures. In the literature, the duration of antimicrobial therapy in *M. marinum* infection varies from 2 weeks to 18 months, depending on several factors, such as the extension and severity of infection, the presence of underlying disorders, and the clinical response (31, 111). In many patients with mild disease, infection improves spontaneously, although complete resolution may take up to several years (31, 38). In our study (5), the duration of therapy

ranged from 1 to 25 months, and the median was 3.5 months. This duration was significantly longer for cases with infection involving deeper structures except for the failure cases.

We may recommend continuing antimicrobial therapy at least until the lesions heal and then for two additional months, especially in cases of deep infection.

Surgery

The place of surgery is controversial. For some authors, surgical debridement along with antimicrobial therapy is usually required for control (38). For others, surgical debridement should be limited to the cases with criteria known to be associated with a poor prognosis, including steroid injections into the lesion, a persistent drainage sinus tract after several months of antimicrobial therapy, and persistent pain (20). Most of the infections spread to deeper structures undergo surgery, which seems reasonable (12). For the infections limited to skin and soft tissue, there is no clear benefit of surgery and surgical side effects are unknown.

Other therapies such as cryotherapy, X-ray therapy, and electrodesiccation have been reported but have not been evaluated (31).

EPIDEMIOLOGY AND PREVENTION

Natural Habitats of *M. marinum*

M. marinum has been reported to affect a wide range of freshwater and marine fish species, suggesting a ubiquitous distribution. *M. marinum* is the main mycobacterium isolated from fish, although very little is known about its prevalence and impact on fisheries (42). Zanoni et al. reported that mycobacteria were found in 46.8% and 29.9% of the fishes imported into Italy which died and that *M. marinum* represented 2.4 to 5.3% of the isolates (110).

M. marinum is transmitted in fishes through the consumption of contaminated feed, cannibalism of infected fish, aquatic detritus, or release of pathogens into the water due to gut or skin lesions or disintegration of infected fishes (28). In this respect, potential sources of infective material are numerous and include the soil and water in which the bacterial cells remain viable for 2 years or more (28).

M. marinum infection in other aquatic vertebrates may be a source of infection to fishes. Frogs, snakes, and turtles may become involved in the transmission cycle. Snails are also thought to be a reservoir (28). Other invertebrate organisms, such as shellfishes or water fleas, have been shown to play a role in the transmission of this agent.

The prevalence of nontuberculous mycobacteria was evaluated in the environment of a swimming pool in Italy. Although 88.2% of pool water samples were positive for *M. gordonae*, *M. chelonae*, and *M. fortuitum*, *M. marinum* was isolated in only 4.5% of the water samples and pool edges (59).

Epidemiology of *M. marinum* Infections

Like other NTM infections, *M. marinum* infections are not contagious from human to human. Before 1962, most cutaneous *M. marinum* infections reported in the literature involved swimming pool-associated injuries, including two large outbreaks involving almost 350 patients (61, 66). A possible explanation of the decline in pool-associated cases is the improvement in swimming pool water disinfection practices in recent decades. *M. marinum* survives only briefly after exposure to free chlorine concentrations of ≥0.6 µg/ml.

M. marinum skin infection is now often acquired from aquarium maintenance and is called "fish tank granuloma" (90). Since *M. marinum* infection is an important zoonosis, there is a significant risk to all personnel working with fishes, aquatic animals, or aquaria. *M. marinum* infection may be an occupational hazard for certain professionals (for example, pet shop workers), but many infections occur in fish fanciers who keep an aquarium at home, hence, the name "fish fanciers' finger syndrome." Although infection may be caused by direct injury from the fish fins or bites, most are acquired during the handling of the aquarium such as cleaning or changing the water (50, 60). Indirect infection has also been described due to a bath that was used to clean out fish tanks (5, 30, 53).

It is anticipated that the incidence of "fish tank granuloma" will increase (30) due to the increase of fish tank hobbyists and aquarium tourism. For example, in France, about 10% of the population has an aquarium at home and business related to fish tank hobbies has increased by 3% per year.

The frequency of *M. marinum* isolation in laboratories is low, and *M. marinum* accounts for less than 1% of the mycobacterial clinical isolates (39). A recent survey involving 21 laboratories in Spain reported 39 cases from 1991 to 1998 (16). Less than half of the cases of *M. marinum* infection are bacteriologically confirmed. The incidence of *M. marinum* infection was estimated to be around 0.09 cases per 100,000 inhabitants per year in France and between 0.05 and 0.27 in the United States.

Prevention Strategies

For the prevention of swimming pool granuloma, the Centers for Disease Control and Prevention recommends that concentrations of free chlorine in swimming pool water should be kept between 0.4 and 1 mg/liter and that concentrations in spa and hot tub water be kept between 2 and 5 mg/liter (66).

Sanitation, disinfection, and destruction of carrier fishes are the primary methods of controlling *M. marinum* infection in fishes. This practice is mostly pursued for food fish; however, in expensive fish species, this practice may be difficult to apply. Antimicrobial treatment is not able to eliminate *M. marinum* from affected fishes (4). Regarding importation of ornamental fish, there is great variation in policy. For example, France requires an EU Directive 2003/858/EC health certificate-derived template for all imported live fish (including tropical ornamentals) (64).

Individual prevention is the first line of defense for anyone involved with aquaria or anyone working or recreating in a marine environment. Preventive strategies should be employed in fish tank-related activities, such as wearing gloves when cleaning the tank (50). Common sense measures could include:

- Bandage or dress any open wound or cut before exposure.
- Wash hands thoroughly before and after exposure to aquarium water and components. Hydroalcoholic solutions may be used instead of hand washing.
- Do not swallow the aquarium water when checking for salinity or siphoning water.
- Do not overcrowd aquaria, since this favors the multiplication of mycobacteria.
- UV germicide lamps to treat aquarium water are efficient for mycobacteria as long as they are used in clean conditions at the correct flow rate (24).
- Do not transfer tank filters or fishes in the bath that is used for humans, or carefully clean it with sodium hypochlorite (63).
- Exposed populations should be educated to recognize signs of *M. marinum* disease in fish and in humans, so they can inform medical staff and expedite the diagnosis.
- Fish salesmen should be educated. Indeed, many tropical fish salesmen ignore "fish tank granuloma." In France, although 20% of them are at risk of *M. marinum* infection, 95% of them immerse their hands without gloves in the fish tanks every day (79).

Some authors recommend not installing ornamental aquaria in hospital units, particularly in units likely to receive immunocompromised patients.

REMAINING PROBLEMS AND CONCLUSION

Treatment evaluation requires large-scale trials, probably at an international level. Infection limited to the skin and soft tissue should be distinguished from infections extended to deeper structures. Antibiotics such as tetracyclines, rifampin, and clarithromycin need to be evaluated along with the new fluoroquinolones and linezolid. Surgery needs evaluation as well.

Surveillance of *M. marinum* infection, which is expected to increase due to the increase in fish tank hobbyists and aquarium tourism, should be undertaken at least in some highly exposed countries. A simple surveillance could be based on culture-confirmed cases. Bacteriology laboratories, dermatologists, and infectious disease physicians should play a crucial role in case finding.

Since there is no human-to-human transmission of *M. marinum*, the prevention of inoculation from the environment is the main strategy for eradicating the disease. Simple recommendations such as hand protection and hygienic measures and fish tank and aquarium maintenance should be disseminated and evaluated.

Professionals should also take *M. marinum* risk into account and apply the recommendation for decreasing *M. marinum* infection among farm fishes and among contamination of professionals handling fishes.

Lastly, diagnosis should be expedited (Fig. 4). Remember to (i) ask "Do you have a fish tank at home? Who cleans it and how?," (ii) sample the lesion for mycobacteriological analysis, (iii) inform the laboratory that there is a suspicion of *M. marinum* infection, and (iv) incubate the sample at 30°C in addition to 37°C and wait for weeks until smooth photochromogenic colonies appear.

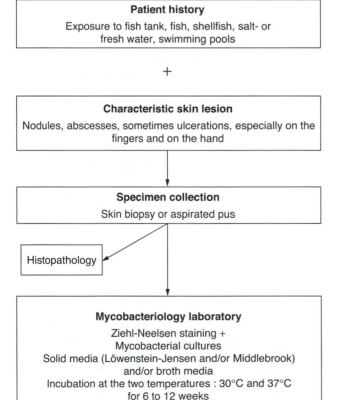

Figure 4. Microbiological diagnosis of human infection due to *M. marinum*.

REFERENCES

1. Ang, P., N. Rattana-Apiromyakij, and C. L. Goh. 2000. Retrospective study of *Mycobacterium marinum* skin infections. *Int. J. Dermatol.* 39:343–347.
2. Arend, S. M., K. E. van Meijgaarden, K. de Boer, E. C. de Palou, D. van Soolingen, T. H. Ottenhoff, and J. T. van Dissel. 2002. Tuberculin skin testing and in vitro T cell responses to ESAT-6 and culture filtrate protein 10 after infection with *Mycobacterium marinum* or *M. kansasii*. *J. Infect. Dis.* 186: 1797–1807.
3. Aronson, J. 1926. Spontaneous tuberculosis in salt water fish. *J. Infect. Dis.* 39:315–320.
4. Astrofsky, K. M., M. D. Schrenzel, R. A. Bullis, R. M. Smolowitz, and J. G. Fox. 2000. Diagnosis and management of atypical *Mycobacterium* spp. infections in established laboratory zebrafish (*Brachydanio rerio*) facilities. *Comp. Med.* 50:666–672.
5. Aubry, A., O. Chosidow, E. Caumes, J. Robert, and E. Cambau. 2002. Sixty-three cases of *Mycobacterium marinum* infection: clinical features, treatment, and antibiotic susceptibility of causative isolates. *Arch. Intern. Med.* 162:1746–1752.
6. Aubry, A., V. Jarlier, S. Escolano, C. Truffot-Pernot, and E. Cambau. 2000. Antibiotic susceptibility pattern of *Mycobacterium marinum*. *Antimicrob. Agents Chemother.* 44:3133–3136.
7. Baker, J., and W. Hagan. 1942. Tuberculosis of a Mexican platyfish (*Platypoecilus maculatus*). *J. Infect. Dis.* 70:248–252.
8. Barker, L. P., D. M. Brooks, and P. L. Small. 1998. The identification of *Mycobacterium marinum* genes differentially expressed in macrophage phagosomes using promoter fusions to green fluorescent protein. *Mol. Microbiol.* 29:1167–1177.
9. Barker, L. P., K. M. George, S. Falkow, and P. L. Small. 1997. Differential trafficking of live and dead *Mycobacterium marinum* organisms in macrophages. *Infect. Immun.* 65:1497–1504.
10. Bataillon, E., A. Moeller, and L. Terre. 1902. Über die identitat des Bacillus des Karpfens (Bataillon, Dubard et terre) und des

bacillus der Blindsschleuche (Moeller). *Zentralbl. Tuberc.* **3:** 467–468.

11. Behr, M. A., and J. O. Falkinham III. 2009. Molecular epidemiology of nontuberculous mycobacteria. *Future Microbiol.* **4:**1009–1020.

12. Bhatty, M. A., D. P. Turner, and S. T. Chamberlain. 2000. *Mycobacterium marinum* hand infection: case reports and review of literature. *Br. J. Plast. Surg.* **53:**161–165.

13. Bonafe, J. L., N. Grigorieff-Larrue, and R. Bauriaud. 1992. Atypical cutaneous mycobacterium diseases. Results of a national survey. *Ann. Dermatol. Venereol.* **119:**463–470.

14. Braback, M., K. Riesbeck, and A. Forsgren. 2002. Susceptibilities of *Mycobacterium marinum* to gatifloxacin, gemifloxacin, levofloxacin, linezolid, moxifloxacin, telithromycin, and quinupristin-dalfopristin (Synercid) compared to its susceptibilities to reference macrolides and quinolones. *Antimicrob. Agents Chemother.* **46:**1114–1116.

15. Brown-Elliott, B. A., C. J. Crist, L. B. Mann, R. W. Wilson, and R. J. Wallace, Jr. 2003. In vitro activity of linezolid against slowly growing nontuberculous mycobacteria. *Antimicrob. Agents Chemother.* **47:**1736–1738.

16. Casal, M., and M. M. Casal. 2001. Multicenter study of incidence of *Mycobacterium marinum* in humans in Spain. *Int. J. Tuberc. Lung Dis.* **5:**197–199.

17. Cernoch, P., R. Enns, and M. Saubolle. 1994. *Cumitech 16A, Laboratory Diagnosis of the Mycobacterioses.* Coordinating ed., Alice C. Weissfeld. American Society for Microbiology, Washington, DC.

18. Chan, K., T. Knaak, L. Satkamp, O. Humbert, S. Falkow, and L. Ramakrishnan. 2002. Complex pattern of *Mycobacterium marinum* gene expression during long-term granulomatous infection. *Proc. Natl. Acad. Sci. USA* **99:**3920–3925.

19. Chemlal, K., G. Huys, P. A. Fonteyne, V. Vincent, A. G. Lopez, L. Rigouts, J. Swings, W. M. Meyers, and F. Portaels. 2001. Evaluation of PCR-restriction profile analysis and IS*2404* restriction fragment length polymorphism and amplified fragment length polymorphism fingerprinting for identification and typing of *Mycobacterium ulcerans* and *M. marinum*. *J. Clin. Microbiol.* **39:**3272–3278.

20. Chow, S. P., F. K. Ip, J. H. Lau, R. J. Collins, K. D. Luk, Y. C. So, and W. K. Pun. 1987. *Mycobacterium marinum* infection of the hand and wrist. Results of conservative treatment in twenty-four cases. *J. Bone Joint. Surg. Am.* **69:**1161–1168.

21. Clark, R. B., H. Spector, D. M. Friedman, K. J. Oldrati, C. L. Young, and S. C. Nelson. 1990. Osteomyelitis and synovitis produced by *Mycobacterium marinum* in a fisherman. *J. Clin. Microbiol.* **28:**2570–2572.

22. Cosma, C., L. Swaim, H. Volkman, L. Ramakrishnan, and J. Davis. 2006. Zebrafish and frog models of *Mycobacterium marinum* infection. *Curr. Protoc. Microbiol.* **10:**10B.2.

23. Daffe, M., M. Laneelle, and C. Lacave. 1991. Structure and stereochemistry of mycolic acids of *Mycobacterium marinum* and *Mycobacterium ulcerans*. *Res. Microbiol.* **142:**397–403.

24. Dailloux, M., C. Laurain, and M. Weber. 1999. Water and nontuberculous mycobacteria. *Water Res.* **33:**2219–2228.

25. Danko, J. R., W. R. Gilliland, R. S. Miller, and C. F. Decker. 2009. Disseminated *Mycobacterium marinum* infection in a patient with rheumatoid arthritis receiving infliximab therapy. *Scand. J. Infect. Dis.* **41:**252–255.

26. Dare, J. A., S. Jahan, K. Hiatt, and K. D. Torralba. 2009. Reintroduction of etanercept during treatment of cutaneous *Mycobacterium marinum* infection in a patient with ankylosing spondylitis. *Arthritis Rheum.* **61:**583–586.

27. Dauendorffer, J. N., I. Guillemin, A. Aubry, C. Truffot-Pernot, W. Sougakoff, V. Jarlier, and E. Cambau. 2003. Identification of mycobacterial species by PCR sequencing of quinolone resistance-determining regions of DNA gyrase genes. *J. Clin. Microbiol.* **41:**1311–1315.

28. Decostere, A., K. Hermans, and F. Haesebrouck. 2004. Piscine mycobacteriosis: a literature review covering the agent and the disease it causes in fish and humans. *Vet. Microbiol.* **99:**159–166.

29. Dionne, M. S., N. Ghori, and D. S. Schneider. 2003. *Drosophila melanogaster* is a genetically tractable model host for *Mycobacterium marinum*. *Infect. Immun.* **71:**3540–3550.

30. Dobos, K. M., F. D. Quinn, D. A. Ashford, C. R. Horsburgh, and C. H. King. 1999. Emergence of a unique group of necrotizing mycobacterial diseases. *Emerg. Infect. Dis.* **5:**367–378.

31. Edelstein, H. 1994. *Mycobacterium marinum* skin infections. Report of 31 cases and review of the literature. *Arch. Intern. Med.* **154:**1359–1364.

32. Even-Paz, Z., H. Haas, T. Sacks, and E. Rosenmann. 1976. *Mycobacterium marinum* skin infections mimicking cutaneous leishmaniasis. *Br. J. Dermatol.* **94:**435–442.

33. Flynn, C. M., C. M. Kelley, M. S. Barrett, and R. N. Jones. 1997. Application of the Etest to the antimicrobial susceptibility testing of *Mycobacterium marinum* clinical isolates. *J. Clin. Microbiol.* **35:**2083–2086.

34. Funakoshi, T., Y. Kazumi, R. Okada, K. Nishimoto, M. Saito, M. Amagai, H. Shimura, and M. Ohyama. 2009. Intractable ulcer caused by *Mycobacterium shinshuense*: successful identification of mycobacterium strain by 16S ribosomal RNA 3'-end sequencing. *Clin. Exp. Dermatol.* **34:**e712–e715.

35. Gao, L. Y., R. Groger, J. S. Cox, S. M. Beverley, E. H. Lawson, and E. J. Brown. 2003. Transposon mutagenesis of *Mycobacterium marinum* identifies a locus linking pigmentation and intracellular survival. *Infect. Immun.* **71:**922–929.

36. Gauthier, D. T., and M. W. Rhodes. 2009. Mycobacteriosis in fishes: a review. *Vet. J.* **180:**33–47.

37. Glickman, M. S. 2008. Cording, cord factors, and trehalose dimycolate, p. 63–73. *In* M. Daffe and J. Reyrat (ed.), *The Mycobacterial Cell Envelope*. ASM Press, Washington, DC.

38. Gluckman, S. J. 1995. *Mycobacterium marinum*. *Clin. Dermatol.* **13:**273–276.

39. Good, R. C. 1980. From the Center for Disease Control. Isolation of nontuberculous mycobacteria in the United States, 1979. *J. Infect. Dis.* **142:**779–783.

40. Hagedorn, M., K. H. Rohde, D. G. Russell, and T. Soldati. 2009. Infection by tubercular mycobacteria is spread by nonlytic ejection from their amoeba hosts. *Science* **323:**1729–1733.

41. Harriff, M. J., L. E. Bermudez, and M. L. Kent. 2007. Experimental exposure of zebrafish, *Danio rerio* (Hamilton), to *Mycobacterium marinum* and *Mycobacterium peregrinum* reveals the gastrointestinal tract as the primary route of infection: a potential model for environmental mycobacterial infection. *J. Fish Dis.* **30:**587–600.

42. Heckert, R. A., S. Elankumaran, A. Milani, and A. Baya. 2001. Detection of a new *Mycobacterium* species in wild striped bass in the Chesapeake Bay. *J. Clin. Microbiol.* **39:**710–715.

43. Helguera-Repetto, C., R. A. Cox, J. L. Munoz-Sanchez, and J. A. Gonzalez-y-Merchand. 2004. The pathogen *Mycobacterium marinum*, a faster growing close relative of *Mycobacterium tuberculosis*, has a single rRNA operon per genome. *FEMS Microbiol. Lett.* **235:**281–288.

44. Hess, S. D., A. S. Van Voorhees, L. M. Chang, J. M. Junkins-Hopkins, and C. L. Kovarik. 2009. Subcutaneous *Mycobacterium marinum* infection in a patient with chronic rheumatoid arthritis receiving immunosuppressive therapy. *Int. J. Dermatol.* **48:**782–783.

45. Ho, M. H., C. K. Ho, and L. Y. Chong. 2006. Atypical mycobacterial cutaneous infections in Hong Kong: 10-year retrospective study. *Hong Kong Med. J.* 12:21–26.

46. Holmes, G. F., S. M. Harrington, M. J. Romagnoli, and W. G. Merz. 1999. Recurrent, disseminated *Mycobacterium marinum* infection caused by the same genotypically defined strain in an immunocompromised patient. *J. Clin. Microbiol.* 37:3059–3061.

47. Huminer, D., S. D. Pitlik, C. Block, L. Kaufman, S. Amit, and J. B. Rosenfeld. 1986. Aquarium-borne *Mycobacterium marinum* skin infection. Report of a case and review of the literature. *Arch. Dermatol.* 122:698–703.

48. Iijima, S., J. Saito, and F. Otsuka. 1997. *Mycobacterium marinum* skin infection successfully treated with levofloxacin. *Arch. Dermatol.* 133:947–949.

49. Jacobs, J. M., M. R. Rhodes, A. Baya, R. Reimschuessel, H. Townsend, and R. M. Harrell. 2009. Influence of nutritional state on the progression and severity of mycobacteriosis in striped bass *Morone saxatilis*. *Dis. Aquat. Organ.* 87:183–197.

50. Jernigan, J. A., and B. M. Farr. 2000. Incubation period and sources of exposure for cutaneous *Mycobacterium marinum* infection: case report and review of the literature. *Clin. Infect. Dis.* 31:439–443.

51. Julian, E., M. Roldan, A. Sanchez-Chardi, O. Astola, G. Agusti, and M. Luquin. Microscopic cords, a virulence-related characteristic of *Mycobacterium tuberculosis*, are also present in nonpathogenic mycobacteria. *J. Bacteriol.* 192:1751–1760.

52. Kim, B. J., S. H. Lee, M. A. Lyu, S. J. Kim, G. H. Bai, G. T. Chae, E. C. Kim, C. Y. Cha, and Y. H. Kook. 1999. Identification of mycobacterial species by comparative sequence analysis of the RNA polymerase gene (*rpoB*). *J. Clin. Microbiol.* 37:1714–1720.

53. King, A. J., J. A. Fairley, and J. E. Rasmussen. 1983. Disseminated cutaneous *Mycobacterium marinum* infection. *Arch. Dermatol.* 119:268–270.

54. Kobashi, Y., K. Mouri, S. Yagi, Y. Obase, N. Miyashita, N. Okimoto, T. Matsushima, T. Kageoka, and M. Oka. 2009. Clinical evaluation of the QuantiFERON-TB Gold test in patients with non-tuberculous mycobacterial disease. *Int. J. Tuberc. Lung Dis.* 13:1422–1426.

55. Kozin, S. H., and A. T. Bishop. 1994. Atypical mycobacterium infections of the upper extremity. *J. Hand Surg. Am.* 19:480–487.

56. Lacaille, F., S. Blanche, C. Bodemer, C. Durand, Y. De Prost, and J. L. Gaillard. 1990. Persistent *Mycobacterium marinum* infection in a child with probable visceral involvement. *Pediatr. Infect. Dis. J.* 9:58–60.

57. Lai, C. C., L. N. Lee, Y. L. Chang, Y. C. Lee, L. W. Ding, and P. R. Hsueh. 2005. Pulmonary infection due to *Mycobacterium marinum* in an immunocompetent patient. *Clin. Infect. Dis.* 40:206–208.

58. Lebrun, L., C. Onody, V. Vincent, and P. Nordmann. 1996. Evaluation of the Etest for rapid susceptibility testing of *Mycobacterium avium* to clarithromycin. *J. Antimicrob. Chemother.* 37:999–1003.

59. Leoni, E., P. Legnani, M. T. Mucci, and R. Pirani. 1999. Prevalence of mycobacteria in a swimming pool environment. *J. Appl. Microbiol.* 87:683–688.

60. Lewis, F. M., B. J. Marsh, and C. F. von Reyn. 2003. Fish tank exposure and cutaneous infections due to *Mycobacterium marinum*: tuberculin skin testing, treatment, and prevention. *Clin. Infect. Dis.* 37:390–397.

61. Linell, F., and A. Norden. 1954. *Mycobacterium balnei*. A new acid fast bacillus occurring in swimming pools and capable of producing skin lesions in humans. *Acta Tuberc. Scand.* 33:1–54.

62. Nikaido, H. 2003. Molecular basis of bacterial outer membrane permeability revisited. *Microbiol. Mol. Biol. Rev.* 67:593–656.

63. Parent, L. J., M. M. Salam, P. C. Appelbaum, and J. H. Dossett. 1995. Disseminated *Mycobacterium marinum* infection and bacteremia in a child with severe combined immunodeficiency. *Clin. Infect. Dis.* 21:1325–1327.

64. Passantino, A., D. Macri, P. Coluccio, F. Foti, and F. Marino. 2008. Importation of mycobacteriosis with ornamental fish: medico-legal implications. *Travel Med. Infect. Dis.* 6:240–244.

65. Pfyffer, G. E., H. M. Welscher, P. Kissling, C. Cieslak, M. J. Casal, J. Gutierrez, and S. Rusch-Gerdes. 1997. Comparison of the Mycobacteria Growth Indicator Tube (MGIT) with radiometric and solid culture for recovery of acid-fast bacilli. *J. Clin. Microbiol.* 35:364–368.

66. Philpott, J., A. Woodburne, and O. Philpott. 1963. Swimming pool granuloma: a study of 290 cases. *Arch. Dermatol.* 88:158.

67. Pourahmad, F., K. D. Thompson, J. B. Taggart, A. Adams, and R. H. Richards. 2008. Evaluation of the INNO-LiPA mycobacteria v2 assay for identification of aquatic mycobacteria. *J. Fish Dis.* 31:931–940.

68. Prouty, M. G., N. E. Correa, L. P. Barker, P. Jagadeeswaran, and K. E. Klose. 2003. Zebrafish-*Mycobacterium marinum* model for mycobacterial pathogenesis. *FEMS Microbiol. Lett.* 225:177–182.

69. Ramakrishnan, L., and S. Falkow. 1994. *Mycobacterium marinum* persists in cultured mammalian cells in a temperature-restricted fashion. *Infect. Immun.* 62:3222–3229.

70. Ramakrishnan, L., H. T. Tran, N. A. Federspiel, and S. Falkow. 1997. A *crtB* homolog essential for photochromogenicity in *Mycobacterium marinum*: isolation, characterization, and gene disruption via homologous recombination. *J. Bacteriol.* 179:5862–5898.

71. Ramos, J. M., M. F. Garcia-Sepulcre, J. C. Rodriguez, S. Padilla, and F. Gutierrez. 2010. *Mycobacterium marinum* infection complicated by anti-tumor necrosis factor therapy. *J. Med. Microbiol.* 59:617–621.

72. Ramsay, J. M., V. Watral, C. B. Schreck, and M. L. Kent. 2009. Husbandry stress exacerbates mycobacterial infections in adult zebrafish, *Danio rerio* (Hamilton). *J. Fish Dis.* 32:931–941.

73. Ranger, B. S., E. A. Mahrous, L. Mosi, S. Adusumilli, R. E. Lee, A. Colorni, M. Rhodes, and P. L. Small. 2006. Globally distributed mycobacterial fish pathogens produce a novel plasmid-encoded toxic macrolide, mycolactone F. *Infect. Immun.* 74:6037–6045.

74. Rhomberg, P. R., and R. N. Jones. 2002. In vitro activity of 11 antimicrobial agents, including gatifloxacin and GAR936, tested against clinical isolates of *Mycobacterium marinum*. *Diagn. Microbiol. Infect. Dis.* 42:145–147.

75. Rogall, T., J. Wolters, T. Flohr, and E. C. Bottger. 1990. Towards a phylogeny and definition of species at the molecular level within the genus *Mycobacterium*. *Int. J. Syst. Bacteriol.* 40:323–330.

76. Ruley, K. M., J. H. Ansede, C. L. Pritchett, A. M. Talaat, R. Reimschuessel, and M. Trucksis. 2004. Identification of *Mycobacterium marinum* virulence genes using signature-tagged mutagenesis and the goldfish model of mycobacterial pathogenesis. *FEMS Microbiol. Lett.* 232:75–81.

77. Russo, C., E. Tortoli, and D. Menichella. 2006. Evaluation of the new GenoType *Mycobacterium* assay for identification of mycobacterial species. *J. Clin. Microbiol.* 44:334–339.

78. Salati, F., M. Meloni, A. Fenza, G. Angelucci, A. Colorni, and G. Orru. 2010. A sensitive FRET probe assay for the selective detection of *Mycobacterium marinum* in fish. *J. Fish Dis.* 33:47–56.

79. Schmoor, P., V. Descamps, F. Bouscarat, M. Grossin, S. Belaich, and B. Crickx. 2003. Tropical fish salesmen's knowledge and behaviour concerning "fish tank granuloma." *Ann. Dermatol. Venereol.* 130:425–427.

80. Sechi, L. A., A. Colorni, I. Dupre, P. Molicotti, G. Fadda, and S. Zanetti. 2002. Strain variation in Mediterranean and Red Sea *Mycobacterium marinum* isolates. *New Microbiol.* 25:351–356.

81. Stahl, D. A., and J. W. Urbance. 1990. The division between fast- and slow-growing species corresponds to natural relationships among the mycobacteria. *J. Bacteriol.* 172:116–124.

82. Stamm, L. M., J. H. Morisaki, L. Y. Gao, R. L. Jeng, K. L. McDonald, R. Roth, S. Takeshita, J. Heuser, M. D. Welch, and E. J. Brown. 2003. *Mycobacterium marinum* escapes from phagosomes and is propelled by actin-based motility. *J. Exp. Med.* 198:1361–1368.

83. Stinear, T. P., G. A. Jenkin, P. D. Johnson, and J. K. Davies. 2000. Comparative genetic analysis of *Mycobacterium ulcerans* and *Mycobacterium marinum* reveals evidence of recent divergence. *J. Bacteriol.* 182:6322–6330.

84. Stinear, T. P., A. Mve-Obiang, P. L. Small, W. Frigui, M. J. Pryor, R. Brosch, G. A. Jenkin, P. D. Johnson, J. K. Davies, R. E. Lee, S. Adusumilli, T. Garnier, S. F. Haydock, P. F. Leadlay, and S. T. Cole. 2004. Giant plasmid-encoded polyketide synthases produce the macrolide toxin of *Mycobacterium ulcerans*. *Proc. Natl. Acad. Sci. USA* 101:1345–1349.

85. Stinear, T. P., T. Seemann, P. F. Harrison, G. A. Jenkin, J. K. Davies, P. D. Johnson, Z. Abdellah, C. Arrowsmith, T. Chillingworth, C. Churcher, K. Clarke, A. Cronin, P. Davis, I. Goodhead, N. Holroyd, K. Jagels, A. Lord, S. Moule, K. Mungall, H. Norbertczak, M. A. Quail, E. Rabbinowitsch, D. Walker, B. White, S. Whitehead, P. L. Small, R. Brosch, L. Ramakrishnan, M. A. Fischbach, J. Parkhill, and S. T. Cole. 2008. Insights from the complete genome sequence of *Mycobacterium marinum* on the evolution of *Mycobacterium tuberculosis*. *Genome Res.* 18:729–741.

86. Stinear, T. P., T. Seemann, S. Pidot, W. Frigui, G. Reysset, T. Garnier, G. Meurice, D. Simon, C. Bouchier, L. Ma, M. Tichit, J. L. Porter, J. Ryan, P. D. Johnson, J. K. Davies, G. A. Jenkin, P. L. Small, L. M. Jones, F. Tekaia, F. Laval, M. Daffe, J. Parkhill, and S. T. Cole. 2007. Reductive evolution and niche adaptation inferred from the genome of *Mycobacterium ulcerans*, the causative agent of Buruli ulcer. *Genome Res.* 17:192–200.

87. Stragier, P., A. Ablordey, W. M. Meyers, and F. Portaels. 2005. Genotyping *Mycobacterium ulcerans* and *Mycobacterium marinum* by using mycobacterial interspersed repetitive units. *J. Bacteriol.* 187:1639–1647.

88. Stragier, P., K. Hermans, T. Stinear, and F. Portaels. 2008. First report of a mycolactone-producing Mycobacterium infection in fish agriculture in Belgium. *FEMS Microbiol. Lett.* 286:93–95.

89. Streit, M., L. M. Bohlen, T. Hunziker, S. Zimmerli, G. G. Tscharner, H. Nievergelt, T. Bodmer, and L. R. Braathen. 2006. Disseminated *Mycobacterium marinum* infection with extensive cutaneous eruption and bacteremia in an immunocompromised patient. *Eur. J. Dermatol.* 16:79–83.

90. Swift, S., and H. Cohen. 1962. Granulomas of the skin due to Mycobacterium balnei after abrasions from a fishtank. *N. Engl. J. Med.* 297:1244–1246.

91. Talaat, A. M., R. Reimschuessel, S. S. Wasserman, and M. Trucksis. 1998. Goldfish, *Carassius auratus*, a novel animal model for the study of *Mycobacterium marinum* pathogenesis. *Infect. Immun.* 66:2938–2942.

92. Talaat, A. M., and M. Trucksis. 2000. Transformation and transposition of the genome of *Mycobacterium marinum*. *Am. J. Vet. Res.* 61:125–128.

93. Tchornobay, A. M., A. L. Claudy, J. L. Perrot, V. Levigne, and M. Denis. 1992. Fatal disseminated *Mycobacterium marinum* infection. *Int. J. Dermatol.* 31:286–287.

94. Tobin, D. M., J. C. Vary, Jr., J. P. Ray, G. S. Walsh, S. J. Dunstan, N. D. Bang, D. A. Hagge, S. Khadge, M. C. King, T. R. Hawn, C. B. Moens, and L. Ramakrishnan. 2010. The lta4h locus modulates susceptibility to mycobacterial infection in zebrafish and humans. *Cell* 140:717–730.

95. Tonjum, T., D. B. Welty, E. Jantzen, and P. L. Small. 1998. Differentiation of *Mycobacterium ulcerans*, *M. marinum*, and *M. haemophilum*: mapping of their relationships to *M. tuberculosis* by fatty acid profile analysis, DNA-DNA hybridization, and 16S rRNA gene sequence analysis. *J. Clin. Microbiol.* 36:918–925.

96. Tortoli, E., A. Nanetti, C. Piersimoni, P. Cichero, C. Farina, G. Mucignat, C. Scarparo, L. Bartolini, R. Valentini, D. Nista, G. Gesu, C. P. Tosi, M. Crovatto, and G. Brusarosco. 2001. Performance assessment of new multiplex probe assay for identification of mycobacteria. *J. Clin. Microbiol.* 39:1079–1084.

97. Trucksis, M. 2000. Fishing for mycobacterial virulence genes: a promising animal model. *ASM News* 66:668–674.

98. Ucko, M., and A. Colorni. 2005. *Mycobacterium marinum* infections in fish and humans in Israel. *J. Clin. Microbiol.* 43:892–895.

99. Ucko, M., A. Colorni, H. Kvitt, A. Diamant, A. Zlotkin, and W. R. Knibb. 2002. Strain variation in *Mycobacterium marinum* fish isolates. *Appl. Environ. Microbiol.* 68:5281–5287.

100. Utrup, L. J., T. D. Moore, P. Actor, and J. A. Poupard. 1995. Susceptibilities of nontuberculosis mycobacterial species to amoxicillin-clavulanic acid alone and in combination with antimycobacterial agents. *Antimicrob. Agents Chemother.* 39:1454–1457.

101. van der Sar, A. M., A. M. Abdallah, M. Sparrius, E. Reinders, C. M. Vandenbroucke-Grauls, and W. Bitter. 2004. *Mycobacterium marinum* strains can be divided into two distinct types based on genetic diversity and virulence. *Infect. Immun.* 72:6306–6312.

102. van Ingen, J., R. de Zwaan, R. Dekhuijzen, M. Boeree, and D. van Soolingen. 2009. Region of difference 1 in nontuberculous *Mycobacterium* species adds a phylogenetic and taxonomical character. *J. Bacteriol.* 191:5865–5867.

103. Vera-Cabrera, L., B. A. Brown-Elliott, R. J. Wallace, Jr., J. Ocampo-Candiani, O. Welsh, S. H. Choi, and C. A. Molina-Torres. 2006. In vitro activities of the novel oxazolidinones DA-7867 and DA-7157 against rapidly and slowly growing mycobacteria. *Antimicrob. Agents Chemother.* 50:4027–4029.

104. Wallace, R., J. Glassroth, D. Griffith, et al. 1997. Diagnostic and treatment of disease caused by nontuberculous mycobacteria. *Am. J. Respir. Crit. Care Med.* 156:S1–S25.

105. Wallace, R. J., Jr., and K. Wiss. 1981. Susceptibility of *Mycobacterium marinum* to tetracyclines and aminoglycosides. *Antimicrob. Agents Chemother.* 20:610–612.

106. Wayne, L. G., and H. A. Sramek. 1992. Agents of newly recognized or infrequently encountered mycobacterial diseases. *Clin. Microbiol. Rev.* 5:1–25.

107. **Werngren, J., B. Olsson-Liljequist, L. Gezelius, and S. E. Hoffner.** 2001. Antimicrobial susceptibility of *Mycobacterium marinum* determined by E-test and agar dilution. *Scand. J. Infect. Dis.* **33**:585–588.

108. **Wolinsky, E.** 1992. Mycobacterial diseases other than tuberculosis. *Clin. Infect. Dis.* **15**:1–10.

109. **Yip, M. J., J. L. Porter, J. A. Fyfe, C. J. Lavender, F. Portaels, M. Rhodes, H. Kator, A. Colorni, G. A. Jenkin, and T. Stinear.** 2007. Evolution of *Mycobacterium ulcerans* and other mycolactone-producing mycobacteria from a common *Mycobacterium marinum* progenitor. *J. Bacteriol.* **189**:2021–2029.

110. **Zanoni, R. G., D. Florio, M. L. Fioravanti, M. Rossi, and M. Prearo.** 2008. Occurrence of Mycobacterium spp. in ornamental fish in Italy. *J. Fish Dis.* **31**:433–441.

111. **Zenone, T., A. Boibieux, S. Tigaud, J. F. Fredenucci, V. Vincent, C. Chidiac, and D. Peyramond.** 1999. Non-tuberculous mycobacterial tenosynovitis: a review. *Scand. J. Infect. Dis.* **31**:221–228.

Chapter 40

Mycobacterium scrofulaceum

EDWARD A. HOROWITZ

INTRODUCTION

Mycobacterium scrofulaceum is a member of the Runyon class II scotochromogenic acid-fast bacilli. It is found widely in nature but is an uncommon human pathogen. It was first described by Prissick and Masson in a preliminary report in 1952 (47) and subsequently in more detail (48, 49). It was they who proposed the name, presumably because of its isolation from cervical lymph nodes.

MICROBIOLOGY

M. scrofulaceum is variable in its length on acid-fast stain preparations and may be either longer or shorter than *Mycobacterium tuberculosis*. It is generally thicker and more coarsely beaded than *M. tuberculosis*. It grows slowly on Löwenstein medium. Although occasional strains may develop visible colonies in as little as 10 days, most require 4 to 6 weeks. Colonies are globular, smooth in consistency, and opaque. Pigmentation is yellow, turning a dark orange with time. Growth is optimal at 37°C, one atmosphere pressure, and under aerobic conditions. Growth is slower at 25° and 35°C. There is no growth at 41°C or higher.

Early work by Wayne and Tsukamura helped to distinguish *M. scrofulaceum* from *Mycobacterium gordonae* (59, 61, 62). The organism is antigenically and biochemically quite similar to *Mycobacterium avium-Mycobacterium intracellulare* (MAI) and for many years was classified with the latter as a complex (*M. avium-M. intracellulare-M. scrofulaceum*). It usually gives a positive urease reaction, which distinguishes it from MAI. Exceptions can occur (19), making distinctions difficult. Recent base sequence analysis of the 16S ribosomal RNA confirms that *M. scrofulaceum* is indeed a unique species (52).

EPIDEMIOLOGY

Sources in Nature

Early reports identified isolates of *M. scrofulaceum* in raw milk, oysters, soil, and water (9, 22, 25, 55, 65). Dunn and Hodgson (14) were able to isolate *M. scrofulaceum*, among other species of nontuberculous mycobacteria (NTM), from raw milk but not from samples of pasteurized milk. Environmental sources have also been identified in Korea (29) and the water supply system of the Czech Republic (34).

In the United States, Brooks et. al. (4) isolated *M. scrofulaceum* from the flood plains of four eastern rivers. The number of organisms increased with more southerly latitudes. A follow-up study (32) confirmed these findings and showed that environmental factors favoring growth include warm temperature, low oxygen tension, lower pH of soils, and higher water concentrations of zinc, humic acid, and fulvic acid. (The authors did not distinguish between strains of *M. scrofulaceum* and those of the MAI complex.) In a study by the same group (42), analysis of stable DNA plasmids in MAI complex and *M. scrofulaceum* strains showed that isolates from humans and aerosols are more likely to carry plasmids than those strains isolated from soil, dust, sediment, and water. The authors suggest that this supports the theory that human disease results from exposure to water aerosols.

HUMAN ISOLATES

M. scrofulaceum is an uncommon isolate from humans. The first national survey of NTM isolates in the United States was organized by the CDC in 1979 (18). The 763 isolates of *M. scrofulaceum* accounted for approximately 2% of all isolates. There

Edward A. Horowitz • Departments of Medicine and Medical Microbiology and Immunology, Creighton University School of Medicine, Omaha, NE 68131.

was a predominance of reports from the South Atlantic region, primarily due to 148 isolates from Florida. A follow-up survey in 1980 (20) had similar results.

The first survey to collect clinical data was carried out between October 1981 and September 1993 (44). *M. scrofulaceum* accounted for 214 (3.9%) of 5,469 overall NTM isolates. Forty-seven (22%) of these 214 were considered to represent clinical disease, or 2.2% of all clinically relevant isolates. Twenty-two of the 47 isolates were from sputum samples, and one was from lung tissue. Eighteen were from lymph nodes, one was from skin, and 5 were from other tissues or fluids. The mean age of the patients was 38.5 years, the lowest for all of the NTM species reported. Fifteen of the 47 were from patients less than 15 years of age. Patients were predominantly urban. No other geographic data were supplied. Of the NTM isolates from lymph nodes, 81% were MAI complex, 16% were *M. scrofulaceum*, and 3% were *Mycobacterium kansasii*. This correlates with the change in distribution of isolates from lymph nodes seen by Wolinsky and others (see below).

Similar data were reported from South Carolina (33) where 2% of NTM isolates from 210 patients between 1971 and 1980 were *M. scrofulaceum*. Only 4 of 269 NTM isolates at the Cleveland Clinic between 1982 and 1985 were *M. scrofulaceum* (66).

A number of recent reports have looked at human exposure to *M. scrofulaceum* by analyzing skin test reactions to purified protein derivative (PPD) sensitins derived from that organism. Bruins et al. (6) found that 7.76% of army recruits in The Netherlands had indurations of 10 mm or greater to *M. scrofulaceum* sensitin. Dascalopoulos et al. (12) analyzed 8,507 Greek armed forces members tested with *M. scrofulaceum* sensitin who lived in or near their birthplaces. Those born in mountainous areas or in seaside areas had positivity rates of 4.1% and 7.1%, respectively. Those born on small Aegean islands or on inland plains near large rivers both had rates described as "greater than 8%." The authors concluded that these data supported the theory that large bodies of water serve as the principal source of infection. Kwamanga et al. (35) tested 1,015 BCG scar-negative children between the ages of 6 and 13 years in 18 randomly selected areas of Kenya; 22.7% reacted to *M. scrofulaceum* sensitin and 6.1% reacted to PPD-RT. Cross reactivity was 23.8% in children who lived at low altitudes. Similarly, Svandova et al. (58) found that approximately 15% of 7-year-old children in two towns in rural Czechoslovakia were skin test reactors to *M. scrofulaceum* sensitin. The reaction was greater than the simultaneous reaction to PPD-RT in approximately 50% of the children.

These data are all subject to certain limitations. Nevertheless, they are consistent with the theory that *M. scrofulaceum* is widely but unevenly distributed in nature, that humans encounter the organism and develop an immune response in a pattern which reflects this distribution, and that clinical disease is much less common than exposure.

CLINICAL SYNDROMES

Lymphadenitis

As mentioned above, *M. scrofulaceum* was originally isolated from cervical lymph nodes of children, and this is the condition most commonly associated with it in the literature (37, 63, 64). Most patients are between 1 and 5 years of age, with occasional cases in patients older than 10 years. In cervical lymphadenitis due to all NTM species, girls outnumber boys by 1.3 to 2.0:1.0. (These data have not been reported specifically for *M. scrofulaceum*.) Most cases involve unilateral nodes in the upper cervical chain or just under the mandible. Occasionally, cases of bilateral disease or peripheral node involvement (axillary, inguinal, epitrochlear, or mediastinal) have been reported. The children have no systemic signs or symptoms and only occasionally have local symptoms. The natural history is variable and probably not completely understood. As Wolinsky and Rynearson noted (63), we do not know how many cases resolve spontaneously and never come to medical attention. Of the cases seen by physicians, those untreated either soften, open, and drain or heal spontaneously with fibrosis or calcification.

The pathophysiology has not been firmly established. The isolation of *M. scrofulaceum* (and also MAI) from tonsils has led to the reasonable speculation that the pharyngeal lymphoid tissue is the portal of entry, with direct drainage into the nodes (64). In cases of peripheral adenopathy, direct inoculation into the skin by trauma has been documented (63).

The distribution of mycobacterial species in childhood cervical lymphadenitis has changed over the years. In the preantibiotic era, most cases were due to *M. tuberculosis* or *Mycobacterium bovis* (24). In the developed countries of the world where tuberculosis has become a rare disease, the NTM species now predominate (2). Following the initial reports (47, 48), *M. scrofulaceum* was the species most commonly identified. Since 1970, MAI has been more commonly identified than *M. scrofulaceum* (44, 63). Whether this represents a true change, reporting artifact, or more reliable identification by laboratories remains unknown but may reflect a decrease in environmental levels of *M. scrofulaceum* and an increase in *M. avium* levels (16).

Skin testing with mycobacterial antigens is a potentially useful diagnostic strategy. Most children with NTM lymphadenitis have a weak reaction to PPD-S (63) but react more strongly to antigens derived from NTM strains (39). The specificity of such comparative testing in this population derives from the relatively small chance that these children have been exposed to *M. tuberculosis*. Unfortunately, these testing agents are not commercially available.

The differential diagnosis includes infection with *M. tuberculosis*, *M. bovis*, other NTM species, and various viruses (e.g., Epstein-Barr virus, cytomegalovirus, and mumps) and deep fungi. Other infections include brucellosis, cat scratch disease, and toxoplasmosis. Noninfectious causes include sarcoidosis, congenital cysts, lymphoma, lipoma, goiter, and drug-induced hyperplasia.

Differentiating NTM lymphadenitis from tuberculosis is usually not difficult. Age from 1 to 5 years, unilateral nodes, lack of systemic illness, no history of contact with active tuberculosis, normal chest radiograph, no or weak response to intermediate-strength tuberculin skin test, nonreactive tuberculin skin tests in siblings, early suppuration, and no response to antituberculous antibiotics are all points which favor NTM disease. There are no clinical clues which will distinguish *M. scrofulaceum* from any other NTM species. Ultimately, culture of biopsy or aspirated material is required for definitive diagnosis.

PULMONARY DISEASE

The vast majority of sputum isolates of *M. scrofulaceum* represent asymptomatic colonization. These are frequently old tuberculosis patients being monitored with serial mycobacterial cultures. True invasive disease is seen occasionally, resulting in an indolent, slowly progressive cavitary pneumonitis. All eight cases reported by Wolinksy (64) had industrial dust or fume exposure, but disease has occurred in the normal host (23). In this report, Gracey and Byrd described a 48-year-old man with an occasionally productive early morning cough and 25-pound weight loss over 1 year. There was no known tuberculosis contact and no industrial exposure. He was afebrile and had posttussive rales over the right lung apex. Chest radiograph had a nodular infiltrate in the right upper lobe, with tomography showing a thin-walled cavity. There was an 8-mm indurated reaction to intermediate-strength PPD skin testing and a 10-mm reaction to PPD-B. Erythrocyte sedimentation rate and routine laboratory values were normal. Three consecutive sputum samples grew a group II scotochromogen, further characterized as falling between

the *M. scrofulaceum* and *Mycobacterium aquae* subgroups. After 3 months of therapy with isoniazid, *para*-aminosalicylic acid, streptomycin, cycloserine, and ethionamide, the sputum remained acid-fast bacillus smear positive but culture negative. After 4 months, the chest radiograph was unchanged. He did well with surgical resection, although the duration of follow-up was not given. Pathology of the lung tissue showed fibrosis with caseating necrosis. There was no underlying pneumoconiosis. Multiple acid-fast bacilli were seen, but mycobacterial and fungal cultures were sterile. This was the only patient of 71 in this series with sputum isolates of group II scotochromogens thought to have invasive disease due to the organism.

LeMense et al. (36) described three pulmonary nodules in a 46-year-old man with a cardiac transplantation for an idiopathic cardiomyopathy. His medications were cyclosporine, azathioprine, trimethoprim-sulfamethoxazole, and acyclovir. He had had episodes of rejection at 7 and 12 months posttransplantation. A routine chest radiograph at 15 months showed a left lower lung nodule. He was asymptomatic but remembered a week-long influenza-like illness 1 month before. Computed tomography disclosed 3 noncalcified nodules. Wedge biopsy of one of the nodules revealed caseating granulomas and acid-fast bacilli, with *M. scrofulaceum* isolated from culture. The remaining two nodules decreased in size during a 6-month course of clarithromycin, ethambutol, and rifampin. Unfortunately, only 3 months of follow-up were reported, during which time the patient remained asymptomatic and the chest radiograph was unchanged.

In a survey of nontuberculous mycobacteria isolated from sputum samples of human immunodeficiency virus (HIV)-negative South African gold miners in the mid-1990s (11) 41 of 297 isolates were *M. scrofulaceum*. Thirty-five of these patients had premorbid chest radiographs for comparison, of which 31 (89%) demonstrated new cavitations. The authors calculated the incidence of *M. scrofulaceum* pulmonary disease to be 12 per 100,000 person-years. It therefore appears that pulmonary disease may be more common than previously thought in at least some selected populations.

EXTRAPULMONARY DISEASE

A small number of extrapulmonary isolates have been reported over the years. Unfortunately, many of the early reports did not identify the organism beyond the level of scotochromogen.

Bojalil (3) reported an isolate from a spinal cord abscess without clinical details. Yamamoto et al. (67)

reported six cases of meningitis due to NTM, five of which were due to scotochromogens. There were four women and one man with an age range of 2 to 32 years. All were said to have had "clinical manifestations of meningitis." In two of the four females, disease started after pregnancy. Chest radiographs showed "fibrocaseous lesions with cavity" in two patients, miliary lesions in one, and no findings in two. The patient with the miliary lesions died. The others were cured with unspecified chemotherapy.

A single case of granulomatous hepatitis has been recognized (45). This was a 39-year-old man with a 3-year history of mild epigastric pain, diffuse aches, fatigue, and night sweats. An abscess of the left groin had been drained during the first year of illness without culture. His temperature was elevated to 101.5°F two to three times per week. Physical examination showed hepatosplenomegaly. Laboratory showed normal SGOT and bilirubin and an elevated alkaline phosphatase. An intermediate strength PPD was "normal." Chest and spinal radiographs were normal. Liver biopsy demonstrated noncaseating granulomas, and culture of the liver tissue grew *M. scrofulaceum*. After 1 year of treatment with isoniazid, rifampin, and cycloserine, the patient was asymptomatic and the alkaline phosphatase level had returned to normal. No long-term follow-up was reported.

A report in 2000 (46) described a case of osteomyelitis/tenosynovitis in the wrist of a 66-year-old diabetic man. He failed to respond to standard antituberculosis therapy. Cultures eventually grew *M. scrofulaceum*, and the infection was controlled with the combination of kanamycin, ethambutol, and ethionamide. A more recent report (8) described a case of flexor tendonitis of the hand in a diabetic male which responded to debridement and a 6-month course of doxycycline.

A number of reports document multisystem disease with the organism isolated from multiple sites, mimicking miliary tuberculosis (7, 10, 13, 15, 17, 26, 30, 38, 40, 41, 50, 53, 54, 56, 60, 69). Some of these patients have had underlying immunodeficiency states (including one adult and one child with gamma interferon receptor 1 deficiency, both of whom developed multifocal osteomyelitis) (17, 38), but others have been apparently normal hosts. In retrospect, one wonders about the HIV status of these apparently normal patients reported before the recognition of AIDS. However, one report (53) documents a patient as being HIV seronegative. That only 14 cases of disseminated disease with *M. scrofulaceum* have been reported in AIDS patients testifies to the low level of the virulence of this organism. Three cases of immune reconstitution syndrome in HIV-positive children have been associated with bacteremia (50).

SKIN DISEASE

There are several reports of cutaneous disease (21, 43). The first (43) was a 32-year-old man with corticosteroid-dependent systemic lupus erythematosis. Multiple painful subcutaneous abscesses appeared over a 3-week period. He was afebrile and otherwise well. His chest radiograph had calcified granulomata. Skin biopsy demonstrated granulomatous inflammation and acid-fast bacilli. The cultures grew *M. scrofulaceum*. The patient received a 9-month course of isoniazid and rifampin despite in vitro resistance to both agents. The lesions healed completely within 5 months, and he remained lesion-free for 2 years of follow-up.

Abbott and Smith (1) listed a single renal transplantation patient on prednisone and chlorambucil as having "skin lesions" positive for *M. scrofulaceum* by microscopy and culture. Sowers (57) described a progressive sporotrichoid skin lesion on both hands of a 77-year-old woman whose hands were chronically exposed to aquarium water. The lesion did not respond to a 5-month course of isoniazid, ethambutol, and topical isoniazid 10% cream. Another aquarium water-associated case (27) grew both *M. scrofulaceum* and *Mycobacterium peregrinum*. This patient responded to successive courses of sparfloxacin and minocycline. Kandyil et al. (31) reported a skin nodule on the index finger of a 59-year-old woman who was 7 months post-autologous bone marrow transplantation for breast cancer. She had exposure to "thorny roses that had been soaking in slimy water" and had sustained a recent paper cut. Her lesion resolved with a course of azithromycin and rifampin of unspecified duration. Most recently, Jang et al. (28) reported an asymptomatic red nodule on the cheek of a previously healthy 4-year-old girl, which grew *M. scrofulaceum*, identified by biochemical and PCR testing. The lesion resolved after 6 months of treatment with clarithromycin (250 mg) daily.

ANTIBIOTIC SENSITIVITY

The sensitivity of *M. scrofulaceum* to antituberculous antibiotics has been reported sporadically. It is one of the most resistant of all NTM species. Unfortunately, few of the reports of clinical isolates describe the methodology used. The organism is resistant to isoniazid, *para*-aminosalicylic acid, and kanamycin. Some strains are sensitive to rifampin, rifabutin, ethambutol, streptomycin, cycloserine, amikacin, ethionamide, viomycin, and capreomycin. Using modern broth dilution methods, the MICs of clarithromycin (5), roxithromycin (51), and sparfloxacin (68) have recently been shown to be within potentially clinically useful ranges.

TREATMENT

No comparative or controlled treatment trials have ever been reported. A large body of anecdotal evidence suggests that antibiotic therapy has no benefit in lymphadenitis and that node resection usually suffices for complete cure (37, 63, 64). It might be noted that this experience predates the advent of the newer macrolide and fluoroquinolone antibiotics which possess promising in vitro activity.

The experience with systemic disease has simply been too scant and variable to allow any strong recommendations to be made. Certainly a trial of two or more agents with demonstrated in vitro activity would seem justified in patients with disease which cannot be surgically removed.

REFERENCES

1. Abbott, M. R., and D. D. Smith. 1981. Mycobacterial infections in immunosuppressed patients. *Med. J. Aust.* 1:351–353.
2. Allen, E. A. 1995. Tuberculosis and other mycobacterial infections of the lung, p. 253–254. *In* W. M. Thurbeck and A. M. Chung (ed.), *Pathology of the Lung*, 2nd ed. Thieme Medical Publishers, New York, NY.
3. Bojalil, L. F. 1961. Frequency and epidemiologic significance of unclassified mycobacteria in Mexico. *Am. Rev. Respir. Dis.* 83:596–599.
4. Brooks, R. W., B. C. Parker, H. Gruft, and J. O. Falkinham III. 1984. Epidemiology of infection by nontuberculous mycobacteria. V. Numbers in eastern United States soils and correlation with soil characteristics. *Am. Rev. Respir. Dis.* 130:630–633.
5. Brown, B. A., R. J. Wallace, Jr., and G. O. Onyi. 1992. Activities of clarithromycin against eight slowly growing species of nontuberculous mycobacteria, determined by using a broth microdilution MIC system. *Antimicrob. Agents Chemother.* 36:1987–1990.
6. Bruins, J., J. H. Gribnau, and R. Bwire. 1995. Investigation into typical and atypical tuberculin sensitivity in the Royal Netherlands Army, resulting in a more rational indication for isoniazid prophylaxis. *Tuber. Lung Dis.* 76:540–544.
7. Campos-Herrero, M. I., H. Rodriguez, J. Lluch, M. Perdomo, M. C. Pérez, and E. Gómez. 1996. Infeccion diseminada por *Mycobacterium scrofulaceum*: a proposito de 3 casos. *Enferm. Infecc. Microbiol. Clin.* 14:258–260.
8. Carter, T. I., P. Frelinghuysen, A. Daluiski, B. D. Brause, and S. W. Wolfe. 2006. Flexor tenosynovitis caused by *Mycobacterium scrofulaceum*: case report. *J. Hand Surg. Am.* 31:1292–1295.
9. Chapman, J. S., J. S. Bernard, and M. Speight. 1965. Isolation of mycobacteria from raw milk. *Am. Rev. Respir. Dis.* 91:351–355.
10. Choonhakarn, C., P. Chetchotisakd, K. Jirarattanapochai, and P. Mootsikapun. 1998. Sweet's syndrome associated with nontuberculous mycobacterial infection: a report of five cases. *Br. J. Dermatol.* 139:107–110.
11. Corbett, E. L., M. Hay, G. J. Churchyard, P. Herselman, T. Clayton, and B. G. Williams. 1999. *Mycobacterium kansasii* and *M. scrofulaceum* isolates from HIV-negative South African gold miners: incidence, clinical significance and radiology. *Int. J. Tuberc. Lung Dis.* 3:501–507.
12. Dascalopoulos, G. A., S. Loukas, and S. H. Constantopoulos. 1995. Wide geographic variations of sensitivity of MOTT sensitins in Greece. *Eur. Respir. J.* 8:715–717.
13. Delabie, J., C. De Wolf-Peeters, H. Bobbaers, G. Bilbe, and V. J. Desmet. 1991. Immunophenotypic analysis of histiocytes involved in AIDS-associated *Mycobacterium scrofulaceum* infection: similarities with lepromatous lepra. *Clin. Exp. Immunol.* 85:214–218.
14. Dunn, B. L., and D. J. Hodgson. 1982. "Atypical" mycobacteria in milk. *J. Appl. Bacteriol.* 52:373–376.
15. Dustin, P., P. Demol, D. Derks-Jacobovitz, N. Cremer, and H. Vis. 1980. Generalized fatal chronic infection by *Mycobacterium scrofulaceum* with severe amyloidosis in a child. *Pathol. Res. Pract.* 168:237–248.
16. Falkinham, J. D., III. 1996. Epidemiology of infection by nontuberculosis mycobacteria. *Clin. Microbiol. Rev.* 91:177–215.
17. Glosli, H., A. Stray-Pedersen, A. C. Brun, L. W. Holtmon, T. Tanjum, A. Chapgier, J. L. Casanova, and T. G. Abrahamsen. 2008. Infections due to various atypical mycobacteria in a Norwegian multiplex family with dominant interferon-γ receptor deficiency. *Clin. Infect. Dis.* 46:e23–e27.
18. Good, R. C., and D. E. Snider, Jr. 1982. Isolation of nontuberculous mycobacteria from the United States, 1980. *J. Infect. Dis.* 146:829–833.
19. Good, R. C. 1980. Isolation of nontuberculous mycobacteria in the United States, 1979. *J. Infect. Dis.* 142:779–883.
20. Good, R. C. 1985. Opportunistic pathogens in the genus *Mycobacterium*. *Annu. Rev. Microbiol.* 39:347–369.
21. Gorse, G. J., R. D. Fairshter, G. Friedly, L. Mela Maza, G. R. Greene, and T. C. Cesario. 1983. Nontuberculous mycobacterial disease. Experience in a southern California hospital. *Arch. Intern. Med.* 143:225–228.
22. Goslee, S., and E. Wolinsky. 1976. Water as a source of potentially pathogenic mycobacteria. *Am. Rev. Respir. Dis.* 113:287–292.
23. Gracey, D. R., and R. B. Byrd. 1970. Scotochromogens and pulmonary disease. Five years' experience at a pulmonary disease center with report of a case. *Am. Rev. Respir. Dis.* 101:959–963.
24. Grzybowski, S., and E. A. Allen. 1995. History and importance of scrofula. *Lancet* 346:1472–1474.
25. Hosty, T. S., and C. I. McDurmont. 1975. Isolation of acid-fast organisms from milk and oysters. *Health Lab. Sci.* 12:16–19.
26. Hsueh, P. R., T. R. Hsiue, J. J. Jarn, S. W. Ho, and W. C. Hsieh. 1996. Disseminated infection due to *Mycobacterium scrofulaceum* in an immunocompetent host. *Clin. Infect. Dis.* 22:156–161.
27. Ishii, N., Y. Sugita, I. Sato, and H. Nakajima. 1998. A case of mycobacterial skin disease caused by *Mycobacterium peregrinum* and *M. scrofulaceum*. *Acta Derm. Venereol.* 78:76–77.
28. Jang, H., J. Jo, C. Oh, M. Kim, J. Lee, C. L. Chang, Y. W. Kwon, and K. S. Kwon. 2005. Successful treatment of localized cutaneous infection caused by *Mycobacterium scrofulaceum* with clarithromycin. *Pediatr. Dermatol.* 22:476–479.
29. Jin, B. W., H. Saito, and Z. Yoshii. 1984. Environmental mycobacteria in Korea. I. Distribution of the organisms. *Microbiol. Immunol.* 128:667–677.
30. Joos, H. A., L. B. Hilty, D. Courington, W. B. Schaefer, and M. Block. 1967. Fatal disseminated scotochromogenic mycobacteriosis in a child. *Am. Rev. Respir. Dis.* 96:795–801.
31. Kandyil, R., D. Maloney, J. Tarrand, and M. Duvic. 2002. Red nodule on the finger of an immunosuppressed woman. *Arch. Dermatol.* 128:689–694.
32. Kirschner, R. A., Jr., B. C. Parker, and J. O. Falkinham III. 1992. Epidemiology of infection by nontuberculous mycobacteria. *Mycobacterium avium, Mycobacterium intracellu-*

lare, and *Mycobacterium scrofulaceum* in acid, brown-water swamps of the southeastern United States and their association with environmental variables. *Am. Rev. Respir. Dis.* **145**: 271–275.

33. **Krajnack, M. A., and H. Dowda.** 1981. Non-tuberculous mycobacteria in South Carolina, 1971-1980. *J. S. C. Med. Assoc.* **77**:551–555.

34. **Kubalek, I., and J. Mysak.** 1996. The prevalence of environmental mycobacteria in drinking water supply systems in a demarcated region in Czech Republic, in the period 1984-1989. *Eur. J. Epidemiol.* **12**:471–474.

35. **Kwamanga, D. O., O. B. Swai, R. Agwanda, and W. Githui.** 1995. Effect of non-tuberculous mycobacteria infection on tuberculin results among primary school children in Kenya. *East Afr. Med. J.* **72**:222–227.

36. **LeMense, G. P., A. B. VanBakel, A. J. Crumbley III, and M. A. Judson.** 1994. *Mycobacterium scrofulaceum* infection presenting as lung nodules in a heart transplant recipient. *Chest* **106**: 1918–1920.

37. **Lincoln, E. M., and L. A. Gilbert.** 1972. Disease in children due to mycobacteria other than *Mycobacterium tuberculosis. Am. Rev. Respir. Dis.* **105**:683–714.

38. **Marazzi, M. G., A. Capgier, A.-C. Defilippi, V. Pistoia, S. Mangini, C. Savioli, A. Dell'Acqua, J. Feinberg, E. Tortoli, and J.-L. Casanova.** 2009. Disseminated *Mycobacterium scrofulaceum* infection in a child with interferon-γ receptor 1 deficiency. *Int. J. Infect. Dis.* **10**:1016–1019.

39. **Margileth, A. M.** 1983. The use of purified protein derivative mycobacterial skin test antigens in children and adolescents: purified protein derivative skin test results correlated with mycobacterial isolates. *Pediatr. Infect. Dis.* **2**:225–231.

40. **McCusker, J. J., and R. A. Green.** 1962. Generalized nontuberculous mycobacteriosis: report of two cases. *Am. Rev. Respir. Dis.* **86**:405–414.

41. **McNutt, D. D., and H. H. Fudenberg.** 1971. Disseminated scotochromogen infection and unusual myeloproliferative disorder: report of a case and review of the literature. *Ann. Intern. Med.* **75**:737–744.

42. **Meissner, P. S., and J. O. Falkinham III.** 1986. Plasmid DNA profiles as epidemiologic markers for clinical and environmental isolates of *Mycobacterium avium, Mycobacterium intracellulare*, and *Mycobacterium scrofulaceum. J. Infect. Dis.* **153**: 325–330.

43. **Murray-Leisure, K. A., N. Egan, and M. R. Weitekamp.** 1987. Skin lesions caused by *Mycobacterium scrofulaceum. Arch. Dermatol.* **123**:369–370.

44. **O'Brien, R. J., L. J. Geiter, and D. E. Snider, Jr.** 1987. The epidemiology of nontuberculous mycobacterial diseases in the United States. *Am. Rev. Respir. Dis.* **135**:1007–1014.

45. **Patel, K. M.** 1981. Granulomatous hepatitis due to *Mycobacterium scrofulaceum*: report of a case. *Gastroenterology* **81**: 156–158.

46. **Phoa, L. L., K. S. Khong, T. P. Thamboo, and K. N. Lam.** 2000. A case of *Mycobacterium scrofulaceum* osteomyelitis of the right wrist. *Ann. Acad. Med. Singapore* **29**:678–681.

47. **Prissick, F. H., and A. M. Masson.** 1952. A preliminary report on a study of pigmented mycobacteria. *Can. J. Public Health* **43**:34.

48. **Prissick, F. H., and A. M. Masson.** 1956. Cervical lymphadenitis in children caused by chromogenic mycobacteria. *Can. Med. Assoc. J.* **75**:798–803.

49. **Prissick, F. H., and A. M. Masson.** 1957. Yellow-pigmented pathogenic mycobacteria from cervical lymphadenitis. *Can. J. Microbiol.* **3**:91–100.

50. **Puthanakit, T., P. Oberdorfer, N. Ukarapol, N. Akarathum, S. Punjaisee, T. Sirisanthana, and V. Sirisanthana.** 2006. Immune reconstitution syndrome from nontuberculous mycobacterial infection after initiation of antiretroviral therapy in children with HIV infection. *Pediatr. Infect. Dis. J.* **7**:645–648.

51. **Rastogi, N., K. S. Goh, and A. Bryskier.** 1993. In vitro activity of roxithromycin against 16 species of atypical mycobacteria and effect of pH on its radiometric MIC. *Antimicrob. Agents Chemother.* **37**:1560–1562.

52. **Rogall, T., T. Wolters, T. Flohr, and E. C. Böttger.** 1990. Towards the phylogeny and definition of species at the molecular level within the genus *Mycobacterium. Int. J. Syst. Bacteriol.* **40**:323–330.

53. **Saad, M. H., V. Vincent, D. J. Dawson, M. Palaci, L. Ferrazoli, and L. D. S. Fonseca.** 1997. Analysis of *Mycobacterium avium* complex serovars isolated from AIDS patients from southeast Brazil. *Mem. Inst. Oswaldo Cruz* **92**:471–475.

54. **Sanders, J. W., A. D. Walsh, R. L. Snider, and E. E. Sahn.** 1995. Disseminated *Mycobacterium scrofulaceum* infection: a potentially treatable complication of AIDS. *Clin. Infect. Dis.* **20**: 549–556.

55. **Schroder, K. H., J. Kazda, K. Muller, and H. J. Muller.** 1992. Isolation of *Mycobacterium simiae* from the environment. *Int. J. Med. Microbiol. Virol. Parasitol. Infect. Dis.* **277**:561–564.

56. **Shafer, R. W., and M. F. Sierra.** 1992. *Mycobacterium xenopi, Mycobacterium fortuitum, Mycobacterium kansasii*, and other nontuberculous mycobacteria in an area of endemicity for AIDS. *Clin. Infect. Dis.* **15**:161–162.

57. **Sowers, W. F.** 1972. Swimming pool granuloma due to *Mycobacterium scrofulaceum. Arch. Dermatol.* **105**:760–761.

58. **Svandova, E., J. Stastna, and M. Kubin.** 1984. Comparative testing of skin reactions to PPD mycobacterins from *Mycobacterium tuberculosis* and *Mycobacterium scrofulaceum* in school-age children. *J. Hyg. Epidemiol. Microbiol. Immunol.* **29**:275–281.

59. **Tsukamura, M.** 1970. Appropriate name for tap water scotochromogens. *Am. Rev. Respir. Dis.* **102**:643–644.

60. **Vinh, L. T., T. V. Duc, P. Nevot, and M. A. St. Thieffry.** 1966. Infection généralisée mortelle due à une mycobactérie atypique. *Arch. Franc. Petiatr.* **23**:1155–1166.

61. **Wayne, L. G., J. R. Doubek, and G. A. Diaz.** 1967. Classification and identification of mycobacteria. IV. Some important scotochromogens. *Am. Rev. Respir. Dis.* **96**:88–95.

62. **Wayne, L. G.** 1970. On the identity of *Mycobacterium gordonae* Bojalil and the so-called tap water scotochromogens. *Int. J. Syst. Bacteriol.* **20**:149–153.

63. **Wolinsky, E., and T. K. Rynearson.** 1968. Mycobacteria in soil and their relation to disease-associated strains. *Am. Rev. Respir. Dis.* **97**:1032–1037.

64. **Wolinsky, E.** 1995. Mycobacterial lymphadenitis in children: a prospective study of 105 nontuberculous cases with long-term follow-up. *Clin. Infect. Dis.* **20**:954–963.

65. **Wolinsky, E.** 1979. Nontuberculous mycobacteria and associated diseases. *Am. Rev. Respir. Dis.* **119**:107–159.

66. **Woods, G., and J. Washington.** 1987. Mycobacteria other than *Mycobacterium tuberculosis*: review of microbiologic and clinical aspects. *Rev. Infect. Dis.* **9**:275–294.

67. **Yamamoto, M., K. Sudo, M. Taga, and S. Hibino.** 1967. A study of diseases caused by atypical mycobacteria in Japan. *Am. Rev. Respir. Dis.* **96**:779–787.

68. **Yew, W. W., L. J. Piddock, M. S. Li, D. Lyon, C. Y. Chan, and A. F. Cheng.** 1994. In-vitro activity of quinolones and macrolides against mycobacteria. *J. Antimicrob. Chemother.* **34**:343–351.

69. **Zamorano, J., Jr., and R. Tompsett.** 1968. Disseminated atypical mycobacterial infection and pancytopenia. *Arch. Intern. Med.* **121**:424–427.

Chapter 41

Mycobacterium bovis and Other Uncommon Members of the *Mycobacterium tuberculosis* Complex

JAIME ESTEBAN AND NOELIA ALONSO-RODRÍGUEZ

Just a few years after Koch's discovery of the tuberculous bacillus in 1882, Theobald Smith found that there were constant phenotypical differences between tuberculous bacilli of human origin and those isolated from cattle, so he subsequently divided the species into human and bovine tubercle bacilli (50). Both species shared common characteristics, but some differences appeared. Probably, the most important one is the low pathogenicity for animals of human strains, while the bovine bacillus could infect both animals and humans and was noted as an important cause of extrapulmonary tuberculosis in humans (15). Moreover, new species of the tuberculous bacillus were described, and some of them also appeared to cause human disease (5, 26; http://www.bacterio.cict.fr/m/mycobacterium.html) (Table 1).

All these organisms, together with the species *Mycobacterium tuberculosis*, form the so-called *Mycobacterium tuberculosis* complex, with important differences among these organisms in epidemiology, microbiology, and even therapy.

EPIDEMIOLOGY AND MOLECULAR TYPING METHODS

Mycobacterium bovis is an ancient pathogen that causes disease in humans and a majority of cases of tuberculosis in cattle and a large number of domesticated and wild mammal species (25, 35, 85). It had long been assumed that *M. tuberculosis*, the principal causative agent of tuberculosis in humans, evolved from *M. bovis* by specific adaptation to the human host around 10,000 to 15,000 years ago, associated with cattle domestication (13). However, recent studies have shown that *M. bovis* (together with other members of *M. tuberculosis* complex such as *M. africanum* and *M. microti*) is part of a separate lineage of bacteria that share a common ancestor with *M. tuberculosis* (13, 47).

M. bovis has a greater number of potential hosts than *M. tuberculosis*. Domestic cattle are considered its natural hosts and the principal reservoir of infection for other animals and humans (19, 50). However, wild animals have a potential role in the maintenance and spread of the disease (36). Some known examples are the European badger in the United Kingdom and the Republic of Ireland (46, 82), the possum and the ferret in New Zealand (20), the red deer and wild boar in Spain (6), the Cape buffalo in parts of South Africa (72), and the white-tailed deer in Michigan (United States) (36).

Some studies have estimated that 0.3 to 1.5% of tuberculosis in humans is due to *M. bovis* in developed countries (23, 27, 50, 84, 92, 93, 115). By contrast, although the percentage of *M. bovis* tuberculosis cases in most developing countries remains unknown due to inappropriate isolation and identification, it is likely to be higher than in the industrialized ones, constituting a major threat to public health (8, 9, 19, 23, 24, 34).

Transmission of *M. bovis* can occur between domestic and wild animals, from animals to humans, and more rarely, from humans to animals or between humans (50, 77, 85, 87, 105). The infection is acquired by aerosol inhalation, ingestion, or direct contact with mucous membranes (35, 50). Bovine tuberculosis in cattle is mainly a disease of the respiratory tract, and dissemination of bacilli in aerosols represents the main source of infection among other animals and humans (70, 77). Human infection has been frequently associated with ingestion of unpasteurized milk and milk products from animals with infected udders. More rarely, it has also been described following ingestion of insufficiently cooked bovine meat. Nowadays, these routes of infections remain only in developing countries where bovine tuberculosis is prevalent, control measures are not applied, and/or pasteurization is rarely practiced (9,

Jaime Esteban and Noelia Alonso-Rodríguez • Department of Clinical Microbiology, IIS-Fundación Jiménez Díaz, Madrid, Spain.

Table 1. Members of the *Mycobacterium tuberculosis* complex

Species	Human pathogen	Yr of description
Mycobacterium tuberculosis	Frequent	1883
Mycobacterium bovis	Frequent	1907
Mycobacterium bovis BCG	Rare	NA[c]
Mycobacterium africanum	Frequent	1969
Mycobacterium caprae	Occasional[a]	2003
Mycobacterium microti	Rare	1957
Mycobacterium pinnipedii	No[b]	2003
"*Mycobacterium canettii*"	Rare	NA[c]

[a]Actual incidence of *M. caprae* is still to be determined in many countries where infection due to *M. bovis* is still of importance.
[b]No human disease due to *M. pinnipedii* has been described, although cases of probable infection secondary to seal disease have been published (58).
[c]NA, not accepted as a different species or subspecies in current classification schemes (http://www.bacterio.cict.fr/m/mycobacterium.html).

23). On the contrary, in developed countries where the implementation of pasteurization of milk is generalized, the incidence of infection was reduced notably and most of the cases occur in older people as reactivation of infections acquired in the past, when animal infection was still common (50, 87). Moreover, the implementation of policies of detection and slaughter in developed countries had reduced the number of contagious animals (22, 35, 50), minimizing the risk of contagion from the usual way. Development of these policies is, however, expensive, and their implementation in developing countries remains difficult for many reasons, including economic ones.

Transmission of *M. bovis* to humans from animals other than cattle occurs only sporadically and is associated with specific occupations like farmers, veterinarians, abattoir workers, animal handlers, or hunters (29, 42, 67, 93, 106, 114). On the other hand, infected humans can also represent a potential source of *M. bovis* infection for animal and human contacts (50, 85). Although evidence of transmission from humans to animals has been reported anecdotally (50, 97), some studies have noted person-to-person transmission associated with nosocomial outbreaks (12, 48, 51, 86, 91, 113) and others sporadically detected in an urban setting (41). In most of these cases, immunosuppression induced by human immunodeficiency virus (HIV) coinfection, cancer therapy, alcohol misuse, and/or insulin-dependent diabetes mellitus could have played an important role by increasing the susceptibility of the host to develop active disease.

The establishment of effective tuberculosis control measures requires understanding of the transmission dynamics of the pathogen and factors involved in disease origin and dissemination. The emergence of molecular epidemiology integrates molecular biology, clinical medicine, and classic epidemiology with this purpose. In this sense, the development of DNA fingerprinting techniques since the 1990s (60) has allowed investigators to identify what cases are infected by strains sharing genotypes and then what cases are involved in the same transmission chain (58, 68).

In contrast to *M. tuberculosis*, restriction fragment length polymorphism (RFLP) typing based on the insertion sequence IS6110 (IS6110 RFLP), the gold standard for *M. tuberculosis* genotyping, provides only limited discrimination among *M. bovis* isolates because this species usually has only one or a few IS6110 copies, especially in isolates from cattle (98). The resolution of the IS6110 RFLP method is inversely proportional to the number of IS6110 copies, due to the existence of IS6110 insertion hot spots. Thus, it has been established that identical RFLP patterns with six or fewer bands are not appropriate to establish recent transmission (60).

Another common epidemiological genotyping method for *M. bovis* strains is spoligotyping. This method analyzes the polymorphisms derived from the presence or absence of 43 spacer sequences found in the direct repeat (DR) region in strains of the *M. tuberculosis* complex (57, 109). The spoligotyping is a fast and reproducible method, and genotypes (based on binary data) can be easily interpreted, computerized, and compared intra- and interlaboratory (www.mbovis.org) (Fig. 1). However, spoligotyping offers a low discriminatory power, and identical patterns are not always related to recent transmission (60). Recently, some studies have included in the analysis a new set of 25 additional spacers, achieving further characterization for *M. bovis*, *M. africanum*, and *M. caprae* isolates (56, 107), although they have not been included in the standardized membrane yet.

In recent years, variable-number tandem repeat (VNTR) sequences have been documented as molecular markers highly discriminative for the genotyping of several bacterial species, especially for genetically homogeneous pathogens such as *M. tuberculosis* complex members (45, 66, 102). Some of the VNTR sequences identified in the *M. tuberculosis* complex were named mycobacterial interspersed

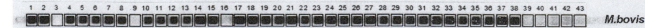

Figure 1. Spoligotyping pattern of *Mycobacterium bovis*. Spacers in the DR locus are indicated by the numbers 1 to 43.

repetitive units (MIRU) (102, 103), and for this reason, the genotyping method is known as both VNTR and MIRU-VNTR. This genotyping method is a PCR-based technique that analyzes the number of repetitions of tandem sequences (from 40 to 120 bp) dispersed in intergenic regions in the genome. The advantages of the MIRU-VNTR method are its high-throughput, discriminatory, and reproducible analysis. Moreover, genotyping profiles are numerical and easily managed and exchanged between laboratories (11, 68).

During the course of evaluation of MIRU-VNTR, different sets of loci have been analyzed, from the early MIRU-12 format (set of 12 loci) to the current more-discriminative MIRU-15 (set of 15 loci) or MIRU-24 (set of 24 loci) format, tested in analyses carried out in different epidemiological contexts (3, 18, 83, 101, 103). However, nowadays, the consensus apparently achieved for the application of the MIRU-24 format in *M. tuberculosis* epidemiological studies seems to not be appropriate for *M. bovis* genotyping. Some authors remarked that the MIRU-24 format does not provide sufficient discrimination power to track *M. bovis* transmission chains and have proposed a new set of loci involving some of those included in the MIRU-24 format and new additional VNTR loci (2, 94, 99). At present, despite efforts invested in standardizing a MIRU-VNTR format for application in *M. bovis* epidemiological studies, this goal has not yet been achieved.

MYCOBACTERIUM BOVIS DISEASE AND ITS DIAGNOSIS

Human disease caused by *M. bovis* is indistinguishable clinically or pathologically from the disease caused by *M. tuberculosis* (14, 23, 30, 39, 41, 54, 73, 84). However, *M. bovis* tuberculosis has been reported by some to have a higher percentage of extrapulmonary syndromes than *M. tuberculosis* disease (14, 23, 30, 54), although other studies showed a higher percentage of lung disease than extrapulmonary disease (39, 41, 85). The explanation for these differences has been related to the route of invasion of the pathogen: *M. bovis* ingested with contaminated milk is usually associated with lymph node or intestinal disease, while respiration-acquired infection is associated with lung disease. Other extrapulmonary forms of tuberculosis due to *M. bovis*, such as genitourinary or osteoarticular disease (Fig. 2), are also found in the same sites affected in *M. tuberculosis* infection but with a lower percentage of pleural disease (30).

In adults, the extrapulmonary forms are usually due to reactivation of older infections, although lung

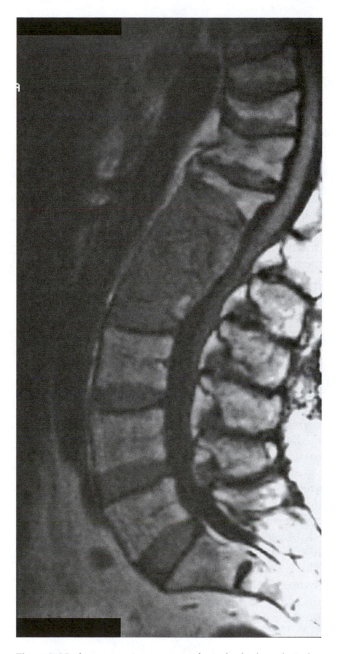

Figure 2. Nuclear magnetic resonance of vertebral tuberculosis due to *Mycobacterium bovis*.

disease remains the most common form of *M. bovis* tuberculosis, with development of disseminated disease especially among immunocompromised hosts, including those with AIDS (30, 39, 95).

Among children, the most common forms of disease are the involvement of cervical lymph nodes and intestinal disease, which probably reflect the most frequent form of acquisition of the bacterium (30). For this reason, it is very important to establish the etiologic cause of the disease, not only for therapeutic but also for epidemiologic and public health reasons.

M. bovis has been described as the causative agent of several outbreaks, most of them caused by drinking infected milk. However, one of these outbreaks with greater relevance was caused by an extremely drug-resistant (XDR) *M. bovis* strain due to airborne transmission between humans (12, 51). These outbreaks present common characteristics with multidrug-resistant (MDR) *M. tuberculosis* outbreaks, including high mortality, high percentage of disseminated disease among the affected patients, and rapid progression of the infected contacts to active forms of disease.

Diagnosis of *M. bovis* disease needs the isolation of the causal organism and its proper identification. Cultural differences between *M. tuberculosis* and *M. bovis* have been known since the discovery of both organisms. *M. bovis* requires pyruvate-supplemented media because it is not able to use glycerol as a carbon source (21). This fact leads to a poor growth of the bacterium in pyruvate-free media like Lowenstein-Jensen, arguably the most commonly used media for mycobacterial culture. In this medium, *M. bovis* showed dysgonic colonies, a feature that must suggest to the microbiologist the possibility of an *M. bovis* isolate. *M. bovis* can be also recovered from different Middlebrook media (both liquid and solid) with good results (53) (Fig. 3), so the implementation of currently automated liquid systems (based on this medium) would allow a higher detection from clinical samples than classical egg-based solid media.

Differential diagnosis between *M. tuberculosis* and *M. bovis* has been performed classically using different biochemical tests (21, 50), such as nitrate reductase (positive for *M. tuberculosis*, negative for *M. bovis*), susceptibility to pyrazinamide (*M. bovis* is resistant, while *M. tuberculosis* is usually susceptible), susceptibility to thiophene-2-carboxylic acid hydrazide (*M. bovis* is susceptible, *M. tuberculosis* is resistant), and niacin accumulation (positive for *M. tuberculosis*, negative for *M. bovis*) (21, 50).

However, these tests are time-consuming, require experience for their proper use and interpretation, and cannot be easily performed in medium- to low-size clinical mycobacteriology laboratories. Another disadvantage based on these phenotypical tests was the identification of *M. bovis* isolates with characteristics similar to *M. tuberculosis* (62). In the last decades, DNA probes became the most common molecular-based tool for identification of pathogenic mycobacterial isolates. However, these probes only provide identification as *M. tuberculosis* complex (78), and additional biochemical tests are necessary for species identification.

The publication of the complete genome sequence of *M. bovis* in 2003 (47) has allowed the search for specific genetic markers associated with *M. tuberculosis* or *M. bovis*. In this way, *M. bovis* strains lack the *mtp40* sequence found in *M. tuberculosis* (112), lack the chromosomal regions RD7, RD8, RD9, and RD10 (13), and carry a particular mutation at position 169 in the *pncA* gene conferring pyrazinamide resistance (96). A specific mutation at position 285 in the *oxyR* gene (100) and the absence of spacers 3, 9, 16, and 39 to 43 in the DR locus (52, 57) have been also described as characteristic for *M. bovis*. However, these markers are not usually analyzed in microbiology diagnostic laboratories but are restricted to reference or research laboratories. Recently, a commercial system based on PCR and hybridization has been introduced in the routine of several clinical laboratories. This system allows an easy identification of the species from the *M. tuberculosis* complex (90). Species identification of the isolates is mandatory for the reasons previously described, and the tools needed for this purpose should be available to all clinical microbiology laboratories which perform species identification of mycobacterial isolates.

SUSCEPTIBILITY AND TREATMENT

M. bovis disease has been treated with antibiotic regimens similar to those used in the treatment of disease caused by *M. tuberculosis*. However, differences between them start with the constitutive resistance to pyrazinamide of *M. bovis* (30, 50). This finding has been used as a key characteristic for microbiological identification of the strains and has great importance in the use of different therapeutic approaches. The current recommended regimen for the treatment of tuberculosis includes the use of isoniazid, rifampin, and pyrazinamide for 2 months (with the addition of ethambutol until sensitivities are known), followed by isoniazid and rifampin for 4 months. This short

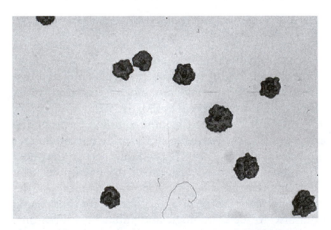

Figure 3. Microcolonies of *Mycobacterium bovis* in Middlebrook 7H11 after 1 week of incubation at 37°C. Magnification, ×10.

protocol is possible because of the introduction of pyrazinamide, a drug useless for the therapy of *M. bovis* because of its resistance (30). Different studies have remarked that in vitro resistance against other drugs seems to be rare, with low rates of isoniazid resistance (30). Otherwise, these rates are similar to that of *M. tuberculosis* in the study of Dankner et al. (30). Other investigators even showed absence of resistant strains, except for pyrazinamide, among a large number of isolates (88), a result confirmed by molecular techniques. However, because of the possibility of infection with resistant strains, susceptibility testing must be done as for *M. tuberculosis*, using the same technology as for *M. tuberculosis*. Treatment should be initiated with isoniazid, rifampin and ethambutol; if the isolate is sensitive to isoniazid and rifampin, these two drugs should be continued for a total of 9 months. If the isolate is isoniazid resistant, rifampin plus ethambutol for 12 months is a reasonable alternative.

MDR *M. bovis* strains, and even XDR *M. bovis* strains, are a rare finding. However, one outbreak of an XDR *M. bovis* strain was described among HIV patients in Spain in the mid-1990s (95). The outbreak started in one hospital in Madrid and extended through different hospitals in Spain and to other countries (39, 95). The strain showed resistance to all first-line antituberculous drugs and also to most second-line drugs. This fact made treatment extremely difficult for these patients, especially for HIV cases, which accounted for the greatest number of patients. Uncommonly used drugs for therapy of tuberculosis, such as linezolid or amoxicillin-clavulanic acid, were used in some cases, with relatively good results, especially among HIV-negative patients (39, 43).

MYCOBACTERIUM BOVIS BCG STRAIN

The BCG strain of *Mycobacterium bovis* is a laboratory-obtained attenuated strain described by Albert Calmette and Camille Guérin (bacille Calmette-Guérin [BCG]) in 1922 (15). It was obtained after many subcultures and showed no pathogenic potential for humans, so it has been used for antituberculous vaccination, being the only current vaccine against tuberculosis even today (38). The strain shows phenotypical characteristics similar to those of other *M. bovis* strains, except that it grows well in pyruvate-free media, with colonies resembling *M. tuberculosis*. The strain is susceptible to first-line antituberculous drugs except pyrazinamide.

Despite its use as an attenuated vaccine, some cases of human disease after vaccination have been described, especially among immunocompromised patients, such as those with primary immunodeficiencies (1), HIV infection (10, 108), or other conditions (16). The disease appears as a broad spectrum of syndromes, from self-limited local complications such as lymphadenitis (1) or local abscesses (104) to severe disseminated disease (1, 10, 16, 104). The last is the most important complication, being a potentially lethal disease (1, 16, 104). It usually starts with local signs, including ulceration, fistulization, and lymphadenopathy. Dissemination appears several weeks/months later, with fever, weight loss, multiorgan disease, and analytical elevation of nonspecific inflammatory markers (1, 16, 104). The disease has an ominous outcome, with mortality higher than 40 to 50% despite proper therapy. Although BCG complications are most frequently observed in children, in recent years, cases have been described among HIV patients several years after vaccination (108). Because of the risk of these severe forms of diseases, BCG vaccination is contraindicated in HIV-positive and other immunosuppressed patients, as with other live vaccines (38, 49).

Another medical use of the BCG strain was developed in 1976, when Morales et al. described the use of BCG strain in intravesical instillations as an adjuvant for the treatment of superficial bladder tumors (75). Its use as immunomodulator became popular, and as happened with BCG vaccination, complications eventually appeared. Lamm et al. described a broad spectrum of complications, including hematuria, cystitis, and fever most commonly, while extravesical complications were rare (65). Osteomyelitis (76, 81), lung and liver involvement, as well as disseminated disease (69) have been described as examples of reactivation following hematogenous spread of the bacterium from the bladder to other organs. Outcomes of these diseases, unlike postvaccination disseminated disease, are good when proper therapy is applied.

M. bovis BCG strains are usually susceptible to first-line antituberculous drugs and resistant to pyrazinamide, a fact that must be taken into account when the proper regimen is selected. Treatment of mild complications of vaccination (like injection abscesses) include drainage, needle aspiration, and use of erythromycin (250 mg/6 hours) or isoniazid (5 mg/kg of body weight daily) for 3 months (49). Uncomplicated cystitis after intravesical instillation can be treated with a quinolone for the same duration (116), though if emerging resistance is a concern, the quinolone could be replaced with isoniazid with or without rifampin. If epididymitis or prostatitis is detected, treatment should be undertaken with isoniazid plus rifampin for 6 months (64). It has been suggested that, in these patients, transient fever which lasts over

12 hours can be treated with isoniazid (300 mg/daily) for 3 months, a regimen that has also been used for hypersensitivity reactions (49).

Disseminated disease—systemic or localized—must be treated like other diseases caused by virulent *M. bovis* strains. Regimens should include isoniazid and rifampin for a minimum of 6 months with the addition of ethambutol, ethionamide, cycloserine, streptomycin, or a quinolone during the first 2 months of therapy; some recommend the addition of ethambutol throughout the entire course (116). The addition of corticosteroids (prednisone, 40 mg daily) has proved useful in severe disease (49, 64, 116). Because of the extreme severity of disseminated forms (both systemic and localized), particularly among immunosuppressed patients, it may be advisable to extend treatment to at least 9 months in such patients, in view of the absence of pyrazinamide from the regimen (16, 69).

MYCOBACTERIUM AFRICANUM

Mycobacterium africanum is a species from the *M. tuberculosis* complex that includes strains which share phenotypic characteristics with *M. bovis* and *M. tuberculosis* (50; http://www.bacterio.cict.fr/m/mycobacterium.html). Strains of this species have been isolated in sub-Saharan African countries, where it is the cause of human tuberculosis with variable percentages (31, 32, 71, 79). However, in developed countries, *M. africanum* isolation is uncommon and is associated with immigrant patients from Africa (4, 37); such patients can infect immigrants from other countries and even autochthonous patients (37).

The species have been classically divided into two groups (from East and West Africa), but recent taxonomic studies have demonstrated that the East strains are *M. bovis* and the West strains are the true *M. africanum* species (79). Finally, the description of the species includes classical phenotypic characteristics and genetic markers, including the lack of RD9, the presence of RD12, and a specific *gyrB* gene polymorphism (79). Currently, a commercial genetic test allows its identification (90).

Disease caused by *M. africanum* is identical to that caused by *M. tuberculosis*. There are reports which evaluate both diseases: one of them showed no differences between the two species, except for less clustering of *M. africanum* cases than *M. tuberculosis* cases, and the appearance of lower lobe lung disease less frequently in *M. africanum* cases (71). Another report showed that *M. africanum* patients are older than *M. tuberculosis* patients and are more frequently HIV infected and malnourished. They also showed more severe disease on chest X ray (31). The association with HIV disease prompted the authors to consider it an opportunistic pathogen (31, 32), but another report did not confirm this association (71). Local differences (the studies were performed in different countries) could be an explanation for such differences.

Treatment for *M. africanum* disease is the same as that for *M. tuberculosis* disease. No MDR *M. africanum* outbreaks have been described as of this writing.

MYCOBACTERIUM CAPRAE

In 1999, strains from the *M. tuberculosis* complex isolated from goats in Spain were described as *M. tuberculosis* subsp. *caprae* (7). The strains shared common phenotypic properties with *M. bovis*, although they were susceptible to pyrazinamide. Other properties differentiate these strains from other members of the *M. tuberculosis* complex. The isolates were subsequently characterized as *M. bovis* subsp. *caprae* (80) and finally as a new species, *M. caprae* (5). Although in the beginning it was described as a cause of tuberculosis in goats, it has been isolated from other mammals in different European countries (89).

Moreover, like *M. bovis*, *M. caprae* has been described as the cause of human disease. Retrospective studies showed that *M. caprae* represents a variable percentage of the strains previously identified as *M. bovis* in different studies (63, 93). Epidemiologic characteristics of both species are similar, with most cases having a previous epidemiological link with animals (28, 93). Treatment is also similar to that for *M. bovis*, although *M. caprae* is susceptible to pyrazinamide.

MYCOBACTERIUM MICROTI, MYCOBACTERIUM PINNIPEDII, AND "MYCOBACTERIUM CANETTII"

Mycobacterium microti is a member of the *M. tuberculosis* complex that has been described as a cause of disease among voles and other animals (61, 111) and was classically considered nonpathogenic for humans. However, recent molecular studies have showed that *M. microti* can be a cause of infection in humans (33, 44, 55, 61, 111, 117), most of them immunosuppressed (44, 55, 111, 117) but also immunocompetent patients (33, 111, 117). Disease seems to be similar to classical tuberculosis, as is the treatment, but the low number of cases makes it difficult to establish general recommendations.

Mycobacterium pinnipedii is the most recently described member of the *M. tuberculosis* complex (26). It has been described as a cause of disease among seals but also among other animals. A recent report suggests the possibility of human infection (59), but no human disease has been described yet.

The name "*Mycobacterium canettii*" has been applied to *Mycobacterium tuberculosis* strains which have glossy and smooth colonies, a rare finding among this species (110). Although cases of human tuberculosis caused by these strains have been described (74, 110), it is not considered a separate species or subspecies in the *M. tuberculosis* complex (http://www.bacterio.cict.fr/m/mycobacterium.html).

REFERENCES

1. Abramowsky, C., B. Gonzalez, and R. U. Sorensen. 1993. Disseminated bacillus Calmette-Guerin infections in patients with primary immunodeficiencies. *Am. J. Clin. Pathol.* 100:52–56.

2. Allix, C., K. Walravens, C. Saegerman, J. Godfroid, P. Supply, and M. Fauville-Dufaux. 2006. Evaluation of the epidemiological relevance of variable-number tandem-repeat genotyping of *Mycobacterium bovis* and comparison of the method with IS6110 restriction fragment length polymorphism analysis and spoligotyping. *J. Clin. Microbiol.* 44:1951–1962.

3. Alonso-Rodriguez, N., M. Martinez-Lirola, M. L. Sanchez, M. Herranz, T. Penafiel, M. D. Bonillo, M. Gonzalez-Rivera, J. Martinez, T. Cabezas, L. F. Diez-Garcia, E. Bouza, and D. Garcia de Viedma. 2009. Prospective universal application of MIRU-VNTR to characterize *Mycobacterium tuberculosis* isolates for fast identification of clustered and orphan cases. *J. Clin. Microbiol.* 47:2026–2032.

4. Alonso-Rodriguez, N., F. Chaves, J. Inigo, E. Bouza, D. Garcia de Viedma, S. Andres, R. Cias, R. Daza, D. Domingo, J. Esteban, J. Garcia, E. Gomez Mampaso, M. Herranz, E. Palenque, and M. J. Ruiz Serrano. 2009. Transmission permeability of tuberculosis involving immigrants, revealed by a multicentre analysis of clusters. *Clin. Microbiol. Infect.* 15:435–442.

5. Aranaz, A., D. Cousins, A. Mateos, and L. Dominguez. 2003. Elevation of *Mycobacterium tuberculosis* subsp. *caprae* Aranaz et al. 1999 to species rank as *Mycobacterium caprae* comb. nov., sp. nov. *Int. J. Syst. Evol. Microbiol.* 53:1785–1789.

6. Aranaz, A., L. De Juan, N. Montero, C. Sanchez, M. Galka, C. Delso, J. Alvarez, B. Romero, J. Bezos, A. I. Vela, V. Briones, A. Mateos, and L. Dominguez. 2004. Bovine tuberculosis (*Mycobacterium bovis*) in wildlife in Spain. *J. Clin. Microbiol.* 42:2602–2608.

7. Aranaz, A., E. Liebana, E. Gomez-Mampaso, J. C. Galan, D. Cousins, A. Ortega, J. Blazquez, F. Baquero, A. Mateos, G. Suarez, and L. Dominguez. 1999. *Mycobacterium tuberculosis* subsp. *caprae* subsp. nov.: a taxonomic study of a new member of the *Mycobacterium tuberculosis* complex isolated from goats in Spain. *Int. J. Syst. Bacteriol.* 49(Pt. 3):1263–1273.

8. Ashford, D. A., E. Whitney, P. Raghunathan, and O. Cosivi. 2001. Epidemiology of selected mycobacteria that infect humans and other animals. *Rev. Sci. Tech.* 20:325–337.

9. Ayele, W. Y., S. D. Neill, J. Zinsstag, M. G. Weiss, and I. Pavlik. 2004. Bovine tuberculosis: an old disease but a new threat to Africa. *Int. J. Tuberc. Lung Dis.* 8:924–937.

10. Azzopardi, P., C. M. Bennett, S. M. Graham, and T. Duke. 2009. Bacille Calmette-Guerin vaccine-related disease in HIV-infected children: a systematic review. *Int. J. Tuberc. Lung Dis.* 13:1331–1344.

11. Barnes, P. F., and M. D. Cave. 2003. Molecular epidemiology of tuberculosis. *N. Engl. J. Med.* 349:1149–1156.

12. Blazquez, J., L. E. Espinosa de Los Monteros, S. Samper, C. Martin, A. Guerrero, J. Cobo, J. Van Embden, F. Baquero, and E. Gomez-Mampaso. 1997. Genetic characterization of multidrug-resistant *Mycobacterium bovis* strains from a hospital outbreak involving human immunodeficiency virus-positive patients. *J. Clin. Microbiol.* 35:1390–1393.

13. Brosch, R., S. V. Gordon, M. Marmiesse, P. Brodin, C. Buchrieser, K. Eiglmeier, T. Garnier, C. Gutierrez, G. Hewinson, K. Kremer, L. M. Parsons, A. S. Pym, S. Samper, D. van Soolingen, and S. T. Cole. 2002. A new evolutionary scenario for the *Mycobacterium tuberculosis* complex. *Proc. Natl. Acad. Sci. USA* 99:3684–3689.

14. Byarugaba, F., E. M. Charles-Etter, S. Godreuil, and P. Grimaud. 2009. Pulmonary tuberculosis and *Mycobacterium bovis*, Uganda. *Emerg. Infect. Dis.* 15:124–125.

15. Calmette, A. 1936. *L'Infection Bacillaire et la Tuberculose*, 4th ed. Masson et Cie, Paris, France.

16. Casanova, J. L., S. Blanche, J. F. Emile, E. Jouanguy, S. Lamhamedi, F. Altare, J. L. Stephan, F. Bernaudin, P. Bordigoni, D. Turck, A. Lachaux, M. Albertini, A. Bourrillon, J. P. Dommergues, M. A. Pocidalo, F. Le Deist, J. L. Gaillard, C. Griscelli, and A. Fischer. 1996. Idiopathic disseminated bacillus Calmette-Guerin infection: a French national retrospective study. *Pediatrics* 98:774–778.

17. Chen, Y., Y. Chao, Q. Deng, T. Liu, J. Xiang, J. Chen, J. Zhou, Z. Zhan, Y. Kuang, H. Cai, H. Chen, and A. Guo. 2009. Potential challenges to the Stop TB Plan for humans in China; cattle maintain *M. bovis* and *M. tuberculosis*. *Tuberculosis* (Edinburgh) 89:95–100.

18. Christianson, S., J. Wolfe, P. Orr, J. Karlowsky, P. N. Levett, G. B. Horsman, L. Thibert, P. Tang, and M. K. Sharma. Evaluation of 24 locus MIRU-VNTR genotyping of *Mycobacterium tuberculosis* isolates in Canada. *Tuberculosis* (Edinburgh) 90:31–38.

19. Cleaveland, S., D. J. Shaw, S. G. Mfinanga, G. Shirima, R. R. Kazwala, E. Eblate, and M. Sharp. 2007. *Mycobacterium bovis* in rural Tanzania: risk factors for infection in human and cattle populations. *Tuberculosis* (Edinburgh) 87:30–43.

20. Coleman, J. D., and M. M. Cooke. 2001. *Mycobacterium bovis* infection in wildlife in New Zealand. *Tuberculosis* (Edinburgh) 81:191–202.

21. Collins, D. M., J. M. Grange, and M. D. Yates. 1997. *Tuberculosis Bacteriology: Organization and Practice*, 2nd ed. Butterworth Heinemann, Oxford, United Kingdom.

22. Collins, J. D. 2006. Tuberculosis in cattle: strategic planning for the future. *Vet. Microbiol.* 112:369–381.

23. Cosivi, O., J. M. Grange, C. J. Daborn, M. C. Raviglione, T. Fujikura, D. Cousins, R. A. Robinson, H. F. Huchzermeyer, I. de Kantor, and F. X. Meslin. 1998. Zoonotic tuberculosis due to *Mycobacterium bovis* in developing countries. *Emerg. Infect. Dis.* 4:59–70.

24. Cosivi, O., F. X. Meslin, C. J. Daborn, and J. M. Grange. 1995. Epidemiology of *Mycobacterium bovis* infection in animals and humans, with particular reference to Africa. *Rev. Sci. Tech.* 14:733–746.

25. Cousins, D. V. 2001. *Mycobacterium bovis* infection and control in domestic livestock. *Rev. Sci. Tech.* 20:71–85.

26. Cousins, D. V., R. Bastida, A. Cataldi, V. Quse, S. Redrobe, S. Dow, P. Duignan, A. Murray, C. Dupont, N. Ahmed, D. M. Collins, W. R. Butler, D. Dawson, D. Rodriguez, J. Loureiro, M. I. Romano, A. Alito, M. Zumarraga, and A. Bernardelli. 2003. Tuberculosis in seals caused by a novel member of the

Mycobacterium tuberculosis complex: *Mycobacterium pinnipedii* sp. nov. *Int. J. Syst. Evol. Microbiol.* **53**:1305–1314.

27. Cousins, D. V., and D. J. Dawson. 1999. Tuberculosis due to *Mycobacterium bovis* in the Australian population: cases recorded during 1970-1994. *Int. J. Tuberc. Lung Dis.* **3**:715–721.

28. Cvetnic, Z., V. Katalinic-Jankovic, B. Sostaric, S. Spicic, M. Obrovac, S. Marjanovic, M. Benic, B. K. Kirin, and I. Vickovic. 2007. *Mycobacterium caprae* in cattle and humans in Croatia. *Int. J. Tuberc. Lung Dis.* **11**:652–658.

29. Dalovisio, J. R., M. Stetter, and S. Mikota-Wells. 1992. Rhinoceros' rhinorrhea: cause of an outbreak of infection due to airborne *Mycobacterium bovis* in zookeepers. *Clin. Infect. Dis.* **15**:598–600.

30. Dankner, W. M., N. J. Waecker, M. A. Essey, K. Moser, M. Thompson, and C. E. Davis. 1993. *Mycobacterium bovis* infections in San Diego: a clinicoepidemiologic study of 73 patients and a historical review of a forgotten pathogen. *Medicine* (Baltimore) **72**:11–37.

31. de Jong, B. C., I. Adetifa, B. Walther, P. C. Hill, M. Antonio, M. Ota, and R. A. Adegbola. 2010. Differences between tuberculosis cases infected with *Mycobacterium africanum*, West African type 2, relative to Euro-American *Mycobacterium tuberculosis*: an update. *FEMS Immunol. Med. Microbiol.* **58**: 102–105.

32. de Jong, B. C., P. C. Hill, R. H. Brookes, J. K. Otu, K. L. Peterson, P. M. Small, and R. A. Adegbola. 2005. *Mycobacterium africanum*: a new opportunistic pathogen in HIV infection? *AIDS* **19**:1714–1715.

33. de Jong, E., R. J. Rentenaar, R. van Pelt, W. de Lange, W. Schreurs, D. van Soolingen, and P. D. Sturm. 2009. Two cases of *Mycobacterium microti*-induced culture-negative tuberculosis. *J. Clin. Microbiol.* **47**:3038–3040.

34. de Kantor, I. N., M. Ambroggi, S. Poggi, N. Morcillo, M. A. Da Silva Telles, M. Osorio Ribeiro, M. C. Garzon Torres, C. Llerena Polo, W. Ribon, V. Garcia, D. Kuffo, L. Asencios, L. M. Vasquez Campos, C. Rivas, and J. H. de Waard. 2008. Human *Mycobacterium bovis* infection in ten Latin American countries. *Tuberculosis* (Edinburgh) **88**:358–365.

35. de la Rua-Domenech, R. 2006. Human *Mycobacterium bovis* infection in the United Kingdom: incidence, risks, control measures and review of the zoonotic aspects of bovine tuberculosis. *Tuberculosis* (Edinburgh) **86**:77–109.

36. de Lisle, G. W., C. G. Mackintosh, and R. G. Bengis. 2001. *Mycobacterium bovis* in free-living and captive wildlife, including farmed deer. *Rev. Sci. Tech.* **20**:86–111.

37. Desmond, E., A. T. Ahmed, W. S. Probert, J. Ely, Y. Jang, C. A. Sanders, S. Y. Lin, and J. Flood. 2004. *Mycobacterium africanum* cases, California. *Emerg. Infect. Dis.* **10**:921–923.

38. Doherty, T. M., and P. Andersen. 2005. Vaccines for tuberculosis: novel concepts and recent progress. *Clin. Microbiol. Rev.* **18**:687–702.

39. Esteban, J., P. Robles, M. Soledad Jimenez, and M. L. Fernandez Guerrero. 2005. Pleuropulmonary infections caused by *Mycobacterium bovis*: a re-emerging disease. *Clin. Microbiol. Infect.* **11**:840–843.

40. Reference deleted.

41. Evans, J. T., E. G. Smith, A. Banerjee, R. M. Smith, J. Dale, J. A. Innes, D. Hunt, A. Tweddell, A. Wood, C. Anderson, R. G. Hewinson, N. H. Smith, P. M. Hawkey, and P. Sonnenberg. 2007. Cluster of human tuberculosis caused by *Mycobacterium bovis*: evidence for person-to-person transmission in the UK. *Lancet* **369**:1270–1276.

42. Fanning, A., and S. Edwards. 1991. *Mycobacterium bovis* infection in human beings in contact with elk (*Cervus elaphus*) in Alberta, Canada. *Lancet* **338**:1253–1255.

43. Fortun, J., P. Martin-Davila, E. Navas, M. J. Perez-Elias, J. Cobo, M. Tato, E. G. De la Pedrosa, E. Gomez-Mampaso, and S. Moreno. 2005. Linezolid for the treatment of multidrug-resistant tuberculosis. *J. Antimicrob. Chemother.* **56**:180–185.

44. Foudraine, N. A., D. van Soolingen, G. T. Noordhoek, and P. Reiss. 1998. Pulmonary tuberculosis due to *Mycobacterium microti* in a human immunodeficiency virus-infected patient. *Clin. Infect. Dis.* **27**:1543–1544.

45. Frothingham, R., and W. A. Meeker-O'Connell. 1998. Genetic diversity in the *Mycobacterium tuberculosis* complex based on variable numbers of tandem DNA repeats. *Microbiology* **144**(Pt. 5):1189–1196.

46. Gallagher, J., R. H. Muirhead, J. M. Daykin, J. A. Smith, S. D. Beavan, J. Kirkham, A. T. Turnball, and J. I. Davies. 2005. Bovine tuberculosis and badgers. *Vet. Rec.* **156**:555–556.

47. Garnier, T., K. Eiglmeier, J. C. Camus, N. Medina, H. Mansoor, M. Pryor, S. Duthoy, S. Grondin, C. Lacroix, C. Monsempe, S. Simon, B. Harris, R. Atkin, J. Doggett, R. Mayes, L. Keating, P. R. Wheeler, J. Parkhill, B. G. Barrell, S. T. Cole, S. V. Gordon, and R. G. Hewinson. 2003. The complete genome sequence of *Mycobacterium bovis*. *Proc. Natl. Acad. Sci. USA* **100**:7877–7882.

48. Gori, A., G. Marchetti, C. Catozzi, C. Nigro, G. Ferrario, M. C. Rossi, A. Degli Esposti, A. Orani, and F. Franzetti. 1998. Molecular epidemiology characterization of a multidrug-resistant *Mycobacterium bovis* outbreak amongst HIV-positive patients. *AIDS* **12**:445–446.

49. Grange, J. M. 1998. Complications of bacille Calmette-Guérin (BCG) vaccination and immunotherapy and their management. *Commun. Dis. Public Health* **1**:84–88.

50. Grange, J. M., and M. D. Yates. 1994. Zoonotic aspects of *Mycobacterium bovis* infection. *Vet. Microbiol.* **40**:137–151.

51. Guerrero, A., J. Cobo, J. Fortun, E. Navas, C. Quereda, A. Asensio, J. Canon, J. Blazquez, and E. Gomez-Mampaso. 1997. Nosocomial transmission of *Mycobacterium bovis* resistant to 11 drugs in people with advanced HIV-1 infection. *Lancet* **350**:1738–1742.

52. Haddad, N., M. Masselot, and B. Durand. 2004. Molecular differentiation of *Mycobacterium bovis* isolates. Review of main techniques and applications. *Res. Vet. Sci.* **76**:1–18.

53. Hines, N., J. B. Payeur, and L. J. Hoffman. 2006. Comparison of the recovery of *Mycobacterium bovis* isolates using the BACTEC MGIT 960 system, BACTEC 460 system, and Middlebrook 7H10 and 7H11 solid media. *J. Vet. Diagn. Investig.* **18**:243–250.

54. Hlavsa, M. C., P. K. Moonan, L. S. Cowan, T. R. Navin, J. S. Kammerer, G. P. Morlock, J. T. Crawford, and P. A. Lobue. 2008. Human tuberculosis due to *Mycobacterium bovis* in the United States, 1995-2005. *Clin. Infect. Dis.* **47**:168–175.

55. Horstkotte, M. A., I. Sobottka, C. K. Schewe, P. Schafer, R. Laufs, S. Rusch-Gerdes, and S. Niemann. 2001. *Mycobacterium microti* llama-type infection presenting as pulmonary tuberculosis in a human immunodeficiency virus-positive patient. *J. Clin. Microbiol.* **39**:406–407.

56. Javed, M. T., A. Aranaz, L. de Juan, J. Bezos, B. Romero, J. Alvarez, C. Lozano, A. Mateos, and L. Dominguez. 2007. Improvement of spoligotyping with additional spacer sequences for characterization of *Mycobacterium bovis* and M. *caprae* isolates from Spain. *Tuberculosis* (Edinburgh) **87**:437–445.

57. Kamerbeek, J., L. Schouls, A. Kolk, M. van Agterveld, D. van Soolingen, S. Kuijper, A. Bunschoten, H. Molhuizen, R. Shaw, M. Goyal, and J. van Embden. 1997. Simultaneous detection and strain differentiation of *Mycobacterium tuberculosis* for diagnosis and epidemiology. *J. Clin. Microbiol.* **35**:907–914.

58. Kanduma, E., T. D. McHugh, and S. H. Gillespie. 2003. Molecular methods for *Mycobacterium tuberculosis* strain typing: a users guide. *J. Appl. Microbiol.* **94:**781–791.

59. Kiers, A., A. Klarenbeek, B. Mendelts, D. Van Soolingen, and G. Koeter. 2008. Transmission of *Mycobacterium pinnipedii* to humans in a zoo with marine mammals. *Int. J. Tuberc. Lung Dis.* **12:**1469–1473.

60. Kremer, K., D. van Soolingen, R. Frothingham, W. H. Haas, P. W. Hermans, C. Martin, P. Palittapongarnpim, B. B. Plikaytis, L. W. Riley, M. A. Yakrus, J. M. Musser, and J. D. van Embden. 1999. Comparison of methods based on different molecular epidemiological markers for typing of *Mycobacterium tuberculosis* complex strains: interlaboratory study of discriminatory power and reproducibility. *J. Clin. Microbiol.* **37:**2607–2618.

61. Kremer, K., D. van Soolingen, J. van Embden, S. Hughes, J. Inwald, and G. Hewinson. 1998. *Mycobacterium microti:* more widespread than previously thought. *J. Clin. Microbiol.* **36:**2793–2794.

62. Kubica, T., R. Agzamova, A. Wright, G. Rakishev, S. Rusch-Gerdes, and S. Niemann. 2006. *Mycobacterium bovis* isolates with *M. tuberculosis* specific characteristics. *Emerg. Infect. Dis.* **12:**763–765.

63. Kubica, T., S. Rusch-Gerdes, and S. Niemann. 2003. *Mycobacterium bovis* subsp. *caprae* caused one-third of human *M. bovis*-associated tuberculosis cases reported in Germany between 1999 and 2001. *J. Clin. Microbiol.* **41:**3070–3077.

64. Lamm, D. L. 2000. Efficacy and safety of bacille Calmette-Guérin immunotherapy in superficial bladder cancer. *Clin. Infect. Dis.* **31:**S86–S90.

65. Lamm, D. L., P. M. van der Meijden, A. Morales, S. A. Brosman, W. J. Catalona, H. W. Herr, M. S. Soloway, A. Steg, and F. M. Debruyne. 1992. Incidence and treatment of complications of bacillus Calmette-Guerin intravesical therapy in superficial bladder cancer. *J. Urol.* **147:**596–600.

66. Le Fleche, P., M. Fabre, F. Denoeud, J. L. Koeck, and G. Vergnaud. 2002. High resolution, on-line identification of strains from the *Mycobacterium tuberculosis* complex based on tandem repeat typing. *BMC Microbiol.* **2:**37.

67. Liss, G. M., L. Wong, D. C. Kittle, A. Simor, M. Naus, P. Martiquet, and C. R. Misener. 1994. Occupational exposure to *Mycobacterium bovis* infection in deer and elk in Ontario. *Can. J. Public Health* **85:**326–329.

68. Mathema, B., N. E. Kurepina, P. J. Bifani, and B. N. Kreiswirth. 2006. Molecular epidemiology of tuberculosis: current insights. *Clin. Microbiol. Rev.* **19:**658–685.

69. McParland, C., D. J. Cotton, K. S. Gowda, V. H. Hoeppner, W. T. Martin, and P. F. Weckworth. 1992. Miliary *Mycobacterium bovis* induced by intravesical bacille Calmette-Guerin immunotherapy. *Am. Rev. Respir. Dis.* **146:**1330–1333.

70. Menzies, F. D., and S. D. Neill. 2000. Cattle-to-cattle transmission of bovine tuberculosis. *Vet. J.* **160:**92–106.

71. Meyer, C. G., G. Scarisbrick, S. Niemann, E. N. Browne, M. A. Chinbuah, J. Gyapong, I. Osei, E. Owusu-Dabo, T. Kubica, S. Rusch-Gerdes, T. Thye, and R. D. Horstmann. 2008. Pulmonary tuberculosis: virulence of *Mycobacterium africanum* and relevance in HIV co-infection. *Tuberculosis* (Edinburgh) **88:**482–489.

72. Michel, A. L., R. G. Bengis, D. F. Keet, M. Hofmeyr, L. M. Klerk, P. C. Cross, A. E. Jolles, D. Cooper, I. J. Whyte, P. Buss, and J. Godfroid. 2006. Wildlife tuberculosis in South African conservation areas: implications and challenges. *Vet. Microbiol.* **112:**91–100.

73. Mignard, S., C. Pichat, and G. Carret. 2006. *Mycobacterium bovis* infection, Lyon, France. *Emerg. Infect. Dis.* **12:**1431–1433.

74. Miltgen, J., M. Morillon, J. L. Koeck, A. Varnerot, J. F. Briant, G. Nguyen, D. Verrot, D. Bonnet, and V. Vincent. 2002. Two cases of pulmonary tuberculosis caused by *Mycobacterium tuberculosis* subsp *canetti. Emerg. Infect. Dis.* **8:**1350–1352.

75. Morales, A., D. Eidinger, and A. W. Bruce. 1976. Intracavitary Bacillus Calmette-Guerin in the treatment of superficial bladder tumors. *J. Urol.* **116:**180–183.

76. Morgan, M. B., and M. D. Iseman. 1996. *Mycobacterium bovis* vertebral osteomyelitis as a complication of intravesical administration of Bacille Calmette-Guerin. *Am. J. Med.* **100:**372–373.

77. Morris, R. S., D. U. Pfeiffer, and R. Jackson. 1994. The epidemiology of *Mycobacterium bovis* infections. *Vet. Microbiol.* **40:**153–177.

78. Musial, C. E., L. S. Tice, L. Stockman, and G. D. Roberts. 1988. Identification of mycobacteria from culture by using the Gen-Probe rapid diagnostic system for *Mycobacterium avium* complex and *Mycobacterium tuberculosis* complex. *J. Clin. Microbiol.* **26:**2120–2123.

79. Niemann, S., T. Kubica, F. C. Bange, O. Adjei, E. N. Browne, M. A. Chinbuah, R. Diel, J. Gyapong, R. D. Horstmann, M. L. Joloba, C. G. Meyer, R. D. Mugerwa, A. Okwera, I. Osei, E. Owusu-Darbo, S. K. Schwander, and S. Rusch-Gerdes. 2004. The species *Mycobacterium africanum* in the light of new molecular markers. *J. Clin. Microbiol.* **42:**3958–3962.

80. Niemann, S., E. Richter, and S. Rusch-Gerdes. 2002. Biochemical and genetic evidence for the transfer of *Mycobacterium tuberculosis* subsp. *caprae* Aranaz et al. 1999 to the species *Mycobacterium bovis* Karlson and Lessel 1970 (approved lists 1980) as *Mycobacterium bovis* subsp. *caprae* comb. nov. *Int. J. Syst. Evol. Microbiol.* **52:**433–436.

81. Nikaido, T., K. Ishibashi, K. Otani, S. Yabuki, S. Konno, S. Mori, K. Ohashi, T. Ishida, M. Nakano, O. Yamaguchi, T. Suzutani, and S. Kikuchi. 2007. *Mycobacterium bovis* BCG vertebral osteomyelitis after intravesical BCG therapy, diagnosed by PCR-based genomic deletion analysis. *J. Clin. Microbiol.* **45:**4085–4087.

82. Nolan, A., and J. W. Wilesmith. 1994. Tuberculosis in badgers (*Meles meles*). *Vet. Microbiol.* **40:**179–191.

83. Oelemann, M. C., R. Diel, V. Vatin, W. Haas, S. Rusch-Gerdes, C. Locht, S. Niemann, and P. Supply. 2007. Assessment of an optimized mycobacterial interspersed repetitive-unit variable-number tandem-repeat typing system combined with spoligotyping for population-based molecular epidemiology studies of tuberculosis. *J. Clin. Microbiol.* **45:**691–697.

84. Ojo, O., S. Sheehan, G. D. Corcoran, K. Okker, K. Gover, V. Nikolayevsky, T. Brown, J. Dale, S. V. Gordon, F. Drobniewski, and M. B. Prentice. 2008. *Mycobacterium bovis* strains causing smear-positive human tuberculosis, Southwest Ireland. *Emerg. Infect. Dis.* **14:**1931–1934.

85. O'Reilly, L. M., and C. J. Daborn. 1995. The epidemiology of *Mycobacterium bovis* infections in animals and man: a review. *Tuber. Lung Dis.* **76**(Suppl. 1):1–46.

86. Palenque, E., V. Villena, M. J. Rebollo, M. S. Jimenez, and S. Samper. 1998. Transmission of multidrug-resistant *Mycobacterium bovis* to an immunocompetent patient. *Clin. Infect. Dis.* **26:**995–996.

87. Palmer, M. 2007. Tuberculosis: a reemerging disease at the interface of domestic animals and wild life. *Curr. Top. Microbiol. Immunol.* **315:**195–215.

88. Parreiras, P. M., F. C. Lobato, A. P. Alencar, T. Figueiredo, H. M. Gomes, N. Boechat, A. P. Lage, R. A. Assis, M. A. Pereira, P. R. Souza, P. M. Mota, and P. N. Suffys. 2004. Drug susceptibility of Brazilian strains of *Mycobacterium bovis* using traditional and molecular techniques. *Mem. Inst. Oswaldo Cruz* **99:**749–752.

89. Prodinger, W. M., A. Brandstatter, L. Naumann, M. Pacciarini, T. Kubica, M. L. Boschiroli, A. Aranaz, G. Nagy, Z. Cvetnic, M. Ocepek, A. Skrypnyk, W. Erler, S. Niemann, I. Pavlik, and I. Moser. 2005. Characterization of *Mycobacterium caprae* isolates from Europe by mycobacterial interspersed repetitive unit genotyping. *J. Clin. Microbiol.* 43:4984–4992.

90. Richter, E., M. Weizenegger, A. M. Fahr, and S. Rusch-Gerdes. 2004. Usefulness of the GenoType MTBC assay for differentiating species of the *Mycobacterium tuberculosis* complex in cultures obtained from clinical specimens. *J. Clin. Microbiol.* 42:4303–4306.

91. Rivero, A., M. Marquez, J. Santos, A. Pinedo, M. A. Sanchez, A. Esteve, S. Samper, and C. Martin. 2001. High rate of tuberculosis reinfection during a nosocomial outbreak of multidrug-resistant tuberculosis caused by *Mycobacterium bovis* strain B. *Clin. Infect. Dis.* 32:159–161.

92. Robert, J., F. Boulahbal, D. Trystram, C. Truffot-Pernot, A. C. de Benoist, V. Vincent, V. Jarlier, and J. Grosset. 1999. A national survey of human *Mycobacterium bovis* infection in France. Network of Microbiology Laboratories in France. *Int. J. Tuberc. Lung Dis.* 3:711–714.

93. Rodriguez, E., L. P. Sanchez, S. Perez, L. Herrera, M. S. Jimenez, S. Samper, and M. J. Iglesias. 2009. Human tuberculosis due to *Mycobacterium bovis* and *M. caprae* in Spain, 2004-2007. *Int. J. Tuberc. Lung Dis.* 13:1536–1541.

94. Roring, S., A. Scott, D. Brittain, I. Walker, G. Hewinson, S. Neill, and R. Skuce. 2002. Development of variable-number tandem repeat typing of *Mycobacterium bovis*: comparison of results with those obtained by using existing exact tandem repeats and spoligotyping. *J. Clin. Microbiol.* 40:2126–2133.

95. Samper, S., C. Martin, A. Pinedo, A. Rivero, J. Blazquez, F. Baquero, D. van Soolingen, and J. van Embden. 1997. Transmission between HIV-infected patients of multidrug-resistant tuberculosis caused by *Mycobacterium bovis*. *AIDS* 11:1237–1242.

96. Scorpio, A., and Y. Zhang. 1996. Mutations in pncA, a gene encoding pyrazinamidase/nicotinamidase, cause resistance to the antituberculous drug pyrazinamide in tubercle bacillus. *Nat. Med.* 2:662–667.

97. Sjogren, I., and O. Hillerdal. 1978. Bovine tuberculosis in man--reinfection or endogenous exacerbation. *Scand. J. Respir. Dis.* 59:167–170.

98. Skuce, R. A., D. Brittain, M. S. Hughes, and S. D. Neill. 1996. Differentiation of *Mycobacterium bovis* isolates from animals by DNA typing. *J. Clin. Microbiol.* 34:2469–2474.

99. Skuce, R. A., T. P. McCorry, J. F. McCarroll, S. M. Roring, A. N. Scott, D. Brittain, S. L. Hughes, R. G. Hewinson, and S. D. Neill. 2002. Discrimination of *Mycobacterium tuberculosis* complex bacteria using novel VNTR-PCR targets. *Microbiology* 148:519–528.

100. Sreevatsan, S., P. Escalante, X. Pan, D. A. Gillies II, S. Siddiqui, C. N. Khalaf, B. N. Kreiswirth, P. Bifani, L. G. Adams, T. Ficht, V. S. Perumaalla, M. D. Cave, J. D. van Embden, and J. M. Musser. 1996. Identification of a polymorphic nucleotide in *oxyR* specific for *Mycobacterium bovis*. *J. Clin. Microbiol.* 34:2007–2010.

101. Supply, P., C. Allix, S. Lesjean, M. Cardoso-Oelemann, S. Rusch-Gerdes, E. Willery, E. Savine, P. de Haas, H. van Deutekom, S. Roring, P. Bifani, N. Kurepina, B. Kreiswirth, C. Sola, N. Rastogi, V. Vatin, M. C. Gutierrez, M. Fauville, S. Niemann, R. Skuce, K. Kremer, C. Locht, and D. van Soolingen. 2006. Proposal for standardization of optimized mycobacterial interspersed repetitive unit-variable-number

tandem repeat typing of *Mycobacterium tuberculosis*. *J. Clin. Microbiol.* 44:4498–4510.

102. Supply, P., J. Magdalena, S. Himpens, and C. Locht. 1997. Identification of novel intergenic repetitive units in a mycobacterial two-component system operon. *Mol. Microbiol.* 26:991–1003.

103. Supply, P., E. Mazars, S. Lesjean, V. Vincent, B. Gicquel, and C. Locht. 2000. Variable human minisatellite-like regions in the *Mycobacterium tuberculosis* genome. *Mol. Microbiol.* 36:762–771.

104. Talbot, E. A., M. D. Perkins, S. F. Silva, and R. Frothingham. 1997. Disseminated bacille Calmette-Guerin disease after vaccination: case report and review. *Clin. Infect. Dis.* 24:1139–1146.

105. Thoen, C., P. Lobue, and I. de Kantor. 2006. The importance of *Mycobacterium bovis* as a zoonosis. *Vet. Microbiol.* 112:339–345.

106. Thompson, P. J., D. V. Cousins, B. L. Gow, D. M. Collins, B. H. Williamson, and H. T. Dagnia. 1993. Seals, seal trainers, and mycobacterial infection. *Am. Rev. Respir. Dis.* 147:164–167.

107. van der Zanden, A. G., K. Kremer, L. M. Schouls, K. Caimi, A. Cataldi, A. Hulleman, N. J. Nagelkerke, and D. van Soolingen. 2002. Improvement of differentiation and interpretability of spoligotyping for *Mycobacterium tuberculosis* complex isolates by introduction of new spacer oligonucleotides. *J. Clin. Microbiol.* 40:4628–4639.

108. van Deutekom, H., Y. M. Smulders, K. J. Roozendaal, and D. van Soolingen. 1996. Bacille Calmette-Guerin (BCG) meningitis in an AIDS patient 12 years after vaccination with BCG. *Clin. Infect. Dis.* 22:870–871.

109. van Embden, J. D., T. van Gorkom, K. Kremer, R. Jansen, B. A. van Der Zeijst, and L. M. Schouls. 2000. Genetic variation and evolutionary origin of the direct repeat locus of *Mycobacterium tuberculosis* complex bacteria. *J. Bacteriol.* 182:2393–2401.

110. van Soolingen, D., T. Hoogenboezem, P. E. de Haas, P. W. Hermans, M. A. Koedam, K. S. Teppema, P. J. Brennan, G. S. Besra, F. Portaels, J. Top, L. M. Schouls, and J. D. van Embden. 1997. A novel pathogenic taxon of the *Mycobacterium tuberculosis* complex, Canetti: characterization of an exceptional isolate from Africa. *Int. J. Syst. Bacteriol.* 47:1236–1245.

111. van Soolingen, D., A. G. van der Zanden, P. E. de Haas, G. T. Noordhoek, A. Kiers, N. A. Foudraine, F. Portaels, A. H. Kolk, K. Kremer, and J. D. van Embden. 1998. Diagnosis of *Mycobacterium microti* infections among humans by using novel genetic markers. *J. Clin. Microbiol.* 36:1840–1845.

112. Vera-Cabrera, L., S. T. Howard, A. Laszlo, and W. M. Johnson. 1997. Analysis of genetic polymorphism in the phospholipase region of *Mycobacterium tuberculosis*. *J. Clin. Microbiol.* 35:1190–1195.

113. Waecker, N. J., Jr., R. Stefanova, M. D. Cave, C. E. Davis, and W. M. Dankner. 2000. Nosocomial transmission of *Mycobacterium bovis* bacille Calmette-Guerin to children receiving cancer therapy and to their health care providers. *Clin. Infect. Dis.* 30:356–362.

114. Wilkins, M. J., P. C. Bartlett, B. Frawley, D. J. O'Brien, C. E. Miller, and M. L. Boulton. 2003. *Mycobacterium bovis* (bovine TB) exposure as a recreational risk for hunters: results of a Michigan Hunter Survey, 2001. *Int. J. Tuberc. Lung Dis.* 7:1001–1009.

115. Wilkins, M. J., J. Meyerson, P. C. Bartlett, S. L. Spieldenner, D. E. Berry, L. B. Mosher, J. B. Kaneene, B. Robinson-Dunn,

M. G. Stobierski, and M. L. Boulton. 2008. Human *Mycobacterium bovis* infection and bovine tuberculosis outbreak, Michigan, 1994-2007. *Emerg. Infect. Dis.* 14:657–660.

116. Witjes, J. A., J. Palou, M. Soloway, D. Lammd, M. Brausi, J. R. Spermon, R. Persad, R. Buckley, H. Akaza, M. Colombel, and A. Böhle. 2008. Clinical practice recommendations for the prevention and management of intravesical therapy–associated adverse events. *Eur. Urol. Suppl.* 7:667–674.

117. Xavier Emmanuel, F., A. L. Seagar, C. Doig, A. Rayner, P. Claxton, and I. Laurenson. 2007. Human and animal infections with *Mycobacterium microti*, Scotland. *Emerg. Infect. Dis.* 13:1924–1927.

Chapter 42

Other Nontuberculous Mycobacteria

MARVIN J. BITTNER AND LAUREL C. PREHEIM

MICROBIOLOGY

The list of clinically important nontuberculous mycobacteria is growing as new species continue to be identified and older ones are found to be pathogenic. More detailed information on these organisms can be found in a number of excellent reviews (9, 15, 21, 23, 92, 97, 98). As a group, these mycobacteria currently cause fewer infections than those species discussed in previous chapters. Some of these organisms are not newly discovered but have heretofore been considered virtually nonpathogenic. Previously, many were regarded as contaminants when isolated from clinical specimens. Timpe and Runyon established that these organisms could cause disease in humans and classified them based on pigment production, growth rate, and colonial characteristics. Photochromogens (group I) grow slowly on culture media (>7 days). Their colonies change from a buff shade to bright yellow or orange after exposure to light. Scotochromogens (group II) also grow slowly but demonstrate pigmented colonies when incubated in the dark or the light. Group III mycobacteria grow slowly and lack pigment in the dark or light. Rapid growers (group IV) also lack pigment, but they grow in culture within 3 to 5 days. Collectively, these four groups have been called the "atypical mycobacteria," nontuberculous mycobacteria (NTM), mycobacteria other than tubercle bacilli, or "potentially pathogenic environmental mycobacteria." Molecular techniques such as real-time PCR and gene amplification and restriction length polymorphism are promising tools for rapid identification of NTM (66, 73).

EPIDEMIOLOGY

Ubiquitous in nature, many NTM have been isolated from ground or tap water, soil, house dust, domestic and wild animals, and birds (65). Despite their wide distribution, some species are more common in certain geographic locations. Most infections, including those that are hospital acquired (56), result from inhalation or direct inoculation from environmental sources. Ingestion may be the source of infection for children with NTM cervical adenopathy and for patients with AIDS whose disseminated infection may begin in the gastrointestinal tract. These infections are not considered contagious, since person-to-person transmission is undocumented (21, 61).

PATHOPHYSIOLOGY

The pathogenic potential for human disease varies among NTM. As a group, these organisms are less virulent for humans than *M. tuberculosis* or *M. bovis* and may colonize body surfaces or secretions without causing disease. However, because of reports of invasive disease with such organisms, all mycobacteria should be considered potentially pathogenic. This is especially true when they are isolated from patients with immunocompromising conditions such as AIDS (21, 75) or cystic fibrosis (18). Other immunologic deficits, such as genetic defects, and other structural lung disease, such as bronchiectasis, may be associated with disease (21). In general, disease is slowly progressive, and histopathologic findings resemble those seen in tuberculosis.

DIAGNOSIS

The steps taken to diagnose tuberculosis generally apply to NTM infections. Standardized, specific skin test antigens for NTM, however, are unavailable. In addition, colonization of asymptomatic individuals and environmental contamination of specimens can yield positive cultures in the absence of clinical infection. Experts have suggested clinical and

Marvin J. Bittner and Laurel C. Preheim • Infectious Diseases Section, VA Medical Center, Omaha, NE 68105, and Departments of Medicine and of Medical Microbiology and Immunology, Creighton University School of Medicine, Omaha, NE 68131.

microbiologic criteria for diagnosis of pulmonary NTM infection. Clinical criteria include, in addition to exclusion of other diagnoses, "pulmonary symptoms, nodular or cavitary opacities on chest radiograph, or a high-resolution computed tomography scan that shows multifocal bronchiectasis with multiple small nodules" (21). Findings needed to meet microbiologic criteria include positive cultures from two expectorated sputum samples or a positive culture from one bronchial wash or lavage fluid. An alternative microbiologic criterion is the combination of a positive culture and characteristic histopathology (21). However, for less common pathogens, such as those discussed in this chapter, the pertinence of these criteria is only "assumed, not proven" (21). Review of 28 specimens from which *Mycobacterium simiae* was isolated, indeed, encountered patients who met accepted criteria for diagnosis yet who remained clinically stable without treatment (87).

Extrapulmonary or disseminated disease is confirmed by isolation of the organism from normally sterile body fluids, closed sites, or lesions, and environmental contamination of specimens is excluded. Owing to the possibility of infection due to fastidious mycobacteria known to cause infections in skin, joints, and bone, specimens from these sources require supplemented media and lower incubation temperatures (21). Radiometric culture systems, DNA probes, and PCR assays have increased the speed and accuracy of laboratory diagnosis of pulmonary and extrapulmonary mycobacterial infections, but susceptibility testing is not standardized (21).

CLINICAL DISEASE

NTM cause a broad spectrum of diseases (Table 1). It should be noted that therapeutic approaches

Table 1. Nontuberculous mycobacterial infection sites and etiologic species

Site of infection	Etiologic species (Runyon group)[a]	
	Common	Less common
Lungs	M. abscessus (IV)	M. celatum (III)
	M. avium complex (III)	M. chelonae (IV)
	M. kansasii (I)	M. fortuitum (IV)
	M. xenopi (II)	M. gordonae (II)
		M. haemophilum (III)
		M. malmoense (III)
		M. simiae (I)
		M. smegmatis (III)
		M. szulgai (I/II)
		M. terrae (III)
Lymph nodes	M. avium complex (III)	M. abscessus (IV)
	M. scrofulaceum (II)	M. chelonae (IV)
		M. fortuitum (IV)
		M. kansasii (I)
		M. malmoense (III)
		M. szulgai (I/II)
Skin or soft tissue	M. abscessus (IV)	M. avium complex (III)
	M. chelonae (IV)	M. gordonae (II)
	M. fortuitum (IV)	M. haemophilum (III)
	M. marinum (I)	M. kansasii (I)
	M. ulcerans (III)	M. malmoense (III)
		M. smegmatis (IV)
		M. szulgai (I/II)
		M. terrae (III)
Disseminated	M. abscessus (IV)	M. celatum (III)
	M. avium complex (III)	M. fortuitum (IV)
	M. chelonae (IV)	M. genavense (III)
	M. haemophilum (III)	M. gordonae (II)
	M. kansasii (I)	M. malmoense (III)
		M. neoaurum (II)
		M. simiae (I)
		M. smegmatis (IV)
		M. terrae complex (III)
		M. xenopi (II)

[a]I, photochromogen; II, scotochromogen; III, nonpigmented; IV, rapid grower.

continue to evolve and therefore remain controversial. Many conventional antituberculous agents have little or no activity against these organisms. Some treatment regimens contain new agents or older antimicrobials newly found to have activity against mycobacteria. Although general guidelines exist for the therapy of infections caused by some of these organisms (19, 21, 75), in most cases, the optimal regimen or duration of therapy has not been firmly established. The results of susceptibility testing may be used to select a therapeutic regimen (90). Immunocompetent patients with clinically significant NTM infections usually should receive 18 to 24 months of therapy. Infected immunocompromised patients, particularly those with disseminated infection and AIDS, probably should receive therapy as long as their immune systems remain impaired.

Mycobacterium celatum

M. celatum is a slowly growing, nonchromogenic species with biochemical and morphologic characteristics resembling those of M. avium-M. intracellulare and M. xenopi. It has been reported as a cause of pulmonary and disseminated infections in patients with AIDS (59, 84, 100). It rarely causes infections in immunocompetent patients (60). M. celatum isolates have shown variable susceptibility to antimicrobial agents, suggesting that different groups of strains may represent separate clones (59). Most isolates are resistant to rifampin. Treatment regimens have included various combinations of clarithromycin, ciprofloxacin, pyrazinamide, ethambutol, rifabutin, clofazimine, and amikacin.

Mycobacterium gordonae

Also known as the "tap water bacillus," the scotochromogen M. gordonae (formerly Mycobacterium aquae) is ubiquitous in the environment. It is commonly isolated from soil and water sources, including tap water. Its presence in water accounts for its association with numerous nosocomial pseudoinfections and pseudoepidemics (53, 79, 80, 94). A molecular probe is commercially available which consists of DNA specific for a sequence of 16S ribosomal RNA (21). M. gordonae has long been considered among the least pathogenic mycobacteria, and its presence in clinical cultures is commonly attributed to specimen contamination or even host colonization. In a review of the literature, Weinberger et al. (94) concluded that 24 published cases met their criteria for a documented infection caused by M. gordonae. These included five cases of disseminated disease with pulmonary and hepatic involvement in four patients, bone marrow involvement in three, and renal and central nervous system involvement in two each. Four of these five patients had no underlying immunodeficiency, and one had AIDS. Localized sites of infection in the remaining 19 patients included the lung (eight cases), soft tissue (seven cases), peritoneum (three cases), and cornea (one case) (94). A small but increasing number of reports suggest that M. gordonae can not only colonize but also cause disease in patients with AIDS (3, 30, 39). Optimal therapy for a documented M. gordonae infection remains undefined. The majority of isolates tested have been resistant in vitro to isoniazid and pyrazinamide, whereas many are susceptible to ethambutol, rifampin, clarithromycin, linezolid, and the fluoroquinolones (21).

Mycobacterium haemophilum

M. haemophilum is nonpigmented, fastidious, and slow growing, and it grows optimally at lower temperatures than most mycobacteria. It requires hemin or ferric ammonium citrate for growth. Initially identified as the cause of cutaneous ulcerating lesions in an Israeli woman with Hodgkin's disease (76), M. haemophilum has been isolated from patients in North America, Europe, Africa, and Australia (72, 82). Many cases have involved patients who are immunocompromised by conditions such as organ or bone marrow transplantation, lymphoma, or AIDS (69). Recent reports have described cases in immunocompetent children (10). Disease can be focal or widespread. Cutaneous and subcutaneous lesions are most common. They frequently overlie joints and can be nodular, cystic, or papular. Typically, they evolve from papules to pustules and can form deep ulcers that may be painful. Other infections have included bacteremia, septic arthritis, osteomyelitis, pneumonitis, sinusitis, endophthalmitis, and lymphadenitis (49, 72). Most M. haemophilum strains demonstrate in vitro susceptibility to first-line antituberculosis drugs (but not ethambutol), sulfonamides, and clarithromycin (21). Immunocompromised adults with multiple cutaneous lesions or osteomyelitis have been successfully treated with regimens that included ciprofloxacin, clarithromycin, and rifampin (62, 82, 96). The addition of granulocyte-macrophage colony-stimulating factor along with a reduction in immunosuppressive treatment was associated with successful treatment of systemic disease in a cardiac transplant patient (49). Immunocompetent children with localized lymphadenitis do well with excisional therapy alone (72).

Mycobacterium malmoense

M. malmoense, first described in 1977, is non-chromogenic and slow growing, often requiring at least 6 weeks for primary isolation. It appears to be distributed worldwide and has been isolated from natural waters in Finland and soil in Japan. This organism was initially linked to chronic pulmonary infection in British and northern European adults who had underlying lung disease (27). An association with coal workers' pneumoconiosis has been described (46). Reports of extrapulmonary disease have described cervical lymphadenopathy, particularly in children, and tenosynovitis (25, 99). Disseminated infection with involvement of the skin, gastrointestinal tract, or lymph nodes has been reported in patients with leukemia or AIDS (99). Most isolates are susceptible to ethambutol, and many are susceptible to rifampin and streptomycin. A regimen effective against M. avium-M. intracellulare is recommended for initial therapy (21). A patient with AIDS and disseminated infection was treated successfully with rifabutin, clofazimine, and isoniazid (99). Success in three cases was reported with rifampin, ethambutol, and clarithromycin (46).

Mycobacterium neoaurum

M. neoaurum is a rapidly growing scotochromogenic mycobacterium found in soil, dust, and water. This organism has been identified as the cause of Hickman catheter infections (13, 29) and meningoencephalitis (24). These isolates frequently show in vitro resistance to conventional antituberculous agents. They may be susceptible to a number of antibiotics, including amikacin, ticarcillin-clavulanate, tetracycline, cefoxitin, imipenem, ciprofloxacin, erythromycin, clarithromycin, and azithromycin.

Mycobacterium simiae

M. simiae was first isolated from a colony of Macacus rhesus monkeys (95). A slowly growing photochromogen, its colonies may be only weakly pigmented even after prolonged exposure to light. Unlike other nontuberculous mycobacteria, it produces niacin and thus may be confused with M. tuberculosis. Unlike all other known mycobacteria, M. simiae contains 16S rRNA sequences that are similar to those found both in slowly growing mycobacteria and in rapidly growing strains. The organism has been isolated from human feces (64) and also from water (37), which has been implicated in pseudo-outbreaks (21).

M. simiae can colonize the respiratory tract, and the lung is the most commonly reported site of infection. Most cases of pulmonary disease have been reported from the United States, Thailand, Israel, and Europe (4, 36, 37, 78). Findings have included caseating granulomas and chronic progressive pulmonary infiltrates with cavitation. Disseminated disease, osteomyelitis, and renal involvement have been reported (70). In AIDS patients, infections can be localized or disseminated, and blood cultures may be diagnostic (31). The value of in vitro susceptibility testing as a guide to therapy has been questioned, with suggested therapy including clarithromycin, moxifloxacin, and trimethoprim-sulfamethoxazole (21).

Mycobacterium smegmatis

The M. smegmatis group includes M. smegmatis, M. wolinskyi, and M. goodii (21). M. smegmatis is a rapidly growing environmental saprophyte that was initially isolated from syphilitic chancres and smegma in the 1880s. The organism was not recognized as a human pathogen for the next hundred years. Although the first known case of human infection involved the lungs and pleura, the majority of subsequent reports have described chronic cutaneous or soft tissue infection following injury or surgery (51, 91). M. smegmatis has been recovered from soil samples, and a history of a soil-contaminated wound should raise the clinical suspicion of infection with this pathogen. The first reported case of disseminated infection due to M. smegmatis involved an 8-year-old girl with inherited gamma interferon receptor deficiency. Cultures of blood and liver tissue were positive, and the patient died despite antimicrobial therapy (58). Patients with cutaneous infection usually require extensive surgical debridement followed by skin grafting. Antimicrobial therapy is indicated for severe infections. Isolates are usually resistant to isoniazid, rifampin, and clarithromycin (21) but may be susceptible to ethambutol, doxycycline, sulfamethoxazole, ciprofloxacin, ofloxacin, streptomycin, amikacin, or imipenem.

Mycobacterium szulgai

M. szulgai is scotochromogenic at 37°C but photochromogenic at 25°C. The organism has been isolated from patients worldwide, but its presumed environmental source has not been identified (42). Most reported cases have involved lung disease indistinguishable from that caused by M. tuberculosis. Other sites of infection have included the bursa, tendon sheaths, bones, lymph nodes, skin, and urinary tract (22, 40, 81). M. szulgai is susceptible to most antituberculous agents in vitro (21). Therapeutic regimens have included combinations of more than two drugs (21, 42). A patient with AIDS who had pulmonary infection caused by multidrug-resistant *M. szulgai* responded to therapy with isoniazid, ethambutol, rifampin, and pyrazinamide. The isolate was resistant in vitro to isoniazid, kanamycin, capreomycin, and cycloserine but susceptible to ethambutol, rifampin, and ciprofloxacin (50). A study performed in The Netherlands found that 12 months of rifampin, ethambutol, and clarithromycin led to favorable outcomes without bacteriological relapse (88). Combination therapy based on in vitro susceptibilities for at least 4 to 6 months is recommended for extrapulmonary *M. szulgai* disease (21).

Mycobacterium terrae Complex

Members of the *Mycobacterium terrae* complex include *M. terrae*, *M. nonchromogenicum*, *M. hiberniae*, and *M. triviale* (21). These slow-growing, unpigmented mycobacteria rarely cause human infection. *M. paraterrae*, a slowly growing scotochromogen, is genetically related to *M. terrae* complex (38). Reports have associated them with pulmonary infection (55, 77, 83, 86). They also may cause bone and joint infections, and *M. nonchromogenicum* should be considered in patients who present with tenosynovitis of the hand that is refractory to routine antibiotics and exacerbated by steroid therapy (67). Although members of the *Mycobacterium terrae* complex are often resistant to many conventional antituberculous agents, susceptibility patterns of isolates vary within and between species. Individual isolates may be susceptible to ethambutol, macrolides, linezolid, sulfonamides, or fluoroquinolones (21). Excision with or without antimicrobial therapy may be curative for cutaneous infections due to *M. nonchromogenicum*.

Mycobacterium ulcerans

M. ulcerans is a slowly growing, unpigmented mycobacterium that grows best at 25 to 33°C, requiring 8 to 12 weeks of incubation and optimally recovered with egg yolk supplementation (21). It produces a heat-stable toxin and is the cause of a chronic necrotizing skin infection (Bairnsdale ulcer or Buruli ulcer). *M. ulcerans* infection was first described in Australia but subsequently has been reported in central and west Africa, Mexico, South America, Southeast Asia, and the central Pacific. Analysis of 16S rRNA sequences of isolates from three continents revealed three subgroups corresponding to the continent of origin (63). Although unproven, it is a generally accepted assumption that the environment is the source of the organism. The majority of reported infections have occurred in persons living near rivers or stagnant bodies of water. Inoculation appears to occur via trauma to the skin. The trauma may be minor and unrecognized by the patient. Infection has followed a snake bite (28), gun shot wound, or vaccination (47).

Most lesions occur on the distal parts of a limb and typically begin as a painless papule or subcutaneous swelling. In several weeks, the lesion becomes a shallow ulcer with a necrotic base and undermined margins. Prominent involvement of subcutaneous tissue follows, and satellite ulcers and nodules can develop. Ulcers vary in severity and size and may involve joints. Healed lesions leave stellate scars with retraction, and patients with large ulcers may have permanent deformity and disability. Most lesions are widely ulcerated when they are detected and require extensive surgical excision and skin grafting.

The pathogenesis of the ulcer is associated with the production of mycolactone, a diffusible cytotoxin with immunomodulating properties. Patients with active ulcers have impaired production of Th1, Th2, and Th17 cytokines upon stimulation with mitogenic agents. These immunological defects are detected early in the disease and resolve after successful therapy (57).

Early diagnosis and treatment improve outcome. Clumps of acid-fast bacilli are usually visible in material taken from skin lesions, but primary culture of *M. ulcerans* may take several months. The efficacy of antimicrobials has been disappointing, particularly when they are used late in the course of disease. They may be helpful early or when coupled with surgical excision. Regimens have included streptomycin and dapsone with or without ethambutol (98) and various combinations of trimethoprim-sulfamethoxazole, rifampin, ethambutol, and clarithromycin (28). Isoniazid, rifampin, and ethambutol for 2 months followed by rifampin and clarithromycin for 5 months was successful therapy in a human immunodeficiency virus-infected patient who had a cutaneous ulcer with infection extending to the underlying fascia (14). A recent open-label randomized trial conducted in Ghana compared two regimens for early, limited *M. ulcerans* infections (52). In this study, 73 of 76 patients who received streptomycin and rifampin for 8 weeks and 68 of 75 patients who received 4 weeks of streptomycin and rifampin followed by 4 weeks of rifampin and clarithromycin had healed lesions at 1 year after the start of treatment. Preventive efforts may help reduce the incidence of disease. Wearing long pants appeared to be protective in a case-control study involving Côte d'Ivoire patients who had lower-extremity lesions (43).

Mycobacterium xenopi

M. xenopi, first isolated from a toad, is a scotochromogen that grows optimally at 43°C. The organism is able to grow at 45°C and has been recovered from hot-water generators and storage tanks. It is frequently found in both cold and hot water samples from taps and showers. Failure to grow at temperatures below 28°C likely explains its absence in samples from water treatment plants, reservoirs, and distribution systems. A cluster of bronchoscopy-associated *M. xenopi* pseudoinfections was linked to use of tap water for cleaning bronchoscopes (5). Human exposure to the organism can occur via aerosolization and inhalation or ingestion. *M. xenopi* appears to have a variable geographic distribution. It has been recovered frequently from clinical specimens in Wales, southern England, the northwest coast of Europe, and Toronto, Canada. It was rarely isolated in the United States prior to the AIDS epidemic (15). Detection of *M. xenopi* in clinical specimens may require prolonged incubation at 37°C or incubation at higher temperatures.

M. xenopi is increasingly recognized as a cause of pulmonary infection. In immunocompetent patients, clinical illness typically occurs as an indolent, often cavitary, lung infection in middle-aged men who have underlying chronic pulmonary diseases (34, 74, 89). Less commonly it may infect the spine (48) or joints (11). In a series of seven cases of arthritis, all patients had a history of invasive procedures, and the authors noted that an earlier outbreak of 58 cases of spinal infection was attributed to contamination of an instrument with tap water (71). *M. xenopi* infections in immunocompromised patients are being reported more frequently. Solid organ transplantation (45, 93) and AIDS increase the risk of pulmonary and disseminated disease (33, 34, 68). Infections with *M. xenopi* have shown variable responses to drug therapy (2). Recommendations for initial therapy include isoniazid, a rifamycin, ethambutol, and clarithromycin with or without an initial course of streptomycin (21). Pyrazinamide and ciprofloxacin have been included in some successful regimens (34, 71).

Rare NTM Pathogens

A growing number of uncommon NTM are being isolated from clinical specimens. Among them are *M. asiaticum*, *M. bohemicum*, *M. branderi*, *M. conspicuum*, *M. flavescens*, *M. gastri*, *M. heckeshornense*, *M. heidelbergense*, *M. interjectum*, *M. intermedium*, *M. lentiflavum*, *M. nebraskense*, *M. phlei*, *M. shimoidei*, *M. thermoresistibile*, *M. triplex*, and *M. tusciae*.

Previously considered nonpathogenic saprophytes or environmental contaminants, many of these strains have been implicated as rare causes of pulmonary, extrapulmonary, or disseminated infections (9, 15, 16, 20, 32, 35, 85, 92, 97, 98). We can expect to see an increase in the clinical significance of these NTM, particularly in patients who have AIDS or other conditions which diminish host defenses.

REFERENCES

1. Andréjak, C., V. Ø. Thomsen, I. S. Johansen, A. Riis, T. L. Benfield, P. Duhaut, H. T. Sørensen, F.-X. Lescure, and R. W. Thomsen. 2010. Nontuberculous pulmonary mycobacteriosis in Denmark. *Am. J. Respir. Crit. Care Med.* **181**:514–521.

2. Banks, J., A. M. Hunter, I. A. Campbell, P. A. Jenkins, and A. P. Smith. 1984. Pulmonary infection with *Mycobacterium xenopi*: review of treatment and response. *Thorax* **39**:376–382.

3. Barber, T. W., D. E. Craven, and H. W. Farber. 1991. *Mycobacterium gordonae*: a possible opportunistic respiratory tract pathogen in patients with advanced human immunodeficiency virus, type 1 infection. *Chest* **100**:716–720.

4. Bell, R. C., J. H. Higuchi, W. N. Donovan, I. Krasnow, and W. G. Johanson, Jr. 1983. *Mycobacterium simiae*. Clinical features and follow up of twenty-four patients. *Am. Rev. Respir. Dis.* **127**:35–38.

5. Bennet, S. N., D. E. Peterson, D. R. Johnson, W. N. Hall, B. Robinson-Dunn, and S. Dietrich. 1994. Bronchoscopy-associated *Mycobacterium xenopi* pseudoinfections. *Am. J. Respir. Crit. Care Med.* **150**:245–250.

6. Reference deleted.

7. Reference deleted.

8. Reference deleted.

9. Brown-Elliott, B. A., D. E. Griffith, and R. J. Wallace, Jr. 2002. Newly described or emerging human species of nontuberculous mycobacteria. *Infect. Dis. Clin. N. Am.* **16**:187–220.

10. Cohen, Y. H., J. Amir, S. Ashkenazi, T. Eidlitz-Markus, Z. Samra, L. Kaufmann, and A. Zeharia. 2008. *Mycobacterium haemophilum* and lymphadenitis in immunocompetent children, Israel. *Emerg. Infect. Dis.* **14**:1437–1439.

11. Coombes, G. M., L. S. Teh, J. Denton, A. S. Johnson, and A. K. Jones. 1996. *Mycobacterium xenopi*—an unusual presentation as tenosynovitis of the wrist in an immunocompetent patient. *Br. J. Rheum.* **35**:1008–1010.

12. Coyle, M. B., L. C. Carlson, C. K. Wallis, R. B. Leonard, V. A. Raisys, J. O. Kilburn, M. Samadpour, and E. C. Bottger. 1992. Laboratory aspects of "*Mycobacterium genavense*," a proposed species isolated from AIDS patients. *J. Clin. Microbiol.* **30**:3206–3212.

13. Davison, M. B., J. G. McCormack, Z. M. Blacklock, D. J. Dawson, M. H. Tilse, and F. B. Crimmins. 1988. Bacteremia caused by *Mycobacterium neoaurum*. *J. Clin. Microbiol.* **26**:762–764.

14. Delaporte, E., S. Alfandari, and F. Piette. 1984. *Mycobacterium ulcerans* associated with infection due to the human immunodeficiency virus. *Clin. Infect. Dis.* **18**:839.

15. Falkinham, J. O., III. 2009. Surrounded by mycobacteria: nontuberculous mycobacteria in the human environment. *J. Appl. Microbiol.* **107**:356–367.

16. Fisher, P. R., J. C. Christenson, A. T. Davis, and G. A. Orme. 1997. Postoperative *M. flavescens* infection in a child. *Infect. Dis. Clin. Pract.* **6**:263–265.

17. Reference deleted.

18. **Gibson, R. L., J. L. Burns, and B. W. Ramsey.** 2003. Pathophysiology and management of pulmonary infections in cystic fibrosis. *Am. J. Respir. Crit. Care Med.* **168:**918–951.

19. **Glassroth, J.** 2008. Pulmonary disease due to nontuberculous mycobacteria. *Chest* **133:**243–251.

20. **Grech, M., R. Carter, and R. Thomson.** 2010. Clinical significance of *Mycobacterium asiaticum* isolates in Queensland, Australia. *J. Clin. Microbiol.* **48:**162–167.

21. **Griffith, D. E., T. Aksamit, B. A. Brown-Eliott, A. Catanzaro, C. Daley, F. Gordin, S. M. Holland, R. Horsburgh, G. Huitt, M. F. Iademarco, M. Iseman, K. Olivier, S. Ruoss, C. Fordham von Reyn, R. J. Wallace, Jr., and K. Winthrop.** 2007. An official ATS/IDSA statement: diagnosis, treatment, and prevention of nontuberculous mycobacterial diseases. *Am. J. Respir. Crit. Care Med.* **175:**367–416.

22. **Gur, H., S. Porat, H. Haas, Y. Naparstek, and M. Eliakim.** 1984. Disseminated mycobacterial disease caused by *Mycobacterium szulgai*. *Arch. Intern. Med.* **144:**1861–1863.

23. **Hale, Y. M., G. E. Pfyffer, and M. Salfinger.** 2001. Laboratory diagnosis of mycobacterial infections: new tools and lessons learned. *Clin. Infect. Dis.* **33:**834–846.

24. **Heckman, G. A., C. Hawkins, A. Morris, L. L. Burrows, and C. Bergeron.** 2004. Rapidly progressive dementia due to *Mycobacterium neoaurum* meningoencephalitis. *Emerg. Infect. Dis.* **10:**924–927.

25. **Henriques, B., S. E. Hoffner, B. Petrini, I. Juhlin, P. Wahlen, and G. Kallenius.** 1994. Infection with *Mycobacterium malmoense* in Sweden: report of 221 cases. *Clin. Infect. Dis.* **18:**596–600.

26. Reference deleted.

27. **Hoefsloot, W., J. van Ingen, W. C. M. de Lange, P. N. R. Dekhuijzen, M. J. Boeree, and D. van Soolingen.** 2009. Clinical relevance of *Mycobacterium malmoense* isolation in the Netherlands. *Eur. Respir. J.* **34:**926–931.

28. **Hofer, M., B. Hirschel, P. Kirschner, M. Baghetti, A. Kaelin, C. A. Siegrist, S. Suter, A. Teske, and E. C. Bottger.** 1993. Disseminated osteomyelitis from *Mycobacterium ulcerans* after a snakebite. *N. Engl. J. Med.* **328:**1007–1009.

29. **Holland, D. J., S. C. Chen, W. W. Chew, and G. Gilbert.** 1994. *Mycobacterium neoaurum* infection of a Hickman catheter in an immunosuppressed patient. *Clin. Infect. Dis.* **18:**1002–1003.

30. **Horsburgh, C., Jr., and R. Selike.** 1989. The epidemiology of disseminated nontuberculous mycobacterial infection in the acquired immunodeficiency syndrome (AIDS). *Am. Rev. Respir. Dis.* **139:**4–7.

31. **Huminer, D., S. Dux, Z. Samra, L. Kaufman, A. Lavy, C. S. Block, and S. D. Pitik.** 1993. *Mycobacterium simiae* infection in Israeli patients with AIDS. *Clin. Infect. Dis.* **17:**508–509.

32. **Iwen, P. C., S. R. Tarantolo, A. M. Mohamed, and S. H. Hinrichs.** 2006. First report of *Mycobacterium nebraskense* as a cause of human infection. *Diagn. Microbiol. Infect. Dis.* **56:**451–453.

33. **Jacoby, H. M., T. M. Jiva, D. A. Kaminski, L. A. Weymouth, and A. C. Portmore.** 1995. *Mycobacterium xenopi* infection masquerading as pulmonary tuberculosis in two patients infected with the human immunodeficiency virus. *Clin. Infect. Dis.* **20:**1399–1401.

34. **Jiva, T. M., H. M. Jacoby, L. A. Weymouth, D. A. Kaminski, and A. C. Portmore.** 1997. *Mycobacterium xenopi*: innocent bystander or emerging pathogen? *Clin. Infect. Dis.* **24:**226–232.

35. **Koukila-Kahkola, P., B. Springer, E. C. Bottger, L. Paulin, E. Jantzen, and M. L. Katila.** 1995. *Mycobacterium branderi* sp.

nov., a new potential human pathogen. *Int. J. Syst. Bacteriol.* **45:**549–553.

36. **Krasnow, I., and W. Gross.** 1985. *Mycobacterium simiae* infection in the United States. A case report and discussion of the organism. *Am. Rev. Respir. Dis.* **111:**357–360.

37. **Lavy, A., and Y. Yoshpe-Purer.** 1982. Isolation of *Mycobacterium simiae* from clinical specimens in Israel. *Tubercle* **63:**279–285.

38. **Lee, H., S.-A. Lee, I.-K. Lee, H.-K. Yu, Y.-G. Park, J. Jeong, S. H. Lee, S.-R. Kim, J.-W. Hyun, K. Kim, Y.-H. Kook, and B.-J. Kim.** 2010. *Mycobacterium paraterrae* sp. nov. recovered from a clinical specimen: novel chromogenic slow growing mycobacteria related to *Mycobacterium terrae* complex. *Microbiol. Immunol.* **54:**46–53.

39. **Lessnau, K. D., S. Milanese, and W. Talavera.** 1993. *Mycobacterium gordonae*: a treatable disease in HIV-positive patients. *Chest* **104:**1779–1785.

40. **Lin, J.-N., C.-H. Lai, Y.-H. Chen, C.-K. Huang, H.-F. Lin, H.-L. Eng, and H.-H. Lin.** 2009. Urinary *Mycobacterium szulgai* infection in an immunocompetent patient. *South. Med. J.* **102:**979–981.

41. Reference deleted.

42. **Maloney, J. M., C. R. Gregg, D. S. Stephens, F. A. Manian, and D. Rimland.** 1987. Infections caused by *Mycobacterium szulgai* in humans. *Rev. Infect. Dis.* **9:**1120–1126.

43. **Marston, B. J., M. O. Diallo, C. R. Horsburgh, Jr., I. Diomande, M. Z. Saki, J. M. Kanga, G. Patrice, H. B. Lipman, S. M. Ostroff, and R. C. Good.** 1995. Emergence of Buruli ulcer disease in the Daloa region of Cote D'Ivoire. *Am. J. Trop. Med. Hyg.* **52:**219–224.

44. Reference deleted.

45. **McDiarmid, S. V., D. A. Blumberg, H. Remotti, J. Vargas, J. R. Tipton, M. E. Ament, and R. W. Busuttil.** 1995. Mycobacterial infections after pediatric liver transplantation: a report of three cases and review of the literature. *J. Pediatr. Gastroenterol. Nutr.* **20:**425–431.

46. **McGrath, E. E., and P. Bardsley.** 2009. An association between *Mycobacterium malmoense* and coal workers' pneumoconiosis. *Lung* **187:**51–54.

47. **Meyers, W. M., N. Tignokpa, G. B. Priuli, and F. Portaels.** 1996. *Mycobacterium ulcerans* infection (Buruli ulcer): first reported patients in Togo. *Br. J. Dermatol.* **134:**1116–1121.

48. **Miller, W. C., M. D. Perkins, W. J. Richardson, and D. J. Sexton.** 1994. Pott's disease caused by *Mycobacterium xenopi*: case report and review. *Clin. Infect. Dis.* **19:**1024–1028.

49. **Modi, D., D. Pyatetsky, D. P. Edward, L. J. Ulanski, K. J. Pursell, H. H. Tessler, and D. A. Goldstein.** 2007. *Mycobacterium haemophilum*. A rare cause of endophthalmitis. *Retina* **27:**1148–1151.

50. **Newshan, G., and R. A. Torres.** 1994. Pulmonary infection due to multidrug resistant *Mycobacterium szulgai* in a patient with AIDS. *Clin. Infect. Dis.* **18:**1022–1023.

51. **Newton, J. A., Jr., P. J. Weiss, W. A. Bowler, and E. C. Oldfield III.** 1993. Soft-tissue infection due to *Mycobacterium smegmatis*: report of two cases. *Clin. Infect. Dis.* **16:**531–533.

52. **Nienhuis, W. A., Y. Stienstra, W. A. Thompson, P. C. Awuah, K. M. Abass, W. Tuah, N. Y. Awua-Boateng, E. O. Ampadu, V. Siegmund, J. P. Schouten, O. Adjei, G. Bretzel, and T. S. van der Werf.** 2010. Antimicrobial treatment for early, limited *Mycobacterium ulcerans* infection: a randomized controlled trial. *Lancet* **375:**664–672.

53. **Panwalker, A. P., and E. Fuhse.** 1986. Nosocomial *Mycobacterium gordonae* pseudoinfection from contaminated ice machines. *Infect. Control* **7:**67–70.

54. Reference deleted.

55. Peters, E., and R. Morice. 1991. Miliary pulmonary infection caused by *Mycobacterium terrae* in an autologous bone marrow transplant patient. *Chest* **100:**1449–1450.

56. Phillips, M. S., and C. F. von Reyn. 2001. Nosocomial infections due to nontuberculous mycobacteria. *Clin. Infect. Dis.* **33:**1363–1374.

57. Phillips, R., F. S. Sarfo, L. Guenin-Macé, J. Decalf, M. Wansbrough-Jones, M. L. Albert, and C. Demangel. 2009. Immunosuppressive signature of cutaneous *Mycobacterium ulcerans* infection in the peripheral blood of patients with Buruli ulcer disease. *J. Infect. Dis.* **200:**1675–1684.

58. Pierre-Audigier, C., E. Jouanguy, S. Lamhamedi, F. Altare, J. Rauzier, V. Vincent, D. Canioni, J. F. Emile, A. Fischer, S. Blanche, J. L. Gaillard, and J. L. Casanova. 1997. Fatal disseminated *Mycobacterium smegmatis* infection in a child with inherited interferon-gamma receptor deficiency. *Clin. Infect. Dis.* **24:**982–984.

59. Piersimoni, C., E. Tortoli, F. de Lalla, D. Nista, D. Donato, S. Bornigia, and G. De Sio. 1997. Isolation of *Mycobacterium celatum* from patients infected with human immunodeficiency virus. *Clin. Infect. Dis.* **24:**144–147.

60. Piersimoni, C., P. G. Zitti, D. Nista, and S. Bornigia. 2003. *Mycobacterium celatum* pulmonary infection in the immunocompetent: case report and review. *Emerg. Infect. Dis.* **9:**399–402.

61. Piersimoni, C., and C. Scarparo. 2009. Extrapulmonary infections associated with nontuberculous mycobacteria in immunocompetent persons. *Emerg. Infect. Dis.* **15:**1351–1358.

62. Plemmons, R. M., C. K. McAllister, M. C. Garces, and R. L. Ward. 1997. Osteomyelitis due to *Mycobacterium haemophilum* in a cardiac transplant patient: case report and analysis of interactions among clarithromycin, rifampin, and cyclosporine. *Clin. Infect. Dis.* **24:**995–997.

63. Portaels, F., P. A. Fonteyene, H. deBeenhouwer, P. de Rijk, A. Guedenon, J. Hayman, and M. W. Meyers. 1996. Variability in 3′ end of 16S rRNA sequence of *Mycobacterium ulcerans* is related to geographic origin of isolates. *J. Clin. Microbiol.* **34:**962–965.

64. Portaels, F., L. Larsson, and P. Smeets. 1988. Isolation of mycobacteria from healthy persons' stools. *Int. J. Lepr.* **56:**468–471.

65. Primm, T. P., C. A. Lucero, and J. O. Falkinham III. 2004. Health impacts of environmental mycobacteria. *Clin. Microbiol. Rev.* **17:**98–106.

66. Richardson, E. T., D. Samons, and N. Banaei. 2009. Rapid identification of *Mycobacterium tuberculosis* and nontuberculous mycobacteria by multiplex, real-time PCR. *J. Clin. Microbiol.* **47:**1497–1502.

67. Ridderhof, J. C., R. J. Wallace, Jr., J. O. Kilburn, W. R. Butler, N. G. Warren, M. Tsukamura, L. C. Steele, and E. S. Wong. 1991. Chronic tenosynovitis of the hand due to *Mycobacterium nonchromogenum*: use of high-performance liquid chromatography for identification of isolates. *Rev. Infect. Dis.* **13:**857–864.

68. Rigsby, M. O., and A. M. Curtis. 1994. Pulmonary disease from nontuberculous mycobacteria in patients with human immunodeficiency virus. *Chest* **106:**913–919.

69. Rogers, P. L., R. E. Walker, H. C. Lane, F. G. Witebsky, J. A. Kovacs, J. E. Parrillo, and H. Masur. 1988. Disseminated *Mycobacterium haemophilum* infection in two patients with the acquired immunodeficiency syndrome. *Am. J. Med.* **84:**640–642.

70. Rose, H. D., G. J. Dorff, M. Lauwasser, and N. K. Sheth. 1982. Pulmonary and disseminated *Mycobacterium simiae* infection in humans. *Am. Rev. Respir. Dis.* **126:**1110–1113.

71. Salliot, C., N. Desplaces, P. Boisrenoult, A. C. Koeger, P. Beaufils, V. Vincent, P. Mamoudy, and J.-M. Ziza. 2006. Arthritis due to *M. xenopi*: a retrospective study of 7 cases in France. *Clin. Infect. Dis.* **43:**987–993.

72. Saubolle, M. A., T. E. Kiehn, M. H. White, M. F. Rudinsky, and D. Armstrong. 1996. *Mycobacterium haemophilum*: microbiology and expanding clinical and geographic spectra of disease in humans. *Clin. Microbiol. Rev.* **9:**435–447.

73. Shin, J.-H., E. J. Cho, J.-Y. Lee, J.-Y. Yu, and Y.-H. Kang. 2009. Novel diagnostic algorithm using *tuf* gene amplification and restriction fragment length polymorphism is promising tool for identification of nontuberculous mycobacteria. *J. Microbiol. Biotechnol.* **19:**323–330.

74. Simor, A. E., I. E. Salit, and H. Vellend. 1984. The role of *Mycobacterium xenopi* in human disease. *Am. Rev. Respir. Dis.* **129:**435–438.

75. Snider, D. E., Jr., P. C. Hopewell, J. Mills, and L. B. Reichman. 1987. Mycobacterioses and the acquired immunodeficiency syndrome. *Am. Rev. Respir. Dis.* **136:**492–496.

76. Sompolinsky, D., A. Lagziel, D. Naveh, and T. Yankilevitz. 1978. *Mycobacterium haemophilum* sp. nov., a new pathogen of humans. *Int. J. Syst. Bacteriol.* **28:**67–75.

77. Spence, T. H., and V. M. Ferris. 1996. Spontaneous resolution of a lung mass due to infection with *Mycobacterium terrae*. *South. Med. J.* **89:**414–416.

78. Sriyabhaya, N., and S. Wongwantana. 1981. Pulmonary infection caused by atypical mycobacteria: a report of 24 cases in Thailand. *Rev. Infect. Dis.* **3:**1085–1089.

79. Steere, A., J. Corrales, and A. von Graevenitz. 1979. A cluster of *Mycobacterium gordonae* isolates from bronchoscopy specimens. *Am. Rev. Respir. Dis.* **120:**214–216.

80. Stine, T. M., A. A. Harris, S. Levin, N. Rivera, and R. L. Kaplan. 1987. A pseudoepidemic due to atypical mycobacteria in a hospital water supply. *JAMA* **258:**809–811.

81. Stratton, C. W., D. B. Phelps, and L. B. Reller. 1978. Tuberculoid tenosynovitis and carpal tunnel syndrome caused by *Mycobacterium szulgai*. *Am. J. Med.* **65:**349–351.

82. Straus, W. L., S. M. Ostroff, D. B. Jernigan, T. E. Kiehn, E. M. Sordillo, D. Armstrong, N. Boone, N. Schneider, J. O. Kilburn, V. A. Silcox, V. LaBombardi, and R. C. Good. 1994. Clinical and epidemiologic characteristics of *Mycobacterium haemophilum*, an emerging pathogen in immunocompromised patients. *Ann. Intern. Med.* **120:**118–125.

83. Tonner, J. A., and M. D. Hammond. 1989. Pulmonary disease caused by *Mycobacterium terrae* complex. *South. Med. J.* **82:**1279–1282.

84. Tortoli, E., C. Piersimoni, D. Bacosi, A. Bartoloni, F. Betti, L. Bono, C. Burrini, G. De Sio, C. Lacchini, and A. Mantella. 1995. Isolation of the newly described species *Mycobacterium celatum* from AIDS patients. *J. Clin. Microbiol.* **33:**137–140.

85. Tortoli, E., and M. T. Simonetti. 1991. Isolation of *Mycobacterium shimoidei* from a patient with cavitary pulmonary disease. *J. Clin. Microbiol.* **29:**1754–1756.

86. Tsukamura, M., N. Kita, W. Otsuka, and H. Shimoide. 1983. A study of the taxonomy of the *Mycobacterium nonchromogenicum* complex and report of six cases of lung infection due to *Mycobacterium nonchromogenicum*. *Microbiol. Immunol.* **27:**219–236.

87. Van Ingen, J., M. J. Boeree, P. N. R. Dekhuijzen, and D. van Soolingen. 2008. Clinical relevance of *Mycobacterium simiae* in pulmonary samples. *Eur. Respir. J.* **31:**106–109.

88. Van Ingen, J., M. J. Boeree, W. C. M. de Lange, P. E. W. de Haas, P. N. R. Dekhuijzen, and D. van Soolingen. 2008. Clinical relevance of *Mycobacterium szulgai* in The Netherlands. *Clin. Infect. Dis.* **46:**1200–1205.

89. **Van Ingen, J., M. J. Boeree, W. C. M. de Lange, W. Hoefsloot, S. A. Bendien, C. Magis-Escurra, R. Dekhuijzen, and D. van Soolingen.** 2008. *Mycobacterium xenopi* clinical relevance and determinants, The Netherlands. *Emerg. Infect. Dis.* **14:**385–389.

90. **Van Ingen, J., T. van der Laan, R. Dekhuijzen, M. Boeree, and D. van Soolingen.** 2010. In vitro drug susceptibility of 2275 clinical non-tuberculous *Mycobacterium* isolates of 49 species in the Netherlands. *Int. J. Antimicrob. Agents* **35:**169–173.

91. **Wallace, R. J., Jr., D. R. Nash, M. Tsukamura, Z. M. Blacklock, and V. A. Silcox.** 1988. Human disease due to *Mycobacterium smegmatis. J. Infect. Dis.* **158:**52–59.

92. **Wayne, L. G., and H. A. Sramek.** 1992. Agents of newly recognized or infrequently encountered mycobacterial diseases. *Clin. Microbiol. Rev.* **5:**1–25.

93. **Weber, J., T. Mettang, E. Staerz, C. Machleidt, and U. Kuhlmann.** 1989. Pulmonary disease due to *Mycobacterium xenopi* in a renal allograft recipient: report of a case and review. *Rev. Infect. Dis.* **11:**961–969.

94. **Weinberger, M., S. L. Berg, I. M. Feuerstein, P. A. Pizzo, and F. G. Witebsky.** 1992. Disseminated infection with *Mycobacterium gordonae*: report of a case and critical review of the literature. *Clin. Infect. Dis.* **14:**1229–1239.

95. **Weiszfeiler, J. G., V. Karasseva, and E. Karczag.** 1981. *Mycobacterium simiae* and related mycobacteria. *Rev. Infect. Dis.* **3:**1040–1045.

96. **White, M. H., E. Papadopoulos, T. N. Small, T. E. Kiehn, and D. Armstrong.** 1995. *Mycobacterium haemophilum* infections in bone marrow transplant recipients. *Transplantation* **60:**957–960.

97. **Wolinsky, E.** 1992. Mycobacterial diseases other than tuberculosis. *Clin. Infect. Dis.* **15:**1–12.

98. **Woods, G. L., and J. A. Washington II.** 1987. Mycobacteria other than *Mycobacterium tuberculosis*: review of microbiologic and clinical aspects. *Rev. Infect. Dis.* **9:**275–294.

99. **Zaugg, M., M. Salfinger, M. Opravil, and R. Luthy.** 1993. Extrapulmonary and disseminated infections due to *Mycobacterium malmoense*: case report and review. *Clin. Infect. Dis.* **16:**540–549.

100. **Zurawski, C. A., G. D. Cage, D. Rimland, and H. M. Blumberg.** 1997. Pneumonia and bacteremia due to *Mycobacterium celatum* masquerading as *Mycobacterium xenopi* in patients with AIDS: an underdiagnosed problem? *Clin. Infect. Dis.* **24:**140–143.

INDEX